The Oxford Textbook of
Clinical Research Ethics

The Oxford Textbook of Clinical Research Ethics

EDITED BY

Ezekiel J. Emanuel
Chair, Department of Bioethics, National Institutes of Health, Bethesda, Maryland

Christine Grady
Head, Section on Human Subjects Research, Department of Bioethics, National Institutes of Health, Bethesda, Maryland

Robert A. Crouch
The Poynter Center for the Study of Ethics and American Institutions, Indiana University, Bloomington, Indiana

Reidar K. Lie
Professor of Philosophy, University of Bergen; Head, Unit on Multinational Research, Department of Bioethics, National Institutes of Health, Bethesda, Maryland

Franklin G. Miller
Bioethicist, National Institute of Mental Health Intramural Research Program, Department of Bioethics, National Institutes of Health, Bethesda, Maryland

David Wendler
Head, Unit on Vulnerable Populations, Department of Bioethics, National Institutes of Health, Bethesda, Maryland

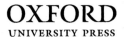
OXFORD
UNIVERSITY PRESS

2008

OXFORD
UNIVERSITY PRESS

Oxford University Press, Inc., publishes works that further
Oxford University's objective of excellence
in research, scholarship, and education.

Oxford   New York
Auckland   Cape Town   Dar es Salaam   Hong Kong   Karachi
Kuala Lumpur   Madrid   Melbourne   Mexico City   Nairobi
New Delhi   Shanghai   Taipei   Toronto

With offices in
Argentina   Austria   Brazil   Chile   Czech Republic   France   Greece
Guatemala   Hungary   Italy   Japan   Poland   Portugal   Singapore
South Korea   Switzerland   Thailand   Turkey   Ukraine   Vietnam

Published by Oxford University Press, Inc.
198 Madison Avenue, New York, New York 10016

www.oup.com

Library of Congress Cataloging-in-Publication Data
The Oxford textbook of clinical research ethics / edited by Ezekiel J. Emanuel ... [et al.].
      p.; cm.
Includes bibliographical references and index.
ISBN 978-0-19-516865-5
1. Human experimentation in medicine—Moral and ethical aspects.   2. Clinical trials—Moral and ethical aspects.
3. Medical ethics. I. Emanuel, Ezekiel J., 1957– II. Title: Textbook of clinical research ethics.
[DNLM: 1. Human Experimentation—ethics.   2. Ethics Committees, Research.   3. Ethics, Research.
4. Research Subjects—legislation & jurisprudence. W 20.55.H9 O98 2008]
R853.H8O96 2008
174.2—dc22   2007016230

9 8 7 6 5 4 3 2

Printed in the United States of America
on acid-free paper

Dedicated to

John I. Gallin, M.D.

Whose vision and continuing support made the Department of Bioethics at the NIH—and, as a consequence, this texbook—possible.

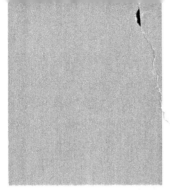

Acknowledgments

A book such as this is a truly collaborative effort, and we have incurred many debts along the way for which we owe thanks. We must first thank those who contributed chapters to our volume. Without their time and effort, this volume would not exist. The contribution of a chapter to an edited volume is often a thankless task, and it is one that does not receive the recognition we believe it deserves. So we here signal our indebtedness to our contributors and give our heartfelt thanks. We hope that the volume is sufficiently well received and widely read such that our contributing authors receive the recognition for their hard work that they deserve.

At the National Institutes of Health, we have many to thank. We are delighted to thank our behind the scenes editor, Bruce Agnew. Bruce read every chapter with his very keen editorial eyes, and offered editorial and substantive suggestions on each chapter. This was an enormous undertaking, and Bruce did it with his characteristic good humor and aplomb. The volume is much better because of his input. Near the end of the process, Rose Murray and Becky Chen stepped in and helped us track down art work and permissions. This, too, was a large undertaking, and Rose and Becky were instrumental in helping us wrap things up. Justine Seidenfeld helped us put together material for one chapter, and we thank her for that. Finally, we gratefully acknowledge the financial assistance provided by the Department of Bioethics, The Clinical Center, National Institutes of Health.

We received a great deal of help from archivists, librarians, and staff at a number of institutions who found material for us and provided us with high-resolution images to include in this volume. To those who helped us at the following institutions, we give our thanks: Bentley Historical Library, University of Michigan, Ann Arbor, Mich.; Chemical Engineering, New York, N.Y.; March of Dimes, White Plains, N.Y.; American Philosophical Society Library, Philadelphia, Penn.; Medical Arts and Photography Branch, National Institutes of Health, Bethesda, Md.; Rutgers University Libraries, Special Collections and University Archives, New Brunswick, N.J.; Indiana University Libraries, Bloomington, Ind.; Frederick L. Ehrman Medical Library Archives, New York University School of Medicine, New York, N.Y.; Royal College of Physicians, Heritage Collections, London, England; United States Holocaust Memorial Museum, Washington, D.C.; and the University of Virginia Library, Special Collections, and Historical Collections, Charlottesville, Va.

Last but not least, we thank our editor at Oxford University Press, Peter Ohlin, for very helpful advice and guidance from day one, as well as tremendous patience.

V   Participant Selection

Section A. Fair Participant Selection

Section B. Special Populations

Contributors

Manish Agrawal, M.D., M.A.
Staff Oncologist, National Cancer
   Institute
National Institutes of Health
Bethesda, Maryland
agrawalm@pol.net

George J. Annas, J.D., M.P.H.
Edward R. Utley Professor and Chair
Department of Health Law, Bioethics
   and Human Rights
Boston University School of Public
   Health;
Professor, Boston University School of
   Medicine, and School of Law
Boston, Massachusetts
annasgj@bu.edu

Paul S. Appelbaum, M.D.
Elizabeth K. Dollard Professor of
   Psychiatry, Medicine, and Law
College of Physicians and Surgeons
Columbia University;
Director, Division of Psychiatry, Law
   and Ethics
New York State Psychiatric Institute
New York, New York
psa21@columbia.edu

John D. Arras, Ph.D.
Porterfield Professor of Biomedical
   Ethics and Professor
Corcoran Department of Philosophy
University of Virginia
Charlottesville, Virginia
jda3a@virginia.edu

Richard E. Ashcroft, Ph.D.
Professor of Bioethics
Queen Mary University of London
School of Law
London, England
r.ashcroft@qmol.ac.uk

Tom L. Beauchamp, Ph.D.
Professor, Department of Philosophy;
Senior Research Scholar
Kennedy Institute of Ethics
Georgetown University
Washington, D.C.
beauchat@georgetown.edu

Justin E. Bekelman, M.D.
Resident, Department of Radiation
   Oncology
Memorial Sloan-Kettering Cancer
   Center
New York, New York
bekelmaj@mskcc.org

Deryck Beyleveld, Ph.D.
Professor of Law and Bioethics
   Department of Law;
Member, Human Rights Centre
Durham University
Durham, England
deryck.beyleveld@durham.ac.uk

Erika Blacksher, Ph.D.
Robert Wood Johnson Health and
    Society Scholar
Columbia University
New York, New York
eb2433@columbia.edu

David Blumenthal, M.D., M.P.P.
Director, Institute for Health Policy;
Physician, Massachusetts General
    Hospital;
Samuel O. Thier Professor of Medicine,
    Professor of Health Care Policy
Harvard Medical School
Boston, Massachusetts
dblumenthal@partners.org

Valerie H. Bonham, J.D.
Office of the General Counsel
Department of Health and Human
    Services
Bethesda, Maryland
bonhamva@mail.nih.gov

Angela J. Bowen, M.D.
President, Western Institutional Review
    Board
Olympia, Washington
abowen@wirb.com

Dan W. Brock, Ph.D.
Frances Glessner Lee Professor of
    Medical Ethics
Department of Social Medicine;
Director, Division of Medical Ethics;
Director, Program in Ethics and Health
Harvard School of Public Health
Harvard Medical School
Boston, Massachusetts
dan_brock@hms.harvard.edu

Eric G. Campbell, Ph.D.
Assistant Professor
Institute for Health Policy
Department of Medicine
Massachusetts General Hospital,
    Harvard Medical School
Boston, Massachusetts
ecampbell@partners.org

Alexander M. Capron, LL.B.
University Professor and
Scott H. Bice Chair in Healthcare Law,
    Policy and Ethics;
Professor of Law and Medicine;
Co-Director, Pacific Center for Health
    Policy and Ethics
University of Southern California
Los Angeles, California
acapron@law.usc.edu

James F. Childress, Ph.D.
John Allen Hollingsworth Professor
    of Ethics
Professor of Medical Education
Department of Religious Studies;
Director, Institute of Practical Ethics
    and Public Life
University of Virginia
Charlottesville, Virginia
jfc7c@virginia.edu

Larry R. Churchill, Ph.D.
Ann Geddes Stahlman Professor of
    Medical Ethics;
Co-Director, Center for Biomedical
    Ethics and Society
Vanderbilt University Medical Center
Nashville, Tennessee
larry.churchill@vanderbilt.edu

Lauren K. Collogan, J.D.
Law student (Class of 2007)
Columbia Law School
New York, New York
lkc2107@columbia.edu

Colleen Denny, B.S.
Pre-Doctoral Fellow
Department of Bioethics
National Institutes of Health
Bethesda, Maryland
dennycc@nih.gov

Neal Dickert, M.D., Ph.D.
Resident, Department of Medicine,
The Johns Hopkins School of Medicine
Baltimore, Maryland
ndicker@jhmi.edu

Rebecca Dresser, J.D.
Daniel Noyes Kirby Professor of Law
Professor of Ethics in Medicine, School
    of Law
Washington University, St. Louis
St. Louis, Missouri
dresser@wulaw.wustl.edu

Alan R. Fleischman, M.D.
Senior Vice President and
    Medical Director
March of Dimes Foundation
White Plains, New York
afleischman@marchofdimes.com

James H. Flory, B.A.
Medical student (Class of 2008)
University of Pennsylvania School of
    Medicine
Philadelphia, Pennsylvania
jflory@mail.med.upenn.edu

Sev S. Fluss, M.S.
Senior Advisor
Council for International Organizations
    of Medical Sciences (CIOMS)
World Health Organization
Geneva, Switzerland
flusss@who.int

Morris W. Foster, Ph.D.
Professor and Acting Chair
Department of Anthropology;
Associate Director, Center for Applied
    Social Research;
Assistant Associate Director, General
    Clinical Research Center
University of Oklahoma
Norman, Oklahoma
morris.w.foster-1@ou.edu

Lawrence M. Friedman, M.D.
Independent Consultant
Rockville, Maryland
l.m.friedman@verizon.net

Nesrin Garan, M.Sc.
Law student (Class of 2008)
Vanderbilt University Law School
Nashville, Tennessee
garan@post.harvard.edu

Grant R. Gillett, M.B., Ch.B., D.Phil., FRACS
Professor, Bioethics Centre;
Consultant Neurosurgeon, Dunedin Hospital;
Clinical Professor, Neurosurgery, Dunedin School of Medicine
University of Otago
Dunedin, New Zealand
grant.gillett@stonebow.otago.ac.nz

Aaron Goldenberg, M.A., M.P.H.
Doctoral student, Department of Bioethics;
Research Associate, Center for Genetic Research Ethics and Law
Case Western Reserve University School of Medicine
Cleveland, Ohio
aaron.goldenberg@case.edu

Sara F. Goldkind, M.D., M.A.
Senior Bioethicist, Office of Critical Path Program
Office of the Commissioner
Food and Drug Administration
Rockville, Maryland
sara.goldkind@fda.hhs.gov

Lawrence O. Gostin, J.D., LL.D. (Hon).
Professor and Associate Dean (Research and Academic Programs)
Georgetown University Law Center
Washington, D.C.;
Professor, Bloomberg School of Public Health;
Director, Center for Law and the Public's Health,
The Johns Hopkins University
Baltimore, Maryland
gostin@law.georgetown.edu

Ronald M. Green, Ph.D.
Eunice & Julian Cohen Professor for the Study of Ethics and Human Values
Department of Religion;
Director, Institute for the Study of Applied and Professional Ethics
Dartmouth University
Hanover, New Hampshire
ronald.m.green@dartmouth.edu

Michael A. Grodin, M.D.
Professor, Department of Health Law, Bioethics and Human Rights
Boston University School of Public Health;
Professor, Boston University School of Medicine
Boston, Massachusetts
grodin@bu.edu

Cary P. Gross, M.D.
Associate Professor
Section of General Internal Medicine
Department of Internal Medicine
Yale University School of Medicine
New Haven, Connecticut
cary.gross@yale.edu

Lindsay A. Hampson, B.A.
Medical student (Class of 2009)
University of Michigan Medical School
Ann Arbor, Michigan
lhampson@med.umich.edu

John Harris, F.Med.Sci., B.A., D.Phil.
Sir David Alliance Professor of Bioethics
Institute of Medicine Law and Bioethics
School of Law, University of Manchester
Manchester, England;
Visiting Professor of Philosophy
Department of Philosophy, Logic and Scientific Method
London School of Economics
London, England;
Editor-in-Chief, Journal of Medical Ethics
john.harris@manchester.ac.uk

Juhana E. Idänpään-Heikkilä, M.D., Ph.D.
Secretary-General
Council for International Organizations of Medical Sciences (CIOMS)
World Health Organization
Geneva, Switzerland
idanpaanj@who.int

James G. Hodge Jr., J.D., LL.M.
Associate Professor, Bloomberg School of Public Health;
Executive Director, Center for Law and the Public's Health
The Johns Hopkins University
Baltimore, Maryland
jhodge@jhsph.edu

Søren Holm, M.D., Ph.D., Dr.Med.Sci.
Section for Medical Ethics, University of Oslo
Oslo, Norway;
Professor, Law School;
Professorial Fellow in Bioethics
Cardiff Institute of Society, Health and Ethics;
Director, Cardiff Centre for Ethics Law and Society
Cardiff University
Cardiff, Wales
holms@cardiff.ac.uk

Steven Joffe, M.D., M.P.H.
Assistant Professor of Pediatrics
Department of Pediatric Oncology
Dana-Farber Cancer Institute;
Department of Medicine, Children's Hospital;
Harvard Medical School
Boston, Massachusetts
steven_joffe@dfci.harvard.edu

Summer Johnson, Ph.D.
Assistant Professor of Medicine (Medical Ethics);
Director, Ethics in Novel Technologies, Research and Innovation,
Alden March Bioethics Institute
Albany Medical College
Albany, New York
summer.johnson@bioethics.net

James H. Jones, Ph.D.
Independent Scholar
San Francisco, California
jones@auwers.com

Albert R. Jonsen, Ph.D.
Professor Emeritus,
Department of Medical History and Ethics
University of Washington
Seattle, Washington
arjonsen@aol.com

Eric T. Juengst, Ph.D.
Associate Professor, Department of Bioethics;
Director, Center for Genetic Research Ethics and Law, School of Medicine
Case Western Reserve University
Cleveland, Ohio
etj2@po.cwru.edu

Jason H. T. Karlawish, M.D.
Associate Professor of Medicine
Division of Geriatric Medicine;
Director, Alzheimer's Disease Center's
    Education and Information Transfer
    Core;
Senior Fellow, Leonard Davis Institute
    of Health Economics;
Fellow, Center for Bioethics
University of Pennsylvania
Philadelphia, Pennsylvania
Jason.Karlawish@uphs.upenn.edu

John Y. Killen Jr., M.D.
Director, Office of International Health
    Research
National Center for Complementary
    and Alternative Medicine
National Institutes of Health
Bethesda, Maryland
jkillen@mail.nih.gov

Nancy M. P. King, J.D.
Professor, Department of Social
    Medicine
University of North Carolina, Chapel
    Hill
Chapel Hill, North Carolina
nmpking@WFUBmc.edu

Greg Koski, Ph.D., M.D., CPI
Senior Scientist, Institute for Health
    Policy;
Associate Professor, Department of
    Anesthesiology and Critical Care
Massachusetts General Hospital and
    Harvard Medical School
Boston, Massachusetts
gkoski@partners.org

James V. Lavery, Ph.D.
Research Scientist
Centre for Research in Inner City Health
Centre for Global Health Research
St. Michael's Hospital;
Assistant Professor
Department of Public Health Sciences
    and
Joint Centre for Bioethics
University of Toronto
jim.lavery@utoronto.ca

Susan E. Lederer, Ph.D.
Associate Professor, Department of
    History;
Section of the History of Medicine,
    School of Medicine
Yale University
New Haven, Connecticut
susan.lederer@yale.edu

Trudo Lemmens, Lic. Jur., LL.M., D.C.L.
Associate Professor, Faculty of Law
University of Toronto
Toronto, Canada
trudo.lemmens@utoronto.ca

Carol Levine, M.A.
Director, Families and Health Care
    Project
United Hospital Fund
New York, New York
clevine@uhfnyc.org

Felice J. Levine, Ph.D.
Executive Director,
American Educational Research
    Association
Washington, D.C.
flevine@aera.net

Robert J. Levine, M.D.
Co-Director, Yale University
    Interdisciplinary Center for
    Bioethics;
Director, Law, Policy and Ethics Core,
    Center for Interdisciplinary Research
    on AIDS;
Professor of Medicine and Lecturer
    in Pharmacology
Yale University School of Medicine
New Haven, Connecticut
levinerj@worldnet.att.net

Charles W. Lidz, Ph.D.
Research Professor, Department of
    Psychiatry;
Director, Center for Mental Health
    Services Research
University of Massachusetts Medical
    School
Worcester, Massachusetts
charles.lidz@umassmed.edu

Bernard Lo, M.D., FACP
Professor, Department of Medicine;
Director, Program in Medical Ethics
University of California at San
    Francisco, School of Medicine
San Francisco, California
bernie@medicine.ucsf.edu

Alex John London, Ph.D.
Associate Professor, Department of
    Philosophy;
Director, Center for the Advancement
    of Applied Ethics and Political
    Philosophy,
Carnegie Mellon University
Pittsburgh, Pennsylvania
ajlondon@andrew.cmu.edu

Ruth Macklin, Ph.D.
Professor of Bioethics
Department of Epidemiology and
    Population Health
Albert Einstein College of Medicine
New York, New York
macklin@aecom.yu.edu

Wendy K. Mariner, J.D., LL.M., M.P.H.
Professor, Department of Health Law,
    Bioethics and Human Rights,
Boston University School of Public
    Health;
Professor, Boston University School of
    Medicine, and School of Law
Boston, Massachusetts
wmariner@bu.edu

Charles R. McCarthy, Ph.D.
Office of Education and Compliance
    Oversight
Virginia Commonwealth University
Richmond, Virginia
c_emcc@wcrichmond.org

Robert E. McKeown, M.Div., Ph.D.
Professor, Department of Epidemiology
    and Biostatistics
Norman J. Arnold School of Public
    Health,
University of South Carolina
Charleston, South Carolina
rmckeown@gwm.sc.edu

Marcia L. Meldrum, Ph.D.
Co-Director, John C. Liebeskind History
  of Pain Collection
University of California, Los Angeles
Los Angeles, California
mlynnmel@earthlink.net

Leslie A. Meltzer, J.D., M.Sc.
Doctoral candidate, Department of
  Religious Studies
University of Virginia
Charlottesville, Virginia;
Greenwall Fellow, Berman Institute of
  Bioethics
The Johns Hopkins University
Baltimore, Maryland
lam3q@virginia.edu

Eric M. Meslin, Ph.D.
Director, Indiana University Center for
  Bioethics;
Assistant Dean for Bioethics, Indiana
  University School of Medicine;
Professor of Medicine, Molecular and
  Medical Genetics, and Philosophy
Indiana University-Purdue University
  Indiana
Indianapolis, Indiana
emeslin@iupui.edu

Jonathan D. Moreno, Ph.D.
David and Lyn Silfen University
  Professor,
Professor of Medical Ethics and the
  History and Sociology of Science
Center for Bioethics, University of
  Pennsylvania
Philadelphia, Pennsylvania;
Senior Fellow, Center for American
  Progress
Washington, D.C.
jmoreno@americanprogress.org

Joan P. Porter, M.Sc., D.P.A., M.P.H, CIP
Associate Director
Office of Research Oversight
Veterans Health Administration
Washington, D.C.
joan.porter@va.gov

**Drummond Rennie, M.D., F.R.C.P.,
  M.A.C.P.**
Adjunct Professor of Medicine
University of California at San
  Francisco;
Deputy Editor, *JAMA*
San Francisco, California
rennie@itsa.ucsf.edu

David B. Resnik, J.D., Ph.D.
Bioethicist
National Institute of Environmental
  Health Sciences
National Institute of Health
Research Triangle Park, North Carolina
resnikd@niehs.nih.gov

Walter M. Robinson, M.D., M.P.H.
Associate Professor of Pediatrics,
  Medicine, and Bioethics,
Dalhousie University Faculty of
  Medicine;
Head, Pediatric Pulmonary Medicine
IWK Health Centre, Halifax
Nova Scotia, Canada
walter.robinson@iwk.nshealth.ca

Donald L. Rosenstein, M.D.
Acting Clinical Director and Chief
Psychiatry Consultation-Liaison Service
National Institute of Mental Health
National Institutes of Health
Bethesda, Maryland
rosenstd@mail.nih.gov

**Eleanor B. Schron, R.N., M.S., FAAN,
  FAHA**
Nurse Scientist, Clinical Trials Scientific
  Research Group
Division of Epidemiology & Clinical
  Applications
National Heart, Lung, and Blood
  Institute
National Institutes of Health
Bethesda, Maryland
schrone@mail.nih.gov

Sebastian Sethe, M.A.
Research Assistant
Sheffield Institute of Biotechnological
  Law and Ethics (SIBLE)
University of Sheffield
Sheffield, England
ssethe@gmail.com

Richard R. Sharp, Ph.D.
Assistant Professor
Department of Bioethics
Cleveland Clinic
Cleveland, Ohio
Sharpr3@ccf.org

Paula R. Skedsvold, J.D., Ph.D.
Senior Legal Research Analyst
International Women's Human Rights
  Clinic
Georgetown University Law Center
Washington, D.C.
pskedsvold@aera.net

Marjorie A. Speers, Ph.D.
Executive Director
Association for the Accreditation of
  Human Research Protection
  Programs, Inc® (AAHRPP®)
Washington, D.C.
mspeers@aahrpp.org

Robert Steinbrook, M.D.
National Correspondent, *New England
  Journal of Medicine;*
Adjunct Professor of Medicine
Dartmouth Medical School
Dartmouth, Vermont
rsteinb@attglobal.net

Robert Temple, M.D.
Director, Office of Medical Policy;
Director, Office of Drug Evaluation I
Center for Drug Evaluation and
  Research
Food and Drug Administration
Silver Spring, Maryland
robert.temple@fda.hhs.gov

Dennis F. Thompson, Ph.D.
Alfred North Whitehead Professor of
  Political Philosophy
Department of Government;
Professor of Public Policy,
John F. Kennedy School of
  Government;
Harvard University
Cambridge, Massachusetts
dennis_thompson@harvard.edu

Robert D. Truog, M.D.
Professor of Medical Ethics,
    Anaesthesia, and Pediatrics
Harvard Medical School;
Senior Associate in Critical Care
    Medicine
Children's Hospital
Boston, Massachusetts
robert_truog@hms.harvard.edu

Takashi Tsuchiya, M.A.
Associate Professor
Department of Philosophy
Osaka City University
Osaka, Japan
tsuchiya@lit.osaka-cu.ac.jp

Brandon T. Unruh, B.A.
Departments of Psychiatry
Massachusetts General Hospital,
    and McLean Hospital
Boston, Massachusetts
unruh@post.harvard.edu

Sumeeta Varma, B.S.
Medical student (Class of 2011)
Washington University of St. Louis
St. Louis, Missouri
sumeeta@standfordalumni.org

Douglas L. Weed, M.D., M.P.H., Ph.D.
Vice President
Epidemiology and Biostatistics
The Weinberg Group
Washington, D.C.
doug.weed@weinberggroup.com

Paul J. Weindling, Ph.D.
Wellcome Trust Research Professor in
    the History of Medicine
The Centre for Health, Medicine and
    Society: Past and Present
Oxford Brookes University
Oxford, England
pjweindling@brookes.ac.uk

Alan Wertheimer, Ph.D.
Professor Emeritus of Political Science
University of Vermont
Burlington, Vermont;
Research Scholar, Department of
    Bioethics
National Institutes of Health
Bethesda, Maryland
wertheimera@cc.nih.gov

Alan Yoshioka, Ph.D.
AY's Edit
Toronto, Canada
ay1@aysedit.com

Pēteris Zilgalvis, J.D.
Deputy Head
Department of Bioethics
Directorate General—Legal Affairs
Council of Europe
Strasbourg, France
peteris.zilgalvis@ec.europa.eu

The Oxford Textbook of
Clinical Research Ethics

Ezekiel J. Emanuel   Robert A. Crouch   Christine Grady
Reidar K. Lie   Franklin G. Miller   David Wendler

Introduction

The last decade has witnessed tremendous controversy surrounding the ethics of clinical research. There have been disagreements over the use of placebos in developing countries when there are effective but costly therapies available in more developed countries; there has been uncertainty over researchers' obligations to participants once trials are complete; there have been disagreements over research with children and mentally incapacitated patients; and there is widespread condemnation of academic researchers' financial conflicts of interest. The deaths of Jesse Gelsinger and Ellen Roche while both were enrolled in clinical research, and the suspension of clinical research at Duke, Johns Hopkins, and other major research institutions has created concern over the safety of clinical research. Suppression of data on adverse drug events by pharmaceutical corporations has created concern over the integrity of both researchers and the research enterprise. Probably nothing signifies this controversy and its public nature better than the April 22, 2002, issue of *Time* magazine, whose cover depicted a human being in a hospital gown inside a cage, under a caption that read, "How Medical Testing Has Turned Millions of Us into . . . Human Guinea Pigs."[1]

Of course, this is not the first era of controversy surrounding clinical research. At least three periods of sustained controversy have occurred before this latest decade. In the late 19th century, there was an important controversy surrounding the search for the cause and a cure of yellow fever. As Susan Lederer describes in Chapter 1, Guiseppe Sanarelli was an Italian researcher working in South America. Working with the legacy of Koch and Pasteur's isolation of microorganisms as causes of disease, he declared that he had isolated the bacillus that caused yellow fever, and was able to induce yellow fever in five people by infecting them with the

agent. (Leave aside that yellow fever is caused not by a bacillus but by a virus.) His work was categorically condemned by many researchers, most importantly by William Osler, at the time the world's most prominent and famed physician and chairman of medicine at Johns Hopkins Medical School and soon to be Regius Professor of Medicine at Oxford. At a professional meeting in 1898, Osler declared, "To deliberately inject a poison of known high degree of virulency into a human being, unless you obtain that man's sanction, is not ridiculous, it is criminal."[2]

After the yellow fever controversy there was the entire episode of Nazi medicine and medical research. As delineated by Paul Weindling in Chapter 2, this period entailed a myriad of the most gruesome and horrific experiments, from placing people in freezing water until they died to subjecting them to very low atmospheric pressures until they exploded, from injecting them with typhoid to Mengele's twin experiments. Part of the horror was how many German researchers were able to use their research samples and data after the war to continue as respected researchers.

Then beginning in the early 1960s, there was a series of research scandals in the United States that culminated in the revelations about the Tuskegee Syphilis Study. This period began in July 1963 with the Brooklyn Jewish Chronic Disease Hospital case, which is described by John Arras in Chapter 6. Prominent cancer researchers "injected live cancer cells into 22 chronically ill and debilitated patients" without informing them that cancer cells were being used. Patients were unaware that this was not a therapeutic intervention to treat their condition, but was rather an experiment to gain scientific knowledge. Furthermore, the patients were not asked for their consent to the study.

Then in 1966, Henry K. Beecher, a prominent anesthesiologist at the Massachusetts General Hospital and professor at Harvard Medical School, published a paper in the *New England Journal of Medicine* entitled "Ethics and Clinical Research."[3] In it, he delineated 22 cases that he claimed were extracted from an original list of 50 cases. He noted that these cases came "from leading medical school, university hospitals, private hospitals, governmental military departments (the Army, the Navy, and the Air Force), governmental institutes (the NIH), Veterans Administration hospitals, and industry." Beecher wrote that these cases represented "troubling practices" in which many of the patients never had the risk satisfactorily explained to them, and further hundreds did not know that they were the subjects of an experiment although they suffered grave consequences as a direct result.

It should be noted that Beecher may not have been careful in all of the 22 cases he criticized. As Walter Robinson and Brandon Unruh note in Chapter 7, although Beecher strongly condemned the Willowbrook hepatitis studies—which left an enduring taint upon its principal investigator, Dr. Saul Krugman—this research seems to have fulfilled ethical requirements and, upon closer examination, to have been conducted in an ethical manner.

As bad as some of Beecher's cases were, worse was revealed in 1972 when the Tuskegee Syphilis Study was disclosed to the public. As described by James Jones in Chapter 8, this study has a great many troubling and unethical aspects. Not only was the scientific justification of the study questionable when it was initiated in the 1930s, the actual trial entailed multiple layers of deception, and trial personnel actively prevented the participants from getting medication—penicillin—to which they were entitled. In the 1960s, a social worker working for the U.S. Public Health Service in San Francisco, Peter Buxton, learned about Tuskegee from coworkers and launched a one man crusade to stop it. As Jones notes, this prompted an internal ethical evaluation of the study, which ultimately sanctioned continuing the study. Only when subjected to public scrutiny through an Associated Press story in 1972 did the trial get halted by the Secretary of the Department of Health Education and Welfare.

Of course, these are not the only scandals or controversies involving clinical research. There were less well known but nonetheless strong condemnations of the appalling research experiments committed by the Japanese military in World War II, well described by Takashi Tsuchiya in Chapter 3. In the 1980s, as John Killen notes in Chapter 9, debate surrounded trials of drugs for HIV/AIDS and whether the research subject protections were excessively paternalistic. Importantly, a big change occurred in this era when research participants were major participants in the debates and, in a surprise to many, challenged the oversight of clinical research as excessively protectionist and paternalistic.

In one sense, such scandals and debates have been quite beneficial. These controversies have forced the reexamination of fundamental issues long deemed settled and produced much of the ethical guidance for clinical research. As Carol Levine has observed, our approach to the ethics of clinical research was "born in scandal and reared in protectionism."[4] Although this may overstate the case a bit, it is certainly true that the condemnation of Sanarelli's claims led Walter Reed to carefully reflect on his yellow fever studies and to delineate five key safeguards: (1) autoexperimentation, with the researchers serving as participants (including the fact that one, Jesse Lazear died as a result); (2) use only of adult participants; (3) signed, written contracts with research

participants; (4) financial payment to the participants; and (5) declaration in the papers that each participant gave his consent, forerunner to the current practice of indicating in published papers that the research was conducted in accord with ethical guidelines. The judicial decision in the post war trial of the Nazi doctors, *United States v. Karl Brandt et al.*, articulated the Nuremberg Code.[5]

In the wake of the Jewish Chronic Disease Hospital case and other scandals, the U.S. Public Health Service required independent review of research studies to assess the risk-benefit ratio and the adequacy of measures to obtain informed consent. The Tuskegee scandal prompted the creation of the National Commission for the Protection of Human Subjects of Biomedical and Behavioral Research by the U.S. Congress. In April 1979, this Commission issued its Belmont Report, which articulated respect for persons, beneficence, and justice as the "broader ethical principles [to] provide a basis on which specific rules may be formulated, criticized, and interpreted."[6] The Commission also induced the Department of Health, Education and Welfare to adopt regulations requiring that institutional review boards review all research protocols before they were begun and other safeguards. Similarly, worries about HIV studies in developing countries led to the International Ethical Guidelines for Biomedical Research Involving Human Subjects promulgated by the Council for International Organizations of Medical Sciences (CIOMS).[7]

Although forcing needed change, these controversies have also stymied clinical research. They have made well-intentioned researchers uncertain of how they can act ethically and how to design an ethical clinical research trial. For instance, ongoing disagreement about the ethics of using placebo controls in developing countries that cannot afford expensive medications or interventions may have inhibited the initiations of studies in developing countries; disagreement about researchers' obligations to health needs of participants that are unrelated to the purposes of research has prevented studies from occurring; different views on what benefits must be provided at the conclusion of trials have generated charges of exploitation; and controversy about the ethics of paying research participants has led many to condemn studies because they are "coercive."

One problem with these controversies is that although bioethicists, research ethics boards, regulatory agencies, international organizations, and others debate what is the ethical thing to do, research must proceed and researchers must make decisions in planning and conducting research studies. This creates challenges for researchers and induces worries that even actions chosen conscientiously and with good intentions may be charged with being unethical. This may cast a chill on research.

Another problem is that the disputes have generated huge amounts of literature—commentaries, conceptual analyses of issues, and empirical research studies. The growth of the literature is not a problem per se. Indeed, good analyses can lead to wider and deeper understanding of many issues. But poor analyses can inappropriately condemn actions and studies as "exploitative," "coercive," or "unjust," thereby inhibiting perfectly ethical research. In addition, a vast literature may make it hard for experts in research ethics, let alone clinical researchers, to be able to know what is the current status of an issue, such as payment to research participants, use of stored biological samples, improving informed consent, or enrollment of people who are mentally incompetent, or what constitutes minimal risk. Although there have been comprehensive review articles on a few relevant topics, there has not been a comprehensive and systematic synthesis and critical analysis of the research ethics literature in all areas. The need for comprehensive reviews is especially critical when it comes to synthesizing empirical studies. Such reviews require collecting large numbers of studies, synthesizing data based on different methodologies, and critically comparing results. The reviews that do exist have generated results that have challenged common assumptions and surprised many people, including experts in the field. For instance, the common assumption that using videos or interactive computer programs will enhance understanding during the informed consent process has been challenged by a comprehensive review. Similarly, the contention that the quality of informed consent is worse in developing countries compared to developed countries was not substantiated when all available studies were analyzed.

A third problem relates to the available ethical guidance. Many codes or declarations were responses to scandals. Walter Reed's five principles were a response to Sanarelli's ethical violations; the Nuremberg Code was a response to the Nazi war crimes; the Belmont Report was a response to Tuskegee Syphilis Study; the ethical guidelines of the Advisory Committee on Human Radiation Experiments was a response to the radiation experiments in the United States; and the latest revision of the Declaration of Helsinki[8] was a response to the controversy surrounding placebo-controlled trials in developing countries. A major problem with such response to scandals is that these guidelines, codes, and declarations focus on the specific issue or issues raised by the scandal and use the scandal as the litmus test for their recommendations. There has been little effort to reflect on a more general ethical framework to guide research ethics, free of the emotional outrage based on the latest egregious violations when, as Bishop Butler put it, "we sit down in a cool hour."

One consequence is that there are contradictions among these various "authoritative" guidelines. For instance, the Nuremberg Code does not permit research with people who cannot consent—children and mentally incapacitated individuals—whereas other guidelines permit such research under certain circumstances; the Declaration of Helsinki seems to prohibit placebo controls whenever there is a proven treatment, whereas most other guidance, including that from CIOMS, the Nuffield Council,[9] and the National Bioethics Advisory Commission,[10] permits such trials under certain circumstances; and CIOMS requires reasonable availability of a drug in a country if it has been proven effective in that country, but this is not required by other guidance including the Declaration of Helsinki and the Nuffield Council.

Further, many of the reviews of ethical issues in clinical research that do exist focus on research work from one country and tend not to be representative of international perspectives. This lacuna prevents comparisons of laws and regulations as well as accepted norms of practice across countries. This has inhibited the identification of areas of agreement and disagreement, and led to claims that upon closer examination seem untenable.

In large measure, this textbook is an effort to remedy these and related lapses. One of its primary aims is to create a comprehensive and systematic synthesis of all the literature relevant to the ethics of clinical research, broadly construed. The textbook addresses all the topics of the ethics of clinical research and attempts to consider all the material written on each topic. It is comprehensive in covering the history of the triumphs of clinical research as well as the scandals—and the formal guidance and scholarship that arose in the wake of these scandals. It analyzes such topics as the various perspectives of different groups of research participants, the assessment of risks and benefits, the operation of institutional review boards, informed consent, and what we know about conflicts of interest. We have tried to define the domain of the ethics of clinical research broadly, encompassing everything that might be relevant to the ethical consideration of a clinical research protocol, from regulations to the social context of research, from fraud and conflict of interest to confidentiality.

The survey is comprehensive in another way: It synthesizes both conceptual work, on issues such as payment to research participants or the involvement of women and children in research, and empirical studies on such topics as informed consent and financial conflicts of interest.

The survey is comprehensive in yet a third way: It focuses not just on the United States but on ethical debates, guidelines, regulations, studies from all over the world. Largely because so much clinical research has been funded by and conducted in the United States, much of the early development of research ethics occurred in the United States. However, with the ongoing and ever accelerating expansion of biomedical research in other countries—that is, with the globalization of research—there will be scandals, guidelines, regulations, and empirical studies from both developed and developing countries outside the United States. Doubtless this will affect research ethics. Although those in the United States often focus on individual rights, autonomy and informed consent, a shift to a global perspective may lead research ethics in new directions, perhaps with a greater emphasis on the impact of research on the wider community. In any case, to reflect and anticipate this globalization, we have tried to include authors from as many countries as possible.

The organization of the textbook is also meant to be instructive. Too often ethical considerations of controversial research trials are chaotic and haphazard, jumping from discussions of informed consent to considerations of risks and potential benefits to posttrial availability of interventions to use of stored tissue samples, and so on. This textbook aims to provide a systematic structure: Parts III through IX follow the logical sequence of development of clinical research protocols, and therefore of the ethical issues that have to be considered along the way. Research begins with defining the questions to be addressed, by what methodologies and in what relevant populations; only toward the end of preparing a research project are the issues of informed consent relevant. The organization and structure of the sections mirror this sequence to provide guidance through the research development process. Our intention is to have the formal structure of the book reemphasize how ethical issues can be addressed in a systematic manner, rather than in a disorganized manner. Hopefully, such an organized manner of analysis will contribute to improving the ethical evaluation of research protocols.

To achieve the goals of the textbook—comprehensiveness, systematic analysis, and wide ranging and international perspectives—we invited the world's leading authorities to contribute chapters. These individuals speak with tremendous knowledge and practical experience. We also sought to identify individuals from many different countries to ensure diverse perspectives and experiences. We believe the collection of over 85 authors from a variety of countries constitutes the very best scholarship on research ethics available.

Furthermore, we asked them to provide comprehensive summaries of their topics. After presenting the diverse perspectives fairly, we expected the authors to inject their own assessments. Why? Because this gives authors an opportunity to provide educated assessments of potential future developments of the ethical issues they have examined. We believe that this combination of comprehensive summaries and editorial perspectives of the author provides the best balance for interesting, informative, and vibrant chapters.

Our aim was to provide a book useful in training researchers and others. Over the last decade, there has been substantial emphasis on capacity development related to research in developing countries. Some of this attention has also focused on improving skills in the ethical review of research. Simultaneously, it has been observed that researchers and members of research review committees in developed countries have lacked training and knowledge in the ethical conduct of clinical research. Consequently, there has been recognition of the needs and efforts in both developed and developing countries to provide training in research ethics. Unfortunately, useful educational materials are lacking. This textbook is part of our efforts to address this deficiency. We hope teachers and students of research ethics will find it useful.

We are acutely aware that at best this textbook provides substantive guidance. This is necessary but not sufficient for ethical clinical research. In 1931, Germany enacted what many believe to be the first systematic, national research ethics guidelines. While these guidelines were in place, the Nazi violations were occurring. Guidelines are not self-enforcing. Researchers, research ethics committees, regulators, and others must enforce the rules. However, enforcers need to know what to enforce. A textbook such as this is absolutely necessary. Before we can enforce, we need to elucidate and specify what needs enforcement. We therefore hope that this is a book that researchers, members of ethics review committees, bioethicists, students, patient advocates, regulators, and others can consult to obtain clear guidance regarding the issues they confront. We hope it becomes a reliable and valued reference work.

In preparing any book, editorial decisions must be made that themselves will be controversial. How broadly or narrowly to define the textbook's subject? What specific topics to include or exclude? How much space to allocate to each topic? Which of several authorities in a particular area should be invited to author a chapter? The editors have wrestled with each of these issues and many others. There is no escaping contentious decisions that will annoy and even offend people. We accept full responsibility for these choices, with the knowledge that this is a work of contemporary reflection and scholarship, not the final account of research ethics. As research proceeds and additional challenges arise, further constructive analyses and refinements will be necessary. This is for future editions.

References

1. *Time*, April 22, 2002.
2. As quoted in: Lederer SE. *Subjected to Science*. Baltimore, Md.: Johns Hopkins University Press; 1995:22.
3. Beecher HK. Ethics and clinical research. *New England Journal of Medicine* 1966;274:1354–60.
4. Levine C. Changing view of justice after Belmont: AIDS and the inclusion of "vulnerable" subjects. In: Vanderpool HY, ed. *The Ethics of Research Involving Human Subjects: Facing the 21st Century*. Frederick, Md.: University Publishing Group; 1996:105–26; p. 106.
5. The Nuremberg Code. In: *Trials of War Criminals Before the Nuremberg Military Tribunals under Control Council Law No. 10. Volume 2*. Washington, D.C.: U.S. Government Printing Office; 1949:181–82 [Online]. Available: http://www.hhs.gov/ohrp/references/nurcode.htm.
6. The National Commission for the Protection of Human Subjects of Biomedical and Behavioral Research. *The Belmont Report: Ethical Principles and Guidelines for the Protection of Human Subjects of Research*. Washington, D.C.: Department of Health, Education and Welfare; DHEW Publication OS 78-0012 1978. [Online] April 18, 1979. Available: http://www.hhs.gov/ohrp/humansubjects/guidance/belmont.htm.
7. Council for International Organizations of Medical Sciences, in collaboration with the World Health Organization. *International Ethical Guidelines for Biomedical Research Involving Human Subjects*. Geneva, Switzerland: CIOMS and WHO; 2002. [Online] November 2002. Available: http://www.cioms.ch/frame_guidelines_nov_2002.htm.
8. World Medical Association. *Declaration of Helsinki: Ethical Principles for Medical Research Involving Human Subjects*. Tokyo, Japan: WMA; October 2004. [Online] 2004. Available: http://www.wma.net/e/policy/b3.htm.
9. Nuffield Council on Bioethics. *The Ethics of Research Related to Healthcare in Developing Countries*. London, UK: Nuffield Council on Bioethics; 2002. [Online] Available: http://nuffieldbioethics.org/fileLibrary/pdf/errhdc_fullreport001.pdf.
10. National Bioethics Advisory Commission. *Ethical and Policy Issues in International Research: Clinical Trials in Developing Countries*. Bethesda, Md.: NBAC; April 2001. [Online] Available: http://www.bioethics.gov/reports/past_commissions/nbac_international.pdf.

A Selected History of Research With Humans

Susan E. Lederer

Walter Reed and the Yellow Fever Experiments

On October 27, 1900, the front page of the *New York Times* brandished the headline "Mosquito Carries Yellow Fever Germ." The special report described how the investigations conducted by U.S. Army surgeon Walter Reed and his colleagues—Aristides Agramonte, James Carroll, and Jesse Lazear—established that the Aedes mosquito served as the "intermediate host" for the so-called parasite of yellow fever.[1] Through a series of elegant and painstaking experiments, the members of the Yellow Fever Commission demonstrated that yellow fever was not transmitted via bodily contact or through infected clothing. Because there was no animal model for yellow fever, these experiments necessarily involved human beings. Two members of the Yellow Fever Commission—Lazear and Carroll—participated in early trials with "loaded" mosquitoes. Later, the members of the Commission secured human subjects, both American soldiers stationed in Havana and recently arrived Spanish immigrants, who agreed to be exposed to infected mosquitoes and to the bed linens and clothing taken from patients dead from yellow fever. Fortunately, after investigator Jesse Lazear succumbed to yellow fever in 1900, no other individuals died as a result of their participation in the yellow fever experiments.[2]

Yellow fever was a major threat to American lives and American commerce in the early 20th century. The successful demonstration of how this often deadly disease was transmitted inspired confidence that the disease could be effectively controlled. United States physicians hailed Walter Reed and his colleagues as scientific heroes and martyrs (both Lazear who died in 1900 from yellow fever and Reed who died following an appendectomy in 1902) for the yellow fever work, which was also taken as a sign of America's growing presence in the world of medical science. With the memory of yellow fever fresh in their minds, Americans initially celebrated Reed as the one "who gave to Man control of that dreadful scourge—yellow fever," as Harvard University president Charles Eliot put it in 1902 when he conferred an honorary degree upon Reed.[3]

As the threat of yellow fever receded, however, the work of the Yellow Fever Commission came to symbolize the willingness of medical researchers to risk their own lives in search of medical knowledge. Reed's willingness to risk life and limb in the name of science—both his own life and those of others—was celebrated, in spite of the fact that he had not actually participated in the yellow fever studies. But Reed was more than a risk-taker; his use of a written contract signed by the experimenter and the research subject offered an example of humane experimentation that in the 1970s could be marshaled to counteract "sweeping moral agitation by earnest and sometimes sentimental and unwise persons" who claimed that all research on human subjects was wrong.[4] This contract, provided in both English and Spanish for the Spanish immigrants who agreed to participate in the studies, outlined the risks of participation in the yellow fever study and the benefits, including medical care and a sum of American gold ($100 for their participation, $200 if they contracted yellow fever). Now touted as "a milestone in the evolution of ethics in medical research" for its introduction of "informed consent," Reed's contract represented a distinct departure from research practices in the early 20th century.[5] But then, as now, social and political factors influenced the meaning of consent and its place in research ethics.

The Problem of Yellow Fever

It would not be exaggeration to describe yellow fever as the scourge of the American South. The disease exerted an effect disproportionate to its relative mortality rate, because even when it failed to kill the patient, it left evidence of its ravages. Signs of classic yellow fever included chills, high fever, muscle aches, liver failure, and jaundice (producing yellow skin). Many patients experienced hemorrhaging from the nose, gums, and stomach, producing what was known as "the black vomit." (In Spanish, the name for the disease was *vomito negro*.) Estimates about mortality from the disease ranged from 10% to 60%.[6] An outbreak of yellow fever led people to abandon their neighborhoods by any means available. The consequences for commerce were often as deadly as the disease; those too poor to flee the city were reduced to begging for food and going without sustenance. In 1898, when the United States declared war against Spain following the sinking of the battleship *Maine,* U.S. officials realized the threat that yellow fever posed to American troops. Their fears were well grounded; although some 400 American soldiers lost their lives in what Secretary of State John Hay memorably dubbed "a splendid little war," more than 2,000 American men fell victim to yellow fever. In the face of the disorder and death caused by yellow fever, it is easy to see why the demonstration of its mode of transmission would be considered front-page news in 1900.

The signs and symptoms of yellow fever were well known, but the cause of the disease remained obscure. With the advent of a new paradigm of disease causation, the germ theory, in the late 19th century, physicians and researchers successfully documented the causes of many diseases, including leprosy (1873), anthrax (1876), and tuberculosis (1882). In 1897, the Italian bacteriologist Giuseppe Sanarelli, working in Montevideo, Uruguay, announced that he had discovered the bacillus that caused yellow fever in the blood of patients with yellow fever. Conforming to Koch's postulates, the conventions identified by German researcher Robert Koch to establish the etiology of disease, Sanarelli claimed to have cultured Bacillus icteroides (a bacterium in the hog cholera group) and to have injected it into five patients at a Montevideo hospital, producing the signs of what he described as "classic yellow fever." Three of his patients reportedly died from the disease. Efforts to replicate Sanarelli's findings failed. Although investigators working with yellow fever epidemics in New Orleans, Havana, Brazil, and Mexico sought to locate the bacillus both in living patients with yellow fever and in yellow fever cadavers, the evidence for Sanarelli's bacillus remained conflicting and unsatisfactory.[7]

Army Surgeon General George M. Sternberg was one of Sanarelli's harshest critics. When he secured from the Secretary of War the appointment of a Board of Medical Officers to investigate yellow fever, Sternberg instructed the officers to evaluate the Italian researcher's report and to explore the possibility of an "intermediate host" in the transmission of the disease. The possibility that the mosquito served as the intermediate host for yellow fever had first been raised in 1881 by Carlos Finlay, a Cuban physician. Finlay not only identified the correct mosquito (Culex, now known as Aedes aegypti) as the vector, but he provided Reed and his colleagues samples with which to start their own mosquito colony. Finlay championed the mosquito theory but he offered little persuasive evidence that this was the only way that the disease could be transmitted. With the successful dem-

onstration in 1898–1899 by Italian researchers Giovanni Grassi and Amico Bignami and English medical officer Richard Ross that anopheline mosquitoes transmitted malaria, the mosquito hypothesis for yellow fever gained currency. It remained for the members of the Yellow Fever Commission to establish that the Aedes mosquito transmitted yellow fever, and that the disease did not spread through clothing, linens, and body fluids of infected individuals.[8]

The Design and Conduct of the Experiments

To establish the etiology of the disease, the members of the Yellow Fever Commission evaluated Sanarelli's claims for Bacillus icteroides. Autopsies on 11 patients dead from yellow fever failed to produce evidence of the bacillus in cultures of blood, liver, spleen, kidney, bile, and small intestine. Using one's own body or that of a colleague was a longstanding convention for many physicians. In August 1900, two of the Commission researchers, Jesse Lazear and James Carroll, undertook experiments on themselves. Lazear, for example, placed an infected mosquito on Carroll's arm to observe the effects. Although unpersuaded at this time of the mosquito's role, Carroll became a supporter when he developed a severe attack of yellow fever following the bite, and came close to death. In September 1900, in circumstances that remain unclear, Jesse Lazear similarly developed yellow fever. Whether the result of a deliberate infection or an accidental inoculation, Lazear died from the disease on September 25, 1900, the first official "martyr" of the Yellow Fever Commission.

Reed and his colleagues were persuaded about the mosquito's role in the transmission of yellow fever, but they also wanted evidence to convince those who resisted the idea. Reed approached Cuba's governor general for permission to solicit approval from the Spanish consul for a plan to recruit recently arrived Spaniards for volunteers in these studies. General Leonard Wood, also a physician, not only endorsed Reed's plan but provided an additional sum of $10,000 to support the research. To demonstrate that the mosquito was solely responsible for transmission of the disease, Reed and his colleagues sought evidence that other traditional routes of infection failed to cause yellow fever. One commonly held theory was that fomites (inanimate objects such as infected bed linen, clothing, and blankets) transmitted yellow fever. To establish that fomites did not play this role in the disease, Reed ordered the construction at Camp Lazear of two frame buildings with wire screen windows and doors to ensure that mosquitoes could not enter (see Figure 1.1). In one experiment, three nonimmune Americans (an assistant surgeon and two privates) entered the infected room where they unpacked boxes filled with sheets, pillow cases, and blankets "purposely soiled with a liberal quantity of black vomit, urine, and fecal matter." Using the soiled linens and wearing the fouled garments of yellow fever patients, the Americans remained in the contaminated room for 20 days and emerged free from yellow fever. In another fomite study, James Hildebrand, a member of the Alabama Infantry and Hospital Corps, spent 20 days sleeping on a towel soaked in the blood of a patient who had died from yellow fever. A series of experiments in the fomite house established that the disease did not spread in this manner.

Reed, Agramonte, and Carroll wanted to demonstrate that yellow fever was a blood-borne disease, either by "loaded mos-

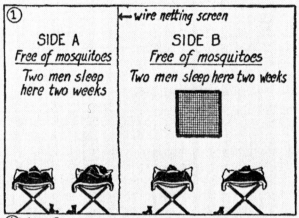

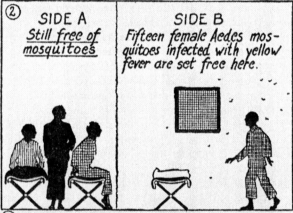

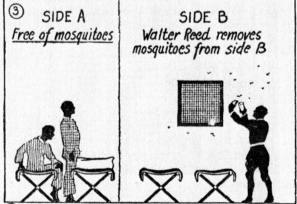

Figure 1.1. Illustrated Depiction of Yellow Fever Experiment. Source: Papers of Jefferson Randolph Kean, MSS 628, Special Collections, University of Virginia Library, Charlottesville, Va. Reproduced with permission.

quitoes" (mosquitoes that fed on patients with active yellow fever) or through experimental injections of blood from patients with active yellow fever. When these "loaded mosquitoes" fed on volunteers who had never had yellow fever, the volunteers developed the disease. Warren Jernegan, for example, an American member of the Hospital Corps, followed his stint in the fomite house by volunteering to be bitten by loaded mosquitoes. He did not develop yellow fever until he subsequently received a subcutaneous injection of blood in January 1901 from a patient with an experimental case of yellow fever. He recovered from the severe case of the disease that the injection caused. In January 1901, when the volunteer who was scheduled to receive an experimental injection refused to participate, Walter Reed apparently volunteered to receive the injection, but Carroll vehemently objected (the disease was regarded as more dangerous to men over 40 such as Reed). Instead, a young American hospital corpsman, John Andrus, volunteered for the injection, received the subcutaneous injection, and developed a severe case of yellow fever, from which he made a slow recovery. A second American volunteer, a civilian related to the wife of an American officer stationed in Cuba, also received two injections of filtered blood from patients with active yellow fever. He developed yellow fever from the second injection, and also recovered. A third American volunteer, Albert Covington, developed a very severe case of yellow fever when he received an injection of the filtered blood serum from an experimental case of yellow fever.[9]

In addition to the 18 Americans (2 civilians, 15 enlisted men, and 1 officer) who participated as research subjects in the yellow fever studies, some 15 Spanish immigrants similarly underwent infection with "loaded" mosquitoes or received subcutaneous injections of the blood taken from yellow fever patients. At least 6 Spanish men developed yellow fever when they were bitten by infected mosquitoes, and one man, Manuel Gutierrez Moran, developed the disease when he received an injection of blood from a yellow fever patient. At least 6 other Spanish immigrants received bites or injections but did not develop the disease. All survived their bouts with experimental infections.

By September 1900, the work of the Reed Commission proved conclusively that the Aedes mosquito was the vector of yellow fever, and that there was an interval of about 12 days between the time that the mosquito took an infectious blood meal and the time it could convey the infection to another human being. In early 1901, the Commission established that the disease could be produced experimentally by the subcutaneous injection of blood taken from the general circulation of a yellow fever patient during the first and second days of his illness.

The establishment of the mosquito's role in the transmission of yellow fever offered a solution to the problem of the disease, namely eradicating the mosquito and the insect's breeding spaces. In December 1900, the Army began an extensive cleanup of the city of Havana, using fumigation (with sulfur, formaldehyde, and insect powder). By the second half of 1901, Havana health authorities reported no cases of the disease for the first time in the memory of many of the citizens. Using similar methods of fumigation, drainage of low lying areas, and larvicides, William Gorgas led the campaign to rid the Panama Canal Zone, Panama City, and Colon of yellow fever. Perhaps not surprisingly, the measures taken against the Aedes mosquito greatly reduced the incidence of malaria, caused by a different mosquito species, in the region.

Contract and Consent

One unusual feature of the yellow fever experiments was the introduction of a written document that outlined the risks involved in the efforts to transmit yellow fever and the reality that there was no effective treatment for the disease. Available in both English and Spanish, the document described how the "contracting party" consented to experiments authorized by the U.S. secretary of war to determine the mode of transmission of yellow fever and acknowledged the risks:

> The undersigned understands perfectly well that in case of the development of yellow fever in him, that he endangers his life to a certain extent[;] but it being entirely impossible for him to avoid the infection during his stay in this island, he prefers to take the chance of contracting it intentionally in the belief that he will receive from the said Commission the greatest care and the most skillful medical service.[4]

Perhaps equally important to the Spanish immigrants (who were desirable subjects, presumed to be nonimmune because of their recent arrival in Cuba) was the paragraph that promised $100 in American gold for two months as an experimental subject, with the further promise of an additional $100 in gold if the subject developed yellow fever. The document explicitly acknowledged the potential for death by explaining that the additional $100 would go to a family member in the event of a subject's death.

Reed's use of a written contract between investigator and research subject was not the first effort by an American physician to identify explicitly the responsibility for participation in research. In 1822, William Beaumont, a U.S. Army physician serving in a remote Michigan outpost, received an urgent request to treat a French Canadian voyageur shot at close range in the abdomen. A musket ball had splintered Alexis St. Martin's rib, and a portion of his lung, "as large as a turkey egg," protruded from the wound. Although Beaumont tried unsuccessfully to close the wound, he soon became convinced that this "accidental orifice" could provide unparalleled information about human digestion. Between 1822 and 1832, Beaumont subjected St. Martin to an extended series of observations and experiments. St. Martin often balked at the doctor's efforts to obtain samples of his stomach fluid, record temperatures of his internal organs, and suspend various foodstuffs into the opening to observe digestion. To ensure St. Martin's compliance, Beaumont engaged attorney Jonathan D. Woodward to draw up a contract that specified St. Martin's duties and his compensation. Adapting the standard legal language for the binding of an indentured servant, Woodward noted that the French Canadian would:

> Submit to, assist and promote by all means in his power, such Physiological and Medical experiments as the said William shall direct or cause to be made on or the stomach of him, the said Alexis, either through or by the means of, the aperture or opening thereto in the side of him, the said Alexis, or otherwise, and will obey, suffer, and comply with all reasonable and proper orders or experiments of the said William, in relation thereto, and in relation to the exhibiting and showing his said Stomach, and the powers and properties thereof, and of the appurtenances and powers, properties, situation and state of its contents.[10]

In exchange for St. Martin's willingness to undergo observations and to be exhibited for the purpose of science, the third paragraph of the contract stipulated that he would receive $150 for one year's service, $40 at the start and the remainder at the end of the year. (In 2005 terms, $150 was worth approximately $2,600.) In addition to this cash payment, Beaumont agreed to provide food, lodging, and clothing. Woodward witnessed the contract; he also signed St. Martin's name on his behalf. Although St. Martin could not write his name, he appended his own mark next to the signature.

This contract has been described as the "first documented instance in the United States where concern for patient welfare was demonstrated, and acknowledgement of human experimentation obtained, via formal written informed consent."[11] Such a characterization, however, is misleading. This was an employment contract drawn up by the employer rather than a written informed consent document. It does not illustrate concern for patient welfare so much as the researcher's concern about obtaining the subject's compliance with the investigations. Nowhere, for example, does the document acknowledge the physical distress or discomfort that accompanied the experiments; there was no discussion of potential and or permanent risk, and there was no provision for withdrawing from the agreement. When St. Martin died in 1880, the Canadian physician William Osler sought to preserve the celebrated stomach for the U.S. Army Medical Museum. Members of St. Martin's family did not welcome this news; to prevent postmortem removal of the organ, his family kept his body in their home longer than usual despite the hot weather to promote the decomposition and render the body less attractive to physicians. To thwart theft of his remains, the family asked that his grave be dug eight feet below the surface "to prevent any attempt at a resurrection."[10]

Unlike the contract between Beaumont and St. Martin, the Reed contracts can be understood as early examples of "informed consent." Reed and his colleagues took pains to ensure that volunteers understood the risks associated with their participation in the experiments. The historical record suggests that Reed's volunteers were able to withdraw from the experiment when they considered the risk of injury or death too great.

Exactly why Reed instituted the practice of contracts is a matter of speculation. Certainly Reed and his superior, Army Surgeon General Sternberg, were aware of the criticism that Sanarelli had received for the experiments in which he infected immigrants, without their consent, with Bacillus icteroides, wrongly thought by Sanarelli to be the cause of yellow fever. Sternberg, for example, was present at the 1898 meeting of the Association of American Physicians wherein University of Michigan physician Victor Vaughan dismissed Sanarelli's experiments as "simply ridiculous." The revered Canadian physician William Osler, the medical educator who introduced bedside teaching for medical students at Johns Hopkins Hospital and the same physician who had attempted to procure St. Martin's viscera, blasted Sanarelli for his experiments. "To deliberately inject a poison of known high degree of virulency into a human being, unless you obtain that man's sanction, is not ridiculous," Osler insisted, "it is criminal."[12] In the 1898 edition of his enormously popular textbook, *The Principles and Practice of Medicine,* Osler took the extraordinary step of censuring the Italian bacteriologist and the "unjustifiable experiments" on yellow fever. In harsh language, Osler demanded that Sanarelli's research receive "the unqualified condemnation of the [medical] profession." Osler offered a similar condemnation of such conduct when he testified on the subject of medical research before the Committee on the District of Columbia of the U.S. Senate in 1900.[2]

Sensitive to the criticism surrounding Sanarelli's exploitation of hospital patients, Sternberg took pains to distinguish the Army Commission's investigations from those conducted by the Italian bacteriologist. In 1901, in a popular article on the mosquito and yellow fever, Sternberg emphasized that nonimmune Spanish immigrants and the American soldiers and civilians who participated in the Reed experiments participated with full knowledge of the risks. "The non-immune individuals experimented upon were all fully informed as to the nature of the experiment and its probable results and all gave their full consent." In addition to being fully informed, Sternberg explained that those who became ill received "the best possible care," and moreover left the experiment with the salutary advantage of being "immune" to the disease which had caused "the death of thousands and tens of thousands of Spanish soldiers and immigrants who have come to Cuba under the orders of their Government or to seek their fortunes."[13]

Sternberg communicated his concern for the human subjects directly to Aristides Agramonte, the Cuban-born physician who served with Reed, Lazear, and Carroll on the Yellow Fever Commission. In May 1900, Sternberg wrote Agramonte about the possibility of resolving whether yellow fever could be transmitted by injecting a healthy man with blood from a yellow fever patient, and emphasized the need to obtain permission: "If you have the opportunity to repeat the experiments and settle this important matter in a definite way," Sternberg noted, "you will bear in mind the fact that they should not be made upon any individual without his full knowledge and consent."[2] Although Agramonte believed that he never received sufficient credit for his role in the yellow fever studies, he similarly emphasized that the volunteers were fully informed about the nature of their participation. Unlike other commentators, Agramonte insisted that newly arrived Spanish men were necessary as subjects, because the American volunteers preferred the fomite tests rather than the bites of infected mosquitoes. As the only Spanish speaker, Agramonte was charged with identifying newly arrived Spaniards and questioning them about their previous exposure to yellow fever. Because the Army had promised the Spanish consul to use only men over the Spanish age of consent (25 years), Agramonte verified the men's ages and also tried to ensure that the men had no wives or children dependent upon them. "When the selection was finally made, the matter of the experiment was put to them," Agramonte explained:

> Naturally they all felt more or less that they were running the risk of getting yellow fever when they came to Cuba and so were not at all averse to allow themselves to be bitten by mosquitoes; they were paid one hundred dollars for this, and another equal sum if, as a result of the biting experiment they developed yellow fever. Needless to say, no reference was made to any possible funeral expenses. A written consent was obtained from each one, so that our moral responsibility was to a certain extent lessened. Of course, only the healthiest specimens were experimented upon.[14]

As Agramonte's explanation makes clear, there was concern about the well-being of the men, as well as recognition that death might result. Although the investigators made no mention of funeral expenses, insisting that the subjects have no dependents may have communicated the threat (together with the information that in case of death from yellow fever, a family member would receive the additional $100).

Sternberg, Reed, Agramonte, and Carroll were also aware that using Spanish immigrants was potentially explosive. At the Pan-American Medical Congress held in Havana in 1901, a Cuban physician criticized the use of the men in dangerous experiments. This criticism echoed the stories in the Havana press, which in November 1900 had denounced the American doctors for injecting poison into unsuspecting immigrants and called on the Spanish consul to investigate these "horrible charges." As a preemptive measure, Reed, Carroll, and Agramonte called on the Spanish official, showed him the signed contracts with the men, and as Agramonte later recalled, the official "being an intelligent man himself" instructed the investigators "to go ahead and not bother about any howl the papers might make."[14]

Reed and his colleagues adopted written contracts with their research subjects for many reasons. The written permission statements, as Agramonte noted, served to lessen the moral responsibility for putting lives at risk, but the risks remained real. Although none of the volunteers died as a result of their participation, the shadow of death had been cast by Lazear's untimely end. In the yellow fever research in Havana that followed the Reed Commission, several volunteers, including a young American nurse, Clara Maas, died from yellow fever.

The Legacy of Walter Reed

Walter Reed died in 1902 from complications following an appendectomy. His death, at the height of his fame, produced an outpouring of remembrances and an also immediate apotheosis into the pantheon of American medical heroes. Reed's death represented a great loss to national medical aspirations, not least because he seemed America's most plausible candidate for a biomedical hero of the stature of European researchers Joseph Lister, Robert Koch, or Louis Pasteur. Moreover, his death meant that American medicine lost its most likely contender for the newly established Nobel Prizes, which then as now were awarded only to the living.

That Reed succumbed to surgical complications rather than yellow fever hardly slowed his commemorators, who quickly glossed over the distinction between medical heroism and martyrdom. Although Lazear lost his life to yellow fever, Reed perished because his prodigious labors in Havana had sapped his energy: "No one will ever know how much of physical expenditure the investigations upon yellow fever cost Dr. Reed," noted one physician, who observed, "There is good reason to believe that Dr. Reed's health was severely shaken by the anxious experiences of this period, and he did not regain his former vigor up to the time of the illness which carried him off."[15]

Despite his untimely end, and perhaps sensitive to the potentially problematic features of experimenting on local individuals, some American physicians adopted the Yellow Fever Commission's use of written contracts with their research subjects. Assigned to the Philippine Bureau of Science in Manila, American physicians Ernest Walker and Andrew Sellards in 1912 obtained written permission from the inmates of Bilibid Prison for their studies of amoebic dysentery. Before feeding the prisoners gelatin capsules containing the pathogens of dysentery, the doctors explained the experiment using the prisoners' "native dialect,"

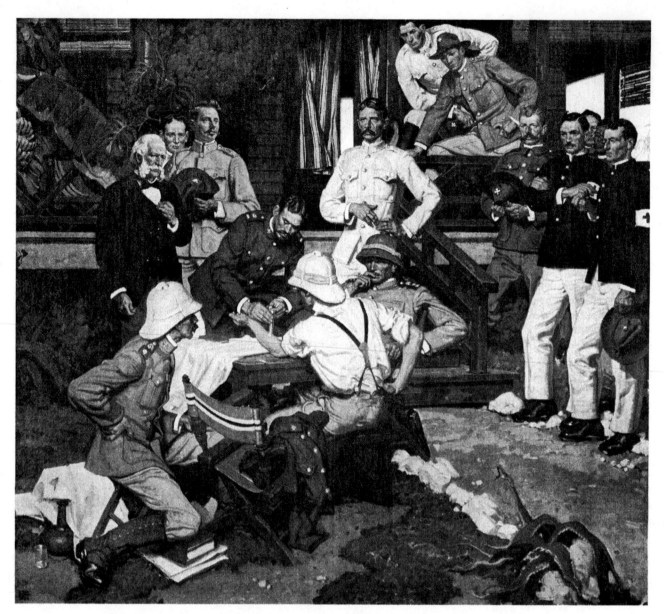

Figure 1.2. Walter Reed, standing in white uniform with colleagues, as Jesse Lazear inoculates James Carroll
with an infected mosquito. Source: Dean Cornwell (1892–1960), *Conquerors of Yellow Fever,* 1939. Reproduced
with permission of Wyeth.

advised the prisoners of the possibility that they would contract
dysentery, and informed them that neither "financial inducement"
nor "immunity to prison discipline or commutation of sentence"
was available. The prisoners gave written permission for their
participation.[2]

Sellards continued this practice when he returned to the
United States. Stationed at the Base Hospital at Camp Meade, Md.,
in 1918, Sellards pursued investigations into the transmission of
measles. The officers and men who volunteered for the study
signed a written statement: "I hereby volunteer as a subject for
inoculation with measles in order to promote the work undertaken in the United States Army for securing a protective inoc-

ulation against this disease." The volunteers, who received "no
reward" for their participation, were informed that the Surgeon
General expressed his appreciation for their "patriotism and de-
votion to duty."[16]

Investigators used written contracts with research subjects
sporadically in the decades between 1920 and 1970. In most
cases, these did not represent efforts at informing subjects; rather
they served as "releases" or "waivers of responsibility" intended
to indemnify the researcher and the institution in case of a bad
outcome. In many cases, investigators were more likely to obtain
written permission from prison inmates than any other group, a
testament to the legal nature of the transaction.

Medical researchers found martyrs like Lazear and near-martyrs like Reed particularly valuable both in their ongoing bid for public esteem and as a tool in battling those who protested animal experimentation. In 1923, when the American Association for Medical Progress was established, the group quickly adopted the cause of volunteers in medical research as a means to undermine antivivisectionist attacks on medical investigators. As one 1927 pamphlet published by the association—titled *How Yellow Fever Was Conquered*—put it, "If the bodies of men like these are not too sacred to dedicate to such work as they performed, is it too much to ask that the bodies of a few rats or rabbits or guinea pigs shall be dedicated to work of equal importance?"[17] The cultural power of medical martyrdom was underscored in 1928 by the yellow fever deaths of three researchers on a Rockefeller mission in West Africa—Hideyo Noguchi, William Young, and Adrian Stokes. The *New York Times,* which reported Noguchi's death on its front page, branded the loss "a sacrifice of medical science in defense of humanity against the great tropic scourge" and eulogized Noguchi as a "martyr of science."[18] Such events reinforced the collective martyrology attached to yellow fever, and with it, the cult of Reed as emblematic of the self-sacrificing scientist.

In the 1950s the formation of the Walter Reed Society demonstrated the Army surgeon's continuing usefulness to the biomedical research community. In 1951, the National Society for Medical Research, an advocacy group established to defend animal experimentation, sponsored the formation of the Reed Society, an "honorary" association composed of men and women who had served medical science as volunteer experimental subjects. Applicants were asked to submit a statement from the investigator who had experimented on them, and (as the printed application form instructed) to describe "in simple, non-technical language the nature of your research and/or experience which qualified you for membership in the Walter Reed Society. Be as colorful, dramatic and specific as possible." By 1953, the Society reported 103 members.[19,20] The Society did not survive the 1960s, when the use of research subjects—mentally retarded children, elderly patients, and others—became the subject of controversy and debate among the research community and the wider public.

That leaders of the National Society for Medical Research selected Reed as their patron illustrated the durable and supple appeal of Reed the investigator. Reed's legacy was significant, in the words of the Society charter, because "he risked his life in a series of brilliant experiments leading to the conquest of yellow fever." In the wake of questions about research ethics prompted by both the Nuremberg Doctors Trial and concerns about American research, Reed's behavior as a researcher became an important symbol for medical investigators. In the literature of the Walter Reed Society and in popular magazines like the *Saturday Evening Post,* Reed became not just a successful researcher, but a self-sacrificing researcher. Major Reed, explained one author in the *Post,* "first dramatized the use of human guinea pigs during the historic yellow fever experiments."[21] These experiments, like those honored by the Reed Society, involved heroic self-experimentation, not the exploitation of involuntary or unsuspecting subjects.

It was Reed's decision to risk life that also attracted admirers. Amid the heightened urgencies of the Cold War, Reed's dedication to finding the solution to the problem of yellow fever could be invoked by military leaders intent on preparing America for the atomic age. In discussions over the feasibility of developing a nuclear-powered airplane, Brigadier General James Cooney, representing the Atomic Energy Commission's Division of Military Applications, deployed Reed in an effort to support the deliberate exposure of military personnel to whole-body radiation to determine its effects on humans. In a transcript about the debate on the need for military-purpose human experimentation, declassified for the Advisory Committee on Human Radiation Experiments in 1995, Cooney stated, "Personally I see no difference in subjecting men to this [whole-body radiation] than I do to any other type of experimentation that has ever been carried on. Walter Reed killed some people. It was certainly the end result that was very wonderful."[22] Cooney argued for the need to recruit "volunteers both officer and enlisted" to undergo exposure to up to 150 rads whole-body radiation to resolve the question and prevent "thousands of deaths" as the result of not knowing the effects of this radiation.[23]

Reed's risk taking also resonated with one of the key figures in the reformulation of research ethics in the 1960s and 1970s, Henry K. Beecher. The Harvard professor of anesthesiology not only conducted human experiments on opiates and analgesics, but also called attention to lapses of professional judgment and morality in mainstream American clinical research in a now famous 1966 article in the *New England Journal of Medicine.*[24] In his 1970 volume *Research and the Individual,* Beecher acknowledged that most patients were unwilling to risk their lives for the sake of science; but there were exceptions, those "rare individuals who perhaps seek martyrdom or devoted investigators such as Walter Reed and his colleagues, whose lonely exploit is still celebrated 70 years or more after the event." When he discussed the regulations that governed the use of volunteers in military experimentation, Beecher noted the irony that the yellow fever experiments would not have been possible at the time he was writing. According to the Special Regulations of the Army adopted in January 1949, "unduly" hazardous or unnecessary experimentation would not be tolerated. Under these rules, Beecher observed, "Walter Reed's triumph would not now be possible!"[25] Perhaps unaware of Reed's written contracts with his research subjects, Beecher did not mention their use in the yellow fever research.

In the 1970s, internist William B. Bean, a prominent medical editor and an experienced clinical investigator (and self-experimenter), was perhaps the first to identify the written contract Reed used with the yellow fever participants. Although he had published earlier articles about Reed and the Yellow Fever Commission in 1952 and 1974, he had made no mention of the written document.[26,27] He first did so when he delivered the Fielding H. Garrison Lecture in 1976 at the American Association for the History of Medicine on Walter Reed and human experimentation, reminding his listeners that concern for individual rights, even amid the groundswell of public concern over unethical human experiments, could be taken too far. Four years after the revelation of the Tuskegee Syphilis Study and two years after the passage of the National Research Act (which required, among other things, the written consent of the research subject), Bean invoked Reed as an exemplar of the relationship of the physician-investigator to the subject and patient. "In our concern for the rights of the individual we must not forget that society has rights too," Bean argued. "Anyone living in society has a debt to it. Experimental biological science is necessary to advance curative medicine and public health. Exclusive focus on individual and

Application Blank

I herewith apply for membership in the Walter Reed Society as a ☐ member; ☐ fellow.

My dues of $1.00 are attached.

My voluntary medical research service [unreadable]

Project _____

Conducted by _____

Purpose _____

Remarks _____

If Published, Name and Date of Journal _____

_____

_____
(unreadable)

_____
(unreadable)

_____

The applicant is qualified for membership in the Walter Reed Society.

_____
(unreadable)

Figure 1.3. Application Form for Membership in the Walter Reed Society. Source: Thomas M. Rivers Papers, box 9, f. National Society for Medical Research, American Philosophical Society, Philadelphia, Penn. Reproduced with permission.

HUMAN VOLUNTEERS IN MEDICAL RESEARCH

personal rights may accelerate the decline of society down the path of its own self-destruction."[4] Bean described Reed's contract as a "sacred scientific document" which gave "substance and symbol of a written agreement to informed consent."[4]

Today most Americans associate Walter Reed with the hospital that bears his name, the Walter Reed Army Medical Center in Washington, D.C. Within the medical research community, perhaps, some trace of Reed's exploits linger. In 1997, for example, as he called on physicians to volunteer as subjects in a HIV vaccine trial, Charles F. Farthing, a member of the International Association of Physicians in AIDS Care, reminded his fellows: "It is time to follow in the tradition of Louis Pasteur, Walter Reed, and hundreds of other colleagues who made the commitment to be the first human subjects in critical clinical trials."[28]

This speaker was doubtless unaware that not only had Reed not participated in clinical trials, but that Pasteur, according to the historian Gerald Geison, had misled his contemporaries about the evidence for his rabies vaccine when he first tested it on a young boy.[29]

Reed's legacy is a complex one, compounded of self-experimentation, heroism and martyrdom, and genuine concern for the men who risked their lives in the yellow fever experiments. The written documents he used to ensure that subjects recognized the risk of their participation illustrate that many American physicians have grappled with the moral and political issues raised by using human beings in research. These issues will no doubt remain with us, so long as human beings are essential to the process.

References

1. Mosquito carries yellow fever germ. *New York Times* Oct. 27, 1900:1.
2. Lederer SE. *Subjected to Science: Human Experimentation in America Before the Second World War.* Baltimore, Md.: Johns Hopkins University Press; 1995.
3. Kelly HA. *Walter Reed and Yellow Fever.* New York, N.Y.: McClure, Philips; 1906:242.
4. Bean WB. Walter Reed and the ordeal of human experiments. *Bulletin of the History of Medicine* 1977;51:75–92.
5. Güereña-Burgueño F. The centennial of the Yellow Fever Commission and the use of informed consent in medical research. *Salud Pública de México* 2002;44:140–44.
6. Humphreys M. *Yellow Fever and the South.* New Brunswick, N.J.: Rutgers University Press; 1992.
7. Reed W. Recent researches concerning the etiology, propagation, and prevention of yellow fever, by the United States Army Commission. *Journal of Hygiene* 1902;2:101–19.
8. Bayne-Jones S. Walter Reed (1851–1902). *Military Medicine* 1967;132:391–400.
9. Pierce JR. In the interests of humanity and the cause of science: The yellow fever volunteers. *Military Medicine* 2003;168: 857–63.
10. Myer JS. *Life and Letters of Dr. William Beaumont.* St. Louis, Mo.: Mosby Co.; 1912:149.
11. Rutkow IM. Beaumont and St. Martin: A blast from the past. *Archives of Surgery* 1998;133:1259.
12. Osler W, Vaughan V. The Bacillus icteroides (Sanarelli) and Bacillus X (Sternberg). *Transactions of the Association of American Physicians* 1898;13:61–72.
13. Sternberg GM. The transmission of yellow fever mosquitoes. *Popular Science Monthly* 1901;59:225–41, p. 233.
14. Agramonte A. The inside story of a great medical discovery. *Scientific Monthly* 1915;1:209–37.
15. Death of Dr. Walter Reed. *Philadelphia Medical Journal* 1902; 10:858.
16. Sellards AW. Insusceptibility of man to inoculation with blood from measles patients. *Bulletin of the Johns Hopkins Hospital* 1919;30:257–68, p. 267.
17. American Association for Medical Progress. *How Yellow Fever Was Conquered.* New York, N.Y.: American Association for Medical Progress, 1927. [Online] Available: http://etext.lib.virginia.edu/etcbin/fever-browse?id=03142011.
18. Dr. Noguchi is dead, martyr of science. *New York Times* May 22, 1928:1.
19. Minutes of the Walter Reed Society, Apr. 8, 1953, Thomas M. Rivers Papers, box 9, f. NSMR, American Philosophical Society Library, Philadelphia, Penn.
20. Rosenbaum JR, Sepkowitz KA. Infectious disease experimentation involving human volunteers. *Clinical Infectious Diseases* 2002;34: 963–71.
21. Koritz LT, with Shubin S. I was a human guinea pig. *Saturday Evening Post* Jul. 25, 1953;226:27,79–80,82.
22. Transcript. *Debate on the Need for Military-Purpose Human Experimentation.* National Archives, Record Group 326, U.S. Atomic Energy Collection: Division of Biology and Medicine, Box 3215, Folder: ACBM Minutes.
23. Advisory Committee on Human Radiation Experiments. *Final Report of the Advisory Committee on Human Radiation Experiments.* New York, N.Y.: Oxford University Press; 1996.
24. Beecher HK. Ethics and clinical research. *New England Journal of Medicine* 1966;274:1354–60.
25. Beecher HK. *Research and the Individual.* Boston, Mass.: Little Brown, 1970;28, 53.
26. Bean WB. Walter Reed. *Archives of Internal Medicine* 1952;89: 171–87.
27. Bean WB. Walter Reed: A biographical sketch. *Archives of Internal Medicine* 1974;134:871–77.
28. Weiss R. Advances inject hope into quest for vaccine. *Washington Post* Sep. 3, 1997:A1.
29. Geison G. *The Private Science of Louis Pasteur.* Princeton, N.J.: Princeton University Press; 1995.

Paul J. Weindling

The Nazi Medical Experiments

Hitler's racial state and racial war provided German doctors and their associates with the opportunity to inflict unparalleled medical atrocities. These involved not only research but also using medical knowledge and resources for a race-based program of public health and genocide. The Nazi government imposed no mandatory professional standards on the conduct of experiments—although Germany had earlier adopted such standards—and no international humanitarian or medical agency intervened to protect the victims. German physicians experimented to advance medical and racial science, and to contribute to the German war effort. They exploited bodies, used body parts and internal organs for research, and drained the blood of Jews and Slavs for use as a cell culture medium and to support transfusion. The exploitation of human beings for medical research occurred within the broader context of how the Nazis harvested hair, gold fillings, and any other usable body parts from victims of the Holocaust.

Physicians and medical and biological researchers took a central role in the implementation of the Holocaust and exploited imprisonment, ghettoization, and killings as opportunities for research. They defined the characteristics of Jews, Gypsies, and Slavs as pathological. They demanded that mental and physical disabilities be eradicated from the German/Aryan/Nordic race by compulsory sterilization, euthanasia, and segregation of racial "undesirables." Doctors and medical ancillaries identified and registered racial "inferiors" in surveys, collecting data on pathological physical and mental traits.

Adjudicating an individual's racial ancestry or deciding on a diagnosis could be a matter of life and death. The killing procedures included poison gas; initially, carbon monoxide was used—first for euthanasia and then in the extermination camps of Belzec, Sobibor, and Treblinka. A modified form of the pesticide Zyklon B was used at Auschwitz.[1] Other methods of killing were by phenol injection and calculated use of starvation. Physicians offered medical support for the mass killing by undertaking selections for the gas chambers and by killing the weak and disabled in the interest of Germany's racial "health."

Research abuses were integral to the Nazi genocide. Doctors were interested in "racial pathology," attempting to prove that Jews responded differently to infections. Because laboratory animals were in increasingly short supply during the war, physician/researchers experimented on racial "inferiors," especially children. In the event, most of the research was found to be scientifically worthless, poorly planned, and often replicating results that had already been established through clinical observation. However, the high status of German medical research meant that U.S. and British researchers expected to find some of the data useful after the war. During that time, researchers screened German research work on aviation physiology and the nerve gas sarin. The scientific value of the German research has been debated since 1945. Some scientists have maintained that the German results were in some cases scientifically valid, but others condemned wholesale such research, calling for destruction of the records.[2-8] The experiments and associated medical war crimes violated the physician's ethic of care to the sick and suffering. Belatedly, the Nuremberg Code with its requirement of "voluntary consent" was promulgated by the presiding judge at the close of the Nuremberg Medical Trial in August 1947[9,10] (see Chapter 12).

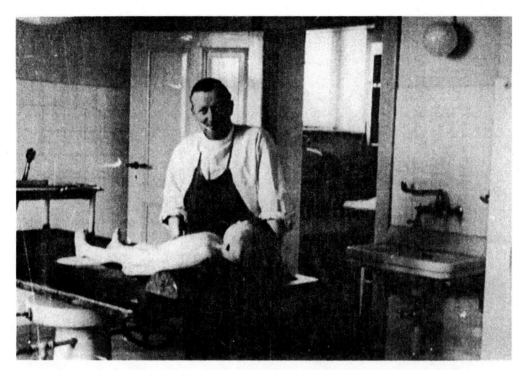

Figure 2.1. Nazi neuropathologist Berthold Ostertag (1895–1975), in his capacity as an associate in Reichsausschusses, during an autopsy on a murdered child. Sources: 1. Klinik für Psychiatrie und Psychotherapie, Akademisches Lehrkrankenhaus der Charité—Universitätsmedizin Berlin. 2. United States Holocaust Memorial Museum Collection. Reproduced with permission.

German Medical Science Before the Nazis

Changing standards of medical ethics and research practices early in the 20th century paved the way for the Nazi medical atrocities. An upswing of experimental medicine and the penetration of racial ideas into biology were predisposing factors.

German medical education had long been science-oriented. A research-based thesis was required for an M.D., and university teaching required an extended Habilitation thesis. Since the era of discoveries by the bacteriologist Robert Koch from the mid-1870s to the 1890s, many German medical researchers had followed an informal ethical code of performing either self-experiments or experiments on their own children before experimenting on others. However, other physicians experimented in orphanages and prisons, and the bodies of executed criminals were routinely delivered to anatomical institutes.[11] Eugenics and the spread of hereditarian medicine gave rise to the idea that the physician should act in the interests of the national community and race, rather than maintaining an inviolable bond of care for the individual patient.

In the years before the Nazi takeover, experimental medicine did raise some public and governmental concern. The case of the hepatologist Hans Eppinger provides a representative example. Eppinger, an innovative experimental researcher and clinician in Germany and then Austria, performed invasive research without consent on patients in public wards in Vienna in the 1930s. When his practices became known, public and political concern increased over "human guinea pigs" in hospitals.[9,12–14]

In 1930, in response to the accidental use of a contaminated batch of BCG vaccine (bacille Calmette-Guérin vaccine, used against tuberculosis) at Lübeck, public protests against therapeutic failures and unethical experiments resulted in the formulating of guidelines on human experiments. The Reich Circular on Human Experimentation of February 28, 1931, laid down some key requirements; at the time, these regulations were the most advanced in the world in safeguarding the patient and research subject. They included the following provisions:

5. Innovative therapy may be carried out only after the subject or his legal representative has unambiguously consented to the procedure in the light of relevant information provided in advance. . . .
6. The question of whether to use innovative therapy must be examined with particular care where the subject is a child or a person under 18 years of age. . . .
12. c. [E]xperimentation involving children or young persons under 18 years of age shall be prohibited if it in any ways endangers the child or young person.

There is no evidence that clinical researchers followed these guidelines, particularly after the Nazis came to power in 1933.[15–17]

Nazism and the Second World War removed civil rights and humane ethics, opening the floodgates to successive waves of unscrupulous experimentation and research abuses. Nazi values stressed the priorities of the nation and race. The sick individual was seen as a burden on the fit, a category defined in physical and racial terms. The state had coercive powers not only to detain and segregate the sick but also to intervene in the body.

After the Nazis achieved power, medical research received increased resources as part of racial health and welfare policies.

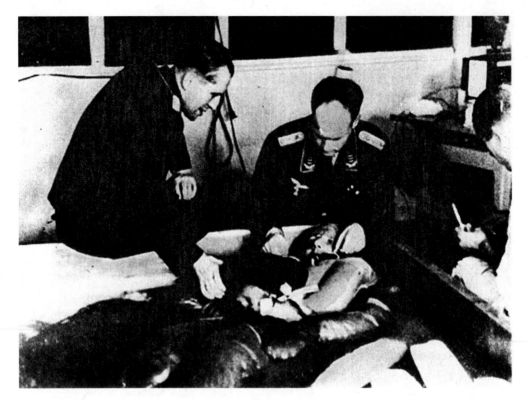

Figure 2.2. Nazi Freezing Experiment at Dachau, September, 1942. SS Sturmbannfuehrer Dr. Sigmund Rascher (right) and Dr. Ernst Holzloehner (left) observe the reactions of a Dachau prisoner who has been immersed in a tank of ice water in an attempt to simulate the extreme hypothermia suffered by pilots downed over frigid seas. Sources: 1. Keystone (Paris); A 1172/14–21.2223; neg. 00977. 2. Yad Vashem Photo Archives; (1595/31A). 3. Sueddeutscher Verlag Bilderdienst; (Deutschland 1933–45: Medizinische Versuche an Haeftlingen). Reproduced with permission of Keystone (Paris).

Researchers constantly lobbied for experimental resources and opportunities. This suggests that the experiments and other medical abuses of the Nazi era were not perpetrated just by a small group of unscientific racial fanatics, who were unrepresentative of the German medical profession, but rather that the atrocities reflected attitudes that were broadly shared in the German medical profession.

Nazification of Medical Values

To understand how researchers viewed their experimental subjects as having lives of lesser value, we have to take account of the Nazi restructuring of medicine and public health on a racialized basis. After the Nazi takeover in 1933, Jewish doctors were purged from universities, hospitals, and public health appointments. They endured harassment and violence from their medical colleagues and students. The Nuremberg laws for racial segregation of 1935 imposed penalties on "Aryan" physicians with a non-Aryan spouse. Despite these restrictions, Jewish doctors retained their right to claim reimbursement of fees from sickness insurance funds. Finally, however, in 1938 Jewish doctors were delicensed: A Jewish physician lost the title of *Arzt* (physician) and was referred to as *Krankenbehändler* (treater of the sick).[18] The Nazi state centralized public health services to implement racial policies, and medical associations (the *Ärztekammer*) were placed under the

Nazi Physicians League. The longstanding German eugenics and racial hygiene movement was Nazified. Roman Catholic, Jewish, and socialist eugenicists were purged from eugenic associations and institutes for hereditary research.[19] "Aryan" physicians obtained the academic posts and contracts of dismissed Jewish and dissident colleagues.[18,20–23]

Research in many branches of medicine intensified in the mid-1930s. Simultaneously, municipal and state health offices were combined; this facilitated compulsory sterilization and the registration of disabilities and malformations, and became a preliminary step toward euthanasia. In addition, many physicians forged alliances with the Nazi system of power, seeing an opportunity to formulate and implement social legislation. In 1930, the human geneticist Fritz Lenz saw the Nazi Party as offering the best hope for a eugenically planned society. The psychiatric geneticist Ernst Rüdin took a leading role in drawing up the sterilization law enacted in July 1933 and implemented from January 1934. Fritz von Wettstein and Hans Nachtsheim, both geneticists at the Kaiser Wilhelm Society (*Gesellschaft*)—later the Max Planck Society—backed the implementation of the sterilization law. Sterilization proved a powerful force in accelerating the shift to a unified state and municipal public health system. It targeted a range of clinical conditions, notably schizophrenia, muscular dystrophy, Huntington's chorea, epilepsy, severe mental defect, and chronic alcoholism. Sexual and mental abnormalities attracted special interest in psychiatric genetics. Otmar von Verschuer led the way in twin studies, using the Frankfurt public health clinic as a base from 1935–42. An estimated 340,000 persons were forcibly sterilized in Germany and in German-annexed Austria between 1933 and 1945.

At the opening of the Nuremberg Medical Trial, Telford Taylor gave a political explanation to the research atrocities: "In the tyranny that was Nazi Germany, no one could give such a consent to the medical agents of the State; everyone lived in fear and acted under duress."[24] The years 1933 to 1939 saw medical researchers stigmatizing ethnic groups and people with disabilities as social burdens of low-grade intelligence. The textbook on human heredity by the botanist Erwin Baur, the anthropologist Eugen Fischer, and human geneticist Lenz endorsed such views.[25,26] Although the sterilization law did not specify race itself as meriting sterilization, ethnic minorities were vulnerable to being sterilized. We see this with the evaluation and sterilization of the children of black French troops and Germans, who were derogatively referred to as *Rheinlandbastarde* ("Rhineland bastards"). A total of 385 mixed-race children were forcibly sterilized in 1937 after extensive evaluations from a psychological, anthropological, and genetic point of view. They would have been between ages 13 and 16.[27]

In June 1936, a Central Office to "Combat the Gypsy Nuisance" opened in Munich. This office became the headquarters of a national data bank on so-called "Gypsies," and atrocities against German and other European Roma ("Gypsies") continued into the war years. Robert Ritter, a medical anthropologist at the Reich Health Office, concluded that 90% of the "Gypsies" native to Germany were "of mixed blood." He described them as "the products of matings with the German criminal asocial sub-proletariat" and as "primitive" people "incapable of real social adaptation." Ritter's views shaped the research by Eva Justin on the "primitive nature" of 148 Roma children raised apart from their families. Justin analyzed the children's psychology at the St. Josefspflege Roman Catholic children's home. At the conclusion of her study, the children were deported to Auschwitz, where all but a few were killed. In 1943, Justin was awarded a doctorate for her life history research on these "racially alien" children.[28,29] Overall, the Germans murdered an estimated 25,000 German and Austrian Sinti and Roma, as well as 90,000 Roma from lands under Nazi occupation. Physicians exploited the mistreatment and murder for research in the "Gypsy Camp" at Auschwitz and at Dachau, where the painful seawater drinking experiments, conducted in 1944, left the Roma victims utterly exhausted.

After Germany annexed Austria in March 1938, a group of energetic medical researchers at the Vienna medical school—notably, Eppinger, the anatomist Eduard Pernkopf, and the psychiatrist Maximinian de Crinis—utilized the opportunity for clinical and racial research on vulnerable groups like the disabled, the racially persecuted, and those with inherited metabolic and physical anomalies. From September 25 to 30, 1939, anthropologists in Vienna took plaster face masks and anthropological measurements of 440 "stateless" Jewish men held in the Praterstadion, the sports stadium. Most were then sent to the concentration camp of Buchenwald and did not survive. This is an early example of coercive research, on terrorized victims in a life-threatening situation, ending in the deaths of many. In June 1941 Austrian anthropologists went to Amsterdam to conduct research on Dutch Sephardic Jews as part of "the comprehensive racial plans." British officers refused to comply with plans for photographing British, Australian, and Maori prisoners of war.[30,31]

Table 2.1

Major Events in the Nazification of German Medical Research

Date	Event
1905	Germany's Racial Hygiene Society is founded.
Oct. 1, 1927	Kaiser Wilhelm Institute for Anthropology, Human Heredity and Eugenics is created.
Feb. 28, 1931	Reich Guidelines on Human Experimentation are issued.
Jan. 31, 1933	Hitler comes to power.
July 1933	Sterilization Law is enacted. Eventually, an estimated 340,000 people are compulsorily sterilized in Germany and Austria.
1937	Mixed-race children in the Rhineland are sterilized.
Sept. 1939	Jews held prisoner in the Vienna Sports Stadium are subjected to anthropological research.
Sept. 1939	Euthanasia programs begin, targeting "worthless lives." Eventually, an estimated 256,000 people are killed.
Feb. 1942	Sigmund Rascher begins lethal aviation medicine experiments at Dachau to test survival and determine the point of death in high altitude and severe cold conditions.
Aug. 1942	Women prisoners at Ravensbrück are deliberately injured for experiments on wound infection.
Mar. 1943	Ravensbrück prisoners protest and manage to sneak information on human experimentation out to the Polish underground.
April 1943	Josef Mengele assigned to Auschwitz as a "Camp Doctor."
April 1944	Roma ("Gypsy") prisoners are subjected to seawater drinking experiments at Dachau.
Nov. 1945	John Thompson identifies "medical war crimes."
July 31–Aug. 1, 1946	International Scientific Commission on War Crimes, and Guidelines on Human Experimentation proposed at Pasteur Institute.
Dec. 1946	Nuremberg Medical Trial begins; 23 Nazi physicians or administrators are accused of war crimes and crimes against humanity.
Aug. 16, 1947	Panel of judges at Nuremberg Medical Trial convicts 16 defendants and pronounces the Nuremberg Code of medical research ethics.

Another early example of coercive experiments were those conducted by Georg Schaltenbrand, a former Rockefeller Foundation fellow, in the neurological clinic at Würzburg. He performed painful lumbar punctures, extracting spinal fluid for research on multiple sclerosis, which he believed was infectious. The victims were German, and at least one was a Nazi Party member. The research was carried out without consent and left victims in pain.[32–34]

German research atrocities included the use of body parts for histological and neurophysiological research. In some cases, research was carried out on living persons who were then killed to obtain their organs to see if there was a defect in the brain accounting for abnormal behavior or psychosis, or to assess the effects of infection on internal organs. This was known as hereditary pathology, or *Erbpathologie*.

The war at first disrupted clinical research. Because of the call-up of research personnel for military service, 1940 marked a low point in the numbers of coercive human experiments. But in 1938, the SS had established a Hygiene Institute in Berlin, supported by SS chief Heinrich Himmler, which was transferred to the Waffen-SS (Armed SS) in the war when it sponsored war-related human experiments. Prime target groups were Soviet and Polish prisoners. Hermann Göring took over as president of the Reich Research Council in July 1942 to remedy the fragmentation of German research and to energize it by setting strategic targets. The SS physicist Rudolf Mentzel aligned research with wartime needs as president of the reorganized *Deutsche Forschungsgemeinschaft* (DFG, or German National Research Council). His deputy, the publisher and SS administrator Wolfram Sievers, was later convicted at the Nuremberg Medical Trial and hanged (see Table 2.2 later in this chapter).

Later phases of the war saw an upsurge of atrocities for scientific research. Often we know about the experiment, but not about the victims. The anatomist August Hirt murdered 86 victims for the collection of Jewish skeletons at the Reich University of Strassburg. The victims were selected in Auschwitz and sent across Germany to Alsace to be killed in the gas chambers of Natzweiler-Struthof.[35]

Euthanasia

A medical lobby around Hitler began pressing for the euthanasia of mentally and physically disabled adults and children in 1935, but the practice was not imposed until Hitler issued a secret degree in 1939. By the end of the war, however, Nazi euthanasia programs had killed an estimated 256,000 people.[36]

Of course, "euthanasia" was a euphemism. The killings did not correspond to conventional notions of "releasing" an individual who so wishes from the pain and suffering of a terminal and incurable illness. Rather, the Nazi euthanasia programs targeted "worthless lives" (*lebensunwertes Leben*)—"undesirables" such as the infirm, non-Aryans, or adolescents who challenged authority. Hitler saw the sick as an economic burden on the healthy, and he wished to rid the German race of the "polluting" effects of the "undesirables." The practice of institutionalized medical murder also allowed deliberate killing to obtain body parts for scientific research and a range of other abusive research practices. Some physician/researchers killed patients to order so that autopsies could be performed.

Standard accounts of Nazi "euthanasia" have claimed that euthanasia arose when a father petitioned the Führer that his malformed child should be killed.[37,38] This account was derived from the exculpatory testimony of Karl Brandt at the Nuremberg Medical Trial. In an important contribution, Benzenhöfer has shown that such an infant indeed existed; but the dates of the child's birth and death mean that any petition to Hitler occurred only after the decision to unleash euthanasia had been reached.[39,40] Brandt, Hitler's escort surgeon, was one of the medical advisers who convinced the Führer of the need for killing of so-called "incurables." Brandt was convicted at Nuremberg of war crimes and crimes against humanity, and was hanged.

Four distinct euthanasia programs were carried out. The first—code-named "T4" after the street address of the central office, Tiergarten Strasse 4—supposedly provided a panel of legal adjudicators to decide individual cases. But instead of a legal procedure of notification and appeal, a doctor at the T4 office made decisions on the basis of cursory scrutiny of clinical records. According to

Nazi records, 70,263 persons were killed in this operation. In its second phase—after a widely publicized sermon attacking the program by the Bishop of Münster, Count Clemens von Galen, in 1941—clinicians ran the killing programs on a decentralized basis, deciding themselves who was to die.

A separate program targeted disabled children: The killings occurred in special pediatric units by means of long-term starvation or lethal medication. Between 1939 and 1945, an estimated 5,000 children were "euthanized." One rationale for this program was the pretense that somehow the killing of severely disabled children could be condoned as in accord with parental wishes and historical precedent. In fact, psychiatrists exercised pressure on parents unwilling to give their children up. Often false promises of therapy were made to overcome parental resistance.

Children were killed in designated clinical wards called *Kinderfachabteilungen* ("special care units for children"). Thirty-eight of these killing wards are known, but the *Kinderfachabteilungen* are far from fully researched. In annexed Czechoslovakia the *Reichsausschuss Kinderverfahrung* (the "Reich Committee for Child Behavior") in Dobrany, near Pilsen, worked in conjunction with T4 and had a hand in the removal of children from the site of the erased village of Lidice. A fourth euthanasia program was carried out in concentration camps: More than 20,000 people were selected from the concentration camps for killing at the euthanasia centers, established in 1939–40 in psychiatric hospitals. By one estimate, there were 216,000 German and Austrian victims of euthanasia. In addition, an estimated 20,000 Polish and 20,000 Soviet victims were killed. A reasonable estimate is a total of 256,000 euthanasia victims.[36]

Euthanasia often was linked to medical research, although there is no comprehensive analysis of such killings. Julius Hallervorden of the Kaiser Wilhelm Institute (KWI) for Brain Research, a component of the Kaiser Wilhelm Society, obtained brain specimens from patients whose clinical records were "of interest." Jürgen Peiffer—a German neuropathologist who discovered that he had unwittingly used the brains of 19 euthanasia victims for publications in 1959 and 1963, and who afterward devoted much effort to documenting the criminal practices and legacy of his specialty—has established that 707 brains stored at Hallervorden's Department of Neuropathology came from euthanasia victims.[41]

Similarly, at the Children's Ward in Wiesengrund in Berlin, the pathologist Ostertag examined 106 brains from killed children. He studied small children with such conditions as microcephaly, had them filmed, and then had them killed. Peiffer observes that brains were delivered to researchers as a result of personal networks rather than any centralized distribution.

Directors of *Kinderfachabteilungen* were invited as guest researchers by the KWI for Brain Research between 1939 and 1942. Researchers at the prestigious Kaiser Wilhelm Society, especially researchers at the KWIs for Psychiatry, Brain Research, Anthropology, and Biochemistry, were involved in human experiments and research on body parts of killed persons.

From August 1943 to 1945, intensive research took place on "mentally defective" children at Heidelberg. A professor of psychiatry, Carl Schneider, was not only an adjudicator for euthanasia but also saw the program as an opportunity for histopathological research. He wanted to determine the difference between inherited and acquired mental deficiency. In one experiment, 52 children were examined, each for six weeks in the clinic. They were subjected to many forms of physical force and terror as part of psychological and psychiatric tests, including a painful X-ray of the brain ventricle. In addition, they were held under cold and warm water to test their reactions. Schneider hoped to correlate the results with anatomical lesions. In the event, 21 of the children were killed deliberately to compare the diagnosis made when they were alive with the postmortem pathological evidence.[42]

Many other children's bodies were also used for research. At the Vienna clinic *Am Spiegelgrund,* where about 800 children were killed, researcher Heinrich Gross examined 417 children's brains.[43] The clinical investigations of the children were often painful. In 1942–43 Elmar Türk carried out tuberculosis immunization experiments at the Vienna General Hospital Children's Clinic and *Am Spiegelgrund* involving the infection, killing, and dissection of the children.[23]

SS Medical Research

Heinrich Himmler, who was commander of the SS and chief of the German police, was ambitious for the SS to control German medicine, transforming universities and medical faculties into centers of racial ideology and practice. In the early 1930s, the geneticist Fritz Lenz evaluated SS officers' racial fitness. The next step was for groups of SS medical officers to take courses of 19 months duration at the KWI for Anthropology in 1934 and 1936. Some undertook various tasks in the SS Race and Settlement Office, which formulated racial policy in the occupied East. The Waffen-SS established medical services that became the Hygiene Institute of the Waffen-SS under the bacteriologist Joachim Mrugowsky, whose holistic approach to infectious disease was critical of genetic determinism. (Mrugowsky also was convicted at Nuremberg and hanged.) In 1936, the SS took control of the German Red Cross through Reichsarzt-SS Ernst Robert Grawitz. Within the SS, medical researchers competed, all seeking to go further than their rivals in their research practices.

The human experiments have often been seen as solely conducted by SS doctors on Himmler's orders. However, other agencies collaborated with the SS. For example, the Luftwaffe (German Air Force) provided pressure chambers and support personnel for Sigmund Rascher's lethal pressure and cold experiments in March–April 1942 at Dachau. Rascher, a Luftwaffe officer, conducted murderous experiments on at least 200 Soviet prisoners and Catholic priests to establish the point of death from cold and low pressure. The research was calculated to be lethal. The experiments came under the control of the Luftwaffe, whereas Rascher's link to the SS was informal. Certainly, Rascher kept Himmler informed about the progress of the experiments.

The SS *Ahnenerbe* (Ancestral Heritage) research organization came under Sievers. Its medical research activities owed much to the initiative of August Hirt, professor of anatomy at Strassburg, who joined the *Ahnenerbe* and the Waffen-SS in April 1942 (he had joined the SS in 1933). The SS anthropologists Bruno Beger and Fleischhacker assisted Hirt in developing an anatomical museum. The *Ahnenerbe* Institute for Military Research supported experiments in Dachau and the concentration camp of Natzweiler in Alsace, where experiments on mustard gas were undertaken. The *Ahnenerbe* authorized Hirt and his assistant to select 29 women and 57 men for transfer from Auschwitz in August 1943 for the human skeleton collection at Strassburg. The *Ahnenerbe* also supported vaccine experiments.

Some professors who held SS rank, such as Karl Gebhardt, developed medical research facilities. Gebhardt established a research facility at the orthopedic clinic of Hohenlychen. (He also was Himmler's personal physician; later, he was convicted at the Nuremberg Medical Trial and hanged.) Importantly, although the SS exerted influence on the medical faculties of Berlin, Munich, Jena, and Marburg, and over the "Reich Universities" of Posen and Strassburg, it did not have unlimited power over academic researchers. There was constant friction in these universities, so that SS influence remained precarious. Rascher could not obtain a Habilitation thesis for experiments on a new type of blood styptic because of opposition within these faculties, indicating academic exclusiveness and a sense that ethical standards had been violated.

However, the concentration camps were under SS control, and scientists came to Himmler and the SS with requests to conduct research on concentration camp prisoners. Erwin Ding-Schuler at Buchenwald, in conjunction with pharmaceutical companies, sought support in the upper echelons of the SS for research on typhus vaccine—circumventing his superior, Mrugowsky, who suggested that experiments be conducted on naturally occurring cases of infection, rather than on cohorts of deliberately infected prisoners. The bacteriologist Gerhard Rose also took this view, and criticized Ding at a military medical conference. Yet later on, both Mrugowsky and Rose were involved in lethal experiments and were convicted at Nuremberg. Mrugowsky was sentenced to death and was hanged; Rose was sentenced to life imprisonment, but the sentence was reduced and he was released in 1955.

Other researchers opportunistically approached the SS for research support and facilities. Gynecologist Carl Clauberg, a Nazi Party member although not an SS officer, conducted cruel and painful experiments on women prisoners at Auschwitz, using various forms of injections to induce sterility. Others, notably the SS doctor Horst Schumann, experimented extensively with X-ray sterilization. The experiments at the concentration camps of Auschwitz, Buchenwald, Dachau, Sachsenhausen, Neuengamme, and Natzweiler-Struthof demonstrate the strong support from the SS and Himmler personally.

Geneticist Hans Nachtsheim (never a member of the Nazi Party), of the KWI for Anthropology, collaborated with SS medical research at the sanatorium of Hohenlychen. Here, the pathologist Hans Klein, an associate of Nachtsheim, dissected glands extracted from 20 children selected by Josef Mengele at Auschwitz. The children were transported to Neuengamme, where they were injected with tuberculosis bacilli and later killed.[33,44–47] Nachtsheim took the view that it was ethically permissible to experiment on persons who were going in any case to be killed.

Yet the SS was not alone in sponsoring such abusive research, and the researchers were not all SS members. Kurt Blome—who disguised intended chemical warfare experiments as "cancer research"—had refused to join the SS, although he was a Nazi, remaining loyal to the SA storm troopers. The malariologist Claus Schilling, who experimented at Dachau from 1942 to 1945, infecting over a thousand victims to test vaccines, was neither an SS officer nor even a Nazi party member. Moreover, not all the experimenters were German. Danish SS doctor Vaernet experimented on homosexuals at Buchenwald, and other researchers were ethnic Germans from the East, such as Fritz Klein from Romania. Overall, we find a great range of types of experiments, perpetrators, and victims.

Many research atrocities were concealed for decades and are only now coming to light. Not long after the war, it became fashionable to presume that only SS-sponsored research was abusive. Ignoring links to non-Nazi researchers reinforced the view that the experiments were carried out by a small number of unscientific fanatics. The West German Medical Chambers made such a claim in a statement in 1949 to the World Medical Association.[48,49] This underestimate has remained until recently the orthodoxy.

Abusive Civilian Research

We are now returning to the view that many German researchers were involved in unethical experiments that were carried out in all sorts of locations. The atrocities were not limited just to human experiments but included a broad range of abuses conducted in support of research, such as killing to obtain body parts, rounding up people in racial groups for human behavior studies before sending them to be killed, tests of X-ray sterilization, and scientifically motivated clinical atrocities like the forcible draining of blood. We therefore find that rather than just a thousand deaths,[50] the Nuremberg Medical Trial focused on "atrocities committed in the name of medical science." Telford Taylor charged that "[t]he victims of these crimes are numbered in the hundreds of thousands."[24] Taylor included both living and dead victims, and all research-related atrocities. His estimate was realistic if the estimated 256,000 euthanasia victims and 340,000 sterilization victims are included, as medical research provided the scientific basis for these programs. Beyond this, racial anthropology took a major role in legitimizing the Holocaust, and eugenically and anthropologically trained experts like Mengele implemented Nazi genocide. Yet, within these broader categories of medically legitimated crimes, the question arises as to how many victims were maimed or killed specifically for research purposes.

We can broadly discern four types of medical research atrocities:

1. *Racial-anthropological research.* These run from the outbreak of war in September 1939, when anthropologists in Vienna took plaster face molds of stateless Polish Jews rounded up in the Vienna Sports Stadium. Josef Mengele's experiments in Auschwitz marked an attempt to demonstrate racial factors in immune responses to infections.
2. *Brain research and neurology.* The victims were mainly German and Austrian. These experiments and research on the brains of euthanasia victims run from 1939 to the war's end in 1945.
3. *Military medical research.* These studies evaluated the wounds caused by explosive bullets, new vaccines for diseases on the eastern front, and research on the treatment of wound infection. The majority of victims were Slav, at first male Russian prisoners of war, and then Polish women prisoners. These experiments extended mainly from 1941 until 1944. The SS dominated military medical research between 1942 and 1944, although here there were significant linkages to the German military and air force.
4. *Medical and genetic experiments and abuses, especially in 1943–44.* This was a final phase of research near the end of the war—commonly described as the era of Mengele at Auschwitz. Many of the victims were Jewish, Sinti, and Roma children.

Some of the experiments and research interventions involved deliberate killing. In other cases, the victims were regarded as disposable once the research had been completed. But the fact that research had been carried out on these victims increased the likelihood of their being killed.

Even 60 years after the close of the war, there is not a full accounting of these atrocities. More experiments and research atrocities come to light as historians comb through the research archives of organizations like the Kaiser Wilhelm Society and the DFG, which is still the main German grant-giving body for research in all branches of science.

Generally, clinical experimentation rose throughout Germany and German-controlled territory, but details of many such experiments are sparse. For example, hepatitis research on British prisoners of war in Crete is known from the scientific literature, rather than from any survivors' accounts.[51] Similarly, there has been a tendency to underestimate numbers of victims, both in terms of numbers who were killed and numbers who survived the debilitating and often traumatizing experiments.

Anatomists continued to use body parts of executed prisoners for teaching and research. Some of these prisoners were condemned for political reasons. The bodies used to create Pernkopf's celebrated anatomical atlas were those of people executed by the Nazi judiciary, which meant that some victims were anti-Nazis. Although anatomical institutes customarily received the bodies of the executed, under Nazism the rate of executions increased and included opponents of the regime.[52] The physiologist in Halle, Gothilft von Studnitz, dilated prisoners' eyes and subjected them to darkness prior to execution. He claimed that he could increase the sensitivity of the eye to low intensity of illumination by using a plant extract. Some prisoners were blindfolded immediately before execution, and their eyes were extracted immediately after execution for comparison with light-adapted eyes.[53] Hermann Stieve, professor of anatomy in Berlin, conducted research on anxiety as manifested in the menstrual cycles of young women executed by the Nazi authorities.[33,54]

The abuses included coercive study of racial characteristics and behavior with measurements, blood tests, casts of the face, histological and anatomical research on murdered victims, and death for dissection. Liters of blood were drained from Auschwitz prisoners for blood transfusion, and living persons incubated pathogenic microorganisms for typhus research. The question also arises as to the demarcation between legitimate and coercive, criminal forms of medical research. In some cases—such as the delivery of typhus vaccines to the Warsaw ghetto in 1941 through the Swiss Red Cross and the bacteriologist Hermann Mooser—it remains unclear whether the research was exploitive or beneficial.[1] SS doctors debated whether clinical research should be limited to naturally occurring cases, although they decided on deliberate infection.

Geneticists at the KWI for Anthropology exploited the situation. In the context of Verschuer's "Hereditary Pathology" program, the psychologist Kurt Gottschaldt studied German twins who were sent to a special observation camp, and Nachtsheim studied epilepsy as genetically inherited in rabbits, developing a cardiazol test for inherited epilepsy. Nachtsheim and the biochemist Ruhenstroh-Bauer saw a parallel between epileptic cramps in rabbits and oxygen deficiency in high-altitude flight. In September 1943 they conducted pressure chamber experiments on at least six children from the *Landesanstalt Brandenburg-Görden—*

an institution that had a significant role in Nazi euthanasia—attempting to induce epileptic seizures in the children. It is certain that one of the six children survived, but the fate of the others remains unclear.[55,56]

The KWI for Anthropology also supported the racial war and genocide in the East. One task was ethnic evaluation, examining individuals as specimens and deciding on their racial ancestry and worth. Nazi medical anthropologists hunted for body parts to support their grotesque views on racial history. Brains, eyes, reproductive organs, internal organs, blood samples, and skeletons were assiduously collected from persons in prisoner of war and concentration camps for comparative anatomical and histological study and teaching. Physical anthropology was an area of considerable interest in anatomy. The racial killing and experimentation had the rationale of isolating and eradicating the carriers of pathogenic genes. Genetics flourished in Nazi Germany in often gruesome research programs and as an incentive to racial policy. The Nazi obsession with race purity provided a favorable climate for genetics and experimental medicine to flourish. A successful career required support from the Nazi Party or the plethora of Nazi agencies.

The Final Phase: Mengele

Josef Mengele was born on March 16, 1911, a Roman Catholic. In 1935 he took a doctorate in anthropology in Munich, before qualifying in medicine in 1938 at Frankfurt with an M.D. thesis on the genetics of cleft palate. At the Institute for Hereditary Biology and Racial Hygiene, he worked as assistant to Otmar von Verschuer, who was interested in the genetics of twins. He joined the Nazi Party in May 1938, the SS in September 1938, and the Waffen-SS in July 1940. In November 1940, Mengele was assigned to the SS Race and Settlement Office on Ethnic German Returnees. In June 1941, he joined a combat unit as a medical officer and received the Iron Cross. From January to July 1942 he was a member of the SS's international Viking Division, and was again decorated for his frontline service. After a further period with the Race and Settlement Office, and visits to Versuchuer, he was sent to Auschwitz as a camp doctor in April 1943. He combined sanitary responsibilities—supervising the "Gypsy Camp," protecting the camp staff from infection—with undertaking racial selections of the newly arrived, sending those deemed "unfit" or simply not needed at the time to their deaths in the gas chambers. Mengele's scientific research was an informal, spare time activity, although his facilities were extensive. He used his position in the selections to find twins and other persons of interest, such as those with growths or other anomalies. Mengele joined the medical anthropologist at Auschwitz, Siegfried Liebau, who also was associated with von Verschuer.

Mengele exemplified the scientific drive to produce outstanding data. About 900 children endured Mengele's twin camp, and he scoured transports for additional subjects. Most but not all of his subjects were twins; children announced they were twins in the hope of surviving. They came from throughout Central and Eastern Europe: Romania, Hungary, Czechoslovakia, and Poland. Most were Jewish, although some were Sinti and Roma who were killed when the Auschwitz "Gypsy Camp" was liquidated, and their bodies were then dissected. Mengele was manipulative; he knew how to calm children when it suited him, but he was re-

lentlessly sadistic. Surviving accounts are fewer than one might expect. Some survivors have no memory; one inmate recalls just a trip to a meadow of flowers by Birkenau. Other twins remember all the procedures done to them, including painless ones, such as the taking of foot sole imprints, and painful, vicious experiments, such as incisions and operations without anesthetic, and often the killing of a beloved sibling.[57] Death was frequent.

Beginning in April 1943, Mengele built up his own research installations with a staff of prisoner pathologists, including Nyiszli and Gisella Perl, working at a number of locations within Auschwitz-Birkenau. Another contact was the physician and political prisoner Ella Lingens. Verschuer obtained a grant from the DFG for research on hereditary pathology, focusing on blood proteins, linking Mengele to the KWI for Anthropology. Mengele injected infective agents to compare their effects, and cross-injected spinal fluid. He would sometimes order the killing of a victim so that internal organs could be analyzed. He assisted in obtaining blood and body parts for Berlin colleagues who would use them for research. Under this DFG project, Mengele assisted in supplying the heterochromic eyes of a Sinto family to Karin Magnussen, a geneticist and Nazi activist in Nachtsheim's Department of Hereditary Pathology in Berlin. Magnussen conducted serial research on iris structure of schoolchildren. When anomalies in the iris of the family of Otto Mechau from Oldenburg came to light, she examined the family members in August 1943 before their deportation to Auschwitz. She then assisted the SS anthropologist Siegfried Liebau in Auschwitz, and made strenuous efforts to secure the Mechaus's eyes through Mengele.[58]

Mengele selected the 20 children sent for TB experiments to Neuengamme camp near Hamburg. These experiments were ostensibly to determine whether there was any natural immunity to tuberculosis and to develop a vaccination serum against TB. Heissmeyer—at the SS Sanatorium of Hohenlychen, a major SS center of research involving coercive experiments—sought to disprove the popular belief that TB was an infectious disease. Heissmeyer claimed that only an "exhaustive" organism was receptive to such infection, most of all the racially "inferior organism of the Jews."[45,47]

Before Auschwitz was liberated on Jan. 27, 1945, Mengele vanished. He moved to the camp of Gross-Rosen, and then evaded detection in the U.S. zone of occupation. In 1948 he used International Red Cross ID to flee to South America and is believed to have died in Brazil in 1979.

The Victims Protest

In a few cases, victims resisted and sabotaged the experiments. In March 1943, some of the 74 Polish women prisoners at the women's concentration camp of Ravensbrück protested against experiments in which the orthopedic surgeon Gebhardt wounded and then infected their legs to test the efficacy of sulphonamide in preventing tetanus. They called themselves "The Rabbits," and they obstructed the experiments, which they also documented. They smuggled news out to Polish resistance networks, which passed the information to Red Cross societies, and—apparently—to the Vatican. The anthropologist Germaine Tillion concealed a film spool with photographs of the sulphonamide and bone transplantation experiments.[9,59,60]

In October 1944 the International Council of Women in London demanded that the International Committee of the Red Cross (ICRC) give "all possible protection" to the women imprisoned at Ravensbrück. The council expressed horror at the "barbarous experiments under the guise of scientific research."[61] But the ICRC offered no protection and never inquired systematically as to the extent of human experiments, although it held substantial documentation.

As the war drew on, animal material—first apes and then even rabbits—was in short supply, and rabbits came to be viewed as foodstuffs. The pressure increased to use imprisoned humans for experiments. As adults resisted, the primary targets changed to "racial inferiors," especially children, and in 1944 especially Jewish, Sinti, and Roma children. The year 1944 marked a high point of the unethical research in the basic medical sciences. This was because German scientists realized that the war was lost, but they believed they could help German science to continue by demonstrating the superiority of its research. They also hoped for academic appointments on the basis of unique research findings. Research for military purposes was rapidly overtaken by the basic medical sciences. German scientists felt that if they held unique data, it ensured continuity of employment after the war, and the survival of German science.

Investigating the Nazi Research Atrocities

After the war, survivors demanded justice, compensation, and a reconsideration of medical ethics to prevent future abuses. Allied scientific intelligence officers realized that the sacrifice of humans as experimental subjects had been widespread in Nazi Germany. One officer was John W. Thompson, an American, born in Mexico, who held an Edinburgh medical degree and conducted aviation medical research with the Royal Canadian Air Force. He demanded comprehensive documentation and ethical analysis of Nazi research. He was convinced that inaction would condone the experiments, and that "there is equally a danger that these practices may continue in Germany or spread to other countries." British officials doubted that medical war crimes were so widespread, but conceded that there should be a special medical trial for the worst offenders. Thompson secured an inter-Allied meeting of war crimes investigators. On May 15, 1946, British, French, and U.S. representatives met "to consider evidence bearing on the commission of war crimes by German scientists believed to be guilty of inhuman experimentation on living men and women." Thompson's achievement was to establish an International Scientific Commission to document German medical war crimes, and he led efforts to assemble a complete databank on all medical atrocities and human experiments.[62] Thompson considered that comprehensive documentation and ethical evaluation of all experiments was necessary because the trials brought only a select number of perpetrators to justice.

The Nuremberg Code

The Nuremberg Medical Trial was one of the war crimes trials that followed the trial of major Nazi war criminals, including Göring, before the International Military Tribunal representing the United States, Britain, France, and Russia in 1945–46. The U.S. prose-

cutors charged 23 interned Nazi medical scientists and administrators with war crimes and crimes against humanity, and brought them to trial before a panel of U.S. judges in December 1946. In August 1947, 16 of the defendants were convicted; 7 were sentenced to death and, after appeals, were hanged in June 1948 (see Table 2.2).

Survivors of experiments were key prosecution witnesses. The U.S. prosecutors selected a representative spectrum of witnesses to achieve maximum impact in court. They included four Polish women from the "Rabbits" as well as priests, Jews, and Roma.[9] At the trial's end, the three judges issued the Nuremberg Code, with its demand for an "enlightened consent" by human subjects of research. This provided the basis for what shortly afterward was referred to as informed consent, which eventually became the ethical prerequisite for all medical research and therapy.

The issue of an ethical code had first been raised at the International Scientific Commission in August 1946. As promulgated at the Nuremberg Medical Trial, the Code required that the experimental subject be informed of the risks and the rationale for the experiment. Its major innovation was to give the experimental subject the right to halt the experiment. The principle of informed consent and the obligations of research workers to ensure the safety and health of their subjects has had—in the long term—profound implications for clinical practice and research. The Nuremberg Code has offered guidelines for genetic counseling, genetic screening, the use of body parts, and therapeutic trials.

Only one associate of the KWI for Anthropology was a defendant at the Nuremberg Medical Trial: Helmut Poppendick of the Race and Settlement office of the SS. He had been seconded to the KWI for Anthropology for a year's course in genetics. No other human geneticist was prosecuted at Nuremberg, and senior researchers were later de-Nazified with just a small financial penalty or wholly acquitted. Evidence against Verschuer was collected for a planned second medical trial during 1946, but this was dropped for various reasons. In 1946, Verschuer claimed that he had not known the true nature of Auschwitz, and contended that using body parts for research was permissible if a person was going to be killed.[19,63] Mengele came to the attention of the British and U.S. war crimes investigators partly through Auschwitz survivors giving testimony at the Belsen Trial, and partly through the prisoner-physician Gisella Perl, who was keen to testify against him.[9,64]

Despite the wave of postwar trials and Thompson's efforts to document medical war crimes, many culpable researchers were only briefly or never interned. Robert Ritter and his assistant Eva Justin, who conducted the research into the psychology of Sinti and Roma, found a postwar niche in public health work.[33] Fritz Lenz, who had been a professor of racial hygiene in Berlin under the Nazis, became professor of human genetics in Göttingen in 1946. Verschuer initially tried to convince the Americans that his expertise was fundamental for solving problems of postwar health. Once he detected their animosity, he made headway in the British zone. Verschuer eventually obtained a chair at the University of Münster. Others who saw themselves rehabilitated included geneticists Wolfgang Lehmann at Kiel in 1948, Hans Grebe, Verschuer's former assistant, with a teaching post in human genetics at Marburg in 1948, and Lothar Loeffler at Hannover in human genetics in 1953.[55]

Karin Magnussen slipped away; she retained the eye specimens while becoming a high school biology teacher in Bremen.[58] The daughter-in-law of Carl Schneider published euthanasia

Table 2.2

Defendants at the Nuremberg Medical Trial

Name	Born	Joined Nazi Party	Role	Sentence (Reduced to)	Released
Karl Genzken	1885	1926	Chief, Medical Dept. of Waffen-SS	Life (20 yrs)	1954
Siegfried Handloser	1885	–	Chief, Armed Forces Medical Services	Life (20 yrs)	Died in custody
Georg August Weltz	1889	1937	Chief, Institute for Aviation Medicine	Acquitted	
Oskar Schröder	1891	–	Chief, Luftwaffe Medical Service	Life (15 yrs)	1954
Paul Rostock	1892	1938	Chief, Office for Medical Science and Research	Acquitted	
Kurt Blome	1894	1922/31	Deputy Reich Health Leader	Acquitted	
Adolf Pokorny	1895	–	Physician, specialist in skin and venereal diseases	Acquitted	
Gerhard Rose	1896	1922/30	Brig. Gen., Luftwaffe Medical Services	Life (15 yrs)	1955
Karl Gebhardt	1897	1933	Himmler's physician; Chief Surgeon, staff of Reich Physician SS and Police	Death	Hanged
Helmut Poppendick	1902	1932	Chief, personal staff of Reich Physician SS and Police	10 yrs	1951
Waldemar Hoven	1903	1937	Chief Doctor at Buchenwald	Death	Hanged
Viktor Brack	1904	1929	Chief Administrative Officer in Hitler's Chancellery	Death	Hanged
Karl Brandt	1904	1932	Reich Commissioner for Health and Sanitation; Hitler's Escort Surgeon	Death	Hanged
Joachim Mrugowsky	1905	1930	Chief Hygienist, Reich Physician SS and Police	Death	Hanged
Wolfram Sievers	1905	1928/9	Reich Manager, SS Ahnenerbe (Ancestral Heritage) Society	Death	Hanged
Wilhelm Beiglböck	1905	1933	Consulting physician to the Luftwaffe	15 (10 yrs)	1951
Siegfried Ruff	1907	1938	Director of Aviation Medicine, German Experimental Institute for Aviation	Acquitted	
Rudolf Brandt	1909	1932	Personal Administrative Officer to Himmler	Death	Hanged
Hermann Becker-Freyseng	1910	1933	Chief, Dept. of Aviation Medicine, Luftwaffe Medical Service	20 (10 yrs)	1952
Herta Oberheuser	1911	1937	Physician at Ravensbrück; Assistant Physician to Gebhardt at Hohenlychen	20 (10 yrs)	1952
Hans Wolfgang Romberg	1911	1933	Doctor, Dept. for Aviation Medicine, Experimental Institute for Aviation	Acquitted	
Konrad Schäfer	1912	–	Doctor, Dept. for Aviation Medicine, Experimental Institute for Aviation;	Acquitted	
Fritz Fischer	1912	1939	Assistant Physician to Gebhardt at Hohenlychen	Life (15 yrs)	1954

results from Heidelberg for her Leipzig M.D. in 1946. Peiffer calculates that of 12,000 victims' brains, at least 2,097 were examined by pathologists resulting in 37 publications after World War II.

One can cite many such cases. Barbara Uiberrak was the pathologist for the Steinhof complex from 1938 until the 1960s. In 1946, she explained to the people's court in Vienna how she found the children's euthanasia cases scientifically significant, taking pride in the 700 brains and gland specimens. Heinrich Gross began to publish in the *Morphologisches Jahrbuch* the first of a long series of neuropathological contributions, in 1952. Between 1954 and 1978 he published 34 research papers on hereditary mental defects. A coauthor, Franz Seitelberger, who had been a member of an SS unit from 1938 to 1945, became director of the Neurological Institute of the University of Vienna in 1959 and eventually was the university's rector. Gross became one of Austria's foremost psychiatrists and neurohistologists.[43]

However, Waldemar Hoven, one of the doctors convicted at Nuremberg was found to have obtained his degree improperly, as prisoners at Buchenwald wrote his M.D. thesis.[9,65] Only in 1961 did the Universities of Frankfurt and Munich annul the doctorates

of Mengele and the euthanasia and Auschwitz sterilization perpetrator, Horst Schumann; the annulled degrees of most Jewish physicians were never restored. The debate on the ethics of Nazi research data, which began in 1945, continues.[66,67] In contrast, the victims of the experiments have remained marginalized, and—ironically—bioethicists have shown little concern with their welfare. The marginalization and underestimate of their numbers has meant that compensation and care have not been—and tragically never will be—adequate. It is extraordinary that 60 years on from the time of the atrocities, we still do not know their full extent or the identities of the victims. The reasons include the decline of interest in war crimes after 1947 and the protracted resistance of the Austrians and Germans to providing compensation for victims of human experiments.

The Cold War facilitated the politics of denial. West German judicial authorities did not accept the Nuremberg verdicts. Thus, SS Obergruppenführer Poppendick, convicted at Nuremberg and sentenced to 10 years imprisonment—although he was released in 1951—obtained a police report that he was free from convictions when (using the alias Poppendiek) he was awarded a doctorate from the University of Münster in 1953.[9,68] This indicates unwillingness of German civil police and academic authorities, as well as the professors (including Verschuer) who affirmed the academic qualities of the thesis, to recognize the Nuremberg verdicts. Judicial ineffectiveness on the part of the U.S. occupation forces and the postwar West German government explains the noncapture and nonprosecution of Mengele, and the continuing citation of Nazi research.[69] The scientific establishment closed ranks; medical leaders wished to retain specimens and to defend the reputation of celebrated teachers. Historians were interested in National Socialism only at a very general level, and failed to analyze medical atrocities.

German medical teaching and research institutes continued to hoard body parts from Holocaust and euthanasia victims until the 1990s. The pendulum swung from retention to disposal. The solution was burial. Examples include clinics in Frankfurt, Heidelberg, Munich, and Vienna, which transferred body parts for religious burial. At Frankfurt, complaints were made that relatives and the public were not invited to attend the ceremony. Neither were full efforts always made to identify the victims, nor to inform relatives. By way of contrast, the sustained efforts of Viennese anthropologists to identify victims remain exemplary.

The number of victims has been underestimated. We need to identify victims at an individual level for commemoration, compensation, and for a full understanding of the chain of tragic events involving scientific networks at the time. The high number of claims for compensation by survivors indicates how our estimates of victims need to revised upward, taking into account not only deaths but also people who were subjected to abusive research but still survived. Given that medical research for typhus and malaria involved thousands of victims, the overall numbers of victims of atrocities conducted for scientific purposes will rise to tens of thousands. Moreover, we need to add the victims of euthanasia killed for medical research purposes, and victims (whether living or dead) of experimental methods of sterilization. No reliable account of the numbers who survived human experiments and those who were killed has ever been made. Close attention to the sources suggests that many groups—children in institutions, prisoners of war, hospital patients, as well as concentration and extermination camp prisoners—were victims of experimental and invasive research. Overall, there were many thousands of victims, possibly in the order of tens of thousands, who were killed or survived.

Victims of human experiments are very much a marginalized group in the history of the Holocaust. Once historians realized that experimental victims were generally not pilots for mass destruction, they lost interest in the often intricate rationales of researchers and their networks, and avoided critical engagement with medical texts indicating genocidal motives. Historians' attention shifted away from experimentation to euthanasia, as a key stage in the Holocaust, whereas the human experiments have been underestimated and neglected. Neither the extent of child experimentation, nor the exploitation of body parts, nor the identities of victims have been fully established. Victims and their families contributed to medical and social insurance, but survivors have never received the medical care they need, let alone adequate compensation beyond that of a single, and belated, small lump sum payment.

The journalist Hans-Joachim Lang, in *Die Namen der Nummern* ("The Names of the Numbers"), has recently identified the victims who were killed for Hirt's skeleton collection. One victim was aged 16. She was Juli Cohen, born in 1927 in Thessaloniki, Greece. The rest of the children in her transport to Auschwitz of April 18, 1943, were killed. In 1967, the journalist Günther Schwarberg set out to identify the 20 children selected by Mengele for fatal TB experiments.[45] His pioneering study remains exemplary as regards the need to reconstruct victims' life histories.

Although Holocaust victims are commemorated on an individual basis, medical victims are often still anonymized. When victims' identities are suppressed on the basis of medical confidentiality, however, it is, in fact, the medical perpetrators who are protected from scrutiny. The identities of the victims need to be established for purposes of both commemoration and medical ethics. Only by knowing the victims can we properly comprehend the Nazi research atrocities. Only then can we unravel the networks of unscrupulous medical researchers to whom the victims fell prey, and restore a measure of justice and ethics to this dark period in the history of scientific medicine.[70]

References

1. Weindling PJ. *Epidemics and Genocide in Eastern Europe*. Oxford, England: Oxford University Press; 2000.
2. Layton TB. A moral problem. *Lancet* 1946;248:882.
3. *The Daily Telegraph* Dec. 14/17, 1946.
4. Byman B. Bitter fruit: The legacy of the Nazi human experiments. *Minnesota Medicine* 1989;62:582–6.
5. Harnett RM, Pruitt JR, Sias FR. A review of the literature concerning resuscitation from hypothermia: Part 1—The problem and general approaches. *Aviation Space and Environmental Medicine* 1983;54: 425–34.
6. U.S. Air Force Surgeon General. *German Aviation Medicine—World War II. Volumes I and II*. Washington, D.C.: U.S. Government Printing Office, 1950.
7. Beecher HK. Ethics and clinical research. *New England Journal of Medicine* 1966;274:1354–60.
8. Schmaltz F. *Kampfstoff Forschung im Nationalsozialismus*. Göttingen, Germany: Wallstein; 2005.
9. Weindling PJ. *Nazi Medicine and the Nuremberg Trials: From Medical War Crimes to Informed Consent*. London, England: Palgrave; 2004.
10. The Nuremberg Medical Trial 1946/47. Transcripts, Material of the Prosecution and Defense. Related Documents. English edition, On Behalf of the Stiftung für Sozialgeschichte des 20. *Jahrhunderts*, edited By Klaus Dörner, Angelika Ebbinghaus and Karsten Linne, in cooperation with Karlheinz Roth and Paul Weindling. Microfiche Edition. Munich, Germany: Saur; 1999.
11. Weyers W. *The Abuse of Man: An Illustrated History of Human Experimentation*. New York, N.Y.: Ardor Scribendi; 2003.
12. Levine C. What's in a name? The Eppinger Prize and Nazi experiments. *Hastings Center Report* 1984;14(4):3–4.
13. Spiro HM. Eppinger of Vienna: Scientist and villain? *Journal of Clinical Gastroenterology* 1984;6:493–7.
14. Reuben A. First do no harm. *Hepatology* 2006;43:243–9.
15. Vollman J, Winau R. Informed consent in human experimentation before the Nuremberg Code. *British Medical Journal* 1996;313:1445–7.
16. Bonah C. Le drame de Lübeck. In: Bonah C, Lepicard E, Roelcke V, eds. *La médecine expérimentale au tribunal: Implications éthiques de quelques procès médicaux du XXe siècle européen*. Paris, France: Editions Scientifiques Gordon Breach; 2003:65–94.
17. Eckart W. Humanexperiment und Probandenrecht in der Medizin des 20 Jahrhunderts. In: Mundt C, Hohendorf G, Rotzoll M, eds.

Psychiatrische Forschung und NS 'Euthanasie': Beiträge zu einer Gedenkveranstaltung an der Psychiatrischen Universitätsklinik Heidelberg. Heidelberg, Germany: Wunderhorn; 2001:247–63.

18. Kater MH. *Doctors Under Hitler.* Chapel Hill, N.C.: University of North Carolina Press; 1989.

19. Weindling PJ. *Health, Race, and German Politics Between National Unification and Nazism, 1870–1945.* Cambridge, England: Cambridge University Press; 1989.

20. Burleigh M, Wipperman W. *The Racial State: Germany 1993–1945.* Cambridge, England: Cambridge University Press; 1994.

21. Labisch A, Tennstedt F. *Der Weg zum 'Gesetz über die Vereinheitlichung des Gesundheitswesens' vom 3. Juli 1934. Entwicklungslinien und -momente.* Düsseldorf, Germany: Akademie für öffentliches Gesundheitswesen; 1985.

22. Fritz Bauer Institut, ed. *"Gerichtstag halten über uns selbst . . ." Geschichte und Wirkungsgeschichte des ersten Frankfurter Auschwitz-Prozesses.* Frankfurt am Main, Germany: Campus Verlag; 2001.

23. Klee E. *Deutsche Medizin im Dritten Reich. Karriere vor und nach 1945.* Frankfurt am Main, Germany: S. Fischer; 2001.

24. Taylor T. Opening statement of the prosecution, December 9, 1946. In: *Trials of War Criminals Before the Nuremberg Military Tribunals Under Control Council Law No. 10.* Nuremberg, October 1946–April 1949. Washington, D.C.: Government Printing Office; 1949–1953.

25. Baur E, Fischer E, Lenz F. *Menschliche Erblichkeitslehre und Rassenhygiene.* München, Germany: Lehmanns; 1921–1940.

26. Fangerau HM. Making eugenics a public issue: A reception study of the first German compendium on racial hygiene, 1921–1940. *Science Studies* 2005;18(2):46–66.

27. Pommerin R. *Die Sterilisierung der Rheinland-Bastarde. Das Schicksal einer farbigen deutschen Minderheit 1918–1937.* Düsseldorf, Germany: Droste; 1979.

28. Stargardt N. *Witnesses of War: Children's Lives Under the Nazis.* New York, N.Y.: Alfred A. Knopf; 2006:74–5.

29. Justin E. *Lebensschicksale artfremd erzogener Zigeunerkinder und ihrer Nachkommen. Veröffentlichungen auf dem Gebiet des Volksgesundheitsdienstes.* M.D. Diss., Berlin, 1944.

30. Teschler-Nicola M, Berner M. *Die Anthropologische Abteilung des Naturhistorischen Museums in der NS-Zeit.* Berichte und Dokumentations von Forschungs- und Sammlungsaktivitäten, 1938–1945. Senatsprojekt der Universität Wien. Untersuchungen zur Anatomischen Wissenschaft in Wien 1938–1945, 1998:333–8. [unpublished report]

31. Spring C. Vermessen, deklassiert und deportiert: Dokumentation zur anthropologischen Untersuchung an 440 Juden im Wiener Stadion im September 1939 unter der Leitung von Josef Wastl vom Naturhistorischen Museum Wien. *Zeitgeschichte* 2005;32:91–110.

32. Schaltenbrand G. *Neurology.* Wiesbaden, Germany: FIAT; 1948.

33. Klee E. *Auschwitz, die NS-Medizin und ihre Opfer.* Frankfurt am Main, Germany: S. Fischer; 1997.

34. Personal information from son of a victim.

35. Lang H-J. *Die Namen der Nummern.* Hamburg, Germany: Hofmann und Campe; 2004.

36. Faulstich H. Die Zahl der "Euthanasie"-Opfer. In: Frewer A, Clemens Eickhoff, eds. *"Euthanasie" und die aktuelle Sterbehilfe-Debatte. Die historischen Hintergründe medizinischer Ethik.* Frankfurt am Main, Germany: Campus Verlag; 2000.

37. Burleigh M. *Death and Deliverance: 'Euthanasia' in Germany 1900–1945.* Cambridge, England: Cambridge University Press; 1995.

38. Friedlander H. *The Origins of Nazi Genocide: From Euthanasia to the Final Solution.* Chapel Hill, N.C.: University of North Carolina Press; 1995:39.

39. Benzenhöfer U. Der Fall "Kind Knauer." *Deutsches Ärzteblatt* 1998;95(19):B954–5.

40. Benzenhöfer U. Genese und Struktur der "NS-Kinder und Jugendlicheneuthanasie." *Monatsschrift Kinderheilkunde* 2003;150:1012–9.

41. Peiffer J. Assessing neuropathological research carried out on victims of the "Euthanasia Programme." *Medizinhistorisches Journal* 1999;34:339–55.

42. Mundt C, Hohendorf G, Rotzoll M, eds. *Psychiatrische Forschung und NS 'Euthanasie': Beiträge zu einer Gedenkveranstaltung an der Psychiatrischen Universitätsklinik Heidelberg.* Heidelberg, Germany: Wunderhorn; 2001.

43. Diehl M. *Endstation Spiegelgrund. Die Tötung behinderter Kinder während des Nationalsozialismus am Beispiel der Kinderfachabteilung in Wien.* Med. Diss., Göttingen, 1996.

44. Klein H, Nachtsheim H. *Hydrops congenitus beim Kaninchen, eine erbliche fetale Erythroblastose.* Abhandlungen der Deutschen Akademie der Wissenschaften. *Mathematisch-Naturwissenschaftliche Klasse* 1947;5:1–71.

45. Schwarberg G. *The Murders at Bullenhuser Damm: The SS Doctor and the Children.* Bloomington, Ind.: Indiana University Press; 1984 [orig. German ed., 1980].

46. Schwarberg G. *Meine zwanzig Kinder.* Göttingen, Germany: Steidl-Verlag; 1996.

47. Weindling PJ. Genetik und Menschenversuche in Deutschland, 1940–1950: Hans Nachtsheim, die Kaninchen von Dahlem und die Kinder von Bullenhuser Damm. In: Schmuhl H-W, ed. *Rassenforschung an Kaiser-Wilhelm Instituten vor und nach 1933.* Göttingen, Germany: Wallstein Verlag; 2003:245–74.

48. Mitscherlich A, Mielke F. *Wissenschaft ohne Menschlichkeit: Medizinische und eugenische Irrwege unter Diktatur, Bürokratie und Krieg—mit einem Vorwort der Arbeitsgemeinschaft der westdeutschen Ärztekammern.* Heidelberg, Germany: Verlag Lambert Schneider; 1949.

49. Report on Medical Ethics. *WMA Bulletin* 1949;1(3):109.

50. Proctor R. *The Nazi War on Cancer.* Princeton, N.J.: Princeton University Press; 1999:344 n.4.

51. Leydendecker B, Klapp B. Deutsche Hepatitisforschung im Zweiten Weltkrieg. In: Aly G, Pross C, eds. *Der Wert des Menscchen: Medizin in Deutschland 1918–1945.* Berlin, Germany: Hentrich; 1989:261–93.

52. Hubenstorf M. Anatomical science in Vienna, 1938–45. *Lancet* 2000;155:1385–6.

53. Weindling PJ. *Sage of Anxiety: On Call to the Human Disasters of the Twentieth Century.* Rochester, NY: University of Rochester Press; forthcoming.

54. Oleschinski B. Der "Anatom der Gynäkologen": Hermann Stieve und seine Erkenntnisse über Todesangst und weiblichen Zyklus. *Beiträge zur Nationalsozialistischen Gesundheits- und Sozialpolitik* 1992, Band 10.

55. Müller-Hill B. *Tödliche Wissenschaft: Die Aussonderung von Juden, Zigeunern und Geisteskranken 1933–1945.* Reinbek, Germany: Rowohlt; 1984.

56. Müller-Hill B. Genetics after Auschwitz. *Holocaust and Genocide Studies* 1987;2:3–20.

57. Sachse C, ed. *Biowissenschaften und Menschenversuche an Kaiser-Wilhelm-Instituten—Die Verbindung nach Auschwitz.* Göttingen, Germany: Wallstein Verlag; 2004.

58. Hesse H. *Augen aus Auschwitz—Ein Lehrstück über nationalsozialistischen Rassenwahn und medizinische Forschung—Der Fall Dr. Karin Magnussen.* Essen, Germany: Klartext Verlag; 2001.

59. Tillion G. *Ravensbrück.* Paris, France: Éditions du Seuil; 1973 [new ed., 1988].

60. Klier F. *Die Kaninchen von Ravensbrück: Medizinische Versuche an Frauen in der NS-Zeit.* Munich, Germany: Knaur; 1994.

61. Weindling PJ. What did the allies know about criminal human experiments in the war and its immediate aftermath? In: Ley A, ed. *Gewissenlos, Gewissenhaft: Menschenversuche im Konzentrationslager: Eine Ausstellung des Instituts für Geschichte der Medizin der Universität Erlangen-Nürnberg in Zusammenarbeit mit dem Stadtmuseum Erlangen.* Erlangen, Germany: Specht-Verlag; 2001:52–66.

62. Weindling PJ. Akteure in eigener Sache: Die Aussagen der Überlebenden und die Verfolgung der medizinischen Kriegsverbrechen nach 1945. In: Sachse C, ed. *Biowissenschaften und Menschenversuche an Kaiser-Wilhelm-Instituten—Die Verbindung nach Auschwitz.* Göttingen, Germany: Wallstein Verlag; 2004:255–82.

63. Kröner H-P. *Von der Rassenhygiene zur Humangenetik: Das Kaiser-Wilhelm-Institut für Anthropologie, menschliche Erblehre und Eugenik nach dem Kriege.* Stuttgart, Germany: Fischer; 1998.

64. Perl G. *I was a Doctor in Auschwitz.* New York, N.Y.: International Universities Press; 1948.

65. Hoven W. Versuche zur Behandlung der Lungentuberkulose. Durch Intulation von Kohlekolloid. Med. Diss., Freiburg i.B., 1943.

66. Weindling PJ. Human guinea pigs and the ethics of experimentation: The BMJ's correspondent at the Nuremberg Medical Trial. *British Medical Journal* 1996;313:1467–70. [Revised version in: Doyal L, Tobias JS, eds. *Informed Consent in Medical Research.* London, England: BMJ Books; 2001:15–9.]

67. Moe K. Should the Nazi research data be cited? *Hastings Center Report* 1984;14(6):5–7.

68. Poppendieck H. *Ueber den Krankheitswert des Pelger-Gens beim Menschen.* Diss., Münster, Feb. 18, 1953.

69. Seidelmann WE. Mengele medicus: Medicine's Nazi heritage. *Milbank Quarterly* 1988;66:221–39.

70. Weindling PJ. Deadly medicine. *Social History of Medicine* (in press).

Takashi Tsuchiya

The Imperial Japanese Experiments in China

Between 1933 and the end of World War II, Japanese researchers—mostly under the aegis of the Japanese Imperial Army—killed thousands of humans in medical experiments. The experiments, which included vivisection, fell broadly into three categories: explanation of diseases, development of therapies, and research into and development of biological and chemical warfare. Most of the human experimentation took place in Japanese-occupied Manchuria and China, although the Japanese army also operated experimental centers in Southeast Asia and on the main Japanese islands. Most of the victims were Manchurian or Chinese criminals, political prisoners, or prisoners of war, although some Allied prisoners of war—such as Americans, Australians, and New Zealanders—were also used and killed in these experiments.

Because of an immunity arrangement with U.S. officials, most of the researchers involved were never brought to trial. In return, the United States got secret access to the results of Japanese biological warfare experiments that had been performed on prisoners. Many of the human experimenters went on to prestigious civilian careers, leaving both Japan and the United States with unresolved ethical issues that now date back more than half a century.

Background

Shiro Ishii, the founder and leader of Japan's network of human experimentation facilities, entered the Army in 1920 upon graduation from Kyoto Imperial University Faculty of Medicine. In 1925, Ishii began to lobby his superiors for research on biological warfare. In 1930, after a two-year trip to Europe and the United States, he became a professor in the Department of Epi-

demic Prevention of the Army Medical College (Rikugun Gun'i Gakko Boeki Bu—Boekigaku Kyoshitsu) in Tokyo. In this position he performed bacteriological studies, conducted research on and development of vaccines, and trained army surgeons. He wanted to improve the prestige of medical officers in the Japanese Army by developing a powerful biological weapons program—even though biological and chemical warfare had been prohibited by the Geneva Convention in 1925. Using the Army's authority and prestige in 1930s Japan, he also envisaged a national network for medical research that would be much more powerful and effective than the existing academic infrastructure, and that would be furnished with state-of-the-art laboratories that could freely use humans for research and development of military medicine.

The takeover of Manchuria by Japan's Kwantung Army in 1931—known as the "Manchurian Incident," or, in China, as the "9/18 Incident"—gave Ishii his opportunity. The following year, he established a large new department specializing in biological warfare in the Army Medical College, and deceptively named it the Epidemic Prevention Laboratory (Boeki Kenkyu Shitsu). This laboratory became the headquarters of his network. Simultaneously, he built a secret facility called the Togo Unit in Beiyinhe, a small town in Manchuria about 70 km southeast of Harbin. This was Ishii's first prison-laboratory, where deadly human experimentation probably began in the fall of 1933. The subjects were mainly Chinese but included some Soviets, Mongolians, and Koreans who were arrested by the Kwantung Army Military Police as spies and resisters and who were scheduled to be executed without trial. Ishii and his colleagues thought it was better to use them as human guinea pigs than merely to execute them.

The facilities of Beiyinhe were insufficient for Ishii's project. The buildings were not strong enough to serve as a prison; in fact, in September 1934, 16 captives revolted and escaped. So Ishii and the army built a much larger, stronger prison laboratory-factory in Pingfang (sometimes written as Ping Fan), about 20 km southeast of downtown Harbin, now one of the districts of Harbin City. Construction at Pingfang began in 1935; residents of four nearby villages were forced to evacuate, and the huge complex was completed around 1938. The Togo Unit became an official unit of the Japanese army in 1936, even before construction was completed. This means that the Japanese Emperor, Hirohito, formally acknowledged Ishii's project, though it seems he was unaware of its details.

The Togo Unit was now known as the Epidemic Prevention Department (Boeki Bu) of the Kwantung Army, and as Unit 731. In addition to medical experimentation, Ishii's units were responsible for water purification for Japanese troops in China from 1937 on, and so the unit was soon renamed the Epidemic Prevention and Water Supply Department (EPWSD) (Boeki Kyusui Bu). Ishii had invented a water purification machine that could be easily carried to the battlefield. During the battles for Beijing and Shanghai, he sent teams to the front to operate it—garnering even more support from army leaders. In 1938, the Japanese army adopted Ishii's machine as standard equipment and organized 18 divisional EPWSDs (Shidan Boeki Kyusui Bu), whose directors were officers of Unit 731. By 1939, Ishii's network included some field water purification units, 18 divisional EPWSDs, and five permanent Epidemic Prevention Departments—in Harbin (Unit 731), Beijing (Unit 1855), Nanjing (Unit 1644), Guangzhou (Unit 8604), and Tokyo (Boeki Kenkyu Shitsu). Altogether, Ishii commanded more than 10,000 people. When the Japanese army occupied Singapore in 1942, another permanent EPWSD was added to the network (Unit 9420). Unit 731 had a proving ground in Anda (about 150 km northwest of Harbin) and five branches located in Mudanjiang, Linkou, Sunwu, Hailar, and Dalian.

In addition, as a leader of army surgeons, Ishii had power over army hospitals in occupied cities in China. His network also had close connections with other biological warfare departments such as the Military Animals Epidemic Prevention Department (Gunju Boeki Shou) in Changchun, Manchuria (Unit 100), and institutions for chemical warfare such as the Army Sixth Technology Institute in Tokyo, the Army Narashino School in the Tokyo suburb of Narashino, the Army Ninth Technology Institute (Noborito Institute) in Noborito, also a Tokyo suburb, and the Kwantung Army Chemical Department in Qiqihar in Manchuria (Unit 516).

Unit 731 probably moved to the new base in Pingfang in 1938. It was a 6-square-kilometer complex of secret laboratory-factories surrounded by trenches and high-voltage electric wires. The whole district became a special military area, which meant anyone approaching without permission was to be shot by the guards. The main building had two special prisons in its inner yard, so that escapees could never get outside. The captives were called *maruta,* which means "logs" in Japanese, and were identified only by numbers.

At a little-noted war crimes trial conducted by Soviet authorities at Khabarovsk in 1949, Surgeon Major General Kiyoshi

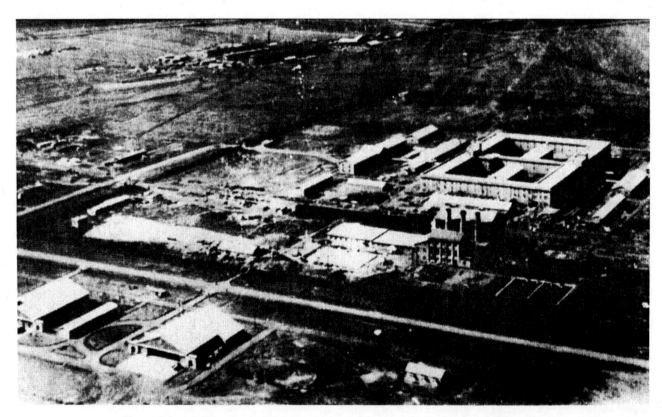

Figure 3.1. Aerial Photograph of Unit 731. Source: Seiichi Morimura. Reprinted with permission.

Kawashima, who was chief of a division of Unit 731, testified that the prisons usually held 200 to 300 captives, including some women and children, but that their maximum capacity was said to be 400.[1] The Military Police sent 400 to 600 captives to Unit 731 every year under the Special Transfer Procedure (Tokui Atsukai), a system the Japanese army developed to supply human subjects.[1] This system for procuring subjects differed from that of Nazi Germany. The Nazi transfer system was not for procuring subjects but for genocide. But in the case of the Japanese medical experiments, victims were purposely selected and sent to Ishii's network to be subjects of experiments.

At least 3,000 people were tortured to death at Unit 731 from 1940 to 1945.[1] But this number does not include victims before 1940 or at other medical experimentation sites. Allied prisoners of war (POWs) may have been subjected to experiments by Unit 731 researchers at the camp in Mukden (now Shengyang).[2,3]

Moreover, the activities of Unit 731 researchers were only a part of the medical atrocities committed by Imperial Japan. According to a large body of testimony, deadly experiments also were performed in other permanent EPWSDs such as Units 1644 and 1855. American, Australian, and New Zealander POWs were forced to participate in experiments by Surgeon Captain Einosuke Hirano of the 24th Field EPWSD in Rabaul, Papua, New Guinea,[4] and eight U.S. airmen were killed in surgical experiments on the Japanese home islands.[5] Table 3.1 presents an approximate timeline of the Imperial Japanese experiments in China, along with other relevant historical dates.

Medical Atrocities

Medical atrocities performed by Imperial Japanese doctors can be classified into three categories:

1. Training of army surgeons.
2. Biological warfare maneuvers.
3. Research with humans.

Training of Army Surgeons

Surgeons at army hospitals performed many vivisections on Chinese captives, with anesthesia. For example, these doctors performed appendectomies and tracheostomies on the prisoners, shot them and took bullets from their bodies, cut open their arms and legs and sewed up the skin around the wounds, and finally killed them. This was purportedly part of training newly assigned army surgeons to treat wounded soldiers at the front lines.

Confessions by many of the surgeons involved are on record.[6,7] At Datong Army Hospital in Datong, Shanxi, in June probably of 1941, Surgeon Major Kazuharu Tanimura and Surgeon Lieutenant Rihei Miura conducted a three-day training program that involved lectures on military surgery and exercise surgeries such as suturing of blood vessels and nerves, thoracotomy, celiotomy, craniotomy, blood transfusion, various anesthetizations, appendectomy, and nephrectomy, performed serially on "six bodies of prepared materials."[8] The trainees were army surgeon officers of the Army Medical College. Judging from confessions about similar cases, the "materials" probably were arrested Chinese resisters who probably were killed in these exercises.

In the summer of 1989, human bones from more than 100 bodies were found in the ground where the Army Medical College had been located in Tokyo from 1929 to 1945. Eleven skulls and most long bones were heavily sawed or drilled. One skull was shot and another one was stabbed. Judging from the condition and technique, they must have been the subjects of test surgeries, preserved as specimens in the Army Medical College, and finally buried when Japan surrendered.[9] They may be the remains of vivisected Chinese prisoners.

Biological Warfare Maneuvers

Hundreds of confessions testify to Imperial Japanese research into the use of biological warfare. Unit 731 used biological warfare during the four-month clash between Japan and the Soviet Union over the Manchukuo-Mongol border in 1939, according to testimonies of former junior assistants of Unit 731.[10,11] Moreover, Japanese army officers themselves wrote about biological warfare against China in their official records. According to these notes, at least three major attacks on Chinese citizens were carried out.

First, in 1940 Lieutenant Colonel Kumao Imoto, then on the general staff of the Japanese Expeditionary Force in China, wrote in his log several times about consultations with army surgeon officers of Unit 731. On October 7, 1940, he wrote that Unit 731 officers reported, "So far six attacks have been completed" on Ningpo City.[12] On October 30, an epidemic of plague suddenly occurred in Ningpo, which is now suspected to have been the result of these attacks. In the log of November 30, 1940, general officer Kaizo Yoshihashi reported, "On November 21 . . . an agreement was reached that next time Jinhua would be attacked" with Ishii's Unit.[13] This coincides with the fact that on November 28 a Japanese bomber sprinkled on the city of Jinhua granules in which plague bacillus was found.[7]

Second, on September 16, 1941, Imoto wrote that "the Imperial Headquarters issued a direction for biological warfare."[14] On November 25 it was reported that Changde was attacked in the morning of November 4 and an epidemic occurred there on November 6.[15]

Third, on August 28, 1942, Imoto noted how army surgeons of Unit 731 had performed biological warfare in Zhegan (Zhejiang-Jianxi) operations. In Guangxin, Guangfeng, and Yushan, plague bacillus was scattered via contaminated fleas, rats, and lice. In Jiangshan and Changshan, vibrio cholerae was thrown directly into wells or smeared on foods and injected into fruits that were left on the streets. In Quxian and Lishui, typhus and paratyphoid were distributed with corrupted fleas. On October 5, Army Surgeon Colonel Tomosada Masuda of Unit 731 told Imoto that the attacks with contaminated fleas and vibrio cholerae in the wells were probably successful.[16]

Fifty-five years later, in August 1997, 180 family members of Chinese victims of the biological attacks filed a complaint in Tokyo District Court demanding an apology and compensation from the Japanese government. On August 27, 2002, the court dismissed the complaint, ruling that individuals cannot sue a country for compensation for wartime suffering. On July 19, 2005, Tokyo Higher Court dismissed it again for the same reason, and so did Japanese Supreme Court on May 9, 2007. But the courts acknowledged that biological warfare had been waged, because the Japanese government never disputed the facts but rather kept silent.

Table 3.1

Timeline of the Imperial Japanese Experiments in China

Date	Event
1925	Shiro Ishii begins to lobby for research on biological warfare.
1930	Ishii becomes a professor of the Army Medical College.
Sept. 1931	Manchurian (9/18) Incident: Japanese army takes over Manchuria.
1932	Japan establishes its puppet state, "Manchukuo."
1932	Ishii establishes both the Epidemic Prevention Laboratory in the Army Medical College in Tokyo, the headquarters of his medical network, and Togo Unit in Beyinhe in Manchuria, the predecessor of Unit 731.
Autumn 1933	Deadly human experiments in Togo Unit begin.
Sept. 1934	Sixteen captives revolt and escape from a prison in Togo Unit.
1935	Construction of a huge prison laboratory-factory begins in Pingfang, near Harbin.
Circa 1935	Satoshi Sugawara of Togo Unit performs distilled water experiments on Chinese captives.
1936	The Togo Unit becomes an official unit of the Japanese army as Unit 731.
1936	Kameo Tasaki of Manchuria Medical College publishes a study of lymphogranuloma with experiments on a condemned guerrilla.
1937	Japan invades the rest of mainland China.
Circa 1938	Unit 731 moves to Pingfang.
1938	The Japanese army adopts Ishii's water purification machine as standard equipment and organizes Units 1855, 1644, and 8604.
Sept. 1939	Nazi Germany invades Poland; World War II begins in Europe.
1939	The Army Science Institute, the Kwantung Army Chemical Department, and Unit 731 appear to perform joint chemical weapon tests with human subjects.
Aug. 1939	Unit 731 conducts biological warfare against Soviet troops in the Japanese-Russian border clash over the Mongolia-Manchukuo border.
May 1940	Toyonori Yamauchi et al. perform cholera vaccine experiments on 20 Chinese captives in Unit 731.
Sept. 1940	Unit 731 performs a large human experiment of mustard gas.
Oct.–Nov. 1940	The Japanese army attacks Ningpo with biological weapons.
1941	Hisato Yoshimura gives a lecture on his frostbite studies with human subjects in Harbin.
Jan.–Feb. 1941	Kazuharu Tanimura et al. perform "winter hygiene studies" in inner Mongolia, abusing and killing 8 Chinese captives in various experiments.
May 1941	Shigeo Ban of the Army 9th Technology Institute performs poison experiments on about 15 humans at Unit 1644.
June 1941 (?)	Kazuharu Tanimura and Rihei Miura conduct a deadly training program for army surgeon officers with 6 human subjects in Datong, Shanxi.
Summer 1941	A plague flea bomb trial on humans is performed at Unit 731's Anda proving ground.
Nov. 1941	The Japanese army attacks Changde with biological weapons.
Dec. 1941	Japan attacks Pearl Harbor, Kota Bahru, and Hong Kong: The Pacific War begins.
Apr. 18, 1942	U.S. bombers launched from an aircraft carrier raid Tokyo and fly to an airbase in Zhejiang, China.
May–Aug. 1942	The Japanese army conducts biological warfare in Zhegan (Zhejiang-Jianxi) Operations.
Aug. 1942	Ishii moves the command post of Unit 731 to Masaji Kitano.
1942	Unit 9420 is established in Singapore.
1942	Naeo Ikeda performs human experiments involving epidemic hemorrhagic fever at Heihe Army Hospital.
1942	Cyanide gas is tested on human subjects, killing them.
1942–43	Vivisections are suspected to have been performed in Manchuria Medical College Anatomy Department.
End of 1943	A typhus vaccine experiment is performed on 50 Chinese prisoners in Unit 731.
End of 1943	An anthrax bomb trial on humans is performed in Anda proving ground.
1944	Kasahara, Kitano, et al. publish a study on epidemic hemorrhagic fever in "ape."
Aug.–Sept. 1944	Tsunetaka Matsui of Unit 100 performs a deadly poison experiment.
1944–45	Einosuke Hirano performs deadly experiments on American, Australian, and New Zealander POWs in Rabaul, Papua, New Guinea.
Jan. 1945	A gas gangrene bomb trial on humans is performed in Anda proving ground.
Jan. 1945	Dr. Muto of Unit 731 performs a salt overdose experiment on Chinese.
Mar. 1945	U.S. Air Force carries out huge air raids on Tokyo, Osaka, Kobe, and Nagoya.
Mar. 1945	Ishii returns as commander of Unit 731.

Table 3.1 *(continued)*

Date	Event
May–June 1945	Fukujiro Ishiyama et al. perform experimental surgeries on 8 U.S. airmen and kill them at Kyushu Imperial University.
Aug. 6, 1945	First atomic bomb is dropped on Hiroshima.
Aug. 8,1945	The Soviet Union declares war against Japan: Japanese army withdraws from Manchuria, destroying evidence of medical atrocities. Ishii's network collapses, and all surviving captives are killed at Unit 731 and other facilities.
Aug. 9, 1945	Second atomic bomb is dropped on Nagasaki.
Aug. 15, 1945	Imperial Japan surrenders.
Sept.–Oct. 1945	Murray Sanders of U.S. Army Chemical Corps investigates Japanese biological warfare R&D: GHQ/SCAP grants immunity from war crime charges to Ishii and his researchers.
Jan.–Mar. 1946	A. T. Thompson of U.S. Army Chemical Corps investigates Ishii and his researchers, but cannot find evidence of deadly experiments.
Dec. 1946	Nazi Doctors Trial opens at Nuremberg Tribunal.
Jan. 1947	The Soviets demand extradition of Ishii and his researchers for investigation of their deadly experiments: U.S. learns the facts of Japanese medical atrocities.
Apr.–June 1947	N. H. Fell of U.S. Army Chemical Corps investigates details of Ishii and his researchers' deadly experiments.
Aug. 1947	The State-War-Navy Coordinating Subcommittee to the Far East approves Ishii and his researchers' immunity from war crimes charges.
Aug. 1947	Medical Trial concludes in Nuremberg: U.S. judges promulgate the Nuremberg Code.
Dec. 1949	The Soviet Union brings officers and soldiers of Units 731 and 100 to trial before a military tribunal at Khabarovsk (the Khabarovsk Trial): The United States brands it as communist propaganda.
1956	The People's Republic of China tries Japanese war criminals before military tribunals, including only one surgeon officer of Unit 731.
1959	Shiro Ishii dies of laryngeal cancer at the age of 67.

Research With Humans

The research by Japanese doctors falls into three categories:

1. Explaining diseases
2. Development of therapies
3. Development of biological and chemical weapons

Explaining Diseases

Doctors in Ishii's network performed lethal experiments on captives in order to gain new scientific knowledge. There were two major kinds of research programs. One group of experiments involved bacteriological studies, including intentional infection in order to observe how the disease occurs and progresses and to search for its pathogen. Another group involved physiological studies, which were similar to the experiments Nazi doctors performed, including observation of the body's reaction to conditions such as extremely low temperature, low pressure such as that experienced at high altitudes, salt overdose, drinking only distilled water, and intravenous air injection. Anthropological-anatomical studies with "fresh human brains" were also performed at Manchuria Medical College.

Bacteriological studies. Shiro Kasahara, a researcher at Kitasato Institute in Tokyo, worked for Unit 731 for several years. In 1944, Kasahara, Surgeon General Masaji Kitano, Commander of Unit 731 from August 1942 to March 1945, and others published a paper concerning the identification of the pathogen of epidemic hemorrhagic fever, the etiology of which was then still unknown. It reads:

> We made an emulsion with 203 ground-up North Manchuria mites and salt water, and injected it into the thigh of an ape

hypodermically. This first ape became feverish with a temperature of 39.4 degrees Celsius on the 19th day after injection and moderately infected. Then we took blood of this feverish ape and injected it into the second ape, which became feverish and produced protein in its urine. Typical epidemic hemorrhagic kidney was found at its autopsy. . . . Epidemic hemorrhagic kidney was never found at autopsy in the most feverish period. . . . But kidney, liver, and spleen of this period are most infective.[17]

This means they vivisected the "ape," because in order for surgeons to "autopsy in the most feverish period," the subject needed to be alive. Moreover, "the ape" must have been a human being, because the normal temperature of an ape is higher than that of a human being; 39.4 degrees Celsius is normal for an ape. In another paper, Kasahara and his colleagues noted that apes do not become feverish from this disease. So it seems probable that they infected humans and vivisected them.[18]

Kasahara himself later confessed:

> My work involved supervising the extraction of blood samples from cases previously injected; they would normally show a slight temperature rise to about 37 deg C. These samples were reinjected into a second spy by members of another section, which had nothing to do with mine, and, after the injection, the second generation of patient became infected with haemorrhagic fever. . . . From the symptoms we were able to discern the transmission of the strain. . . .
>
> Only on rare occasions did patients die of EHF [epidemic hemorrhagic fever]; normally, they would recover. I have heard rumour that in extremely rare cases, military surgeons,

anxious to perform an autopsy, had injected critical and terminal cases with morphine. . . .

. . . when I went to the Unit for the second time in 1942 I had to participate in the experiments of Kitano and the military doctors that were already in progress, namely, injecting people, spies; this was the result of orders and simply had to be obeyed.

I feel very guilty about what I have done and I think I did wrong. There were very few instances but, when a spy did die as a result of human experiment . . . I felt terribly sad and I always arranged for a memorial service to be held in the main hall of the Ishii Unit, which was given by a Buddhist priest from among the soldiers . . . but that's how deeply I was disturbed, and I think I was the only person in the Ishii Unit to arrange such a memorial service.[2]

In the late 1960s former Surgeon Lieutenant Colonel Naeo Ikeda, who practiced medicine in Osaka after the war, published papers reporting his Unit 731 experiments on epidemic hemorrhagic fever, in which the "fatality rate was 15% in 1941."[19] Ikeda wrote that in 1942, at Heihe Army Hospital, he injected blood taken from a feverish patient into two "volunteers," who became infected, in order to confirm that this disease was infectious.[19] At the same time, he infected another two "healthy volunteers" with contaminated lice and four "volunteers" with contaminated fleas.[20] Later Ikeda said in an interview that these volunteers were "coolies" at Heihe Army Hospital, and insisted that he sent them back there after treatment at Unit 731.[21]

However, Ikeda evidently killed subjects in a study of tetanus. To measure muscle chronaxie of tetanic patients, he injected 14 with tetanus toxin or spore. All died, but before their deaths, Ikeda and Army Engineer Saburo Araki measured chronaxie of their masseter, nasal muscle, orbicular muscle of eye, papillary muscle, intercostal muscles, anterior tibial muscle, and musculus gastrocnemius.[22]

Extensive data regarding the dose at which 50% of those exposed would develop various diseases, the so-called minimum infectious dose for 50% (MID50), were described in a U.S. investigator's report.[23] A determination of the MID50 was thought to be very important for the development of biological weapons. Japanese researchers infected humans to learn the MID50 of anthrax, plague, typhoid, paratyphoid A and B, dysentery, cholera, and glanders. Experiments were performed to determine the MID50 for a variety of pathogens that were introduced into humans subcutaneously, orally, and through respiration of infected air samples. Some of the infections were not fatal, but many of those exposed died.

Experiments with human captives also were performed at medical schools in Manchuria. Kameo Tasaki, a research associate of the Department of Dermatology and Urology of Manchuria Medical College, then the top medical school in Manchuria, described his "human experiment" of lymphogranuloma in a 1936 paper. Tasaki wrote that he injected emulsion of grated brain tissue of an infected mouse to the condemned "guerrilla's" prepuce. A papula grew at the focus, but the subject was executed two weeks after the injection.[24] Judging by other anatomical-anthropological studies, using "the condemned" for medical studies seems to have been a not uncommon practice in Manchuria.

Physiological studies. Hisato Yoshimura was a lecturer at Kyoto Imperial University Faculty of Medicine when his head professor ordered him to go to Unit 731 in 1938. He stayed there until

Unit 731 collapsed in 1945, and he used captives in studies of frostbite. At the Khabarovsk Trial, many officers and soldiers testified about the cruelty of Yoshimura's experiments. Satoru Kurakazu, a Sergeant Major of Military Police at Unit 731, testified:

I saw experiments performed on living people for the first time in December 1940. I was shown these experiments by researcher Yoshimura, a member of the 1st Division. These experiments were performed in the prison laboratory.

When I walked into the prison laboratory, five Chinese experimentees were sitting on a long form [bench]; two of these Chinese had no fingers at all, their hands were black; in those of three others the bones were visible. They had fingers, but they were only bones. Yoshimura told me that this was the result of freezing experiments.[1]

Naoji Uezono, who had worked for the Printer Division of Unit 731, described another grisly scene in an interview in the 1980s: "Two naked men were put in an area 40–50 degrees below zero and researchers filmed the whole process until they died. They suffered such agony they were digging their nails into each other's flesh."[2]

Yoshimura himself gave a lecture on his frostbite studies in Harbin in 1941, although he said nothing about cruel experiments.[25] After the war, he and his colleagues published three papers in Japanese medical journals—in English—reporting part of the studies.[26–28] We know that these papers concern their studies at Unit 731, because they themselves wrote that outlines of the papers were read at the 21st and 22nd annual meetings of Japanese Physiological Society in 1942–43. They wrote, "The experiments were made on about 100 male subjects (laboratory workers, students, soldiers and laborers)."[26] They explained their methods as follows:

To examine the temperature reaction of blood vessels to cold, the authors chose the tip of the left middle finger of humans as the site of examination, and the finger was dipped in ice water of 0°C up to its base for 30 minutes. The skin temperature of the back of its tip was then measured every one minute after immersion. To determine the skin temperature, a thermopile of Lewis' type made with copper and constantan wire of 0.02 mm. [sic] diameter was applied on the tip of the finger with adhesive plaster, and protected against water with vaseline. E.M.F. of the junction on the finger was measured potentiometrically against its cold junction in ice water. The water in which the finger is [sic] immersed was stirred frequently and the room temperature was usually maintained at about 20°C.[26]

Women, children, and even an infant were included in the experiments:

The temperature reaction in ice water was examined on about 100 Chinese coolies from 15 to 74 years old and on about 20 Chinese pupils of 7 to 14 years. . . . Though detailed studies could not be attained on children below 6 years of age, some observations were carried out on a baby. . . . [T]he reaction was detected even on the 3rd day after birth, and it increased rapidly with the lapse of days until at last it was nearly fixed after a month or so.

As to sexual difference of the reactivity, only an outlining aspect was obtained from the observation on Orochon subjects. . . . The reactivity of the female subject was a little lower than the male's in adult age, while they were nearly the same with each other in childhood.[27]

After the war, Yoshimura became a professor at Hyogo Prefectural School of Medicine and finally became president of Kyoto Prefectural University of Medicine. In 1978, Emperor Hirohito gave him the Order of the Rising Sun-Third Class for pioneering work in "environmental adaptation science."[2]

Frostbite experiments with Chinese captives were also performed elsewhere. Surgeon Major Kazuharu Tanimura of Datong Army Hospital organized a detachment and went on an expedition into Inner Mongolia from January 31 to February 11, 1941, to study frostbite, field surgeries, hemostatis, blood transfusion, and other procedures.[29] He took eight "living bodies"—male Chinese captives—as "material" for experiments. At dawn on February 6, researchers performed frostbite experiments on six people in various conditions such as wearing wet socks or gloves, drunk, hungry, and after administration of atropine. Their report, reprinted in 1995, describes the results precisely with sketches and photographs.[29] The eight captives were also used in other experiments and operations, and finally were shot or vivisected to death. The report includes the names of the subjects, direction for their confinement, a log of their killing, the program of their memorial service, and Tanimura's condolences.[29]

Sadao Koshi, a driver of Unit 731, described a shooting experiment performed in an airtight chamber designed to study gunshot wounds in low pressure conditions. When a fighter pilot was shot in a dogfight and parachuted at very high altitude, his wounds would gape in low pressure.[30]

According to the testimony at the Chinese investigation of Japanese war criminal Masauji Hata, Dr. Muto of Yoshimura's division performed a salt overdose experiment on a Chinese captive in January 1945 in order to confirm that salt increases basal metabolism.[7]

Yoshio Kurihara, an assistant in the Togo Unit at Beiyinhe from 1935 to 1936, described a torture test with distilled water:

> I was ordered to help civilian Dr. Satoshi Sugawara's experiment to learn how long man can live only on distilled water. The subject lived for 45 days with ordinary water and 33 days with distilled water. A subject forced to drink distilled water asked me, "Mister, please give me tasty water." The subject who lived for 45 days was a physician called Zuo Guangya, a very intelligent man, not a bandit.[31]

Yoshitoshi Omino, a corporal of the Shinkyo (now Changchun) Military Police, testified that Surgeon Captain Takeshi Ogasawara intravenously injected air into a Chinese worker arrested for alleged stealing. The subject did not seem to be harmed, but was decapitated with two other captives by Omino.[7] According to the testimony by an assistant, Yataro Ueda, doctors of Unit 731 seemed to know the lethal dose of an air injection.[10]

Anthropological-anatomical studies.   Doctors of the Department of Anatomy of Manchuria Medical College performed anthropological-anatomical studies with specimens of seemingly vivisected Chinese brain. According to an accusation by a Chinese assistant at the department, Zhang Buqing, vivisections were performed about five times from the autumn of 1942 to the spring of 1943. About 25 male captives were killed.[7] The doctors prepared many brain tissue specimens, which have been found in China

Medical University in Shengyang, which took over the facilities of Manchuria Medical College. Zhang concluded that vivisections had been performed because he saw fresh blood on the floor of the dissection room and the color of the corpses indicated that they had recently died.

The doctors published anatomical studies of the brain experiments with figures and photographs of these specimens in academic journals. For example, Naokiti Suzuki et al. wrote: "The present work on the cytoarchitectural structure of the regio frontalis was based upon the study of serial sections of the fresh human brains. Each of them was the brain of an adult Chinese man with no history of mental or physiological disease."[32] They then expressed their gratitude to army surgeons in a footnote: "We are greatly indebted to Surgeon-Colonel Dr. Kizima, the director of Mukden Garrison Hospital and Surgeon-Captain Dr. Watanabe who acted so kindly and satisfactily [*sic*] in performing the delicate operations desired."[32] These passages seem to confirm Zhang's accusation.

Development of Therapies

The second category of human experiments in Ishii's network was for development of therapies, including vaccines, surgical techniques both in hospital and on the battlefield, hemostasis, and transfusion of blood or its substitute.

Vaccine experiments.   Yoshio Shinozuka, a former junior assistant of Unit 731 whose birth name was Yoshio Tamura, wrote in 2004:

> Unit 731 was developing an envelope vaccine of plague . . . Karasawa Division, to which I belonged, also performed human experimentation and vivisection on five Chinese under the pretext of a virulence test of the germ. First we collected blood from them and measured their immunity. On the next day, we injected four kinds of plague vaccines to each of four subjects. No vaccine was given to one subject as control. A week later, vaccines were given again. A month later, we injected 1.0 cc liquid with the same number of plague germs in every subject. All five were infected with plague. . . . The man that had no vaccine was infected first. Two or three days later he became feverish and pale. On the next day he was dying and his face grew darker. He was still alive but the members of the Special Division, which administered the special prison of "Maruta" ["logs"] brought him naked on the stretcher to the dissection room where we awaited him. . . . Lieutenant Hosoda auscultated his heartbeat on his chest. At the moment the auscultation finished, Surgeon Colonel Ohyama ordered "Let's begin!"[33]

Shinozuka's superiors vivisected the subject and took organs as specimens. Shinozuka testifies that even his friend, junior assistant Mitsuo Hirakawa, was vivisected when infected with plague.[33]

Masauji Hata, who testified about the salt overdose experiment, also testified that in January 1945 Surgeon Major Masahiko Takahashi of the First Division of Unit 731 injected plague bacteria into three Chinese people and infected them with severe pneumonic and bubonic plague. Takahashi then tried to treat them with Japanese sulfa drug but failed. All of these subjects died.[7]

Toyonori Yamauchi, a researcher at Kanagawa Prefectural Hygiene Laboratory, and his superiors studied manufacturing vaccine with ultrasonic devices (vaccine made with virus attenuated by exposure to ultrasound). Their study drew Ishii's attention, and Ishii hired them in 1938. One of their papers was found in the journal of Ishii's headquarters.[34] Yamauchi and his superiors were sent to Unit 731 in June 1939, and performed cholera vaccine experiments on 20 Chinese captives in the special prison in May 1940. He was told that the subjects were "guerrillas convicted to death." Eight people were given vaccine made with ultrasonic devices, eight were given vaccine made at the Army Medical College, and four served as controls and received nothing. They were then forced to drink milk contaminated with cholera bacteria that had been developed as a weapon. The eight subjects who received ultrasound-attenuated vaccine did not become seriously ill, but those who received the other vaccine had severe diarrhea, and one of them died. All four controls died. Ishii ordered Yamauchi and his superiors to produce ultrasound-attenuated vaccine on a large scale.[7]

Medical orderly Furuichi of Unit 731 also testified at Khabarovsk about a typhus vaccine experiment:

[T]his was at the end of 1943. To test the effectiveness of vaccines 50 Chinese and Manchurians were used as experimental material. First these 50 men were given preventive inoculations, but these were differentiated inoculations—some prisoners were given one, others were given two. Furthermore, different men were inoculated with different quantities of vaccine, and some of these 50 men were not inoculated at all.

Thus, these 50 men were divided into five different groups. All these men were forced to drink water contaminated with typhoid germs and then observation was kept to see what effect these pathogenic germs had in the different cases, depending on whether preventive inoculations had been performed on the man or not, how many times, and in what quantities. . . . Most of these men contracted typhoid. Exactly what percentage I do not remember, at all events 12 or 13 of the men died. . . . I myself know of one other case of such infection, this was at the end of 1944 or beginning of 1945, when infection was caused by similar methods.[1]

Human vaccine experiments were also performed at Manchuria Medical College. Masaji Kitano, then a professor of microbiology at that College and later the Commander of Unit 731, and his colleagues wrote in an unpublished paper found in China after the war, "In Linjiang area we performed human experiments with 10 volunteers and 3 condemned. . . . They were healthy men of 32–74 years old with no anamnesis of typhus and other acute fever."[35] Kitano and his colleagues injected Typhus bacteria into 11 people who had been vaccinated and into two condemned without vaccination as controls. The condemned subjects both developed fever and were vivisected on the 11th and 19th day, respectively. Of the 11 who were vaccinated, five became feverish, and one was vivisected.

Surgical innovation.   Deadly experimental surgeries were performed on captives to develop new surgical methods, not to train beginning surgeons. At least two studies are documented. One set of experiments aimed at developing hospital techniques was performed on U.S. Army Air Force crews in mainland Japan. The other experiments, to develop field surgical procedures, were performed on Chinese captives in Inner Mongolia.

From May to June 1945, Professor Fukujiro Ishiyama of the First Department of Surgery, Apprentice Army Surgeon Taku Komori, and other Ishiyama subordinates performed experimental surgeries on eight U.S. crewmen at Kyushu Imperial University Faculty of Medicine. The American airmen were captured when their B-29s were downed. The Japanese Western District Army decided to execute them and handed them over to Komori and Ishiyama. On May 17, 1945, Ishiyama removed a lung from two POWs. On May 22, Ishiyama and his team performed total gastric resection and heart surgery on a POW, and removed the gall bladder and half of the liver of another POW. On May 25, they performed trigeminal rhizotomy (severing the facial nerve roots) on a POW. Finally, on June 2 Ishiyama performed surgery on the mediastinum and removed the gall bladder of two of three POWs. The last POW had a blood substitute transfusion later. All eight American POWs died during these operations.[5]

After the war, GHQ/SCAP brought this case to the military tribunal in Yokohama. Komori had already died; he had been badly injured in a U.S. air raid on Fukuoka in July 1945. Ishiyama hanged himself in prison in July 1946. On August 28, 1948, the Yokohama tribunal condemned two army officers and three university doctors to death by hanging, and sentenced another officer and two doctors to life imprisonment. Five other officers, eight doctors, and a head nurse were ordered to hard labor. However, their sentences were reduced in 1950 when the Korean War broke out and none among the convicted was executed.

Surgeon Major Kazuharu Tanimura and his colleagues experimented with field surgery during their expedition to Inner Mongolia. They wrote in their log that on February 4, 1941, they performed enteroanastomosis (intestinal bypass) on "living material No. 1." On the next day, "In order to follow up wounds, using living material No. 3, we amputated the left thigh, cut and sewed right thigh skin, and cut open the skin of the left hypogastrium. Treatments of dummy perforate gunshot wounds were performed on the left arm and right thigh of living material No. 7, and on the left waist and left chest of No. 6." On February 6, they shot No. 8 to make perforate wounds, then performed transfusion and tracheostomy on him.[29]

Hemostasis experiments.   Tanimura and his colleagues also performed hemostasis experiments to develop methods to save lives of bleeding soldiers on the battlefield. On February 5, they experimented on an arm wound on subject No. 6 and a thigh wound on subject No. 7. On February 6, they cut No. 5's arteries in the leg and performed hemostasis with clamps. On February 8, they performed various experiments with tourniquets on the same person.[29]

Transfusion experiments.   Tanimura's detachment performed various transfusion experiments, also to develop battlefield treatments. On February 5, 1941, they wrote that subjects No. 1 and No. 3 had transfusions of blood and Ringer solution at room temperature. On February 7 they transfused blood kept in a thermos bottle, blood that had been frozen and then thawed, and sheep blood. On February 8, they transfused blood taken from the heart of a corpse.[29]

At Unit 731, transfusion experiments with different blood groups were performed. Naeo Ikeda wrote:

In my experience, when A type blood 100 cc was transfused to an O type subject, whose pulse was 87 per minute and temperature was 35.4 degrees C, 30 minutes later the temperature rose to 38.6 degrees with slight trepidation. Sixty minutes later the pulse was 106 per minute and the temperature was

39.4 degrees. Two hours later the temperature was 37.7 degrees, and three hours later the subject recovered. When AB type blood 120 cc was transfused to an O type subject, an hour later the subject described malaise and psychroesthesia in both legs. When AB type blood 100 cc was transfused to a B type subject, there seemed to be no side effect.[36]

At Kyushu Imperial University Faculty of Medicine, sterilized and diluted brine was transfused into U.S. airmen as a blood substitute in the experimental operations described above. On May 17, 1945, Professor Ishiyama and his aides transfused 2,000 cc of blood substitute into the POW whose lung was removed. On June 2, they drew about 500 cc of blood from the right thigh artery of another POW and transfused 300 cc of blood substitute.[5]

Development of Biological and Chemical Weapons

The third research category related to weapons development. The aim of those engaged in this kind of research was to find ways to kill people more effectively and efficiently. Doctors in Ishii's medical network performed both biological and chemical weapon experiments on humans.

Biological weapon experiments.   U.S. investigator N. H. Fell described many biological weapon trials in his report. Regarding anthrax bomb trials he noted:

> In most cases the human subjects were tied to stakes and protected with helmets and body armor. The bombs of various types were exploded either statically, or with time fuses after being dropped from aircraft. . . . The Japanese were not satisfied with the field trials with anthrax. However, in one trial with 15 subjects, 8 were killed as a result of wounds from the bombs, and 4 were infected by bomb fragments (3 of these 4 subjects died). In another trial with a more efficient bomb ("Uji"), 6 of 10 subjects developed a definite bacteremia, and 4 of these were considered to have been infected by the respiratory route; all four of these latter subjects died. However, these four subjects were only 25 meters from the nearest of the 9 bombs that were exploded in a volley.[23]

Fell's description corresponds with testimony by Japanese officers and soldiers at the Khabarovsk Trial and the Chinese investigation. For example, Surgeon Major Tomio Karasawa, who was the chief of the Production Division of Unit 731, testified at Khabarovsk:

> I was present on two occasions at experiments in infecting people under field conditions at the Anta [sic] Station proving ground. The first experiment was made towards the end of 1943 with anthrax bacteria. Ten persons were used for these experiments. They were brought to the proving ground and tied to stakes five metres apart from one another. A fragmentation bomb was used for the purpose, placed 50 metres from the people to be infected. The bomb was exploded by electric current. Some of the experimentees were infected as a result of these experiments. They were given certain treatments and then sent back to the detachment. I later learned from the report that the persons who had got infected with anthrax subsequently died.[1]

Surgeon Major Hideo Sakakibara, who was the Chief of Linkou Branch of Unit 731, testified at the Chinese investigation that he took part in a similar anthrax experiment at the Anda Proving Ground.[10] Masauji Hata of Unit 731 testified that he saw a film that recorded this kind of experiment.[7]

Fell reported the following about plague trials:

> d. Bomb trials
> A summary of 3 or 4 of the best trials is given below (in these trials the concentration of bacilli on the ground around the subjects was measured with plates). . . . The conclusions from all the bomb trials was that plague [bacilli] were not a satisfactory B.W. weapon due to their instability but that it was much more practical to spread plague by means of fleas.

> e. Spraying experiments
> The results indicated that this method was highly effective, both with subjects held within a room and also exposed to bacilli spread from aircraft at low altitudes. 50–100 per cent of the subjects used in various trials became infected and the mortality was at least 60 per cent.

> f. Stability
> No success was attained in stabilizing plague bacilli either in suspensions or by drying.

> g. Infected fleas
> . . . It was found that infected fleas survived for about 30 days under the best conditions and were infective for that length of time. It was also found that one flea bite per person usually caused infection. It was also found that if subjects moved freely around a room containing a concentration of 20 fleas per square meter, 6 of 10 subjects became infected and of these 4 died. Bomb trials were carried out using the "UJI" porcelain bomb with primacord explosive. The fleas were mixed with sand before being filled into the bomb. About 50 per cent of the fleas survived the explosion which was carried out in a 10 meter square chamber with 10 subjects. 8 of the 10 subjects received flea bites and became infected and 6 of the 8 died.[23]

Surgeon Major General Kiyoshi Kawashima of Unit 731 testified at Khabarovsk about an experiment in the summer of 1941:

> The persons used for these experiments, fifteen in number, were brought from the detachment's inner prison to the experimental ground and tied to stakes which had been driven into the ground for the purpose. Flags and smoke signals were used to guide the planes and enable them to find the proving ground easily. A special plane took off from Pingfan [sic] Station, and when it was over the site it dropped about two dozen bombs, which burst at about 100 or 200 metres from the ground, releasing the plague fleas with which they were charged. The plague fleas dispersed all over the territory.
> A long interval was allowed to pass after the bombs had been dropped in order that the fleas might spread and infect the experimentees. These people were then disinfected and taken back by plane to the inner prison at Pingfan Station, where observation was established over them to ascertain whether they had been infected with plague.[1]

Fell also reported a trial of spreading glanders by bombing: "Only one trial was conducted using 10 human subjects and 10 horses. Three of the horses and one of the men became infected, but there are no data on cloud concentration or density of the organisms on the ground."[23]

Surgeon Lieutenant Colonel Toshihide Nishi, who was the chief of the Training and Education Division of Unit 731, testified at the Khabarovsk Trial about gas gangrene bomb experiments in Anda:

In January 1945, by order of the Chief of Detachment 731, I went to Anta [sic] Station. There I saw experiments in inducing gas gangrene, conducted under the direction of the chief of the 2nd Division, Ikari, and the researcher Futaki. Ten prisoners were used for the purpose. They were tied [to] facing stakes, five to ten metres apart from one another. The prisoners' heads were covered with metal helmets, and their bodies with screens.

Each man's body was fully protected, only the naked buttocks being exposed. At about 100 metres away a fragmentation bomb was exploded by electricity, this being the means of causing the infection. All ten men were wounded in the exposed part. The experiment over, the ten men were put in a special automobile and sent back to the prison at Pingfan Station. I later asked Ikari and researcher Futaki what the results had been. They told me that all ten men had been injured and died of gas gangrene.[1]

Chemical weapon experiments.   A report authored by unknown researcher in the Kamo Unit (Unit 731) describes a large human experiment of yperite gas (mustard gas) on September 7–10, 1940. Twenty subjects were divided into three groups and placed in combat emplacements, trenches, gazebos, and observatories. One group was clothed with Chinese underwear, no hat, and no mask, and was subjected to as much as 1,800 field gun rounds of yperite gas over 25 minutes. Another group was clothed in summer military uniform and shoes; three had masks and another three had no mask. They also were exposed to as much as 1,800 rounds of yperite gas. A third group was clothed in summer military uniform, three with masks and two without masks, and were exposed to as much as 4,800 rounds. Then their general symptoms and damage to skin, eye, respiratory organs, and digestive organs were observed at 4 hours, 24 hours, and 2, 3, and 5 days after the shots. Injecting the blister fluid from one subject into another subject and analyses of blood and soil were also performed. Five subjects were forced to drink a solution of yperite and lewisite gas in water, with or without decontamination. The report describes conditions of every subject precisely without mentioning what happened to them in the long run.[37]

There are other documents describing similar chemical weapon experiments. In his log of April 21, 1939, Surgeon Colonel Setsuzo Kinbara wrote about a "Report of Special Tests in Manchuria" that was presented at the Department of Army by Surgeon Lieutenant Colonel Kondo of the Army Science Institute. These "tests" seem to have been performed jointly by the Army Science Institute, the Kwantung Army Chemical Department, and Unit 731. Kondo reported results as follows. About cyanide fume, he noted that "subjects became unconscious in 4–6 minutes. Since the results of human being and guinea pig are the same, we can bring latter."[38] About yperite and lewisite, he wrote that "treatments are effective if done in 30 seconds. Direct disinfection causes heat and burn."[38]

Similarly, on November 19, 1942, Lieutenant Colonel Kumao Imoto wrote in his log about "A Study of 'Cha' "—meaning cyanide gas. Imoto wrote, "50 kg blow guns were placed at 25 m intervals for 1000 m in width. When a total of 17.5 tons of cyanide fume was blown from these guns and covered the area of 4 km in depth, death rate of the subjects placed at 2 km away from the guns was 100%, while that at 4 km away was 50%. With a density of 1500 mg/m^3, subjects died within two minutes."[39]

Williams and Wallace report this description of a cyanide bomb experiment by an anonymous researcher of Unit 731 Dalian Branch:

They used a gas bomb newly developed by Unit 516 for human experiments conducted at Hailar. Nearly 100 marutas [subjects] were used and, except one, all of them were killed. Their bodies were carried by truck, ten or twenty at a time, and transported to Haruarushan where tents had been erected for a pathologist to carry out a pathological autopsy. I wasn't involved in the dissection. The person who actually did the dissection was Dr. Okamoto. I had to wait outside the tent to obtain the blood that had been recovered from various organs of the autopsies and placed in tubes, and took these to the military hospital in Hailar. There I checked the contents of cyanide in the blood. That was my job.[2]

At the Khabarovsk trial, Senior Sergeant Kazuo Mitomo of Unit 100 described poison experiments in which he helped researcher Tsunetaka Matsui:

Experiments on human beings were performed in August–September 1944. These experiments took the form of giving experimentees, without their knowledge, soporific drugs and poisons. The experimentees included 7–8 Russians and Chinese. Korean bindweed, heroin and castor-oil seed were among the poisons used in the experiments. These poisons were put in the food.

The poisoned food was given to the experimentees five or six times over a period of two weeks. Korean bindweed was used mostly in soups, I think heroin in porridge, while tobacco was mixed with heroin and bactal. After eating the soup mixed with Korean bindweed the experimentees dropped off into a deep five-hour sleep 30 minutes or an hour later. After two weeks the experimentees were so weak that they could no longer be used. . . .

For purposes of secrecy all the experimentees were put to death. . . . There was the case of a Russian experimentee who, on the orders of Matsui, a researcher, was put to death with an injection of one-tenth of a gram of potassium cyanide. . . . I made the injection of potassium cyanide. . . . I dissected the body at the detachment's cattle cemetery.[1]

Poison experiments were also performed at other EPWSDs. Engineer Major Shigeo Ban of the Army 9th Technology Institute (Noborito Institute) confessed to performing poison experiments at Unit 1644 in Nanjing. Early in May 1941, the Army General Staff Corps ordered Ban and his eight colleagues to visit Unit 1644 to test the toxicity of a newly developed poison, acetone cyanhydrin, in humans. In 1993, Ban wrote:

Director Shinoda of Noborito Institute met Commander Shiro Ishii of Unit 731 at the General Staff Corps and asked for cooperation with this experiment. Ishii freely agreed. Unit 731 was established as the Japanese Army's secret biological warfare unit, but in its pharmacological division cyanide compounds were also studied. . . . According to the program, the experiment would continue for about a week, the experimenter would be an army surgeon of Unit 1644, and researchers of Noborito Institute would support him. The subjects were captive soldiers of Chinese Army or the condemned for general crimes. The number of the subjects was about fifteen. . . .

The aims of the experiment were to determine lethal dose of acetone cyanhydrin, to observe symptoms, and to compare it with potassium cyanide. The results of deglutition and injection experiments demonstrated that, as had been predicted, both forms of cyanide made almost the same progress from administration to death and showed almost the same effects at dissection. Injection was most effective, hypodermic injection was enough.

The lethal dose of acetone cyanhydrin was about 1 cc (1 g), whose effect appeared in a few minutes and led to death in 30 minutes. But it depends on constitution, sex, and age, in some cases it took from several to more than ten hours to die. We could not determine it precisely. Anyway, acetone cyanhydrin begins to take effect in seconds, though it takes a little more time than potassium cyanide.[40]

These passages show that the Ishii medical network had close connections with other science and technology institutes, and that the Army used Ishii's EPWSDs as laboratories for human experimentation.

Ban, who died soon after writing these passages in November 1993 at the age of 87, expressed deep remorse about this experiment:

Even though it was on captive soldiers and the condemned, inhumane and horrible human experimentation was performed. Belonging to the dark side of wartime, this fact has been passed over in silence. But now I want to disclose it. By revealing this historic fact now I want to offer my sincerest prayer for the repose of their soul and for world peace.[40]

Cover-Up

Ishii's medical network suddenly collapsed in August 1945 when the Soviet Union declared war on Japan and advanced into Manchuria. The Japanese Army immediately decided to withdraw all human experimentation units from China and to destroy evidence of medical atrocities. At Unit 731, all the surviving captives were killed, cremated, and cast into the Songhuajiang River. The main building with its special prisons was totally destroyed by artillery. Its surgeon officers, researchers, workers, and soldiers were hurriedly evacuated in specially chartered trains and ships. Most succeeded in escaping and returned to Japan. In Tokyo, the Epidemic Prevention Laboratory, headquarters of Ishii's network, had already been destroyed by U.S. air raids in March and May of 1945. But Ishii and his colleagues held onto their biological warfare data.

Although the United States occupied Japan after Japan's surrender on August 15, 1945, General Headquarters/Supreme Command for the Allied Powers (GHQ/SCAP) did not investigate medical crimes. Instead, investigators from the U.S. Army Chemical Corps in Camp Detrick, Maryland, which oversaw U.S. chemical and biological warfare efforts, sought the biological warfare data that Ishii and his colleagues had accumulated—so

that the United States could catch up with the Soviet Union and other countries in biowar research and development.[3,31,41,42] The Soviets had begun research in biological warfare in 1928, but the United States had not started it until 1942. The Cold War had already begun to emerge, and U.S. officials were under pressure to surpass Soviet capabilities in all fields.

In return for the Japanese data, Lieutenant Colonel Murray Sanders, the first Chemical Corps investigator, asked General Douglas MacArthur and General Charles Willoughby, a close MacArthur aide, to promise Ishii and his researchers immunity from war crimes charges in September 1945. Ishii and his colleagues gave up some data, but they concealed from Sanders and his successor, Lieutenant Colonel Arvo T. Thompson, that the data were from experiments with humans. The United States did not obtain evidence of deadly human experiments until 1947.

Early in January 1947, the Soviet Union sought the extradition of Ishii and his researchers for investigation of their experiments, which the Soviets had learned about from captured officers and soldiers of Ishii's network. The Soviets also wanted the biowar data and threatened to reveal the Japanese medical atrocities at the International Military Tribunal for the Far East—the Tokyo Tribunal, which conducted the war crimes trial of top Japanese leaders from 1946 to 1948—if the United States did not share the information. United States officials dismissed this threat—the United States controlled the Tokyo Tribunal—but then began to investigate the Japanese researchers more closely.

At this point, U.S. officials recognized that human experiments had occurred, and the immunity that they had granted to Ishii and others now became a problem. In Nuremberg, the United States was prosecuting Nazi doctors for their human experiments (see Chapters 2 and 12). MacArthur's headquarters discussed the dilemma repeatedly with officials in Washington, and an interagency task force in the U.S. capital finally concluded:

Information of Japanese BW [biological warfare] experiments will be of great value to the U.S. research program. . . . The value to the U.S. of Japanese BW data is of such importance to national security as to far outweigh the value accruing from "war crimes" prosecution. . . . The BW information obtained from Japanese sources should be retained in Intelligence channels and should not be employed as "war crimes" evidence.[43]

This conclusion was based on close examination of the data that was finally provided by Ishii and his colleagues. The last investigator, Edwin V. Hill, reported to the chief of the U.S. Army Chemical Corps:

Evidence gathered in this investigation has greatly supplemented and amplified previous aspects of this field. It represents data which have been obtained by Japanese scientists at the expenditure of many millions of dollars and years of work. Information has accrued with respect to human susceptibility to these diseases as indicated by specific infectious doses of bacteria. Such information could not be obtained in our own laboratories because of scruples attached to human experimentation. These data were secured with a total outlay of ¥250,000 to date, a mere pittance by comparison with the actual cost of the studies.[44]

Who in the United States ultimately made the decision on immunity from war crimes prosecution? The fact that the

State-War-Navy Coordinating Subcommittee to the Far East approved immunity indicates that both the armed forces and the Department of State were involved. But no documents have been found that determine how much President Harry S. Truman knew about the medical atrocities.

Most officers and researchers involved in Japan's human experimentation program, including Ishii himself, never faced war crimes charges. Ishii died of laryngeal cancer in 1959, at the age of 67. Many army surgeon officers and researchers gained positions in medical schools, national institutes, or hospitals. Some practiced in their own clinics; some others established pharmaceutical companies.[2]

Although failing to get custody of Ishii or access to his data, the Soviet Union brought 12 captured officers and soldiers to trial before an open military tribunal at Khabarovsk in December 1949, commonly called the Khabarovsk Trial.[1] The accused included the Captain General of the Kwantung Army, Otozo Yamada, six army surgeon officers, and two veterinarian officers. Six of the accused were from Unit 731 and two from Unit 100. They were all sentenced to confinement in a labor correction camp for sentences that ranged from 2 to 25 years, but they returned to Japan by 1956 when the Soviet Union and Japan resumed diplomatic relations.

The Soviets had intended to spread the news of the medical atrocities worldwide, but because the prosecutors, lawyers, and judges were all Russian, and there were no reporters from abroad, the proceedings drew little attention. The United States succeeded in branding the trial as communist propaganda.

The People's Republic of China also tried Japanese war criminals before military tribunals in 1956, but only one surgeon officer of Ishii's network was included. None of these defendants received a death sentence, and all returned to Japan by 1964.

Causes

Racism, ethnic prejudice, anticommunism, and lack of respect for individual rights are often blamed for creating the atmosphere in which such human experimentation could take place. But there were other causes, too.

First, Imperial Japan had become more and more dominated by the military in the 1930s. As the invasion of China grew wider and deeper, militarism became more powerful in the Japanese parliament, known as the Diet. For example, the National Mobilization Law in 1938 enabled the government to call out any resources necessary for operations without the Diet's permission. Because the Emperor officially commanded the Imperial Japanese Armed Forces, army leaders claimed to be acting with the authority of the Emperor even when they really were operating on the basis of their own judgment. In these circumstances, army surgeons might gradually have convinced themselves that everything was justifiable when it was done for the sake of the country and the Emperor.

Second, Japanese military rule in China was known to be very cruel. Chinese people who were forced to work in Japanese factories were treated violently and often killed. The murders during the experiments were only one part of a huge massacre by the Japanese army. Doctors in Ishii's network might have gotten used to treating foreigners harshly, too.

Third, because human experimentation was performed strictly behind closed doors, researchers might have lost a common sense of humanity. The Imperial Japanese Government was in part afraid of severe international condemnation if such atrocities became widely known overseas. Therefore, the fact of deadly human experimentation was treated as the "secret of secrets." The existence of the laboratories was completely hidden from the public, making it possible for researchers to ignore the constraints of medical ethics.

Most of the doctors who performed the deadly experiments were academic researchers who had already been professors at leading medical schools. They were temporarily employed by the army. Why did they join Ishii's network? Was it impossible to avoid participation?

In Imperial Japan, pressure for their participation was high. As militarism grew powerful, cooperation with the military was common. Researchers would be considered traitors ("Hikokumin") if they refused to participate. Most accepted their fate without trying to resist, even when they knew what they would be assigned to do. Former Army Surgeon Ken Yuasa, who performed deadly surgical training at Luan Army Hospital, recalls the moment when he was ordered to perform a vivisection:

> When I was told that, I felt tense and thought, "Ah, this is it." It was whispered among students in my schooldays at Jikeikai Medical University that an army surgeon sent to China risked having to perform vivisection. Students knew that most of those who became army surgeons and went to China did it. Since I became an army surgeon, I recognized that I couldn't escape from it.[6]

In addition, many researchers were ordered to go to China by their academic superiors. In Japanese medical schools, even now, head professors exercise supreme power over their staffs. Usually, there is only one professor in each "Ikyoku"—roughly speaking, a department, but with much more authority than university departments in most countries. The Ikyoku system is unique to the Japanese medical profession. The Ikyoku functions as an office of clinical practice, a faculty for graduate education, and a research laboratory. Even after earning a doctoral degree, researchers devote themselves to the Ikyoku, hoping to be nominated by the head professor as his successor. They cannot oppose their professor because refusal to follow the professor's order (for example, to go to a certain facility) would result in their excommunication from the Ikyoku and the destruction of their academic careers.

With research facilities and funding in short supply, head professors were willing to cooperate with the army and Ishii. They promised to send their best disciples to Ishii's factories; in return, the army supplied research equipment to the professors. The medical atrocities would have been impossible without the support of the leading medical professors. Therefore, not only the army but also the Japanese medical profession was guilty of the crimes.

But some researchers assigned to Unit 731 seemed to hate being there and strenuously asked their head professors for another position in Japan. In some cases, the professors accepted such appeals, probably because they valued their disciples' talents. Thus, a head professor's order seems to have been sufficient reason to go to the Ishii network, but not necessarily a strong enough reason to stay over the long term.

However, Ishii's facilities were luxurious places for the researchers. For example, the annual budget of Unit 731 was 10 million yen—equal to about 9 billion yen in modern currency

($80 million U.S.). Half of this budget was for research, and the other half was for labor costs for about 3,000 employees.[1] The salaries were high, and the food served there was wonderful. In fact the laboratories of Unit 731 were among the most luxurious in the Japanese Empire.

Moreover, researchers in Ishii's network could study diseases that were hardly ever observed in the Japanese homeland—such as epidemic hemorrhagic fever, plague, typhus, and severe frost-bite. The researchers could thus produce brilliant scientific achievements. That's why they could gain good positions in the Japanese medical establishment after the war.

Enduring Legacy

In cooperation with the United States, Japan hid the medical atrocities from both the international and domestic public for decades. Testimony from the Khabarovsk trial was regarded as false communist propaganda. Researchers who confessed to conducting such experiments in China were considered to have been brainwashed. But in 1981, popular writer Seiichi Morimura published a bestselling book about Unit 731 that included testimony by many of its anonymous soldiers.[45] In the same year, historian Keiichi Tsuneishi published his first extensive study of Unit 731.[18] Because of this, these atrocities became widely known in Japan, and historical studies have advanced greatly since then as significant documents have been found in Japan, the United States, China, and the former Soviet Union.

Outside Japan, the Imperial Japanese medical atrocities did not become widely known until even later. In Britain and the United States, the first comprehensive book in English was published at the end of the 1980s[2] and another essential study was published in the mid-1990s.[3] Even in China, there was little modern research into the human experiments before the testimony of Japanese war criminals was published in 1989.[7]

Today, more than 60 years after the end of World War II, the U.S. government is no longer closing its eyes to the record of human experimentation. The government has refused to allow former employees of Unit 731 into the country on the ground that they are war criminals. In 1998, Yoshio Shinozuka was denied entry, and deported to Japan from Chicago's O'Hare International Airport, even though he had been invited to the country and intended to confess his Unit 731 crimes in public symposia. This attitude is hypocritical because the U.S. government must share in the responsibility for keeping these experiments secret because of its immunity deals with the researchers.

On the other hand, the Japanese government is still keeping silent on this issue. It acknowledged in the Diet in 1982 that Unit 731 surely existed, but has never explained what was done there. The government and conservative nationalists in Japan are still hiding the historical truth. Moreover, it seems they wish the truth would be forgotten. One of the most enduring legacies of these experiments is therefore the silence that continues to surround them.

Within the Japanese medical profession, the subject of *Jintai Jikken* (human experimentation) became taboo after the end of World War II. Many of the researchers who performed these experiments became prominent figures in academia. If junior researchers speak of human experimentation, they might touch on their head professors' "secret of secrets" and wreck their own academic careers. Therefore, not only Ishii's researchers themselves but also their disciples have hardly mentioned this issue publicly.

On the other hand, most of the public has thought it unnecessary to discuss human experimentation seriously. Because the Japanese and U.S. governments have been fairly successful in covering up the experiments, even today most people find it hard to believe that medical doctors, who devote themselves to saving lives, really treated human beings like guinea pigs. Those who found the Khabarovsk trial to be credible and who appealed for public inquiry were often sneered at.

This failure to examine history publicly permits most Japanese citizens to regard human experimentation as a barbarism performed by mad doctors—totally different from typical medical procedures carried out by normal doctors. As a matter of fact, many cases of abuse of humans in research have been reported in newspapers, journals, and TV in postwar Japan.[46] However, these were presumed to be exceptional deviations. The Japanese public has avoided reflection on human experimentation in both military and civil medicine.

These circumstances are reflected in the field of medical ethics. The failure to confront reality means that Japanese medical ethics lack a framework for critically discussing and evaluating human experimentation. Medical ethicists have seldom tried to draw from historical cases of abuse the guiding principles that should regulate medical research. There has been little discussion, publication, or teaching about protection of humans in research. Even in postwar cases of abuse, journalists and ethicists have focused discussion on a case-by-case basis and failed to derive general principles. Consequently, politicians have never proposed a blanket law to govern medical research, and the government has never articulated a general policy for the protection of humans in research. So far, Japanese guidelines for medical research are only patchworks of articles transferred from international guidelines such as the Declaration of Helsinki. They have not been derived from the lessons of history, especially of the past medical massacre performed by our own doctors.

This is a poor ethical state for a country boasting of its economic development and trying to lead world medical science. Looking into and evaluating one's own past is one of the prime imperatives of ethics. In order to be acknowledged as an ethical country, Japan must admit its past deeds, inquire into the truth, apologize to and compensate the victims for their suffering. This will surely lead to the establishment of true clinical research ethics in Japan.

Note on Translation of Sources

In this chapter, Japanese names are written in Western form, given name first and family name last. In many East Asian languages, including Japanese and Chinese, names are spoken and written in the opposite order, family name first and given name last. Some Western publications and references follow the Eastern style. All quotations from Japanese documents in this chapter were translated into English by the author.

Acknowledgments

A draft of this chapter was read at the symposium "Japanese Human Experimentation in Wartime China: Inquiries into its

Historical, Political, Cultural and Ethical Issues," at the 22nd International Congress of History of Science in Beijing, China, on July 29, 2005. I am grateful to its participants for valuable comments. I also greatly thank the editors of this volume for advice on improving the chapter.

References

1. *Materials on the Trial of Former Servicemen of the Japanese Army Charged with Manufacturing and Employing Bacteriological Weapons.* Moscow, U.S.S.R.: Foreign Languages Publishing House; 1950.

2. Williams P, Wallace D. *Unit 731: Japan's Secret Biological Warfare in World War II.* New York, N.Y.: The Free Press; 1989.

3. Harris SH. *Factories of Death: Japanese Biological Warfare, 1932–45, and the American Cover-Up,* revised ed. New York, N.Y.: Routledge; 2002 [1994].

4. Tanaka Y. *Hidden Horrors: Japanese War Crimes in World War II.* Boulder, Colo.: Westview Press; 1996.

5. Supreme Command for the Allied Powers (SCAP): Legal Section: ADM. DIV. MISC. File. Trial Case #394: Record of Trial in the Case of *United States v. Kajuro Aihara.* 1940–1948. NARA, Record Group 331, Stack Area 290, Row 11, Compartment 34, Shelf 4, Boxes 1331–1332.

6. Yoshikai N. *Kesenai Kioku: Yuasa Gun'i Seitaikaibo no Kiroku [Unforgettable Memory: A Document of Army Surgeon Yuasa's Vivisection],* expanded ed. Tokyo, Japan: Nitchu Shuppan; 1996 [1981].

7. Chinese Central Archive et al., eds. *Seitai Kaibo [Vivisection], Jintai Jikken [Human Experimentation],* and *Saikin Sakusen [Germ Warfare].* Tokyo, Japan: Dobunkan, 1991–1992. (These three volumes are a Japanese translation of *Xijunzhan yu Duqizhan [Biological and Chemical Warfare].* Beijing, China: Zhonghua Shuju [Chinese Printing Office], 1989.)

8. Daido Rikugun Byoin [Datong Army Hospital]. Chumogun Gun'i Shoko Rikugun Gekagaku Syugo Kyoiku Katei Hyo [A Program of a Group Education of Military Surgery for Army Surgeon Officers of the Occupation Forces in Mongolia]. In: Toki Eisei Kenkyuhan [The Detachment for Hygiene Studies in Winter]. *Chumougun Toki Eisei Kenkyu Seiseki [The Report of Hygiene Studies in Winter by the Occupation Forces in Mongolia],* March, 1941. Tokyo, Japan: Gendai Syokan; 1995:Appendix.

9. Tsuneishi K. *Hone Wa Kokuhatsu Suru [The Bones Are Accusing].* Tokyo, Japan: Kaimeisha; 1992.

10. Takidani J. *Satsuriku Kosho—731 Butai [Murderous Factory Unit 731].* Tokyo, Japan: Niimori Shobo; 1989.

11. 731 Kenkyukai [Society for Investigation of Unit 731], eds. *Saikinsen Butai [Germ Warfare Units].* Tokyo, Japan: Bansei Sha; 1996. See esp. pp. 64–67.

12. Imoto K. Gyomu Nisshi [Operation Log], Vol. 9. Collection of the Military Archives, Japan Defense Agency, 23 vols., circa Sept. 1940–Dec. 1942. Cited in: Yoshimi Y, Iko T. Nihon No Saikinsen (Japanese Biological Warfare). *Senso Sekinin Kenkyu (Studies in Responsibility for War)* December 1993;2:8–29.

13. Imoto K. Gyomu Nisshi [Operation Log], Vol. 10. Collection of the Military Archives, Japan Defense Agency, 23 vols., circa Sept. 1940–Dec. 1942. Cited in: Yoshimi Y, Iko T. Nihon No Saikinsen (Japanese Biological Warfare). *Senso Sekinin Kenkyu (Studies in Responsibility for War)* December 1993;2:8–29.

14. Imoto K. Gyomu Nisshi [Operation Log], Vol. 13. Collection of the Military Archives, Japan Defense Agency, 23 vols., circa Sept. 1940–Dec. 1942. Cited in: Yoshimi Y, Iko T. Nihon No Saikinsen (Japanese Biological Warfare). *Senso Sekinin Kenkyu (Studies in Responsibility for War)* December 1993;2:8–29.

15. Imoto K. Gyomu Nisshi [Operation Log], Vol. 14. Collection of the Military Archives, Japan Defense Agency, 23 vols., circa Sept. 1940–Dec. 1942. Cited in: Yoshimi Y, Iko T. Nihon No Saikinsen (Japanese

16. Imoto K. Gyomu Nisshi [Operation Log], Vol. 19. Collection of the Military Archives, Japan Defense Agency, 23 vols., circa Sept. 1940–Dec. 1942. Cited in: Yoshimi Y, Iko T. Nihon No Saikinsen (Japanese Biological Warfare). *Senso Sekinin Kenkyu (Studies in Responsibility for War)* December 1993;2:8–29.

17. Kasahara S, Kitano M, et al. Ryukosei Syukketsunetsu no Byogentai no Kettei [Identification of the pathogen of epidemic hemorrhagic fever]. *Nihon Byori Gakkai Kaishi [Japanese Journal of Pathology]* 1944;34(1–2):3–5, esp. 3.

18. Tsuneishi K. *Kieta Saikinsen Butai [The Germ Warfare Unit That Disappeared],* expanded ed. Tokyo, Japan: Kaimeisha; 1989 [1981].

19. Ikeda N. Ryukosei Syukketsunetsu no Ryukogakuteki Chosa Kenkyu [Epidemiological studies of epidemic hemorrhagic fever]. *Nihon Densenbyo Gakkai Zasshi [The Journal of the Japanese Association for Infectious Diseases]* 1967;41(9):337–47.

20. Ikeda N. Ryukosei Syukketsunetsu no Shirami, Nomi ni yoru Kansen Jikken [Experimental studies of epidemic hemorrhagic fever: Pediculus vestimenti and Xenopsylla chepis as suspected vectors of the disease]. *Nihon Densenbyo Gakkai Zasshi [The Journal of the Japanese Association for Infectious Diseases]* 1968;42(5):125–30.

21. Asano T, Tsuneishi K. *Kibyo—Ryukosei Syukketsunetsu [Weird Disease—Epidemic Hemorrhagic Fever].* Tokyo, Japan: Shincho Sha; 1985. See esp. p. 96.

22. Ikeda N, Araki S. Hashofu Dokuso narabini Gaho Sesshuji ni okeru Kin Chronaxie ni tsuite [Muscle chronaxie of patients injected with toxin and spore of tetanus]. Date unknown. In: Tanaka A, Matsumura T, eds. *731 Butai Sakusei Shiryo [Documents Made by Unit 731].* Tokyo, Japan: Fuji Shuppan; 1991:45–57, esp. 52.

23. Fell NH. Brief summary of new information about Japanese B. W. activities. HHF/ars/3, 20 June 1947. Dugway, Utah: Dugway Proving Ground, File No. 005. In: Kondo S, ed. *731 Butai Saikinsen Shiryo Shusei [Japanese Biological Warfare; Unit 731: Official Declassified Records].* CD-ROM, 8 Discs. Tokyo, Japan: Kashiwa Shobo; 2003:Disc 3.

24. Tasaki K. Sokei Rimpa Nikugasyu Sho ("N. F." Byo) no Kenkyu, Dai 1 Hou [A study of lympho granuloma ("N.F. disease"), Part 1]. *Manshu Igaku Zasshi [Manchuria Medical Journal]* 1936;24:785–804, esp. 790.

25. Yoshimura H. Tosho ni Tsuite [On frostbite]. Manuscript of the special lecture at the 15th Meeting of the Harbin Branch of Manchu Medical Society, October 26, 1941. In: Tanaka A, Matsumura T, eds. *731 Butai Sakusei Shiryo [Documents Made by Unit 731].* Tokyo, Japan: Fuji Shuppan; 1991:225–88.

26. Yoshimura H, Iida T. Studies on the reactivity of skin vessels to extreme cold. Part 1. A point test on the resistance against frost bite. *The Japanese Journal of Physiology* 1950–1951;1:147–59.

27. Yoshimura H, Iida T. Studies on the reactivity of skin vessels to extreme cold. Part 2. Factors governing the individual difference of the reactivity, or the resistance against frost bite. *The Japanese Journal of Physiology* 1951–1952;2:177–85.

28. Yoshimura H, Iida T, Koishi H. Studies on the reactivity of skin vessels to extreme cold. Part 3. Effects of diets on the reactivity of skin vessels to cold. *The Japanese Journal of Physiology* 1951–1952;2:310–15.

29. Toki Eisei Kenkyuhan [The Detachment for Hygiene Studies in Winter]. *Chumougun Toki Eisei Kenkyu Seiseki [The Report of Hygiene Studies in Winter by the Occupation Forces in Mongolia],* March 1941. Tokyo, Japan: Gendai Syokan; 1995.

30. Takasugi S. *Nippon no Auschwitz wo Otte [Searching for the Japanese Auschwitz].* Tokyo, Japan: Kyoiku Shiryo Shuppankai; 1984.

31. Tsuneishi K. *Igakusha Tachi no Soshiki Hanzai [The Conspiracy of Medical Researchers].* Tokyo, Japan: Asahi Shimbun Sha; 1994.

32. Suzuki N, Terui S, Takenaka Y, Ohno K, Juh S. Histological study of the Chinese brain. Part 1. On the cytoarchitectural structure of the regio frontalis. *Arbeiten aus dem Anatomischen Institut der Kaiserlich-Japanishen Universtitat zu Sendai* 1942;25:139–86.

33. Shinozuka Y, Takayanagi M. *Nihon nimo Senso ga Atta: 731 Butai Moto Shonen Taiin no Kokuhaku* [*There Was a War in Japan: A Confession of a Former Junior Assistant of Unit 731*]. Tokyo, Japan: Shin Nihon Shuppansha; 2004.

34. Watanabe H, et al. Cho-onpa Cholera Yobosesshueki no Jintai Sesshugo ni okeru Kakushu Shojo oyobi Kesseigakuteki Hanno ni tsuite [On various symptoms and serologic reactions of injection of ultrasonic cholera vaccine to human body]. *Rikugun Gun'i Gakko Boeki Kenkyu Hokoku* [*Bulletin of the Epidemic Prevention Laboratory in the Army Medical College*] 1939; 2(36):1–16.

35. Kitano M, Iwata S, Watanabe S. Hasshin Typhus no Yobosesshu ni kansuru Kenkyu: Yo ra no Chosei seru Hasshin Typhus Vaccine no Jintai Kansen Bogyoryoku Shiken [A Study of Vaccination of Typhus: On An Immunity Test of Our Typhus Vaccine]. Unpublished. Abridged Chinese translation in: Yang Y, Xin P, eds. *Xijunzhan* [*Biological Warfare*]. Harbin, China: Heilongjiangxing Renmin Chubanshe [Heilongjiang People's Press]; 2002:333–46.

36. Ikeda N. Ketsuekigata no Futekigo Yuketsu no Kiken [Risk of Different Blood Type Transfusion]. *Osaka Hoken'i Shimbun* [*Newspaper for Practitioner in Osaka*] Jan. 21, 1966.

37. Kamo Butai [Kamo Unit]. Kiidan Shageki ni yoru Hifu Shogai narabini Ippan Rinshoteki Shojo Kansatsu [An observation of skin injuries and general clinical symptoms occurred by shots of yperite shell]. Date unknown. In: Tanaka A, Matsumura T, eds. *731 Butai Sakusei Shiryo* [*Documents Made by Unit 731*]. Tokyo, Japan: Fuji Shuppan; 1991: 1–42.

38. Kinbara S. Rikugun Gyomu Nisshi Tekiroku [Summary of the Army Operation Log]. Collection of the Military Archives, Japan Defense Agency, 35 vols., circa Aug. 1937–Nov. 1941: esp. Part 1, 1-a. Cited in: Yoshimi Y, Iko T. Nihon No Saikinsen (Japanese Biological Warfare). *Senso Sekinin Kenkyu* [*Studies in Responsibility for War*] December 1993;2:8–29.

39. Imoto K. Gyomu Nisshi [Operation Log], Vol. 22. Collection of the Military Archives, Japan Defense Agency, 23 vols., circa Sept. 1940–Dec. 1942. Cited in: Yoshimi Y, Iko T. Nihon No Saikinsen (Japanese Biological Warfare). *Senso Sekinin Kenkyu* (Studies in Responsibility for War) December 1993;2:8–29.

40. Ban S. *Rikugun Noborito Kenkyujo no Shinjitsu* [*The Truth about the Noborito Institute*]. Tokyo, Japan: Fuyo Shobo Shuppan, 2001.

41. Ohta M. *731 Menseki no Keifu* [*The Pedigree of 731 Immunity*]. Tokyo, Japan: Nihon Hyoronsha; 1999.

42. Regis E. *The Biology of Doom: The History of America's Secret Germ Warfare Project.* New York, N.Y.: Henry Holt and Company, 1999.

43. State-War-Navy Coordinating Subcommittee for the Far East. Interrogation of Certain Japanese by Russian Prosecutor. Enclosure. SFE 188/2, 1 August 1947. SWNCC 351/2/D. NARA, Record Group 165, Entry 468, Box 428. In: Kondo S, editor. *731 Butai Saikinsen Shiryo Shusei* [*Japanese Biological Warfare; Unit 731: Official Declassified Records*]. CD-ROM, 8 Discs. Tokyo, Japan: Kashiwa Shobo; 2003: Disc 3.

44. Hill EV. Summary Report on B. W. Investigations. December 12, 1947. Dugway, Utah: Dugway Proving Ground, APO 500. In: Kondo S, ed. *731 Butai Saikinsen Shiryo Shusei* [*Japanese Biological Warfare; Unit 731: Official Declassified Records*]. CD-ROM, 8 Discs. Tokyo, Japan: Kashiwa Shobo; 2003:Disc 6.

45. Morimura S. *Akuma no Hoshoku* [*The Devils' Gluttony*], new ed. Tokyo, Japan: Kadokawa Shoten; 1983 [1981].

46. Tsuchiya T. In the shadow of the past atrocities: Research ethics with human subjects in contemporary Japan. *Eubios: Journal of Asian and International Bioethics* 2003;13(3):100–2.

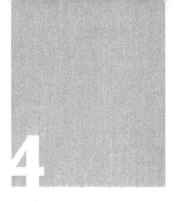

Alan Yoshioka

The Randomized Controlled Trial of Streptomycin

Background

In 1946, as word spread throughout the British Isles about a new and potentially life-saving substance called streptomycin, patients and doctors began besieging the government with requests for the drug. The vast majority of requests were for treatment of tuberculosis, which in that era was killing some 25,000 Britons each year. In July 1945, the Labour Party had swept to its first majority government, on the slogan "Fair Shares for All." Though patients did not speak in terms of a "right to treatment," even after the passage of the National Health Service Act establishing universal health care for the first time, the mood of the country was such that to have the old webs of influence carry too much weight in the distribution of streptomycin would have been politically intolerable. The medical authorities needed a fair and equitable means of distributing the drug. But knowledge about which patients, if any, were most likely to benefit in the long term was still very limited. And would it be worthwhile for British pharmaceutical firms, still operating under industrial controls remaining in place from the war effort, to be allowed to produce the drug?

Thus it was that the Medical Research Council (MRC) of the United Kingdom began planning in 1946 for a series of clinical trials of streptomycin. Of these experiments, by far the best known is the trial of streptomycin in pulmonary tuberculosis, published by the *British Medical Journal* (*BMJ*) in October 1948.[1] This trial was a model of meticulousness in design and implementation, with systematic enrollment criteria and data collection compared with the ad hoc nature of much other contemporary research, even other trials conducted under the auspices of the MRC.

A landmark because of both its methods and its findings, it conclusively confirmed streptomycin as the first effective chemotherapy for pulmonary tuberculosis, as a number of U.S. studies had been suggesting. By 1950, the MRC was trumpeting it as the first statistically controlled study of its kind.[2] It is generally recognized as the first randomized curative trial;[3] even if subsequent historical research should some day uncover an obscure earlier trial fitting that description, the MRC's pulmonary tuberculosis trial will remain among the most methodologically influential clinical experiments ever conducted.

It is commonly stated that because of a shortage of dollars for imports, only a small amount of U.S. streptomycin could be used in the trial, and that therefore it was ethically justifiable to provide streptomycin to only half the patients.[2,4–10] Such a picture of the ethics of the trial is incomplete: Although the research was conducted before principles of informed consent had been fully articulated, the MRC may be criticized for withholding from patients the information that they were part of a controlled trial, and the government's streptomycin program as a whole involved deception of the British public.

Tuberculosis and Experimental Methods

The annual rate of mortality from tuberculosis in England and Wales declined dramatically and fairly steadily from roughly 330 deaths per 100,000 population in the middle of the 19th century to roughly 60 per 100,000 just before streptomycin was introduced in the mid-20th century, aside from increased rates during the two world wars[11] (see Figure 4.1). The reasons for this decline have been hotly dis-

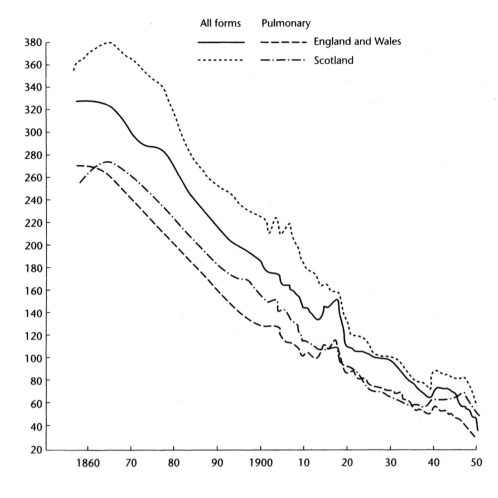

All forms   Pulmonary

———————   – – – – –   England and Wales

·············   –·–·–·–   Scotland

Figure 4.1. Standardized Death Rates from Tuberculosis (All Forms and Pulmonary) per 100,000 Population, England and Wales, and Scotland, 1850–1950. Source: Linda Bryder, *Below the Magic Mountain*, New York, N.Y.: Clarendon Press, 1988, p. 7. Reproduced with the permission of Linda Bryder and Oxford University Press.

puted by epidemiologists and demographers; what is clear, though, is that it occurred in the absence of effective drug treatment.

Because tuberculosis, especially in its pulmonary forms, exhibited spontaneous recoveries, numerous treatments were adopted on the basis of rather slim clinical evidence, only to be discredited later.[12–14] Perhaps most notorious of these was sanocrysin, a gold compound discovered in 1923. In 1931, a team in Detroit, Mich., divided 24 patients into two groups, with patients paired as closely as possible according to criteria such as age and severity of disease. A single flip of a coin decided which group would receive sanocrysin and which group injections of distilled water. The control group fared better.[12,15,16] Despite this experiment and continuing evidence of toxicity, sanocrysin remained popular until about 1935 and was still used occasionally as late as 1947. A survey published in 1940 showed some specialists continuing to use it "because one must do something" rather than because they believed in it.[11]

Sanatorium treatment was widespread. In Britain it often involved "work therapy" along with a variety of social interventions, but bed rest was also common. The latter enjoyed greater favor in the United States. Artificial pneumothorax, one form of "collapse therapy," consisted of collapsing one lung by the injection of air into the chest cavity outside the lung.[11] The theory was that without the continual movement of breathing, the lung tissue would have a better chance to heal, and there was some evidence,

albeit not conclusive, that this was effective.[17,18] Only one lung of a patient could be treated in this way at a time, of course, so patients with tuberculosis in both lungs were considered less promising candidates for pneumothorax.[11]

In 1944, William Feldman and Corwin Hinshaw, leading tuberculosis researchers at the Mayo Clinic in Rochester, Minn., presented numerous techniques to reduce the possibility of erroneous claims from antituberculosis trials in human patients. Their concepts of clinical trial design attempted to extend controlled laboratory conditions to the bedside. Their guidelines included careful definition of eligible cases to ensure a homogeneous group of cases, X-ray interpretation blinded as to whether patients had received treatment, and "some procedure of chance" in allocating patients[19]—ideas all implemented in the MRC's trial. Feldman and Hinshaw referred to an unidentified study of their own, then under way, which used the toss of a coin to select one member from each of several pairs of patients who had been matched for clinical condition.

In Britain, meanwhile, researchers such as those involved with the MRC's Therapeutic Trials Committee, which had been created in 1931, were likewise developing controlled clinical experiments. In 1937, *The Lancet* carried a series of articles by Professor (later Sir) Austin Bradford Hill in which he attempted to explain to medical practitioners some introductory principles of medical statistics.[20]

Hill promoted the use of random allotment primarily to reduce bias by balancing the known and unknown characteristics of the treatment groups.[21] This rationale was distinct from that of statistician R. A. Fisher, whose theory of randomization emphasized estimation of the uncertainty of experimental findings.[22] Uncertainty is now familiar, of course, in the context of opinion polls mentioning the margin of error within which, 19 times out of 20, they are likely to be accurate. As the historian Harry Marks has emphasized, though, statistical estimation of uncertainty has taken hold only slowly and partially within clinical medicine.[22]

Hill's 1937 series in *The Lancet* presents alternation—that is, alternating between treatment groups by order of admission to a trial—as simply one way of randomly allocating patients. There is no sign, in other words, of a distinction that would eventually emerge between alternation and randomization. Late in his career, Hill suggested that he had wished to avoid scaring off his audience by discussing more complicated techniques such as the random sampling numbers he would use in the streptomycin trial;[7] contemporary evidence on this question would be welcome.[23]

A procedure of alternation is theoretically open to bias. If the admitting physician knows that the next patient to be entered in the trial at his or her site would definitely fall into the control group, then a prospective patient might conceivably be encouraged to come back a few days later so as to have a better chance to receive the new treatment. Even so, during the Second World War such alternation was considered a satisfactory way of balancing the treatment groups, and indeed Peter Armitage has argued that strict alternation is no more prone to bias than randomization.[24] An MRC study of the antibiotic patulin in treatment of the common cold and a Royal Army Medical Corps study of a sulphonamide in bacillary dysentery used alternation; two of the organizers of those trials, Philip Hart and J. G. Scadding, went on to organize the MRC's streptomycin trials.[3,25–28] Alternation was also used in certain streptomycin trials that followed the famous pulmonary trial.

Intriguingly, the streptomycin trial was not the first to use randomization of individual patients, as Iain Chalmers has pointed out.[21] In a comparative trial of vitamin supplements published late in 1937, patients randomly assigned themselves to treatment groups by drawing beads from a box.[29] No evidence has been presented, though, that this vitamin study had any influence on the subsequent development of experimental design.

The Development of Streptomycin

The antibiotic streptomycin, like penicillin before it, was subject to extraordinary commercial and public pressures.

Penicillin was discovered in 1928 by Alexander Fleming at St. Mary's Hospital in London, England.[30] Its therapeutic potential lay largely unexplored, though, until a decade later, when a team of researchers at Oxford University, led by Howard Florey and Ernst Chain, tested the substance in animals and described how to produce it in significant quantities. The first clinical trial, in six patients, was completed in June 1941. At the Oxford researchers' suggestion, the U.S. government and selected U.S. pharmaceutical firms collaborated on production. Under wartime conditions, proprietary rights were set aside and competing manufacturers exchanged information freely. Production increased from 425 million units in June 1943 to about 460 billion units in March 1945, at which time the drug became generally available to civilian patients in the United States; during the same interval, the cost per 100,000 units (roughly 100 milligrams) plummeted from $20 to less than $1.[31]

The U.S. Committee on Medical Research rationed civilian supplies of penicillin in the name of science.[16,32] Centralized control of research during wartime allowed some medical scientists the opportunity to try implementing innovative approaches they had long favored on methodological grounds, though cooperative trials were not without their difficulties. In a large trial of penicillin in syphilis, many of the physicians deviated from the protocol, leaving data that could not be analyzed. After extensive internal debate, the U.S. National Research Council agreed to test a new sulfonamide drug, sulfathiazole, on prison volunteers experimentally infected with gonorrhea, only to abandon the study partway through when it appeared that technical problems would keep it from yielding sound conclusions.[16] Chester Keefer of the U.S. Committee on Chemotherapeutics initially ruled that penicillin should not be used in subacute bacterial endocarditis, in which long-term treatment at high dosages would be required—supposing that the drug was effective at all. Some clinicians disregarded this restriction and showed that penicillin did often control this previously fatal infection, as was also later confirmed by one of the MRC's penicillin studies;[31] MRC insiders have pointed to this study as a methodologically sound use of historical controls.[6,33]

In the late 1930s, Selman Waksman's microbiology laboratory at Rutgers University in New Brunswick, N.J., began systematically screening antibiotic substances for possible therapeutic activity. A large manufacturer of pharmaceuticals and fine chemicals, George Merck and Company, based in nearby Rahway, N.J., agreed with Waksman in 1940 to develop any promising substances. Streptomycin was isolated around November 1943 by Albert Schatz, a Ph.D. student in Waksman's department[34,35] (see Figure 4.2). (A bitter dispute over royalties and scientific credit for the discovery broke out in 1949 between Schatz and Waksman and was fully resolved only after several decades.) On the strength of clinical findings in tularemia (rabbit fever), influenzal meningitis, and gram-negative urinary tract infections, the U.S. War Production Board decided in June 1945 to permit Merck to proceed with a new plant in Elkton, Va., in which the company invested $3.5 million[36] (see Figures 4.3 and 4.4). In the month of October 1945, before this plant became operational, Merck made three kilograms of streptomycin. A year later, it was making 100 kilograms per month. Some 10 or 12 other firms belonging to the U.S. streptomycin consortium tried to produce the drug—most with reportedly little success.[37]

In December 1944, Feldman and Hinshaw showed "striking" results of streptomycin in tuberculosis in experimentally infected guinea pigs, the animal model of choice. A subsequent study, published in October 1945, examined 20 animals treated with streptomycin and 10 untreated controls and showed the drug to effectively resolve or suppress established experimental infections in guinea pigs.[38] In September 1945, the Mayo Clinic reported preliminary clinical trials in tuberculosis, with cautiously optimistic conclusions.[39]

Meanwhile, research elsewhere in the United States was proceeding apace. In September 1946, Keefer and his colleagues from the Committee on Chemotherapeutics published their findings from 1,000 cases of disease treated with streptomycin.[40,41] In the summer of 1946, the U.S. Veterans Administration, with 9,000 tuberculosis patients in its hospitals, began a large trial of streptomycin in treatment of men with pulmonary tuberculosis.[42] Fearful of the political repercussions of using an untreated control

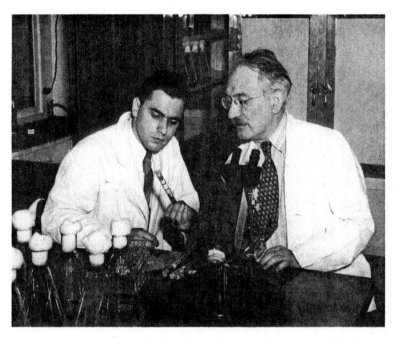

Figure 4.2. Albert Schatz and Selman Waksman at Martin Hall, New Jersey College of Agriculture, circa 1944. Source: Special Collections and University Archives, Rutgers University Libraries. Reproduced with permission.

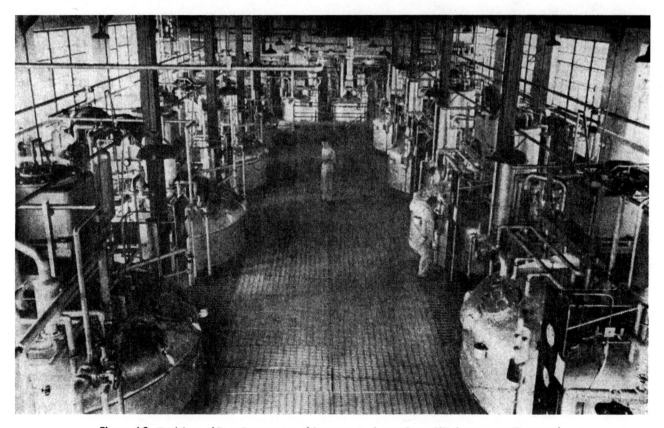

Figure 4.3. Final Stage of Deep Fermentation of Streptomycin. Source: Porter RW. Streptomycin: Engineered into commercial production. *Chemical Engineering* 1946;53(10)94–8, 142–5. Reproduced with permission.

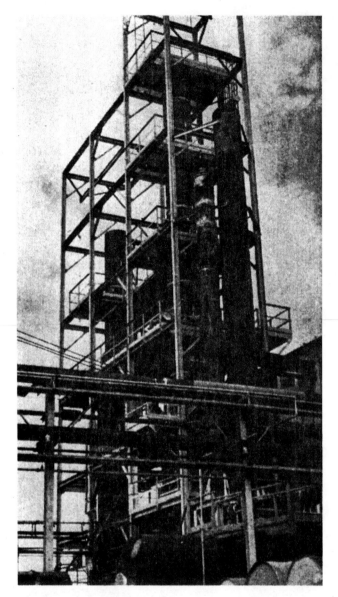

Figure 4.4. Distillation Towers to Recover Solvents Used in Streptomycin Extraction, Elkton, VA. Source: Porter RW. Streptomycin: Engineered into commercial production. *Chemical Engineering* 1946;53(10)94–8, 142–5. Reproduced with permission.

group, the researchers proceeded without one. In contrast, the U.S. Public Health Service agreed in May 1947 that patients in its study would be randomly allocated to the streptomycin treatment group or a control group without the drug.[16]

Early in 1946, two British pharmaceutical firms were hoping to begin large-scale manufacture of streptomycin: Glaxo Laboratories, based in Ware, north of London, and the Boots Pure Drug Company, based in Nottingham in the Midlands. They approached the Ministry of Supply, the wartime ministry that continued to oversee virtually all industrial activity in the country. Only if the Ministry of Supply granted them "priorities" would the companies be permitted to allocate to the project the necessary building materials, steel tanks, industrial solvents, and skilled laborers, all of which were in short supply. There was thus a key industrial

incentive to know how effective streptomycin was. Then, between July 15 and 20, William Feldman's lecture tour through London and Oxford stirred up medical interest—much to the consternation of the Ministry of Health, which foresaw a public demand that could not be met. The Mayo Clinic experimentalist's presentation included a highly persuasive graphic illustration of the laboratory evidence of the effectiveness of streptomycin in tuberculosis in guinea pigs[38] (see Figure 4.5).

The Planning of the British Program of Streptomycin Research

The MRC first became involved with streptomycin in September 1945, when one of the members of its Penicillin Clinical Trials Committee, L. P. Garrod, read of the first clinical use of streptomycin, in a typhoid outbreak in Philadelphia. The mortality in streptomycin-treated patients was 40%, considerably higher than the 9% in untreated patients.[43] Garrod remarked dryly, "The evidence of curative action is not wholly convincing,"[44] but he nonetheless requested a supply of streptomycin to try treating a patient of his who was described as an intractable typhoid carrier. At the time, though, the drug was not to be found in the United Kingdom, and Garrod's request was deferred.

In March 1946 the MRC Secretary, Sir Edward Mellanby, tried to procure streptomycin for one of his close relatives, himself a medical man. He asked pharmacologist A. N. Richards at the University of Pennsylvania, who was an adviser to Merck. Richards at first agreed to help Mellanby but then was forced to retract his offer because of the restrictions imposed on streptomycin distribution in the United States.[45]

The Ministry of Supply and Ministry of Health decided in June 1946 that clinical trials of British streptomycin needed to be run, but the health official in charge dawdled for weeks, until finally Harold Raistrick, the Ministry of Supply representative, took action himself. Four days after Feldman's final lecture in Oxford, Raistrick collared the MRC Secretary. Suddenly under pressure to say how much of the drug would be needed, Mellanby came up with the idea of using 100 patients. To treat that many patients for six months, he told Raistrick, 75 kilograms of streptomycin would suffice.[46] Boots, Glaxo, and a third manufacturer, the Distillers Company (which had been brought into the British penicillin project because of its expertise in fermentation technology), were expected to have the drug ready soon for clinical testing.

Geoffrey Marshall (Figure 4.6), a respected consultant at the Brompton Hospital, Britain's most prestigious institution for the treatment of tuberculosis, chaired a hastily assembled conference of clinicians, all of them with experience in the treatment of tuberculosis. Not surprisingly, they decided that the main trial would focus on pulmonary tuberculosis, though consideration was also given to leprosy.[47] Hill was not present at this conference, nor at a meeting of a few physicians a few days later at Marshall's home, at which time it was suggested that control cases were "highly desirable, if not essential, for the main group of broncho-pneumonic cases."[48] A few more men, including Hill, were invited to a second streptomycin conference, which was held on August 27.[49]

The Streptomycin Clinical Trials (Tuberculosis) Committee, as it was formally known, was created in October 1946,[50] with Marshall as chairman and Philip Hart, who later directed the MRC's tuberculosis research unit, as secretary.[51] Marc Daniels, as the "registrar," coordinated the clinicians at participating hospitals.

CONTROLS

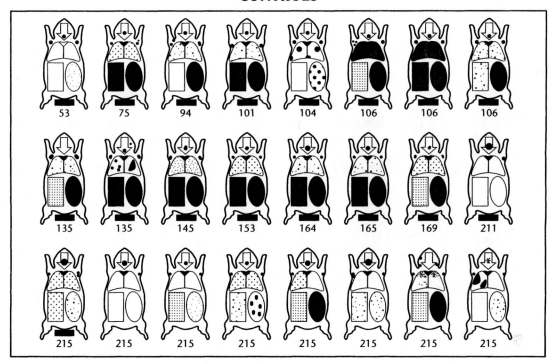

STREPTOMYCIN SERIES

TREATED AFTER 49 DAYS

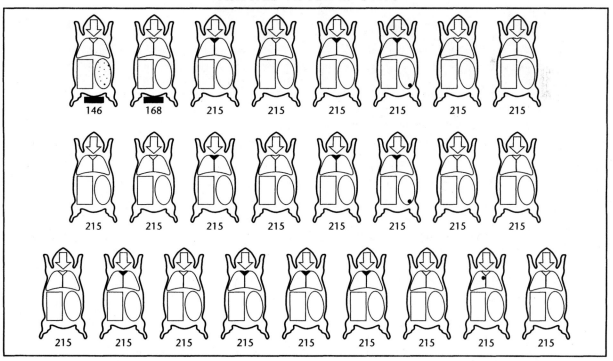

Figure 4.5. Controlled Study of Streptomycin Treatment of Tuberculous Guinea Pigs. Amount of tuberculosis, shown schematically, noted grossly at necropsy in treated and untreated groups of guinea pigs. The number beneath an animal represents the length of life in days after inoculation. A black bar above a numeral indicates that the animal died (third experiment). Source: Feldman WH, Hinshaw HC, Mann FC. Streptomycin in experimental tuberculosis. *American Review of Tuberculosis* 1945;52:269–98, p. 281. © American Thoracic Society. Reproduced with permission.

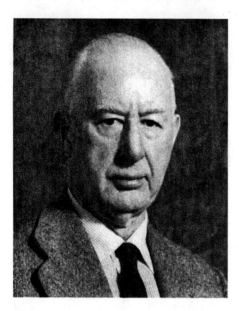

Figure 4.6. Sir Geoffrey Marshall (1887–1982).
Source: Heritage Collections, Royal College of
Physicians (London), *Munk's Roll*, Volume VII,
p. LIII. Reproduced with permission.

British regulations permitted the importation of streptomycin for private use, so unknown quantities of the drug circulated around the country. A black market emerged.[52] In addition, the BBC began broadcasting a series of appeals to the public for streptomycin to be used in medical emergencies it highlighted—typically, cases of tuberculous meningitis in children.[53] In the first of many such incidents, in November 1946, one company donated a tiny amount of the drug in the vain hope of saving a young boy who was critically ill in hospital.

In order to manage public demand, MRC officials wanted their research program to absorb any supplies that would be entering the country. The MRC's staff repeatedly told the public that supplies had to be fully restricted to the clinical trials.[54] These officials reasoned that the scarce and potentially life-saving drug would be used inefficiently if allowed into untrained hands, and they had ample reason to be wary. For example, in one of many poignant cases, a prominent banker had sought the MRC's help in procuring the antibiotic to treat his young grandson, who was dying of leukemia[55]—an indication for which there was no laboratory or clinical evidence to suggest the drug would be effective.[46]

Streptomycin was difficult to manufacture, even more so than penicillin. The process was quite complex and demanded huge amounts of raw materials (see Figure 4.7). Also, contamination from airborne organisms could reduce the yield. The British firms experienced continual production delays, so when a large U.S. shipment became available in mid-November 1946, the MRC leapt at the chance to purchase it.[46]

Research Study Events

The trial was designed "to give a negative or affirmative answer to the question, is streptomycin of value in the treatment of pulmonary tuberculosis?"[1] That is, as the *BMJ* paper emphasizes, it

was not meant to find the ideal dosage or to find the best treatment regimen. Later the tuberculosis committee would investigate, for example, whether pulsed treatment, with several weeks on and several weeks off, in alternation, might help to avoid the development of resistant strains of bacteria.[1] Hill subsequently made a point of recommending that clinical trials test the efficacy (as it has now come to be called) of a strictly controlled treatment regimen, rather than the effectiveness of a treatment in a wide variety of less easily compared circumstances.[56,57]

The duration of treatment was originally set up to be six months. Once the trial got underway, however, evidence from the Mayo Clinic and from the trial clinicians themselves suggested that the greatest benefit would result during four months of treatment. A shorter course of treatment was therefore implemented as of July 1947. Patients remained in hospital under observation for their final two months in the study.[1]

One of the Committee's most important decisions was to restrict admission to a homogeneous set of cases: "acute progressive bilateral pulmonary tuberculosis of presumably recent origin, bacteriologically proved, unsuitable for collapse therapy, age group 15 to 25 (later extended to 30)."[1] Previous clinical evidence suggested that such patients would be more likely to benefit than those with long-established disease, and the similarity of cases meeting these criteria lent credibility to the comparison between the treatment and control group. As it happened, the initial entry criteria were loosened because not enough eligible patients could be found.

The enrollment of control patients who did not receive streptomycin was justified explicitly in the study paper, on the ground that there was not enough of the drug to go around. The control patients did receive bed rest, the then standard treatment.

The story is often repeated that a controlled trial could be run because there were not enough U.S. dollars to import streptomycin.[2,6–9] The evidence does not really support this after-the-fact explanation. Although supplies of streptomycin in the United Kingdom fell short of demand until 1949, the British government's problems with its balance of payments did not become serious until the MRC's controlled trial was well underway. Export quotas set by the U.S. government, not limits imposed by the British Treasury, determined the quantity of streptomycin that the MRC could obtain. A substantial 50 kilograms (enough to fully treat more than 135 patients) were offered to the British government in November 1946, at a cost of $320,000, for which the spending of dollars was not an obstacle. It was in April 1947, months after the trial had begun, that the Treasury first implemented procedures requiring high-level approval of the spending of dollars, and even then, the import of a further 50 kilograms of streptomycin was approved with little delay.[46]

The clinicians in the pulmonary tuberculosis trial were not blinded as to the treatment assignment. Patients were not told they were in an experiment at all.[56] Use of placebo injections was considered at the meeting at Marshall's home but was ruled out by the Committee at its first meeting in November.[48,51] The Committee's rationale for considering placebos unnecessary was that four-times-daily injections of saline would cause too much discomfort relative to the value they would provide in safeguarding the validity of the study, in that the main comparisons relied upon objective measures: deaths and changes in radiological condition. Patients' X-rays were assessed independently by two radiologists

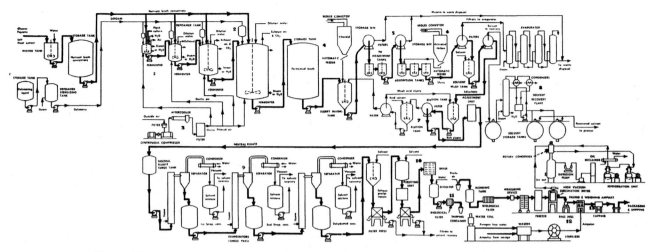

Figure 4.7. Schematic Diagram of the Streptomycin Manufacturing Process. Source: Porter RW. Streptomycin: Engineered into commercial production. *Chemical Engineering* 1946;53(10)94–8, 142–5. Reproduced with permission.

and a clinician, all of whom were blinded with regard to the treatment assignment.

Randomization Versus Alternation

As is well known, Hill instituted a new method in the pulmonary trial, which the tuberculosis committee's report in the *BMJ* describes in detail:

> Determination of whether a patient would be treated by streptomycin and bed-rest (S case) or by bed-rest alone (C case) was made by reference to a statistical series based on random sampling numbers drawn up for each sex at each centre by Professor Bradford Hill; the details of the series were unknown to any of the investigators or to the co-ordinator and were contained in a set of sealed envelopes, each bearing on the outside only the name of the hospital and a number. After acceptance of a patient by the panel, and before admission to the streptomycin centre, the appropriate numbered envelope was opened at the central office: the card inside told if the patient was to be an S or C case, and this information was then given to the medical officer of the centre. Patients were not told before admission that they were to get special treatment; C patients did not know throughout their stay in hospital that they were control patients in a special study; they were in fact treated as they would have been in the past, the sole difference being that they had been admitted to the centre more rapidly than was normal. Usually they were not in the same wards as S patients, but the same regimen was maintained.[1]

Subsequent accounts have differed somewhat in their characterizations of what was novel about this system.[6,8,9,33,58–60] Chalmers praises Hart for making clear that a key advantage of Hill's system over alternation was "allocation concealment" at the time patients entered the study.[3,21,28] That is, randomization permitted, though it did not ensure, concealment from the admitting physician of the treatment group to which a prospective patient entering the

study would be assigned. Marks, following Chalmers, suggests that this was intended "to prevent physicians from cream skimming—selectively assigning healthier patients to the experimental drug."[22]

There is room for further research and reflection on the topic, but, given that access to treatment was such a sensitive issue, it may be that the key issue was centralization of the experimental "decision"—impersonal as it had become—to assign any individual patient to the control group. Surely some observers would have seen this as consigning some patients in the trial to inferior care, despite the existing uncertainties about the value of the new drug and despite the point, brought out in the *BMJ* report, that most control patients were admitted to hospital within a week. Thus it may be that the main significance of Hill's scheme lay in keeping treatment allocation out of the hands of those who came face to face with patients and were responsible for their care. In the words of the *BMJ* leading article that introduced the report, the new method of random allocation "removed personal responsibility from the clinician."[61]

Conduct of the Trial

By September 1947, when admission to the pulmonary trial was closed, 109 patients had been accepted. Two died during a preliminary observation week during which all patients received only standard clinical care. Of the 107 patients analyzed, 52 were in the control group (21 men and 31 women), and 55 in the group receiving streptomycin (22 men and 33 women).[1]

When the condition of some patients deteriorated, they received collapse therapy if this was judged medically advisable. With such pressure on the resources of the trial, it made sense to restrict admission to those patients who were least likely to benefit from the alternative of collapse therapy. Even so, it did happen that 11 patients from the control group (5 during the first four months of the trial and 6 during the last two months of observation) were judged to require collapse therapy, which was duly applied. Another 11 patients in the streptomycin group also were treated with collapse therapy, all during the two-month observation period in hospital that followed active treatment under the revised treatment schedule.[1]

Though there were a number of what would now be called protocol amendments, the fundamental design of the trial was adhered to remarkably closely, which was no minor accomplishment.[62]

Study Drug Supplies and the Other Streptomycin Trials

It is all but forgotten that two other streptomycin trials began under the same MRC committee around the same time. One was in acute miliary tuberculosis; the other, tuberculous meningitis. Both trials are mentioned as examples in which it would have been unethical to use a control group.[6,8] With essentially 100% mortality to that point (for example, in tuberculous meningitis, only some 60 recoveries had ever been recorded worldwide, and not all of these cases had been diagnosed conclusively),[63] there was no need for a concurrent control group. All of the MRC researchers' patients who had these conditions were given streptomycin. Hospitals in the MRC scheme admitted 25 patients with miliary tuberculosis between March and September 1947,[64] and 105 patients with proven tuberculous meningitis before August 18, 1947.[65]

The pulmonary tuberculosis paper justified the control group partly through "the fact that all the streptomycin available in the country was in any case being used," the rest of the supply being taken up for these two hitherto fatal conditions.[1] This was a convenient gloss: The Committee's decision to run a controlled trial was made before the trials in miliary tuberculosis and tuberculous meningitis were approved. And although the Committee decided to treat all the patients in these other trials with streptomycin—and hindsight has declared that to do otherwise would have been unjustifiable[6]—remarkably, the MRC's second streptomycin conference during the summer of 1946 had not been equally definite, declaring only that the use of a control group in miliary and meningeal tuberculosis was "possibly not" essential.[49]

Still more obscure was the trial of streptomycin in nontuberculous conditions. A few weeks after the MRC set up the tuberculosis committee, it created a committee to conduct clinical trials of streptomycin in nontuberculous conditions. Sir Alexander Fleming, who enjoyed great scientific prestige because of his discovery of penicillin, chaired this body, which had no statistical representative. This lesser-known committee tested streptomycin in *Haemophilus influenzae* meningitis, whooping cough, and several other conditions including—satisfying L. P. Garrod's request at last—typhoid fever (see Table 4.1). It allowed the participating clinicians to gain experience in treating patients with the drug. And in this trial, as with the others run by the MRC, careful bacteriological testing examined the development of resistance.

The trial in nontuberculous conditions illustrates a different style of research from that of the tuberculosis trials—similar in fact to what Hill's lectures on clinical trial design would criticize in the years to come. For most of the conditions studied, the small numbers of cases made it difficult to draw firm conclusions. The minutes from the meetings during the committee's first year make no mention at all of the possibility of using control groups for any of the diseases; in 1948 a trial using alternating controls was approved for infantile gastroenteritis.[66] Initially the record keeping was left to the discretion of investigators,[67] though after several months a standard clinical report form was adopted, at least for the meningitis cases.[68]

Among the reasons for setting up this committee was to help ensure that all of the MRC's supplies were allocated to research. For uniformity, all the streptomycin given to patients with pulmonary or meningeal tuberculosis came from a single manufacturer, Merck, whereas all of the streptomycin given to patients with miliary tuberculosis came from another firm. The nontuberculous conditions trial was crucial to the success of the three tuberculosis trials, in that it used up allotments of streptomycin for which the latter had no use, for example an initial 540 grams in December 1946.[67] Courses of treatment sometimes involved much smaller quantities of the drug than were needed for pulmonary tuberculosis; for example, in March 1947, several centers for influenzal meningitis each received a 50-gram supply that was expected to treat 5 to 10 cases.[69] In May 1947, Fleming's committee requested an additional 20 kilograms over the next year.[70] Streptomycin could not be released to the general public without causing chaos, so the committee quietly treated more than 227 patients by September 1948 and gained some useful knowledge along the way.

Outcomes

The Streptomycin Clinical Trials (Tuberculosis) Committee told the Ministry of Health in April 1947 that streptomycin definitely prolonged the lives of patients with tuberculous meningitis.[71] The ministry hastened to make streptomycin treatment available for this condition (and also, as of June 1947, for miliary tuberculosis) throughout the country through a network of teaching hospitals.[72] Its scheme was running by September. The MRC's tuberculous meningitis report was published in *The Lancet* in April 1948. Of 105 proved cases admitted between early January and August 18, 1947, there were 38 patients surviving as of December 15, 1947, after 120 or more days' treatment and observation. Of these, 30 (28% of the original total) were said to be making good progress.[65]

An interim report on streptomycin in nontuberculous conditions[73] was summarized in both the *BMJ* and *The Lancet* in September 1948.[74,75] It described some success in controlling infections due to gram-negative bacteria such as *H. influenzae*. In 1950, though, when Fleming's committee was concluding its work, MRC headquarters advised its secretary not to go to the trouble of publishing a final report if there was "nothing very fresh to say."[76]

The landmark report on pulmonary tuberculosis was published in the *BMJ* on October 30, 1948. In this trial, four of the 55 patients in the S group (7%) and 14 of the 52 patients in the C group (27%) died by the end of the sixth month. The probability that this difference between groups would occur by chance was said to be less than one in a hundred.[1] The report documented the emergence of streptomycin-resistant strains of the tubercle bacillus, a phenomenon that Mayo researchers had first described in a clinical setting in 1946.[77]

The Ministry of Health scheme for treating meningeal and miliary tuberculosis progressively widened to cover other tuberculous conditions, and the MRC began testing streptomycin in conjunction with surgical procedures and the new drug para-aminosalicylic acid. The report on the miliary tuberculosis trial was not published until 1950, by which time of course many other studies had appeared, though the MRC paper did provide lengthier follow-up than the others cited: By October 1949, at the end of at least 24 months of observation, there were 14 survivors (56%) out of the original 25 patients.[64]

Table 4.1

Features of the Initial MRC Clinical Trials of Streptomycin

Committee	Streptomycin Clinical Trials (Tuberculosis) Committee			Streptomycin Clinical Trials (Non-Tuberculous Conditions) Committee
Chair	Geoffrey Marshall			Sir Alexander Fleming
Disease(s) (number of cases)	Pulmonary tuberculosis (109)[1]	Tuberculous meningitis (138)[65]	Acute miliary tuberculosis (25)[64]	H. influenzae meningitis (43), other meningitis (14), septicaemias with or without subacute bacterial endocarditis (8), urinary tract infection (61), local sepsis (45), chronic lung infection due to bronchiectasis and lung abscess (14), whooping cough (not stated), infantile diarrhea (42), ulcerative colitis or typhoid fever (not stated)[71,72]
Admission criteria	Predefined	Predefined	Predefined	Generally not specified—subject to the restriction that, in most of the conditions studied, the infection should be resistant to penicillin and sulphonamides
Record keeping	Standard case record forms	Standard case record forms	Standard case record forms	Discretionary at first,[67] then standardized for at least meningitis[68]
Controls	Randomized	Historical, due to near 100% mortality	Historical, due to near 100% mortality	None for most conditions; alternating for a 1948 study of infantile gastroenteritis
Duration of treatment	6 months initially (changed to 4 months treatment followed by 2 months observation in hospital)	Initially planned as 3 months or more	Initially planned as 3 months or more	Dependent on the condition; many patients for between 4 and 14 days, and very few patients for as many as 28 days
Dosage in treatment group	2 g daily, given in four intramuscular injections at 6-hour intervals	Some combination of intramuscular injections of up to 2 g daily (depending on age and body weight), and intrathecal injections of between 50 mg and 100 mg daily	Intramuscular injections of up to 2 g daily (depending on age and body weight), given as four intramuscular injections at 6-hour intervals; plus intrathecal injections if showing evidence of meningitis	Depending on age, body weight, and disease category; intrathecal injections of between 50 and 100 mg daily in meningitis
Form of drug	Streptomycin hydrochloride	Streptomycin hydrochloride	Streptomycin sulphate	Not stated

Once Glaxo's large new plant at Ulverston began producing the drug, the supply of streptomycin ceased to be a problem. On November 1, 1949, the drug became available to anyone in the United Kingdom with a valid prescription (see Table 4.2).[78]

Ethical Issues

Discussion of the ethics of the MRC's streptomycin research has remained curiously one-sided. More than half a century after the publication of the pulmonary tuberculosis paper, there is no shortage of literature reiterating the Committee's rationale for using a control group without streptomycin.[2,4–10] Sir Richard Doll, who worked closely with Hill for decades, has written, "No one has questioned the Committee's contention that it would have been unethical not to conduct the trial, nor the way the trial was carried out."[8] Yet this seems surprising: It is hard to imagine that anyone would put forward the MRC's arguments so explicitly and so per-

sistently if the ethical objections they answered had remained purely hypothetical.

One can only wonder where any contrary views, or even any questioning views, are expressed. A symposium at Oxford in 2002 represents a rare published dialogue touching on the subject.[79] As researchers continue their recent foray into the archives, the "official story" may finally receive the scrutiny and debate it deserves.

According to several members of the MRC committee for streptomycin in tuberculosis, the greatest contribution of its chairman, Geoffrey Marshall, lay in persuading the clinicians around the country that the pulmonary tuberculosis trial was a respectable venture.[80] The MRC files do not spell out, though, quite which clinicians had to be won over or from what positions. Here the MRC's archival records stand in contrast to those of, for example, the U.S. Committee on Medical Research and the U.S. National Research Council, in which frank methodological and ethical exchanges are amply documented, as Marks describes.[16]

Table 4.2

Timeline of the Context of British Clinical Trials of Streptomycin

1918–19	The Medical Research Committee (later Medical Research Council) is formed.
1925–35	The "gold decade." The gold compound sanocrysin is used frequently to treat tuberculosis, despite evidence of toxicity.
1929	Fleming publishes first paper on penicillin, describing its bactericidal properties.
1931	Amberson discredits sanocrysin through a controlled trial with group assigned to treatment by a single flip of a coin.
1935	Domagk publishes paper on the antibacterial action of prontosil, the first of the sulphonamides.
1937	*The Lancet* publishes Hill's series on medical statistics.
1940–41	Florey and Chain demonstrate chemotherapeutic potential of penicillin.
Aug. 1940	Merck and Rutgers sign agreement on commercialization of substances derived from Waksman's research program.
Nov. 1943	Schatz isolates streptomycin.
Jan. 1944	Schatz, Bugie, and Waksman publish first paper on streptomycin.
1944	Merck begins manufacturing streptomycin on a pilot scale using surface-culture process.
Dec. 27, 1944	Feldman and Hinshaw prove that streptomycin arrests tuberculosis in guinea pigs.
Mar. 1945	Penicillin becomes commercially available in United States.
June 20, 1945	Civilian and military researchers at streptomycin conference conclude that it is effective against tularemia, influenzal meningitis, and gram-negative urinary tract infections.
July 1945	Labour Party wins British general election with a majority. Aneurin Bevan becomes Minister of Health.
Aug. 1945	U.S. War Production Board approves large-scale production of streptomycin.
Sept. 1945	MRC receives its first proposal for streptomycin research from Garrod.
Sept. 1945	Feldman and Hinshaw publish first clinical report on streptomycin in tuberculosis.
Dec. 1945	Fleming, Florey, and Chain win Nobel Prize for discovery of penicillin.
Jan. 1946	Glaxo decides to invest in streptomycin production plant.
Jan. 1946	MRC first tries to procure streptomycin for clinical trial, in treatment of plague.
Jan. 5, 1946	Lehmann publishes paper in *The Lancet* on para-aminosalicylic acid (PAS) against clinical tuberculosis.
Mar. 1946	Ministry of Supply consults with MRC about streptomycin manufacture.
Mar. 1946	U.S. Committee on Chemotherapeutics decides that no further patients should be started on streptomycin therapy until supplies increase.
Mar. 1946	Bevan introduces National Health Service Bill in Parliament.
June 1946	Penicillin becomes available by prescription in the United Kingdom.
July 1946	Feldman's lectures stir up medical interest in streptomycin in the United Kingdom.
July 29, 1946	MRC convenes First Streptomycin Conference, which agrees to study streptomycin in tuberculosis.
Aug. 27, 1946	MRC convenes Second Streptomycin Conference, which decides to run a pilot trial using streptomycin to be manufactured in the United Kingdom by surface culture.
Sept. 1, 1946	Streptomycin becomes commercially available in the United States. Export restrictions remain in effect.
Oct. 1946	MRC creates its Streptomycin Clinical Trials (Tuberculosis) Committee under chairmanship of Geoffrey Marshall.
Oct. 1946	Feldman and Hinshaw demonstrate recovery of four patients with tuberculous meningitis treated with streptomycin.
Nov. 1946	MRC creates its Streptomycin Clinical Trials (Non-Tuberculous Conditions) Committee under chairmanship of Fleming.
Nov. 12–15, 1946	British Treasury approves import of 50 kg of streptomycin at a cost of $320,000.
Nov. 21, 1946	MRC Streptomycin in Tuberculosis Committee holds first meeting, approves randomized design, abandons idea of pilot trial.
Dec. 14, 1946	*BMJ* publishes statement on danger of streptomycin treatment.
Jan. 1947	MRC streptomycin trials admit first patients.
April 1947	Early findings from the MRC tuberculous meningitis trial justify making treatment more widely available. Treasury approves import of a further 50 kg of streptomycin for the MRC's research and subsequently allocates $500,000, which is sufficient for about 160 kg.
May 1947	Bevan and other key cabinet ministers agree to grant highest possible priority for the development of streptomycin, including the Ulverston plant.
July 1947	MRC committee shortens course of treatment in pulmonary tuberculosis to four months.
Apr. 17, 1948	MRC committee publishes paper in *The Lancet* on streptomycin treatment of tuberculous meningitis.
Sept. 18, 1948	MRC Streptomycin Clinical Trials (Non-Tuberculous Conditions) Committee publishes interim report in *The Lancet* and *BMJ*.
Oct. 30, 1948	MRC publishes landmark paper in *BMJ* on streptomycin treatment of pulmonary tuberculosis.
1949	Glaxo's streptomycin plant at Ulverston begins producing enough streptomycin to supply the United Kingdom's needs.
Nov. 1949	MRC officially establishes the long-awaited Tuberculosis Research Unit, with Philip D'Arcy Hart as director.
Nov. 1, 1949	Streptomycin becomes available by prescription throughout the United Kingdom.
1950	MRC committee publishes paper in *The Lancet* on streptomycin treatment of acute miliary tuberculosis.
1952	Robitzek and Selikoff publish paper on isoniazid against tuberculosis.
1952	Waksman wins the Nobel Prize for discovery of streptomycin.

Marks has coined the term *therapeutic reformers* for "individuals who sought to use the science of controlled experiments to direct medical practice."[16] He points out that such therapeutic reformers were indeed driven by an ethical concern: that physicians be guided rationally by evidence from properly controlled trials.[16] Thus first and foremost the MRC hoped to obtain reliable evidence of whether the new drug was of value. Looking back in 1963 on the circumstances of the streptomycin trial, Hill wrote, "It would, the Committee believed, have been unethical *not* to have seized the opportunity to design a strictly controlled trial which could speedily and effectively reveal the value of the treatment."[5]

Access to Treatment

The pulmonary tuberculosis report took pains to defend the use of a control group, a familiar but still ethically contentious research design. It argued, understandably, that the effectiveness of the drug was still uncertain, no controlled trial in pulmonary tuberculosis having been conducted in the United States as of 1946.[1] Marks has rightly pointed out that there was great concern about the clinical variability and unpredictability of pulmonary tuberculosis.[79] Even so, a condition of equipoise, as it later came to be called by ethicists, did not really exist at the time of the trial, in that a rational, informed person would have had good grounds for preferring to receive streptomycin relative to bed rest alone. But it has been argued, quite independently of the streptomycin scenario, that randomization in the absence of personal equipoise is "permissible, indeed desirable, when access to treatment is in any case limited as a result of inadequate resources."[81] Given the shortage that existed, then, a requirement for equipoise does not stand as a barrier to the use of a control group.

"Additional justification," the MRC report said, "lay in the fact that all the streptomycin available in the country was in any case being used, the rest of the supply being taken up for two rapidly fatal forms of the disease, miliary and meningeal tuberculosis."[1] As explained above, this glossed over a substantial program in non-tuberculous conditions. The MRC steadfastly told external inquirers that all of its supplies were being devoted to large-scale clinical trials and that requests for individual allocations could not be entertained. Quietly, though, MRC officials made exceptions for certain insiders. It has been reported, for instance, that a senior physician fell ill with tuberculosis and was provided with streptomycin outside the MRC's trial so as not to compromise the allocation scheme.[52] It should be noted that the MRC did not have a complete monopoly but controlled only the supplies in government hands: Because of private imports, which were quite legal, others could and did use streptomycin outside the MRC trials. In February 1948, for example, the U.S. royalties from *Animal Farm* provided the dollars to import a supply of the drug for author George Orwell, in an unsuccessful attempt to treat the pulmonary tuberculosis that would eventually take his life.[82] In April 1948 the U.S. Red Cross donated supplies for 10 patients who were treated in an uncontrolled case series.[83]

Informed Consent

Some instances of attention to informed consent have been identified from before the Second World War—for example, an MRC policy dating from 1933,[84] as well as German guidelines enacted in 1931 and U.S. case law from early in the 20th century.[85] It is not altogether clear, though, how successful these examples were in identifying a standard against which we, looking back, might judge researchers who simply took their ethical cues from prevailing practice. Overall, it is probably fair to characterize the dominant ethos of the British medical profession at the time of the streptomycin research as a duty of beneficence toward patients rather than respect for patient autonomy.[85] Whatever the circumstances, it was remarked only briefly in the pulmonary tuberculosis paper that control patients were not made aware that they were being enrolled in a trial.[1] The study files do not document what, if anything, the streptomycin patients were told about the identity of their injections or about the risks their treatment entailed. Strikingly, Hill wrote in 1951 that precautions were taken to keep both groups of patients in ignorance of their participation in a controlled trial.[56]

The U.S. Public Health Service trial, begun around the same time as the MRC's, likewise did not inform control patients that they were part of an experiment.[16] Hill later acknowledged the value of having an independent ethical committee oversee the experimenting doctors (which was not a consideration in the 1940s), but he continued to view it as wrong to shift onto patients the responsibility of giving informed consent.[7]

Transparency

Arguably the greatest ethical lapse in the MRC's streptomycin program lay in the handling of public relations. In statements to the British public, the MRC repeatedly framed the current state of knowledge in terms so pessimistic as to be deliberately deceptive.[86] Although evidence continued to accumulate from the United States to the effect that streptomycin was effective in a number of conditions and fairly safe,[87] the British authorities left inquirers to imagine that brain damage in patients who survived tuberculous meningitis might be the result of the drug rather than an effect of the disease itself. In the face of overwhelming public demand for the drug, the MRC's press officer, Frank Green, and the Ministry of Health arranged for alarming statements to appear in the *BMJ* and *The Times*.[88–90] The latter warned in January 1947, "In the very small number of patients with tubercular meningitis whose life has been prolonged by the treatment there has nearly always been permanent derangement, blindness or deafness."[90] *The Lancet,* however, did not cooperate with this campaign.[91] One paper published by *The Lancet* presented evidence that toxicity was inversely proportional to purity; noting that the purity of streptomycin preparations had been steadily improving over time, the authors declared themselves convinced that the drug could be used safely at the dose levels they had adopted.[92] Waksman, writing from New Jersey, objected to the scare. Green explained unrepentantly to the British Foreign Office in April 1947 that the statement "was intended to discourage broadcast appeals for the drug, by indicating these cannot be met from British sources at the present time."[93]

The adverse publicity evidently left many British medical practitioners confused about the true benefit of streptomycin.[11,94] In 1950 the Ministry of Health belatedly (and disingenuously) tried to correct the apparently common belief that the treatment did no more than "prolong life or produce 'recovery' as a physical and mental wreck."[95]

Given the lack of transparency with which information was presented to the public, readers of the MRC's publications on the streptomycin program may be excused for wondering whether other statements should be accepted at face value.

Enduring Legacy

The MRC's trial of streptomycin in pulmonary tuberculosis is significant in several ways. In terms of tuberculosis treatment, it was one of several studies that established the efficacy of streptomycin. The MRC study supported other observations of the rather rapid emergence of drug resistance. Together these findings led to the investigation of pulsed treatment and the continued push to develop new therapies that, alone or in combination, would minimize acquired resistance. Along with these other newer drugs, streptomycin contributed greatly to the declining prevalence of tuberculosis in developed countries over the next several decades and the shortening of stays in hospitals and sanatoria. As for the initial industrial question the research program had been intended to settle, it was mainly evidence from the United States (though also the British interim findings in meningitis early in 1947) that would guide decisions about production priorities.[96]

As founding director of the MRC's Tuberculosis Research Unit, which was formally established in 1949,[97] Hart went on to organize much important research, ably assisted by Daniels until the latter's untimely death in 1953. Notably the unit demonstrated that vaccines substantially reduced the incidence of tuberculosis and, later, that chemotherapy could be effective against tuberculosis even in outpatients living in very difficult circumstances in developing countries.[98,99]

The greatest influence of the pulmonary tuberculosis trial, though, lay in its methods, which have affected virtually every area of clinical medicine. The trial quickly came to be recognized as a model of design and implementation.[100] Hill was invited to the United States to lecture on clinical trials and became a great popularizer of randomized controlled trials.[5,56,57] Daniels also wrote on clinical trial methods.[62] Over the years, as the discipline of controlled clinical trials grew in sophistication and influence, the streptomycin trial continued to be referred to as groundbreaking.[101–103] Two notable features were the concealment of the allocation schedule and the use of objective measures such as interpretation of X-ray films by experts who were not aware of patients' treatment assignment.

Advocates of randomized controlled trials have had considerable success in changing the culture and policies of medical journals and regulatory agencies.[104,105] A now vast body of evidence gathered from randomized controlled trials is disseminated globally by The Cochrane Collaboration, named in honor of a leading promoter of such trials, British health-care researcher Archie Cochrane.[106]

To some observers, however, the push for greater methodological rigor has come at a price. In the 1980s, for example, AIDS activists objected to the use of placebo controls when treatments for life-threatening conditions were being tested.[107] Placebo controls—which were not used in the MRC study—have continued to evoke controversy.

The MRC's trials illustrate a recurring quandary about how to allocate treatment fairly under conditions of uncertain knowledge

and short supply. To their credit, the MRC researchers answered their main clinical questions conclusively, and health officials then extended treatment as broadly and quickly as resources allowed. Ethical reservations may remain, though, about the approach that scientists and government officials took to the sharing of information with experimental patients and members of the public.

References

1. Medical Research Council. Streptomycin treatment of pulmonary tuberculosis. *British Medical Journal* 1948;2:769–82.
2. Report of the Medical Research Council for the years 1945–48, Cmd 7846. *Parliamentary Papers* 1948–49;xviii:1–283.
3. Hart PD'A. A change in scientific approach: From alternation to randomised allocation in clinical trials in the 1940s. *British Medical Journal* 1999;319:572–3.
4. Reid DD. Statistics in clinical research. *Annals of the New York Academy of Sciences* 1950;52:931–4.
5. Hill AB. Medical ethics and controlled trials. *British Medical Journal* 1963;1:1043–9.
6. Thomson AL. *Half a Century of Medical Research. 2. The Programme of the Medical Research Council (UK)*. London, UK: HMSO; 1975.
7. Hill AB. Memories of the British streptomycin trial in tuberculosis: The first randomized clinical trial. *Controlled Clinical Trials* 1990;11:77–9.
8. Doll R. Development of controlled trials in preventive and therapeutic medicine. *Journal of Biosocial Science* 1991;23:365–78.
9. Doll R. Sir Austin Bradford Hill and the progress of medical science. *British Medical Journal* 1992;305:1521–6.
10. Ryan F. *Tuberculosis: The Greatest Story Never Told*. Bromsgrove, UK: Swift Publishers, Ltd.; 1992.
11. Bryder L. *Below the Magic Mountain: A Social History of Tuberculosis in Twentieth-Century Britain*. Oxford, England: Clarendon Press; 1988.
12. Hart PD'A. Chemotherapy of tuberculosis: Research during the past 100 years. Part I. *British Medical Journal* 1946;2:805–10.
13. Hart PD'A. Chemotherapy of tuberculosis: Research during the past 100 years. Part II. *British Medical Journal* 1946;2:849–55.
14. Smith B. Gullible's travails: Tuberculosis and quackery, 1890–1930. *Journal of Contemporary History* 1985;20:733–56.
15. Amberson JB, McMahon BT, Pinner M. A clinical trial of sanocrysin in pulmonary tuberculosis. *American Review of Tuberculosis* 1931;24:401–35.
16. Marks HM. *The Progress of Experiment: Science and Therapeutic Reform in the United States, 1900–1990*. New York, N.Y.: Cambridge University Press; 1997.
17. Trail RR, Stockman GD. After history and artificial pneumothorax: Comments on 91 successful and 31 unsuccessful cases. *Quarterly Journal of Medicine* 1932;1:415–24.
18. Brand W, Edwards PW, Hawthorne CO, Jessel G, Vere Pearson S, Powell DA, Sutherland DP, Watt J, Trail RR. The results of artificial pneumothorax treatment: Report to the Joint Tuberculosis Council on artificial pneumothorax. *Tubercle* 1937;18(suppl.).
19. Hinshaw HC, Feldman WH. Evaluation of chemotherapeutic agents in clinical tuberculosis: A suggested procedure. *American Review of Tuberculosis* 1944;50:202–13.
20. Hill AB. Principles of medical statistics: The aim of the statistical method. *Lancet* 1937;1:41–3.
21. Chalmers I. Comparing like with like: Some historical milestones in the evolution of methods to create unbiased comparison groups in therapeutic experiments. *International Journal of Epidemiology* 2001;30:1156–64.
22. Marks HM. Rigorous uncertainty: Why RA Fisher is important. *International Journal of Epidemiology* 2003;32:932–7.

23. Chalmers I. MRC Therapeutic Trials Committee's report on serum treatment of lobar pneumonia, BMJ 1934. The James Lind Library. [Online] 2002. Available: http://www.jameslindlibrary.org/trial_records/20th_Century/1930s/MRC_trials/mrc_commentary.pdf.

24. Armitage P. Quoted in: Chalmers I. Comparing like with like: Some historical milestones in the evolution of methods to create unbiased comparison groups in therapeutic experiments. *International Journal of Epidemiology* 2001;30:1156–64.

25. MRC Patulin Clinical Trials Committee. Clinical trial of patulin in the common cold. *Lancet* 1944;2:373–5.

26. Scadding JG. Sulphonamides in bacillary dysentery. *Lancet* 1945;2:549–53.

27. Chalmers I, Clarke M. The 1944 patulin trial: The first properly controlled multicentre trial conducted under the aegis of the British Medical Research Council. *International Journal of Epidemiology* 2004;32:253–60.

28. Chalmers I. Statistical theory was not the reason that randomization was used in the British Medical Research Council's clinical trial of streptomycin for pulmonary tuberculosis. In: Jorland G, Opinel A, Weisz G, eds. *Body Counts: Medical Quantification in Historical and Sociological Perspective.* Montreal & Kingston, Canada: McGill-Queen's University Press; 2005:309–34.

29. Theobald GW. Effect of calcium and vitamin A and D on incidence of pregnancy toxaemia. *Lancet* 1937;2:1397–9.

30. Fleming A. On the antibacterial action of cultures of a penicillium, with special reference to their use in the isolation of H influenzae. *British Journal of Experimental Pathology* 1929;10:226–36.

31. Hobby GL. *Penicillin: Meeting the Challenge.* New Haven, Conn.: Yale University Press; 1985.

32. Adams DP. *"The Greatest Good to the Greatest Number": Penicillin Rationing on the American Home Front, 1940–1945.* New York, N.Y.: Peter Lang; 1991.

33. Green FHK. The clinical evaluation of remedies. *Lancet* 1954;2:1085–90.

34. Schatz A, Bugie E, and Waksman SA. Streptomycin, a substance exhibiting antibiotic activity against gram-positive and gram-negative bacteria. *Proceedings of the Society for Experimental Biology and Medicine* 1944;55:66–9.

35. Wainwright M. *Miracle Cure: The Story of Penicillin and the Golden Age of Antibiotics.* Oxford, U.K.: Blackwell; 1990.

36. Porter RW. Streptomycin: Engineered into commercial production. *Chemical Engineering* 1946;53(10):94–8, 142–5.

37. [Raistrick H, Keep TB.] Streptomycin. Unpublished [circa May 1946]. MH58/636, Public Record Office (PRO), London.

38. Feldman WH, Hinshaw HC, Mann FC. Streptomycin in experimental tuberculosis. *American Review of Tuberculosis* 1945;52:269–98.

39. Hinshaw HC, Feldman WH. Streptomycin in treatment of clinical tuberculosis: A preliminary report. *Proceedings of the Weekly Staff Meeting of the Mayo Clinic* 1945;20:313–8.

40. Keefer CS. Streptomycin in the treatment of infections: A report of one thousand cases. Part 1. *JAMA* 1946;132:4–11.

41. Keefer CS. Streptomycin in the treatment of infections: A report of one thousand cases. Part 2. *JAMA* 1946;132:70–7.

42. Veterans Administration. The effect of streptomycin upon pulmonary tuberculosis: preliminary report of a cooperative study of 223 patients by the Army, Navy, and Veterans Administration. *American Review of Tuberculosis* 1947;56:485–507.

43. Reimann HA, Elias WF, Price AH. Streptomycin for typhoid: A pharmacologic study. *JAMA* 1945;128:175–80.

44. Garrod LP to Green FHK, 10 Sep 1945, FD1/6760, PRO.

45. Richards AN to Mellanby E, 13 Apr 1946, FD1/6751, PRO.

46. Yoshioka A. *Streptomycin, 1946: British Central Administration of Supplies of a New Drug of American Origin, with Special Reference to Clinical Trials in Tuberculosis* [PhD thesis]. London, UK: Imperial College, London; 1998.

47. Minutes of Conference, 29 Jul 1946, FD1/6756, PRO.

48. Minutes of meeting, 4 Aug 1946, FD1/6756, PRO.

49. Minutes of Conference, 27 August 1946, FD1/6756, PRO.

50. Extract from Council minutes, 18 Oct 1946, FD1/6764, PRO.

51. Minutes of Streptomycin Clinical Trials (Tuberculosis) Committee, 21 November 1946, FD1/6756, PRO.

52. Holme CI. Trial by TB: A study into current attempts to control the international upsurge in tuberculosis. *Proceedings of the Royal College of Physicians of Edinburgh* 1997;27(suppl. 4):1–53.

53. Distribution of streptomycin [leading article]. *Lancet* 1947;1:833.

54. Streptomycin. Stencilled statement, 8 Oct 1946, FD1/6760.

55. Cable to H.M. Representative, 11 Oct 1946, copied in FD1/6760, PRO.

56. Hill AB. The clinical trial. *British Medical Bulletin* 1951;7:278–82.

57. Hill AB. The clinical trial. *New England Journal of Medicine* 1952;247:113–9.

58. Doll R. Clinical trials: Retrospect and prospect. *Statistics in Medicine* 1982;1:337–44.

59. Armitage P. The role of randomisation in clinical trials. *Statistics in Medicine* 1982;1:345–52.

60. Yoshioka A. Use of randomisation in the Medical Research Council's clinical trial of streptomycin in pulmonary tuberculosis in the 1940s. *British Medical Journal* 1998;317:1220–3.

61. The controlled therapeutic trial [editorial]. *British Medical Journal* 1948;2:791–2.

62. Daniels M. Clinical evaluation of chemotherapy in tuberculosis. *British Medical Bulletin* 1951;7:320–6.

63. Krafchik LL. Tuberculous meningitis treated with streptomycin. *JAMA* 1946;132:375–6.

64. Medical Research Council Streptomycin in Tuberculosis Trials Committee. Streptomycin in acute miliary tuberculosis. *Lancet* 1950;1:841–6.

65. Medical Research Council Streptomycin in Tuberculosis Trials Committee. Streptomycin in tuberculous meningitis. *Lancet* 1948;1:582–96.

66. Streptomycin Clinical Trials (Non-Tuberculous) Conditions Committee, minutes of sixth meeting, 26 Jan 1948, FD1/7943, PRO.

67. Streptomycin Clinical Trials (Non-Tuberculous) Conditions Committee, minutes of first meeting, 6 Dec 1946, FD1/7943, PRO.

68. Case record summary, MRC.47/241A, 8 May 1947, FD1/7943, PRO.

69. Streptomycin Clinical Trials (Non-Tuberculous) Conditions Committee, minutes of second meeting, 4 Mar 1947, FD1/7943, PRO.

70. Streptomycin Clinical Trials (Non-Tuberculous) Conditions Committee, minutes of fourth meeting, 2 May 1947, FD1/7943, PRO.

71. Note of a meeting held at the Treasury on 29 Apr 1947, FD1/6752, PRO.

72. Green FHK to Everett FC, 10 Jun 1947, FD1/6752, PRO.

73. Interim Report of the M.R.C. Sub-Committee for Therapeutic Trials of Streptomycin in Non-Tuberculous Infections, MRC.48/190, 1 Apr 1948, FD1/7943, PRO.

74. Wilson C. Streptomycin in non-tuberculous conditions. *British Medical Journal* 1948;2:552–3.

75. Wilson C. Streptomycin in non-tuberculous conditions. *Lancet* 1948;2:445–6.

76. Ware M to Wilson C, 19 May 1950, FD1/7944, PRO.

77. Youmans GP, Williston EH, Feldman WH, Hinshaw HC. Increase in resistance of tubercle bacilli to streptomycin: A preliminary report. *Proceedings of the Weekly Staff Meeting of the Mayo Clinic* 1946;21:126–7.

78. Ministry of Health. Streptomycin available on prescription. *British Medical Journal* 1949;2:752.

79. Chalmers I, chair. Fisher and Bradford Hill: A discussion. *International Journal of Epidemiology* 2003;32:945–8.

80. Scadding JG. Address for memorial service for Geoffrey Marshall, unpublished; 1983.

81. Lilford RJ, Jackson J. Equipoise and the ethics of randomization. *Journal of the Royal Society of Medicine* 1995;88:552–9.

82. Bastian H. Down and almost out in Scotland: George Orwell, tuberculosis and getting streptomycin in 1948. The James Lind Library. [Online] 2004. Available: http://www.jameslindlibrary.org/trial_records/20th_Century/1940s/MRC_bmj/bastian.pdf.

83. Keers RY. Streptomycin in pulmonary tuberculosis: report on ten cases. *Lancet* 1948;2:449–51.

84. Weindling P. Human guinea pigs and the ethics of experimentation: The BMJ's correspondent at the Nuremberg medical trial. *British Medical Journal* 1996;313:1467–70.

85. Faden RR, Beauchamp TL, with King NMP. *A History and Theory of Informed Consent.* New York, N.Y.: Oxford University Press; 1986.

86. Yoshioka A. Streptomycin in postwar Britain: A cultural history of a miracle drug. In: van Heteren GM, Gijswijt-Hofstra M, Tansey EM, eds. *Biographies of Remedies: Drugs, Medicines and Contraceptives in Dutch and Anglo-American Healing Cultures* (Clio Medica/The Wellcome Series in the History of Medicine, Vol. 66). Amsterdam, The Netherlands: Rodopi; 2002:203–27.

87. Hinshaw HC, Feldman WH, Pfuetze KH. Treatment of tuberculosis with streptomycin: A summary of observations on one hundred cases. *JAMA* 1946;132:778–82.

88. Streptomycin: The present position [annotation]. *British Medical Journal* 1946;2:906.

89. Green FHK to Murphy GE, 10 Dec 1946, FD1/6756, PRO.

90. Streptomycin. *Times of London* Jan. 23, 1947.

91. Streptomycin in tuberculosis [leading article]. *Lancet* 1947;1:144–5.

92. Madigan DG, Swift PN, Brownlee G. Clinical and pharmacological aspects of the toxicity of streptomycin. *Lancet* 1947;1:9–11.

93. Green FHK to Under-Secretary of State, Foreign Office, 16 Apr 1947, FD1/6769, PRO.

94. Waksman SA. *The Conquest of Tuberculosis.* Berkeley, Calif.: University of California Press; 1964.

95. Ministry of Health. Streptomycin in tuberculous meningitis: Ministry report. *Lancet* 1950;2:230–1.

96. Streptomycin in Tuberculous Trials Committee, minutes of second meeting, 18 Apr 1947, FD1/6756, PRO.

97. Report of the Medical Research Council for the years 1948–50, Cmd 8387. *Parliamentary Papers* 1950–51;xvi:1–218.

98. Tansey EM. Philip Montagu D'Arcy Hart, CBE, FRCP, Hon FmedSci. The James Lind Library. [Online] 2004. Available: http://www.jameslindlibrary.org/trial_records/20th_Century/1940s/MRC_lancet_1944/hart_biog.pdf.

99. Hart PD'A. The MRC and tuberculosis research. *MRC News* 1988;41:19–21.

100. Marshall EK, Merrill M. Clinical therapeutic trial of a new drug. *Bulletin of the Johns Hopkins Hospital* 1949;85:221–30.

101. Dowling HF. *Fighting Infection: Conquests of the Twentieth Century.* Cambridge, Mass.: Harvard University Press; 1979.

102. Armitage P. Bradford Hill and the randomized controlled trial. *Pharmaceutical Medicine* 1992;6:23–37.

103. Armitage P. Before and after Bradford Hill: Some trends in medical statistics. *Journal of the Royal Statistical Society A* 1995;158:143–53.

104. Moher D, Schulz KF, Altman DG, for the CONSORT Group. The CONSORT statement: Revised recommendations for improving the quality of reports of parallel-group randomised trials. *Lancet* 2001;357:1191–4.

105. International Conference on Harmonisation. E9: Statistical principles for clinical trials. *Federal Register* 1998;63(179):49583–98.

106. Clarke M. Systematic reviews and the Cochrane Collaboration. [Online] 22 April 2004. Available: http://www.cochrane.org/docs/whycc.htm.

107. Epstein S. *Impure Science: AIDS, Activism, and the Politics of Knowledge.* Berkeley, Calif.: University of California Press; 1996.

Marcia L. Meldrum

The Salk Polio Vaccine Field Trial of 1954

Epidemiology of Polio

In the first half of the 20th century, poliomyelitis meant long summers of fear and suffering for families living in the United States. The disease, hardly recognized before the 20th century, had become a significant danger to children and to general quality of life, especially in the post–World War II era. The epidemiological work of John Paul, Thomas Francis, Dorothy Horstmann, and others had only recently shown that the apparent increased danger of the infection was directly related to modern American affluence. In less prosperous, less sanitized times and places, babies usually contracted the polio, or infantile paralysis, virus early in life, while still protected by their mother's immune system. In the postwar United States, a whole generation was growing up healthy, well nourished and often bottle-fed, protected from infection until they began nursery school. But these practices left them defenseless against polio virus.[1] Although the incidence of the paralytic form of the disease was quite low, it was disproportionately high among young, middle-class children. As prosperity increased, so did crippling and death; for Americans, polio took on the face of a fearful plague. In 1948, polio incidence had risen to 19 per 100,000 people in the population, the highest since the horrible epidemic of 1916. In 1949, it rose again to 28.3 per 100,000.[2]

Early Research on Vaccines

The most famous polio victim had been Franklin D. Roosevelt, who contracted the disease in the 1920s, before becoming president. In the mid-1930s, he had launched an annual Birthday Ball

to raise funds for his favorite rehabilitation resort in Warm Springs, Ga., and recruited his former law partner, Basil O'Connor, to head the effort. The Birthday Ball Commission proved far more successful than anticipated; in 1934, the event brought in more than $1 million, much more than was needed for Warm Springs. O'Connor recruited some scientific advisers to help disburse the surplus. Some of the windfall funds were given to William H. Park, the respected director of the Bureau of Laboratories of the New York Health Department, and his young associate Maurice Brodie, for development of a killed-virus poliomyelitis vaccine—even though the virus had not been fully identified and cultured at this time.[3,4]

Park and Brodie produced their vaccine by exposing infected monkey tissue to formalin to inactivate its pathogenicity. In 1935, it was tested on more than 7,000 children without ill effects, except for some localized reactions to the injection.[5] In the same year, another experimenter, John Kolmer of Temple University, referred to his polio vaccine as "attenuated." He chopped the monkey tissue very fine and treated it with what some called a chemical "witch's brew."[6] At the same meeting of the American Public Health Association where Brodie presented his data, Kolmer reported on the vaccination of 10,725 people, mostly children. He stated that the vaccine was "probably safe." Yet 10 of the children given his preparation had contracted polio and 5 had died, an incidence higher than that of the natural disease.[7]

Both Brodie and Kolmer met with scathing attacks from the small community of U.S. virologists, led by Thomas Rivers of the Rockefeller Institute and James Leake of the U.S. Public Health Service (PHS). In their view, killed-virus polio vaccine was scientifically impossible. Any such preparation would either be "reasonably safe but ineffective," as Rivers described the Park-Brodie product, or itself pathogenic, as Kolmer's appeared to be.[8,9] As Rivers' Rockefeller colleagues, Peter Olitsky and Herald Cox, had reported, "If these chemicals did not act a sufficient time, the vaccine by itself could produce polio in monkeys; if they . . . killed the virus, no immunity, except rarely, was induced."[4]

Despite these discouraging events, O'Connor did not stop supporting research, but he shifted the focus away from vaccines. In 1938, the Birthday Ball Commission was reorganized as the National Foundation for Infantile Paralysis (NFIP), popularly nicknamed the March of Dimes, "to lead, direct, and unify the fight on every phase of this sickness," Roosevelt announced.[3,10] Volunteer chapters, established in each of the nation's 3,608 counties, organized the annual "Mothers' March" to collect dimes and quarters from their neighbors. Half of the funds raised were returned to the chapters to be used primarily for the care of polio victims.[3] The emphasis on grass roots organization built strong loyalties to the NFIP. The volunteers said of it, "It's always the little people" and "you have the feeling of belonging . . . that it's *our* organization."[11]

Foundation Sponsorship of Basic Research

What funds were left, after the costs of medical care, publicity, and administration were covered, were given to research. O'Connor set up a new Committee on Scientific Research in 1938, later the Committee on Virus Research and Epidemiology, with Rivers at its head. Under his leadership, the Committee emphasized gradual progress through basic virological research. Rivers said later:

> We actually knew very little about the nature of poliovirus. . . . [O]ften we didn't know what questions to ask. . . . [I]f we wanted answers to problems in polio and they were not forthcoming, it might be to our advantage to study related viruses where we had better information and techniques. . . . I never minded broad gauged grants if they in any way furthered our knowledge of virus disease.[4]

The NFIP was the only major sponsor of poliomyelitis research in the 1940s and 1950s, although never able to offer more than $1 million in one year before 1949. This crucial funding made possible several major achievements.[12] One of these was the demonstration, by David Bodian of Johns Hopkins University, that there were in fact three distinct types, or strains, of polio virus. In the late 1940s, the Foundation supported the painstaking type identification of each of the several hundred polio cultures maintained in various laboratories around the country.[4]

A few years later, in 1949, John Enders, Thomas Weller, and Frederick Robbins at Harvard University cultured polio virus for the first time in nonnervous tissue; if the virus could grow outside the nervous system, then a vaccine that generated antibodies in the blood prior to infection could theoretically prevent the disease from reaching the brain and causing paralysis.[13] At the same time, Isabel Morgan of Johns Hopkins reported to the NFIP Research Committee that she had inactivated all three types of polio virus with formalin and successfully immunized monkeys against a pathogenic dose injected directly into the brain.[14] About Morgan's results Rivers said, "Most virologists believed that you couldn't immunize against poliomyelitis with a formalin-inactivated poliovirus. She converted us, and that was quite a feat."[4]

The subject of polio vaccines had now been reopened at the Committee's regular round table conferences. By 1951, a number of experiments were in progress: inactivation with formalin and ultraviolet light; passive immunization through the use of gamma globulin prepared from the blood of convalescent cases, urged by William Hammon of the University of Pittsburgh; and culturing of live virus to try to isolate an "attenuated" mutant that, in a vaccine preparation, would confer lasting immunity through a subclinical infection. This live-virus work was pursued by Hilary Koprowski and Herald Cox, then at Lederle Laboratories, and by Albert Sabin at the University of Cincinnati.[15] The Foundation created a special Immunization Committee, with the immediate objective of advising O'Connor on Hammon's trials of gamma globulin.[4,16,17] The year that followed, 1952, was the worst polio year in a series of "worsts." The disease struck 57,879 people, an incidence of 37.2 per 100,000, and 2,500 people died.[2]

Jonas Salk's Killed-Virus Vaccine

Jonas Salk had been supported by NFIP grants since completing his medical residency, first working on influenza with Thomas Francis at the University of Michigan, then in his own lab at Pittsburgh, where he had participated in the exacting and tedious "scut work" of poliovirus typing.[4,11] He had become convinced that rigorous treatment with heat and formalin could produce a viral culture that was no longer pathogenic but still triggered the production of antibodies, which he argued were not just the by-products, but the agents of immunity.[18] During 1952, he tested an inactivated vaccine on 161 children: first on paralyzed polio survivors living at the Watson Home near Pittsburgh, then on mentally retarded children at the Polk State School. These tests were done with parental and institutional consent; all the children's guardians thought it appropriate for the unfortunates to make their small contribution to society. "We just enjoyed being part of the project," said the Watson Home administrator.[19] Salk had given injections to himself, his staff, and his own young sons as well (see Figure 5.1). On January 23, 1953, he presented his results to the NFIP's Immunization Committee. The vaccinated children had shown no ill effects; their antibody titers had risen demonstrably.[20]

Events then moved swiftly. On January 26, 1953, the Foundation announced to the press and public that it would conduct field trials of this new vaccine within a year.[21] On February 26, a special meeting chaired by Rivers recommended as a first step that Salk begin safety trials on another 500 to 600 children in the Pittsburgh area.[22] On May 25, O'Connor appointed a new seven-member Vaccine Advisory Committee to take over supervision of the field trial project; it included only three members of the Immunization Committee and only two virologists, Rivers and Joseph Smadel of Walter Reed Army Medical Center.[4]

The decision to proceed to a national field trial was considered precipitous by many members of the Immunization Committee, particularly Enders and Sabin.[23] Enders called Salk's work "most encouraging" but argued that "the ideal immunizing agent against any virus infection should consist of a living agent exhibiting a degree of virulence so low that it may be inoculated without risk."[24] Cox agreed: "The most logical and practical way to immunize infants and children against poliomyelitis is to follow the pattern that seems to take place so universally under natural conditions."[25] In their view, Salk should continue with limited

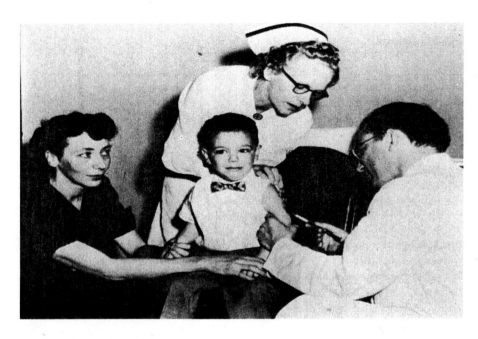

Figure 5.1. Donna Salk, Jonas Salk's wife (at left), and an unidentified nurse, help as Jonas Salk administers his polio vaccine to their son, Jonathan, on May 16, 1953. Source: © The March of Dimes. Reproduced with permission.

tests that would contribute to the growing fund of knowledge on polio vaccine. But only an attenuated or live-virus preparation, developed through natural mutation, would possess the essential attributes of safety and lasting efficacy for use in a mass vaccination program.

Salk, his mentor Francis, and Bodian, among others, disagreed. Killed-virus vaccine stimulated antibody production and, if there were no remaining trace of live virus, it was clearly safer than any natural variant that could mutate in succeeding generations. The live-virus advocates were arguing, Francis said, for "some undesignated advantage derived from apparently harmless infection" that they could not define.[26] To his biographer, Richard Carter, Salk spoke with more passion: "What had once been skepticism about attempts to develop an effective killed vaccine was now becoming ideological conflict. . . . How could a killed vaccine contain the magical life force of the natural disease—its élan vital?"[19] But proof that killed-virus vaccine would be both safe and effective would require what Isabel Morgan had called "a vast human experiment" in which "no risk whatsoever would be justified."[27]

O'Connor and Rivers recognized that they were in fact taking a significant risk, against the counsel of many of their own expert advisers. But by June 30, 1953, the World Health Organization had reported that polio incidence in the United States was 17% above the 1952 figure.[28] The National Foundation was answerable first to its grass roots base, its volunteers and small contributors. They wanted their children protected against polio and they did not care if killed-virus vaccine was not "the ideal immunizing agent." If Salk's further tests provided sufficient evidence of safety, then the gamble had to be taken.[4,19]

Debates Over the Field Trial Design

The National Foundation faced many hurdles in designing its massive field trial. The major tasks involved were: (1) selection of the trial design; (2) selection of the field trial population; (3) obtaining parental consent; (4) production of a consistently safe vaccine product in sufficient quantity; (5) recruitment and coor-

dination of the volunteers needed to vaccinate the children, screen for signs of polio, and maintain records; and, (6) systematic collection and accurate tabulation of the outcome data. Of these, the trial design was the most crucial and problematic.

The NFIP's Vaccine Advisory Committee supported a randomized and blinded clinical trial with a control group receiving an injection of placebo.[4] However, both Salk and O'Connor thought that such a trial would be too complicated and risky. Salk wrote an emotional letter to O'Connor on October 16, 1953: "The use of a placebo control, I am afraid, is a fetish of orthodoxy and would serve to create a 'beautiful epidemiologic' experiment over which the epidemiologist could become quite ecstatic but would make the humanitarian shudder."[19] No such trial had ever been carried out on healthy children and there were no government regulations prescribing the methodology. The first large-scale, randomized, placebo-controlled trial had been carried out with streptomycin in British tuberculosis patients in 1947, and the relative scarcity of the drug in the United Kingdom at that time had forestalled ethical concerns over the design[29,30] (see Chapter 4). A placebo-controlled trial on many thousands of children was considered to be difficult to administer and to present to anxious parents.

O'Connor announced on November 9, 1953, that the vaccine would be given to second grade children, whereas their first and third grade schoolmates would serve as unvaccinated "observed-controls."[31,32] Ten days later, Hart van Riper, the NFIP medical director, wrote to the chief public health officers in every state, requesting information on the numbers of children, of schools, and of recent polio cases by age in counties of historic high incidence.[33] By December 9, he had received enthusiastic responses from 38 states and the District of Columbia, as well as "a large volume of unsolicited offers of assistance."[34] Through January 1954, the plan continued to call for the use of observed controls.

However, Rivers and the Vaccine Advisory Committee knew that this study design would not achieve their goal. Such a trial might establish that the Salk vaccine was *safe,* but not that it was definitely effective against polio. The disease might be light among second-graders that year, or physicians might misdiagnose doubtful cases, based on their knowledge that the child had or had not

Table 5.1
Salk Polio Vaccine Field Trial Timeline

Date	Event
1789	First clinical description of polio by British physician Michael Underwood
1894	First small epidemic in the United States, in Vermont
1908	Polio virus isolated by Karl Landsteiner and Erwin Popper
1916	Major epidemic kills several thousand in United States
1921	Franklin D. Roosevelt stricken and left paralyzed
1934	First "President's Birthday Ball" for Polio
1935	Kolmer and Park-Brodie vaccines fail to prevent paralysis
1938	National Foundation for Infantile Paralysis established, led by Basil O'Connor; Research Committee chaired by Thomas Rivers
1948	Polio incidence is 19/100,000
1948	Isabel Morgan first reports immunization of monkeys with killed-poliovirus vaccine
1949	Polio incidence is 28.3/100,000
1949	Enders, Weller and Robbins culture poliovirus in non-nervous human tissue
1951	Polio incidence is 18.5/100,000
1951–52	Gamma globulin field trials carried out by William Hammon
1952	Polio incidence is 37.2/100,000; 2500 die
1952	Jonas Salk tests his killed-virus vaccine at Watson Home and Polk State School
1953	Polio incidence is 22.5/100,000
Jan. 1953	Salk reports his tests to NFIP Immunization Committee
Jan. 1953	Foundation announces plans for national field trial of new vaccine
May 1953	Foundation creates new Vaccine Advisory Committee
Oct. 1953	Target counties selected for field trial
Nov. 1953	Foundation announces field trial will take place in spring 1954
Jan. 1954	Thomas Francis meets with state health officers
Feb. 1954	Francis appointed to head Vaccine Evaluation Center
Feb. 1954	Salk begins testing commercial vaccine in Pittsburgh
Mar. 1954	"Manual of Suggested Procedures" goes out to state health departments and to Foundation volunteers
Mar. 1954	Parents receive request form and O'Connor letter
Apr. 4 1954	Walter Winchell broadcast warns that vaccine may *cause* polio
Apr. 25 1954	Vaccine Advisory Committee recommends that field trial proceed
Apr. 26 1954	Vaccinations begin in first 8 states
June 1954	Vaccinations end and observation period begins
Jan. 1955	Codes broken at VEC
Mar. 9 1955	Last completed report on suspected polio case arrives at VEC
Apr. 12 1955	Francis presents summary report and announces vaccine is 80–90% effective against paralytic polio; Public Health Service immediately licenses vaccine
Apr. 25 1955	First child falls ill after receiving Cutter-manufactured vaccine
May 7 1955	Vaccination programs suspended
May 14 1955	Vaccinations resume with Parke-Davis vaccine
June 7 1955	Surgeon General Leonard Scheele appears on national television to announce new manufacturing standards and continuation of vaccinations
1956	Polio incidence is 9.1/100,000 (15,140 cases)
Late 1956	75% of children ages 5–12 have received injections of Salk vaccine
1958–59	Albert Sabin's attenuated-virus vaccine in field trials outside the United States
1961	Sabin vaccine licensed and quickly replaces Salk in clinical practice
2000	CDC recommends return to sole use of improved killed-virus vaccine

been vaccinated. Only a placebo-controlled trial would be strong enough evidence to pacify the scientific critics and to get the vaccine licensed and widely distributed. Several state health officers were supportive of a placebo-control design, but they were also doubtful of the Foundation's ability to evaluate its own field trial objectively.

On November 16, 1953, O'Connor and van Riper asked Francis, a highly respected virologist and backer of the killed-virus concept, to direct an independent evaluation of the field trial, supported by NFIP funds.[35,36] "I think I shall do it," Francis wrote in a letter on Dec. 29, but before he took the job, he recruited the support of key state health officers for a randomized, placebo-controlled study.[37] He identified those states that had well-organized and professionally respected health departments. In January 1954, he convened a series of crucial meetings in which leading officials of these health departments endorsed a placebo-control plan in 12 states and agreed that those areas would have "priority on available vaccine" if supplies should run short.[38,39] He was formally appointed director of the Vaccine Evaluation Center (VEC) to be established at the University of Michigan, on February 9, 1954.[40] Five days later, the Foundation announced that both observed-control and placebo-control trials would be conducted, and that "a combination of the two procedures [would] assure a valid evaluation of the trial vaccine."[41] "The best Departments are committed to this [placebo-control] plan," Francis noted.[42] The placebo-control study remained his primary focus throughout the three years that followed.

The Field Trial Protocol

But the observed-control trials were not a sideshow to the main event. Thirty-six states were tied to that plan, and they, too, were necessary to the field trial. To succeed in legitimizing killed-virus vaccine, the Foundation needed both scientific evidence and widespread public support. It was essential that the trial be a massive national event, ensuring a high level of public participation and commitment.

The field trial population had to be large and demographically diverse, to ensure a representative sample. Moreover, because natural polio incidence was quite low but disproportionately high in children aged 6 to 11, these were the only individuals in whom a trial was likely to be statistically valid. In October 1953, Gabriel Stickle, the Foundation's statistician, and medical consultant Thomas Dublin had made a careful selection of those U.S. counties with total populations above 50,000 that had the highest case rates (at least 2.6 cases per 10,000) for the previous five years. These 272 counties, at least 1 in every state, were targeted as trial areas.[43,44]

To be eligible for the trial, the targeted children in the selected counties would have to be identified, recruited, and delivered to central locations for vaccination; the most efficient way to accomplish this was through the primary schools. Consequently, Van Riper excluded preschool children from the study, although they were a higher risk group than their older siblings. He may also have thought the younger children would entail a higher emotional cost.[45]

In the observed-control areas, only those in the second grade would be recruited for vaccination; parents of first- and third-graders would be asked to sign forms requesting that their children participate as controls. In the placebo-control areas, parents of children in all three grades would be asked to allow their children to participate. This arm of the trial was to be double-blinded. Enrolled children would receive injections of vaccine or placebo from one of a pair of coded vials on "V-Day," and follow-up shots at one and five weeks. None of the teachers leading the children, the physicians giving the shots, nor the NFIP volunteers checking off the names, would know which vials contained vaccine.[46] The codes were not broken at the VEC until January 1955.[47]

The health officers at the January meetings had drawn up the full protocol with the guidance of Francis and statisticians William Cochran and Hugo Muench. A randomly chosen 2% of each group, including the observed-controls, would have blood samples drawn before and after the injections, and again in the fall, to check antibody levels. The health departments, with Foundation assistance, would keep track of suspected polio cases among all the different groups of children. Because many illnesses could resemble a nonparalytic case of polio, each small patient was to be evaluated by a complex set of diagnostic procedures, including blood samples for antibody titers, fecal testing for virus, and muscle evaluation for paralysis. Ten regional laboratories were enlisted to conduct the blinded analyses of the blood and stool samples.[39,47]

Volunteer Collaborators in the Vaccine Field Trial

The National Foundation had been built on volunteer contributions and public support; these were O'Connor's greatest assets and he intended to capitalize on them to ensure the success of the field trial. Foundation staff lavished the same concern on the observed-control trials as on the placebo-control series, which Francis preferred. Planning and publicity endlessly highlighted the importance of the local volunteer chapters, local schools, local parents' groups, and local health departments. The "Manual of Suggested Procedures," issued to the local NFIP chapters and health departments in March 1954, stressed that "the Local Health Officer who wisely utilizes the many volunteers [sic] services [of the chapters] will not only relieve himself and his staff of many burdens but . . . make it possible for many devoted chapter volunteers to have a rewarding satisfaction that comes from taking an intimate part in this great scientific undertaking."[46]

Similarly, when Foundation staff met with state chapter representatives that month, they emphasized that the volunteers' role was to defer to and assist the health officers as needed, while working "to ensure maximum public acceptance and participation in the test areas."[48] The volunteers were to coordinate all the local publicity, the distribution and collection of patient permission forms, and the organization of vaccination centers at the schools. The health departments would give the injections, collect the blood samples, and oversee the evaluation of possible polio cases in the study population.[39,47]

O'Connor's Letter to Parents

The most crucial support needed for the field trials was the consent of the children's parents. Each child brought home from school, four to five weeks before "V-Day," a request form with a carefully worded one-page message from Basil O'Connor. "A vaccine which may protect children against polio is now being tested by your National Foundation for Infantile Paralysis," the letter to the observed-control areas began. "Thousands of children in selected communities will be given the chance of receiving this vaccine. . . . Your child and his classmates have been selected to take part in this great scientific test."[48] O'Connor's letter explained that some children would be vaccinated, whereas others would simply be observed, and that some blood samples would be taken; that the choice of children for each part of the trial "will conform to a nation-wide plan"; and that all roles were "equally important to the study." The strongest emphasis was laid on the fact that "THE VACCINE WILL BE GIVEN ONLY ON REQUEST OF PARENTS"; but the letter also stated that parental request did not guarantee that a child would receive any vaccine. No specific risks or benefits of participation were mentioned. "This is one of the most important projects in medical history. . . . We feel sure you will want your child to take part."[46] The request form itself briefly outlined the procedures again and emphasized the importance of all participants. It described the vaccine as "chemically killed poliomyelitis virus of all three known types." Parents were asked to request that their child "be vaccinated if selected, or otherwise be permitted to participate in the procedures described above without cost to me."[46]

Vaccine Supply Issues

The remaining major concern for the organizers was an adequate supply of safe vaccine. Vaccine produced in Salk's own laboratory had been tested by this time on many people without ill effect. Albert Milzer and Sidney Levinson of the University of Chicago, however, reported that they were unable to inactivate polio virus using Salk's guidelines. NFIP Medical Director van Riper, speaking for the Foundation, said that Milzer and Levinson could not have been using Salk's "exact methods."[49] But the five commercial firms chosen to manufacture vaccine for the field trial also found it difficult to replicate his results, particularly as Salk kept revising his process to get a better balance between safety and antigenicity. Each commercial batch was tested on monkeys three times for live virus: at the manufacturing plant, at Salk's Pittsburgh lab, and by the PHS.[50] Several animals sickened and died after injection with commercial vaccine in these tests. Only Parke–Davis and Eli Lilly had managed to produce several consecutive batches that passed the safety screenings before the trials began. The other firms selected were Cutter, Pitman-Moore, and Wyeth.[4]

The Vaccine Advisory Committee insisted that Salk test the commercial products on a pilot group of 5,000 Pittsburgh children, causing further delays. The trials were postponed until late March and then to late April.[4,51] Anxieties persisted until the day before the field trials began; some state health officers wavered about the risks, whereas others were unsure whether there would be sufficient vaccine supplies.[52]

April 1954: The Acid Test

On April 4, 1954, citing the reports of live virus found in the commercial batches, Walter Winchell made his famous announcement on nationwide radio that the Salk vaccine "may be a killer!" Anxious letters and telegrams arrived in Ann Arbor and in Washington from one state health department and medical society after another.[53–55] Salk, O'Connor, and Francis did their best to placate the fearful. The PHS laboratory insisted indignantly that it would never release any batch of vaccine if live virus were found. Minnesota was the only state to withdraw from the trials as a result of this incident; some individual counties also declined. North Carolina tried to withdraw, but public pressure forced state officials to re-enlist. Most of the states and counties, and all the NFIP volunteer chapters, remained committed to proceed.[52,56–59]

On Sunday, April 25, 1954, the NFIP's Vaccine Advisory Committee met in Washington and nervously but unanimously approved the Salk vaccine for "carefully controlled vaccine studies," noting that it was the result of "a broad program of scientific research . . . supported financially by the American people." The Vaccine Advisory Committee also recommended that the National Foundation "assume the administrative and financial responsibility for the trials."[4,60] The following day, April 26, 1954, Dublin confirmed to Francis by telegram that vaccinations had begun in 4 observed-control sites and 10 placebo-control areas.[61] Arizona, Maryland, and the District of Columbia had to withdraw when early school closings ended easy access to the student population. Georgia also left the ranks when polio broke out there before vaccinations could begin. The remaining 44 states, with 84 placebo-control and 127 observed-control areas, stayed with the research design, namely, three injections at zero, one, and five weeks, with blood samples drawn from 2% of both test subjects and consenting controls for antibody titers.[62]

Overall, as calculated and detailed in Francis's Summary Report, the field trials also passed the acid test of parent support for participation. The eligible population of the first three grades in the 11 placebo-control states was 749,236. The parents of 455,474, or 60.8%, returned the request forms, asking that their children participate as "Polio Pioneers." A small percentage of these did not attend the first clinic, missed follow-up injections, or received in error a mixed series of vaccine and placebo. Ultimately, 401,974 children, or 53.7% of the study population, completed the full series of coded injections, divided almost precisely between vaccine (200,745) and placebo (201,229).[47]

The study population in the 33 observed-control states was 1,080,260 in the first three grades; 355,527 were in the second grade, the group designated for vaccination. The parents of this group requested participation at a higher rate, 69.2%, or 245,895 children, than did those in the placebo-control study. Of those whose parents made the request, 221,998 children, 62.4% of the second graders in the 33 areas, and 20.5% of the total observed-control population, received the full three injections of vaccine.[47]

Collecting the Data

As the trials continued into June, momentum and morale seemed to build. Several states arranged for special school openings for the second and third shots.[63] Health officers were impressed by "the remarkable cooperation of the public"; the willingness of so many to participate "instilled complete confidence in the field trial."[64] Press reports noted that the children themselves were enjoying their important role: "They were glad to be shot as pioneers."[65]

THE NATIONAL FOUNDATION FOR INFANTILE PARALYSIS
FRANKLIN D. ROOSEVELT, FOUNDER

120 BROADWAY
NEW YORK 5, N.Y.

BASIL O'CONNOR   BEEKMAN 3-0500
PRESIDENT

A MESSAGE TO PARENTS:

A vaccine which may protect children against polio is now being tested by your National Foundation for Infantile Paralysis with the cooperation of local health and educational authorities and of the medical profession.

Thousands of children in selected communities will be given the chance of receiving this vaccine to test its effectiveness. At least an equal number of children who do not receive the vaccine will be observed so that a comparison can be made between the two groups.

In certain instances it will be necessary to test small samples of blood before and after the vaccine is given to determine its effect. Samples from some of the children who are not vaccinated will also be necessary for comparison.

Your child and his classmates have been selected to take part in this great scientific test.

After the next polio season, records of all the children will be studied to determine whether those who received the vaccine were protected against infantile paralysis.

The choice of the children in your community who are to be vaccinated will conform to a nation-wide plan. Some children will receive the vaccine and some will not. The children in each group, those who receive the vaccine and those who do not, are equally important to the study.

Please read and sign the enclosed request form and return it promptly to your child's teacher. If you request participation, your child may be among those receiving the vaccine.

THE VACCINE WILL BE GIVEN ONLY ON REQUEST OF PARENTS. Remember that the vaccine must be given three times. One or two doses will not be enough to test its effectiveness.

This is one of the most important projects in medical history. Its success depends on the cooperation of parents. We feel sure your will want your child to take part.

Sincerely yours,

Basil O'Connor
President

Figure 5.2. Letter From Basil O'Connor to Parents. Source: Thomas Francis Papers, Manual of Suggested Procedures for the Conduct of the Vaccine Field Trial in 1954, Bentley Historical Library, University of Michigan. Reproduced with permission of the March of Dimes, White Plains, N.Y.

The enthusiasm of the volunteers and participants did not ensure complete and accurate data. Despite visits of Francis and his VEC statistical staff to 32 states during the trials and numerous instructional memoranda, the completed vaccination and blood sampling schedules were late in arriving in Ann Arbor.[47,66] By the end of September, 8,000 schedules were still outstanding and many that had been submitted were sketchily and erratically completed, necessitating revisits to 35 field trial areas.[47,48]

Collection of data on the 1,013 cases of suspected poliomyelitis that occurred among the study population during the relevant period also proved troublesome. Children diagnosed with polio were to be reported weekly to the VEC as of May 1, 1954. However, not every case was reported promptly or even at all. The staff was forced to check its lists against the Foundation's hospitalization reports and to insist on immediate notification by collect telegram. Once a case was identified, the protocol required that the diagnosis be verified by physical examination, blood, and fecal tests.[47] Only after all records of vaccinations, blood samplings, and polio case evaluations for a field trial area had been submitted to the VEC could the evaluation begin. Head statistician Robert Voight wrote plaintively in mid-October, "We have received only six completed areas. . . . Without a flow of completed tabulations, our personnel will be out of work in the very near future."[68]

Some data were never collected or were unusable for analysis. Records were very nearly complete for the children whose parents requested participation and who were inoculated; more than 96% of these reported and received three injections. In addition, strict randomization and blinding had been well maintained in the placebo-controlled study population.[47,67] Randomized selection of children for blood sampling, particularly among the observed-controls, however, had proven impossible.[67] "The actual collections were made pretty much as the local areas saw fit. The ideal distribution was not achieved in most areas."[69] Antibody levels in the field trial population were therefore difficult to compare with accuracy.

Another element of uncertainty was the history of previous polio infection among the children. This information was requested on the schedules but the answers "were so inadequately filled out in the field that we believe the data are highly unreliable."[69] And the NFIP itself introduced a possible major element of bias through free administration of gamma globulin to areas with high polio incidence during the summer of 1954. The health officers' group had endorsed the withholding of the blood serum from the study population when they met in January 1954.[39] But the policy proved to be difficult to adhere to as the summer wore on, according to reports from local doctors in Virginia, Florida, Ohio, Utah, and many other states that were both placebo and observed-control sites.[70] "We are having a terrible time withholding gamma globulin in the field trial areas," Mason Romaine of Richmond told Francis;[71] his colleague L. L. Parks of Jacksonville added in a plaintive letter that, "[T]he poor health officer is placed in a difficult spot."[72] Francis and his staff pleaded with them to "hold the line," but were not always successful.[73]

The long-anticipated results of the trial were announced in a much publicized ceremony at the University of Michigan on April 12, 1955, and reported in print in a special supplement to the May issue of the *American Journal of Public Health*. As summarized in Tables 5.2 and 5.3, the vaccine was shown to be 80%–90% effective

Table 5.2
Poliomyelitis in the Placebo-Control Trial

Experimental Group	Paralytic Polio Cases (rate/10,000)	Nonparalytic Polio Cases (rate/10,000)
Vaccinated (series of 3)	33 (1.6)	24 (1.2)
Placebo (series of 3)	115 (5.7)	27 (1.3)
Incomplete vaccine series	1 (1.2)	1 (1.2)
Not vaccinated*	121 (3.6)	36 (1.1)

*Includes children whose parents refused to allow participation, children not present on V-Day, or children who received one or two injections of placebo only. Children who received one or two injections of vaccine or a mixed series of vaccine and placebo are listed under "Incomplete series of vaccine." (Table adapted from Francis 1955.)[74]

in preventing the paralytic form of the disease in the placebo-controlled study population. Francis did not minimize the procedural and statistical problems noted above, nor did he try to draw unwarranted generalizations from the data in these or later reports.[47] About cases of polio among nonvaccinated children in the placebo-control areas, for example, he stated in an article for *JAMA*: "The populations receiving vaccine or placebo are strictly comparable in every characteristic; they are equal parts of one population, while those who refused participation are distinctly different. . . . The nonparticipating portions of the populations . . . are not additional controls."[74]

Francis was similarly candid in his Summary Report: "From these data it is not possible to select a single value giving numerical expression . . . to the effectiveness of vaccine as a total experience."[47] The rates of nonparalytic polio in vaccinated children and placebo children were almost identical. There appeared to be a significant difference in rates of paralytic polio between the vaccinated children and the large group of controls in the observed-control population, but the latter was so ill-defined that it was not possible to interpret these results. Whatever the observed-control trials had contributed to the Foundation's goals, they did not provide the needed statistical verification of efficacy. But the painstakingly confirmed rates of diagnosed paralytic polio in the placebo-control groups showed striking differences between the vaccinees and the controls. "It may be suggested," Francis concluded, on the basis of "the results obtained from the strictly controlled and almost identical test populations of the placebo areas," that the vaccine was indeed highly effective against paralytic poliomyelitis.[47]

Table 5.3
Poliomyelitis in the Observed-Control Trial

Experimental Group	Paralytic Polio Cases (rate/10,000)	Nonparalytic Polio Cases (rate/10,000)
Vaccinated (series of 3)	38 (1.7)	18 (.8)
Controls*	330 (4.6)	61 (.8)
Incomplete vaccine series	4 (4.0)	—
Second-graders not vaccinated	43 (3.5)	11 (.9)

*Total population of first and third grades. (Table adapted from Francis 1955.)[74]

From Research Protocol to Clinical Practice

The PHS, with the approval of Oveta Culp Hobby, secretary of the new Department of Health, Education, and Welfare, immediately licensed the vaccine on the strength of the April 12, 1955, report, and mass vaccinations began under NFIP auspices.[75] On April 25, 1955, a child who had received some of the new vaccine made by Cutter Laboratories fell ill with what appeared to be polio. Other cases followed; 11 deaths and 153 cases of paralysis were eventually attributed to "the Cutter crisis." Surgeon General Leonard Scheele stopped the vaccination programs and appointed a Technical Advisory Committee, which met for many hours and released multiple reports.[76] Sabin and Enders, testifying before a House Subcommittee in June, again raised serious doubts that killed-virus vaccine could ever be both harmless and effective.[77] As the technical data eventually made clear, and as Paul Meier would later explain, neither Salk's very precise inactivation procedures nor tissue-culture tests guaranteed that any batch of the vaccine was free of live virus. The PHS found that such batches could still infect cortisone-treated monkeys, and presumably susceptible humans, with the paralytic disease. All the batches released for the field trials had undergone triple testing, including monkey trials; no such requirement had been imposed on the commercial firms when the PHS licensed the vaccine.[78]

Vaccinations, however, resumed almost immediately, under new manufacturing and testing standards that Scheele asserted would ensure "negligible" risk.[79] Public support had been shaken but in large part recovered. By late 1956, 75% of American children aged 5–12 had received Salk vaccine, although only 40% of the nation's teenagers and fewer than 12% of adults had followed suit.[80] The following year, polio incidence had diminished to 3 per 100,000 in the United States.[2] The summers of fear and suffering had ended.

Ethical Issues

The Salk vaccine field trials pose a number of interrelated ethical questions: issues of adequate pretesting, full informed consent, and the social versus the scientific justification for seeking clarity in therapeutic choice. In an era when ethical decisions were normally entrusted to the wisdom of investigators, and medical progress was considered an unquestioned social good, the National Foundation, as a lay volunteer group, invited an unusual amount of consultation and debate—from its scientific advisers, the state health officers, and the PHS—in formulating the trial design and procedures. Yet core issues remained unresolved and are still debated today. Did the Foundation act precipitately and without adequate scientific justification in deciding to hold a sizable field trial? Were the organizers justified in claiming safety for the experimental vaccine? Given that the final evaluation rested on the findings of the placebo-control trials, involving just over 400,000 children, was it ethical to expose the additional children in the observed-control areas to the possible risks of vaccination? Were the children's parents fully informed of the risks of the trial? Was their consent based on a rational assessment of the situation or did the trial organizers rely on their fear of polio, their faith in the Foundation, and the national excitement fueled by constant publicity?

The Foundation throughout this period used the press and its volunteer network to build the idea of an alliance between scientists and laypeople, to stress the importance of the trials, and to describe participation as a special privilege earned by the participants through their long-term financial support of polio research. The letter accompanying the request (not consent) form conveyed this idea of an earned reward: "Your child and his classmates have been selected to take part in this great scientific test." O'Connor's editorial in *Today's Health* in 1954 struck a similar note: "If an effective vaccine emerges from these studies . . . the layman—who furnished the original impetus for this effort—will have been instrumental in dealing the disease its final blow."[81]

It was this idea of a nationwide alliance that mandated the continuance of the observed-control plan, so that there would be at least one trial area in every possible state, and that impelled the blitz of publicity which surrounded the advance planning, the trials themselves, and the announcement of the results. O'Connor, Francis, and their colleagues also relied on the fear of the disease to maintain public support, deciding, for example, that the placebo-control plan "would not be difficult to sell as there is a high attack rate in the three grades."[39]

The confidence and enthusiasm with which participating families responded is evident in the statistics, as well as the many letters sent to the Foundation and the VEC. The letters make clear that many, perhaps most, of the parents in the placebo-control areas were informed about trial procedures. They understood the 50% chance that their children had not received "the real shot" and that they were participating in a test of the efficacy of an experimental vaccine.[82] "No one is more anxious for the success of your venture than [nine-year-old son] and I," wrote one physician from Detroit. "It was with that idea that we decided on the trial of the vaccine."[83]

What the parents probably did not understand, and what neither the Foundation nor the PHS made clear, was the risk-benefit ratio entailed in exposure to the experimental vaccine. They did not realize, in all probability, the tenuousness of Salk's hypothesis of a steady inactivation rate linked to the time of exposure to formalin;[78] the likelihood of persistence of live virus in any batch; the extent of the manufacturers' failure to produce virus-free batches; and the uncertainty as to whether a decisively killed-virus vaccine could confer lasting immunity. Experimental risks were not commonly outlined for experimental subjects in 1954, as is the standard today.

What the parents knew was that Salk had given his vaccine to many children without ill effect. They had faith in the National Foundation and they had faith in modern science, which had already given them insulin, penicillin, streptomycin, and cortisone. On the basis of that past experience and of the rhetoric that described medical advances emerging from research, they anticipated a "breakthrough." That confidence and anticipation persisted, despite Winchell's warning broadcast, through a year of waiting, and even through the frightening "Cutter crisis."

O'Connor and Rivers certainly recognized, as did their scientific advisers, that they were taking a calculated gamble. The trial participants were taking some risk in receiving an experimental vaccine, but this could be balanced against their existing risk of contracting paralytic polio. The Foundation was staking its reputation, its solvency, and its very existence, which depended on public confidence. Salk himself could make a safe vaccine; there was a triple-testing procedure in place for all batches to be used;

but Rivers and O'Connor knew that the margin of safety of the commercial products was relatively narrow. If the live-virus advocates were correct, moreover, and the vaccine did not prove to be very effective, the field trial would be seen as a great waste of time and money. Worse, even a few vaccine-associated cases of polio would be seen as a great waste of lives.

Against these risks, O'Connor and Rivers had to set the likelihood of several more summers of fear and an unknown additional number of paralyzed and dead children, while the work on an "ideal immunizing agent" continued. Yet the natural incidence of this frightening disease was still quite low. Their impetus to act rather than wait was a function of the Foundation's philanthropic bias toward activism, rather than the result of a systematic assessment of risk versus benefit. The decision may be considered as socially, if not scientifically, justified.

Caught between its volunteer constituency and its scientific advisers, and in an era when research ethics were less well-defined and regulated than they are today, the Foundation may be considered culpable on several counts. The field trial organizers failed to inform parents fully of the potential risks of the vaccine; exposed children in the observed-control areas to some risk for political, not scientific, reasons; publicized every aspect of the great experiment, but glossed over the difficulty of manufacturing safe, but antigenic, vaccine; and moved into a national field trial without fully adequate scientific justification. On the positive side, the organizers chose to use a rigorous experimental design in the placebo-control areas, one of which parents were fully informed, and to employ a screening process that proved to be effective in producing safe experimental vaccine. The Foundation also provided financial and emotional support for all U.S. polio victims that year, within the trial areas or elsewhere.

The most serious ethical lapse was an error not in research procedures but in translating research results into practice. The PHS was cognizant of all the risks and caveats, including the evidence produced by its own laboratories of manufacturing failures. But in the excitement of the public announcement of the field trial results, Hobby, Scheele, and their advisers failed to accurately assess the risks of blanket licensing and mass vaccinations with the commercial product, versus a phased-in and prescreened program. The PHS had no authority at that time to regulate research ethics, but the agency was responsible for the safety of U.S. vaccines.

Enduring Legacy

The 1954 Salk polio vaccine trials, despite the many scientific and ethical criticisms leveled at the time and in the half-century since, were a masterpiece of trial design and organization. They proved that a randomized and blinded design could be effectively used on a large scale to provide a rigorous demonstration of therapeutic efficacy. Most large-scale, multisite randomized, controlled trials since 1954 probably owe some debt to the polio vaccine trials.

Although the statistical results of the trials made possible a mass vaccination program with killed-virus vaccine, the virological community continued to support the idea of a live-virus preparation as "the ideal agent." The Sabin oral live-virus vaccine, after being tested in the Soviet Union, Mexico, and Czechoslovakia, was introduced into the United States in 1961 and remained the standard for polio prevention for more than 30 years. There were 8 to 10 cases of polio each year associated with the use of this virus, however; and as the wild virus was gradually eliminated from the U.S. population, the live-virus vaccine presented a greater threat than the disease to most Americans. In 1997, the Centers for Disease Control and Prevention (CDC) approved a mixed vaccination schedule of two killed-virus injections and two live-virus doses, and in 2000, the CDC recommended the sole use of killed-virus vaccination (an improved preparation with greater antigenic content than Salk's original vaccine was developed in 1978).[84]

The ethical choice at the heart of the Salk field trials confronts the researcher in every such case; at some point, he or she must choose action over caution, must decide to take a calculated risk. The polio vaccine story throws into high relief the interests and concerns surrounding many experimental innovations today—the researcher's interest in clear and replicable results; the manufacturer's concern for production efficiency, costs, and profit; and the desperation and hope of the individuals and families at risk—and it reminds us how easily those interests can be conflated or misrepresented. That the outcome proved to justify the decision the National Foundation made should not obscure the dimensions of the risk taken or the ethical complexities of the choice.

References

1. Paul JR. Historical and geographical aspects of the epidemiology of poliomyelitis. *Yale Journal of Biology and Medicine* 1954;27:101–13.
2. U.S. Bureau of the Census. *Historical Statistics of the United States From Colonial Times to 1970.* Washington, DC: United States Government Printing Office; 1975:38.
3. Cohn V. *Four Billion Dimes.* White Plains, N.Y.: National Foundation for Infantile Paralysis; 1955.
4. Benison S. *Tom Rivers: Reflections on a Life in Medicine and Science.* Cambridge, Mass.: The MIT Press; 1967.
5. Brodie M, Park WH. Active immunization against poliomyelitis. *American Journal of Public Health* 1936;26:119–25.
6. Paul JR. *A History of Poliomyelitis.* New Haven, Conn.: Yale University Press; 1971.
7. Kolmer JA. Vaccination against acute anterior poliomyelitis. *American Journal of Public Health* 1936;26:126–33.
8. Rivers TA. Immunity in virus diseases with particular reference to poliomyelitis. *American Journal of Public Health* 1936;26:126–42.
9. Leake JP. Discussion. *American Journal of Public Health* 1936;26:148.
10. *New York Times* Sep. 23, 1937:3, 23.
11. Carter R. *The Gentle Legions.* New York, N.Y.: Doubleday, 1961.
12. Deignan SL, Miller E. The support of research in medical and allied fields for the period 1946 through 1951. *Science* 1952;115: 321–43.
13. Enders JF, Weller TH, Robbins FC. Cultivation of the Lansing strain of poliomyelitis virus in cultures of various human embryonic tissues. *Science* 1949;109:85–7.
14. Morgan IM. Immunization of monkeys with formalin-inactivated poliomyelitis viruses. *American Journal of Hygiene* 1948;48:394–406.
15. Minutes of the Round Table Conference on Immunization in Poliomyelitis, Hershey, Pennsylvania, March 15–17, 1951. Thomas Francis Papers, Michigan Historical Collections, Bentley Historical Library, University of Michigan (hereafter TF-BLUM), Box 27, Folder, Proceedings, Round Table Conference, March 1951.
16. Weaver H to Salk JE, May 3, 1951. Jonas Salk Papers, University of California at San Diego Library Special Collections (hereafter JS-UCSD), Box 253, Folder 7.

17. Hammon WM, Coriell LL, Stokes J Jr. Evaluation of Red Cross gamma globulin as a prophylactic agent for poliomyelitis. 1. Plan of controlled field tests and results of 1951 pilot study in Utah. *JAMA* 1952;150:739–49.

18. Salk JE. Principles of immunization as applied to poliomyelitis and influenza. American *Journal of Public Health* 1953;43:1384–98.

19. Carter R. *Breakthrough: The Saga of Jonas Salk.* New York, N.Y.: Trident Press; 1966.

20. Minutes of the Committee on Immunization, Hershey, Pennsylvania, January 23, 1953. JS-UCSD, Box 254, Folder 2.

21. Plumb RK. New polio vaccination treatment offers hope in curbing paralysis. *The New York Times* Jan. 27, 1953:1, 28.

22. Rivers TM. Vaccine for poliomyelitis. [letter] *JAMA* 1953;151:1224.

23. Meldrum ML. The historical feud over polio vaccine: How could a killed vaccine contain a natural disease? *Western Journal of Medicine* 1999;171:271–3.

24. Enders JF. Some recent advances in the study of poliomyelitis. *Medicine* 1954;33:87–95.

25. Cox HR. Active immunization against poliomyelitis. *Bulletin of the New York Academy of Medicine* 1953;29:943–60.

26. Francis T. Summary and review of poliomyelitis immunization. *Annals of the New York Academy of Sciences* 1955;61:1057–8.

27. Morgan IM. Mechanism of immunity in poliomyelitis and its bearing on differentiation of types. *American Journal of Medicine* 1949;6:556–62.

28. This year's poliomyelitis rate. *The New York Times* June 30, 1953:25.

29. Medical Research Council. Streptomycin treatment of pulmonary tuberculosis. *British Medical Journal* 1948;2:769–82.

30. Marks HM. *The Progress of Experiment: Science and Therapeutic Reform in the United States, 1900–1990.* New York, NY: Cambridge University Press; 1997.

31. New tests on polio to dwarf old ones. *The New York Times* Nov. 10, 1953:32.

32 Laurence WL. Mass polio tests will start February 8. *The New York Times* Nov. 17, 1953:34.

33. Van Riper H to Neupert CN, November 19, 1953. TF-BLUM, Box 18, Folder, NFIP—Van Riper.

34. Dublin to Van Riper H, December 9, 1953. Response from State Health Officers Regarding Selection of Field Trial Areas. TF-BLUM, Box 18, Folder, NFIP—Memos.

35. Barlow S to Van Riper H, November 16, 1953. TF-BLUM, Box 6, Folder, National Foundation—Van Riper.

36. Van Riper H to Francis T, January 11, 1954. TF-BLUM, Box 6, Folder, National Foundation—Van Riper.

37. Francis T to Weaver H, December 29. 1953. TF-BLUM, Box 6, Folder, National Foundation—Weaver.

38. Minutes of the Meeting of Advisory Group on Evaluation of Vaccine Field Trials, January 11, 1954. TF-BLUM, Box 18, Folder, Meeting—New York, January 11, 1954.

39. Minutes of the Advisory Committee on Technical Aspects of the Poliomyelitis Field Trials, January 30–31, 1954. TF-BLUM, Box 18, Folder, Meeting—Atlanta, Advisory Committee, January 30–31, 1954.

40. Named to direct study on polio vaccine tests. *The New York Times* Feb. 10, 1954:16.

41. School tests set for polio vaccine. *The New York Times* Feb. 15, 1954:25.

42. Francis T. For Discussion with Van Riper, typed notes, n.d. (early 1954). TF-BLUM, Box 18, Folder, Meeting—Detroit, February 23–24, 1954.

43. Stickle G. October 22, 1953. Epidemiological Considerations for the Selection of Areas for Vaccine Field Trial. TF-BLUM, Box 21, Folder, Vaccine—Selection of Counties.

44. Dublin T to Van Riper H. Predicting Poliomyelitis Incidence for the 1954 Field Trial, n.d. (1953). TF-BLUM, Box 21, Folder, Vaccine—Selection of Counties.

45. Van Riper H to NFIP Staff, December 1, 1953. Brief Background Statement for the Vaccine Field Trial. TF-BLUM, Box 18, Folder, NFIP—1954.

46. Manual of Suggested Procedures for the Conduct of the Vaccine Field Trial in 1954, March 1, 1954. TF-BLUM, Box 14, Folder, Field Trial—Manual.

47. Francis T Jr, et al. An evaluation of the 1954 poliomyelitis vaccine trials. *American Journal of Public Health* 1955;45(5 Part 2): 1–63.

48. Voight R to Francis T, March 9, 1954. TF-BLUM, Box 17, Folder, Francis—Daily Memos.

49. Laurence WL. Anti-polio vaccine defended as safe. *The New York Times* November 11, 1953:28.

50. Specifications and Minimal Requirements for Poliomyelitis Vaccine Aqueous (Polyvalent) as Developed by Dr. Jonas E. Salk, Virus Research Laboratory, University of Pittsburgh, Pittsburgh, Pennsylvania (To Be Used in Field Studies to Be Conducted During 1954 Under the Auspices of the National Foundation for Infantile Paralysis), February 1, 1954. TF-BLUM, Box 21, Folder, Vaccine—Specifications.

51. Polio fund defers trial for vaccine. *The New York Times* Jan. 29, 1954:21.

52. Meldrum ML. *Departures From the Design: The Randomized Clinical Trial in Historical Context, 1946–1970.* Ph.D. dissertation, State University of New York, Stony Brook, 1994.

53. Voight R to Francis T, April 6, 1954, TF-BLUM, Box 17, Folder, Francis—Daily Memos.

54. Van Riper H to Osborn SN, April 7, 1954. TF-BLUM, Box 21, Folder, Vaccine—Safety.

55. Telegram, Sullivan JA to Scheele L, April 10, 1957. Public Health Service Reports on the Salk Polio Vaccine, National Library of Medicine, MS. C251.

56. Smith J. *Patenting the Sun: Polio and the Salk Vaccine.* New York, N.Y.: William Morrow & Co., 1990.

57. Health units call polio vaccine safe. *The New York Times* Apr. 5, 1954:27.

58. Plumb RK. Vaccine for polio affirmed as safe. *The New York Times* Apr. 6, 1954:33.

59. Minnesota Defers Polio Test Action. *The New York Times* Apr. 16, 1954:22.

60. Action Taken by Vaccine Advisory Committee on April 25, 1954. TF-BLUM, Box 18, Folder, Meeting—Washington, Advisory Committee, April 1954.

61. Dublin T to Francis T, April 25, 1954. TF-BLUM, Box 21, Folder, Vaccine—Schedules.

62. Dublin TD. 1954 poliomyelitis vaccine field trial: Plan, field operations, and follow-up observations. *JAMA* 1955;158:1258–65.

63. Voight R to Francis T, May 19, 1954. TF-BLUM, Box 17, Folder, Francis—Daily Memos.

64. Markel IJ to Korns R, October 2, 1954. TF-BLUM, Box 17, Folder, Gamma Globulin.

65. O Pioneers! *New Yorker* May 8, 1954;30:24–5.

66. Additional Field Observation and Review of Follow-Up Procedures, June 1, 1954. TF-BLUM, Box 17, Folder, Francis—Travel.

67. Voight R. Obtaining and Processing Records, November 4, 1954. TF-BLUM, Box 83, Folder VEC Advisory Committee, November 4, 1954.

68. Robert Voight to Nern JL, October 13, 1954. TF-BLUM, Box 21, Folder, Bureau of Census.

69. Hemphill F to Francis T, July 29, 1955. TF-BLUM, Box 19, Folder, Technical Committee—General.

70. Francis T. Dear Doctor letter, August 6, 1954. TF-BLUM, Box 17, Folder, Gamma Globulin.

71. Romaine M to Francis T, October 8, 1954. TF-BLUM, Box 17, Folder, Gamma Globulin.

72. Parks LL to Korns R, July 22, 1954. TF-BLUM, Box 17, Folder, Gamma Globulin.

73. Korns R to Parks LL, July 28, 1954. TF-BLUM, Box 17, Folder, Gamma Globulin.

74. Francis T Jr. Evaluation of the 1954 poliomyelitis vaccine field trial: Further studies of results determining the effectiveness of poliomyelitis vaccine (Salk) in preventing paralytic poliomyelitis. *JAMA* 1955;158:1266–70.

75. Laurence WL. Salk polio vaccine proves success; millions will be immunized soon. *The New York Times* Apr. 13, 1955:1, 20.

76. Scheele LA, Shannon JA. Public health implications in a program of vaccination against poliomyelitis. *JAMA* 1955;158: 1249–58.

77. Brandt AM. Polio, politics, publicity, and duplicity: Ethical aspects in the development of the Salk vaccine. *International Journal of Health Services* 1978;8:257–70.

78. Meier P. Safety testing of poliomyelitis vaccine. *Science* 1957;125: 1067–71.

79. Blair WM. U.S. lays defects in polio program to mass output. *The New York Times* June 10, 1955:1, 24.

80. A Study of the Public's Acceptance of the Salk Vaccine Program. Prepared by the American Institute of Public Opinion, Princeton, New Jersey, for the National Foundation for Infantile Paralysis, January, 1957. JS-UCSD, Box 138, Folder 5.

81. O'Connor B. Those mighty dimes of ours. *Today's Health* 1954;32:13.

82. G.J.H. to Francis T, May 20, 1955. TF-BLUM, Box 21, Folder, Vaccine—Correspondence.

83. W.K.T. to Francis T, January 18, 1955. TF-BLUM, Box 21, Folder, Vaccine—Reactions.

84. Advisory Committee on Immunization Practices. Poliomyelitis Prevention in the United States. *MMWR Recommendations and Reports* 2000;49(5):1–22.

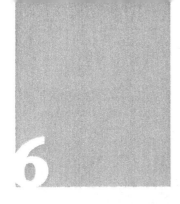

John D. Arras

The Jewish Chronic Disease Hospital Case

During the summer of 1963, Chester M. Southam and Deogracias B. Custodio together injected live, cultured cancer cells into the bodies of 22 debilitated patients at the Jewish Chronic Disease Hospital (JCDH) in Brooklyn, New York. Custodio, a Philippine-born, unlicensed medical resident at JCDH, was participating in a medical experiment designed by Southam, a distinguished physician-researcher at the Sloan-Kettering Institute for Cancer Research, an attending physician at Memorial Hospital in New York City, and associate professor of medicine at Cornell University Medical College. The purpose of the research was to determine whether the previously established immune deficiency of cancer patients was caused by their cancer or, alternatively, by their debilitated condition. Southam thus looked to a group of noncancerous but highly debilitated elderly patients who might bear out his guiding hypothesis that cancer, not old age, was the cause of the previously witnessed immune deficiency. Importantly, he believed on the basis of long experience that the injection of cultured cancer cells posed no risk to these patients, and that all of the cells would eventually be rejected by their immune systems. Although Southam's professional credentials were impeccable, and although his work was deemed by his peers to be of the utmost scientific importance, the JCDH experiment soon erupted in a major public controversy. Critics denounced Southam's methods as being morally comparable to those of the Nazi physicians tried at Nuremburg, whereas his defenders countered that he was a distinguished physician-researcher, and by all accounts an honorable man, who merely had the bad luck to be caught in the shifting rip tides of history.

Curiously, although the JCDH case has gone down in history as one of the most important milestones in the development of contemporary ethical and regulatory approaches to biomedical research, the case is not nearly as well known as similar scandals, such as the Willowbrook hepatitis experiments or the Tuskegee syphilis study (see Chapters 7 and 8). And although the JCDH case is almost always briefly mentioned in published litanies of important research scandals, including Henry Beecher's landmark study of medical science run amok,[1] it has never been the exclusive subject of any full-length scholarly paper, let alone a book. (It has, however, been the focus of two very helpful short papers in recent years, on which I have been happy to draw.)[2,3]

Basic Chronology

Southam's research project focused on the relationship between the body's immune system and cancer. Beginning in 1954, Southam had performed numerous studies on more than 300 cancer patients at Memorial Hospital and on hundreds of healthy prison volunteers at the Ohio State Penitentiary. Southam had noticed that cancer patients exhibit a delayed immunological response to injected cancer cells. He had chosen cultured cancer cells for these experiments because they possessed the necessary uniformity, reproducibility, comparability, and growth potential to cause a measurable reaction in patients. Whereas the immune systems of healthy volunteers would normally reject such foreign tissue completely and promptly in roughly 4 to 6 weeks, it took cancer patients much longer, often 12 weeks or longer, to finally reject the injected cells. Southam worried about a gap in his data. Was the delayed immune response in cancer patients due to their cancer, or was it due instead to the fact that most such patients were elderly, debilitated, and chronically ill? In order to fill this gap in knowledge, Southam proposed to repeat his immunological study on a group of noncancerous but elderly and debilitated patients. He hypothesized that this study population would reject the injected material at the same rate as normal, healthy volunteers. He hoped that studies such as this would ultimately lead to progress in our ability to boost the human immune system's defenses against cancer, but he was also aware of possible applications in the area of transplant immunology. This, then, was important research.

To test his hypothesis, Southam contacted Emanuel Mandel, who was then director of the department of medicine at the JCDH. Eager to affiliate his modest hospital with the work of a famous doctor at a prestigious medical institution, Mandel immediately agreed to provide the requisite number of chronically ill patients for Southam's study. Like many of the studies criticized in Henry Beecher's famous whistle-blowing exposé in the *New England Journal of Medicine,* this project was to be funded by eminently respectable sources, including the American Cancer Society and the U.S. Public Health Service. At their first meeting to discuss the study, Southam explained to Mandel that his proposal was not related to the care and treatment of patients; that it was, in other words, a pure example of "nontherapeutic" research. Southam also informed Mandel that it would not be necessary to obtain the written informed consent of patients at JCDH, because these immunological studies had become "routine" at Memorial Hospital. He also noted that there was no need to inform these elderly patients that the injected material consisted of live, cultured cancer cells, because that would be of "no consequence" to them. On the basis of his considerable prior experience of such studies with patients and prisoners, which easily included more than 600 subjects, Southam was convinced that the injection of cultured cancer cells from another person posed no discernible risk of transmitting cancer. In his opinion, it would simply be a question of when, not whether, such injected cells would eventually be rejected by the patients' immune systems. Because in his view the subjects would not be placed at risk by his study, Southam saw no need to inform them specifically that live cancer cells would be injected into their bodies. The whole point of using cancer cells had to do with their special properties within the context of his research project; no one, he opined, was actually at risk of getting cancer.

Prior to initiating the study at JCDH, Mandel hit a snag. He had asked three young staff physicians at the hospital—Avir Kagan, David Leichter, and Perry Fersko—to help with the injections of live cancer cells into the hospital's debilitated patients. All three had refused to cooperate on the ground that, in their view, informed consent could not be obtained from the potential subjects that Mandel and Southam had in mind for the study. Undeterred, Mandel and Southam forged ahead, eventually settling upon the unlicensed and comparatively vulnerable house officer, Custodio, to help with the injections.

On July 16, 1963, Custodio, Southam, and Mandel met at the JCDH to initiate the study. Custodio and Mandel had already selected the 22 chronically ill patients to be asked to participate. Southam demonstrated the injection procedure on the first three patients, and then Custodio proceeded to inject the remaining 19 with two separate doses of tissue-cultured cells. According to Southam and Custodio, each patient was told that the injections were being given to test their immune capacity—there was no mention of research—and that a small nodule would likely form at

the site of the injections but would eventually disappear. In the investigators' view, this constituted sufficient "oral consent" to participate in the study. At the end of just two hours, 22 elderly and debilitated patients on six floors of two separate hospital buildings had received injections, and this first crucial phase of the research was complete.[4] With the passage of a few weeks, Southam's hypothesis would be fully vindicated: With the exception of patients who had died shortly after receiving their injections, all of the JCDH patients rejected the foreign tissue as completely and at the same rate as the prior group of physically healthy individuals. The gap in the data was thus filled: It was cancer, not debilitation and chronic illness, that was responsible for the impaired immune reaction of Southam's patients at Memorial Hospital. None of the JCDH patients, moreover, experienced any long-lasting physical harms attributable to the study.

The Battle Within the JCDH

News of the Southam-Mandel study spread quickly along the corridors of the JCDH. Samuel Rosenfeld, chief of medicine at the Blumberg Pavilion of JCDH for the previous seven years, was outraged both by the nature of the study, which he regarded as immoral and illegal, and by the fact that he had not even been consulted about it.[5] The three young physicians who had rebuffed Southam and Mandel—Kagan, Fersko, and Leichter—fearing that their silence might be construed as condoning the research, resigned en bloc on August 27, 1963, less than six weeks after the injections.[2,5] All three were Jewish; Leichter was a Holocaust survivor, and the other two had lost many family members to Nazi violence during the catastrophe of World War II. Each subsequently attributed his negative response to this study to a visceral revulsion at the thought of using such debilitated and helpless patients in experiments without their consent. None had had any training in ethics or law during their medical studies, and Kagan subsequently admitted that none of them had even heard of the Nuremberg Code.[2]

In order to quiet the gathering storm, authorities at the JCDH assembled the hospital's Grievance Committee on September 7, 1963. After hearing testimony from the hospital's executive director, Solomon Siegel, and Southam, the Committee judged that the resignations of Kagan, Fersko, and Leichter were "irresponsible" and should therefore be accepted by the hospital. The Committee then fully and enthusiastically endorsed the scientific and medical importance of Southam's research and concluded that the allegations of the three young doctors and of the medical director, Rosenfeld, against Mandel and Southam were baseless.[5] Later that month, the JCDH's Board of Directors approved the Grievance Committee's report, and four months later the hospital's Research Committee approved the continuation of Southam's study at the JCDH, but only on the condition that he obtain the written consent of all subjects in the study.

Growing increasingly desperate, the three young doctors turned to William A. Hyman, an internationally recognized lawyer who had helped to found JCDH in 1926 and had sat on its Board ever since. Hyman had many reasons to be furious with his fellow Board members and with the medical authorities at the hospital, who, in his view, had aided, abetted, and then whitewashed this sordid story of human experimentation. One reason for his fury was, however, based upon the erroneous belief that the purpose of

Southam's research was to determine whether cancer could be induced by the injection of live cancer cells.[5] Against the backdrop of this factual misunderstanding, it's no wonder that Hyman promptly accused Southam, Mandel, and Custodio of acting like Nazi doctors: "I don't want Nazi concentration camps in America. I don't want Nazi practices of using human beings as experimental guinea pigs."[2]

Fearing that the JCDH could be subject to legal liability for providing Southam with patients for his experiment, Hyman, in his capacity as Board member, sought the minutes of the Grievance Committee meeting of September 9, 1963, as well as the medical records of all the patients enlisted in the study. Rebuffed by the hospital authorities and ignored by the New York State Department of Education, Hyman then took his case to the Supreme Court of Brooklyn (a terminological oddity, because this is a *trial* court, not in appeals court in New York State), where he argued that, as a member of the JCDH Board of Directors, he had a legal right and responsibility to inspect committee minutes and patient records in response to allegations of wrongdoing and threats of potential legal liability. It is important to note at this point in the story that Hyman's quixotic legal quest was actually directed at a very narrowly focused topic. His case, *Hyman v. Jewish Chronic Disease Hospital*,[6] was not an investigation into the substantive moral or legal issues raised by Southam's research. That would come later. The case was, rather, focused exclusively on the narrowly construed procedural question bearing on a Board member's right to see certain documents and patients' countervailing rights to the privacy of their medical records. Hyman's procedural claims were ultimately vindicated at the level of the state's highest court,[5] but the real significance of his legal odyssey lay elsewhere. Although the New York State Department of Education, whose Board of Regents controlled medical licensure, had dithered and effectively ignored Hyman's original allegations, it was finally drawn into this case by the high public visibility and news accounts of the legal proceedings in Brooklyn. The Grievance Committee of the Board of Regents would henceforth provide the crucible for the ethical and legal implications of Southam's research at the JCDH.

Arguments in the Case of Chester Southam

In its 1965 inquiry into the JCDH case, the Grievance Committee of the Board of Regents focused on two major issues: the assessment of risk and the quality of informed consent. Southam offered strong arguments on both fronts, at least when viewed in the context of social and medical assumptions of the time.

The Inquiry Into Risk

With regard to the presence or absence of risk in this study, Southam argued that the injection of cultured cancer cells from an extraneous source into the human body posed no appreciable risk. His 10 years of prior experience with more than 600 subjects—including cancer patients at Memorial Hospital in New York and healthy prison volunteers in Ohio—had led him to conclude that "it is biologically and medically impossible to induce cancer by this means."[5] The Regents concurred in this conclusion. As reported in the *New York Times*, the Regents established to their own satisfaction that prior to the JCDH study in July 1963, "medical opinion was unanimous that the patients were running no risk of contracting cancer and hence need not be cautioned that there was any such risk."[7]

Medical opinion at the time was not, however, entirely unanimous on the question of risk, as it hardly ever is on any question worthy of public debate. One reputable physician, Bernard Pisani, past president of the Medical Society of the County of New York and director of obstetrics and gynecology at St. Vincent's Hospital, testified during the Supreme Court hearing that "the known hazards of such experiments include growth of nodules and tumors and may result in metastases of cancer if the patient does not reject these cells."[5] In addition, according to a recent account based upon an interview with Kagan many years after the fact, "Kagan, Leichter, and Fersko . . . disagreed with Southam's contention that the injections posed no risk to the patients involved."[2]

Another reason to doubt Southam's unequivocal denial of any risk in this experiment is the fact that in one of his own previous studies, the injected cancer cells had migrated 10 inches up the arm of a subject from the injection site to a nearby lymph node. The patient in question had died shortly thereafter, but there was some speculation at the time that, had the patient lived, cancer cells that had migrated that far might then have been subsequently disseminated throughout the body via the lymphatic system. Although Southam claimed that the cells would not have traveled beyond the lymph node if the patient had lived, he admitted that he could not settle the matter with a "statement based on fact."[5]

But perhaps the most telling and unintentionally humorous admission that Southam made regarding the possibility of risk came during his cross-examination before the Board of Regents. Mr. Calanese, an attorney for the Regents, was quizzing Southam about an apparent contradiction in an article based upon an interview with him in the journal *Science*.[8] Although emphasizing Southam's confidence that there was "no theoretical likelihood" that the injections of live cancer cells would cause cancer, the article also noted Southam's unwillingness to inject himself or his colleagues. Calanese then quoted the following line from the interview: "But, let's face it, there are relatively few skilled cancer researchers, and it seemed stupid to take even the little risk." To which Southam responded: "I deny the quote. I am sure I didn't say, 'Let's face it.' "[5] In retrospect, we can grant Southam the objective truth of the proposition that those live cancer cells posed zero appreciable risk to the residents of the JCDH. But we can also question his assertion that any right-minded physician *at the time* would have corroborated this claim. This doubt, plus Southam's own admission that the injections posed "little risk"—which suggests at least *some* risk—to himself and his staff, leads me to conclude that the doctor was being somewhat disinguous and misleading in his outright denials of risk. Even if he believed that the likelihood of those injections causing cancer was vanishingly small, it is not obvious, even judging by the louche standards of informed consent operative at the time, that Southam did not owe these elderly residents of the JCDH some mention of the possibility of risk.

Informed Consent and Professional Norms

The historical importance and personal poignancy of Southam's story are both due in large measure to the fact that his case played out against a backdrop of changing societal and professional mores with regard to the physician-patient relationship. Southam was obviously brought up and trained within a system of medical education that was deeply and pervasively paternalistic. In those days, there were no "strangers at the bedside,"[9] no institutional review boards, lawyers, bioethicists, patient advocates, or hospital risk managers to second-guess the experienced judgments of physicians. Although the nascent doctrine of informed consent was beginning to percolate through the medical and research establishments, at the time of the JCDH case in 1963 most physician-researchers believed that obtaining the subject's consent was a matter of individual professional discretion. If one were doing research on healthy subjects in nontherapeutic experiments, then one might well ask for the subjects' written informed consent, as Southam did in his trials with state prisoners in Ohio. But research on sick patients was another matter, and here researchers were more likely to cloak themselves in the mantle of the traditional ethic governing relationships between patients and physicians.

In the clinical setting, truthful information regarding risks was regarded less as an ethical or legal matter and more as a matter of therapeutics. If the risks were small, physicians would likely conclude that informed consent was not necessary, especially if they believed that the information in question would upset or depress the patient. But if the risks were great, or if physicians needed the patient to be informed in order to better collaborate on recovery, then information would be "medically indicated." According to this paternalistic physician ethic, information regarding risks was viewed as essentially one more tool in the physician's black bag. Truth-telling was a matter of individual physician discretion, and the relevant yardstick for disclosure was the perceived benefit or harm of disclosing information bearing on the patient's medical condition. Even though medical researchers were primarily interested in producing knowledge rather than in the traditional physician's goal of advancing the best interests of particular patients, they felt free to avail themselves of this traditional physician ethic in their research.

Against the background of this professional practice, Southam's duty seemed clear. The risk of injecting cancer cells into the bodies of frail, elderly patients was, in his view, infinitesimally small, perhaps even nonexistent. Were he to announce to these patients that he was about to inject them with *live cancer cells*, such a disclosure would have advanced no legitimate medical purpose while only serving to make the elderly residents very upset and anxious. In those days, physicians tended to avoid the dreaded word *cancer* when talking to their patients, preferring instead to speak cryptically of *nodes, cysts,* or *growths*.[10] It was standard medical practice to envelop patients in a conspiracy of silence in order to shield them from information that was perceived to be alarming, depressing, or otherwise harmful.[11] Contrary to Board member Hyman's misguided allegation, Southam was not trying to determine if cancer could be induced through the injection of live, foreign cancer cells; his choice of live, cultured cancer cells was dictated solely by methodological and comparative purposes. So, because using the word *cancer* was irrelevant to the actual state of affairs, because there was little to no risk, and because the dreaded word would only serve needlessly to alarm patients, Southam believed disclosure of the cells' derivation to be medically "contraindicated." In reaching this conclusion, Southam insisted that he was merely acting in the "best tradition of responsible clinical practice."[5] It is important to note that the notion of medical relevance advanced here by Southam was purportedly "objective" and scientific rather than subjective, and that the arbiter of what

counts as medically relevant, objective information was, in his view, the physician (who also just happens to be a researcher), not the individual patient-subject.

Southam's paternalistic view of researchers' obligations to subjects was confirmed by a parade of distinguished witnesses on his behalf before the tribunal of the Board of Regents. High-ranking medical officers and practitioners at such prestigious institutions as Memorial Hospital, Cornell University, West Virginia Medical Center, the University of Pennsylvania, and the Roswell Park Memorial Institute of Buffalo, New York, a cancer research center, all expressed their complete agreement with Southam's central contentions: specifically that his research was of high scientific and social merit; that there was no appreciable risk to subjects; that informed consent was a matter for individual physician discretion; that disclosure of information should be "titrated" according to the level of risk posed by research; that the word *cancer* was generally avoided so as not to upset patients, and would in any case not accurately and objectively represent the true nature of the injected materials; and, finally, that Southam's conduct toward the subjects in the JCDH trial was in complete conformity with the prevailing standards of medical practice. As one of Southam's lawyers remarked at the time, "If the whole profession is doing it, how can you call it 'unprofessional conduct'?"[5]

Even journalists chimed in on behalf of the beleaguered Southam. At a time when the authority of the legal and medical professions was still largely unchallenged, the press tended to echo the larger society's unbridled enthusiasm for medical progress while ignoring, if not denigrating, what we today would call the rights of patients and research subjects. Thus, journalist Earl Ubell, writing in the *New York Herald Tribune,* conjured images of "enormous pay-offs" from Southam's research, including a possible vaccine against cancer, in dismissing the controversy over the JCDH case as a mere "brouhaha." He concluded, "It would be a shame if a squabble over who-told-what-to-whom should destroy a thrilling lead in cancer research."[5]

The Judgment of the New York State Board of Regents

The ultimate arbiters of professional medical norms in New York, the State Board of Regents, did not view Southam's case as a mere squabble over who-told-what-to-whom. On the contrary, the Board summoned Southam before its Grievance Committee as it heard evidence and eventually passed judgment on whether his license to practice medicine should be revoked. The Regents considered two related charges: (1) that Southam was guilty of fraud or deceit in the practice of medicine, and (2) that he was guilty of unprofessional conduct. The first charge focused on Southam's alleged failure to obtain informed consent from the patients at the JCDH, while the second implied that violating patient-subjects' rights of informed consent constituted a violation of professional norms.

Consent at the JCDH

The charge bearing on informed consent had two distinct components: the competency of the research subjects and the extent of information disclosure. Before discussing the adequacy of consent obtained at JCDH on these two indicia, let us recall what transpired on that day in the summer of 1963. Twenty-two residents were selected for this experiment. All were frail elderly residents of a long-term care hospital, and many were Holocaust survivors whose primary language was Yiddish. Following Southam's initial demonstration of the injection procedure on the first 3 subjects, Custodio proceeded during the next two hours to obtain "consent" from the remaining 19 residents in two separate buildings and to inject them all with the cancer cells. None of the residents was told the purpose of the injections or that they were about to participate in a research project having nothing to do with their own health and well-being. Each was told, however, that they were about to receive an injection designed to test their immune capacity, and that soon a nodule would form that would go away in a short time.

The first question, then, is whether all of these frail, debilitated elderly were "competent" to make an informed decision whether or not to hold out their arms to Southam and Custodio—that is, were they of "sound mind," capable of understanding complex medical information and coming to a decision on whether or not to participate? The evidence and testimony on this question were mixed. Custodio testified that all the patients were fully competent to make their own decisions, and that he had no trouble communicating with any of them. On the other hand, Samuel Rosenfeld, chief of medicine at the Blumberg Pavilion of the JCDH for many years, testified that many of the 18 patients injected on his ward were mentally incapable of giving consent.[5] Mendel Jacobi, the consultant pathologist at JCDH, added considerable specificity to this charge through an examination of the charts of 5 of the 22 patients. He painted the following picture: Chart No. K-14397 described a 67-year-old patient with "poor cerebration" who had been in a depressive state for a year. Chart No. 2290 showed a 63-year-old patient with advanced Parkinson's disease, low mentality, and lack of insight and judgment. Patient No. 8183 had a history of depressive psychosis and had been diagnosed at JCDH as suffering from dementia praecox and unsound judgment. And the chart of patient No. 3762 recorded a diagnosis of postencephalitic Parkinson's, difficulty in communicating, constant falling, suicidal ideation, and considerable sedation throughout the years. Although it's at least theoretically conceivable that each one of these debilitated patients was lucid during his or her brief interview with Custodio on that summer day, Saul Heller, one of the Regents who heard testimony and rendered a judgment in the case, concluded that under such conditions these debilitated patients could not possibly have understood such complex matters in a mere one- to five-minute encounter.[5]

The Regents' deliberations on the nature and extent of disclosure required for genuine consent were of far greater philosophical, legal, and historic importance than their findings on the issue of competency; indeed, the Board's deliberations on this subject take us to the heart of the matter. Whereas Mandel, Custodio, and Southam were entirely satisfied with the amount of information disclosed to the residents, the Regents concluded that the patients' consent was woefully inadequate. In the first place, none of the residents was told that they were about to participate in a research project. The Regents reasoned that in order for consent to be valid, it had to be informed; and for consent to be adequately informed, subjects had to understand that they were being asked to participate in nontherapeutic research. For all these patients knew, the good doctors in white coats were merely run-

ning routine tests on their immune responses; they had every reason to think that the nature of the impending injections was entirely therapeutic and had nothing to do with research. A mere signature, mere verbal assent, or, worse yet, the resigned nod of a confused patient's head, were not enough. In the Regents' judgment, "[d]eliberate nondisclosure of the material fact [i.e., that the injections were done for research purposes] is no different from deliberate misrepresentation of such a fact."[5] They concluded that such misrepresentation constituted a serious deception and fraud perpetrated upon the JCDH subjects.

Secondly, the Regents were genuinely scandalized by Southam's deliberate omission of the word *cancer*. Gauging his duties to research subjects through the lens of a paternalistic medical ethic, Southam had claimed that disclosure of the nature of the cells would have been both medically, objectively irrelevant and needlessly upsetting to frail, elderly patients. The Regents concluded, by contrast, that physician-researchers had a legal duty to disclose all information "material" to a patient-subject's decision whether or not to participate. In contrast to Southam's belief that any negative reaction on the part of potential subjects to the word *cancer* would have been irrational, the Regents held that "any fact which might influence the giving or withholding of consent is material," whether or not physicians might consider such influence to be irrational. The bottom line for the Regents was that *the decision is the patient's to make,* not the physician's.[5] The patient's subjectivity (or at least that of a "reasonable person") was henceforth to be the touchstone of researchers' duty of disclosure, not physicians' estimates of objective truth. In taking this step, the Regents explicitly repudiated the entrenched paternalism of the traditional Hippocratic ethic in the domain of research on which Southam and his supporters had relied.

In response to Southam's additional claim that withholding the word *cancer* was dictated by a genuine concern for patients' well-being—a concern in keeping with "the best tradition of responsible clinical practice"—the Regents pointed out the obvious fact that in this particular case there was no preexisting doctor-patient relationship. Southam may well have professed a concern to shield these patients from any undue emotional distress during a time when doctors often shielded patients from bad news, particularly about cancer; but they were not *his* patients. He was essentially an interloper at the JCDH who had never previously met the 22 injected residents, let alone had a long-standing professional relationship with them. The Regents concluded that, at least with regard to the kind of nontherapeutic research involved at the JCDH, Southam, Custodio, and Mandel were acting primarily as researchers who also just happened to be physicians. They thus had no right to help themselves to the wide-ranging discretion normally allowed at that time to physicians charged with pursuing the best interests of their patients.

Viewing the charges against them through the lens of traditional (paternalistic) medical ethics, Custodio, Mandel, and Southam had focused narrowly on the question of physical harm. They contended that in the absence of a serious risk of harm, failure to disclose the experimental nature of the injections or the true nature of the cells injected could not possibly constitute a valid reason to reproach their behavior. As we currently say with good humor in the rough and tumble world of U.S. professional basketball, "No harm, no foul." The Regents concluded, however, that Southam and colleagues, although not physically harming anyone, had robbed the JCDH residents of their "basic human right" to make their own decisions whether or not to participate in research.[5] In the language of the law of torts, under which violations of informed consent would soon be subsumed,[11] Southam's failure adequately to inform his subjects constituted a "dignitary insult" and a legal wrong, quite apart from the question whether anyone was physically harmed.

After considering and sharply rejecting all of Southam's and Mandel's justifications for withholding vital information bearing on the nature, rationale, and conduct of the JCDH trial, the Board of Regents issued its final verdict in the case: Both physicians were guilty of fraud, deceit, and unprofessional conduct in the practice of medicine. They had allowed their zeal for research to override "the basic rights and immunities of a human person."[5] Having rendered their verdict, the Regents then considered the nature and severity of the punishment for the physicians' misdeeds. Fifteen of the 17 members of the Regents' Grievance Committee, meeting on June 10, 1965, voted for censure and reprimand, whereas the remaining 2 members, apparently believing that being dragged before that tribunal was punishment enough, voted for no further action. In its final action in this case, the Board voted to suspend the medical licenses of both Southam and Mandel for one year, a stinging rebuke especially to Southam, who was at the time a prominent leader of the New York and national communities of cancer researchers. The Regents softened this punishment considerably, however, by staying the license suspensions on the condition that the physicians stayed out of trouble for the next year, during which time they would remain on probation.

Dénouement

Events subsequent to the resolution of the JCDH case proved just as freighted with ambiguity as the evidence presented before the Regents' tribunal. Kagan and Fersko, two of the three courageous young residents who had refused to cooperate, were rewarded for their efforts with exclusion from the American College of Physicians. As Preminger reports, their exclusion was doubtless prompted by their refusal to cooperate in the experiment and their subsequent "irresponsible" resignations from the staff of the JCDH. They appealed, and their exclusion was eventually reversed on the ground that their "overreaction" to Southam's experiment was excusable in light of their families' "Holocaust situations."[2] These all-too-rare profiles in courage were thus trivialized by the governors of the American College of Physicians, reduced to the status of merely exculpatory psychological pathology. The three dissenters had refused to cooperate in wrongdoing, apparently, not because of any allegiance to an ethical principle or the "basic rights of the human person," but rather because Mandel's proposal had triggered their memories of the Holocaust, which, in turn, caused their "irresponsible" behavior.

William Hyman, the founding Board member of the JCDH whose protracted lawsuit to view the subjects' charts eventually brought the Regents into the case, was refused perfunctory re-election to the hospital's Board of Trustees in 1966. Even though he had won his narrowly focused lawsuit, and even though the larger issues for which he fought were eventually vindicated by the Regents, his fellow trustees of the JCDH expelled him from the Board of a hospital he helped to found.

But the most remarkable historical irony was reserved for Southam himself. Having been publicly humiliated by an inqui-

sition before the New York State Board of Regents; having been found guilty of fraud, deceit, and the unprofessional conduct of medicine, and having had his medical license suspended and been placed on probation, as his lawyer put it, like some "low-brow scoundrel," Chester M. Southam was elected president of the American Association for Cancer Research in 1968.[5] Although his case both reflected and helped to bring about profound changes in the ethos and rules governing biomedical research, those changes had not yet percolated down into the rank and file of the research community, which still clung to its paternalistic ways and duly rewarded Southam with one of its greatest honors. In most researchers' view, apparently, the JCDH case was nothing more than a mere "brouhaha," a mere "squabble over who-told-what-to-whom." For them, there were no lessons to be learned, but as we know now, history was on the side of Hyman and the brave young residents. The days of untrammeled physician discretion in research ethics were numbered, and strangers were indeed gathering at the bedside. It would not be long before the revelations at Tuskegee would explode once and for all any lingering doubts about the desirability and necessity of imposing strict rules on the practice of biomedical research.

Ethical Legacy

What is the legacy and verdict of history on Chester Southam? In his own eyes, Southam might well have considered himself the victim of a cruel historical joke. In the process of doing important research in the usual way according to the regnant Hippocratic canons of medical ethics, he became enmeshed in a wrenching chapter in the development of contemporary research ethics. At one moment he was nobly pursuing research that promised "enormous pay-offs" for millions of future patients, the next he was accused of fraudulent actions befitting a Nazi doctor in the dock at Nuremburg. Indeed, the fact that Southam could muster so many distinguished physicians and researchers in his defense, and that he was subsequently given high honors by his peers in the cancer research establishment, suggests that the verdict in his case had a certain ex post facto quality about it. Many years later his daughter reported that Southam viewed his election to the presidency of the American Association of Cancer Research as vindication for his having been unfairly singled out by the Board of Regents.[3]

However, it would be an exaggeration to say that Southam's perspective on the obligations of researchers was the only one available at the time, and that he was therefore completely blindsided by history. Several physicians at the JCDH—and not just Kagan, Leichter, and Fersko—strenuously objected to the terms of Southam's proposed research. It says something that Mandel had to settle for an unlicensed and highly vulnerable Philippine medical resident to do his bidding in facilitating Southam's study. It should be noted, moreover, that Southam's cavalier attitude toward informed consent directly contradicted contemporary standards as articulated by one of the study's sponsors, the U.S. National Institutes of Health (NIH). As the attorney general of New York pointed out in his charges, the NIH's Clinical Center had explicitly required principal investigators to "personally provide the assigned volunteer, in lay language and at the level of his comprehension, with information about the proposed research project. He outlines its purpose, method, demands, inconveniences and discomforts, to enable the volunteer to make a mature judgment as to his willingness and ability to participate."[3]

Clearly, Southam's behavior does not measure up very well to this contemporaneous standard. He basically left the selection of subjects to Mandel and Custodio, an unlicensed physician, whom he then left to their own devices in dealing with the remaining 19 resident-subjects. True, there may well be some ambiguity regarding the official reach of the NIH regulations. It is unclear whether they governed only intramural research within the NIH's Clinical Center in Bethesda, Maryland, or also extended to all extramural research funded by the NIH, such as the JCDH case. Similarly, those regulations may only have applied to competent volunteers, whom they surely covered, and not to hospitalized patients, a more doubtful category. It should nevertheless be obvious that there were other, more demanding interpretations of the researcher's duties in play at the time this case transpired.

The ethical assessment of Southam's behavior in this case should also take note of the fact that he was unwilling to expose himself and his colleagues to the same, admittedly small risks to which he was willing to subject the residents of the JCDH. Whether or not he uttered or wrote the words, "Let's face it," Southam admitted on cross-examination before the Board of Regents that there might after all be a small risk associated with the injection of live cancer cells into one's body, and that he was unwilling to subject himself to that small risk. In refusing on principle to share the fate of his elderly, debilitated subjects at the JCDH, Southam appears to be a man who, because of his exalted status as a medical researcher, believed himself to exist on a higher plane than the human beings whom he conscripted into his studies. However, it should be noted that Southam and colleagues were not physically debilitated and therefore would not have been suitable subjects, given the aim of the research.

This last point touches on what for many is perhaps the most galling aspect of Southam's behavior in this case. This man apparently believed that because he was a medical researcher whose study aimed at truth and posed no lasting harm to subjects, *he was thereby entitled to a special dispensation from ordinary morality to conscript the bodies and lives of whomever he pleased.* Although this

must have seemed to Southam to be a most natural assumption to make, it is in actuality a presumption exhibiting remarkable, albeit all-too-common hubris. Writing in 1970, just four years after the Regents' judgment in the JCDH case, one of the great forerunners of contemporary bioethics, the distinguished moral theologian Paul Ramsey offered a new bioethical gloss on Lincoln's famous proclamation that "no man is good enough to govern another without his consent." Referring explicitly to then-recent scandals in research ethics, Ramsey wrote that "[n]o man is good enough to experiment upon another without his consent."[12] In 1972, the public reaction to the Tuskegee syphilis study would finally put a decisive end to the freewheeling discretion enjoyed by Southam and his peers in the medical establishment. The era of heavily regulated biomedical research was about to begin.

References

1. Beecher HK. Ethics and clinical research. *New England Journal of Medicine* 1966;274:1354–60.
2. Preminger BA. The case of Chester M. Southam: Research ethics and the limits of professional responsibility. *The Pharos* 2002;65(2):4–9.
3. Lerner BH. Sins of omission—Cancer research without informed consent. *New England Journal of Medicine* 2004;351:628–30.
4. Lear J. Do we need new rules for experiments on people? *Saturday Review* Feb. 5, 1966;49:68.
5. Katz J, with Capron AM, Glass ES, eds. *Experimentation With Human Beings.* New York, N.Y.: Russell Sage Foundation; 1972.
6. 42 Misc. 2d 427, 248 N.Y.S.2d 245 (Sup.Ct. 1964).
7. *The New York Times* Jan. 22, 1964; 38.
8. Langer E. Human experimentation: Cancer studies at Sloan-Kettering stir public debate on medical ethics. *Science* 1964;143:551–3.
9. Rothman DJ. *Strangers at the Bedside: A History of How Law and Bioethics Transformed Medical Decision Making.* 2nd ed. New York, N.Y.: Aldine; 2003.
10. Oken D. What to tell cancer patients: A study of medical attitudes. *JAMA* 1961;175:1120–8.
11. Katz J. *The Silent World of Doctor and Patient.* New York, N.Y.: The Free Press; 1984.
12. Ramsey P. *The Patient as Person.* New Haven, Conn.: Yale University Press; 1970:6–7.

Walter M. Robinson   Brandon T. Unruh

The Hepatitis Experiments at the Willowbrook State School

The hepatitis experiments performed at the Willowbrook State School are routinely cited as one of the most serious breaches of research ethics of the post–World War II period.[1–3] This determination is principally due to the inclusion of the experiments in Henry K. Beecher's 1966 article "Ethics and Clinical Research" in the *New England Journal of Medicine*.[4] Beecher's criticism set off a decade of debate about the ethics of clinical research at Willowbrook, with sharply differing opinions from leaders in the field.[5,6] Beecher extended his critique of the experiments at Willowbrook in his book *Research and the Individual* in 1970.[7]

Willowbrook was an institution for the mentally retarded operated in Staten Island, New York, from 1947 to 1987. For many, Willowbrook is seen today as a symbol of both the improper institutionalization of the retarded and the successful use of the legal system to force state governments to improve the conditions for retarded citizens under their care.[8] For the research ethics community, Willowbrook has become a potent symbol of unethical research. The experiments are often referred to in the same litany as the Jewish Chronic Disease Hospital case and the Tuskegee syphilis experiments (see Chapters 6 and 8). Indeed, Willowbrook is seen by many as the "pediatric Tuskegee," and the principal scientist involved in the studies, Saul Krugman, is routinely vilified.

The reality of the experiments at Willowbrook is more complicated. What really happened at Willowbrook? What are the real lessons of Willowbrook for contemporary research ethics?

Hepatitis Before Willowbrook

Krugman began his work at Willowbrook in 1954. At the time, the causative agent for hepatitis was thought to be a virus and the

disease was characterized by two related clinical patterns. The first pattern was *infectious* hepatitis, thought to be transmitted by the ingestion of infectious material from feces. Transmission of infectious hepatitis by food workers through inadequate sanitation facilities, or by person-to-person contact without good hand-washing, had been documented. The second pattern was *serum* hepatitis, in which the infection was transmitted through inadequately sterilized needles or blood transfusions.

The diagnosis of hepatitis was made by observation of a clinical pattern of vomiting, anorexia, jaundice, and liver tenderness. Blood enzyme assays to detect liver damage were just being introduced. Reliance on the clinical symptoms alone for diagnosis meant that the infection might go undetected or be misdiagnosed. In the mid-1950s, it was unclear whether these "subclinical" cases of hepatitis could still lead to the spread of the infection.[9,10]

Previous research by Joseph Stokes at the University of Pennsylvania had demonstrated that injections of gamma globulin, an antibody-rich distillate of human serum, could modulate the clinical course of hepatitis by means of "passive" immunity. Stokes theorized that if hepatitis infection occurred during the period of passive immunity produced by gamma globulin, the clinical disease would be mild and long-lasting immunity to future infection might result.[11] He called this theory "passive-active" immunity.

The Initial Studies at Willowbrook

Krugman came to the Willowbrook State School as a consultant in infectious disease from New York University and Bellevue Hospital. He described his intentions at Willowbrook in the *New England Journal of Medicine* in February of 1958:

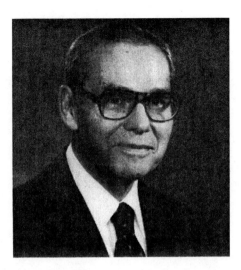

Figure 7.1. Saul Krugman (1911–1995). Source: Ehrman Medical Library Archives, New York University School of Medicine. Reproduced with permission.

The present report is concerned with an attempt to control the high prevalence of infectious hepatitis in an institution for mentally defective patients. Its purpose is threefold: to describe the circumstances under which the disease occurred, and the effect of gamma globulin in reducing its occurrence; an attempt to induce "passive-active immunity" by feeding virus to persons protected by gamma globulin; and [to describe the] excretion of virus during the incubation period of the disease.[12]

The investigations, funded in part by the Armed Forces Epidemiology section of the U.S. Surgeon General's Office, began with an epidemiologic survey of hepatitis at the school. Krugman demonstrated that the majority of hepatitis cases were acquired while at the institution, rather than as the result of infection prior to admission. By surveying the sewer and water systems, the growth and preparation of food, and the clinical histories of those who prepared and served the food, he also demonstrated that the source of hepatitis at the school was contact among infected students rather than infection from the food supply.

The Willowbrook strain of hepatitis was mild compared with other reported cases. Indeed, there were no deaths from hepatitis either in the patient population or in the attendants from 1953 to 1957. Krugman documented the rate of clinically apparent hepatitis among children and attendants at the school. The rate of acquisition of hepatitis among children at the school was to become a source of much contention, but Krugman's estimate at the time was that 40 to 50 patients per 1,000 per year contracted hepatitis.

Krugman and his coinvestigators set out to explore the protective effects of gamma globulin on the children at Willowbrook. After an initial trial with what was shown to be an inadequate dose, a second trial compared hepatitis rates between two groups of recently admitted students, only one of which was given gamma globulin injections. The results were startling. The children given gamma globulin appeared to be protected against clinical hepatitis for 39 weeks. The duration of the protection against infection was unexpected, because in the work by Stokes and others the pro-

tective effects of gamma globulin had lasted only 6 weeks. In order to explain the difference, Krugman asked whether the prolonged protection against hepatitis in persons injected with gamma globulin might be due to Stokes' passive-active immunity: "If so, it might be induced artificially by feeding virus to patients protected by an injection of gamma globulin."[12]

This hypothesis is the essential aspect of Krugman's experimental program, namely, that infection of children with a mild form of hepatitis could be an effective strategy to confer long-lasting immunity. In a report in 1957, Krugman wondered,

> Would gamma-globulin prevent [the] spread [of hepatitis], and if prevention occurred, would the effect be transitory or would it be prolonged in such a way as to suggest "passive-active" immunity (Stokes)? Could "passive-active" immunity be induced experimentally in small isolated groups by injecting gamma-globulin and then feeding hepatitis virus?[13]

The idea that infection with a mild form of a viral agent could induce immunity was well established by the time of Krugman's work, and in 1957 Krugman directly refers to his research as "immunization."[13] Much of the work on infectious diseases of childhood focused on just this approach. The polio trials[14] are perhaps the most famous example, but the work to induce immunity to measles also followed a similar pattern at precisely the same time, the mid-1950s[15] (see Chapter 5).

Ethical Issues Considered Before Beginning the Research

In outlining their intention to initiate the research, Krugman and colleagues wrote that "[t]he decision to feed hepatitis virus to patients at Willowbrook was not undertaken lightly."[12] The depth of planning for the trial and the lengthy list of ethical considerations prior to beginning the research are clearly enumerated in the 1958 *New England Journal of Medicine* article:

> It is well recognized that infectious hepatitis is a much milder disease in young children. Hepatitis was especially mild at Willowbrook; it was even benign in adults and there were no deaths. . . . Only the local strain or strains of virus already disseminated at Willowbrook would be used. . . . Since the annual attack rates of jaundice were high, for example 20 to 25 per 1000, and since in all probability cases of hepatitis without jaundice were occurring with the frequency equal to overt forms, it was apparent that most of the patients at Willowbrook were naturally exposed to hepatitis virus. . . . The advantages were considered of inducing the infection under the most favorable circumstances such as special isolation quarters with special medical and nursing personnel to provide close observation and extra care. . . . The study was planned so as to begin with very small and obviously ineffective doses of virus and to increase the dosage level gradually, in accordance with the results obtained. . . . The study group would contain only patients whose parents gave consent. . . . A serious uncontrolled endemic situation existed in the institution, and knowledge obtained from a series of suitable studies could lead to its control. . . . These factors were instrumental in the decision to proceed with the plan for titrating virus and inducing so-called passive active immunity.

The plan was sanctioned by the authorities of the New York State [D]epartment of Mental Hygiene, by the Armed Forces Epidemiologic Board of the [O]ffice of [S]urgeon [G]eneral.[12]

From today's perspective, this list of considerations mimics those presented in protocol applications to an institutional review board. Krugman designed an experiment that presented the least risk possible to those enrolled. He began with a low dose to observe side effects, created a specialized system for monitoring the children, and used an agent known to produce a mild form of the disease. He took into account the risks that the children faced in the absence of participating in the research. He considered the benefit to those enrolled as well as to other children facing the same circumstances. He obtained consent from the parents of every child who participated. And he obtained an independent review of the study design from experts in the field.

One result of the research program at Willowbrook was a reduction in the incidence of hepatitis among patients and employees by "80 to 85 percent."[16] Yet a beneficial outcome does not justify unethical research.

Criticisms of the Willowbrook Studies

Criticism of the Willowbrook experiments was first published in the *New England Journal of Medicine* in 1966 by Beecher, who continued his attack in 1970 in his *Research and the Individual*. Beecher set the tone for all subsequent condemnations of the experiments, and the legacy of his errors can be seen not only in the literature[2,3] but also in a brief unsuccessful attempt to outlaw all pediatric research in New York.[17] Beecher and later critics have made seven interlocking charges against the experiment.

1. Research that is done not for the benefit of the children involved in the study, but for others, is unacceptable. One of Beecher's primary concerns in writing the 1966 article was to criticize experimentation on one group of individuals solely to benefit another group. He cites the World Medical Association's draft code on ethics—which was to become known as the Declaration of Helsinki—and concludes, "[t]here is no right to risk injury to one person for the benefit of others."[4]

Beecher's criticism misses the mark at Willowbrook. Krugman had been clear in each report of the Willowbrook research that the goal of the research was to induce immunity in the children participating in the research so as to afford them protection against future infection.[12,13] Hepatitis was a problem at Willowbrook. Were Krugman to have performed the experiments on children who were not in an institution, and therefore not at an increased risk of acquiring hepatitis, then a case could be made that the experiment would place the children at risk only to benefit other children or adults. In the modern parlance, there was a "prospect of a direct benefit" to the children participating in the study, although this wording was unavailable to either Beecher or Krugman.

This is, of course, not to say that only the children at Willowbrook would benefit from the experiment; if Krugman were correct, then the induction of "passive-active" immunity might provide a boon to others who lived in crowded conditions with an increased potential for acquiring hepatitis. It is likely that the prospect of effective immunization against hepatitis that might be used with military recruits was the reason for the funding provided for the experiments. But the prospect of benefiting others does not exclude the prospect of benefit to the children at Willowbrook.

2. Deliberate infection of a person with an infectious agent as a part of research is unacceptable. Beecher's argument is that the intentional induction of an infectious disease is an unacceptable practice as part of research, regardless of the reason or the potential benefits of the research. Although he does not elaborate his concern, it appears that he has a principled objection to making someone sick when they are part of an experiment.

Beecher's objection is not very persuasive. There is no ethical weight that should be attached to the use of an infectious agent in a study independent of the effect that the infectious agent has on the study's risk. Beecher's rhetoric of "infection" carries with it undertones of dirt or pestilence when none is reasonably present. Beecher's argument appears to rest on a view of the human body as being irrevocably damaged by contact with infectious agents, and this is simply not the case, as the history of immunization programs amply demonstrates. The ethical issue is the harm done by the infection, not the mere fact of infection itself.

3. The parents who consented were unaware of the risks of participation. Beecher's claim is not that parents did not consent, but that there was inadequate disclosure of the details of the trial to the parents. His argument is that the research was so risky that no reasonably informed parent ought to have consented, and he takes the fact that the parents did consent as evidence that the consent process must have been inadequate.

Not much is known about the specific information provided to parents of children approached to participate in the Willowbrook experiments. In 1967, Joan Giles, Krugman's longtime collaborator in the hepatitis studies, described the consent process in the following way:

> I explain that there is no vaccine against infectious hepatitis, that the disease is always present here, and that their child is quite likely to come in contact with it by the intestinal-oral route common to a close quartered group of this type. I also tell them that we can modify the disease with gamma globulin but we can't provide lasting immunity without letting them get the disease. I explain that we use blood serum taken from Willowbrook patients who had hepatitis and that experience has shown a minimum dosage that can induce the disease in a form even less severe than occurs naturally in patients outside the hepatitis unit.[20]

In *Research and the Individual* Beecher responds to Giles' comments by arguing that "it was not clear whether any or all of the parents were told that hepatitis sometimes progresses to fatal liver destruction or that there is a possibility that cirrhosis developing later in life may have had its origin in earlier hepatitis."[7] Beecher's criticism boils down to a concern that there was a failure to focus on the serious but small risk of death due to hepatitis with liver failure. His criticism ignores that this complication had not been seen during the survey of hepatitis carried out at Willowbrook before the studies began: "Hepatitis was especially mild at Willowbrook; it was even benign in adults and there were no deaths."[12] In considering the overall quality of the consent process described by Giles, and acknowledging that she may have been explaining it in the best possible light considering Beecher's criticism, it is hard to argue convincingly that the parental consent was so insufficiently informed as to make the entire process unethical and the consents invalid.

4. Parents were coerced into enrolling their children in the research by the lack of available space at the school.   Beecher's criticism is based on events that were reported in 1967 but that occurred in 1964. Admissions to Willowbrook were halted due to overcrowding, yet space remained for additional children in the separate hepatitis research building. At that time, letters were sent by Dr. Jack Hammond, the medical director of Willowbrook and a coauthor on several reports of the hepatitis experiments, to the parents of children who were on the waiting list informing them that there was space in the research building.[20] Beecher's conclusion was that the investigators could not ethically be allowed to benefit, in the form of new children in their trial, from the lack of space at the school, and that enrollment should have ceased once parents had only the option of enrolling their children in the study or of not placing their children in Willowbrook at all.

The grounds for Beecher calling this letter unacceptably coercive are unclear: Parents clearly did want to admit their children in the school before they heard of the hepatitis experiments, and there is no evidence that the clinical standards for admission to the school were manipulated for those parents willing to enroll their children in the experiments. Parents were offered a set of options, neither of which was by itself unethical. There was no evidence of monetary or other incentives that induced the parents to choose enrollment in the studies. It is not prima facie unacceptable to require consent to research participation as a prerequisite for entry into a specialized care facility. Under such a reading of coercion, one might conclude that all institutions such as the NIH Clinical Center, where patients are admitted by agreeing to participate in a research program, systematically engage in unacceptable coercion. Such a reading abuses the meaning of the term coercion.[21]

5. Infection with hepatitis was not "inevitable" for children admitted to Willowbrook as Krugman had argued.   The rate of hepatitis infection among the children at Willowbrook has been the subject of enduring debate. Krugman and others argued that if infection with hepatitis were "inevitable" for children admitted to Willowbrook, then it would be acceptable to infect them under controlled conditions.

It is now clear that Krugman's rhetoric inflated the risk of infection with hepatitis. He reported in 1958 that the rate of hepatitis with jaundice was 25 per 1,000 per year, and that the rate of infection without jaundice was likely to be twice that, or 50 per 1,000 per year. Yet a recent best estimate using data available to Krugman at the time concludes that between 30 and 53% of the children admitted to Willowbrook would have acquired hepatitis during a childhood spent at the institution.[23] These estimates are below the claim of "inevitability" cited by Krugman and his supporters. Although all children in the experiments would contract hepatitis, only half—using a "generous" estimate[23]—of the children not participating in the trial would contract the disease. There may have been a subpopulation of children in whom the risk of infection was greater—perhaps those with a greater degree of disability or those exhibiting specific behaviors—and if so, then there may have been a subset of children for whom infection was "inevitable." But as these characteristics were not used in selecting children for the trial, the claim that infection was "inevitable" for the children in the general population does not withstand close scrutiny.

How much does this matter to the overall assessment of the experiment? If the goal of the trial were to study the effects of infection per se—or if the goal were, as Beecher suggests, simply to

determine the period of infectivity—then the lack of "inevitability" damns the trial, because the risk to the children not enrolled in the trial is less than that to those enrolled. Yet this was not the case, because there was the prospect of direct benefit to the children participating in the experiments.

If we correctly recognize that the experiments were done in an attempt to confer long-lasting immunity, then we can ask at what threshold of risk for an infectious illness in a given population should we begin immunization trials. We can get a sense of the acceptable threshold at the time by comparing Krugman's work to the other immunization research of his era. Using the 30% figure, the risk of contracting hepatitis as a child at Willowbrook was substantially greater than the risk of contracting polio as a child in the general population.[14] The point is that we ought to use a threshold risk in the population substantially lower than "inevitable" for the comparison of the risks of trial participation. Compared to other trials at the time, a risk of 30% was certainly over the acceptable threshold.

6. The experiments were unacceptable "experiments in nature."   Some have criticized Krugman for participating in a problematic "experiment in nature," a situation in which something bad is known to be happening to a group of people, and rather than preventing the bad event, a researcher exploits the situation by studying those negatively affected by it.[3] Rather than study hepatitis in children, the argument goes, Krugman had a moral duty to change the institutional conditions that led to the infection.

Calling the research at Willowbrook an "experiment in nature" rests on a mistaken idea that infection of the children was done in a convenient population simply to understand the consequences of infection. As Krugman explained in 1967, "Willowbrook was not chosen because its population is mentally retarded, but because it had endemic infectious hepatitis and a sufficiently open population so that the disease [hepatitis] could never be quieted by exhausting the supply of susceptibles."[20] Krugman was intervening in an epidemic situation, not simply standing by and observing. More importantly, his goal was to help those afflicted or likely to be afflicted by the illness in the very institution where the study was being done. Krugman's aim was to remedy the situation he found, not just to use it for an experiment. Again, the criticism that the studies were "experiments in nature" rests on a failure to see them as a program of immunization designed to address the problem of hepatitis in the institution.

7. The researchers should have cleaned up the conditions that led to the increased risk of infection rather than studied how to protect the children via immunization.   At Willowbrook, the increased hepatitis risk faced by the children was a consequence of the decision to gather children with mental disabilities and incontinence together in an institution, rather than a consequence of the children's disabilities per se. It can thus be argued that the conditions leading to the increased risk of hepatitis at Willowbrook were artificially created, because they were a result of a policy of institutionalization, and that by halting the institutionalization of children, the risk of hepatitis would be greatly reduced without the children having to undergo the risk of participation in research. If so, did the investigators have a moral duty to change the policy and to thereby decrease the risk of hepatitis faced by the children?

In order to answer this question, we must first know whether there were steps short of closing the institution (and not involving immunization) that might have prevented the risk of hepatitis infection. Preventing the fecal-oral spread of infectious agents among incontinent children in an institution is not a simple matter, even in a resource-rich environment. Control of hepatitis A outbreaks in neonatal intensive care units remain difficult even today.[23,24] Effective cohorting of children to prevent cross infection takes strict measures, with quarantining of all infectious children. Prior to the work of Krugman and his colleagues, such cohorting within the institution would have proven ineffective, because identification of those who were infectious was not possible. Nor would it have been clear what the duration of quarantine should be. In the context of a long-term residential program, physical measures to prevent infection would likely have meant the end of interactions among the children, with the indefinite closing of play groups and other measures thought to be therapeutic. Faced with those options, an attempt to discover an effective means of conferring immunity seems an appropriate means to address the medical risk to the children while preserving their ability to participate in the life of the institution.

So, were the investigators ethically bound to close the institution, or was it ethically viable instead to study how to make the institution safer? At the time of the hepatitis experiments, parents and physicians were eager to get children admitted to Willowbrook because institutionalization was thought to be the best thing for the children and for their families.[25] Placement in Willowbrook—that is, placement in a specialized school where retarded children could have access to the services of experts—was at the time seen by many as a symbol of an enlightened approach to the plight of retarded children.[26] Objecting to the institutionalization of children at Willowbrook in the 1950s and early 1960s, based on our contemporary approach to mental retardation in children, is open to a charge of anachronism, as well as of a certain arrogance that we are more ethically evolved than those who preceded us. Given the view that institutionalization was a beneficial policy for children and their families, Krugman and colleagues did what they could to improve the chances that institutions were safer for their child residents. Accusing Krugman of ignoring the suffering of the children at Willowbrook only to further his own agenda makes no sense in this context.

Correcting the Distorted Legacy

Because of the mistaken views of Beecher and others about the scientific objectives of the hepatitis research, Krugman's studies at Willowbrook are persistently cited as an example of unethical pediatric research. Yet many in the medical community who correctly understood the scientific and social context of the research have honored Krugman's work at Willowbrook, as have many of the families of the children in the research.

The mistakes of Beecher's analysis should be held to account for much of the continued misunderstanding. The errors are not simply of historical interest, because Willowbrook continues to be invoked in order to cast doubt on the ethics of researching the medical and social problems of retarded or otherwise socially vulnerable children. The use of Willowbrook in such a manner dangerously discourages research as a means to ameliorate health conditions for vulnerable populations of children.

Participation in medical research can be a powerful vehicle by which we devote social resources toward understanding the med-

ical problems of specific populations, as the parallel example of women in clinical research makes clear. Excluded from participating in research, in part by misplaced ethical concerns over the effect of research on a possible pregnancy, women were assumed to benefit from the products of research if men were shown to have benefited from this research. The result was twofold: The unique medical issues of women were ignored, and different physiological responses of women to standard care were rendered invisible. It is a similar mistake to continue to allow the experiments at Willowbrook to cast a restrictive ethical pall over the participation of vulnerable children in medical research.

References

1. Grodin MA, Glantz LH, eds. *Children as Research Subjects: Science, Ethics, and Law.* New York, N.Y.: Oxford University Press; 1994.
2. Guerrini A. *Experimenting With Humans and Animals: From Galen to Animal Rights.* Baltimore, Md.: Johns Hopkins University Press; 2003:140.
3. Rothman DJ. Were Tuskegee and Willowbrook "studies in nature"? *Hastings Center Report* 1982;12(2):5–7.
4. Beecher HK. Ethics and clinical research. *New England Journal of Medicine* 1966:274;1354–60.
5. Goldby S. Experiments at the Willowbrook State School. *Lancet* 1971;1:749.
6. Ingelfinger FJ. The unethical in medical ethics. *Annals of Internal Medicine* 1975:83;264–9.
7. Beecher HK. *Research and the Individual: Human Studies.* Boston, Mass.: Little, Brown & Co.; 1970.
8. Rothman DJ, Rothman SM. *The Willowbrook Wars.* New York, N.Y.: Harper & Row; 1984.
9. Paul H. *The Control of Communicable Diseases.* London, England: Harvey and Blythe; 1952:149–52.
10. Sodeman W. Infective (non-spirochetal) hepatitis. In: Pullen RL, ed. *Communicable Diseases.* Philadelphia, Penn.: Lea and Febiger; 1950:596–606.
11. Stokes J Jr, Farquhar JA, Drake ME. Infectious hepatitis: Length of protection by immune serum globulin (gamma globulin) during epidemics *JAMA* 1951:147:714–9.
12. Ward R, Krugman S, Giles JP, Jacobs AM, Bodansky O. Infectious hepatitis: Studies of its natural history and prevention. *New England Journal of Medicine* 1958:258;407–16.
13. Krugman S, Ward R, Giles JP, Jacobs AM. Experimental transmission and trials of passive-active immunity in viral hepatitis. *A.M.A. Journal of Diseases of Children* 1957;94:409–11.
14. Francis T Jr, Korns RF, Voight RB, et al. An evaluation of the 1954 poliomyelitis vaccine trials: Summary report. *American Journal of Public Health* 1955;45(5 Suppl 2):1–63.
15. Katz SL, Enders JF, Holloway A. Studies on an attenuated measles virus vaccine II: Clinical, virologic and immunologic effects of vaccine in institutionalized children. *New England Journal of Medicine* 1960;263:159–61.
16. Charges focus on ethics in institutional setting. *Medical Tribune* Feb. 15, 1967;8:24.
17. Smith T. "Smear and scare" charged to Thaler by city's doctors. *New York Times* Jan. 13, 1967.
18. Lederer SE. *Subjected to Science.* Baltimore, Md.: Johns Hopkins University Press; 1995.
19. Miller FG, Grady C. The ethical challenge of infection-inducing challenge studies. *Clinical Infectious Diseases* 2001;33:1028–33.
20. Studies with children backed on medical, ethical grounds. *Medical Tribune and Medical News* Feb. 20, 1967;8:1.

21. Hawkins JS, Emanuel EJ. Clarifying confusions about coercion. *Hastings Center Report* 2005;35(5):16–9.

22. Howell JD, Hayward RA. Writing Willowbrook, reading Willowbrook: The recounting of a medical experiment. In: Goodman J, McElligott E, Marks L, eds. *Useful Bodies: Humans in the Service of Medical Science in the Twentieth Century.* Baltimore, Md.: Johns Hopkins University Press; 2003:190–213.

23. Klein BS, Michaels JA, Rytel MW, et al. Nosocomial hepatitis A: A multinursery outbreak in Wisconsin. *JAMA* 1984;252;2716–21.

24. Watson JC, Fleming DW, Borella AJ, et al. Vertical transmission of hepatitis A resulting in an outbreak in a neonatal intensive care unit. *Journal of Infectious Diseases* 1993:167;567–71.

25. Shorter E. *The Kennedy Family and the Story of Mental Retardation.* Philadelphia, Penn.: Temple University Press; 2000:1–34.

26. Wolfensberger W. The origin and development of our institutional models. In: President's Committee on Mental Retardation, Kugel RB, Wolfensberger W, eds. *Changing Patterns in Residential Service for the Mentally Retarded.* Washington, D.C.: DHEW; 1969:63–161.

James H. Jones

The Tuskegee Syphilis Experiment

The Tuskegee Syphilis Experiment, commonly called The Tuskegee Study, was a peculiarly American tragedy, and it ultimately played a key role in creating the institutions and practices that today govern the use of human volunteers in U.S. biomedical research.[1-3] From 1932 until 1972, the U.S. Public Health Service (PHS), aided and abetted by a number of partners, conducted a nontherapeutic study of the effects of untreated syphilis on more than 400 black men in Macon County, Alabama, in and around the county seat of Tuskegee. Although PHS officers and other participating physicians performed a variety of tests and medical examinations on the men over the years, the Tuskegee Study in essence was a 40-year deathwatch. Only men with advanced cases of syphilis were selected for study, and the men were left largely untreated. Instead, the Tuskegee Study's basic procedures called for periodic blood tests and routine autopsies to supplement the information obtained through regular clinical examinations. The fact that only men with advanced syphilis were selected for the study indicated that the PHS officers were eager to learn more about the serious complications that the disease inflicts on its victims. To comprehend the magnitude of the risks to the men from denying them adequate treatment, it is useful to know a few basic facts about the disease.

Syphilis

Syphilis is a highly contagious disease caused by the *Treponema pallidum*, a delicate bacterium that is microscopic in size and resembles a corkscrew in shape. The disease may be acquired or congenital. In acquired syphilis, the spirochete (as the *Treponema*

pallidum is also called) enters the body through the skin or mucous membrane, usually during sexual intercourse, though infection may also occur from other forms of bodily contact, such as kissing. Congenital syphilis is transmitted to the fetus from the infected mother when the spirochete penetrates the placental barrier.

From the onset of infection, syphilis is a generalized disease involving tissues throughout the entire body. Once they wiggle their way through the skin or mucous membrane, the spirochetes enter the lymph capillaries, where they are hurried along to the nearest lymph gland. There they multiply at a rapid rate and work their way into the bloodstream. Within days the spirochetes invade every part of the body.

Three stages mark the natural history of the disease: primary, secondary, and tertiary. The primary stage lasts from 10 to 60 days starting from the time of infection. During this first incubation period, the primary lesion of syphilis, the chancre, appears at the point of contact, usually on the genitals. The chancre, typically a slightly elevated, round ulcer, rarely causes personal discomfort and may be so small as to go unnoticed. If it does not become secondarily infected, the chancre will heal without treatment within a month or two, leaving a scar that persists for several months.

While the chancre is healing, the second stage begins. Within six weeks to six months, a rash appears, signaling the onset of secondary syphilis. The rash may resemble measles, chicken pox, or any number of skin eruptions, though occasionally it is so mild as to evade notice. Bones and joints often become painful, and circulatory disturbances, such as cardiac palpitations, may develop. Fever, indigestion, headaches, or other nonspecific symptoms may accompany the rash. In some cases skin lesions develop into moist ulcers teeming with spirochetes, a condition that is especially severe when the rash appears in the mouth and causes open sores that are viciously infectious. Scalp hair may drop out in patches, creating a "moth-eaten" appearance. The greatest proliferation and most widespread distribution of spirochetes throughout the body occur in secondary syphilis.

Secondary syphilis gives way in most cases, with or without treatment, to a period of latency that may last as little as a few weeks or as long as 30 years. As if by magic, all symptoms of the disease seem to disappear, and the syphilitic patient does not associate the disease's early symptoms with the occasional skin infections, periodic chest pains, eye disorders, and vague discomforts that may follow. But the spirochetes do not vanish once the disease falls silent. They bore into the bone marrow, lymph glands, vital organs, and central nervous systems of their victims. In some cases the disease seems to follow a policy of peaceful coexistence, and its hosts are able to enjoy full and long lives. Even so, autopsies in such cases often reveal syphilitic lesions in vital organs as contributing causes of death. For many syphilitic patients, however, the disease remains latent only 2 or 3 years. Then the illusion of a truce is shattered by the appearance of signs and symptoms that denote tertiary syphilis, the disease's final and most deadly stage.

It is during late syphilis, as the tertiary stage is also called, that the disease erupts into a merciless killer. Gummy or rubbery tumors (so-called gummas), the characteristic lesion of late syphilis, appear. They are the stigmata from the concentration of spirochetes in the body's tissues, with deadly destruction of vital structures. The tumors often coalesce on the skin, forming large ulcers covered with crust consisting of several layers of exuded matter. Their assaults on bone structure produce deteriorations resembling osteomyelitis or bone tuberculosis. The small tumors may be absorbed, leaving slight scarred depressions, or they may cause wholesale destruction of the bone, such as the horrible mutilation that occurs when nasal and palate bones are eaten away. The liver may also be attacked; here the results are scarring and deformity of the organ that impede circulation from the intestines.

The cardiovascular and central nervous systems are frequent (and often fatal) targets of late syphilis. The tumors may attack the walls of the heart or the blood vessels. When the aorta is involved, the walls become weakened, scar tissue forms over the lesion, the artery dilates, and the valves of the heart no longer open and close properly. Instead, they start to leak. Then the stretching of the vessel walls often produces an aneurysm, a balloon-like bulge in the aorta. If the bulge bursts, the result is sudden death.

The results of neurosyphilis are equally devastating. Syphilis spreads to the brain through the blood vessels, and while the disease can take several forms, the best known is paresis, a general softening of the brain that produces progressive paralysis and, eventually, insanity. Tabes dorsalis, another form of neurosyphilis, produces a stumbling, foot-slapping gait in its victims due to the destruction of nerve cells in the spinal cord. Syphilis can also attack the optic nerve, causing blindness, or can invade the eight cranial nerves, inflicting deafness. Because nerve cells lack regenerative power, all such damage is permanent.

The Social Context

The germ that causes syphilis, the stages of the disease's development, and the complications that can result from untreated syphilis

were all known to medical science in 1932, the year the Tuskegee Study began. Indeed, among the many diseases that plagued mankind, syphilis was the most exhaustively studied, the most richly documented, the most elegantly described, and the best understood. So why would the U.S. PHS decide to launch a study of the effects of untreated syphilis in 1932, and why would PHS officials limit the study to black males?

The South in the 1930s was the section of the United States that most resembled the underdeveloped nations of the world. Its people, white and black, remained mostly rural; they were less educated than other Americans; and they made decidedly less money.

As a group, black Americans in the South were among the poorest of the poor. Indeed, they were virtual paupers—chronically unemployed or underemployed, many living in shacks without benefit of sanitation, adequate diet, or the rudiments of hygiene. As a group, they did not enjoy good health. Many suffered from a host of diseases, including tuberculosis, syphilis, hookworm, pellagra, rickets, and rotting teeth, and their death rate far exceeded that of whites.

Despite their chronic need, few blacks received proper medical care. In fact, many blacks lived outside the world of modern medicine, going from cradle to grave without ever seeing a physician. There was a severe shortage of black physicians throughout the South, and many white physicians refused to treat black patients. In addition, there were only a handful of black hospitals in the South, and most white hospitals either denied blacks admission or assigned them to segregated wings that were often overcrowded and understaffed.

But poverty was as much to blame as racism for the medical neglect of black Americans during the 1930s. The United States was in the depths of a bleak economic depression, and blacks, always the last to be hired and the first to be fired, were especially hard hit by the collapse of the economy. Medical care in the United States was offered on a fee-for-service basis, and the truth was that many black Americans simply did not have the money to pay for health care.

The Rise and Role of the PHS

During the Progressive Era, that period of social, economic, and political reform in the United States that began around 1890 and ended around 1920, the federal government took steps to ease the hardships on the poor, and part of these efforts centered on medical care. In 1912 the federal government united all its health-related activities under the PHS. Over the next few decades, the PHS distinguished itself by launching attacks on hookworm, pellagra, and a host of other illnesses. In no field was the PHS more active than in its efforts to combat venereal diseases.

Health reformers knew that syphilis, in particular, was a killer, and that the disease was capable of inflicting blindness, deafness, and insanity on its victims. Furthermore, they regarded syphilis as a serious threat to the family because they associated it with prostitution and with loose morals in general, adding a moral dimension to their medical concerns.

Taking advantage of the emergency atmosphere of World War I, progressive reformers pushed through Congress in 1918 a bill to create a special Division of Venereal Diseases within the PHS. The PHS officers who worked in the VD Division called themselves "syphilis men," so great was their personal identification with their vocations. They were crusaders, true believers. Safeguarding the public's health was their mission and, as zealots, they had a tendency to overstate the challenges they confronted. Labeling syphilis "the great killer," they proclaimed the gospels of prophylaxis, prompt diagnosis, and early treatment. To them syphilis was the most insidious of diseases, and they worked night and day to drive it from the land. The offensive they launched began with high hopes, and their initial successes were impressive. By 1919, they had established over 200 health clinics, which treated over 64,000 patients who otherwise could not have afforded health care.

To their credit, PHS officers did not ignore the health of black Americans. In the late 1920s, the PHS joined forces with the Rosenwald Fund, a private, philanthropic foundation in Chicago named in honor of its benefactor, Julius Rosenwald, who had made a fortune as one of the founders of Sears, Roebuck and Co. Together, the PHS and the Rosenwald Fund developed a syphilis control program for blacks in the South. In 1929, Michael M. Davis, the director of the Rosenwald Fund's Medical Division, asked the PHS to assign one of its officers to the Fund in order to advise the Fund on health issues that would benefit blacks living in the South. Julius Rosenwald had a special interest in uplifting blacks, and he was eager to see his foundation's medical division develop programs that would improve their health. In response, the PHS seconded a physician named Taliaferro Clark to the Rosenwald Fund, with instructions to provide advice and assistance in the Fund's efforts to develop new programs to improve the health of blacks living in the South. Clark, who had served as the director of the PHS Division of Venereal Diseases, immediately recommended that the Rosenwald Fund develop a syphilis control program for blacks in the South.

Most white physicians believed the racial stereotypes that permeated white society, including the notion the blacks were libidinous creatures who could not control their sexual behavior. As a result, many white physicians assumed that blacks suffered a much higher infection rate than whites because blacks abandoned themselves to sexual promiscuity. And once infected, the argument held, blacks remained infected because they were too poor and too ignorant to seek medical care. In short, many physicians despaired of being able to treat syphilis in the black community, creating a powerful rationale for inactivity in the face of a health crisis that public health officials and private physicians alike agreed had reached epidemic portions.

Armed with money from the Rosenwald Fund, the PHS devised a health study designed to establish the incidence of syphilis in blacks and to learn whether blacks could be treated successfully for syphilis if treatment programs were made available to them. To answer these questions, the PHS selected communities in six different southern states, each chosen because of the different demographic profiles it offered for representing a continuum of the living conditions and circumstances of blacks in the South. In each of the six communities, the PHS dispatched health professionals into the field to ascertain the incidence of syphilis by administering Wassermann tests to a representative sample of the local black residents and then to offer free treatment to those who tested positive and were found to be infected.

The results of this pilot program were at once informative and impressive. Based on the data from the six southern communities, the PHS learned that the rate of infection varied greatly from community to community, ranging from a low of roughly 7% in

Albemarle County, Virginia, to a high of 36% in Macon County, Alabama. In large measure, PHS officers pointed to different socioeconomic conditions to explain the jarring variations they discovered among the communities. In communities where blacks enjoyed higher incomes, better housing, and affordable health care, the incidence of syphilis was relatively low, whereas blacks who suffered higher rates of infection were much more likely to live in communities where living wages, decent housing, and affordable health care were rare. In addition, the data from this pilot program demonstrated conclusively that black patients not only wanted medical treatment for syphilis but returned to the clinics in large numbers to complete the extended program of therapy required to cure the disease.

This program had to be abandoned, however, soon after the stock market collapse of 1929 forced the Rosenwald Fund to terminate its support, leaving the PHS without sufficient funds to follow up its syphilis control work among blacks in the South.

The Tuskegee Syphilis Study

The PHS was reluctant to take leave of one of its pilot programs in particular, the one in Macon County, Alabama. Its county seat, Tuskegee, was the home of the Tuskegee Institute, the famed school founded by Booker T. Washington in 1882 to uplift blacks in the South. It was in and around Tuskegee that the PHS discovered an infection rate of 36%, the highest incidence in the six communities studied. In fact, despite the presence of the Tuskegee Institute, which boasted a well-equipped hospital that might have provided low-cost health care to blacks in the region, Macon County was home to the worst poverty and the most sickly residents that the PHS uncovered anywhere in the South.

It was precisely this ready-made laboratory of human suffering that prompted the PHS to return to Macon County in 1932. Because the PHS could not afford to treat syphilis, Clark decided to document the disease's damages on its victims by launching a scientific study of the effects of untreated syphilis on black males. (The reason he decided to limit the study to males was his belief that it was easier to get a reliable clinical history from males than it was from females because men were more likely to observe and remember the date of the appearance of the primary chancre, a crucial piece of data for pinpointing how long each person had suffered from the disease.) Many white Southerners, including many white physicians, believed that although syphilis was widespread among blacks, the disease did not harm them as severely as it did whites. PHS officials thought that this was nonsense because they knew that syphilis was a serious threat to the health of black Americans, and they intended to use the results of the study to pressure Southern state legislatures into appropriating funds for syphilis control work among rural blacks. By denying the men treatment, the PHS intended to document the ravages of the disease in black people, build a case for treatment programs sponsored by state governments, and force state health officials to develop and fund treatment programs for Southern blacks modeled after the recently completed Rosenwald Fund syphilis control demonstrations. Here, the irony was palpable: By withholding treatment from the men in Tuskegee, the PHS hoped to secure treatment for blacks throughout the South.

Still, whatever social value might accrue from encouraging state legislatures to appropriate funds to diagnose and treat syphilis in their black citizens, the fact remains that these "hoped for" benefits in no way justified withholding treatment for a deadly disease from people who believed they were being helped.

There was another motive for the proposed study. For decades medical scientists and clinical physicians alike had accepted as an article of faith the notion that advanced syphilis affected whites and blacks differently. Blacks were believed to suffer a much higher incidence of cardiovascular syphilis, whereas whites were thought to suffer a higher incidence of brain damage and related neuro-

logical disease. The Oslo Study of untreated syphilis in a select group of Caucasians, a retrospective study that dated back to the 1890s, had provided medical science with a controlled experiment on whites, and the PHS officers wanted to develop comparable data on blacks. In other words, the Tuskegee Study was intended to provide a black counterpoint to the Oslo Study, supplying data that would permit scientists to test the notion that advanced syphilis affected blacks and whites differently. Here again, the social value of determining whether the disease affected the races differently

Table 8.1

Tuskegee Syphilis Study Timeline

Date	Event
Nov. 1929	The Rosenwald Fund, a private philanthropic foundation, appropriates $50,000 to finance syphilis control demonstrations by the U.S. Public Health Service (PHS) with African Americans in six different communities in six different southern states, one of which is the town of Tuskegee, the county seat of Macon County, Ala.
Jan. 1930	The PHS begins its syphilis control demonstrations in Tuskegee and other communities in the South.
Oct. 1932	The PHS returns to Tuskegee, where it previously uncovered an infection rate of 35% among those tested, to study the effects of untreated syphilis in a select group of African American males. The men are not told the purpose of the study nor the effects of syphilis on human beings.
May 1933	Spinal taps are performed on the subjects of the study without the procedure or its effects being explained to them.
June 1933	Taliaferro Clark, who originated the study, retires from the PHS. Raymond Vonderlehr, who is intent on continuing the study, succeeds him.
Nov. 1933–Mar. 1934	PHS officers return to Tuskegee and add a group of approximately 200 African American men to serve as controls for the study, again without explaining the study to them.
May 1935	The Milbank Memorial Fund, another private philanthropic foundation, gives the PHS a grant of $500 to pay burial stipends to the men as an incentive for them and their families to consent to autopsies on the men when they die. The grant is extended in subsequent years.
1937–1938	The PHS sends mobile units into Macon County to treat people for syphilis, but treatment is withheld from the men in the study.
1942–1943	The PHS intervenes with the local draft boards in and around Macon County to secure deferments for the men in the study in order to prevent them from receiving treatment from the armed services upon induction into military service.
1943	The PHS starts treating patients who have syphilis with penicillin in several medical centers in the United States.
1947	The Nuremberg Code is articulated to protect human subjects from unethical and illegal medical experiments and studies.
1952	The PHS attempts to improve its record keeping and diagnostic standards for the study.
1958	The PHS distributes certificates of appreciation and small cash payments to the men in the study.
1964	The Declaration of Helsinki, which stipulates that researchers must obtain informed consent from their subjects, is issued by the World Medical Association.
1966, 1968	Peter Buxtun, a PHS employee in San Francisco, Calif., raises strong moral objections to the Tuskegee Study.
Feb. 1969	The PHS convenes a blue-ribbon panel to review the Tuskegee Study, and the panel recommends that the study be continued, with one panelist in dissent.
July 1972	Peter Buxtun tells a newspaper reporter about the Tuskegee Study and the press breaks the story.
Aug. 1972	In response to public outrage, the Department of Health, Education and Welfare (HEW) appoints a panel to investigate the Tuskegee Study.
Feb./Mar. 1972	The U.S. Senate holds hearings on human experimentation; the Tuskegee Study is given prominent attention.
Mar. 1973	HEW officially ends the Tuskegee Study by authorizing treatment for the survivors.
July 1973	Attorney Fred Gray files a $1.8 billion class action lawsuit against the United States, HEW, the State of Alabama, the State Board of Health of Alabama, and the Milbank Fund, as well as certain individuals in their private capacity.
Dec. 1974	A settlement is reached in the lawsuit.
1975	The U.S. government agrees to treat the wives and children of the men in the Tuskegee Study.
1997	President Bill Clinton apologizes for the Tuskegee Study.

must be weighed against the risks to the men from lack of treatment for a disease that medical authorities agreed was a killer.

The Design of the Tuskegee Study

In 1932, Clark dispatched two of his best officers from the Division of Venereal Disease, Oscar C. Wenger and Raymond Vonderlehr, to Alabama to conduct the study. As part of their preparations, Wenger and Vonderlehr briefed state health officials, the chief administrators and medical officials at the Tuskegee Institute, local doctors in the region, and other concerned parties on the proposed study and secured their full cooperation and support. In addition, they hired a black nurse, Eunice Rivers, to help with the study. Once these preparations were completed, the PHS officers went through Macon County and the surrounding counties with a Wassermann dragnet. Based on the test results of the men they examined, the PHS officers selected approximately 400 men who would serve as subjects in the study group. In 1933 and 1934, the PHS officers selected an additional 200 men who were free of the disease to serve as controls.

From the outset, the Tuskegee Study was a nontherapeutic scientific experiment. It had nothing to do with treatment; its overriding purpose was to document the natural history of disease in black males. In order to secure their cooperation, Wenger and Vonderlehr told the local residents and the men who were selected for study that the PHS had returned to Macon County to resume the treatment program that had been started under the Rosenwald Fund syphilis control demonstrations. The PHS did not inform the men that they had syphilis. Instead, the men were told only that they had "bad blood," a catchall phrase that rural blacks used to describe a host of ailments. In short, the PHS did not obtain informed consent from the men in study. Rather, the PHS deceived them by withholding critical information about the nature of their illness and the true purpose of the study.

Although the PHS had no intention of treating the men, J. N. Baker, the ranking state health officer, demanded as the price for the Alabama Health Department's cooperation that the men in the study be given treatment—not enough to cure them, to be sure, but enough to render them noninfectious. Consequently, all of the men in the study received at least some treatment with arsphenamine by injection and mercury by inunction—the drugs and treatment methods of choice in the 1930s.

No one worried much at the time about the glaring contradiction of treating subjects in a study of untreated syphilis because the men did not receive enough treatment to cure them. Treatments against syphilis did exist at the time, although they were not as effective as current therapies. Any amount of treatment, however, was fatal to the scientific integrity of the experiment. Flawed beyond redemption, the Tuskegee Study had no scientific validity because it was hopelessly contaminated from the outset. In addition to being morally bankrupt, it was bad science.

The original plan called for the Tuskegee Study to last from six months to a year. After Vonderlehr started examining the men, however, he was fascinated by the high incidence of cardiovascular syphilis he believed he had discovered in the subjects. He urged Clark to extend the study for several more years so that science could learn more about the effects of untreated syphilis. Clark refused his request, explaining that the Division of Venereal Diseases did not have enough money to continue the study. Within the year, however, Clark retired and Vonderlehr succeeded him as the director of the Division. Vonderlehr's promotion settled the matter. He decided to continue the Tuskegee Study, stipulating that its time frame would be open-ended.

Vonderlehr's decision to continue the study anticipated one of the most important reasons why the Tuskegee Study would last for 40 years. Over and over again during the next four decades, the PHS policy of promoting from within would bring to the directorship of the Division of Venereal Diseases officers who had worked in one capacity or another on the Tuskegee Study earlier in their careers. Often they had been sent to Tuskegee as young PHS recruits to sharpen their diagnostic skills by examining the men, and over the years they became not only knowledgeable about the study but comfortable with it. On those rare occasions when questions were asked regarding the study, these officers found it difficult to be objective. Time after time, they brushed aside scientific challenges and moral objections to continuing the study. In effect, they were co-opted by familiarity and they found it impossible to bring an unbiased assessment to the study.

The Tuskegee Study was not a difficult experiment to run. The PHS officers had only to monitor the progress of the disease in the subjects and perform autopsies on them when they died. To accomplish these tasks, the PHS sent teams of officers back to Tuskegee at regular intervals to perform what they called "annual round-ups." Nurse Rivers was responsible for transporting the men in her automobile from their homes either to the Andrews Hospital on the campus of the Tuskegee Institute or to the nearby Veterans Hospital, the two facilities where most of the clinical examinations were performed. Men who were discovered to be in poor or declining health were followed closely until they died, at which time Nurse Rivers negotiated with their families to secure permission for doctors to perform autopsies.

The PHS offered the families of the deceased men a powerful incentive to allow the autopsies. Because most of these families did not have any kind of burial insurance, they were hard pressed to come up with the money for decent burials. The PHS offered the families burial stipends if they would consent to autopsies. Most did. To finance the burial stipends, the PHS turned directly to the Milbank Memorial Fund, a medical philanthropic foundation. Over the years, the Milbank Memorial Fund provided a series of grants to the PHS for the explicit purpose of providing burial stipends to the families that permitted autopsies.

Burial stipends were not the only incentives offered by the PHS. In order to make the men think they were being treated for their "bad blood," Wenger, at the beginning of the study, started handing out pink-colored aspirin tablets to them. This "pink medicine," as the doctors dubbed the aspirin, became an instant hit. Most of the men had never taken aspirin before and they marveled at how quickly it relieved their aches and pains. From then on, the "government doctors" routinely dispensed little bottles of "pink medicine" every time they examined the men. A few years later, the "government doctors" also started dispensing iron tonic to the men. It, too, became much in demand. Perhaps no better placebos could have been used.

It is striking how little the PHS offered the men. Indeed, it is difficult to imagine a risk-benefit ratio that was more lopsided. Small amounts of syphilis therapy at the beginning of the study, aspirin, iron tonics, and burial stipends were the only benefits the men received in the early years of the study. In the 1950s, the PHS sweetened the deal by giving the men official-looking certificates

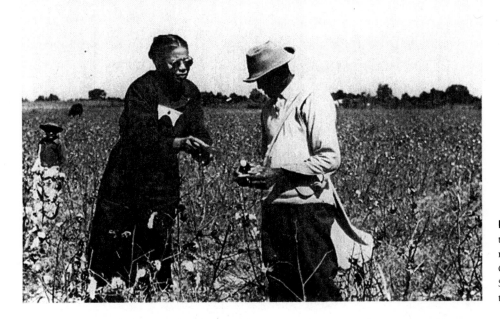

Figure 8.1. Nurse Eunice Rivers in the cotton fields with an unidentified man. Source: Centers for Disease Control Papers, Tuskegee Syphilis Study Administrative Records, National Archives—Southeast Region.

of appreciation and a dollar a year for every year they had remained in the study (see Figure 8.2). Added together, the benefits can only be described as paltry. As a group, the men saw their life expectancy decline by 20%, and one estimate placed the number of men who died from complications from syphilis at 100, fully a quarter of the men with the disease. Meager as the benefits were, they had their intended effect. They kept the men in the study, illustrating to perfection two crucial factors that the PHS counted on to keep the study going: deception and inducements to the poor.

Originally, the Tuskegee Study was supposed to last for only six months to a year. But because there was no formal protocol at the beginning, the time frame proved to be remarkably elastic. As the years passed, it became open-ended, and PHS officials simply assumed that the study would continue until the last man had died. It was as though the PHS had converted Macon County and the surrounding areas into its own private laboratory—in effect, a "sick farm"—where diseased and dying subjects could be maintained without further treatment and herded together for inspection at the yearly roundups. One of the health officers who conducted an "annual roundup" even spoke of "corralling" the men, as though they were so many sheep or cattle. In truth, the Tuskegee Study made no emotional demands on the PHS officers who conducted it because the little contact they had with the subjects did not require them to develop person-to-person relationships. They never got to know the men as patients or as people.

Instead, the PHS officers behaved like absentee landlords, issuing orders from afar, demanding strict accountings for day-to-day affairs, and appearing in Tuskegee only when needed. From their standpoint, the operation of their sick farm in Alabama was ideal. They were free to analyze data and to write scientific papers about the effects of untreated syphilis in black males; a few weeks of frantic work each year during the roundups was all they had to do in Alabama. Time, disease, and Nurse Rivers took care of the rest.

Potential Challenges to the Tuskegee Study

During the first few years of the experiment, there was no real danger that the men would receive medical treatment; poverty and ignorance decreed that they would remain untreated. That situation changed dramatically in 1937. In that year, the Rosenwald Fund decided to renew its support of syphilis control programs in the South and sent a black physician, William B. Perry of the Harvard School of Public Health, to Macon County. Fearing that the resumption of treatment activities might endanger the experiment and aware that Perry badly needed help, Vonderlehr shrewdly arranged to have Nurse Rivers assigned as his assistant. Perry agreed to cooperate fully with the experiment by not treating any of the subjects. Nurse Rivers worked closely with him to make certain that none of the subjects, all of whom she knew by name and on sight, received treatment.

Although withholding treatment from the subjects had always been standard operating procedure, this episode marked a sea change. Before the study began, the men were in no real danger of being treated because they were too poor and too ignorant to seek medical care. In a sense, then, all the Tuskegee Study did was to take a de facto situation and place it under a microscope so that science could compile data from the men's plights. By denying the subjects in the study therapy when treatment became widely available in the late 1930s and early 1940s, however, the PHS actually prevented the men from benefiting from therapy that they otherwise would have received.

Nor was this the only time when the PHS took steps to deny the men treatment. Until World War II erupted, Nurse Rivers, with the aid of local and state health authorities, had successfully cut the men off from treatment programs, but the war created a situation in which representatives of the lay public were making certain that syphilitic men in Macon County received treatment. Approximately 250 of the syphilitic subjects were under 45 years

U. S. PUBLIC HEALTH SERVICE

This certificate is awarded to

In grateful recognition of 25 years

of active participation in the

Tuskegee medical research study.

Figure 8.2. U.S. Public Health Service
Tuskegee Syphilis Study Certificate of
Recognition, 1958. Source: Centers for
Disease Control Papers, Tuskegee
Syphilis Study Administrative Records,
National Archives—Southeast Region.

Awarded 1958

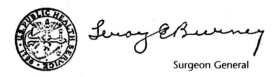

Surgeon General

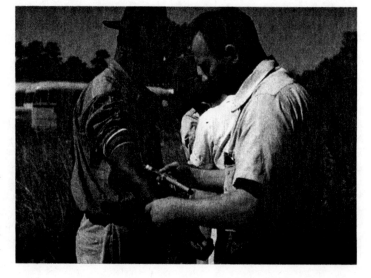

Figure 8.3. Dr. Walter Edmondson drawing blood from
unidentified man, early 1950s. Source: Centers for Disease Control
Papers, Tuskegee Syphilis Study Administrative Records, National
Archives—Southeast Region.

of age (the cutoff age for the draft) in 1941, and they became "1-A" registrants, the group first in line for induction into the armed services. Once their physical examinations revealed syphilis, the men in the study started receiving letters from their local draft boards ordering them to take treatment. To prevent them from being treated and from being inducted into the armed services, the PHS intervened with the local drafts and obtained deferments for all of the men in the study. Thanks to the PHS intervention, a significant number of the subjects were denied treatment once again, for the PHS had no intention of losing men from the study. If the men were to be placed in harm's way, the PHS meant for them to do so as "soldiers of science," not as soldiers who fought the nation's enemies on foreign battlefields.

Preventing the men from receiving treatment had always been a violation of Alabama's public health statutes requiring public reporting and prompt treatment of venereal disease cases. In 1943 these regulations were superseded by the Henderson Act, an extremely stringent public health law inspired by the wartime emergency. The law pertained to tuberculosis as well as venereal diseases and required state and local health officials to test everyone in the state between the ages of 14 and 50 and to treat those who were found to be infected. Under the auspices of the law, health officials conducted the largest state-level testing and treatment program in the history of the nation. But just as the men in the Tuskegee Study were cut off from earlier treatment programs, the Henderson Act was never applied to them. State and local health officials deferred to the PHS policy of keeping the men untreated and continued to cooperate with the study.

The Tuskegee Syphilis Study After World War II

Two developments associated with World War II might have impinged on the study, but did not do so. The first was the discovery of penicillin and the drug's mass production during the last part of the war. Yet penicillin did not produce any soul searching or second thoughts within the PHS. It was withheld for the same reason that other drugs had been denied to the men from the beginning of the experiment: Treatment would have ended the Tuskegee Study. In the view of the PHS, the men were subjects, not patients; clinical material, not sick people.

The other development associated with World War II that might have given the PHS officers pause was the Nuremberg trials and the Nuremberg Code, the 10 basic conclusions or principles on human experimentation that emerged from the trials (see Chapter 12). The PHS officers associated with the Tuskegee Study during and immediately after World War II saw no connection whatsoever between the atrocities committed by Nazi scientists and their own actions in the Tuskegee Study. Indeed, there is no evidence that the Tuskegee Study was ever discussed in light of the Nuremberg Code.

And yet there was a similarity between the Nazi experiments and the Tuskegee Study, one that transcended their racist and medical natures. Just as the chain of command within the military hierarchy of Nazi Germany blunted individual responsibility and failed to frame moral issues, the Tuskegee Study's firm entrenchment within the PHS bureaucracy reduced the sense of personal responsibility and ethical concerns. Like the Nazi doctors who pleaded that they were simply following orders, the PHS

officers, state health officials, the medical staff of the Tuskegee Institute, and the staff from the Veterans Hospital in Tuskegee all felt that they were simply doing their jobs. Some spoke of merely "following orders," whereas others insisted that they had worked to advance science.

Black professionals in and around Tuskegee showed no more concern for the men than did the white doctors and health officials who launched and sustained the experiment. Over the decades, a procession of black doctors, health officials, educators, and nurses all lent their support, knowing full well the details of the study and its goals. Robert Russa Moton, who succeeded Booker T. Washington as the principal of the Tuskegee Institute; Eugene Dibble, the head of the Andrews Hospital at the Tuskegee Institute; William B. Perry, who conducted the second Rosenwald Fund syphilis treatment program in Macon County; Jerome J. Peters, who performed many of the autopsies at the Veterans Hospital in Tuskegee, all cooperated with the Tuskegee Study. Indeed, they and other black professionals lent a powerful element of biracial support to the Tuskegee Study. For at every stage of the study, the black professionals worked side-by-side with their white counterparts, and their very presence served to reassure the subjects that they were being helped by their participation in the Tuskegee Study. Indeed, it seems doubtful that the Tuskegee Study could have kept going without the black professionals. Yet as a group, they went largely unnoticed by the later pundits who saw the experiment as a simple morality play that cast white people in the familiar role of exploiters and oppressors of black people. It was far easier to keep things simple than to explore class divisions, based largely on education and income, within the black community, or to ponder how those same class divisions and professional identities could ally black professionals with white professionals.

Exposing the Tuskegee Study

Despite its powerful element of biracial support, the Tuskegee Study was a bellwether for race relations in the United States. Only 35 miles from Tuskegee, Rosa Parks and Martin Luther King were launching historic protests against racial injustice in the United States.

At one level, the civil rights movement made it difficult for the PHS to conduct business as usual with regard to the Tuskegee Study. Previously, PHS officers had always published their scientific reports on the experiment like scientists who had nothing to hide. By the 1960s and early 1970s, however, the self-confidence of their predecessors had been replaced by self-consciousness. For beneath the façade of "business as usual" there was a growing uneasiness, a perception that things had changed. It was not that the PHS officers had come to the conclusion that the Tuskegee Study was morally wrong. Rather, they feared dire consequences if the experiment became known. In other words, they regarded the Tuskegee Study as a potential public relations disaster waiting to happen. The day had passed when medical researchers could ignore the public's concern over the protection of human subjects, and they knew it. They understood, at least at some level, that race added a volatile issue.

In the years following the appearance of the Nuremberg Code and the Declaration of Helsinki (see Chapter 13), pressure gradually grew within the United States for the government to regulate human experimentation. In 1966, the Surgeon General's office issued Policy and Procedure Order Number 129, outlining the PHS's first guidelines on grants for clinical research and training. The guidelines established a system of peer review conducted by a standing panel of colleagues at an investigator's institution. Members of the committee had the responsibility of reviewing all proposals from their institution and submitting an "assurance of compliance" to the PHS.

Significantly, none of the guidelines contained provisions that applied to the PHS's own research programs. And nothing in the guidelines—except, of course, their spirit—obliged the PHS to meet the same standards as its grantees. Thus, none of the PHS health officers connected with the Tuskegee Study felt bound by these guidelines, and none expressed any ethical concern about the experiment in the light of these guidelines.

Peter Buxtun was different. He thought the Tuskegee Study was a moral disaster, and he said as much to anyone within the PHS who would listen. In the mid-1960s, Buxtun, a psychiatric social worker by training, was employed by the PHS at the Hunt Street Clinic in San Francisco, California, where he worked as a venereal disease interviewer and investigator. Buxtun learned about the Tuskegee Study from discussions with coworkers, and he researched the topic for a short paper he was required to prepare as part of his training. Disturbed by what he learned from his research, Buxtun launched a one-man crusade within the PHS to protest the bankrupt morality of the Tuskegee Study. He wrote letters, met with officials, and did everything in his power to persuade them to end the study.

As a result of Buxtun's protests, the PHS conducted a full-scale review of the Tuskegee Study in 1969. The review was held at the Communicable Disease Center (now the Centers for Disease Control and Prevention, or CDC) in Atlanta, Georgia, and the committee consisted of several high-ranking PHS officials, three medical professors, the state health officer of Alabama, and a senior representative of the Milbank Memorial Fund, the philanthropic foundation that had provided the money to pay small stipends to cover the burial expenses of deceased subjects in exchange for their families' permission to perform autopsies. No one with training in medical ethics was invited to the meeting, none of the participants was black, and at no point during the discussions did anyone mention the PHS's own guidelines on human experimentation or those of other federal agencies. Equally noteworthy, all the members of the committee except one had been directly involved with the Tuskegee Study in one capacity or another in the past. And precisely because all of them but one had been implicated by familiarity, it was difficult for them to bring an objective, fresh perspective to their task. Instead, as group, they were hostages of the same attitudes and values that had allowed them to work on the study for years.

During the course of the review, the committee members discussed whether to stop the study and offer the surviving subjects treatment. In the end, however, they decided to continue the study and recommended steps to improve it scientifically. In addition, they concluded that it would be an excellent idea to seek some type of "informed consent" for the study. Following a discussion, they agreed that the subjects were incapable of giving "informed consent" due to their meager educations and advanced ages. In place of the subjects, the committee members recommended that the PHS consult with state health authorities and the members of the local medical societies in and around Tuskegee, explain the study to these officials, and seek their cooperation and approval—obtaining, as it were, a kind of "surrogate informed consent" from the local medical establishment.

The committee's recommendation settled the fate of the Tuskegee Study, at least for the time being. It would continue. All of the committee members were physicians, and they approached the experiment as a medical matter. And once a medical judgment had been made against treating the men, the members of the committee saw no point in stopping the study. As a group, they did not perceive a conflict between their own scientific interests in continuing the experiment and attempting to decide what was best for the subjects. As physicians and men of science, they felt fully capable of deciding both. In their professional judgment, the Tuskegee Study was important to science, and they agreed that much remained to be learned from its continuation. Therefore, they decided to follow the men until the last subject had died and all the data had been analyzed and reported in scientific articles.

The members of the committee obviously felt comfortable deciding the fate of the men as a group, without bothering to examining a single subject. For although they expressed concern for the men and discussed whether any might benefit from treatment, they did not recommend that the PHS monitor the men and care for their well-being.

The PHS paid more attention to building alliances with medical groups in Alabama than it did to the subjects. In 1970, the PHS followed up on its plans to meet with state and county health officials in Alabama and with the membership of the local medical societies in and around Tuskegee. During those conferences the PHS officials reviewed the history of the Tuskegee Study, outlined their plans for continuing the study, asked for suggestions, and requested the cooperation of the health officials and private physicians with whom they met. In each instance, the PHS officials were pushing against an open door. Not only did the state health authorities and the local doctors fail to question or criticize the experiment, they offered to help in any way they could. Their response was all the more noteworthy for the fact that the Macon County Medical Society included many black physicians among its members. Thus, from beginning to end, the Tuskegee Study enjoyed the support of white and black doctors and health officials alike.

The Final Disclosure of Tuskegee

Had the PHS been left to its own devices, there is no doubt that the Tuskegee Study would have continued until the last subject had died, all the data had been analyzed, and the final article had been published. Instead, Peter Buxtun suddenly reappeared on the scene. Aided by the press, he moved with dispatch and purpose to end the experiment. Buxtun had resigned from the PHS in 1967 to attend law school, and during his years as a law student, he had attempted to interest several different law professors in the Tuskegee Study, all to no avail. After finishing law school, he finally told his story early in 1972 to someone who was willing to do something more than listen politely—Edith Lederer, a longtime friend who worked as an international affairs reporter for the Associated Press. After Buxtun showed her published articles and copies of his correspondence with PHS officials regarding the experiment, Lederer forwarded these materials to her superiors at the Associated Press, asking to be assigned to the story. Instead, the Associated Press gave the story to a highly regarded young reporter named Jean Heller, largely because she was based in Washington, D.C., and was familiar with government agencies.

A little digging on Heller's part uncovered additional medical articles on the experiment, but her best source proved to be the officials at the CDC. Heller recalls that in numerous telephone interviews, she received straightforward, matter-of-fact answers to her questions—however sensitive or potentially damaging to the PHS. Spokesmen there even provided estimates of the number of men who had died from the various complications of late syphilis, placing the figure between 28 and 100.

True to their goal of pursuing the study until the last subject had died, PHS officers were still conducting the experiment when Heller broke the story on July 25, 1972. In a series of hard-hitting articles that followed in rapid succession, Heller did a brilliant job of laying out the bare facts of the study. Her articles were only the beginning. All across the country television news shows and newspapers bombarded the public with facts and commentary on the Tuskegee Study. At first PHS officials tried to defend the experiment, but public outrage quickly silenced them, and the PHS officials announced that they had given orders for the experiment to be ended—effective immediately.

Fallout

Suddenly, the 40-year deathwatch was over, but the fallout from the experiment continued unabated. In the wake of the experiment's abrupt ending, Fred Gray, a black attorney and civil rights leader in Tuskegee, brought a class action lawsuit on behalf of the Tuskegee Study's surviving subjects and the estates of the deceased subjects. Rather than go to trial, the government settled the case. As part of the out-of-court settlement, the surviving subjects were finally treated with penicillin for syphilis. In addition, the men and the families of the deceased subjects received small cash payments.

In 1973, Senator Edward Kennedy of Massachusetts held hearings on the Tuskegee Study and other human experiments, and the next year the National Commission for the Protection of Human Subjects of Biomedical and Behavioral Research was created to explore the full range of issues involved in the use of humans in biomedical research. In response to the public uproar and the National Commission's recommendations, the government issued new guidelines for research projects that used federal funds in the United States. Drafted for the explicit purpose of protecting human subjects in scientific and medical experiments, these guidelines established and strengthened institutional review boards in universities and hospitals throughout the United States (see Chapter 14).

The Tuskegee Legacy

But the Tuskegee Study's troubled legacy did not end there. No scientific experiment in history inflicted more damage on the collective psyche of black Americans than the Tuskegee Study. In the

years after the experiment's disclosure, news of the tragedy spread in the black community. In addition to what they read in newspapers and magazines or heard on the radio and television, many blacks learned about the study by word of mouth, replete with the sorts of embellishments and distortions that usually attend oral traditions. Many blacks and whites were told that the federal government deliberately inoculated black sharecroppers with syphilis, whereas others were given to understand that the experiment was conducted on black prisoners.

Despite such errors, most black Americans got the gist of the story right: They understood that for 40 years, an agency of the federal government had withheld treatment from men with syphilis so science could learn what the disease, if left untreated, would do to people. Many of the men, the black public learned, had died from syphilis, whereas others had gone blind or insane. Confronted with the experiment's moral bankruptcy, many blacks lost faith in the government and in the medical establishment and no longer trusted health officials who spoke to them on matters of public concern.

This problem came into stark relief when the HIV epidemic struck the United States. Predisposed to distrust health authorities, many black Americans believed the rumors that circulated in the black community charging that HIV was a man-made virus created to perpetrate genocide on African Americans. Although these charges had no scientific basis, many of the people who heard them believed that they were true. And many of these same people did not believe the government's official explanations and theories about the causes of HIV. Suspicious and mistrustful of the government's reports on HIV, they felt deeply alienated from the experts who purported to have their best interests at heart.

Not surprisingly, then, many health officials encountered opposition when they tried to study HIV in black communities. In 1988, federal health authorities were forced to abandon a planned study of HIV infections in the District of Columbia. As designed, the scrapped project proposed to ask the residents of a black neighborhood to submit to household blood tests and complete a questionnaire to determine the feasibility of a national survey to gather data on the incidence of HIV. According to the *New York Times,* city officials "expressed concern that Washington's black community was being used as a 'guinea pig' in a project that would stigmatize the city and its minority communities."[4] The meaning of this and similar episodes across the country was clear: The legacy of the Tuskegee Study was hampering the government's efforts to control HIV in the black community.

In an effort to address this problem, President Bill Clinton held a public ceremony at the White House on May 16, 1997, and officially apologized for the Tuskegee Study. Speaking to the handful of Tuskegee Study survivors who had been brought to the White House at government expense to hear the apology— and speaking, by extension, to the nation—Clinton delivered an apology that constituted a masterly performance of the politics of symbolism. Aware that blacks have long placed great faith in symbols to express their hopes that they would one day enjoy true freedom and equality in the "land of the free," Clinton used the moral authority of his office to attempt to make amends for the Tuskegee Study and to begin the healing process within the black community.

Despite Clinton's best efforts, however, the Tuskegee Study remains today what it has been ever since the public became aware of it in 1972: a symbol of research malfeasance in which virtually every principle underlying the ethical treatment of human subjects of research was violated.

Acknowledgment

This essay is based on my book *Bad Blood: The Tuskegee Syphilis Experiment*, expanded ed. New York, N.Y.: The Free Press; 1993 [1981].

References

1. James H. Jones, *Bad Blood: The Tuskegee Syphilis Experiment,* expanded ed. New York, N.Y.: The Free Press; 1993 [1981].
2. Susan M. Reverby, ed. *Tuskegee's Truths: Rethinking the Tuskegee Syphilis Study*. Chapel Hill, N.C.: University of North Carolina Press; 2000.
3. Fred D. Gray. *The Tuskegee Syphilis Study: The Real Story and Beyond*. Montgomery, Ala.: NewSouth Books; 1998.
4. Boffey PM. U.S. drops AIDS study in community protests. *The New York Times* Aug. 17, 1988:A14.

John Y. Killen Jr.

HIV Research

In the 26 years since its first recognition, the AIDS epidemic has had a profound impact on human history. The Joint United Nations Programme on HIV/AIDS estimates that in 2006 there were 39.5 million people worldwide living with HIV, 4.3 million became newly infected, and 2.9 million died. "In addition to the untold grief and human misery caused by AIDS, the epidemic is wiping out development gains, decreasing life expectancy, increasing child mortality, orphaning millions, setting back the situation of women and children, and threatening to undermine national security in highly-affected societies."[1]

Since 1981, an enormous, worldwide biomedical research response has been mounted. For example, U.S. government funding of AIDS research by the National Institutes of Health (NIH) totaled $2.902 billion in fiscal year 2006, an amount representing over 10% of the total NIH budget.[2] Although much remains to be accomplished, the output of that investment has been spectacular. Indeed, as Anthony Fauci has written, "the extraordinary research effort devoted to AIDS during the first two decades of the pandemic and the rapidity with which advances have been realized surpass those associated with any other life-threatening infectious disease in history and certainly any newly recognized disease."[3]

The epidemic has also had a profound impact on virtually every facet of research ethics. I will examine just one of those facets in this chapter—how activism and other events in the early history of the HIV epidemic in the United States have caused the field to look anew at the principles of autonomy and justice, as they were articulated in the Belmont Report and implemented in regulation and policy that followed from it. In particular, I will focus on the following:

1. How advocacy for access to promising experimental therapy and clinical trials has:

   • Broadened the concept of autonomy to include the notion that humans with life-threatening diseases are entitled to an important role in assessing the potential risks and benefits of their participation in clinical research.
   • Broadened the concept of justice by giving specific form to the notion that the potential benefits of participation in research must be fairly and equitably shared.

2. How extensive involvement of the HIV/AIDS community has shaped scientific progress and altered the general landscape of clinical biomedical research.

Other facets of the epidemic will be considered in detail in other chapters. Of necessity, this examination is neither chronological nor comprehensive. More complete historical assessments are available.[3–7] Furthermore, because the epidemic continues to unfold at this writing and is likely to do so for many years to come, the story and its legacy for research ethics are both works in progress. Table 9.1 presents a timeline of selected events in HIV/AIDS treatment research.

Overview: The HIV/AIDS Epidemic in the United States

The disease that was to become known as AIDS was first identified in 1981 in the form of independent outbreaks of Kaposi's sarcoma (KS) and *Pneumocystis carinii* pneumonia (PcP) in homosexual

Table 9.1
Timeline of Selected Events in HIV/AIDS Treatment Research

Date	Event
1981	Recognition of AIDS (initially known as GRID) in homosexual men
1982	Identification of AIDS in intravenous drug users, hemophiliacs, women, transfusion recipients, and children
1983	Identification of causative virus Identification of AIDS cases in Africa
1984	Recognition of pre-AIDS conditions (AIDS-related complex) Establishment of relationship between high-risk sex and HIV transmission
1985	Licensure of diagnostic test for HIV Initiation of routine HIV screening and heat treatment of blood products
1986	AZT enhances survival of patients with advanced AIDS Establishment of AIDS Clinical Trials Group AZT treatment IND provides AZT to 4,000 patients in four months
1987	Approval/licensure of AZT
1988	Association between cervical dysplasia and HIV infection in women established Enactment of Health Omnibus Programs Extension (HOPE) Act
1989	AZT delays disease progression in patients with early HIV infection ACTG Community Constituency Group
1990	First guidelines for use of antiretroviral therapy Initiation of first trials of combinations of antiretroviral chemotherapy National Conference on Women and HIV Infection Demonstration: "Storm the NIH"
1991	Start of ACTG 076, a study of AZT to prevent mother-to-infant transmission of HIV
1992	FDA announces Parallel Track and Accelerated Approval Initiatives Start of first clinical trial testing a protease inhibitor
1993	Establishment of Women's Interagency Health Study
1994	AZT reduces mother-to-infant transmission of HIV by 70% (ACTG 076)
1995	First demonstration of effectiveness of combinations of highly active antiretroviral therapy (HAART) in treating HIV-infected patients at various stages of disease Licensure and approval of first protease inhibitor
1996	AZT dramatically reduces mother-to-infant transmission in the general population Combination HAART dramatically reduces morbidity and mortality in clinical trials
1997	Huge decreases in U.S. AIDS mortality, attributed to HAART
1998	Identification of lipodystrophy and other long-term complications of HAART Treatment Action Campaign launched by AIDS activists in South Africa to promote greater access to effective treatment
1999	Interruption of HAART explored as strategy for reducing long-term side effects
2000	13th International AIDS Conference ("Break the Silence") in Durban, South Africa, focuses attention on the unavailability of state-of-the-art HIV/AIDS care in the developing world World Medical Association revises Declaration of Helsinki, endorsing the concept that clinical trial participants everywhere must receive worldwide best standard of care
2002	Global Fund to Fight AIDS, Tuberculosis, and Malaria established to fund locally driven strategies to combat the three pandemics World Health Organization releases guidelines for antiretroviral therapy in resource-poor settings
2004	15th International AIDS Conference in Bangkok, Thailand, under the theme "Access for All," includes major activist protests highlighting global disparities in availability of care and heavy emphasis on programs to deliver care in resource-poor settings

men in New York and Los Angeles. Prior to these reports, the two diseases were virtually unknown in healthy young adults. Immunological evaluation of the affected individuals revealed severely compromised immune systems. The syndrome was initially referred to as gay related immune deficiency (GRID). In 1982, the identification of new cases among people with hemophilia, re-

cipients of blood transfusions, and intravenous drug users (IV-DUs) and their children confirmed the presence of an epidemic. The term GRID was soon replaced by the term acquired immunodeficiency syndrome (AIDS).

AIDS was initially defined by the coexistence of certain clinical conditions (e.g., PcP or KS) and specific laboratory findings in-

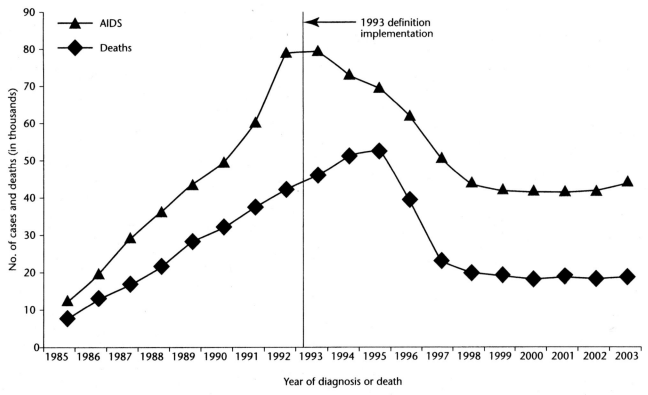

Figure 9.1. Estimated Number of AIDS Cases and Deaths Among Adults and Adolescents With AIDS in the United States, 1985–2003. Note: Data adjusted for reporting delays. Source: U.S. Department of Health and Human Services, Centers for Disease Control and Prevention.

dicative of immune deficiency. Further epidemiological investigation led to the identification of various pre-AIDS conditions and with that, the understanding that progressive deterioration of immune function occurred over a number of years. Thus, it became clear that the clinical disease known as "AIDS" was only the tip of the iceberg of an epidemic of unknown size. Gay and bisexual men remained the most heavily affected group. The cause remained unknown until 1983 when investigators in France and the United States independently isolated a previously unknown retrovirus from affected individuals. Although scientific disputes regarding their respective discoveries continued for years, the virus they identified became known as human immunodeficiency virus 1 (HIV-1). This pivotal discovery led directly to the licensure of the first diagnostic test for HIV two years later, in turn paving the way for better elucidation of the course of infection, as well as for routine screening and securing of the safety of blood and blood products. It also connected HIV-1 with "slims disease," a fatal AIDS-like syndrome characterized by wasting and bouts of severe infection that had been recognized among eastern and central Africans for a number of years before.

In 1986, five years and thousands of U.S. deaths after the first cases of AIDS were identified, the first major advance in treatment occurred. A placebo-controlled clinical trial sponsored by the Burroughs Wellcome Company demonstrated the effectiveness of azidothymidine (AZT), a drug that had been explored but abandoned years earlier as a potential treatment for cancer, in reducing mortality among patients with AIDS.[8] Over the ensuing decade,

advances in pathogenesis and treatment research led to dramatic improvements in morbidity and mortality through development of potent, multidrug chemotherapy regimens, and strategies for their use.[9] Striking evidence of the public health impact of these advances in the United States, which parallel those seen in many developed countries, is seen in Figures 9.1 and 9.2.

The Emergence of U.S. HIV/AIDS Activism

The history of HIV/AIDS research is bound together with the story of AIDS activism, which arose in the peculiar social and political milieu of the gay communities of several major metropolitan areas of the United States. Much has been written about the tactics, mechanisms, dynamics and sociopolitical factors involved.[4,6] The essential point here is that AIDS first appeared in a community that was simultaneously and rapidly emerging, through social and political activism, from a long history of persecution, repression, and marginalization by government, society, and medicine. As a consequence, there existed strong, highly motivated, and politically savvy leadership, with grass roots organizational abilities and powerful communication networks. Unfortunately, the concomitant sexual freedom of the time in general, and of gay liberation in particular, created conditions that permitted the epidemic to spread silently for years. This convergence of biology and sociology was hugely important in shaping the U.S. epidemic and the scientific and activist responses to it.

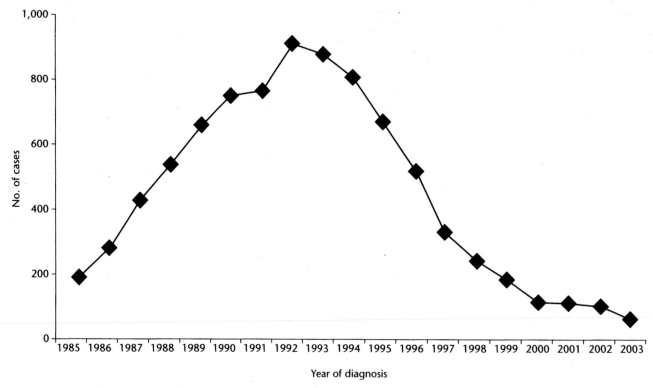

Figure 9.2. Estimated Number of AIDS Cases Resulting From Mother-to-Infant Transmission, 1985–2003. Note: Data adjusted for reporting delays and for estimated proportional redistribution of cases in persons initially reported without an identified risk factor. Source: U.S. Department of Health and Human Services, Centers for Disease Control and Prevention.

In this context, AIDS activism was fueled by anger and fear, which grew with scientific insights into the epidemic that included the following: (1) the understanding that there was an initial phase of clinically silent infection that spanned years or decades; (2) estimates that the true scope of the epidemic of viral infection (as opposed to clinical illness manifest as AIDS) included 5 to 10 times as many asymptomatic as symptomatic individuals; (3) proof that transmission of virus from infected to uninfected could occur throughout the asymptomatic phase; (4) an inability to quantify the risk of specific sexual practices known to place gay and bisexual men at increased risk of infection; (5) the rapidly escalating numbers of deaths among friends and sexual partners; (6) frustration and desperation at the lack of effective treatment; and (7) the perceived (often real) indifference of government and the biomedical research establishment to the rights and welfare of gay people.

From this milieu during the mid-1980s emerged a vocal and effective AIDS activist movement that, in the United States, encompassed "a wide range of grassroots activists, lobbying groups, service providers, and community-based organizations [representing] the diverse interests of people of various races, ethnicities, genders, sexual preferences, and HIV 'risk behaviors.'"[4] The movement employed all manner of classic and novel activist tactics. The initial focus was on expediting the development of promising experimental AIDS therapies and increasing access to clinical trials in which they were being studied.

Activism and Advocacy for Access

Access to Experimental Therapy

Immediately upon release of the results of the Burroughs Wellcome clinical trial showing effectiveness of AZT, activists demanded that the thousands of people with AIDS in the United States be given access to the drug. This created difficult scientific and regulatory problems because the trial was the first and only controlled study of the drug.[10] Furthermore, it was a relatively small study, its eligibility criteria defined a small subset of infected individuals with advanced disease, the improvement in mortality was short term, side effects were significant, and long-term efficacy and safety were unknown.

Nonetheless, because of the desperate situation at hand and the lack of proven therapeutic options, the U.S. Food and Drug Administration (FDA) followed the advice of its Anti-Infective Advisory Committee and quickly granted approval for marketing of AZT for use by individuals with disease similar to that of the clinical trial population. In the interval between trial results and marketing, the U.S. Department of Health and Human Services and the Burroughs Wellcome Company jointly launched a massive and creative access program, utilizing the regulatory mechanism known as a "treatment IND." Until that time, access to experimental drugs outside of clinical trials by terminally ill patients was limited, typically entailing case-by-case review by the

FDA. In contrast, under the AZT treatment IND, physicians registered with the FDA as investigators on a protocol designed to collect safety data. Once registered, they submitted information documenting the eligibility of each patient for participation in the program. Drugs for patients deemed eligible were shipped to a registered pharmacy to be administered under the physician's care in accordance with and according to the protocol.

The AZT treatment IND marked the beginning of a major shift in attitude about access to and regulation of experimental drugs for life-threatening diseases that was quite remarkable, given the uncertainties inherent in the results of the relatively small, short-term clinical trial on which it was based and the massive scale of expedited access that resulted. AZT was provided to more than 4,000 people during the six months between advisory committee recommendation and ultimate licensure for marketing by the FDA.[11] As other new drugs began to move through the early clinical pipeline of development, activist testimony and advocacy contributed substantially to other important access initiatives that became known as the parallel track policy and accelerated approval.

The parallel track policy permitted limited access to certain investigational drugs by patients with HIV/AIDS who could not participate in clinical trials by virtue of ineligibility or lack of geographic proximity to a clinical trial site.[12] Like the treatment IND, it required that there be substantive preliminary evidence of efficacy from earlier studies, and that research toward ultimate marketing approval be underway. Drugs were supplied free of charge by the pharmaceutical company sponsor to patients.

More sweeping change was seen in the accelerated approval initiative, designed to expedite the approval of a new drug for serious and life-threatening diseases when the drug provides meaningful therapeutic benefit over existing products.[12] Until that time approval by the FDA for marketing required proof of significant improvement in one or more important clinical endpoints such as increased survival or disease-free interval, or shortened duration of clinical illness. (AIDS activists referred to such studies as "body count trials."[13]) Accelerated approval effectively lowered this threshold and allowed sponsors to seek marketing approval on the basis of changes in surrogate measures that reasonably predict clinical benefit (e.g., decreases in tumor size in cancer or increases in measures of immune function in HIV infection). Again, the policy required that research to establish clinical efficacy be continued after marketing approval was granted. It also contained provisions for removal of the drug from the market if those studies failed to confirm clinical benefit.

Access to Clinical Trials

Although it originated in the gay community, the agenda of the U.S. AIDS activist movement was diverse and inclusive from the start. Thus, access to promising experimental therapies also included demands for fair and equitable access to clinical trials by *all* individuals affected by the epidemic. Activists worked diligently to diminish scientific, logistical, and ethical barriers to participation in clinical trials by women and minorities. This focus coincided and was synergistic with parallel emerging government initiatives on a number of fronts to address underrepresentation of women and minorities in clinical research, a problem that compromised the amount and quality of health information available to them.[14]

For example, the routes of access to cutting-edge experimental treatment led mainly to clinical trials at academic research centers. These, of course, were not evenly distributed among the U.S. population. AIDS activists demanded that special efforts be taken to ensure opportunities for access to clinical trials among minority communities affected by AIDS. Although it seemed to many a confusion between the goals of research and access to care, clinical research sites (with variable enthusiasm) devoted increased resources to minority community outreach, and progress in accruing underrepresented populations became an important benchmark for evaluation of the performance of clinical trial sites.

AIDS activists also demanded an end to exclusion of women of childbearing potential from participation in experimental drug trials, which had become routine practice following the thalidomide tragedy of the 1960s. Instead they helped bring about regulatory change by the FDA, as well as a general shift in ethical review toward more inclusive approaches such as allowing participation by women if pregnancy testing was negative, and encouragement for all research participants enrolled in a clinical trial to utilize effective birth control measures.[15]

Problems with serious adverse events have occurred under these access initiatives but fortunately have been infrequent. For instance, pancreatitis emerged as a severe toxicity of unexpectedly high frequency when the antiretroviral drug didanosine (ddI) was made available under the parallel track mechanism.[16] In retrospect it became clear that patients who received the drug under expanded access had, on average, more advanced disease than those who had been included earlier clinical trials. Surveillance detected the problem quickly, and appropriate changes in labeling were instituted. For other important scientific and ethical concerns with expanded access in interesting and informative analyses, consult discussions by Rebecca Dresser, David Rothman, and Harold Edgar.[17,18] Of particular importance for research ethics is the potential to exacerbate the therapeutic misconception (see Chapter 58).

Legacy for Research Ethics

The scientific and ethical debate behind these sweeping changes in social attitude, policy, and regulation was intense. The activist argument for change was passionate and straightforward. For example, Martin Delaney, a leader of the AIDS movement from San Francisco, stated the case before the 26th annual meeting of the Infectious Diseases Society of America, and also in the pages of the *Journal of Infectious Diseases*.[19] First, he summarized the three main arguments made by those opposing change: "(1) that patients must be protected from their own desperation, (2) that the experimental drugs might do more harm than good, and (3) that public access to experimental drugs would render it impossible to conduct clinical studies, since no one would bother participating if they could have the drugs any other way."

Focusing on the first two points, he argued that in the "broad gray area" between no evidence for efficacy and "fully proven to FDA standards," there comes a time when evidence of effectiveness, although not conclusive, emerges. "[It] is in this area that we believe life-threatened patients and their physicians must have the handcuffs removed." He went on to acknowledge that the multiphase steps of clinical research were a proven way to quantify the effects of a drug, but questioned "whether those steps should be equally required when seeking to restrain a contagious, world-wide epidemic as when judging a new cold tablet or pain remedy." He also asked, "Who gets to decide what risks are acceptable: the bureaucracy in Washington or the patient whose life is on the line?" With similar lucidity he dismissed the concern that easier access during the development phase might slow the drug development process by "siphoning off" potential research participants.[19] Such arguments, emanating from the community of people most affected, were powerful and compelling forces in the scientific and regulatory debate, and since that time proponents for expanded access and accelerated approval have prevailed, repeatedly, and on the fronts of many life-threatening conditions in addition to AIDS.[12]

In the process, they have challenged the manner in which principles articulated in the Belmont Report had been translated into clinical practice in the United States. Given the context of scandal and abuse from which Belmont and its offspring arose, it is not surprising that there existed a more-or-less explicit assumption that researchers and participation in research (and therefore access to investigational drugs) should be considered dangerous to patients, who must be protected from them. Thus the regulation and practice of ethical review—including institutional review board (IRB) oversight and FDA regulation of investigational drug research—erected substantial protective barriers around all human experimentation. In this context, autonomy was regarded largely a matter of ensuring fully informed consent and voluntary participation throughout the course of the study. Similarly, justice was considered largely in terms of ensuring that burdens of research were not unfairly carried by the vulnerable of society.

AIDS activists, on the other hand, did not see protection from uncertain and unacceptable risk. Instead, they saw insurmountable barriers blocking access to their only source of medical hope and potential survival, with no opportunity for discussion or appeal. Their argument was poignantly and succinctly summarized on an activist poster that read, "Stop Protecting Us to Death." In effect, they asserted that paternalistic protectionism did not constitute respect in the case of persons whose lives were in imminent jeopardy and who had available to them no known effective alternative interventions. Instead, respect required that those persons be permitted a substantial role in autonomous and informed choice regarding the interpretation and meaning of the potential risks and benefits of participation in experimental drug trials.

Furthermore, AIDS activists viewed access to clinical trials as a matter of social privilege. The AIDS Coalition to Unleash Power (ACT UP) used the phrase *medical apartheid* to describe "the routine exclusion of women, children, people of color, and IV drug users from most AIDS research."[20] Rhetoric aside, they argued in effect that the principle of justice required equitable distribution of the opportunity to benefit from participation in experimental drug research as well as protection of the vulnerable from exploitation.

In summary, the realities of the AIDS epidemic presented the field of research ethics with an entirely new set of issues and concerns regarding access to experimental interventions. It demanded a new look at and added new depth to the meaning of basic principles. This legacy is clearly etched in sweeping U.S. regulatory reform regarding human experimentation in the case of treatments for life-threatening conditions and in the processes of ethical review of clinical research that is integral to research and development of new therapy for them.

Community Involvement in the Research Enterprise

Perhaps even more far-reaching than the legacy of expanded access and accelerated approval has been the legacy of involvement of the community of people affected by AIDS in more "upstream" aspects of the biomedical research enterprise. Elements of this involvement, which has truly altered the entire landscape of clinical biomedical research, include the following:

1. The establishment of numerous formal and informal opportunities for direct involvement of people with or affected by HIV/AIDS in all aspects of the federal HIV/AIDS research program.
2. Important involvement of the community in shaping the science that has been carried out under those programs.
3. Use of the political process to change important aspects of oversight, management, administration, and funding of the federal HIV/AIDS research effort.

A few highly selected examples illustrate these three themes.

Direct Involvement in the Research Enterprise

The AIDS Clinical Trials Group (ACTG) is a national multicenter clinical research network that was established in 1987 by the U.S. National Institute of Allergy and Infectious Diseases (NIAID), a part of the NIH, to study treatments for the disease.[21] AZT had just been approved by the FDA for marketing as the ACTG began work, and the Group's initial scientific efforts focused on research aimed at extending knowledge of the usefulness and toxicity of the drug for other AIDS-related indications, for example, in earlier stages of infection than the original Burroughs Wellcome study. Because AZT was the only proven treatment option and research was synonymous with state-of-the-art care, many observers and AIDS patients viewed the ACTG as a key route of access to AIDS treatment. For the ACTG's first several years, the number of people entered in trials was the benchmark by which many activists and congressional observers judged the Group's progress and success.

Others, however, grew increasingly critical of the ACTG's science and its scientific leadership, "in part because of growing concerns about the ethics of clinical research, and in part because activists recognized that it was no good fighting for faster approval of drugs if there were few such drugs to be approved."[4] Rapidly mounting criticism focused on the slow pace of progress in treatment research; the small number of new drugs that were being studied; the methodology used to study them (e.g., placebo-controlled trials); the heavy emphasis on studies of AZT-based antiretroviral therapy; the inadequacy of research on treatments for opportunistic complications of the disease; the failure to study a variety of "underground" alternative treatments that were not approved by the FDA but were nonetheless being used in the community by people with HIV; the organizational structure put in place to administer the Group and carry out the trials; and the seemingly secretive processes of prioritization, study development, and execution.

Scientists were in the bull's eye of activist frustration and anger. The leadership of the ACTG—internationally prominent researchers in infectious diseases, virology, microbiology, and immunology—became known to many as "the Gang of Five," a phrase borrowed from Chinese political activists, referring to their "control of most U.S. AIDS research." A flier from a chapter of the activist organization ACT UP stated: "They are not the sole source of all the ACTG's problems, but they symbolize and embody them: obsession with AZT, excessive ties with the large pharmaceutical companies, conflicts of interests, disdain for community concerns, lack of interest in opportunistic infections, opposition to expanded access, and love of secrecy, decision-making behind closed doors." The flier concluded with the statement: "These are the people who are killing us!"[22]

Scientists in general were surprised and bewildered. Accustomed to less incendiary approaches to discourse and debate, they were ill-equipped and unprepared for protest, demonstrations, and ad hominem attacks. They were also stunned and hurt by accusations of greed, selfishness, or that they were working for any goal other than the best interests of their patients and people with AIDS in general. For example, virologist Martin Hirsch described a 1988 activist protest during a presentation he was giving at a national medical conference in Boston. An activist carried a sign which read, "Marty Hirsch and Clinical Trials = Jim Jones and Jamestown." Another sign read, "The blood of 19 is on your hands" (referring to the 19 placebo recipients in the trial he was describing). He recalled:

> What was even more troubling was that one of my own patients was carrying the sign. When asked about it later by one of my colleagues, the patient responded casually, "Hirsch shouldn't take it personally." What was seen by the medical community as a major triumph . . . was seen by some in the patient advocate community as a needless waste of life. Where had these different perceptions arisen? Clearly, the protesters and I came from different backgrounds and had different expectations concerning the proper conduct of clinical investigation. We had failed to communicate with each other concerning our different expectations.[23]

Anthony Fauci, Director of NIAID and a frequent activist target, borrowed from Mario Puzo in counseling scientists and staff who became the subject of such attacks: "It's nothing personal; it's strictly business."[24] Many, however, had a difficult time distancing themselves from the rhetoric, and there was talk at the time of researchers leaving the field because of it all. The activist-science relationship hit a low point during the 1990 International AIDS Conference in San Francisco, when leading government scientists were provided with bodyguards because of anonymous threats.

In the midst of such turmoil, a group of activists demanded admittance to and participation in ACTG meetings.[25] They asserted a right to be directly involved in a publicly funded program that directly affected them and their communities, with which they had many disagreements and which they could neither understand nor influence from the "outside." Not surprisingly, most ACTG scientists and NIH staff resisted, arguing that open and healthy scientific debate would be either misinterpreted or stifled by the presence of scientifically naive and hostile "outsiders"; that the inherently difficult and deliberative process of establishing research priorities and implementing studies to address them would be slowed even further by the need to explain complex matters of science to lay people; and that proprietary, privileged, or preliminary scientific data would be "leaked" to the public

inappropriately or before it was adequately reviewed and analyzed. In retrospect it is easy to see that raw emotions were just beneath the surface of such rational arguments.

To the chagrin of many of his staff and scientists in the field, Fauci was moved by the substance of the activists' arguments. He listened carefully and at length to both sides of the debate, determined that more good than bad would come from openness, and assigned to his Division of AIDS the task of working with ACTG researchers and activists to implement his decision to open the ACTG to participation by the HIV/AIDS community.

During the next several years, avenues were created for membership and participation in all aspects of the ACTG by people with HIV and representatives of their communities. The centerpiece of the process was the Community Constituency Group (CCG), a new permanent ACTG committee.[26] The job of the CCG and its members was to bring direct community perspective and expertise to all aspects of the ACTG. Over time, individual CCG members and the CCG as a whole have developed and contributed indispensable expertise in many areas including science as well as community relations, information dissemination, advocacy, and inclusion. From the beginning, the CCG aspired to a level of diversity in representation that reflected the full scope of the HIV epidemic and the communities affected by it. Members of the CCG choose their peers and successors, and they sit as full members on every ACTG scientific operational committee, task force, and governing body. Together with the Group's scientists and operational staff, they participate directly in the establishment of research priorities, plan and implement studies, and analyze and disseminate study results. NIAID and the ACTG leadership also mandated the establishment of Community Advisory Boards (CABs) at each clinical trial site.[21] CABs play a role analogous to the CCG at the locations where the clinical trials actually take place. Many CAB members are also part of the CCG.

This paradigm of ongoing, direct community involvement has become a feature of virtually all other NIH-sponsored HIV/AIDS clinical research programs, scientific meetings and workshops, and both formal and informal HIV/AIDS advisory bodies of the NIH. Analogous types of involvement have also become standard practice in much pharmaceutical company-sponsored HIV/AIDS research.

This is not to say that the process was easy for either scientists or activists. Scientists' hopes that such involvement would end protest were quickly dashed when, only six months following the first meeting of the newly "opened" ACTG, more than 1,000 demonstrators descended on the NIH in Bethesda, Md., in a protest called "STORM THE NIH." They demanded that President George H. W. Bush and Congress increase funding for AIDS research and that the NIH "study the whole disease, test all AIDS treatments immediately, and end medical apartheid."[20] *The Washington Post* reported that 83 demonstrators were arrested for trespassing or resisting arrest as they occupied offices, hung red streamers in the trees to symbolize bureaucratic red tape, and left mock gravestones around the campus[27] (see Figure 9.3).

The CCG members, too, faced challenges reconciling their role with their activist roots. Their more militant counterparts charged that CCG members were being co-opted and did not really represent people with AIDS. In addition, there were several bitter disputes within the CCG on important scientific and policy directions, such as the design of studies to prevent mother-to-infant transmission of HIV. Several CCG members were also

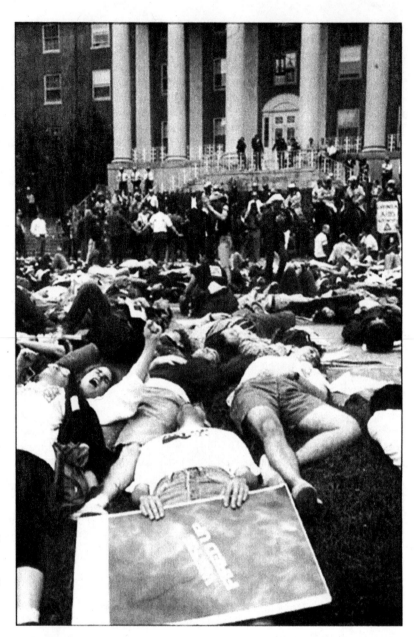

Figure 9.3. Protesters "storm the NIH" and conduct a "die-in" in front of the Office of the Director of the NIH, May 21, 1990. Source: *NIH Record*, 5/29/1990, page 1; Office of NIH History, Office of Communication and Public Liaison. Credit: Ernie Branson, NIH Medical Arts and Photography Branch. Reproduced with permission.

"Storm" demonstrators as well as parties to a consensus statement endorsed by an ad hoc coalition of 25 AIDS-related organizations released only four days before the demonstration.[28] Its critically thoughtful approach to the same issues stood in stark counterpoint to the tactics and rhetoric of the demonstration.

Shaping Science From Within and Without

Over time, however, this new and important perspective has been assimilated at the table of science and has evolved to a more stable, collegial partnership. Epstein provides an insightful, detailed, and well-balanced account in which he posits that AIDS activists were effective because they established credibility by studying and understanding the science, and speaking with scientists on scientific terms.[4]

Activist Publications, Studies, and Reports

AIDS activists have subjected virtually all aspects of the research enterprise to independent scientific analysis. Their critiques, conclusions, and recommendations are contained in innumerable reports such as those listed in Table 9.2. Far from activist diatribe, these were important sources of AIDS activists' credibility. First, they staked out clear positions that could be debated and discussed. Second, they were often informed by, or facilitated alignments with, the agenda of subsets of scientists within the research enterprise. Such activist-scientist alliances were critical in facilitating change toward mutual objectives. Third, the scope of topics goes far beyond the immediate, specific, and applied interests in treatment research of the community of people with HIV. Finally, they served as an important resource for a virtual industry of periodical publications written by or for people with HIV/AIDS. Such pub-

Table 9.2

Selected Reports and Publications Produced by AIDS Activists
and Treatment Advocates

Reports

- A Glossary of AIDS Drugs, Treatments, and Trials (ACT UP, 1988)
- National AIDS Treatment Research Agenda (ACT UP, 1989, 1990, 1991)
- The Countdown 18 Months Plan (ACT UP, 1990)
- A Critique of the AIDS Clinical Trials Group (ACT UP, 1990)
- AIDS Research at the NIH: A Critical Review (TAG 1992)
- Basic Research on HIV Infection: A Report From the Front (TAG, 1993)
- The Crisis in Clinical AIDS Research (TAG, 1993)
- Rescuing Accelerated Approval: Moving Beyond the Status Quo (TAG, 1994)
- Problems With Protease Inhibitor Development Plans (TAG, 1995)
- AIDS Research at the National Cancer Institute: An Analysis and Call to Action (GMHC, 1995)
- Structured Treatment Interruptions Workshop Report (FAIR and TAG, 1999)
- NIH Funded Vaccine Research: A Critical Review (TAG, 2000)

National Periodicals

- *TAGline*. The Treatment Action Group's monthly publication of research and policy.
- *AIDS Treatment News*. Reports on mainstream and alternative treatment, access to care, Web resources, public policy, and political action.
- *GMHC Treatment Issues*. The Gay Men's Health Crisis Newsletter of Experimental AIDS Therapies.
- *Women Alive Newsletter*. Women Alive Coalition. Los Angeles, CA.
- *Bulletin of Experimental Treatment for AIDS (BETA)*. San Francisco AIDS Foundation. San Francisco, CA.
- *Project Inform Perspective*. Project Inform, San Francisco, CA.
- *Research Initiative/Treatment Action (RITA)*. The Center for AIDS Information and Advocacy, Houston, TX.
- *AIDS Community Research Initiative of America (ACRIA) Update*. Treatment Education Newsletter. New York, NY.

---

lications served an invaluable role in building an informed constituency of unprecedented scientific sophistication.

Engaging Science on Science's Terms

An illustrative, early example is "Countdown 18 Months," a well-researched, thoughtful, and passionate critique of the state of clinical research on treatment of opportunistic infections (OIs). Released in late 1990 by a group associated with chapters of ACT UP, the report challenged prevailing scientific priorities that focused on the long-term goal of controlling the underlying cause of AIDS through antiretroviral drug development. It argued that such research must be balanced by research addressing the immediate needs of thousands of patients with life-threatening complications of the disease. The report contained a detailed scientific agenda for OI research and drug development, recommendations aimed at multiple federal agencies and the pharmaceutical industry for specific new research and policy/regulatory initiatives, benchmarks for measuring progress during its 18-month timeline, and

explicit notice that progress would be scrutinized closely and regularly. The report, in turn, triggered a congressional investigation which, not surprisingly, came to many of the same conclusions.[29]

Many of the report's arguments resonated with groups of scientists within the research enterprise. The resulting activist-scientist alliance advocated successfully for increased attention to OI treatment and prevention research within the ACTG and industry—although the same activists continued to criticize the pace. Their efforts contributed directly to the fact that by 2005, at least 30 drugs had been approved for marketing by the FDA specifically for treatment or prevention of AIDS-related OIs and other complications. Several of the activists responsible for the report became important and highly respected contributors to the efforts of the ACTG OI Committee.

Activists became increasingly important participants in complex deliberations about significant matters of science, such as acceptance of the validity of "surrogate markers" as endpoints in antiretroviral drug research and development.[30] In a somewhat ironic convergence of interests, activists found themselves aligned with scientists in the pharmaceutical industry who advocated use of CD4+ cell counts as more efficient routes to licensure through quicker answers in studies with fewer research participants. Advocacy from this activist-scientist coalition led to a large, coordinated, retrospective analysis of clinical trial data from previously completed studies. This analysis established that changes in CD4+ cell counts following treatment correlated well with subsequent morbidity and mortality. In turn, subsequent clinical trials relied increasingly on CD4+ cell count and other surrogate endpoints as primary measures of treatment effect. There can be no doubt that answers to clinical trials accrued more quickly as a result. However, there was intense debate for years about the wisdom of this scientific leap of faith. Scientifically conservative opponents argued that it would create a "house of cards" of short-term data that then would become the standard by which the next intervention was judged, a concern that subsequently gained traction for a number of years. In fact, a subset of the same activists who were instrumental in the push for surrogate markers reversed course several years later and argued for larger clinical endpoint studies because, in their judgment, pharmaceutical companies failed to follow through on their obligation to pursue postlicensing research documenting clinical benefit.[31]

To a large degree, this concern has been mitigated as highly effective antiretroviral chemotherapy and better surrogate markers, such as precise, reliable quantitative measures of viral load, have been validated and become more widely available. However, such phenomenal advances have brought with them complex management decisions for people with HIV and their care providers. As people with HIV live longer, new complications of the disease or long-term side effects of therapy have emerged, engendering complex management problems for patients and their health-care providers. Activists have kept these matters squarely on the table of problems requiring scientific attention. More importantly, they have become parties to the process of grappling with vexing methodological challenges and clinical dilemmas of research to address them, such as the following:

- Management of a syndrome of metabolic dysfunction causing disfiguring changes in body fat distribution
- When, in the course of HIV infection, to begin antiretroviral therapy

- Indications and optimal strategies for antiretroviral therapy when relapse appears
- The possibility that effective treatment can be safely interrupted for periods of time as a way of decreasing unacceptable long-term side effects

HIV/AIDS Research Addressing the Needs of Women

Activism of a different sort played a pivotal role in increasing the attention of the research enterprise to the specific problems of women infected with HIV. Because the early epidemic in the United States was overwhelmingly among men, specific manifestations of the disease in women went unrecognized and were not included in the Centers for Disease Control (CDC) case definition of AIDS. As a result, women were undercounted in national case figures that provided the basis for many AIDS service programs around the country. Furthermore, most research involving women with HIV addressed the problem of mother-to-infant transmission. Activists banded together with concerned scientists and spearheaded the first National Conference on Women and HIV Infection, held in 1990. Research and other presentations at that conference led directly to changes in the national case definition of AIDS to include conditions that specifically affected women.[32] The conference also led to federal funding in 1993 of a national multicenter cohort study of women with HIV, and to a number of more specific clinical and basic research studies addressing pathogenesis, prevention, and care of HIV infection in women.[33]

Engaging the Political Process: The HOPE Act

AIDS activists have been widely recognized for their success in lobbying for increased federal funding for prevention, care, and research. They have also used the legislative process in other ways to directly influence science and science policy.

A particularly far-reaching example was the Health Omnibus Programs Extension (the "HOPE" Act, PL 100–607), signed into law by President Ronald Reagan on November 4, 1988.[34] Among its provisions, Title II contained language that affected the structure and design of the federal HIV/AIDS research enterprise. Of particular note for the purposes of this discussion were requirements that NIH do the following:

- Establish a clinical research review committee within NIAID.
- Establish community-based clinical trials.
- Provide the public with information on HIV/AIDS treatments and options for participating in clinical trials.
- Expedite the review process for all AIDS-related grants.
- Create an Office of AIDS Research within the Office of the Director of NIH.

Establishing a Clinical Research Review Committee

This legislative requirement was notable for several reasons. First was the striking level of detail in the Clinical Research Review Committee's mandate—a virtual charter addressing specific concerns of the activist community at the time. Second was the unusual requirement that NIH develop what amounted to treatment guidelines—essentially recognition of the need for intimate connection between such an important national resource and the rapidly changing state of science. Finally, was a requirement to provide recommendations to FDA regarding drugs that should be made available under the parallel track policy, clearly indicating explicit congressional intent to facilitate access to promising experimental therapies.

Establishing Community-Based Clinical Trials

The community-based clinical trial "movement" was borne of the frustration of many activists and primary care providers. It rested on impressions that mainstream clinical trials programs were isolated in academia and skewed toward populations that did not fully represent the epidemic; addressed the scientific questions and needs of academic researchers rather than the everyday issues confronted by physicians and patients in the course of routine primary care; and utilized study designs with restrictive and narrowly defined eligibility requirements that led to results of limited or uncertain generalizability. In at least some activist and clinician circles there existed the attitude that "If they can't do research that has meaning to us, we'll do it ourselves."

Thus, community-based HIV/AIDS research was strongly shaped by activist initiatives. Perhaps the boldest was the establishment of independent research networks based in primary care settings. Two prominent examples were the County Community Consortium in San Francisco and the Community Research Initiative in New York City. An explicit goal of both was to carry out community-relevant research on potential new AIDS treatments in community settings as an alternative to the academic base of most clinical research at the time.

In this context, the HOPE Act articulated specific congressional direction for NIAID's then-emerging Community Programs for Clinical Research on AIDS (CPCRA).[35] The objectives of the CPCRA, indicative of those of the community-based research movement in general, are to do the following:

- Conduct research in HIV primary-care settings.
- Reach underserved populations.
- Conduct clinical studies that answer questions about the day-to-day medical management of HIV disease.
- Generate data about therapies and treatment strategies that can be used in a wide range of patients.
- Provide research results concerning new therapies and treatment strategies to clinicians, clinical researchers, pharmaceutical companies, and patient advocates.

It is beyond the scope of this chapter to assess either the validity of the assumptions behind the community-based research movement or the ultimate impact of such organizations on the current state of HIV/AIDS research and care. It is fair to say that novel and alternative models for clinical research were created and tested, and that important, useful, and interesting studies have been carried out. For example, an early trial established the efficacy of aerosolized pentamidine in preventing PcP, an approach first advocated by prominent community practitioners[36]; and a recently published study demonstrated that intermittent administration of antiretroviral treatment (with the hope of diminishing side effects) results in increased morbidity and mortality and does not reduce adverse events compared to standard continuous administration.[37] It is also fair to say that community-based research programs have faced many challenges, including the involvement of critical masses of creative scientific talent and the development of systems for data collection and quality control in primary care medical practices. The important point for this discussion is that these networks were, in part, activist-inspired and driven alternatives to mainstream clinical research.

Providing Public Information on AIDS Clinical Trials

With an explicit goal of facilitating access to experimental treatment by people with HIV, the HOPE legislation mandated that NIH create a publicly available resource of information on NIH-sponsored clinical trials. In the process, Congress signaled support for the regulatory reform concerning investigational drug access already underway at the time and discussed above, as well as for a nascent, joint NIH-CDC initiative to establish the AIDS Clinical Trials Information Service (ACTIS).[38] ACTIS began as a toll-free telephone-based service. It has since expanded in scope and sponsorship to become AIDSinfo, a federally supported, authoritative and comprehensive source for information on HIV prevention and treatment. It contains tools for locating federally and privately supported clinical trials, trial results, educational resources, treatment guidelines, and extensive data on HIV/AIDS drugs and vaccines. (ACTIS later served as a prototype for www.clinicaltrials.gov, a congressionally mandated "registry of clinical trials for federally and privately funded trials of experimental treatments for serious or life-threatening diseases or conditions.")

Expediting the Review of Grants

Two other provisions of the HOPE legislation related to the management and organization of the NIH itself. One specifically mandated that NIH expedite peer review and award of HIV-related grant applications, a process that typically takes nine months or more from grant submission to award (if successful). Activists joined many scientists who argued that "business as usual" was unacceptable in a public health emergency. The HOPE legislation reduced review and processing time to six months, concerns about cost, logistics, and perceived unfairness by other scientists of such "AIDS exceptionalism" notwithstanding. The legislative mandate stands intact as of this writing.

Creating an Office of AIDS Research

The final provision affecting the organization of the NIH established an Office of AIDS Research (OAR) within the Office of the NIH Director. The OAR was charged with coordinating the AIDS activities of the various NIH Institutes and Centers supporting HIV research. Many activists and scientists were critical of the traditional decentralized and primarily investigator-initiated research grant activities that constituted a substantial proportion of the basic HIV research portfolio. Some even called for an AIDS "Manhattan Project."[39,40] The HOPE legislation compromised on this matter and created a locus of accountability toward a more directed program, but stopped short of central government direction of science. The OAR quickly became the focal point for heated debate between proponents of centralized management on the one hand, and decentralized management on the other. The culmination was a massive independent review of the entire NIH AIDS research effort and a report, released in 1996.[41] One of the most hotly contested of the many recommendations of the "Levine Report"—named for the cochair of the panel that produced it,

Arnold Levine of Princeton University—led directly to additional congressional legislation that took another step toward centralization. It significantly increased the authority of the Director of the OAR over the establishment of overall NIH AIDS research priorities, the creation and submission of the NIH AIDS budget to Congress, and the allocation of the appropriated NIH AIDS budget.

Legacy for Research Ethics

Even from this limited overview, it should be evident that the field of HIV research has been shaped to an unprecedented degree by involvement of the community of people directly affected by the disease. It should also be evident, as Epstein notes, that it has usually been the case that movement on specific issues has been the result of alliances involving activists and groups of scientists within the research or political establishments. Rarely, if ever, has it been the case that the entire scientific establishment was completely on one side of an issue whereas the entire activist community was on the other. Epstein correctly notes, "This is a complicated history in which no party has had all the answers. All players have revised their claims and shifted their positions over time; all have had to wrestle with the unintended consequences of their own actions."[4]

Thus, the almost overwhelming temptation to look in these events for heroes and villains diminishes the real story and its larger lessons. Clearly, the enduring legacy of this fascinating history is the extraordinary scientific progress that has occurred, almost in spite of the extreme mistrust, anger, fear, and divisiveness that characterized the early relationship between science and the community of people affected by HIV. To the mutual credit of both activists and scientists, a relatively stable and productive democracy has evolved and made this scientific progress possible. Through diligent advocacy from their perspective as the people most directly affected by the disease, and in coming to understand the scientific method and the complexities of the scientific challenge posed by HIV, activists have become essential partners in the scientific enterprise. Similarly, most scientists have come to value understanding of the priorities and perspectives of the people most directly affected by HIV, and they acknowledge that better studies are launched that involve well-educated and savvy participants. Most important, to a vastly greater extent than any could have imagined in 1989, most activists and scientists have, in general, come to see each other as allies who know they share the same goals, even if they sometimes disagree on the path to pursue them. It is impossible to overstate just how remarkable the transformation has been.

Indeed, Lo views the events associated with AIDS activism as a stringent and highly successful test of the concept of partnership between community and science.[42] In that vein, another enormously important legacy of these events lies in the contribution of this paradigm of partnership in the sometimes difficult matter of determining whether research has social and scientific value. In other words the perspectives of the community have become an integral part of the scientific process. Although it does not prevent disagreement, it helps ensure that a richer variety of practical and immediate perspectives on social and scientific relevance are in the forefront of discussion about the science that is planned and undertaken.

One might question whether this paradigm has relevance to other situations, given the unique milieu in which it arose. The model of U.S. AIDS activism has been adopted in other countries with vastly different social and cultural contexts, most notably South Africa. Advocates for conditions as diverse as breast cancer, Alzheimer's disease, and Parkinson's disease frequently credit the model of AIDS activism.[17,24,43–45] Furthermore, increasing attention is being devoted on a variety of fronts to the importance of including a public perspective in scientific processes.[46] Although neither necessary nor sufficient, the AIDS model surely represents a proven approach to contentious situations that should bolster confidence that the first requirement for ethical research—social and scientific relevance[47]—is satisfied.

Epilogue

The very limited history discussed here mainly concerns events in the early years of the HIV epidemic in the United States, and focuses on sentinel events of particular relevance to one enduring legacy of the U.S. HIV epidemic on research ethics—activism and community involvement in science. The focus on this aspect of the story also lays a foundation for better understanding of another enduring and more troubling legacy—some of the ethical controversies concerning exploitation, considered at length elsewhere in this volume, that have come to dominate the arena of international research ethics for more than a decade. At the core of those controversies is the juxtaposition of tremendous progress in treatment that has occurred in wealthier countries of the world (in association with activism and community involvement) on the one hand, and the fact that this progress is beyond the reach of most people with HIV infection, who live in the developing world, on the other (see Part X). Two practical and vexing questions related to this problem have fueled the current environment of suspicion and mistrust:

1. Are researchers obligated to ensure that study participants receive state-of-the-art care, regardless of the objectives of the study or the level of care available in the setting in which the study is carried out?
2. What are the obligations of researchers to study participants after a study is completed?

That this ethical controversy has persisted for so long suggests that answers cannot be derived solely from either the fundamental principles of research ethics or in the abundance of existing guidelines and frameworks. One must hope that creative attempts to apply the HIV/AIDS partnership paradigm to this global health research issue[48] might bring about movement toward solutions that help identify research that is important and fair to the communities concerned, and has impact on the broadest possible global scale.

References

1. Joint United Nations Programme on HIV/AIDS. [Online] Available: http://www.unaids.org/en/default.asp.
2. National Institutes of Health. Estimates of funding for various diseases, conditions, research areas. [Online] March 10, 2006. Available: http://www.nih.gov/news/fundingresearchareas.htm.
3. Fauci AS. The AIDS epidemic: Considerations for the 21st century. *New England Journal of Medicine* 1999;341:1046–50.
4. Epstein S. *Impure Science.* Berkley and Los Angeles, Calif.: University of California Press; 1996.
5. Folkers GK, Fauci AS. The AIDS research model: Implications for other infectious diseases of global health importance. *JAMA* 2001;286:458–61.
6. Wachter RM. AIDS, activism, and the politics of health. *New England Journal of Medicine* 1992;326:128–33.
7. Fauci AS. HIV and AIDS: 20 years of science. *Nature Medicine* 2003;9:839–43.
8. Fischl MA, Richman DD, Grieco MH, et al. The efficacy of azidothymidine (AZT) in the treatment of patients with AIDS and AIDS-related complex. A double-blind, placebo-controlled trial. *New England Journal of Medicine* 1987;317:185–91.
9. U.S. Public Health Service. AIDSinfo. *Clinical Guidelines.* [Online] Available: http://aidsinfo.nih.gov/guidelines/.
10. Kolata G. Imminent marketing of AZT raises problems. *Science* 1987;235:1462–3.
11. Fleiger K. FDA consumer special report: FDA finds new ways to speed treatments to patients. [Online] January 1995. Available: http://www.fda.gov/fdac/special/newdrug/speeding.html.
12. Greenberg MD. AIDS, experimental drug approval, and the FDA new drug screening process. *Legislation and Public Policy* 2000;3:295–350.
13. Anonymous. ACTG 320: Last of the body count trials? *Project Inform Perspective* 1997;21:7.
14. Public Health Service Task Force on Women's Health Issues. *Report of the Public Health Task Force on Women's Health Issues.* Public Health Reports 1985;100:73–106.
15. Food and Drug Administration, Department of Health and Human Services. Guideline for the study and evaluation of gender differences in the clinical evaluation of drugs. *Federal Register* 1993;58(139): 39406–16.
16. Seidlin M, Lambert JS, Dolin R, Valentine FT. Pancreatitis and pancreatic dysfunction in patients taking dideoxyinosine. *AIDS* 1992; 6:831–5.
17. Dresser R. *When Science Offers Salvation.* New York, N.Y.: Oxford University Press; 2001.
18. Rothman DJ, Edgar H. AIDS, activism, and ethics. *Hospital Practice* 1991;26:135–42.
19. Delaney M. The case for patient access to experimental therapy. *Journal of Infectious Diseases* 1989;159:416–9.
20. ACT UP. An open letter to all NIH employees concerning the May 21 AIDS demonstration, 1990.
21. AIDS Clinical Trials Group. [Online] Available: http://www.aactg .org/.
22. ACT UP. Who are the Gang of Five? AIDS Coalition to Unleash Power; 1990.
23. Hirsch MS. Reflections on the road to effective HIV therapy. *Infectious Diseases in Clinical Practice* 1998;7:39–42.
24. Fauci AS. The AIDS model: Scientific and policy lessons for the 21st century. *Journal of Clinical Investigation* 2000;106:S23–S27.
25. Harrington M. In the belly of the beast: ACT UP crashes the ACTG. *OutWeek* 1989: 34–5.
26. ACTG opens meeting to advocates, who pledge to learn, provide input. *AIDS Update* 1990;3(44):1–3.
27. Jennings VT, Gladwell M. 1,000 rally for more vigorous AIDS effort. *Washington Post* May 22, 1990:B1.
28. Ad-Hoc Coalition of AIDS and Health Organizations. HIV/AIDS Biomedical Research Priorities. Recommendations to the National Institutes of Health. 1990.
29. Committee on Government Operations. The Obstacles to Drug Development for HIV-Related Opportunistic Infections. (Seventh Report from the Committee on Government Operations, 102nd Congress, December 1991).

30. Epstein S. Activism, drug regulation, and the politics of therapeutic evaluation in the AIDS era: A case study of ddC and the "surrogate markers" debate. *Social Studies of Science* 1997;27:691–726.

31. Wyatt EA. Rushing to judgment. *Barron's* 1994;74(33):23.

32. Centers for Disease Control and Prevention. 1993 Revised classification system for HIV infection and expanded surveillance case definition for AIDS among adolescents and adults. *Morbidity and Mortality Weekly Report* 1992;41(RR-17):961–2.

33. National Institute of Allergy and Infectious Diseases. *HIV Infection in Women*. [Online] Available: http://www.niaid.nih.gov/factsheets/womenhiv.htm.

34. National Institutes of Health. *The NIH Almanac—Historical Data*. [Online] Available: http://www.nih.gov/about/almanac/historical/legislative_chronology.htm.

35. Community Programs for Clinical Research on AIDS. [Online] Available: http://www.cpcra.org/about_overview.htm.

36. Leoung G, Feigal D, Montgomery A, et al. Aerosolized pentamidine for prophylaxis against Pneumocystis carinii pneumonia: The San Francisco community prophylaxis trial. *New England Journal of Medicine* 1990;323:769–75.

37. TheStrategies for Management of Antiretroviral Therapy (SMART) Study Group. *New England Journal of Medicine* 2006;355:2283–96.

38. U.S. Department of Health and Human Services. AIDSinfo. [Online] Available: http://aidsinfo.nih.gov/.

39. Delaney M. Future directions in AIDS research. Project Inform Briefing Paper #4; Feb. 1994:1–3.

40. Paul WE. Reexamining AIDS research priorities. *Science* 1995;267:633–6.

41. Office of AIDS Research Advisory Council. *Report of the NIH AIDS Research Program Evaluation Working Group of the Office of AIDS Research Advisory Council*. [Online] March 16, 1996. Available: http://www.oar.nih.gov/public/pubs/levine.pdf.

42. Lo B. Personal communication. 2005.

43. Houyez F. Active involvement of patients in drug research, evaluation, and commercialization: European perspective. *Journal of Ambulatory Care Management* 2004;27:139–45.

44. McCormick S, Brody J, Brown P, Polk R. Public involvement in breast cancer research: An analysis and model for future research. *International Journal of Health Services* 2004;34:625–46.

45. Rabeharisoa V. The struggle against neuromuscular diseases in France and the emergence of the "partnership model" of patient organisation. *Social Science and Medicine* 2003;57:2127–36.

46. National Institutes of Health. Director's Council of Public Representatives. [Online] Available: http://copr.nih.gov/.

47. Emanuel EJ, Wendler D, Grady C. What makes clinical research ethical? *JAMA* 2000;283:2701–11.

48. Chase M. AIDS scientists, activists fail to fully resolve rift over trials. *Wall Street Journal* May 24, 2005.

Robert Steinbrook

The Gelsinger Case

Background

The death of Jesse Gelsinger in September 1999 is one of the defining cases in the recent history of research with humans. Gelsinger, 18, died during a gene transfer experiment at the University of Pennsylvania School of Medicine.[1] His death—the first directly attributed to gene transfer—raised profound questions about the protection of patients in this high-profile research field, as well as in other clinical studies. It also raised questions about adherence to research protocols, the reporting of adverse events, informed consent, and financial conflicts of interest. It shook the confidence of the public and the federal government in the competence and ethics of clinical researchers and the institutions where they work, and led to efforts to improve the protection of research participants.

Although the terms gene transfer and gene therapy are often used interchangeably, gene transfer is more precise. Gene transfer refers to the transfer to a person of recombinant DNA, or the transfer of DNA or RNA derived from recombinant DNA. The aim is to modify or manipulate the expression of a gene in the body or to change the biological properties of cells. Although the promise of gene transfer is great, progress has been slow. A 1995 review of the investment in the field by the National Institutes of Health (NIH) advocated caution: "Significant problems remain in all basic aspects of gene therapy. Major difficulties at the basic level include shortcomings in all current gene transfer vectors and inadequate understanding of the biological interaction of these vectors with the host."[2]

As of February 2000, several months after Gelsinger's death, more than 4,000 patients had participated in gene transfer studies.

Of the 372 clinical trials that were registered with the NIH, 89% were Phase I studies of safety and toxicity.[3] For many years, the public and scientists have been concerned about the potential environmental and infectious disease risks of recombinant DNA technology. This is one reason that the federal government has treated gene transfer studies differently from other clinical research. Extensive data about all trials registered with the NIH are publicly available—far more than for most other studies. Investigators who are funded by the NIH or who conduct their work at institutions that receive NIH support for any type of recombinant DNA research must comply with specific NIH guidelines. In addition to this, a Recombinant DNA Advisory Committee (RAC) was established within the NIH in 1974. The RAC is a public forum for discussion of novel and substantial issues related to gene transfer trials, including the review of specific protocols. Although the guidelines and the specific duties of the RAC have changed over time, it has a critical role in the oversight of this research.[4] The Food and Drug Administration (FDA) also regulates clinical gene transfer trials.

Gene Transfer for Ornithine Transcarbamylase Deficiency

Ornithine transcarbamylase (OTC) deficiency is a recessive X-linked autosomal genetic defect that interferes with the metabolism of ammonia by the liver. Although the mutations that lead to this enzyme deficiency are rare—affecting 1 in 40,000 to 1 in 80,000 people—they are the most common of the inborn errors of urea synthesis. Correction of this single gene enzyme deficiency has been viewed as a model for gene transfer directed at the liver.[5] The reason is that restoration of the enzyme activity should treat the disorder, as has been demonstrated by treatment with liver transplantation.[6] Gene transfer for OTC deficiency has been studied in the sparse fur mouse, which is deficient in the enzyme. Studies in this animal model suggest that the gene defect can be corrected.[1]

People with OTC deficiency can develop profound hyperammonemia. Excessive levels of ammonium ion in the brain can lead to life-threatening encephalopathy, coma, and brain damage. Complete deficiency usually leads to death during infancy. Without a liver transplant, only about half of those born with OTC deficiency will survive to age 5, and many survivors have profound mental impairment. For people with partial enzyme deficiency, a low protein diet supplemented with oral medications (sodium benzoate and sodium phenylacetate/sodium phenylbutyrate) can be used to minimize the risk of complications or death. Such treatment eliminates excess urea and precursors of ammonia. However, adherence to diet and medical therapy is difficult, and only partially effective.

Background to the Research Study at the University of Pennsylvania

A chronology of events leading up to and following Gelsinger's death is shown in Table 10.1. In 1993, James M. Wilson was recruited to the University of Pennsylvania from the University of Michigan. At the time of Gelsinger's death, Wilson was widely considered to be one of the leading gene transfer researchers in the world. He was director of the Institute for Human Gene Therapy and professor and chair of the Department of Molecular and Cellular Engineering in the university's School of Medicine. In 1992, while working in Michigan, Wilson was a founder of Genovo, Inc., which had the rights to market his discoveries related to gene transfer. Wilson held patents related to the use of vectors derived from the adenovirus for gene transfer.

There were many financial links between Genovo, whose principal offices were in a Philadelphia suburb, Wilson, the Institute for Human Gene Therapy, and the University of Pennsylvania. By 1999, Genovo provided more than $4 million a year to the institute, a substantial portion of its budget. Wilson and his immediate family had a 30% nonvoting equity stake in Genovo, and the University of Pennsylvania had a 3.2% equity stake.[7] Other shareholders included past and present employees of the university and the institute. In the late 1990s, Penn was aggressively seeking to profit from the discoveries of its professors. The *Philadelphia Inquirer* quoted the managing director of Penn's Center for Technology Transfer: "For years, Penn wasn't even in the game. Now we're in the game and we're looking for some home runs"[8] (see Chapters 68–71).

In December 1994, Penn's Center for Technology Transfer had officially requested that the Conflict of Interest Standing Committee at the University of Pennsylvania Medical Center review Wilson's involvement with Genovo. The committee had the authority to review the case and to make recommendations for managing potential conflicts of interest. The committee considered the case of great importance and conducted a detailed review. For example, according to the minutes of the committee's February 6, 1995, meeting, many comments and questions were considered.

Members were concerned that Wilson's multiple roles would "conflict" with his responsibilities at Penn and "create conflicts" for the medical school in allocating resources or implementing ethical and academic policies. According to the minutes, "Since Dr. Wilson's research efforts will be directed towards the solution of a problem in which he has a financial interest in the outcome, how can Dr. Wilson assure the University that he will not be conflicted when making decisions that could have an impact on either Genovo, Biogen [another biotechnology company that had invested in Genovo], or the further development of his intellectual property?" Another question appeared in the draft version of the minutes, but not in the final version: "How can Dr. Wilson and the University avoid liability for damages if a patient died from any products produced or studied at the University?"

The Conflict of Interest Standing Committee recognized the potential conflicts of interest involving Wilson's commitments to Genovo and to the University of Pennsylvania. It also recognized that his research program could lead to important medical advances that might benefit the public. In 1995, it did not seek to end his financial arrangements with the company. Instead, it recommended actions to manage the conflicts by reducing his managerial and scientific control. These included making Wilson's stock nonvoting and prohibiting him from being a member of the company's scientific advisory board.

The Research Study

Between 1997 and 1999, Gelsinger and 17 other subjects participated in the clinical protocol, "Recombinant Adenovirus Gene Transfer in Adults With Partial Ornithine Transcarbamylase Deficiency."[5,9] Wilson was a coinvestigator and the sponsor of the research. His main collaborators were Steven E. Raper, a surgeon at the University of Pennsylvania, who was the principal investigator, and Mark L. Batshaw of the Children's National Medical Center in Washington, D.C., who was the coprincipal investigator. Batshaw had pioneered the drug and diet treatment that was widely used for OTC deficiency. On June 21, 1997, Wilson signed FDA form 1572, in which he agreed to conduct the study in accordance with the investigational plan and applicable federal regulations.

The adenovirus-derived vector contained a functional OTC gene. The vector was rendered incapable of replicating by the deletion of two adenoviral genes; it was designed to be safer than earlier versions of the vector. The purpose of the research was "to establish a safe dose of recombinant adenovirus to serve as a treatment for adults with partial OTC [deficiency]."[5] Like most gene transfer studies at the time, the trial was a Phase I safety study of escalating doses of the vector, not a study of the effectiveness of the treatment. Thus, subjects were not expected to benefit directly from their participation. The protocol was reviewed and approved by many oversight bodies, including the RAC, the FDA, and human subjects review boards at the University of Pennsylvania Medical Center and the Children's Hospital of Philadelphia. The NIH and Genovo, the company that Wilson had helped to found and in which he held equity, were the major funders of the research and of Wilson's laboratory.

The protocol called for groups of three or four participants to be assigned to one of six dosing regimens; each group received a progressively higher dose of the vector, with adjustment for their body weight. The genetically altered adenovirus was administered

Table 10.1

Timeline of Events Leading Up To and Following the Death of Jesse Gelsinger

Date	Event	Date	Event
1992	While at the University of Michigan, James M. Wilson is a founder of Genovo, Inc., a company involved in gene transfer research and development. The company has rights to market Wilson's discoveries related to gene transfer.	Apr. 2000	An independent, external panel appointed by the president of the University of Pennsylvania reports on the Institute for Human Gene Therapy.
1993	Wilson is recruited to the University of Pennsylvania to be the director of the Institute for Human Gene Therapy.	May 2000	The University of Pennsylvania announces that the Institute for Human Gene Therapy will stop conducting clinical studies and sponsoring clinical trials.
1995	The Recombinant DNA Advisory Committee (RAC) at the National Institutes of Health approves a clinical protocol from the Institute for Human Gene Therapy, "Recombinant Adenovirus Gene Transfer in Adults With Partial Ornithine Transcarbamylase [OTC] Deficiency." The principal investigator is Steven E. Raper, also of the University of Pennsylvania. The coprincipal investigator is Mark L. Batshaw of the Children's National Medical Center in Washington, D.C. Wilson is a coinvestigator.	Aug. 2000	Targeted Genetics Corp. of Seattle agrees to acquire Genovo, Inc. Wilson receives stock valued at about $13.5 million and the University of Pennsylvania stock valued at about $1.4 million.
		Sept. 2000	Gelsinger's family files a civil lawsuit against Wilson, other researchers, and the University of Pennsylvania.
		Nov. 2000	The lawsuit is settled out of court; details are not disclosed.
1997	Enrollment of patients in the gene transfer protocol begins. The informed consent document includes a one-sentence statement about the financial interest of the University of Pennsylvania, Wilson, and Genovo, Inc., in "a successful outcome of the research involved in this study."	Nov. 2000	The FDA, citing six violations of federal regulations, begins proceedings to disqualify Wilson from performing clinical research with investigational drugs.
1998	Jesse Gelsinger, an 18-year-old man with partial OTC deficiency and a resident of Tucson, Ariz., learns about the Penn study from his physician.	Sept. 2001	The Office for Human Research Protections, in the Department of Health and Human Services, accepts Penn's corrective actions with regard to the OTC deficiency protocol and the University's system for protecting human subjects.
June 1999	Gelsinger and his father go to the Institute for Human Gene Therapy. Blood tests to determine his eligibility for the gene transfer trial are performed.	Feb. 2002	The FDA concludes that Wilson's explanations "fail to adequately address the violations."
Sept. 9, 1999	Gelsinger returns to Philadelphia to begin the trial.	Apr. 2002	Wilson announces that he will step down as director of the Institute for Human Gene Therapy.
Sept. 13, 1999	Gelsinger receives an infusion of 3.8×10^{13} particles of the adenoviral vector through a femoral catheter into the right hepatic artery. He is the 18th, and last, subject in the study.	Summer 2002	The Institute for Human Gene Therapy closes.
		Apr. 2003	The University of Pennsylvania revises its conflict of interest policies for faculty participating in clinical trials.
Sept. 17, 1999	Gelsinger dies. After his death, the study is halted.	Oct. 2003	A report on Gelsinger's death, "Fatal Systemic Inflammatory Response Syndrome in a Ornithine Transcarbamylase Deficient Patient Following Adenoviral Gene Transfer," is published in the medical literature.[1]
Sept. 29, 1999	*The Washington Post* reports on Gelsinger's death. Serious problems with the conduct of the OTC deficiency trial and the financial relationships between Wilson, Penn, and Genovo subsequently become widely known.		
Dec. 1999	The RAC considers Gelsinger's death at a public meeting.	Feb. 2005	Resolving investigations by the Office of Criminal Investigations at the FDA and the Office of Inspector General of the Department of Health and Human Services, the Department of Justice reaches civil settlements with the University of Pennsylvania, the Children's National Medical Center, Wilson, Raper, and Batshaw.
Jan. 2000	After conducting multiple inspections at Penn, the FDA closes down all clinical trials at the Institute for Human Gene Therapy.		

as a single two-hour infusion of one ounce of fluid through a femoral catheter into the right hepatic artery. Participants were not compensated.

The informed consent document cited three major risks:

1. The possibility that the adenovirus would inflame the liver. "It is even possible that this inflammation could lead to liver toxicity or failure and be life-threatening," the consent document stated.

2. The possibility that the adenovirus would provoke an immune response that would damage the liver.

3. The possibility that receiving the vector would prevent the research participants from receiving it as part of a therapy in the future. If used again, the vector would likely trigger an immune response and the body would eliminate it.

The consent document also stated that if a subject developed liver failure, "a liver transplant could be required." Participants were to undergo a liver biopsy; the document stated that this procedure was associated with a "very small risk (1 in 10,000) of serious unpredicted complications which can include death."[10]

A particularly controversial aspect of the study was the decision to enroll adults with mild disease, rather than children with severe disease. The investigators had initially planned to use dying newborn infants as subjects but changed their minds.[11] According to the informed consent document, "Because this is a study of safety and long-term metabolic improvement is not expected, we felt it most appropriate to study adults (ages 18–65) who have a mild deficiency of OTC rather than children."[10]

One reason for the switch was that adults without mental impairment were better able to provide informed consent than the parents of children with terminal illness. Another was that it would be difficult to recognize adverse or life-threatening events in children who were already dying from their disease. Arthur L. Caplan, a leading bioethicist, a professor of bioethics at Penn, and a member of Wilson's department, advocated this approach.[11] Wilson has stated that the decision to use adults "was based on the collective input and recommendations from the University of Pennsylvania's own bioethicists, as well as from families of diseased children and other metabolic disease experts not associated with the study."[12] In some ways, the choice between enrolling adults with mild disease or children with severe disease represented a no-win situation for the investigators. Although this was a Phase I safety study, terminally ill newborns potentially had the most to gain.[13] Both positions can be justified, and both can be criticized.

The enrollment of subjects with only mild disease was criticized before and after Gelsinger's death. The RAC (which at the time had to approve gene transfer studies) had approved the protocol in December 1995.[14] The approval, by a vote of 12 to 1, with 4 abstentions, followed a lengthy discussion during which some members questioned the safety and wisdom of the proposed experiment. One concern was the enrollment of patients with mild disease. Another was the infusion of large quantities of the vector directly into the blood supply of the liver. For example, one reviewer of the protocol said that it would "be more acceptable if the vector can be repeatedly delivered by the less invasive intravenous route" and if the treatment was "given to affected children with life threatening OTC deficiency."[14] At the time, the researchers agreed to infuse the vector into the bloodstream, not directly into the liver. This decision was subsequently reversed, as the FDA requested when it approved the protocol in 1997. The rationale was that because the vector would travel through the circulation to the liver anyway, it was safer to put it directly where it was needed with the hope that it would not travel elsewhere. The RAC was not informed of this change.[15]

The informed consent document also included a one-sentence statement about the financial interests of the sponsors: "Please be aware that the University of Pennsylvania, Dr. James M. Wilson (the Director of the Institute for Human Gene Therapy), and Genovo, Inc. (a gene therapy company in which Dr. Wilson holds an interest), have a financial interest in a successful outcome from the research involved in this study."[10] Such a statement was highly unusual at the time. The form did not specify what the financial interests were, or their potential magnitude. According to the University, Wilson had no role in recruiting patients, obtaining informed consent, or treating patients, including Gelsinger. Wilson, however, was a coinvestigator. As the director of the Institute for Human Gene Therapy, he was the sponsor of the study. It was

his gene transfer research that made the trial possible. Wilson was extensively involved in activities such as the preclinical animal work, the development of the gene transfer vector and its mode of delivery, the design of the trial, protocol modifications, laboratory work during the trial, and the analysis of the results.

Jesse Gelsinger

Jesse Gelsinger was diagnosed with partial OTC deficiency when he was a young child. He was subsequently found to have a unique mutation. Some of his cells had a defective OTC gene with a large deletion, whereas others had a normal gene—a condition known as mosaicism.[16] Despite diet and drug therapy, he developed serious hyperammonemia many times, including an episode of hyperammonemic coma in December 1998 that required treatment with mechanical ventilation. He recovered from this episode without apparent adverse effects. In 1999, his disease was considered generally controlled.

Gelsinger lived in Tucson, Arizona. He was the 18th subject in the study and, at age 18, the youngest person enrolled. He had learned about the trial in 1998 from his physician. His father said after his death that he "was doing this for other people."[17] Jesse Gelsinger set aside his personal life to participate, and took an unpaid leave from his job.[18] According to his father, "One night he even said, 'The worst that could happen is that I could die and maybe help doctors figure out a way to save sick babies.' I've never been more proud of my son than the moment he decided to do this experiment."[17]

The doses of the vector in the study ranged from 2×10^9 to 6×10^{11} particles/kg of body weight. (The second-highest dose was 2×10^{11} particles/kg.) On September 13, 1999, Gelsinger became the second subject to receive the highest dose of 6×10^{11} particles/kg; his total dose, based on his weight, was 3.8×10^{13} particles. In the other study participants, including the first to receive the highest dose, the adverse effects were transient muscle aches and fevers and laboratory abnormalities such as thrombocytopenia, anemia, hypophosphatemia, and elevated levels of the liver enzymes known as transaminases. The adverse events in other study participants, however, were not life threatening.

About 18 hours following infusion of the adenovirus vector, Gelsinger developed altered mental status and jaundice—neither of which had been seen in the first 17 study participants. He subsequently developed the systemic inflammatory response syndrome, disseminated intravascular coagulation and multiple organ system failure, and the acute respiratory distress syndrome.[1] Gelsinger died on September 17, 1999, 98 hours following gene transfer.

An autopsy and subsequent studies indicated that his death was caused by a fulminant immune reaction (with high serum levels of the cytokines interleukin-6 and interleukin-10) to the adenoviral vector.[1] Substantial amounts of the vector were found not only in his liver (as expected) but also in his spleen, lymph nodes, and bone marrow. According to an NIH report on adenoviral safety and toxicity that was prompted by Gelsinger's death, "The data suggested that the high dose of Ad [adenoviral] vector, delivered by infusion directly to the liver, quickly saturated available receptors . . . within that organ and then spilled into the circulatory and other organ systems including the bone marrow, thus inducing the systemic immune response."[19] The report added, "Although the Ad vector used in the OTC trial was incapable of replicating, the capsid

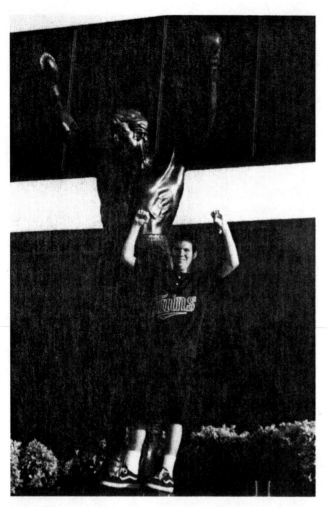

Figure 10.1. Jesse Gelsinger, June 22, 1999. "Having just been screened for participation in the Ornithine Transcarbamylase Deficiency clinical trial, Jesse Gelsinger was ready, just like Rocky Balboa was ready for battle, to help advance treatments for his disease," says Jesse's father, Paul Gelsinger. "Jesse had no real idea of the concealed dangers involved in what he was about to do, nor of the ethical awareness his death would bring." Source: Mickie Gelsinger and Paul Gelsinger. Reproduced with permission.

proteins encoating the vector [the shell of the vector] likely contributed to the participant's immune response."

In October 2003, the research team published a report on "the unexpected and tragic consequences of Jesse Gelsinger's participation in this trial."[1] They concluded that his death pointed to "the limitations of animal studies in predicting human responses, the steep toxicity curve for replication defective adenovirus vectors, substantial subject-to-subject variation in host responses to systemically administered vectors, and the need for further study of the immune response to these vectors."[1]

Subsequent Developments at Penn

After Gelsinger's death, the study was halted. Although a Tucson newspaper had reported on his death a few days earlier, the events were not widely known until an article appeared in the *Washington Post* on September 29, 1999.[20,21] The FDA, the NIH, and the Office for Protection from Research Risks at NIH began intensive reviews of the protocol and other gene transfer research.

Serious deficiencies in the conduct of the study soon became widely known.[22] One was that Gelsinger should not have been allowed into the study, because his liver was not functioning at the minimal level required for inclusion on the day he received the infusion. Another was that the researchers failed to immediately notify the FDA when earlier participants had "Grade III" liver toxicity. Their liver enzyme abnormalities were sufficiently severe that the study should have been put on hold, as the research protocol required. Still another was that the FDA was not promptly informed about the results of tests in laboratory animals that suggested a significant risk of the adenoviral vector for human subjects. When given higher doses of the vector (1×10^{13} particles/kg), rhesus monkeys developed disseminated intravascular coagulation and liver failure; some died. However, at the dose administered to Gelsinger (6×10^{11} particles/kg), which was about 15-fold less, only minor toxicities to the liver were observed in the monkeys. Yet another deficiency was that the researchers had changed the protocol multiple times without notifying the FDA, and failed to make changes they had agreed to make. These included tightening the exclusion criteria in a way that would have made more potential subjects ineligible, because they were at risk for liver toxicity on the basis of their medical histories. Other questions had to do with Wilson's and Penn's financial interest in the study's success, deficiencies in the informed consent process, including downplaying the risks by failing to give potential participants all the relevant safety information, such as the monkey deaths and the serious side effects in other subjects, failure to follow the protocol, failure to maintain complete and accurate records, and the adequacy of the review of the trial by Penn's institutional review board (IRB).[22–29]

In January 2000, after conducting multiple inspections at Penn, the FDA issued a "list of inspectional observations" and closed down all clinical trials at the Institute for Human Gene Therapy.[25] Neither the FDA nor the Office for Protection from Research Risks sought to halt all clinical research at Penn.

Although acknowledging mistakes and extending its sympathy to the Gelsinger family, the research team vigorously defended its work, and Penn defended its researchers.[30] According to Wilson, "the alleged lure of potential financial gain played no role in any clinical decisions."[12] Penn's position has been that "as deeply regrettable as Gelsinger's death was, it was simply not foreseeable based on informed medical judgment and the best scientific information available at the time," according to a written statement in October 2003 by Rebecca Harmon, the chief public affairs officer for the University's School of Medicine.

After Gelsinger's death, Penn initially sought to reopen its gene transfer program. Soon, however, it changed its mind. In early 2000, Judith Rodin, then the president of the university, appointed an independent, external panel to evaluate the issues. William H. Danforth, former chancellor of Washington University in St. Louis, chaired the panel. In April 2000, the panel recommended that the university do a better job of evaluating and monitoring clinical trials and ensuring that informed consent is properly obtained.[31] The panel also recommended that Penn review its policies on conflict of interest, especially with regard to clinical trials. For clinical trials, the panel found that

[E]quity positions by an investigator and/or the University may be ill advised, even if, in reality, there is no practical effect whatsoever. Given that the overriding responsibility of the University and its investigators is to the welfare of patients, the avoidance of conflict of interest that even remotely might detract from putting the needs of patients first becomes paramount. In that regard, investments in new therapies differ from those in other ventures, such as computer technology, which involve no responsibility for patient care.

The panel also questioned whether it made sense "to have an entire Institute devoted to gene therapy."

Rodin also requested a second report, an internal review by Penn faculty of all aspects of research involving human subjects at the university. In an interim report, also in April 2000, the internal Committee on Research Using Humans recommended that Rodin carry out a comprehensive review of the university's IRB system, and develop formal monitoring mechanisms for clinical trials as well as "standard operating procedures" that apply to human subjects research.[32] At the time, Penn had more than 3,900 ongoing research protocols involving humans, of which more than 750 involved the use of investigational drugs. The committee also recommended that the IRB "act expeditiously to require that principal investigators and coinvestigators disclose on the forms requesting IRB approval any proprietary interest in the product or procedure under investigation, including potential future compensation both for themselves and their immediate family. The IRB should then determine on a case-by-case basis whether disclosures in the patient consent document or other protections are required."[32] The committee never issued a final report, as the university quickly implemented changes.

In May 2000, the University of Pennsylvania announced that the Institute for Human Gene Therapy would stop conducting clinical studies and sponsoring clinical trials. Instead, it would conduct animal experiments and preclinical research. The university also announced other changes, including reforms in its IRB system, educational programs for researchers, and a more comprehensive infrastructure to protect research subjects.[33] According to a university publication, the work of the internal review committee and other efforts by faculty and administrators "have generated unprecedented change in Penn's research infrastructure and culture."[34]

In August 2000, Targeted Genetics Corp. of Seattle agreed to acquire Genovo, the company that Wilson had helped to found.[35] The acquisition enriched Wilson and the University of Pennsylvania. Under the agreement, Wilson was to receive Targeted Genetics stock that was then valued at about $13.5 million. The University of Pennsylvania was to receive stock valued at about $1.4 million.[7] Although the actual amount of money that Wilson and the university received is not known, it may have been considerably less, because the value of the stock plummeted.

In September 2001, the Office for Human Research Protections of the Department of Health and Human Services (DHHS), which had replaced the Office for Protection from Research Risks at the NIH, accepted Penn's corrective actions with regard to the OTC deficiency protocol and the University's system for protecting research participants.[36] In April 2002, Wilson announced that he would step down as director of the Institute for Human Gene Therapy. He continued as chairman and professor of the Molecular and Cellular Engineering Department. The institute closed in the summer of 2002.

The University of Pennsylvania also revised its conflict of interest policies. In April 2003, a policy on "financial disclosure and presumptively prohibited conflicts for faculty participating in clinical trials" became effective.[37] An earlier version had been used as an interim policy. The policy prohibited clinical investigators from maintaining certain "significant financial interests" such as service on the board of directors or as an officer of a company or entity that sponsors a clinical trial, significant equity interest in the sponsor, or ownership of a proprietary interest in the tested product. The policy defined "significant equity interest" as

[A]ny ownership interest, stock options, or other financial interest whose value cannot be readily determined through reference to public prices (generally, interests in a non-publicly traded corporation), or any equity interest in a publicly traded corporation that exceeds $10,000 (or exceeds 5% ownership) during the time the clinical investigator is carrying out the study and for 1 year following the completion of the study. Interest in any publicly traded mutual fund is excluded.

Like policies at many academic medical centers, Penn's policy allowed for exceptions on a case-by-case basis when there are "compelling circumstances." The policy defined "compelling circumstances" as "facts that convince the [Conflict of Interest Standing Committee] that an investigator should be permitted to participate in a specific trial in spite of a Significant Financial Interest." Relevant information "includes the nature of the research; the magnitude of the financial interest; the extent to which the financial interest could be influenced by the research; the degree of risk to human subjects; and whether the interest is amenable to management."[37]

The Response of Gelsinger's Family

Following his son's death, Paul Gelsinger became an outspoken advocate of improved protection for research participants. In the first months after the death, he continued to support his son's doctors—"believing that their intent was nearly as pure as Jesse's"—even as the news media exposed the flaws in their work.[18] However, while attending the discussion of his son's death at a RAC meeting in December 1999, he became convinced that he and his son had not been given all the relevant information. He changed his mind. "It wasn't until that three-day meeting that I discovered that there was never any efficacy in humans," he later wrote. "I believed this was working based on my conversations with Mark Batshaw and that is why I defended Penn for so long." At a meeting with FDA and NIH officials and the Penn doctors during the RAC meeting, "after touching on many issues I let them know that I had not to this point even spoken to a lawyer, but would be in the near future. Too many mistakes had been made and unfortunately, because of our litigious society, it was the only way to correct these problems."[18] In September 2000, Gelsinger's family filed a civil lawsuit against the lead researchers, the University of Pennsylvania, and others.[38] In November 2000, the suit was settled out of court; details have not been disclosed.[39,40]

The Response of the Federal Government

At the time of Gelsinger's death, adenoviral vectors were used in one quarter of the 372 gene transfer trials that were registered with the NIH. After reviewing safety and toxicity data from these trials, the RAC recommended that human gene transfer research with adenoviral vectors continue, but with greater caution.[19] The committee also recommended a centralized data base for collecting and organizing safety and toxicity data on gene transfer vectors, greater standardization of the experimental data collected during trials, improved informed consent documents, and more extensive monitoring of research participants.

Prompt and complete reporting of serious adverse events was a particular concern. After Gelsinger died, the NIH and the FDA both reminded researchers of their obligations to report adverse events in gene transfer trials. The NIH soon received nearly 700 such reports, including reports of deaths that occurred before Gelsinger's.[41] For example, the NIH learned that a gene transfer trial at another academic medical center had been suspended in June 1999 after three of the first six participants died and a seventh became seriously ill. The study participants were terminally ill cancer patients. The NIH also had not been promptly notified of two deaths at a third institution during trials involving genes for a vascular endothelial growth factor aimed at growing new blood vessels in patients with coronary or peripheral artery disease. In 2000, the FDA halted the experiments.[42] The FDA and the NIH subsequently tightened the monitoring procedures for gene transfer trials, increased federal oversight and public access to information about the trials, increased inspections of gene transfer clinical investigators, and improved the reporting of serious adverse events. In March 2004, the agencies launched the Genetic Modification Clinical Research Information System, known as GeMCRIS. This Web-accessible database on human gene transfer (http://www.gemcris.od.nih.gov) provides information about clinical gene transfer trials. It also allows investigators and sponsors to report adverse events using a secure electronic interface, thus improving and centralizing reporting procedures.

In March and July 2000, the FDA sent warning letters to Wilson, outlining what the agency viewed as widespread deficiencies in the conduct of the research.[26,27] In November 2000, the FDA sent warning letters to Batsaw[43] and Raper[44] and began proceedings to disqualify Wilson from performing clinical research with investigational drugs.[28] It is unusual for the FDA to seek such a disqualification. In a 15-page letter, the FDA detailed the evidence that Wilson had "repeatedly or deliberately violated regulations governing the proper conduct of clinical studies involving investigational new drugs."[28] It cited six violations: failure to fulfill the general responsibilities of investigators; failure to ensure that an investigation was conducted according to the investigational plan; failure to submit accurate reports about the safety of the study to the University of Pennsylvania IRB; failure to accurately and completely identify changes in the research for review and evaluation by the review board; failure to properly obtain informed consent; and failure to maintain accurate case histories of the research subjects. Wilson contested many of the allegations.

In February 2002, the FDA concluded that Wilson's written explanations failed "to adequately address the violations."[45] The agency told Wilson that, although he was assisted by "several subinvestigators," as "the clinical investigator you were responsi-

ble for all aspects of the study." It added, "While you assert that you delegated many aspects of the subject recruitment and subject management to others, you were the responsible leader of the investigational team. Indeed, you were present when prospective subjects' cases were discussed, and when protocol modifications were considered at the OTCD team meetings."[45]

Following investigations by the Office of Criminal Investigations at the FDA and the Office of Inspector General at the DHHS, the Department of Justice brought civil charges against the University of Pennsylvania, the Children's National Medical Center, Wilson, Batshaw, and Raper. The government alleged that the investigators and their institutions violated the federal False Claims Act by making false statements and claims in connection with grant applications and progress reports to the NIH, submissions to the FDA, information supplied to the IRBs that had oversight over the research, and by failing to obtain proper informed consent.

In February 2005, the government reached civil settlements with the investigators and institutions.[40] The institutions and investigators did not acknowledge the government's allegations and maintained that they acted appropriately and within the law at all times. The investigators did not take responsibility for Gelsinger's death. The University of Pennsylvania agreed to pay a fine of $517,496 and to increase IRB oversight of clinical research and training for investigators and clinical coordinators. The settlement agreement outlined the steps the university had taken to promote safety in clinical research. For example, between fiscal years 1998 and 2005, the number of full-time employees of the University's Office of Regulatory Affairs, which is responsible for staffing the IRBs, increased from 5 to 23. In a written statement, the university said, "Out of this tragedy has come a renewed national effort to protect the safety of those who help to advance new treatments and cure through clinical research." The Children's National Medical Center agreed to pay $514,622 and to increase its IRB budget and staff.

Wilson continued to work at the University of Pennsylvania. The agreement terminated the FDA's administrative proceedings against him. Wilson agreed not to serve as a sponsor of a clinical trial regulated by the FDA or to participate without restriction in research with humans until February 2010. (He already had not been involved with human research participants since January 2000.) Wilson also agreed to meet specified educational, training, and monitoring requirements related to his research and to lecture and write an article on the lessons of human research participants protections learned from the OTC deficiency trial. In a written statement released by Penn, Wilson said, "In the last few years, I have focused my research on the discovery and design of new gene-transfer vectors for gene therapy and genetic vaccines. Reaching this agreement means that I may continue to devote myself fully and without restriction to my laboratory and that I may conduct clinical research when it would be appropriate for scientific advancement." Batshaw and Raper agreed to lesser restrictions.

Enduring Legacy

More than eight years after Gelsinger's death, the case remained sensitive for the University of Pennsylvania. Despite repeated requests, neither Wilson nor any of the university officials with extensive knowledge of the case were willing to speak about it; Wilson has granted no interviews for many years.

According to Donna Shalala, Secretary of DHHS during the Clinton administration, "The tragic death of Jesse Gelsinger focused national attention on the inadequacies in the current system of protections for human research subjects."[46] In a better world, improved protection for research subjects would be less dependent on responses to tragedy. Nonetheless, the protection of research subjects has often improved after crises, such as the Tuskegee syphilis experiment in the 1970s (see Chapter 8). In an article in the *New England Journal of Medicine* in 2000, Shalala wrote that "the American people expect that clinical researchers will never compromise or neglect the safety of human subjects." She also cited practical considerations: "To put it simply, if we cannot guarantee sound research in general—and patients' safety in particular—public support for gene therapy and other potentially lifesaving treatments will evaporate."[46]

Reports from the DHHS Office of Inspector General, some of which were completed before Gelsinger's death, documented problems with IRBs in the United States. The review boards have been criticized for reviewing too many protocols, working too quickly, having insufficient expertise, and providing too little training for investigators and board members.[47] The National Bioethics Advisory Commission and the Institute of Medicine examined these and additional problems with assuring the safety of subjects.[48,49] A common theme was that broader and more effective federal oversight of clinical research was needed.

In 2000, DHHS established the Office for Human Research Protections. The office replaced the NIH Office for Protection from Research Risks, which had less visibility and stature. In 2001, the FDA established the Office for Good Clinical Practice to coordinate its efforts to protect research subjects. As indicated above, in 2004, the NIH and the FDA launched the GeMCRIS to provide information about clinical gene-transfer trials and allow prompt reporting of adverse events. Institutions that have corrected serious problems with their programs for protecting subjects, such as Johns Hopkins University and Duke University as well as Penn, have markedly increased their spending for these programs, and have increased the number of review boards.[47]

Lawsuits against investigators, IRBs, and academic institutions are increasingly common.[50] Traditionally, litigation in clinical research was based on allegations about failure to obtain informed consent. For example, investigators may not have given research participants sufficient information to permit meaningful consent. In the Gelsinger case and other recent actions, new types of claims have been made. These include product liability claims against a drug manufacturer and fraud claims against investigators for not revealing their financial ties or problems encountered by previous subjects. The number and types of defendants have also expanded.

The allegations in the civil lawsuit filed by Gelsinger's family included wrongful death, product liability, lack of informed consent, and fraud. The initial defendants included William N. Kelly, the former dean of the School of Medicine and the chief executive of its health system, who had recruited Wilson to Penn and had patent interests related to gene transfer research. They also included Caplan, who had been consulted about the trial, the trustees of the University, the main investigators, and Genovo, the company that Wilson had helped to found.[38] When the lawsuit was settled, Kelly and Caplan were dismissed from the suit.[40] According to an analysis of these trends by Mello, Studdert, and

Brennan, litigation may help injured subjects obtain compensation. However, it is also likely to lead IRBs to adopt "a more legalistic, mechanistic approach to ethical review that does not further the interests of human subjects or scientific progress."[50]

In response to the Gelsinger case, the American Society of Gene Therapy revised its conflict of interest policies.[51] The Association of American Medical Colleges issued guidelines for oversight of both individual and institutional financial interests in human subjects research.[52,53] In 2004, after years of consideration, DHHS issued guidance on financial relationships and interests and human subject protection.[54] The department recommended that "IRBs, institutions, and investigators consider whether specific financial relationships create financial interests in research studies that may adversely affect the rights and welfare of subjects." Among the questions to be addressed were, "What financial relationships and resulting financial interests could cause potential or actual conflicts of interest?" and "At what levels should those potential or actual financial conflicts of interest be managed or eliminated?"[54]

Despite the various reports and institutional changes following Gelsinger's death, it can be argued that nothing has really changed. Review boards and other oversight mechanisms can do only so much. As of 2007, Congress had enacted no legislation to make the system for protecting research participants more efficient and effective. There had been no new federal regulations. For example, according to David Blumenthal, the guidance from DHHS about financial relationships is "notable for the qualified nature of its recommendations, which are not backed by any regulatory authority."[55] In addition, improvements in the federal oversight of research primarily affect federally funded programs. With the exception of research involving new drugs and medical devices that is under the jurisdiction of the FDA, there is no requirement that participants in privately sponsored research receive the same protection that federal regulations provide.[47] The National Bioethics Advisory Commission concluded in 2001 that the difference in protection was "ethically indefensible" and "a fundamental flaw in the current oversight system."[48] This situation remains unchanged. Although it might seem that that research subjects should be safer than they were before Gelsinger's death, there is no way to know for sure.

Ethical Issues

The issues raised by the Gelsinger case have a common theme. In their zeal to help patients with a life-threatening disease, leading researchers at one of the premier academic medical centers in the United States lost their focus. They overlooked warning signals that the experimental intervention was not safe, with tragic, fatal consequences. The ethical issues relate to the selection of the research subjects, informed consent, adherence to the research protocol, and financial conflicts of interest.

The concerns about the selection of research subjects are discussed earlier in this chapter. Although adults with mild OTC deficiency and no mental impairment could provide informed consent, participation in the trial may have placed them at unnecessary risk. New treatments for OTC deficiency were urgently needed for patients with severe disease, not mild disease. Both the enrollment of adults with mild disease or newborns with the lethal form of the disease can be justified, and both positions can be criticized. As a Phase I study of dosage and safety, the Penn experiment was not intended to evaluate the therapeutic effectiveness of gene transfer for OTC deficiency. It is easy to criticize decisions after a tragedy. There was a rationale for the enrollment criteria, and many oversight groups approved the protocol.

The case underscores the responsibilities of investigators to properly obtain informed consent, to clearly disclose all the risks of research, to adhere to the research protocol, to keep good records, and to communicate promptly and completely with IRBs and regulatory agencies.[13] It also underscores the obligations of review boards and regulatory agencies to provide effective oversight of research.

There is no evidence that the financial interests of the University of Pennsylvania and Wilson in the success of the research had any relation to Gelsinger's death. Nonetheless, the existence of their financial interests inherently created uncertainty about their motives. Even if their motives had nothing to do with making money and their financial incentives had nothing to do with the conduct of the study, there was no way that either Penn or Wilson could effectively respond to the charge that the research was pursued for financial gain. The informed consent document included a statement about the financial interests of Penn, Wilson, and Genovo "in a successful outcome from the research involved in this study," although it did not indicate what the financial interests were, or their magnitude.[10] It can be argued that although disclosing this information to subjects was preferable to not disclosing it, the conflicts did not have to exist in the first place. A key question is whether Penn or Wilson should have been allowed to have these financial interests at all, or if the clinical trial should have been conducted by other investigators or at another institution. An IRB or a conflict of interest committee could require that financial conflicts be eliminated.

Cooperation between academic medical centers and industry can advance medical knowledge and speed the development of new treatments and technologies. Financial relations, however, complicate this cooperation. Some experts consider a presumption that financial conflicts should be eliminated, not managed, to be too draconian because it will impede vital research. Others argue that less radical approaches are doomed to fail. According to Marcia Angell, a former editor-in-chief of the *New England Journal of Medicine,*

> [O]ur society is now so drenched in market ideology that any resistance is considered quixotic. But medicine and clinical research are special, and I believe we have to protect their timeless values of service and disinterestedness. Patients should not have to wonder whether an investigator is motivated by financial gain, and the public should not have to wonder whether medical research can be believed. The only way to deal with the problem is to eliminate it as much as possible.[56]

Gene transfer is still in its infancy. It continues to hold great promise, but the risks and benefits are still being discovered. For example, encouraging results with gene transfer in the treatment of X-linked severe combined immunodeficiency (X-SCID), a devastating disease of young children, were followed by reports of a leukemia-like disorder in some of the research participants. One of these children died in 2004. According to Philip Noguchi of the FDA, the developments are a reminder that "the manipulations needed to create gene therapy add enormous complexity to con-

siderations of safety and preclinical toxicity testing, and for every intended consequence of a complex biological product, there are unintended consequences."[57] In March 2005, an advisory committee to the FDA recommended that gene transfer for X-SCID be restricted to children who have no alternative. As of that month, the FDA had received 472 investigational new drug applications for gene transfer; 123 had been withdrawn, 92 were inactive, 14 had been terminated, and 243 remained active. As of October 18, 2007, the FDA had received 562 applications; 150 had been withdrawn, 101 were inactive, 15 had been terminated, and 296 remained active. The agency had approved no gene therapies.

The death of Jesse Gelsinger has taught the medical community and society about how to make clinical research safer. Research, however, is still research. Only a minority of clinical trials will show benefit. Adverse events are inevitable. Some will continue to be unexpected, and tragic.

References

1. Raper SE, Chirmule N, Lee FS, et al. Fatal systemic inflammatory response syndrome in a ornithine transcarbamylase deficient patient following adenoviral gene transfer. *Molecular Genetics and Metabolism* 2003;80:148–58.
2. Orkin SH, Motulsky AG (co-chairs). Report and Recommendations of the Panel to Assess the NIH Investment in Research on Gene Therapy. [Online] December 7, 1995. Available: http://www4.0d.nih.gov/oba/rac/panelrep.htm.
3. Statement of Amy Patterson, M.D., Office of Biotechnology Activities, National Institutes of Health, Before the Subcommittee on Public Health, Committee on Health, Education, Labor and Pensions, U.S. Senate. [Online] February 2, 2000. Available: http://www4.0d.nih.gov/oba/rac/patterson2–00.pdf.
4. National Institutes of Health. Guidelines for Research Involving Recombinant DNA Molecules. [Online] April 2002. Available: http://www4.0d.nih.gov/oba/rac/guidelines/guidelines.html.
5. Batshaw ML, Wilson JM, Raper S, et al. Clinical protocol: Recombinant adenovirus gene transfer in adults with partial ornithine transcarbamylase deficiency (OTCD). *Human Gene Therapy* 1999;10:2419–37.
6. Whittington PF, Alonso EM, Boyle JT, et al. Liver transplantation for the treatment of urea cycle disorders. *Journal of Inherited Metabolic Disease* 1998;21(Suppl 1):112–8.
7. Hensley S. Targeted Genetics' Genovo deal leads to windfall for researcher. *Wall Street Journal* Aug. 10, 2000:B12.
8. Fernandez B. Penn engineering new profits from school's scientific work. *Philadelphia Inquirer* June 21, 1998:A19.
9. Raper SE, Yudkoff M, Chirmule N, et al. A pilot study of *in-vivo* liver-directed gene transfer with an adenoviral vector in partial ornithine transcarbamylase deficiency. *Human Gene Therapy* 2002;13:163–75.
10. Raper SE, Batshaw ML, Wilson JM, et al. Consent to act as a subject in an investigational study (January 1999), CHOP IRB #1994–7–794, Penn IRB #366–0, "Recombinant adenovirus gene transfer in adults with partial ornithine transcarbamylase deficiency."
11. Sisti, DA, Caplan AL. Back to basics: Gene therapy research ethics and oversight in the post-Gelsinger era. In: Rehmann-Sutter C, Muller H, eds. *Ethik und Gentherapie: Zum praktischen Diskurs um die molekulare Medizin.* Stuttgart, Germany: Francke Verlag; 003:135–49.
12. Wilson JM. Risks of gene therapy research. *Washington Post* Dec. 6, 1999:A26.
13. Friedmann T. Principles for human gene therapy studies. *Science* 2000;287:2163–5.

14. Department of Health and Human Services, National Institutes of Health, Recombinant DNA Advisory Committee. Minutes of Meeting, December 4–5, 1995. [Online] December 5, 1995. Available: http://www4.0d.nih.gov/oba/rac/meeting.html.

15. Stolberg SG. The biotech death of Jesse Gelsinger. *New York Times Magazine* Nov. 28, 1999.

16. Maddalena A, Sosnoski DM, Berry GT, Nussbaum RI. Mosaicism for an intragenic deletion in a boy with mild ornithine trans-carbamylase deficiency. *New England Journal of Medicine* 1988;319: 999–1003.

17. Newton C. Story of first gene therapy death began with ambitious doctor, hopeful teen. *Associated Press Newswires* May 21, 2000.

18. Gelsinger P. Jesse's Intent. [Online] Available: http://www.sskrplaw.com/gene/jessieintent.html.

19. National Institutes of Health, Recombinant DNA Advisory Committee. Assessment of Adenoviral Vector Safety and Toxicity: Report of the National Institutes of Health Recombinant DNA Advisory Committee. *Human Gene Therapy* 2002;13:3–13.

20. Miller H. Sick teen who died in research called hero. *Arizona Daily Star* Sept. 26, 1999:1B.

21. Weiss R, Nelson D. Teen died undergoing experimental gene therapy. *Washington Post* Sept. 29, 1999:A1.

22. Nelson D, Weiss R. Hasty decisions in the race to cure? Gene therapy proceeded despite safety, ethics concerns. *Washington Post* Nov. 21, 1999:A1.

23. Marshall E. Gene therapy on trial. *Science* 2000;288: 951–7.

24. Department of Health and Human Services, National Institutes of Health, Recombinant DNA Advisory Committee. Minutes of Symposium and Meeting, December 8–10, 1999. [Online] December 10, 1999. Available: http://www4.0d.nih.gov/oba/rac/minutes/1299rac.pdf.

25. Rashti MM, Eggerman TL. FDA Form 483 Inspectional Observations. Philadelphia: Food and Drug Administration; January 19, 2000.

26. Masiello SA. Warning letter to James M. Wilson, University of Pennsylvania. Rockville, Md.: Food and Drug Administration; March 3, 2000.

27. Masiello SA. Warning letter to James M. Wilson, University of Pennsylvania. Rockville, Md.: Food and Drug Administration; July 3, 2000.

28. Masiello SA. Notice of initiation of disqualification proceeding and opportunity to explain. Letter to James M. Wilson, University of Pennsylvania Health System. Rockville, Md.: Food and Drug Administration; November 30, 2000.

29. Borror KC. Human research subject protections under multiple project assurance (MPA) M-1025. Letter to Neal Nathanson, University of Pennsylvania. Rockville, Md.: Office for Human Research Protections, Department of Health and Human Services; May 7, 2001.

30. Nelson D, Weiss R. Gene researchers admit mistakes, deny liability. *Washington Post* Feb. 15, 2000:A3.

31. Danforth WH, Benz EJ, Callahan D, et al. Report of Independent Panel Reviewing the University of Pennsylvania's Institute for Human Gene Therapy. [Online] April 27, 2000. University of Pennsylvania Almanac 2000;46(34):4–6. Available: http://www.upenn.edu/almanac/v46pdf/000530/053000.pdf.

32. University of Pennsylvania, Committee on Research Using Humans. Interim Report. University of Pennsylvania Almanac 2000;46(30):2. [Online] April 25, 2000. Available: http://www.upenn.edu/almanac/v46pdf/000425/042500.pdf.

33. Rodin J. Action by the University of Pennsylvania in Response to the "Report of the Independent Panel Reviewing the Institute for Human Gene Therapy." *University of Pennsylvania Almanac* 2000;46(34):6. [Online] May 30, 2000. Available: http://www.upenn.edu/almanac/v46pdf/000530/053000.pdf.

34. Bonett JB. Changing the culture of research. *Penn Medicine* 2002; XV(2):6–11. [Online] October 1, 2002. Available: http://www.uphs.upenn.edu/prnews/publications/Penn_Medicine/PennMedicine%20Fall%202002.pdf.

35. Hensley S. Targeted Genetics agrees to buy Genovo. *Wall Street Journal* Aug. 9, 2000:B2.

36. Borror KC. Human research subject protections under multiple project assurance (MPA) M-1025. Letter to Neal Nathanson, University of Pennsylvania. Rockville, Md.: Office for Human Research Protections, Department of Health and Human Services; September 26, 2001.

37. University of Pennsylvania Senate Executive Committee. Financial Disclosure and Presumptively Prohibited Conflicts for Faculty Participating in Clinical Trials. (Approved: April 2, 2003). University of Pennsylvania Almanac 2003;49(32):8–9. [Online] May 6, 2003. Available: http://www.upenn.edu/almanac/v49pdf/030506/050603.pdf.

38. *Gelsinger* v. *University of Pennsylvania* (Pa. C., No. 001885, complaint filed September 18, 2000). [Online] September 18, 2000. Available: www.sskrplaw.com/links/healthcare2.html.

39. Weiss R, Nelson D. Penn settles gene therapy suit; university pays undisclosed sum to family of teen who died. *Washington Post* Nov. 4, 2000:A4.

40. United States Attorney's Office, Eastern District, Pennsylvania. Press Release: U.S. Settles Case of Gene Therapy Study That Ended with Teen's Death. [Online] February 9, 2005. Available: http://www.usdoj.gov/usao/pae/News/Pr/2005/feb/UofPSettlement%20release.html.

41. Nelson D, Weiss R. Earlier gene test deaths not reported; NIH was unaware of "adverse events." *Washington Post* Jan. 31, 2000:A1.

42. Nelson D, Weiss R. FDA stops researcher's human gene therapy experiments. *Washington Post* Mar. 2, 2000:A8.

43. Masiello SA. Warning letter to Mark L Batshaw, Children's National Medical Center. Rockville, Md.: Food and Drug Administration; November 30, 2000.

44. Masiello SA. Warning letter to Steven E. Raper, Institute for Human Gene Therapy. Rockville, Md.: Food and Drug Administration; November 30, 2000.

45. Baker DE. Notice of opportunity for hearing. Letter to James M. Wilson, University of Pennsylvania Health System. Rockville, Md.: Food and Drug Administration; February 8, 2002.

46. Shalala D. Protecting research subjects—What must be done. *New England Journal of Medicine* 2000;343:808–10.

47. Steinbrook R. Improving protection for research subjects. *New England Journal of Medicine* 2002;346:1425–30. [Erratum: *NEJM* 2002;346:1838.]

48. National Bioethics Advisory Commission. *Ethical and Policy Issues in Research Involving Human Participants, Volume I.* Bethesda, Md.: NBAC; 2001. [Online] August, 2001. Available: http://www.georgetown.edu/research/nrcbl/nbac/human/overv011.pdf.

49. Institute of Medicine. *Responsible Research: A Systems Approach to Protecting Research Participants.* Washington, D.C.: National Academies Press; 2003.

50. Mello MM, Studdert DM, Brennan TA. The rise of litigation in human subjects research. *Annals of Internal Medicine* 2003;139:40–5.

51. American Society of Gene Therapy. Policy of the American Society of Gene Therapy on Financial Conflict of Interest in Clinical Research. *Molecular Therapy* 2000;1:384.

52. Association of American Medical Colleges, Task Force on Financial Conflicts of Interest in Clinical Research. *Protecting Subjects, Preserving Trust, Promoting Progress: Policy and Guidelines for the Oversight of Individual Financial Interests in Human Subjects Research.* [Online] December 2001. Available: http://www.aamc.org/members/coitf/firstreport.pdf.

53. Association of American Medical Colleges, Task Force on Financial Conflicts of Interest in Clinical Research. *Protecting Subjects, Preserving*

Trust, Promoting Progress II: Principles and Recommendations for Oversight of an Institution's Financial Interests in Human Subjects Research. [Online] October 2002. Available: http://www.aamc.org/members/coitf/2002coireport.pdf.

54. Department of Health and Human Services. Financial Relationships and Interests in Research Involving Human Subjects: Guidance for Human Subject Protection. *Federal Register* 2004;69(92):26393–7.

55. Blumenthal D. Academic-industrial relationships in the life sciences. *New England Journal of Medicine* 2003;349:2452–9.

56. Remarks of Marcia Angell, M.D., DHHS Human Subject Protection and Financial Conflicts of Interest Conference. [Online] August 16, 2000. Available: http://aspe.hhs.gov/sp/coi/angell.htm.

57. Noguchi P. Risks and benefits of gene therapy. *New England Journal of Medicine* 2003;348:193–4.

Codes, Declarations, and Other Ethical Guidance for Research With Humans

Ezekiel J. Emanuel   David Wendler   Christine Grady

11

An Ethical Framework for Biomedical Research

Over the last 60 years or so, there has been myriad guidance on the ethical conduct of research with humans[1–13] (see Table 11.1). Despite the profusion, the extant guidance seems flawed in several respects. First, most guidance was "born in scandal."[14] That is, the guidelines or reports were a response to a specific controversy, and therefore tend to focus on what was perceived to be the transgression of that scandal. The Nuremberg Code directly addressed the atrocities of the Nazi physicians;[2] the Belmont Report was a response to the Tuskegee Syphilis Study and other scandals;[4] and the Advisory Committee on Human Radiation Experiments responded to covert radiation experiments during the Cold War and therefore emphasized deception.[15] Second, regulatory guidance tends not to examine the overall ethics of research but to have a specific practical purpose. For instance, the International Conference on Harmonisation has the purpose of creating common rules across developed countries for the "registration of pharmaceuticals for human use."[8] The aim is more to enhance the efficiency of drug approval than to protect research participants, for which it defers to the Declaration of Helsinki.[3] In general, these regulatory guidelines emphasize the procedural safeguards of informed consent and independent review by an institutional review board or research ethics committee because these leave "paper trails" that can subsequently be audited.

Both of these deficiencies contribute to a third: existing guidance is neither comprehensive nor systematic. The guidelines tend to be lists of claims or principles. For instance, the Nuremberg Code with its 10 statements and the Declaration of Helsinki, originally with 22 principles subsequently expanded to 32, contain no elaboration.[2,3] Such sparse, oracular statements lack an overarching framework to ensure that all relevant ethical issues are

addressed. They also lack justifications for their claims, implying that the ethical guidance is either self-evident or beyond debate. Consequently, when controversies arise about whether the principle itself is valid or how a principle should be applied to a case, there is nothing to appeal to other than the authority of these documents. Agreement can frequently be secured on the broad principles, but this often hides deep disagreements about how they should be interpreted and applied to specific situations.[16]

Finally, and maybe most important, the existing guidance seems mistaken on some important issues. For instance, the Nuremberg Code's strong statement that "the voluntary consent of the human subject is absolutely essential" seems to prohibit all pediatric research.[2] Yet this seems wrong. Similarly, the 1993 Council for International Organizations of Medical Sciences (CIOMS) guidelines recommended that Phase I or II studies of drugs and vaccines should be conducted first in sponsoring countries before being done in developing countries.[17] Because of strong objections, especially by developing countries, a decade later this was deleted from the revision.[6] The most recent version of the Declaration of Helsinki addresses conflicts of interest through disclosure, requiring that potential research participants be adequately informed about "any possible conflict of interest" and that these "should be declared in the publication."[3] The value and importance of disclosing conflicts of interest to research participants is controversial.[18] More important, exclusive reliance on disclosure in the absence of prohibitions on certain conflicts of interest seems inadequate.[19,20]

Because of the deficiencies of existing research ethics guidance, there is a need for a broader, systematic, and comprehensive framework that includes an ethical justification and specification

Table 11.1

Selected Guidelines on the Ethics of Biomedical Research With Humans

Guideline	Source	Year Issued, Revised, or Amended	Chapter and Reference
Nuremberg Code	Nuremberg Military Tribunal decision in *United States* v. *Brandt et al.*	1947	Chapter 12 http://www.hhs.gov/ohrp/ references/nurcode.htm
Declaration of Helsinki	World Medical Association	1964; revised: 1975, 1983, 1989, 1996, 2000; amended: 2002, 2004	Chapter 13 http://www.wma.net/e/ policy/b3.htm
Belmont Report	National Commission for the Protection Human Subjects of Biomedical and Behavioral Research	1979	Chapter 14 http://www.hhs.gov/ohrp/ humansubjects/guidance/ belmont.htm
45 CFR 46 (Common Rule)	U.S. Department of Health and Human Services (DHHS) and 16 other U.S. federal agencies	DHHS guidelines: 1981 Common Rule: 1991	Chapter 16 http://www.hhs.gov/ohrp/ humansubjects/guidance/ 45cfr46.htm
International Ethical Guidelines for Biomedical Research Involving Human Subjects	Council for International Organizations of Medical Sciences in collaboration with World Health Organization	1982 [draft]; revised: 1993, 2002	Chapter 15 http://www.cioms.ch/frame _guidelines_nov_2002.htm
Good Clinical Practice: Consolidated Guidance	International Conference on Harmonisation (ICH) of Technical Requirements for Registration of Pharmaceuticals for Human Use	1996	http://www.fda.gov/cder/ guidance/959fnl.pdf
Resolution 196/96: Rules on Research Involving Human Subjects	National Health Council, Brazil	1996	
Convention on Human Rights and Biomedicine	Council of Europe	1997; revised: 2005	Chapter 17 http://conventions.coe.int/ treaty/ en/treaties/html/ 164.htm [1997]; http:// conventions.coe.int/treaty/ en/treaties/html/195.htm [2005]
Medical Research Council Guidelines for Good Clinical Practice in Clinical Trials	United Kingdom	1998	http://www.mrc.ac.uk/ pdf-ctg.pdf
Guidelines for the Conduct of Health Research Involving Human Subjects in Uganda	Uganda National Council for Science and Technology	1998	
Tri-Council Policy Statement: Ethical Conduct for Research Involving Humans	Tri-Council Working Group, Canada	1998; amended: 2000, 2002, 2005	http://www.pre.ethics.gc.ca/ english/policystatement/ policystatement.cfm
National Statement on Ethical Conduct in Research Involving Humans	National Health and Medical Research Council, Australia	1999	http://www.nhmrc.gov.au/ publications/_files/e35.pdf
Ethical Guidelines for Biomedical Research on Human Subjects	Indian Council on Medical Research, New Delhi	2000	http://www.icmr.nic.in/ bioethics.htm
Guidelines on Ethics for Health Research in Tanzania	Tanzania National Health Research Forum	2001	
Guidelines on Ethics in Medical Research: General Principles	Medical Research Council of South Africa	1977; revised: 1987, 1993, 2002	http://www.sahealthinfo.org/ ethics/ethicsbook1.pdf
Guidelines for Good Clinical Practice in the Conduct of Clinical Trials in Human Participants in South Africa	Department of Health, South Africa	2000	http://www.doh.gov.za/ docs/index.html

for how each principle is to be fulfilled in practice.[21,22] Among other goals, this framework should incorporate those concerns that overlap in the existing guidance and organize them into a coherent whole.

Fundamental Ethical Purpose

Informing this overarching framework is the understanding that the fundamental ethical challenge of all research with humans is to avoid exploitation.[21,22] Research aims at obtaining generalizable knowledge that can be used to improve health and health care. Participants in research are a necessary means to obtaining this knowledge. Consequently, participants are used in the research process for the benefit of others and are at risk of being exploited. The fundamental purpose of research guidelines is to minimize the possibility of exploitation in clinical research.

There are two distinct conceptions of exploitation. Both are important in protecting research participants. One is the traditional, Kantian notion of exploitation as using an individual merely as a means and not simultaneously as an end in itself.[23,24] This Kantian conception of exploitation is grounded in the use of individuals for an end they do not agree with or to which they have not consented. Using individuals without their consent violates their autonomy.[25] The remedy for the Kantian type of exploitation is obtaining informed consent and sometimes ensuring collaborative partnership with a larger community that agrees to the research.

A second conception of exploitation elaborated by Alan Wertheimer rests on the unfair distribution of the benefits and burdens of an interaction.[26,27] This is distinct from the Kantian conception because it concerns the distribution of benefits—who benefits and how much they benefit—rather than autonomy. Importantly, this type of exploitation can occur even when the interacting parties provide valid consent.[26] Minimizing this type of exploitation is more complex, requiring the fulfillment of multiple principles.[27]

Principles and Benchmarks of Ethical Clinical Research

The following eight ethical principles provide a comprehensive and systematic framework to guide the ethical conduct of clinical research and thereby minimize the possibility of exploitation[21,22] (see Table 11.2). These principles are general and identify considerations necessary to justify research as ethical. They are conceptually included in most of the previously mentioned guidance, although existing guidelines do not necessarily include all of them. In addition, they are presented sequentially, going from the development of research proposals to the conduct of research to monitoring during research.

Each principle is specified by benchmarks that offer a specific elaboration and understanding of each principle.[22] The benchmarks are practical interpretations of what is required to fulfill each principle.[22,28,29] In this sense, the benchmarks should clarify and focus the kinds of values and considerations at stake in fulfilling each principle. No matter how specific and detailed, the benchmarks cannot eliminate all controversy over the principles.[16,22] However, by specifying and clarifying the eight principles, these benchmarks should help to narrow any disagreement related to specific cases, making it easier to focus on the substance of the disagreement, assess the importance of the problems and concerns, and even identify potential solutions.[22]

Collaborative Partnership

Clinical research is meant to serve a social good, to enhance the health and health care of people. It is part of the way people collectively improve their well-being. Clinical research is not meant to be done *to* people but done *with* people.[30] The principle of collaborative partnership recognizes that the community in which research is conducted should collaborate in the research endeavor.[22,27] Seeking the community's agreement and input helps ensure that the particular community will not be exploited.[27] In addition, collaboration helps ensure—although it does not guarantee—that the community will receive fair benefits from the conduct of the research.[27,31] Collaborative partnership helps ensure that the community determines for itself whether the research is acceptable and responsive to its health problems. Finally, collaborative partnership is practically important. Without the engagement of researchers and community members, research is unlikely to have any lasting impact. Without the investment of health policy makers, the research results are unlikely to influence policy making and the allocation of scarce health-care resources.[22]

Collaborative partnership can be fulfilled through myriad formal and informal mechanisms. For instance, establishment of community advisory boards, consultations with advocacy groups, public meetings with community members, and advocacy for funding of research are approaches to developing collaborative partnerships.[30,32] Which method is preferred depends upon the nature of the particular research study. Because many of these mechanisms exist in the background without the need to launch explicit initiatives or are just part of "doing business," collaborative partnership has infrequently been included as an explicit ethical requirement of clinical research.[21] One example of research that fails on collaborative partnership grounds includes "helicopter research" in which researchers arrive in a community, take samples, and leave, never to return.

Several benchmarks are essential to fulfilling the principle of collaborative partnership.[22] First, collaborative partnership obviously requires partners. This means identifying representatives of the target community to be involved in the research. Second, it requires collaboration. This entails sharing responsibility for assessing the importance of the health problem and the value of the research to the community, as well as for planning and conducting the study, disseminating the results, and ensuring that the results are used for health improvements.

Third, a collaborative partnership requires mutual respect. This entails recognition of and respect for a community's distinctive values, circumstances, culture, and social practices.[30] Importantly, respect does not mean uncritical acceptance of practices that might be oppressive or coercive. Indeed, some of these practices may be challenged in research. A true collaborative partnership based on respect also aspires toward equality between the partners. In this sense, collaborative partnership aspires to minimize the deprived circumstances of the involved community. Research aims to ameliorate deprivations usually of disease and sometimes of social circumstances. This could occur through a number of interventions directly related to the goals of the research

Table 11.2

Principles and Benchmarks for Ethical Clinical Research

Principles	Benchmarks
Collaborative partnership	• Which community representatives will be partners, involved in helping to plan and conduct the research, disseminate the results and use the results to improve health?
	• How will responsibility be shared with these partners for planning and conducting the research, disseminating the results and using the results to improve health?
	• How will respect for the community's values, circumstances, culture, social practices, and so forth, be demonstrated?
	• How will fair benefits for the community from the conduct and results of the research be assured?
	• How will the tangible benefits of the research, such as authorship credit and intellectual property rights, be distributed to ensure fairness?
Social value	• Who will benefit from the conduct and results of research?
	• What is the potential value of the research for each of the prospective beneficiaries?
	• How will the social value of the research be enhanced?
	• How can adverse impacts, if any, of conducting the research be minimized?
Scientific validity	• Do the scientific and statistical design and methods satisfy generally accepted standards and achieve the objectives of the study? If not, is there clear justification for the deviations?
	• Will the research results be interpretable and useful in the context of the health problem?
	• Does the study design ensure participants health-care services they are entitled to? If not, are there methodologically compelling reasons and are participants protected from serious harm?
	• Is the research design practically feasible given the social, political, economic, and cultural environment?
Fair participant selection	• Is the research population selected to ensure that the research complies with scientific norms and will generate valid and reliable data?
	• Is the research population selected to minimize risks to the participants?
	• Are the individual research participants selected to maximize social value and enhance the possibility of benefits to the participants?
	• Are the participants vulnerable based on age, clinical status, social marginalization, economic deprivation, and so forth? If so, what safeguards are included to protect the participants?
Favorable risk-benefit ratio	• Are the potential physical, psychological, social, and economic risks of the research for the individual participants delineated and their probability and magnitude quantified to the extent possible given the available data?
	• Are the potential physical, psychological, social, and economic benefits of the research for the individual participants delineated and their probability and magnitude quantified to the extent possible given the available data?
	• When compared, do the potential benefits to the individual participants outweigh the risks? If not, does the knowledge gained from the study for society justify the net risks to the individual participants?
Independent review	• Are the procedures for independent review established by law and regulation being properly followed?
	• Is the review body both independent and competent?
	• Is the review process transparent, and are reasons given for the review committee's decisions?
	• Are multiple reviews minimized and reconciled if they conflict?
Informed consent	• Are recruitment procedures and incentives consistent with cultural, political and social practices of the potential participants and their community?
	• Are disclosure forms and verbal disclosure procedures sensitive to participants' culture, language, and context?
	• Is the information presented to participants complete, accurate, and not overwhelming?
	• Are there appropriate plans in place for obtaining permission from legally authorized representatives for individuals unable to consent for themselves?
	• Are supplementary consents or permissions, for example, from spouses or community leaders, obtained? If so, are there ways to ensure that the individual participant can still decide whether to participate independent of the spouse or community leader?
	• Are the mechanisms to symbolize consent consistent with participants' culture and context?
	• How will individual participants be made aware of their right to refuse to participate and are they actually be free to refuse?
Respect for participants	• How will the health and well-being of participants be monitored to minimize harms? Are the criteria for changing doses or procedures for stopping the study for the health of participants adequate?
	• How will the confidentiality procedures actually be implemented?
	• How will it be ensured that participants who want to withdraw can withdraw without penalty?
	• How will results of the research be disseminated?
	• What are the plans for care of the participants after the research is completed?

project or ancillary mechanisms such as developing the general infrastructure necessary to actually conducting ethical research.

Fourth, the community in which the research is being conducted should receive fair benefits from the conduct and/or results of the research.[27,31] What level of benefits is fair depends upon the burdens the community bears for the conduct of the research.[26] Such benefits might include direct benefits to the research participants as well as more indirect benefits such as employment and training for community members to augment health care services for the entire community.[27,31]

Finally, collaborative partnership requires a fair distribution of the tangible and intangible rewards of research among the partners. Very little can generate more resentment, mistrust, and sense of exploitation than an unfair distribution of the benefits of collaboration. This may require agreements regarding sharing intellectual property rights, royalties, and other sources of financial profit as well as appropriate authorship and other credit for contributions to the research.[27,31]

Social Value

Clinical research is not an end in itself. It has instrumental value because it generates knowledge that leads to improvement in health or health care.[33,34] It is such improvements in health that ultimately constitute the social value of research. Unfortunately, the emphasis on protection of research participants has displaced the importance of assessing research's social value. Without social value, research exposes participants to risks for no good reason and wastes resources.[21,22,33–35] However, the process of translating research results into health improvements is complex, incremental, and haphazard.[36] Typically, early studies are valuable because the data they generate informs additional research that ultimately could improve health. Priorities may change while a study is being conducted, and the cooperation of diverse groups is often needed to make changes based on research results. This makes the process of going from research to health improvement uncertain and arduous. Assessment of the value of research is made prospectively before any data are collected. Consequently, determinations of social value are uncertain and probabilistic, entailing judgments about the usefulness of a sequence of research and chances of implementing the results.[35,36] Even in wealthy countries with well-established research studies and health system infrastructures, research results are imperfectly incorporated into clinical practice.

Certain kinds of research clearly lack social value: for example, research that is nongeneralizable, that addresses a problem of little relevance to anyone, that will not enroll sufficient numbers of patients, that assesses proven or empirically well-established results, and research that could never be practically implemented to improve health or health care even if effective in the research setting.[37,38]

Consideration of four benchmarks helps to ensure fulfillment of the principle of social value.[21,22] First, to whom will the research be valuable? It is important to delineate both the short-term and long-term prospective beneficiaries of the research study, specifying whether they include a specific group, similarly situated groups, a larger community from which research participants will be recruited, the country hosting the research, or people outside the host country.[22]

Second, what is the potential value of the research for each of the prospective beneficiaries? Potential beneficiaries may rank the health problem's importance differently and may receive different benefits from the research results. Factors to be considered might include how widespread the disease or condition is, the impact of the disease on individuals and communities, and the extent to which the research is likely to offer an intervention or information useful to the beneficiaries. For example, because malaria is a substantially greater health problem for certain developing countries than for developed countries, research on cerebral malaria may be of substantial value to people in developing countries. Conversely, research on prophylactic medications for malaria is likely to be more valuable for tourists, whereas research on a malaria vaccine may be perceived as valuable to everyone, but to a different degree. Similarly, research on new HIV/AIDS medications in a developing country, although needed in that country, could benefit those outside the host country more than the community in which the research is being conducted if the ultimate cost of the medication is high.

Third, it is important to develop mechanisms to enhance the social value of research. Through collaborative partnerships, strategies should be devised to disseminate results in appropriate ways to key stakeholders including people with the disease, practicing clinicians, advocacy groups, health policy makers, and sometimes international health-care organizations.[22,30] In addition to presentations at scientific conferences and journal publications, this may require novel forms of dissemination such as letters to patients, articles in advocacy publications, presentations at community gatherings, public service announcements in the media, or letters to clinicians. Social value can also be enhanced when research is integrated into a long-term collaborative strategy, so that one research project forms part of a more comprehensive research and health delivery strategy to address significant health problems.[27]

Finally, consideration should be given to the impact of the research on the existing health-care infrastructure. The conduct of the research should not undermine a community's existing health-care services or social structures and leave it worse off at the end of the research. Supplementing the existing system and contributing to sustainable improvements in health through the provision of additional resources, equipment, medications, or training appropriate to the research can enhance value.

Scientific Validity

Contrary to many claims, in research, science and ethics do not conflict.[21,22,34] Valid science is a fundamental ethical requirement.[21,22,35] Unless research generates reliable and valid data that can be interpreted and used by the specified beneficiaries of the research, it will have no social value and participants may be exposed to risks for no benefits.[39,40] Research must be designed in a way that provides valid and reliable data.

Four benchmarks are important in fulfilling the principle of scientific validity. First, the scientific and statistical design and methods of the research must plausibly realize the objectives of the research and must also satisfy the generally accepted norms of research. Research must have clear, justifiable objectives, an adequate sample size, and unbiased and reliable outcome measures and statistical analyses. Deviations from such standards, such as innovative designs, must be plausibly justifiable to the research community.

Second, a research study must be designed to generate results that will be interpretable and useful in the context of the health problem.[15] Interventions should be selected to ensure that the design is useful in identifying ineffective or appropriate interventions; implementing socially, culturally, and economically appropriate changes in the health-care system; or providing a reliable foundation for conducting subsequent research. Interventions should be selected to ensure that the design will realize social value and that the data are generalizable.[21,22,41]

Third, the study design must realize the research objectives while neither denying health-care services that participants are otherwise entitled to nor requiring services that are not feasible to deliver in the context.[37,38,42] However, studies can be ethically designed yet not provide a service or intervention individuals are entitled to under certain, restrictive conditions.[41,43–45] Specifically, it is ethical to use placebo or less than the diagnostic tests or treatments to which individuals are entitled when two conditions are fulfilled: (1) there is a methodologically compelling reason to do so, and (2) there is only minimal chance of serious harm—such as suffering irreversible morbidity or disability, or reversible but serious injury.[41,43–45]

Determining entitlement to medical services in studies is challenging because entitlements differ among countries, and may differ among groups within a country.[46,47] Even in wealthy countries, participants are not entitled to every available or effective medical service, because justice necessitates establishing priorities for the distribution of scarce resources.[46,48] For instance, some developed countries may not guarantee expensive drugs when inexpensive but more inconvenient yet effective drugs are available. Similarly, it is widely accepted that cardiac research conducted in developing countries need not be designed to require a coronary care unit because participants would not necessarily be entitled to this service under a just distribution of scarce resources in those countries.[37,38,42,46,49] Conversely, in a study evaluating interventions to reduce mortality from cerebral malaria conducted in rural settings in which travel to hospitals is impracticable, provision of bed nets may be part of a valid design even if participants may not otherwise have them.[50] However, even if the study's objective is deemed socially valuable, especially to the enrolled participants' community, it is not ethically necessary to provide more comprehensive interventions beyond those to which participants are entitled, especially interventions that may not be feasible and sustainable. Doing so may even be unethical if it undermines the scientific objectives or makes the results irrelevant to the enrolled participants' community.

Finally, the study must be designed in a way that is practically feasible given the social, political, and cultural environment in which it is being conducted.[51] Ensuring feasibility might require extensive community education and outreach as well as sustainable improvements to the health-care infrastructure, such as training of personnel, construction of additional facilities, or provision of an affordable drug. Feasibility also requires that it be possible to achieve the sample size in a reasonable time frame.

Fair Participant Selection

Historically, populations that were poor, uneducated, or powerless to defend their own interests were targeted for high-risk research, whereas promising research was offered to more privileged individuals.[15,34,52] Fair selection of participants requires that the research objectives be the primary basis for determining eligibility.[4,15,21,22,34] Once a target group is identified based on scientific objectives, considerations of minimizing risk, enhancing benefits, minimizing vulnerability, feasibility, as well as facilitating collaborative partnership, become determinative.[22] Factors extraneous to the objectives, risks, benefits, and feasibility of conducting the research should not be the basis for selecting target communities or excluding individuals or communities.[4,15,22,34]

Four benchmarks are necessary to fulfill the principle of fair participant selection. First, the study population should be selected to ensure valid science.[21,22,34,53] Scientific reasons for choosing a particular group of individuals or a community might be high prevalence or incidence of a disease, the magnitude of harms caused by the disease, high transmission rates of an infection, special drug resistance patterns, deprived social circumstances that increase susceptibility to a disease, or particular combinations of diseases. Social status that is irrelevant to the research objectives should not influence selection. Scientific considerations alone, however, will usually underdetermine which community or individuals are selected.

Second, selecting participants in a way that minimizes risk is essential.[54] For instance, in selecting a target population for an HIV vaccine study, the extent to which a community protects HIV-infected persons against discrimination and provides treatment for opportunistic infections are important considerations to minimize risk. Similarly, individuals with high creatinine clearance may be appropriately excluded from a trial of a potentially renal toxic drug in order to reduce risk.

Third, individuals should be selected in order to enhance both the social value of the research and the possibility of benefits to participants.[22,55–57] For example, assuring an adequate number of women in a study of a disease largely affecting women enhances benefits to women. Selecting individuals who are able to comply with the study's requirements will enhance the chances that they will benefit from the intervention and that the study will yield valid data. Communities should be selected in which a collaborative partnership can be developed and in which social value can be realized. Consequently, it is preferable to select communities that have, or can establish, a system for identifying legitimate representatives and that will share responsibility for planning and conducting the study and ensuring that results are implemented through health system improvements or additional research.

Finally, factors such as cognitive ability, age, clinical status, familial relationships, social marginalization, political powerlessness, and economic deprivation should be considered in order to determine the vulnerability of individuals or groups.[58] For instance, if health policy makers suggest a particular group for research participation, the researchers should determine whether the group has been selected for good reasons, such as a high incidence of disease, or because of social subjugation. If scientifically appropriate individuals or groups are identified as vulnerable, specific safeguards to protect the population should be implemented, such as consent monitoring or independent capacity assessment, independent clinical monitoring, ensuring confidentiality, and ensuring that potential research participants are free to decline joining the study.

Favorable Risk-Benefit Ratio

Like life itself, all research entails some risks. However, clinical research typically should offer individual participants a favorable net risk-benefit ratio.[21,22,34] In cases in which potential risks outweigh benefits to individual participants, the social value of the study must be sufficient to justify these net risks.[4,59] Because clinical research involves drugs, devices, and procedures about which there is limited knowledge, uncertainty about the degree of risks and benefits is inherent. And the uncertainty is greater in early phase research.

The principle of a favorable net risk-benefit ratio requires fulfilling three benchmarks. First, the risks of the research should be delineated and minimized. Researchers should identify the type, probability, and magnitude of the risks of the research. The risks are not limited to physical risks, but should also encompass potential psychological, social, and economic risks. To the extent possible, the assessment of risks should be based on available empirical data, not intuition or speculation. Within the context of good clinical practice, these risks should be minimized "by using procedures which are consistent with sound research design and which do not unnecessarily expose subjects to risk, and whenever appropriate, by using procedures already being performed on the subjects for diagnostic or treatment purposes."[5] In addition, research procedures should be performed by trained and competent individuals who adhere to the standards of clinical practice.[3]

Second, the type, probability, and magnitude of the benefits of the research should be identified. The benefits to individual participants, such as health improvements, are relevant. The specification of potential benefits to individual participants should consider only health-related potential benefits derived *from the research intervention itself.*[21,22,34] The benefits to society through the generation of knowledge are assumed if the research is deemed to be of social value and scientifically valid. Secondary benefits, such as payment, or adjunct medical services, such as the possibility of receiving a hepatitis vaccine not related to the research, should *not* be considered in the risk-benefit evaluation; otherwise simply increasing payment or adding more unrelated services could allow the benefits to justify even the riskiest research.[22,60] Furthermore, although participants in clinical research often receive some health services and benefits, the purpose of clinical research is not the provision of health services. Services directly related to clinical research are necessary to ensure scientific validity and to protect the well-being of the individual participants.

As a matter of general beneficence, consideration should be given to enhancing benefits to participants and their community, especially when such benefits can be provided easily and will not compromise the scientific validity of the study. However, such enhancements of benefits are not to be considered in the assessment of the risk-benefit ratio—or even of the social value—of the research study itself.

Third, the risks and potential benefits of the clinical research interventions to individual participants should be compared. In general, the more likely and/or more severe the potential risks, the greater in likelihood and/or magnitude the prospective benefits must be; conversely, research entailing potential risks that are less likely and/or of lower severity can have more uncertain and/or circumscribed potential benefits. Importantly, this comparison of risks and benefits should take into account the context in which the participants live and the risks they actually face. The underlying risks of a particular disease can vary because of differences in incidence, drug resistance, genetic susceptibility, or social or environmental factors. When participants confront a higher risk of disease, riskier research may be justifiable.[61] Similarly, the net risk-benefit ratio for a particular study may be favorable in communities in which the social value of the research is high, yet may be unfavorable in communities in which the potential value is lower.

When potential benefits to participants from the research are proportional to the risks they face, then the additional social value of the research, assured by the fulfillment of the value and validity requirements, implies that the cumulative benefits of the research outweigh its net risks.

The notions of "proportionality" and potential benefits "outweighing" risks are metaphorical.[4] Yet the absence of a mathematical formula to determine when the balance of risks and potential benefits is proportionate does not connote that such judgments are inherently haphazard or subjective. Instead, assessments of risks and potential benefits to the same individuals can appeal to explicit standards, informed by existing data on the potential types of harms and benefits, their likelihood of occurring, and their long-term consequences.[4] Evaluations of the quality of books are not quantifiable either, but neither are they merely matters of subjective taste; comparing the quality of Shakespeare or Dostoevsky with Danielle Steel entails judgments based on shared standards that can be justified to others. Similarly, people routinely make discursively justifiable intrapersonal comparisons of risks and benefits for themselves, and even for others, such as children, friends, and employees without the aid of mathematical formulae.[62]

Finally, a more complex evaluation is necessary when clinical research presents no or few potential benefits to individual participants, such as in Phase I safety and pharmacokinetic studies, and even in some epidemiology research, or when the risks outweigh the potential benefits to individual participants. In this case, a more complex evaluation, what Charles Weijer calls a " 'risk-knowledge' calculus," is necessary.[57] This calculus assesses whether the societal benefits in terms of knowledge gained justify the "excess" risks to individual participants.[63] Determining when potential social benefits outweigh net risks to individual participants requires interpersonal comparisons that are conceptually and practically more difficult than intrapersonal comparisons.[62] However, policy makers are often required to make these kinds of comparisons, for example, when considering whether pollution and its attendant harms to some people are worth the potential benefits of higher employment and tax revenues to others. There is no settled framework for how potential social benefits should be "balanced" against individual risks. Indeed, the appeal to a utilitarian approach of maximization, as in cost-benefit analysis, is quite controversial both morally and because many risks and benefits of research are not readily quantifiable on commensurable scales.[64–66] Nevertheless, these comparisons are made,[67] and regulations mandate that investigators and research review committees make them with respect to clinical research.[4,5] When research risks exceed the combination of potential medical benefits to individuals and the benefit of useful knowledge to society, clinical research is not justifiable.

Independent Review

Independent ethical review of all clinical research protocols is necessary for two reasons: (1) to minimize concerns regarding researchers' conflicts of interest and (2) to ensure public accountability.[21,22] Investigators inherently have multiple, legitimate interests—interests to conduct high quality research, to complete the research expeditiously, to protect research participants, to obtain funding and advance their careers, and so forth.[18,19] Even for well-intentioned investigators, these diverse interests can generate conflicts that may unwittingly distort or undermine their judgments regarding the design, conduct, and analysis of research, as well as adherence to ethical requirements.[19,68–70] Wanting to complete a study quickly may lead to the use of questionable scientific methods or to the use of readily available participants rather than fairer participant selection criteria; enthusiasm for and commitment to the research project may lead to overemphasis of potential benefits and underemphasis of potential harms to participants. Independent review by individuals unaffiliated with the clinical research study helps to minimize the potential impact of such conflicts of interest.[21,22,34,71] In this way, independent reviewers can assure potential research participants that the study they are considering is ethical—that is, it will generate socially valuable information, and the risk-benefit ratio is favorable.

Independent review of clinical research is also important for a second, less emphasized, reason: social accountability.[21] Clinical research imposes risks on participants for the benefit of society. An independent review of a study's compliance with ethical requirements assures members of society that people who enroll in trials will be treated ethically. Based on this review, members of society can have confidence that they will not benefit from the exploitation of other humans.

Four benchmarks help in fulfilling this principle. First, procedures established by law and regulation should be followed. Research has not revealed the best mechanism to conduct independent review.[72] Consequently, the actual review mechanisms are usually determined by laws and regulations that vary both internationally and locally. For instance, some countries and institutions separate scientific and ethical review, whereas others integrate scientific and ethical assessments into a single review. Similarly, some countries have ethics review committees composed only of laypersons, whereas others have committees dominated by medical scientists and physicians. Nevertheless, prevailing laws and regulations establish the standards that should be followed for independent review. They should be amended as better processes are identified.

Second, whatever the process, the review must be independent and competent. Members of the review committees must be free of any conflicts with the researchers or the research study. The reviewers should not be collaborators on the research or with the researchers, and should not have any financial interests in the outcomes of the study. Similarly, reviewers should be excluded from the review if they have other conflicting interests, such as responsibility for the financial interests of the institution in which the research is conducted, that might preclude them from evaluating the protocols according to ethical principles and without bias. Similarly, the reviewers should have sufficient expertise—or be able to access advice—in the scientific, clinical, and statistical areas necessary to assess the research protocol. Training in research ethics for the reviewers may be necessary.

Third, the review should be transparent. This is especially important in multinational research in which differences in culture, practices, and understandings may yield different judgments. One fundamental aspect of transparency is that the reasons for decisions of the independent review committee are explained. This allows observers to assess whether the reasons are appropriate and relevant considerations have been addressed.

Finally, given the increasing complexity of research, multiple independent reviews frequently occur.[73–75] Multiple independent reviews may seem to be required by law or regulation for multisite studies or studies conducted by investigators from multiple institutions. Importantly, however, the ethical principle of independent review does not require multiple reviews.[76] The only requirement is that the reviewers competently and independently assess relevant scientific and ethical considerations. Indeed, multiple reviews may have no added value or may even be counterproductive, by taking time and requiring adjudication without added protections.[72] Such situations are unethical—resources are expended that produce no value or even waste value.[40]

If there is disagreement among such reviews, it is important to clarify its nature. Disagreement may reflect different ways of balancing various principles and benchmarks, or the appropriateness of different ways of fulfilling them. That is, disagreement might reflect *how* the ethical principles are met, rather than *whether* they are met.[77] Conflicts may also arise because of different guidelines or regulatory requirements, which themselves may not have good ethical justification or may be insensitive to particular cultural or social circumstances.[78] Only rarely are there fundamental disagreements about whether ethical principles and benchmarks are fulfilled. Unfortunately, there is no widely accepted procedure for adjudicating such conflicts. In practice, the requirements specified by the sponsor's review board are often determinative. This contravenes the principle of collaborative partnership and the notion that the community that assumes the risks of the research should make the assessment about the research protocol.[79]

Informed Consent

No requirement has received as much explication as informed consent. The purpose of informed consent is to show respect for the autonomy of individuals.[4,6,15,25,34,80–85] To enroll individuals in clinical research without their authorization is to treat them merely as a means to purposes and ends they may not endorse or even know about, denying them the opportunity to choose what projects they will pursue and subjecting them to Kantian-type exploitation.[23–25] By allowing individuals to decide if—and how—they contribute to research, informed consent respects persons and their autonomy.[4,25]

Valid informed consent requires that the consenting person has the capacity to understand and make decisions, receives relevant information about the research study, understands that information, and consents voluntarily and without coercion.[4,15,25,34,80–84] Each of these elements is necessary to ensure that individuals make rational and free determinations of whether the research trial is consonant with their interests.[86]

Seven benchmarks are necessary to fulfill the principle of informed consent. First, recruitment procedures and incentives for participants should be consistent with *cultural, political and social practices of the potential participants*. In some communities, compensation for participation in research may be expected, whereas in others, it may be considered offensive. The appropriate form and level of compensation depends upon the local economic and social context.[87] Although concerns about undue inducement are frequently raised,[4,5,84] high potential social value and a favorable risk-benefit ratio—implying minimal net risks to the participants—dispel these concerns.[88–91] Indeed, worry about undue inducement could reduce compensation and some other benefits for participants and host communities. Paradoxically, balancing fair compensation and undue inducement may result in less compensation for members of impoverished communities and raise the specter of exploitation.[26,88]

Second, both written and verbal disclosure of information should be sensitive to participants' culture and context. Disclosures should use the language, culturally appropriate idioms, and analogies of the prospective participants at a level they can understand. This entails a need for collaborative partnership. After disclosure, investigators should feel confident that participants understand the information and are consenting without any pressure or major misconceptions. In some cases, a formal assessment of understanding, monitoring of the consent process, or independent assessment of participants' capacity to consent may be warranted.[92]

Third, the disclosure of information relevant to the research study must be complete and accurate, but not overwhelming. Providing less than complete and accurate information raises concerns about potential deception of participants. However, complete information does not imply lengthy or exhaustive disclosure forms detailing every aspect of the research study, which may be overwhelming to the participants. Indeed, shorter, more focused forms, without repetition and boilerplate disclosures, may be more effective.[93] Disclosure forms must balance completeness with not being overwhelming.

Fourth, some research entails enrollment of individuals unable to consent because of their age, permanent mental incapacity, an acute loss of mental functions, or other reasons. In these cases, researchers must have a strategy for obtaining permission from legally authorized representatives of the potential participants.[15,83,84,94–99]

In some cases, "spheres of consent" ranging from spouses to heads of households to school principals to village elders or community leaders may be required before researchers can invite individual participation.[30,100,101] With a few exceptions, such as emergency research, it is unacceptable to supplant individual consent of competent adults by family or community consent.[102] The family or community gives permission only to approach individuals. When family or community permission to approach individuals is reasonable, special care should be given to assure that the individual can still refuse participation—that is, that there is no coercion.

Sixth, researchers should utilize consent procedures that are acceptable within the local context, while ensuring that an independent observer could verify voluntary participation by the individuals. For instance, U.S. regulations require a written signature.[5] In many cases, this is an acceptable and efficient way to document consent authorization. However, in some cases, because of limited literacy or cultural differences, such requirements may be inappropriate and unethical.[77] Alternative methods to express consent, such as handshakes, embracing, or sharing a meal, are known.[77] Appropriate alternative procedures for documenting informed consent might include tape recordings or witnessed written documentation of these methods of consent.

Finally, special attention must be given to ensure that individuals are aware of their right to, and are actually free to, refuse to participate or to withdraw from research. A key element of informed consent is the ability to refuse or withdraw participation without penalty.[103] Prorating offered compensation and other research-related benefits may help to obviate possible familial or community coercion or retribution.

Respect for Participants

The ethical conduct of clinical research does not end when informed consent is obtained.[21,22,104] Researchers have ongoing obligations to treat individuals with respect from the time they are approached—even if they refuse enrollment—throughout their participation and even after their participation ends. Respecting potential and enrolled participants entails multiple activities. First, and arguably most important, this principle requires monitoring the health and well-being of participants, and intervening to prevent or treat harms that might result from the adverse reactions, untoward events, or changes in clinical status associated with the research.[104] In some cases, research studies need to include procedures to adjust drug doses and even withdraw study participants because of adverse events. Furthermore, specific stopping rules may be necessary if excessive adverse events or benefits are identified.

Second, pledges of confidentiality should be honored and procedures to protect confidentiality implemented. Such procedures include securing databases, locking file cabinets containing data, coding specimens and data forms, as well as interviewing participants in private spaces where they cannot be overheard. In addition, it is important to alert participants that despite researchers' best efforts, absolute confidentiality cannot be guaranteed.

Third, respect includes permitting participants to change their minds, to decide that the research does not comport with their interests or preferences, and to withdraw without penalty. Fourth, as new information about the impact of the intervention or about the participant's clinical condition is gained during the course of the research, respect requires providing this new information to the participants. Researchers should also develop explicit strategies to inform participants and host communities of the results of the research. Having participated in research and assumed risks, the participants and host communities have a right to know what was found and its implications for public health and health-care policies.

Finally, plans should be made regarding the care of participants when the trial is over. In some cases, this may simply involve referral to a primary care provider. In other cases, this may require researchers to find creative strategies for providing access to treatments benefiting the participants, even when these interventions are unlicensed.

Characteristics of the Principles

The eight general principles and the benchmarks delineate a systematic and comprehensive way of assessing the ethics of particular clinical research.[21,22] They provide a coherent and organized way for researchers, ethics reviewers, participants, and others to evaluate a research protocol and to determine whether it fulfills ethical standards. They should not be seen as adding ethical requirements, but rather distilling and coherently articulating the ethical norms underlying much of the prevailing guidance. These principles and benchmarks offer a more organized and systematic delineation of what many researchers, ethics reviewers, and others already do.

Importantly, these principles are not independent of all other ethical principles. They operate within and presume compliance with more general moral norms, such as honesty and promise keeping.[22] Similarly, these principles focus on what is required to evaluate research studies, not on the enforcement or proper conduct of the research itself. Having ethical researchers is important for implementation of the framework but not a requirement for evaluating the research protocol. Determining *what* is ethical and what needs to be enforced must be done prior to and should not be confused with *how* to implement an ethical protocol or to enforce the requirements.[21,22]

These eight principles are necessary. The presumption is that they must all be fulfilled for a research protocol to be ethical. There is no picking and choosing. However, in specific cases, such as emergency research, informed consent may be legitimately waived. These principles are justified by ethical values that are widely recognized and accepted, that reasonable people would want to be treated in accordance with—avoidance of exploitation, the just distribution of benefits and burdens, beneficence, respect for persons, and so forth.[105,106] These requirements are precisely the types of considerations that would be invoked to justify clinical research if it were challenged. The benchmarks provide more practical considerations for discerning satisfaction of the general principles.

The principles are sufficient. Fulfilling these eight principles means the research is ethical. Failing on any one principle—except for waiving informed consent in specific cases, in which waiving consent must be justified—makes the research unethical. The proposed benchmarks, however, may not be sufficient, and may need revision with experience and time. They certainly provide a useful first estimation of the kind of specific elements that need to be fulfilled.

These eight principles are universal; they apply in all countries and contexts, regardless of sponsorship. The principles are general statements of value; they must be elaborated by traditions of interpretation and require practical interpretation and specification. The benchmarks offer a first level of specification, indicating how to fulfill these principles. However, the details of this specification will inherently be context and culture dependent. This does not make them relativistic or less universal. It simply recognizes that applying ethical principles in the world requires taking facts into account, and these facts depend upon the context.

> Moral arguments take place in context, and they therefore depend at least implicitly on matters of fact, estimates of risk, suppositions about feasibility, and beliefs about human nature and social processes. . . . Even those who rely on what they regard as universal moral principles do not presume that their practical conclusions are independent of reliable facts and plausible assumptions about particular societies. The arguments begin from where we are, and appeal to those with whom we now live. This is why moral relativism is seldom as important an issue in practical as it is in theoretical ethics.[107]

Importantly, that there are eight principles suggests that the ethics of research is complex. Adherence to a single ethical principle rarely provides a complete solution; most situations implicate multiple principles.[48,62,64,105,107–110] Consequently, the various principles and benchmarks will sometimes conflict. What is fair participant selection could at times increase risk; what is required for informed consent may sometimes compromise scientific validity. Unfortunately, there is no simple algorithm for determining how to balance or weigh these principles when they conflict. Different researchers and communities will balance the principles in different ways, some emphasizing informed consent, others the importance of minimizing risks or enhancing social value. Ignoring or rejecting basic principles in designing or conducting a research study could render it unethical. Conversely, accepting the principles and benchmarks, yet disagreeing about how to balance them in a particular case, highlights the intricacies of ethical judgments entailing multiple considerations. Disagreement on the balancing of the various benchmarks does not necessarily make one assessment ethical and the other unethical. Rather, it reflects different, but perhaps legitimate, ways of resolving competing ethical claims.[107] In fact, this framework can help narrow disagreements and elucidate the different underlying views. When conflicts between principles and benchmarks occur, or when different groups weigh the principles differently, the important point is to be clear about the reasons for the evaluation and the differences. Ultimately, a thoughtful process of balancing ethical considerations can be as important as any particular judgment in the effort to ensure that research is conducted ethically.

References

1. Fluss S. *International Guidelines on Bioethics.* Geneva, Switzerland: European Forum on Good Clinical Practice/CIOMS; 1998.
2. The Nuremberg Code. In: *Trials of War Criminals Before the Nuremberg Military Tribunals Under Control Council Law No. 10. Volume 2.* Washington, DC: U.S. Government Printing Office; 1949:181–2. [Online] Available: http://ohsr.od.nih.gov/guidelines/nuremberg.html.
3. World Medical Association. *Declaration of Helsinki: Ethical Principles for Medical Research Involving Human Subjects.* Tokyo, Japan: WMA; October 2004. [Online] 2004. Available: http://www.wma.net/e/policy/b3.htm.
4. The National Commission for the Protection of Human Subjects of Biomedical and Behavioral Research. *The Belmont Report: Ethical Principles and Guidelines for the Protection of Human Subjects of Research.* Washington, DC: Department of Health, Education and Welfare; DHEW Publication OS 78-0012 1978. [Online] April 18, 1979. Available: http://www.hhs.gov/ohrp/humansubjects/guidance/belmont.htm.
5. Department of Health and Human Services, National Institutes of Health, and Office for Human Research Protections. *The Common Rule, Title 45 (Public Welfare), Code of Federal Regulations, Part 46 (Protection of Human Subjects).* [Online] June 23, 2005. Available: http://www.hhs.gov/ohrp/humansubjects/guidance/45cfr46.htm.
6. Council for International Organizations of Medical Sciences, in collaboration with the World Health Organization. *International Ethical Guidelines for Biomedical Research Involving Human Subjects.* Geneva, Switzerland: CIOMS and WHO; 2002. [Online] November 2002. Available: http://www.cioms.ch/frame_guidelines_nov_2002.htm.
7. Council of Europe, Directorate of Legal Affairs. *Convention for the Protection of Human Rights and Dignity of the Human Being With Regard*

to the Application of Biology and Medicine: Convention on Human Rights and Biomedicine. Strasbourg, France: Council of Europe; 1997. [Online] April 4, 1997. Available: http://conventions.coe.int/treaty/en/treaties/html/164.htm.

8. International Conference on Harmonisation of Technical Requirements for Registration of Pharmaceuticals for Human Use. *The ICH Harmonised Tripartite Guideline—Guideline for Good Clinical Practice.* Geneva: ICH; 1996. [Online] Available: http://www.ich.org/LOB/media/MEDIA482.pdf.

9. U.K. Medical Research Council. *Guidelines for Good Clinical Practice in Clinical Trials.* London, England: MRC; 1998. [Online] Available: http://www.mrc.ac.uk/pdf-ctg.pdf.

10. Uganda National Council of Science and Technology (UNCST). *Guidelines for The Conduct of Health Research Involving Human Subjects in Uganda.* Kampala, Uganda: UNCST; 1998.

11. Canadian Institutes of Health Research, the Natural Sciences and Engineering Research Council, and the Social Sciences and Humanities Research Council. *Tri-Council Policy Statement: Ethical Conduct for Research Involving Humans.* [Online] 1998 (with 2000, 2002 and 2005 amendments). Available: http://www.pre.ethics.gc.ca/english/policystatement/policystatement.cfm.

12. National Health and Medical Research Council, Commonwealth of Australia. *National Statement on Ethical Conduct in Research Involving Humans.* Canberra: NHMRC; 1999. [Online] Available: http://www.nhmrc.gov.au/publications/_files/e35.pdf.

13. Department of Health and Human Services, Office for Human Research Protections. *International Compilation of Human Subject Research Protections.* 2nd ed. [Online] October 1, 2005. Available: http://www.hhs.gov/ohrp/international/HSPCompilation.pdf.

14. Levine C. Has AIDS changed the ethics of human subjects research? *Law Medicine and Health Care* 1988;16:167–73.

15. Advisory Committee on Human Radiation Experiments. *Final Report of the Advisory Committee on Human Radiation Experiments.* New York, N.Y.: Oxford University Press; 1996.

16. Macklin R. After Helsinki: Unresolved issues in international research. *Kennedy Institute of Ethics Journal* 2001;11:17–36.

17. Council for International Organizations of Medical Sciences, in collaboration with the World Health Organization. *International Ethical Guidelines for Biomedical Research Involving Human Subjects.* Geneva, Switzerland: CIOMS and WHO; 1993.

18. Forster HP, Emanuel E, Grady C. The 2000 revision of the Declaration of Helsinki: A step forward or more confusion. *Lancet* 2001;358:1449–53.

19. Thompson DF. Understanding financial conflicts of interest. *New England Journal of Medicine* 1993;329:573–6.

20. American Society of Clinical Oncology. Revised Conflict of Interest Policy (adopted on November 7, 2002, by the American Society of Clinical Oncology). *Journal of Clinical Oncology* 2003;21:2394–6.

21. Emanuel EJ, Wendler D, Grady C. What makes clinical research ethical? *JAMA* 2000;283:2701–11.

22. Emanuel EJ, Wendler D, Killen J, Grady C. What makes clinical research in developing countries ethical? The benchmarks of ethical research. *Journal of Infectious Diseases* 2004;189:930–7.

23. Wood AW. Exploitation. *Social Philosophy and Policy* 1995;12:135–58.

24. Buchanan A. *Ethics, Efficiency and the Market.* Lanham, Md.: Rowman & Littlefield; 1985.

25. Beauchamp TL, Childress J. *The Principles of Biomedical Ethics.* 5th ed. New York, N.Y.: Oxford University Press; 1996.

26. Wertheimer A. *Exploitation.* Princeton, N.J.: Princeton University Press; 1996.

27. Participants in the 2001 Conference on Ethical Aspects of Research in Developing Countries. Moral standards for research in developing countries: From "reasonable availability" to "fair benefits." *Hastings Center Report* 2004;34(3):17–27.

28. Daniels N, Bryant J, Castano RA, et al. Benchmarks of fairness for health care reform a policy tool for developing countries. *Bulletin of the World Health Organization* 2000;78:40–50.

29. Daniels N, Light DW, Caplan RL. *Benchmarks of Fairness for Health Care Reform.* New York, N.Y.: Oxford University Press; 1996.

30. Weijer C, Emanuel EJ. Protecting communities in biomedical research. *Science* 2000;289:1142–4.

31. Participants in the 2001 Conference on Ethical Aspects of Research in Developing Countries. Fair benefits for research in developing countries. *Science* 2002;298:2133–4.

32. Diallo DA, Doumbo OK, Plowe CV, et al. Community permission for research in developing countries. *Clinical Infectious Diseases* 2005;41:255–9.

33. Vanderpool HY, editor. *The Ethics of Research Involving Human Subjects: Facing The 21st Century.* Frederick, Md.: University Publishing Group; 1996.

34. Levine RJ. *Ethics and Regulation of Clinical Research,* 2nd ed. New Haven, CT: Yale University Press; 1988.

35. Freedman B. Scientific value and validity as ethical requirements for research. *IRB: A Review of Human Subjects Research* 1987;9(6):7–10.

36. Black N. Evidence based policy: Proceed with care. *British Medical Journal* 2001;323:275–8.

37. Grady C. Science in the service of healing. *Hastings Center Report* 1998;28(6):34–8.

38. Crouch RA, Arras JD. AZT trials and tribulations. *Hastings Center Report* 1998;28(6):26–34.

39. President's Commission for the Study of Ethical Problems in Medicine and Biomedical and Behavioral Research. *Summing Up.* Washington, DC: U.S. Government Printing Office; 1983. [Online] Available: http://www.bioethics.gov/reports/past_commissions/summing_up.pdf.

40. Rutstein DD. The ethical design of human experiments. In: Freund PA, ed. *Experimentation With Human Subjects.* New York, N.Y.: George Braziller; 1970:383–401.

41. Emanuel EJ, Miller FG. The ethics of placebo-controlled trials—A middle ground. *New England Journal of Medicine* 2001;345:915–9.

42. Freedman B. Placebo-controlled trials and the logic of clinical purpose. *IRB: A Review of Human Subjects Research* 1990;12(6):1–6.

43. Temple R, Ellenberg SS. Placebo controlled trials and active control trials in the evaluation of new treatments. I. Ethical and scientific issues. *Annals of Internal Medicine* 2000;133:455–63.

44. Wendler D, Emanuel EJ, Lie RK. The standard of care debate: Can research in developing countries be both ethical and responsive to those countries' health needs? *American Journal of Public Health* 2004;94:923–8.

45. Nuffield Council on Bioethics. *The Ethics of Research Related to Healthcare in Developing Countries.* London, England: Nuffield Council on Bioethics; 2002. [Online] Available: http://nuffieldbioethics.org/fileLibrary/pdf/errhdc_fullreport001.pdf.

46. Emanuel EJ. *The Ends of Human Life.* Cambridge, Mass.: Harvard University Press; 1991:chapters 4 and 5.

47. Daniels N, Sabin JE. *Setting Limits Fairly.* New York, N.Y.: Oxford University Press; 2002:chapter 2.

48. Walzer M. *Spheres of Justice.* New York, N.Y.: Basic Books; 1983.

49. Faden RR, Kass N. HIV research, ethics and the developing world. *American Journal of Public Health* 1998;88:548–50.

50. Kidane G, Morrow RH. Teaching mothers to provide home treatment of malaria in Tigray, Ethiopia: A randomized trial. *Lancet* 2000;356:550–5.

51. Bloom BR. The highest attainable standard: Ethical issues in AIDS vaccines. *Science* 1998;279:186–8.

52. Lederer SE. *Subject to Science.* Baltimore, Md.: Johns Hopkins University Press; 1995.

53. National Institutes of Health. NIH policy and guidelines on the inclusion of children as participants in research involving human

subjects. [Online] March 6, 1998. Available: http://grants2.nih.gov/grants/guide/notice-files/not98–024.html.

54. Weijer C, Fuks A. The duty to exclude: Excluding people at undue risk from research. *Clinical and Investigative Medicine* 1994;17: 115–22.

55. DeBruin D. Justice and the inclusion of women in clinical studies. *Kennedy Institute of Ethics Journal* 1994;4:117–46.

56. Mastroianni AC, Faden RR, Federman DD. *Women and Health Research: Ethical and Legal Issues of Including Women in Clinical Studies.* Washington, D.C.: National Academies Press; 1994.

57. Weijer C. Evolving issues in the selection of subjects for clinical research. *Cambridge Quarterly of Healthcare Ethics* 1996;5: 334–5.

58. Kipnis K. Vulnerability in research subjects: A bioethical taxonomy. In: National Bioethics Advisory Commission. *Ethical and Policy Issues in Research Involving Human Participants, Vol. II.* Rockville, Md.: NBAC; 2001. [Online] Available: http://www.georgetown.edu/research/nrcbl/nbac/human/overv012.pdf.

59. Weijer C. The ethical analysis of risk. *Journal of Law, Medicine and Ethics* 2000;28:344–61.

60. Freedman B, Fuks A, Weijer C. Demarcating research and treatment: A systematic approach for the analysis of the ethics of clinical research. *Clinical Research* 1992;40:653–60.

61. Weijer C. The future of research into rotavirus vaccine. *British Medical Journal* 2000;321:525–6.

62. Anderson E. *Value in Ethics and Economics.* Cambridge, Mass.: Harvard University Press; 1993:chapter 9.

63. Weijer C. Thinking clearly about research risks: Implications of the work of Benjamin Freedman. *IRB: A Review of Human Subjects Research* 1999;21(6):1–5.

64. Sen A, Williams B. Introduction. In: Sen A, Williams B, eds. *Utilitarianism and Beyond.* New York, N.Y.: Cambridge University Press; 1982:1–22.

65. Leonard H, Zeckhauser R. Cost-benefit analysis and the management of risk: Philosophy and legitimacy. In: MacLean D, ed. *Values at Risk.* Totowa, N.J.: Rowman & Littlefield Publishers; 1986:31–48.

66. Gold MR, Siegel JE, Russell LB, Weinstein MC, editors. *Cost-Effectiveness in Health and Medicine.* New York, NY: Oxford University Press; 1996.

67. Sen A. Interpersonal comparisons of welfare. In: Sen A. *Choice, Welfare, and Measurement.* Cambridge, Mass.: Harvard University Press; 1982:264–84.

68. Relman AS. Economic incentives in clinical investigations. *New England Journal of Medicine* 1989;320:933–4.

69. Porter RJ, Malone TE. *Biomedical Research: Collaboration and Conflicts of Interest.* Baltimore, Md.: Johns Hopkins University Press; 1992.

70. Spece RG, Shimm DS, Buchanan AE, eds. *Conflicts of Interest in Clinical Practice and Research.* New York, N.Y.: Oxford University Press; 1996.

71. National Commission for the Protection of Human Subjects of Biomedical and Behavioral Research. *Institutional Review Boards: Report and Recommendations.* Washington, D.C.: U.S. Government Printing Office; 1978.

72. Emanuel EJ, Wood A, Fleischman A, et al. Oversight of human participants research: Identifying problems to evaluate reform proposals. *Annals of Internal Medicine* 2004;141:282–91.

73. McWilliams R, Hoover-Fong J, Hamosh A, et al. Problematic variation in local institutional review of a multicenter genetic epidemiology study. *JAMA* 2003;290:360–6.

74. Roberts LM, Bowyer L, Homer CS, Brown MA. Multicentre research: Negotiating the ethics approval obstacle course [letter]. *Medical Journal of Australia* 2004;180:139.

75. Stair TO, Reed CR, Radeos MS, et al., for the MARC Investigators. Variation in Institutional Review Board responses to a standard protocol for a multicenter clinical trial. *Academic Emergency Medicine* 2001;8:636–41.

76. Wood A, Grady C, Emanuel EJ. Regional ethics organizations for protection of human research participants. *Nature Medicine* 2004;10: 1283–8.

77. Mulholland K, Smith PG, Broome CV, et al. A randomized trial of a Haemophilus influenzae type b conjugate vaccine in a developing country for the prevention of pneumonia—Ethical considerations. *International Journal of Tuberculosis and Lung Disease* 1999;3: 749–55.

78. Wendler D, Rackoff JE. Informed consent and respecting individual autonomy: What's a signature got to do with it? *IRB: Ethics and Human Research* 2001;23(3):1–4.

79. White MT. Guidelines for IRB review of international collaborative medical research: A proposal. *Journal of Law, Medicine and Ethics* 1999;27:87–94.

80. Freedman B. A moral theory of informed consent. *Hastings Center Report* 1975;5(4):32–9.

81. President's Commission for the Study of Ethical Problems in Medicine and Biomedical Research. *Making Health Care Decisions: Ethical and Legal Implications of Informed Consent in the Physician-Practitioner Relationship.* Washington, DC: U.S. Government Printing Office; 1982. [Online] Available: http://www.bioethics.gov/reports/past_commissions/making_health_care_decisions.pdf.

82. Donagan A. Informed consent in therapy and experimentation. *Journal of Medicine and Philosophy* 1977;2:318–29.

83. Faden RR, Beauchamp TL, with King NMP. *A History and Theory of Informed Consent.* New York, N.Y.: Oxford University Press; 1986: chapters 5–9.

84. Berg JW, Applebaum PS, Lidz CW, Parker LS. *Informed Consent: Legal Theory and Clinical Practice.* 2nd ed. New York, N.Y.: Oxford University Press; 2001: chapters 2, 3, 11, and 12.

85. Dworkin G. *The Theory and Practice of Autonomy.* New York, N.Y.: Cambridge University Press; 1988:chapters 1, 6, and 7.

86. Sreenivasan G. Does informed consent to research require comprehension? *Lancet* 2003;362:2016–8.

87. Dickert N, Grady C. What's the price of a research subject? Approaches to payment for research participation. *New England Journal of Medicine* 1999;341:198–203.

88. Emanuel EJ, Currie XE, Herman A, on behalf of Project Phidisa. Undue inducement in clinical research in developing countries: Is it a worry? *Lancet* 2005;366:336–40.

89. Emanuel EJ. Ending concerns about undue inducement. *Journal of Law, Medicine and Ethics* 2004;32:100–5.

90. Harris J. *Wonderwoman and Superman: The Ethics of Human Biotechnology.* New York, NY: Oxford University Press; 1992:chapter 6.

91. Wilkinson M, Moore A. Inducement in research. *Bioethics* 1997;11: 373–89.

92. Grisso T, Applebaum PS. *Assessing Competence to Consent to Treatment.* New York, N.Y.: Oxford University Press; 1998.

93. Flory JH, Emanuel EJ. Interventions to improve research participants' understanding in informed consent for research: A systematic review. *JAMA* 2004;292:1593–1601.

94. National Bioethics Advisory Commission. *Research Involving Persons With Mental Disorders That May Affect Decisionmaking Capacity.* Rockville, Md.: NBAC; 1998. [Online] Available: http://www.georgetown.edu/research/nrcbl/nbac/capacity/TOC.htm.

95. Buchanan AE, Brock DW. *Deciding for Others: The Ethics of Surrogate Decision Making.* New York, N.Y.: Cambridge University Press; 1990:chapter 2.

96. Dresser R. Mentally disabled research subjects: The enduring policy issues. *JAMA* 1996;276:67–72.

97. Michels R. Are research ethics bad for our mental health? *New England Journal of Medicine* 1999;340:959–61.

98. Capron AM. Ethical and human-rights issues in research on mental disorders that may affect decision-making capacity. *New England Journal of Medicine* 1999;340:1430–4.

99. Wendler D, Prasad K. Core safeguards for clinical research with adults who are unable to consent. *Annals of Internal Medicine* 2001;135:514–23.

100. Weijer C, Goldsand G, Emanuel EJ. Protecting communities in research: Current guidelines and limits of extrapolation. *Nature Genetics* 1999;23:275–80.

101. Macaulay AC, et al. Participatory research with native community of Kahnawake creates innovative code of research ethics. *Canadian Journal of Public Health* 1998;89:105–8.

102. IJsselmuiden CB, Faden RR. Research and informed consent in Africa: Another look. *New England Journal of Medicine* 1992;326:830–4.

103. Karim QA, Karim SSA, Coovadia HM, Susser M. Informed consent for HIV testing in a South African hospital: Is it truly informed and truly voluntary? *American Journal of Public Health* 1998;88:637–40.

104. Weijer C, Shapiro S, Fuks A, Glass KC, Skrutkowska M. Monitoring clinical research: An obligation unfulfilled. *Canadian Medical Association Journal* 1995;152:1973–80.

105. Scanlon TM. *What We Owe to Each Other*. Cambridge, Mass.: Harvard University Press; 1999:chapters 1 and 8.

106. Kymlicka W. *Liberalism, Community and Culture*. New York, N.Y.: Oxford University Press; 1989.

107. Gutmann A, Thompson D. *Democracy and Disagreement*. Cambridge, Mass.: Harvard University Press; 1996:chapter 1.

108. Nagel T. The fragmentation of value. In: Nagel T. *Mortal Questions*. New York, N.Y.: Cambridge University Press; 1979:128–41.

109. Temkin L. *Inequality*. New York, N.Y.: Oxford University Press; 1993:chapter 2.

110. Richardson HS. Specifying norms as a way to resolve concrete ethical problems. *Philosophy and Public Affairs* 1990;19:279–310.

George J. Annas   Michael A. Grodin

12

The Nuremberg Code

History

The Nuremberg Code is a primary foundational document informing all ethical codes on research with humans. Many consider it the most authoritative legal and human rights code on the subject of human experimentation. Its significance cannot be appreciated without a basic knowledge of its historical origins: It is a legal and ethical code promulgated by U.S. judges at the trial of the Nazi doctors at Nuremberg after World War II.

Immediately after World War II, the Allies prosecuted the major surviving Nazi war criminals at the International Military Tribunal (IMT) before judges from the United States, the United Kingdom, France, and the former Soviet Union. The IMT made new international law and can properly be seen, together with the promulgation of the 1948 Universal Declaration of Human Rights, as the birth of the international human rights movement. The IMT produced the Nuremberg Principles, which recognize that there are crimes against peace, war crimes, and crimes against humanity, and that individuals can be punished for committing these crimes even if their actions were consistent with the laws of their own country, and even if they were "obeying orders."

The subsequent Doctors Trial (1946–47) opened on December 9, 1946. During this trial, U.S. physicians, especially Leo Alexander and Andrew Ivy,[1,2] worked together with U.S. prosecuting attorneys, especially Telford Taylor and James McHaney, to present evidence of murder and torture under the guise of medical experimentation to a panel of U.S. judges.

Chief prosecutor Taylor, who held the Army rank of Brigadier General, set the tone for the trial in his opening statement:

The defendants in the dock are charged with murder, but this is no mere murder trial. We cannot rest content when we have shown that crimes were committed and that certain persons committed them. To kill, to maim, and to torture is criminal under all modern systems of law. These defendants did not kill in hot blood, nor for personal enrichment. Some of them may be sadists who killed and tortured for sport, but they are not all perverts. They are not ignorant men.[3]

Taylor also warned that "[t]he perverse thoughts and distorted concepts which brought about these savageries are not dead. They cannot be killed by force of arms. They must not become a spreading cancer in the breast of humanity." And he echoed the declaration of U.S. Supreme Court Justice Robert Jackson, chief prosecutor at the IMT, that "[t]he wrongs which we seek to condemn and punish have been so calculated, so malignant, and so devastating, that civilization cannot tolerate their being ignored because it cannot survive their being repeated."[3]

The 23 defendants, including 20 physicians, faced varying charges including conspiracy, war crimes, crimes against humanity, and membership in a criminal organization, the SS. Sixteen were found guilty. Seven were hanged.

The Evidence

The Doctors Trial documented that Nazi medicine was formed and nurtured by a symbiosis of National Socialist ideology and social Darwinism, mixed with a theory of racial hygiene and eugenics that viewed some racial and ethnic groups as subhuman and gave physicians an ideological excuse to use their medical skills to harm people in the name of the state (see Chapter 2). This transformed murder and mayhem into legally endorsed medical euthanasia and sterilization. Physicians rose in power and prestige to the extent that they agreed to treat the racial "sickness" that threatened the health of the German *Volk*. In this sense, physicians and the German state used each other: The Nazis used physicians to perform horrific tasks to implement Nazi racial hygiene theories—which would have been much harder to accomplish without the use of physicians—and physicians were granted privileges and power in the Nazi regime. These physicians were able to accept the pseudoscientific Nazi ideology that labeled certain humans, like Jews, gypsies, Slavs, homosexuals, and the disabled, as subhuman (*Untermenschen*) and thus not entitled to basic human rights. In its verdict, the Nuremberg court recognized that Nazis are not the only human beings who are vulnerable to seduction by social, political, or economic organizations that seek to corrupt medicine for their own agendas. No one is immune.

A number of themes recur in Nazi medicine: the devaluation and dehumanization of defined segments of the community; the medicalization of social and political problems; the training of physicians to identify with the political goals of the government; fear of the consequences of refusing to cooperate with civil authority; the bureaucratization of the medical role; and a lack of concern for medical ethics and human rights. Nazi physicians failed to see themselves as physicians first, with a calling and an ethic dedicated to healing and caring for the welfare of human beings. Instead they were seduced by power and ideology to view the state as their "patient" and to see the extermination of an entire people as "treatment" for the state's health.

Nazi Medical Experiments

The Doctors Trial centered on what Taylor described as "crimes committed in the guise of scientific research."[3] One of the most notorious was the so-called high-altitude or low-pressure experiments at Dachau concentration camp, in which prisoners were placed in a pressure chamber to simulate conditions that German pilots might encounter when bailing out of their planes without oxygen and without pressure suits. One Nazi document gave this description of the experiments:

> Some of the experimental subjects died during a continued high altitude experiment; for instance, after one-half hour at a height of 12 kilometers. After the skull had been opened under water, an ample amount of air embolism was found in the brain vessels and, in part, free air in the brain ventricles. . . . [In another experiment,] in order to find out whether the severe psychic and physical effects, as mentioned [elsewhere] are due to the formation of embolism, the following was done: After relative recuperation from such a parachute descending test had taken place, however before regaining consciousness, some experimental subjects were kept under water until they died. When the skull and cavities of the breast and of the abdomen were opened under water, an enormous volume of air embolism was found in the vessels of the brain, the coronary vessels, and the vessels of the liver and the intestines.[3]

"The victims who did not die in the course of such experiments surely wished that they had," Taylor told the court. He introduced the report of another experiment in which the subject was given an oxygen mask, raised to a simulated altitude of 47,000 feet, and then deprived of oxygen and subjected to a simulated parachute jump. As described by the report, the victim's reaction was "spasmodic convulsions," "agonal convulsive breathing," "clonic convulsions, groaning," "yells aloud," "convulses arms and legs," "grimaces, bites his tongue," "does not respond to speech," "gives the impression of someone completely out of his mind."[3]

Other "experiments" with death as their planned endpoint included immersing victims in freezing water or subjecting them to open-air freezing to test various rewarming techniques, with the objective of developing treatments for German aviators who were forced to parachute into the icy North Sea. The Nazi doctors also subjected prisoners to experiments involving malaria, mustard gas, bone transplant, sea-water drinking, epidemic jaundice, typhus, poison, and sterilization.

"The Nazis were searching for methods of extermination, both by murder and sterilization, of large population groups by the most scientific and least conspicuous means," Taylor told the court. "They were developing a new branch of medical science which would give them the scientific tools for the planning and practice of genocide. The primary purpose was to discover an inexpensive, unobtrusive, and rapid method of sterilization which could be used to wipe out Russians, Poles, Jews, and other people."[3]

The Trial

During the trial, which spanned 139 trial days from December 9, 1946, to August 20, 1947, 32 witnesses gave oral testimony for the prosecution, and 53 witnesses, including the 23 defendants themselves, gave oral evidence for the defense. In addition, 570 affidavits, reports, and documents were introduced into evidence by the prosecution and 901 by the defense, for a total of 1,471. All English-language documents were translated into German, and each defendant was represented at trial by a lawyer of his own choosing.

The Doctors Trial was the first of 12 separate and so-called "subsequent" trials conducted at Nuremberg by the U.S. Army. It was based on international law, but because of the military jurisdiction of the occupying power and the U.S. composition of the court, the trial could produce definitive law directly applicable only to Germany and the United States. The trial judges, who were appointed by President Harry S Truman, were Walter B. Beals, a justice of the Supreme Court of Washington, as presiding judge; Harold L. Sebring, a justice of the Supreme Court of Florida; Johnson Tal Crawford, an Oklahoma District Court judge and Victor C. Swearingen, alternate judge, a former assistant attorney general of Michigan. Hundreds of other Nazis, including some physicians, were tried before military tribunals made up exclusively of military officers, including trials at Dachau, Mauthausen, and Buchenwald.[4–6]

The charges in the Doctors Trial primarily involved war crimes and crimes against humanity committed in concentration camp experiments. The judges based their conclusion on universal human rights principles and, as the prosecution requested, they saw themselves as speaking as the "voice of humanity."

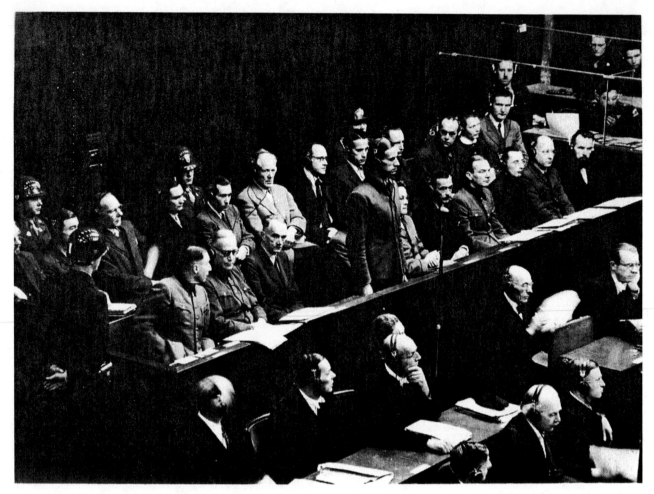

Figure 12.1. Karl Brandt and his fellow defendants in the dock at the Doctors Trial. Source: United States Holocaust Memorial Museum Collection. Courtesy of John W. Mosenthal. Reproduced with permission.

The Nuremberg Code

The final judgment, which was delivered in August 1947, also set forth the Nuremberg Code, a 10-point statement of rules designed to protect the rights and welfare of research subjects[7] (see Box 12.1). The court prefaced its enunciation of the Code as follows:

> The great weight of the evidence before us is to the effect that certain types of medical experiments on human beings, when kept within reasonably well-defined bounds, conform to the ethics of the medical profession generally. The protagonists of the practice of human experimentation justify their views on the basis that such experiments yield results for the good of society that are unprocurable by other methods or means of study. All agree, however, that certain basic principles must be observed in order to satisfy moral, ethical and legal concepts.[7]

The Code's Strengths

The most significant strength of the Nuremberg Code is that it is a legal code based on principles of natural law and human rights that have universal application. Another central strength is its articulation of the principle of informed consent, insisting that the voluntary, competent, informed, and understanding consent of the research subject is a necessary (but not sufficient) prerequisite for lawful human experimentation, and requiring that a person retain the right to withdraw his or her consent at any time during the experiment.

Although discussions and debates continue about the use as research subjects of individuals who are incapable of providing informed consent on their own behalf, there is worldwide agreement that the voluntary and informed consent of those capable of giving it is a prerequisite to lawful and ethical experimentation with humans. This proposition has become a central principle of medical ethics, in both the research and therapeutic settings, and has been enshrined in international human rights law, including the International Covenant on Civil and Political Rights, which states in Article 7: "[N]o one shall be subjected without his free consent to medical or scientific experimentation."[8] The Nuremberg Code's eight other provisions relate to the welfare of research subjects and the obligation of researchers to protect subjects' welfare when conducting research.

The Code has been invoked and endorsed by a variety of U.S. courts.[9] A U.S. district court in Ohio has ruled that it applies to

BOX 12.1
The Nuremberg Code

1. The voluntary consent of the human subject is absolutely essential. This means that the person involved should have legal capacity to give consent; should be so situated as to be able to exercise free power of choice, without the intervention of any element of force, fraud, deceit, duress, over-reaching, or other ulterior form of constraint or coercion; and should have sufficient knowledge and comprehension of the elements of the subject matter involved as to enable him to make an understanding and enlightened decision. This latter element requires that before the acceptance of an affirmative decision by the experimental subject there should be made known to him the nature, duration, and purpose of the experiment; the method and means by which it is to be conducted; all inconveniences and hazards reasonably to be expected; and the effects upon his health or person which may possibly come from his participation in the experiment.

    The duty and responsibility for ascertaining the quality of the consent rests upon each individual who initiates, directs or engages in the experiment. It is a personal duty and responsibility which may not be delegated to another with impunity.

2. The experiment should be such as to yield fruitful results for the good of society, unprocurable by other methods or means of study, and not random and unnecessary in nature.

3. The experiment should be so designed and based on the results of animal experimentation and a knowledge of the natural history of the disease or other problem under study that the anticipated results will justify the performance of the experiment.

4. The experiment should be so conducted as to avoid all unnecessary physical and mental suffering and injury.

5. No experiment should be conducted, where there is an *a priori* reason to believe that death or disabling injury will occur; except, perhaps, in those experiments where the experimental physicians also serve as subjects.

6. The degree of risk to be taken should never exceed that determined by the humanitarian importance of the problem to be solved by the experiment.

7. Proper preparations should be made and adequate facilities provided to protect the experimental subject against even remote possibilities of injury, disability, or death.

8. The experiment should be conducted only by scientifically qualified persons. The highest degree of skill and care should be required through all stages of the experiment of those who conduct or engage in the experiment.

9. During the course of the experiment, the human subject should be at liberty to bring the experiment to an end if he has reached the physical or mental state where continuation of the experiment seems to him to be impossible.

10. During the course of the experiment the scientist in charge must be prepared to terminate the experiment at any stage, if he has probable cause to believe, in the exercise of the good faith, superior skill and careful judgment required of him that a continuation of the experiment is likely to result in injury, disability, or death to the experimental subject.

both civil and criminal cases in federal courts.[10] The Maryland Court of Appeals, the state's highest court, has adopted it as a common law standard; the Maryland court noted in 2001 that the Code "at least in significant part, was the result of legal thought and legal principles, as opposed to medical or scientific principles, and thus should be the preferred standard for assessing the legality of scientific research on human subjects."[11] The U.S. Supreme Court's view is complex. It has recognized the Nuremberg Code as part of U.S. law, and yet by a 5 to 4 vote in 1987 it refused to permit members of the U.S. military to use the Code as a basis to sue the U.S. government for money damages for violating its provisions.[12]

The Nuremberg Code has also informed every other major code of conduct regarding human experimentation developed since its promulgation in 1947.

The Code's Limitations

The Code's deficiencies are directly related to its strengths and its origin. Perhaps its major problem has been its origin as an American response to Nazi medicine. The Code originated in a U.S. Army tribunal. It was formally adopted by the U.S. Defense Department as doctrine in 1953. Incredibly, it was classified "top secret" and not declassified until 1975. For decades, physicians around the world, but U.S. physicians especially, treated Nazi medicine as such an aberration that the Nuremberg Code was marginalized and seen as having nothing to teach non-Nazi physicians. Some even argued that the Nuremberg Code itself is a good code for barbarians, but not for civilized physicians.

Furthermore, the emphasis on consent did not really fit the Nazi crimes. Yale law professor Robert Burt correctly observes that the "basic problem" of the murders and tortures by the Nazis in the name of medical research was not that "the subjects did not agree to participate." Thus the emphasis on consent in this setting, he writes, seems "peculiar."[13] Unlike many others, however, Burt recognizes that the judges at Nuremberg were forward-looking in their judgment and that they sought to craft a document to provide some assurance against a repetition, not only in Germany but around the world, including the United States. Because the judges could not rely on physicians to police themselves, Burt writes, "The Nuremberg judges established, as their first line of defense against recurrence of these barbarities, the individual subject-patient armed with the principle of self-determination."[13]

A related problem has been what has sometimes been seen as the Code's "rigid" insistence on informed consent as the most important aspect of ethical research. Jay Katz of Yale Law School, the world's leading authority on informed consent, argued in 1963, and again in the *Final Report of the Advisory Committee on Human Radiation Experiments*,[14] that:

> [O]nly when the Nuremberg Code's first principle on voluntary consent is firmly put into practice can one address the claims of . . . society to benefit from science. Only then can one avoid the dangers that accompany a balancing of one principle against the other that assigns equal weight to both; for only if one gives primacy to consent can one exercise the requisite caution in situations where one may wish to make an exception to this principle for *clear and sufficient* reasons.[14]

Katz acknowledges that exceptions could be made to the Code's consent principle, but he argues that such exceptions must be democratically arrived at by society at large, not determined by researcher-dominated institutional review boards (IRBs) or by researchers themselves. The judges at Nuremberg, although upholding research on humans as a legitimate activity, nonetheless considered that using individuals for the benefit of others by testing a hypothesis on them and putting them at risk of harm is inherently a suspect activity. In the absence of the informed consent of the research subject, research on human beings is (and should be) extremely difficult to justify.

As influential as the Code is, it is incomplete as guidance for research ethics. The Nuremberg judges made no attempt to deal with clinical research on children, patients, or mentally impaired people. More importantly, the Code fails to address many issues related to international research trials, including the questions of care for research subjects after the trial's end and benefit to the host community.[15,16]

Enduring Legacy

The year 2007 marks the 60th anniversary of the Nuremberg Code. On the 50th anniversary of the Code, many people offered commentaries.[17] We wrote: "Human rights law is similar to medical ethics in that both are universal and aspirational, and since the Nuremberg Trials, both have been unenforceable. A critical challenge is to make both meaningful, and this may be the most important legacy of the Nuremberg trials."[18] We proposed that physicians and lawyers work together to make the promise of the Code as a human rights document a reality, just as physicians and lawyers worked together at Nuremberg to bring the Nazi physicians to justice.

Ten years later, what have we learned? Informed consent continues to be recognized as the core ethical and legal requirement for legitimate medical research, but the globalization of research has made the realization of this principle even more difficult in practice. Nonetheless, the continued distancing of time from the Nazi horrors has permitted the Nuremberg Code to gain new adherents, and its universal aspiration is gaining in reality.

In 2005, on the 60th anniversary of the signing of the World War II surrender of Germany, Berlin finally was able to build a memorial to the Holocaust.[19,20] Consisting primarily of 2,700 concrete slabs constructed in the former no man's land where the Berlin Wall once stood, it is meant to symbolize the bureaucratic processes that allow human beings to accept evil as a normal part of the world. The question that the memorial failed to ask, according to Paul Spiegel of Germany's Center Council of Jews, is, "Why were members of a civilized people in the heart of Europe capable of planning and carrying out mass murder?"[21] This question echoes one that Elie Wiesel has asked over and over again about the Nazi doctors: "How is it possible?"[21] How is it possible that physicians could turn into mass murderers?

Of course, memorials can't do everything and can't speak to everyone. In a real sense the Nuremberg Code can be seen as a living memorial to the suffering and deaths of the concentration camp victims of the Nazi doctors. And the more we are distanced temporally from the crimes of the Nazi doctors, the more we may be able to see our relationship not just with the victims, but with the U.S. judges and physicians at Nuremberg who were able to confront this evil and attempt to imagine a way to prevent its repetition.[22] In this regard, we may come to see the legacy of Nuremberg as a U.S. legacy, not a Nazi legacy; and as a profound human rights code, not a Nazi relic.

References

1. Grodin MA. Historical origins of the Nuremberg Code. In: Annas GJ, Grodin MA, eds. *The Nazi Doctors and the Nuremberg Code: Human Rights in Human Experimentation.* New York, N.Y.: Oxford University Press; 1992:121–44.
2. Schmidt U. *Justice at Nuremberg: Leo Alexander and the Nazi Doctors' Trial.* New York, N.Y.: Palgrave Macmillan; 2004.
3. Taylor T. Opening statement of the prosecution, December 9, 1946. In: Annas GJ, Grodin MA, editors. *The Nazi Doctors and the Nuremberg Code: Human Rights in Human Experimentation.* New York, N.Y.: Oxford University Press; 1992:67–93.
4. Greene JM. *Justice at Dachau.* New York, N.Y.: Broadway Books; 2003.
5. Proctor R. *Racial Hygiene: Medicine Under the Nazis.* Cambridge, Mass.: Harvard University Press; 1988.
6. Lifton RJ. *The Nazi Doctors: Medical Killing and the Psychology of Genocide.* New York, N.Y.: Basic Books; 1986.
7. The Nuremberg Code. In: *Trials of War Criminals Before the Nuremberg Military Tribunals Under Control Council Law No. 10. Volume 2.* Washington, D.C.: U.S. Government Printing Office; 1949:181–2. [Online]. Available: http://www.hhs.gov/ohrp/references/nurcode.htm.
8. United Nations, Office of the High Commissioner for Human Rights. *International Covenant on Civil and Political Rights* (adopted and opened for signature, ratification and accession by General Assembly resolution 2200A [XXI] of 16 December 1966; entry into force 23 March 1976, in accordance with Article 49). [Online] Available: http://www.unhchr.ch/html/menu3/b/a_ccpr.htm.
9. Annas GJ. Mengele's birthmark: The Nuremberg Code in United States courts. *Journal of Contemporary Health Law and Policy* 1991;7:17–45.
10. *In re Cincinnati Radiation Litigation,* 874 F. Supp. 796, 822 (S.D. Ohio 1995).
11. *Grimes v. Kennedy Krieger Institute,* 782 A.2d 807 (Md. 2001).
12. *U.S. v. Stanley,* 483 U.S. 669 (1987).
13. Burt RA. *Death Is That Man Taking Names.* Berkeley, Calif.: University of California Press; 2002.
14. Katz J. Statement by Committee member Jay Katz. In: Advisory Committee on Human Radiation Experiments. *Final Report of the Advisory Committee on Human Radiation Experiments.* New York, N.Y.: Oxford University Press; 1996:543–8.
15. Glantz LH, Annas GJ, Grodin MA, Mariner WK. Taking benefits seriously in developing countries. *Hastings Center Report* 1998;28(6):38–42.
16. Annas GJ, Grodin MA. Human rights and maternal-fetal HIV transmission prevention trials in Africa. *American Journal of Public Health* 1998;88:560–3.
17. Shuster E. Fifty years later: The significance of the Nuremberg Code. *New England Journal of Medicine* 1997;337:1436–40.
18. Grodin MA, Annas GJ. Legacies of Nuremberg: Medical ethics and human rights. *JAMA* 1996;276:1682–3.
19. Czuczka T. Germany dedicates Holocaust Memorial. *Boston Globe* May 11, 2005:A13.
20. Ouroussoff N. A forest of pillars, recalling the unimaginable. *New York Times* May 9, 2005:Bl.
21. Wiesel E. Without conscience. *New England Journal of Medicine* 2005;353:1511–3.
22. Annas GJ. Human rights outlaws: Nuremberg, Geneva, and the global war on terror. *Boston University Law Review* 2007;87:427–66.

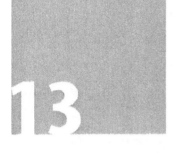

Richard E. Ashcroft

The Declaration of Helsinki

The Declaration of Helsinki is arguably the most widely known and influential guideline in medical research worldwide. Titled the "World Medical Association Declaration of Helsinki: Ethical Principles for Medical Research Involving Human Subjects," it is an official policy of the World Medical Association (WMA). Initially promulgated in 1964, it has been revised five times, most recently in 2000. The 2000 revision was greatly controversial before, during, and after its publication, and subsequently two "clarificatory" notes have been added, in 2002 and 2004. This chapter reviews the history of the Declaration, describes its current contents, discusses its strengths and deficiencies, and gives a prognosis for its future importance and influence.

History of the Declaration

The Declaration of Helsinki was adopted by the WMA at its annual General Assembly in Helsinki in 1964. The WMA had been founded in Paris in 1947 as an association for national medical associations.[1] Its mission, as currently stated, is "to serve humanity by endeavoring to achieve the highest international standards in Medical Education, Medical Science, Medical Art and Medical Ethics, and Health Care for all people in the world."[2]

When it was established, its member institutions were particularly concerned with the violations of human rights and medical ethics that had taken place in Germany and elsewhere during the Nazi period. The establishment of the WMA was roughly contemporaneous with the Nuremberg doctors' trial, the establishment of the United Nations, and the adoption of the Universal Declaration of Human Rights. The Association adopted a declaration on fun-

damental medical ethics, the Declaration of Geneva, in 1948 and an International Code of Medical Ethics in 1949. However, medical research was not formally discussed by the WMA until 1953, when a position paper on human experimentation was discussed by the WMA's Ethics Committee. This became a "Resolution on Human Experimentation: Principles for Those in Research and Experimentation," adopted by the WMA's Eighth General Assembly in Rome in 1954.[3] The then president of the WMA, Lambert Anthonie Hulst, a Dutch specialist in internal medicine who had attended the Nuremberg Doctors' Trial, was a member of the drafting committee for the 1954 resolution.[4] Discussion of these issues continued within the WMA, leading to a draft Declaration in 1961 and, finally, the adoption of the original Declaration in 1964.[5]

It is not clear why the Resolution was proposed in 1953, or why once the Resolution had been adopted in 1954, a further draft Declaration was proposed in 1961. Nor is it clear why it took a further three years for the Declaration finally to be adopted. Historians generally have been able only to speculate: None seems to have had full access to public or private papers, or to interviews with participants in the process. The WMA itself implies that the whole process was a natural development of the founding documents of the Association, and that the process involved "discussion and research."[5,6] Scholars, such as David Rothman and Jay Katz, have focused on the role of Henry Beecher's exposés of unethical medical research in 1966 to explain the reception of the Declaration, but this obviously does not explain its production. Beecher's revelations brought about a great explosion of concern with the ethics of medical research and the realization that unethical research was not merely a pathology of totalitarian regimes, but could also be found in liberal democracies.[7,8]

More recent scholarship suggests that discussion of the ethics of medical research was widespread in funding agencies, government research institutes, and elsewhere even before 1964, but that this discussion was not part of mainstream medical debate.[9] Paul McNeill suggests that the long delays between 1954 and 1961, and between 1961 and 1964, are evidence of internal dissent and debate.[10] He cites George Annas and Leonard Glantz to the effect that one of the main drivers for the adoption of the Declaration was the U.S. Food and Drug Administration's need to tighten drug registration regulations after the thalidomide disaster.[11] Annas elsewhere suggests that the Declaration was an attempt on the part of doctors to refashion the Nuremberg Code in terms that were more physician-friendly and more facilitative of research.[12] Recent works by Gerald Kutcher and Wolfgang Weyers lend further weight to this interpretation.[3,13] These issues are complex, and further detailed historical scholarship will be necessary to untangle them.

The 1954 Resolution

Comparison of the 1954 Resolution with the Nuremberg Code and the 1964 Declaration is instructive. The Nuremberg Code commenced with an insistence on voluntary consent of the individual research subject, and went on to consider the utility of the research for human health, the necessity for research to be based on sound medical knowledge and research in animals, minimization and control of risk of harm, and the need for medical oversight at all times (see Chapter 12). It set out 10 strict norms. The 1954 Resolution, however, stated only 5 principles (see Box 13.1). It started with the need for scientific and moral justification for the research, then considered the need for "prudence and discretion" in the publication of results.[3] The third and fourth principles referred to the differing requirements of research on healthy volunteers and sick patients, and the final principle stated the need for written informed consent, either from the subject him- or herself, or—if the subject is "irresponsible" (lacks the capacity to decide)—from his or her legal representative.

The Resolution is clearly focused on the conduct of the physician-investigator, rather than the rights of patients. Interestingly, the Resolution addressed experimentation in sick subjects in terms of heroic medical or surgical interventions rather than in terms of clinical trials under uncertainty. In many respects the Resolution was a poorly drafted document, particularly in comparison with the Nuremberg Code. However, in introducing a distinction between the healthy volunteer and the patient-subject, and in considering that experimentation may be a form of medical care, the Resolution did contain the seeds of the later Declaration, and represented an important revision of the approach contained in the Nuremberg Code.

The 1964 Declaration

The Declaration of Helsinki in its 1964 version was a much more formal document than the earlier Resolution. It had a formal preamble, relating it to the WMA's Declaration of Geneva and International Code of Medical Ethics, and stating the rationale behind its promulgation:

BOX 13.1
Code of the World Medical Association, 1954: Principles for Those in Research and Experimentation[3]

I. Scientific and Moral Aspects of Experimentation

The word experimentation applies not only to experimentation itself but also to the experimenter. An individual cannot and should not attempt any kind of experimentation. Scientific qualities are indisputable and must always be respected. Likewise, there must be strict adherence to the general rules of respect for the individual.

II. Prudence and Discretion in the Publication of the First Results of Experimentation

This principle applies primarily to the medical press and we are proud to note that in the majority of cases, this rule has been adhered to by the editors of our journals. Then there is the general press, which does not in every instance have the same rules of prudence and discretion as the medical press. The World Medical Association draws attention to the detrimental effects of premature or unjustified statements. In the interest of the public, each national association should consider methods of avoiding this danger.

III. Experimentation on Healthy Subjects

Every step must be taken in order to make sure that those who submit themselves to experimentation be fully informed. The paramount factor in experimentation on human beings is the responsibility of the research worker and not the willingness of the person submitting to the experiment.

IV. Experimentation on Sick Subjects

Here it may be that, in the presence of individual and desperate cases, one may attempt an operation or a treatment of a rather daring nature. Such exceptions will be rare and require the approval either of the person or his next of kin. In such a situation it is the doctor's conscience which will make the decision.

V. Necessity of Informing the Person Who Submits to Experimentation of the Nature of the Experimentation, the Reasons for the Experiment, and the Risks Involved

It should be required that each person who submits to experimentation be informed of the nature of, the reason for, and the risk of the proposed experiment. If the patient is irresponsible, consent should be obtained from the individual who is legally responsible for the individual. In both instances, consent should be obtained in writing.

Because it is essential that the results of laboratory experiments be applied to human beings to further scientific knowledge and to help suffering humanity, the World Medical Association has prepared the following recommendations as a guide to each doctor in clinical research. It must be stressed that the standards as drafted are only a guide to physicians all over the world. Doctors are not relieved from criminal, civil and ethical responsibilities under the laws of their own countries.[14]

This statement expressed the essential feature of all subsequent versions of the Declaration—balancing the need to generate useful medical and therapeutic knowledge with the need to protect the health and interests of research participants, especially the health and interests of ill patients participating in research. In this regard, the Declaration differed fundamentally from the Nuremberg Code, which was essentially a statement of the need to protect the rights and welfare of individuals, with an implicit assumption that scientific research is "experimentation in man" which is contrary to human dignity. The shift in language from the language of "experimentation"—still present in the 1954 Resolution—to the language of "clinical research" in the 1964 Declaration marked this shift in emphasis.

The language of the 1964 Declaration was more carefully crafted than the language of the 1954 Resolution. Some features merit particular attention. First, there was a strong shift back toward the categorical language of the Nuremberg Code. Although the 1964 Declaration presented itself as merely offering guidance, each of its 14 numbered paragraphs stated some requirement which "must" or "should" be met. Second, although these requirements were categorical, the 1964 Declaration frequently reverted to a language of "proportion" and "comparison," particularly in relating the risks of research to the benefits the subject, the patient, or society will gain from the research. Yet, as Charles Weijer has argued, the 1964 Declaration contained no principled account of risk, or of "proportionality."[15] Thus, principle I.3 reads: "Clinical research cannot legitimately be carried out unless the importance of the objective is in proportion to the inherent risk to the subject"[14]

Although this is where the concept of benefit in proportion to risk is introduced, no guidance is given on how to assess this proportionality, and no qualitative or quantitative concept of risk is defined. Addressed as it is to the physician-investigator, it appears that what is "in proportion" must be judged by the physician in accordance with his or her professional judgment and sense of good conduct, rather than being subject to external technical evaluation.

Third, the 1964 Declaration, like the 1954 Resolution, concerned the responsibilities of doctors toward their patients or their research subjects, rather than the rights or wishes of patients. In particular, the 1964 Declaration continued to distinguish between therapeutic and nontherapeutic research and to give a higher priority to the assessment of risk than to the obtaining of consent. Unlike the 1954 Resolution, the 1964 Declaration did stress that consent is a requirement in research with both healthy volunteers and patients, but it qualified this requirement in the case of patients. The second paragraph of principle II.1. reads:

> If at all possible, consistent with patient psychology, the doctor should obtain the patient's freely given consent after the patient has been given a full explanation. In case of legal incapacity, consent should also be procured from the legal guardian; in case of physical incapacity, the permission of the legal guardian replaces that of the patient.[14]

This is a complex paragraph, with particular difficulties attending what was meant by "physical" and "legal" incapacity, the role of legal guardians, and what was meant by "also" obtaining consent from the legal guardian in the case of legal incapacity. The qualification "consistent with patient psychology" is particularly significant. It is clear that in 1964, it was possible to override the obligation to obtain consent from some patients who had the legal capacity to decide, if obtaining consent was "inconsistent" with the patients' psychology. Obviously this was a serious departure from the Nuremberg Code's insistence that consent is "absolutely

essential," even if it may not have been a serious departure from widely understood clinical practice according to concepts of "therapeutic privilege." In context, this paragraph related to "clinical research combined with professional care," and would have been consistent with the then applicable ethos relating to informed consent in routine clinical care. This, in a nutshell, is the still vexed debate over whether standards of consent in clinical research should be lowered to be consistent with the standards of consent in routine clinical medicine, or whether the standards of consent in clinical medicine should be raised to the level of the standards applicable in clinical research.[16]

The difficulty of interpreting this paragraph from today's standpoint is great. Given 40 years of bioethics and health law scholarship on notions of mental capacity, patient autonomy, and research ethics, it is difficult now to step back and read the paragraph as it may have been intended in 1964. Further, issues such as the limits of informed consent remain controversial now, so that some ambiguity or vagueness in 1964 should not unduly surprise the reader in the 21st century. A critical ambiguity in interpretation here is that it is possible to read the 1964 Declaration as a weakening of the Nuremberg Code (with the Declaration's references to proportionality and to making allowances for patient psychology, as I have discussed) or instead as a humanization of a legalistic code (with the Declaration's emphasis on research as part of patient care and the norms of ordinary clinical medicine).

The 1964 Declaration also contained some inconsistencies and ambiguities. For example, the provisions in part III of the 1964 Declaration for "non-therapeutic clinical research" included the following paragraphs:

> 3a. Clinical research on a human being cannot be undertaken without his free consent, after he has been fully informed; if he is legally incompetent, the consent of the legal guardian should be procured.
>
> 3b. The subject of clinical research should be in such a mental, physical, and legal state as to be able to exercise fully his power of choice.
>
> 3c. Consent should as a rule be obtained in writing. However, the responsibility for clinical research always remains with the research worker; it never falls on the subject, even after consent is obtained.[14]

Paragraph 3b is clearly inconsistent with 3a, because 3b seems to require full mental and legal capacity, whereas 3a implies that if potential research subjects are legally or mentally incapacitated, a legal guardian can give consent. This is particularly striking because for many commentators, the rationale behind the 1964 Declaration was to develop standards consistent with the spirit of Nuremberg for research involving the mentally or legally incapable, such as young children, the seriously mentally ill, or the unconscious. Moreover, these commentators contended that placing responsibility for risks and benefits on the researchers created a test that could substitute for the consent of the patient when the patient was legally, mentally, or physically incapable of consenting.[10,17] Whether 1964 Declaration did, in fact, create such a loophole was unclear, however. The inconsistency between paragraphs 3a and 3b suggests that this substitute test would not be applicable, and that the strict bar on nontherapeutic research with incompetent subjects remained in force.

In addition, it can be argued that a prisoner or a member of the armed forces is not in a "legal state" to exercise her or his choice, and therefore could be considered incapable of giving informed consent. Depending on the interpretation of the conflict between 3a and 3b, the 1964 Declaration either banned research on prisoners and military personnel, or permitted it on the authorization of their "legal guardian"—the prison authorities or superior officers. Of course, theoretically such permission would only be sought if the research met the risk/benefit tests of the Declaration. But this dilemma, or inconsistency, would prove to be of great significance over the following decades, as controversies involving research with vulnerable subjects took place fairly regularly, notably the controversial research at Willowbrook, Tuskegee, and Holmesburg Prison[18,19] (see Chapters 7, 8, and 43).

The 1975 Declaration

Eleven years after the adoption of the original version, the Declaration was revised again.[20] Povl Riis, a Danish researcher, physician, and ethicist who was a coauthor of the 1975 version, argues that the motivation behind this second version of the Declaration was to strengthen the protections for research subjects in response to revelations of a range of shocking disclosures about research on the dying, the mentally disabled, and other socially or medically vulnerable groups in the United States and elsewhere.[21] A revised Declaration was adopted at the 1975 WMA General Assembly in Tokyo, shortly after the establishment of the U.S. National Commission for the Protection of Human Subjects of Biomedical and Behavioral Research (see Chapter 14). The history of the 1975 revision has received considerably less discussion than the 1964 Declaration, but for most commentators, the 1975 version is in fact the classical text of the Declaration.[22] The revision was led by the Danish, Norwegian, and Swedish medical associations. Riis believes that their role was primary because of the mutual interests of the democratic political institutions in the Nordic countries, and the response to the democratizing movements in the United States (the civil rights movement) and in Europe (the "events" of May 1968, the month-long French riots and strikes that threatened the government of President Charles de Gaulle).[21]

The 1975 revisions to the text were substantial, although much of the language of the 1964 text was retained. The preamble was extended, with new paragraphs setting out the rationale for biomedical research (the word *biomedical* entered the Declaration for the first time here). The 1975 Declaration emphasized that the risks of research should be weighed in the light of the risks of treatment and that medical progress depends on medical research—that is, that current treatments depend for their success on earlier research. This seemed to imply that we should not be overly cautious about research risks and also, perhaps, that we have a duty to participate in research, if we are willing to benefit from its results. But, as the Declaration was addressed to researchers, it is not clear what the implications of making these statements are, or why they are there. Persuading patients of the merits of medical research can hardly have been a function of the Declaration. In addition, as McNeill argues, the Declaration's rationale justifying research was specifically tied to the need to develop knowledge of pathology, physiology, and therapeutics for diagnosis and treatment, rather than the vaguer purpose of advancing science generally.[10]

Interestingly, the 1975 Declaration also contained a single-sentence paragraph in the preamble urging that "Special caution must be exercised in the conduct of research which may affect the environment, and the welfare of animals used for research must be respected."[20]

This nod to bioethics beyond human bioethics may reflect contemporary concerns about the environmental impact of the use of technologies to protect human health, such as DDT. It also reflects a wider appreciation of the types of experiment used in drug development, as later picked up in Basic Principle 1: "Biomedical research involving human subjects must conform to generally accepted scientific principles and should be based on adequately performed laboratory and animal experimentation and on a thorough knowledge of the scientific literature."[20]

The final paragraph of the preamble stressed, as in 1964, that the guidelines were only recommendations, but added that the Declaration should be "kept under review in future."

The 1975 Declaration also introduced the statement that "concern for the interests of the subject must always prevail over the interests of science and society." Although this was part of the statement of Basic Principles, it is buried about halfway down the document, rather than making its appearance in the Introduction (as in the 2000 revision). The 1975 Declaration made much more detailed statements than had the 1964 Declaration and 1954 Resolution about the interests of research participants in privacy, informed consent, management of the hazards of research, and protection from the abuse of dependency on one's doctor. Although the 1975 document was not a statement of research subjects' rights, it placed more emphasis on the interests of human subjects than on the duties of doctors. This is a delicate nuance, yet it marked an important change. The most important indicator of this change was the Declaration's requirement, for the first time, of a clearly stated research protocol and review of that protocol by an independent committee.

The remainder of the 1975 Declaration continued to observe the 1964 distinction between therapeutic and nontherapeutic research, and its statement on therapeutic research was no longer concerned solely with heroic "experimental" interventions, but implicitly focused on clinical trials. The famous requirement that "every patient—including those of a control group, if any—must be assured of the best proven diagnostic and therapeutic method" made its appearance in section II.3. There was now a presumption in favor of informed consent, strengthening the position of the 1964 document, and requiring, in section II.5, that "if the doctor considers it essential not to obtain informed consent, the specific reasons for this proposal should be stated in the experimental protocol for transmission to the independent committee." Thus, doctors were no longer free to judge for themselves whether informed consent could be waived if a patient's "psychology" did not permit it. Similarly, in section III.2, on nontherapeutic research, the confused language of 1964 was replaced with the much clearer statement that "the subjects should be volunteers—either healthy persons or patients for whom the experimental design is not related to the patient's illness." This clearer statement apparently ruled out nontherapeutic research in the legally, mentally, or physically incompetent.

Other Revisions Before 2000

The Declaration continued to evolve, being revised again at the Venice assembly of 1983, the Hong Kong assembly of 1989, and the Somerset West, Republic of South Africa, assembly of 1996. Most of the revisions were minor, and continued in the spirit of the 1975 revisions. The Declaration commanded wide support across the worlds of medical research in academia and industry, and was taken up as the normative statement of research ethics standards in the rapidly developing system of research ethics committees and institutional review boards in the developed world. It had wide influence in policy, for example, in the development of bioethics standards such as those elaborated in the U.S. Belmont Report. One key example of the influence of the Declaration is that, as Riis argues, the 1975 Declaration's requirement for ethical review introduced greater transparency and openness on the part of both the pharmaceutical industry and academic researchers.[21] In combination with the development of drug regulations over the same period, this led to the adoption of the Good Clinical Practice guidelines in 1996.[23] The emphasis of the Declaration became more and more clearly directed toward the ethical governance of clinical trials of drugs. By 1996, reference to the responsibilities of sponsors, duties regarding publication (not seen since the 1954 Resolution), and "the use of inert placebo in studies where no proven diagnostic or therapeutic method exists" had appeared. The other main development was more detailed consideration of risk assessment, including an emphasis on the predictability of hazards. Interestingly, the exclusion from nontherapeutic research of subjects who are unable to volunteer for such research remained.

Current Content of the Declaration

By the late 1990s, the Declaration had become widely criticized among regulators and within the research community and industry. Many academic and patient groups felt that the Declaration was too weak. They contended that it should bar the use of placebo in trials in which a proven effective treatment exists, require the publication of research results (in order to improve the reliability of the evidence base), ensure that patients who benefit from trial treatments could continue to receive treatment after the trial, and demand that trials conducted in the developing world (or in resource-poor settings) are held to the same standards as trials in the developed world, in terms of treatment of controls and availability of treatment after the trial. Academic and industry groups argued that placebo controls could be justified even in many situations in which active treatment had been proven effective, and that the "standard of care" in resource-poor settings should be the "best available" treatment, not the "best proven" (see Chapters 64–67). In addition to this controversy, some critics had argued for many years that the Declaration's distinction between therapeutic and nontherapeutic research was incorrect. Instead, these critics contended that the Declaration should distinguish between therapeutic and nontherapeutic procedures done in the context of treatment for research purposes.[17] This controversy led to a very significant redrafting of the Declaration in 2000, together with the addition of "Notes of Clarification" in 2002 and 2004.[24]

The revision process for the eventual 2000 Declaration proved controversial. A revision process began in 1997, only one year after the adoption of the 1996 revision. A draft revision got as far as the 1999 meeting of the WMA before being rejected, and a new working party was established in 1999 under the chairpersonship of Nancy Dickey of the American Medical Association, which then initiated a consultation in February 2000.[25] As the debate developed, it progressed on two fronts—the debate about the ethical norms of the Declaration itself, and the debate on the authority of the WMA and of its Declarations to regulate clinical research worldwide. An important feature of the latter debate concerned the authority of doctors who were (or were not) active clinical researchers to shape the Declaration, and the authority of those who were (or were not) citizens or residents of the developing world to prescribe norms for the conduct of research in developing world settings.[26] As with the overlapping debate about the revision of the Council for International Organizations of Medical Sciences (CIOMS) guidelines, a lot of discussion turned on how far such norms were universal or situation-relative, and on how transparent and accountable the revision process was. That the debate coincided with the dramatic explosion of the Internet made this a far more open debate than on previous occasions, but also may have heightened the impression that the consultation mechanisms used were neither democratic nor transparent. Given the international importance of the Declaration, many commentators felt that the process of revision and its accountability were of crucial importance for its legitimacy. Yet the WMA as a membership association is not accountable to anyone save its membership, and the Declaration is not law. It is not clear that the WMA was obliged to be accountable in the way its critics suggested.

The current structure of the Declaration is as follows. The 1964–1996 distinction between therapeutic and nontherapeutic research has been dropped, and the Declaration is now in three parts: Introduction; Basic Principles for All Medical Research; and Additional Principles for Medical Research Combined With Clinical Care.

The introductory section begins (paragraphs 1–3) by setting out the scope of the document and relating it to other WMA policy (the Declaration of Geneva and the International Code of Medical Ethics). The scope of the document, for the first time, includes not only experimental procedures on the body and mind of subjects but also the use of human tissue or data that can be identified with a particular individual. This reflects the role of epidemiology, pathology, and genetic research in modern biomedicine. The next four paragraphs (paragraphs 4–7) set out the rationale for medical research, as in the 1975–1996 versions, placing the statement about the priority of the interests of the individual over those of science and society at paragraph 5. Paragraph 8 is a detailed statement of the need to protect the "health and rights" of human beings, and describes different types of vulnerability, both of individuals and of populations. This is a significant change both in its reference to populations and in its suggestion that vulnerability may take the form of "economic vulnerability" or "economic and medical disadvantage." Paragraph 9 states the relationship between the Declaration and national laws, reversing the relationship established in 1964 by holding that "no national ethical, legal or regulatory requirements should be allowed reduce or eliminate any of the protections for human subjects set forth in this Declaration." Whereas in 1964 the Declaration was seen as guidance that helped researchers in areas in which the law was silent, now it is seen as a human rights document that takes moral and jurisprudential priority over national laws that are seen as compromised.[27]

The next section sets out the basic principles for all medical research. It starts by stating the duty of the physician to protect the "life, health, privacy and dignity of the human subject" (paragraph

10). It requires research to be founded on accepted scientific principles and prior research, including both animal research and literature review (paragraphs 11–12). It then requires the research protocol to be reviewed by an independent ethics committee, for the research to be open to external monitoring, and for the researcher to state compliance with the Declaration as part of the protocol (paragraphs 13–14). The next paragraphs (15–19) relate the responsibilities of the physician to supervise the research, to control and monitor risks, and to ensure that the research risks are reasonable in the light of the importance of the research objective.

There are two controversial elements here. First, the necessity for biomedical research to be supervised by a "clinically competent medical person" has been queried by nurse researchers as well as by basic scientists, who do not see why a doctor must be in charge, as opposed to merely assisting. Second, the Declaration states that, among other considerations, research risks are justified only "if there is a reasonable likelihood that the populations in which the research is carried out stand to benefit from the results of the research." Here it could be argued that this excludes some people from participation simply on the ground that others (in the same population) will not be able to benefit. Further, it could be argued that this paragraph places the responsibility for providing treatment on the researcher, rather than on government, sponsor, patient, or other purchasers. This issue arises again at paragraph 30.

Paragraphs 20–26 set out the requirements of informed consent. Here, controversial issues include the relationship between paragraph 20, which requires subjects to be volunteers, and paragraphs 24, 25, and 26, which discuss alternatives to consent when the subject is legally incompetent. Paragraph 22 requires disclosure of the source of funding for the research. Paragraph 23 requires research participants to have access to a physician who is not involved in the research, in order to protect them from duress due to dual relationships (researcher-subject and physician-patient). Paragraphs 24–26 allow research on incompetent subjects, including minor children, provided that "the research is necessary to promote the health of the population represented and this research cannot instead be performed in legally competent persons," which is accepted in some jurisdictions but not in others (as was demonstrated in the debates over the Council of Europe's Convention on Human Rights and Biomedicine).

All of these paragraphs are controversial to some extent. Some of the Declaration's requirements are criticized as impractical in resource-poor settings, in which an independent physician may be hard to find. Some of the guidelines are viewed as inconsistent, and industry officials consider them unduly restrictive or motivated by "industry bashing." This criticism has also been leveled at paragraph 27, which requires the publication of research data, positive and negative, and states that research in breach of the Declaration should not be published.

The final section delineates principles for research combined with medical care. Paragraph 28 justifies such research provided the procedure has potential diagnostic, prophylactic, or therapeutic value. Paragraphs 29 and 30 are the most controversial elements of the whole Declaration. Paragraph 29, as amended by a "Note of Clarification" in 2002, requires that new methods of treatment, prophylaxis, or diagnosis should be tested against "the best current . . . methods." Placebo control is not ruled out if there is no proven method in existence. This is qualified by the Note of Clarification, which states that placebo controls may be used even when a proven method does exist, provided that placebo controls are necessary "for compelling and scientifically sound methodological reasons," or when the disease is "a minor condition and the patients who receive placebo will not be subject to any additional risk of serious or irreversible harm."

The controversial points here are whether placebo controls can be justified even if this means that patients are denied effective treatment, whether placebo can be justified if patients normally would not receive the best standard treatment for economic reasons, and whether a moral obligation to provide the best possible care (if there is such an obligation) can be trumped by a scientific or methodological requirement.[28]

Paragraph 30 states that every participant, at the end of the study, should receive the best proven prophylactic, diagnostic, and therapeutic methods identified by the study (if they need them). This again is controversial: For how long should they continue to be provided with care? By whom? Paid for by whom? In a vaccine trial, does this mean providing long-term treatment for a disease they might have caught anyway? Most supporters of the Declaration in its current form accept that there are problems with the way this guideline is formulated, but would argue that the underlying principle of nonabandonment of patients in whom a relationship of dependency has been created is sound.[29] The Note of Clarification added at the Tokyo meeting of the WMA in 2004 reads:

> The WMA hereby reaffirms its position that it is necessary during the study planning process to identify post-trial access by study participants to prophylactic, diagnostic and therapeutic procedures identified as beneficial in the study or access to other appropriate care. Post-trial access arrangements or other care must be described in the study protocol so the ethical review committee may consider such arrangements during its review.[24]

This allows, but does not require, ethics committees to require researchers to consider and describe their position on posttrial access, and give reasons for it, even if it stops short of obliging researchers to provide such access themselves.

Paragraph 32 describes the principles relating to attempts to use unproven or experimental interventions on patients in the interests of "saving life, re-establishing health or relieving suffering" if everything else has failed. This is a return to some of the concerns of the 1964 Declaration. However, it requires that such experiments be made the object of research, and thus subject to the provisions of the Declaration.

Strengths, Weaknesses, and Prospects for the Declaration

Strengths

The undoubted strength of the Declaration is its standing as the most well known and widely available guideline on medical research ethics. Its historical status as the preeminent guideline for doctors conducting medical research, and its international status placing it over and above national legal and policy questions, vest it with considerable authority. The basic structure of the Declaration—attempting to define the moral status of clinical research, the importance of balancing risk and benefit to subjects and to society, the role of informed consent, and the importance of considerations of justice for patients, subjects, and populations—

is undoubtedly sound. Although every version of the Declaration has contained contradictions, vague formulations, and some controversial elements, in general terms it is a clear and helpful document that can be cited by researchers wishing to avoid unethical practice and by ethical committees wishing to enforce ethical standards. Some of the provisions of the recent Declaration reflect a welcome concern with the scope of biomedical research today, both in terms of the resources it requires (data, population participation, tissue, as well as patient participation in clinical research) and in terms of the way modern research is sponsored and conducted (commercial and multinational multisite research are a large component). Particularly welcome is the Declaration's recognition of the need to ensure that research is conducted in a way that produces genuine medical advance, rather than repetitious or imitative work (through the requirement of prior literature review and publication of both positive and negative results). This shift is due largely to the growing importance of meta-analysis and systematic review in medicine and health policy. The current Declaration sees research as only one part in a more complex process of medical progress and health-care quality improvement.

Weaknesses

The greatest weakness of the Declaration now is the way it has become highly contested—some would say, "politicized." Some critics of the original WMA Resolution and Declaration argued that these were a medical attempt to soften the Nuremberg Code, by weakening the centrality of informed consent in order to permit a wider range of medical research to take place. They see the Declaration as always a political document framed with doctors' interests at its heart. Although this is an extreme view, it cannot be doubted that the 2000 Declaration and the attempts to "clarify" it were highly contested, especially in the context of the overlapping debates about intellectual property rights and access to treatment. However, the precise nature of the contest is hard to specify simply. Although some critics felt that this was a struggle between U.S. interests and developing world interests, many developing world participants in the debate shared "U.S." views, and many U.S. and European commentators argued from a "developing world" perspective.[21,30] In this respect, the debate over the revision of the Declaration overlapped both chronologically and intellectually with the debate over access to essential medicines that took place during the debate about compulsory licensing and parallel generic production of patented pharmaceuticals in the context of the World Trade Organization's Trade Related Intellectual Property rights framework at the beginning of the 2000s.

There were in both cases debates about principle and about practice. A developing world physician might insist that placebo-controlled trials were in his population's interest, whereas a developed world human rights activist might insist that this created an indefensible relativism about moral standards. This could be seen as a debate about moral universals, but was equally a debate about how best in practice to promote international justice in the health and development contexts. Hence it is perhaps better to see this as a debate about political interests and strategy than as purely a debate about moral philosophy and practice.

Internally, the main weaknesses of the Declaration remain persistent internal contradictions and vagueness of statement, as illustrated by the debates over paragraphs 29 and 30 and their interpretation. Perhaps the main difficulty is the problem of producing a comprehensive ethical guideline that covers everything from in silico genetic research to clinical trials of surgical procedures, and applies everywhere from Washington to rural Africa. The Declaration has no explanatory notes and no discussion points, so its interpretation is always somewhat controversial. The text of the Declaration states that it is for guidance, rather than a set of strict rules, yet in its 2000 version it places itself above national legal norms, suggesting that where legal norms conflict with it, the Declaration should take priority. This claims for the Declaration of Helsinki a moral standing equivalent such documents as the Universal Declaration of Human Rights, or similar conventions. Yet it was produced by the World Medical Association and ratified by the WMA's General Assembly, which has only a small membership (fewer than half of the world's nations have a member association). Moreover, very few individual members of national medical associations have any influence over what happens at the WMA, because it is constituted as an association of associations. The drafting of the Declaration and its revisions has normally been done by a small group of doctors (usually three or four).

Given the structure and working methods of the WMA it is perhaps unsurprising that the Declaration has become complex in statement and controversial in content and in authority. In many countries, however, the Declaration has been enacted as law, and adherence to its principles (if not its exact letter) is a requirement of many national and international guidelines, such as the International Conference on Harmonisation's Good Clinical Practice guidelines. Many groups clearly have a powerful interest in influencing the formulations adopted by the Declaration.

Prospects

The Declaration of Helsinki probably will continue to be the central international guidance document on research ethics, and it probably will continue to be revised, and each revision undoubtedly will remain controversial. In a sense these three predictions are all of a piece: Each explains the other. Nonetheless, it is arguable that since 2000 the authority of the Declaration has weakened, and it is an open question whether this is because the latest revision could not command consensus, or because its vagueness and internal contradictions became less tenable, or because it set ethical standards that are too high for most to be able to follow—and therefore are useless—or whether its standards are high but appropriate, and vested interests are trying to discredit it. Be that as it may, it is hard to see how any other international organization could produce guidelines with a similar authority and importance to replace the Declaration. Certainly much could be done to improve the quality of the drafting of the Declaration, but the underlying ethical principles will continue to guide and inspire, however controversial they may be.

References

1. World Medical Association. WMA History: Background and Preliminary Organisation. [Online] Available: http://www.wma.net/e/history/background.htm.
2. World Medical Association. About the WMA. [Online] Available: http://www.wma.net/e/about/index.htm#mission.

3. Weyers W. *The Abuse of Man: An Illustrated History of Dubious Medical Experimentation*. New York, N.Y.: Ardor Scribendi; 2003.

4. Weindling PJ. *Nazi Medicine and the Nuremberg Trials: From Medical War Crimes to Informed Consent*. Basingstoke, England: Palgrave MacMillan; 2004:327.

5. World Medical Association. WMA History: Declaration of Helsinki. [Online] Available: http://www.wma.net/e/history/helsinki.htm.

6. Human D, Fluss SS. The World Medical Association's Declaration of Helsinki: Historical and Contemporary Perspectives. [Online] 2001. Available: http://www.wma.net/e/ethicsunit/pdf/draft_historical _contemporary_perspectives.pdf.

7. Rothman DJ. Ethics and human experimentation: Henry Beecher revisited. *New England Journal of Medicine* 1987;317:1195–9.

8. Katz J. The consent principle of the Nuremberg Code: Its significance then and now. In: Annas GJ, Grodin MA, eds. *The Nazi Doctors and the Nuremberg Code: Human Rights in Human Experimentation*. New York, N.Y.: Oxford University Press; 1992:227–39.

9. Advisory Committee on Human Radiation Experiments. *Final Report of the Advisory Committee on Human Radiation Experiments*. New York, N.Y.: Oxford University Press; 1996.

10. McNeill PM. *The Ethics and Politics of Human Experimentation*. Cambridge, England: Cambridge University Press; 1993.

11. Annas GJ, Glantz LH. *Informed Consent in Veterans Administration Cooperative studies: Legal and Ethical Issues*. Washington, D.C.: Veterans Administration Cooperative Studies Program; 1987:8.

12. Annas GJ. Mengele's birthmark: The Nuremberg Code in the United States courts. Journal of Contemporary *Health Law and Policy* 1991; 7:17–45.

13. Kutcher GJ. *Clinical Ethics and Research Imperatives in Human Experiments: A Case of Contested Knowledge*. Unpublished doctoral dissertation, Department of History and Philosophy of Science, University of Cambridge; 2002.

14. World Medical Association. *Code of Ethics of the World Medical Association: Declaration of Helsinki*. Helsinki, Finland: WMA; June 1964. *British Medical Journal* 1964;2:177.

15. Weijer C. The ethical analysis of risk. *Journal of Law, Medicine, and Ethics* 2000;28:344–61.

16. Chalmers I, Lindley RI. Double standards on informed consent to treatment. In: Doyal L, Tobias JS, eds. *Informed Consent in Medical Research*. London, England: BMJ Books; 2001:266–75.

17. Schüklenk U, Ashcroft RE. International research ethics. *Bioethics* 2000;14:158–72.

18. Moreno JD. *Undue Risk: Secret State Experiments on Humans*. New York, N.Y.: W. H. Freeman; 1999.

19. Hornblum AM. *Acres of Skin: Human Experiments at Holmesburg Prison*. New York, N.Y.: Routledge; 1998.

20. World Medical Association. *Declaration of Helsinki: Recommendations Guiding Medical Doctors in Biomedical Research Involving Human Subjects*. Tokyo, Japan: WMA; October 1975. *Medical Journal of Australia* 1976;1:206–7.

21. Riis P. Thirty years of bioethics: The Helsinki Declaration 1964–2003. *New Review of Bioethics* 2003;1(1):15–25.

22. Carlson RV, Boyd KM, Webb DJ. The revision of the Declaration of Helsinki: Past, present and future. *British Journal of Clinical Pharmacology* 2004;57:695–713.

23. International Conference on Harmonisation of Technical Requirements for Registration of Pharmaceuticals for Human Use. *The ICH Harmonised Tripartite Guideline—Guideline for Good Clinical Practice*. Geneva: ICH; 1996. [Online] Available: http://www.ich.org/ LOB/media/MEDIA482.pdf.

24. World Medical Association. *Declaration of Helsinki: Ethical Principles for Medical Research Involving Human Subjects*. Tokyo, Japan: WMA; October 2004. [Online] 2004. Available: http://www.wma.net/e/ policy/b3.htm.

25. Beecham L. WMA begins consultation on Declaration of Helsinki. *British Medical Journal* 2000;320:585.

26. Forster HP, Emanuel EJ, Grady C. The 2000 revision of the Declaration of Helsinki: A step forward or more confusion. *Lancet* 2001; 358:1449–53.

27. Andreopoulos GJ. Declarations and covenants of human rights and international codes of research ethics. In: Levine RJ, Gorovitz S, Gallagher J, eds. *Biomedical Research Ethics: Updating International Guidelines*. Geneva, Switzerland: CIOMS; 2001: 181–203.

28. Nuffield Council on Bioethics. *The Ethics of Research Related to Healthcare in Developing Countries*. London, England: Nuffield Council on Bioethics; 2002. [Online] Available: http:// nuffieldbioethics.org/fileLibrary/pdf/errhdc_fullreport001 .pdf.

29. Greenwood B, Hausdorff WP. After a trial is over: The ethical issues. SciDev.Net [Online] October, 2003. Available: http://www.scidev .net/dossiers/index.cfm?fuseaction=policybrief&dossier=5& policy=41.

30. European Group on Ethics in Science and New Technologies. *Opinion No. 17 to the European Commission: Ethical Aspects of Clinical Research in Developing Countries*. Brussels, Belgium: EGE; 2003. [Online] Feb. 4, 2003. Available: http://ec.europa.eu/european_group _ethics/docs/avis17_en.pdf

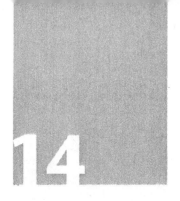

Tom L. Beauchamp

The Belmont Report

The Belmont Report is a short document on moral principles that was published in 1978 by the National Commission for the Protection of Human Subjects of Biomedical and Behavioral Research (National Commission). Since that time it has provided a basic framework for analyzing ethical issues that arise during medical research in the United States and in many other countries.

History

The National Commission was established in 1974 by the U.S. Congress with a charge to identify ethical principles and develop guidelines to govern the conduct of research involving humans. It was hoped the guidelines would ensure that the basic ethical principles would become embedded in the U.S. research oversight system, so that meaningful protection was afforded to research participants. Another mandated goal was to distinguish the boundaries between the accepted and routine practice of medicine, on the one hand, and biomedical and behavioral research, on the other.

The Commission held its first meeting on December 3–4, 1974, and its 43rd and final meeting on September 8, 1978.[1] It completed a draft of the Belmont Report in late 1977, and issued it in final form on September 30, 1978. The report was published in the *Federal Register* on April 18, 1979—the date now commonly cited as the original date of publication.

The National Commission also published 16 other reports and appendix volumes, most focused on ethical issues in research involving vulnerable populations. Its more than 100 recommendations for reform went directly to the Secretary of the Department

of Health, Education and Welfare (DHEW)—now the Department of Health and Human Services (DHHS)—and many of these were eventually codified as federal regulations.[2] The Belmont Report itself was not written in the style of federal regulations and was never so codified. It was the National Commission's statement of a general, principled moral framework. The foundation of this "analytical framework," as it is called in the report, was a collection of moral principles appropriate for research that first emerged during discussions at a retreat the National Commission held on February 13–16, 1976, at the Smithsonian Institution's Belmont Conference Center in Elkridge, Md. There had been no draft or planning for this framework prior to the retreat. This conference center's name was then appropriated, and the report was published under the full title of *The Belmont Report: Ethical Principles and Guidelines for the Protection of Human Subjects of Research.*

The National Commission came into existence in the aftermath of public outrage and congressional uncertainty over the Tuskegee syphilis experiments and other questionable uses of humans in research (see Chapter 8). The socioeconomic deprivation of the African American men who were enrolled in the Tuskegee experiments made them vulnerable to overt and unjustifiable forms of manipulation at the hands of health professionals, as had been widely reported in news media and widely circulated in the report of an advisory panel to DHEW in 1973.[3] Other reports of the abuse of fetuses, prisoners, children, and "the institutionalized mentally infirm" appeared in the news media.

The law that created the National Commission specified that no more than 5 of the Commission's 11 members could be research investigators (see Table 14.1). This stipulation testified to congressional determination at the time that research activities of

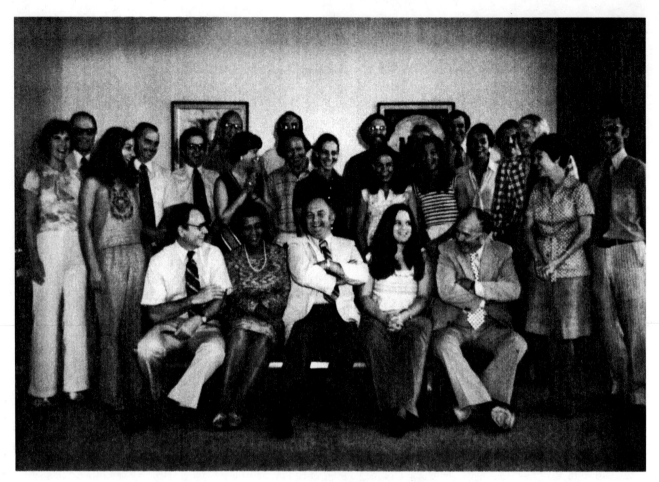

Figure 14.1. Members of the National Commission for the Protection of Human Subjects of Biomedical and Behavioral Research, 1977. Source: Tom L. Beauchamp. Reproduced with permission.

the biomedical and behavioral sciences be brought under the critical eye, and possibly the control, of persons outside of the sciences. At that time, the research system generally placed responsibility for the protection of humans in research on the shoulders of individual investigators. That is, federal policies relied on the discretion and good judgment of investigators to determine the conditions under which research should be conducted. Federal involvement and review committees were then in the formative stages. They were destined to undergo rapid change toward protectionism under the guidance of the National Commission.

Carol Levine offers the following sobering, but accurate, statement of the context in which the National Commission deliberated:

> The Belmont Report . . . reflected the history of the 30 years immediately preceding it. This emphasis is understandable, given the signal event in the modern history of clinical-research ethics [Nazi experimentation]. American public opinion was shaped by the revelations of unethical experiments such as the Willowbrook hepatitis B studies . . . ; the Jewish Chronic Disease Hospital studies . . . ; and, especially, the Tuskegee Syphilis Study. . . . Our basic approach to the ethical conduct of research and approval of investigational drugs was born in scandal and reared in protec-

tionism. Perceived as vulnerable, either because of their membership in groups lacking social power or because of personal characteristics suggesting a lack of autonomy, individuals were the primary focus of this concern.[4] [see Chapters 6 and 7]

Content and Core Strengths

The Belmont Report is especially well known for its framework of basic moral principles, which are still today referred to as the "Belmont principles." The National Commission identified three general principles as underlying the conduct of research: respect for persons, beneficence, and justice. The key organizing conception underlying the Commission's presentation of these principles and their use was the following: Respect for persons applies to informed consent; beneficence applies to risk-benefit assessment; and justice applies to the selection of research participants. The following abstract schema represents this conception: In this way, each moral principle makes moral demands in a specific domain of responsibility for research—a general conception of the relationship between abstract moral principles and research ethics. This conception of the connection between abstract moral

Table 14.1

Members of the National Commission for the Protection
of Human Subjects of Biomedical and Behavioral Research

- Kenneth John Ryan, M.D., Chairman, Chief of Staff, Boston Hospital for Women
- Joseph V. Brady, Ph.D., Professor of Behavioral Biology, Johns Hopkins University
- Robert E. Cooke, M.D., President, Medical College of Pennsylvania
- Dorothy I. Height, President, National Council of Negro Women, Inc.
- Albert R. Jonsen, Ph.D., Associate Professor of Bioethics, University of California at San Francisco
- Patricia King, J.D., Associate Professor of Law, Georgetown University Law Center
- Karen Lebacqz, Ph.D., Associate Professor of Christian Ethics, Pacific School of Religion
- David W. Louisell, J.D., Professor of Law, University of California at Berkeley
- Donald W. Seldin, M.D., Professor and Chairman, Department of Internal Medicine, Southwestern Medical School, University of Texas
- Eliot Stellar, Ph.D., Provost of the University and Professor of Physiological Psychology, University of Pennsylvania
- Robert H. Turtle, LL.B., Attorney, VomBaur, Coburn, Simmons and Turtle, Washington, D.C.

principles and applied bioethics has been enduring. Many engaged in research ethics carry this general conception with them today.

Principle of	Respect for persons	Applies to	Informed consent
	Beneficence		Risk/benefit assessment
	Justice		Selection of research participants

The principle of respect for persons demands that the choices of autonomous persons not be overridden or otherwise disrespected and that persons who are not adequately autonomous be protected by the consent of an authorized third party likely to appreciate their circumstances and who will look after their best interests. This principle in effect requires valid permission before investigators can proceed with research. To achieve this goal, the principle insists on the individual's informed consent, analyzed in terms of the conditions of information disclosure, comprehension, and voluntariness. The National Commission proposed "the reasonable volunteer" as an appropriate standard for judging the adequacy and clarity of information disclosure. Investigators are held responsible for ascertaining that research participants have comprehended the information they have been given about the proposed research. The purpose of consent provisions is not protection from risk, as earlier federal policies seemed to imply, but protection of autonomy and personal dignity, including the personal dignity of incompetent persons incapable of acting autonomously. The report went on to suggest that third parties be encouraged to follow the research as it proceeds, retaining the right to withdraw an incompetent person from his or her research participation.

The principle of beneficence is an abstract norm that includes rules such as "Do no harm," "Balance benefits against risks," and "Maximize possible benefits and minimize possible harms." This principle is satisfied in the research context by refraining from intentionally causing injury and by assuring that risks are reasonable in relation to probable benefits. The National Commission required that there be an arrayal of data pertaining to benefits and risks and of alternative ways of obtaining the benefits (if any) sought from involvement in research. It demanded that, if possible, systematic and nonarbitrary presentations of risks and benefits be made to research participants as part of the informed consent process and that the assessment of risks and safeguards be considered by an institutional review board (IRB) in weighing the justifiability of research protocols. The National Commission stated that participants ought not to be asked or allowed to consent to more risk than is warranted by anticipated benefits and that forms of risk incommensurate with participants' previous experience should not be imposed in the case of groups such as children, who might be overburdened and possibly disturbed or terrified. However, the report recognized that risks must be permitted during the course of many forms of research in order for investigators to be positioned to distinguish harmful from beneficial outcomes.

The principle of justice requires fairness in the distribution of both the burdens and the benefits of research. The National Commission insisted that this principle requires special levels of protection for vulnerable and disadvantaged parties. This principle demands that researchers first seek out and select persons best prepared to bear the burdens of research (e.g., healthy adults) and that they not offer research only to groups who have been repeatedly targeted (e.g., mentally retarded children). The National Commission noted that, historically, the burdens of research were placed heavily on the economically disadvantaged, the very sick, and the vulnerable, owing to their ready availability. This conclusion was not based on a systematic review, but was based more on impressions from published data, reports in the media, public testimony to the Commission, and some onsite visits to places such as prisons. Yet the advantages of research benefit all in society. The overutilization of readily available, often compromised, segments of the U.S. population was a matter of deep moral concern to the National Commission. The theme of justice and proper selection of research participants was the Belmont Report's way of saying that because medical research is a social enterprise for the public good, it must be accomplished in a broadly inclusive and participatory way. If participation in research is unwelcome and falls on a narrow spectrum of citizens because of their ready availability, then it is unwarranted. Likewise, the National Commission recommended that persons who are already burdened by some form of disability or institutionalization should not be asked to accept the burdens of research—unless, as occurs in some cases, other participants cannot be located or are otherwise inappropriate.

The Belmont Report includes not only these three abstract principles and their analysis, but also a moral view that moves modestly in the direction of an applied research ethics. Just as there is a distinction between theoretical or general ethics and applied or practical ethics, so the National Commission thought of the Belmont Report as its theoretical framework. However, because of its objectives, the explanation of the principles had a noticeably applied character. Nonetheless, the National Commission had no ambition to make the report itself specific and practical for institutions that conduct research. This objective was to be accomplished by the other 16 volumes on problems of research ethics that the National Commission issued. The Belmont Report itself was intended to provide only a general framework of basic principles for research ethics.

National Commission members and staff were keenly aware that this framework was too indeterminate by itself to decide practice or policy or to resolve moral conflicts. The process of molding the general principles in the Belmont Report so that they become sufficiently concrete is a process of reducing the indeterminateness and abstractness of the principles to give them increased action-guiding capacity. The report looks to educational institutions, professional associations, government agencies and IRBs to provide the more specific rules and judgments required for research ethics.

The works of philosophers such as W. D. Ross and William Frankena were often consulted in the drafting of the Belmont Report, but the moral principles featured in the report should not be read as deriving from the writings of philosophers. The Belmont Report made reference to values "generally accepted in our cultural tradition" as the basis of its principles. These principles derived from National Commission members' understanding of social morality. What the commissioners meant by our "tradition" is unclear, but the import of the Belmont principles is not to be tied to the unique views of a particular tradition or nation. The National Commission apparently conceived of its principles as universally valid norms. That is, the principles were taken to be applicable to all contexts of human research, not merely to some local region, such as an institution or a nation. The presumption is that no responsible research investigator could conduct research without reference to these principles; these principles form the core of any policy worthy of the name "research ethics."

Weaknesses, Deficiencies, and Unclarities

Despite the Belmont Report's wide acceptance, several issues have been or can be raised about the adequacy of the Belmont principles. Here are six possible problems.

1. The way the principles are delineated is arguably confused, especially the principle of respect for persons. This appears to confusingly blend two principles: a principle of respect for autonomy and a principle of protecting and avoiding harm to incompetent (nonautonomous) persons. The National Commission said that it was attempting to protect both autonomous persons and those with "diminished autonomy," those who are incapable of self-determination. Both are persons, it said, and both are entitled to protection.

The question is whether protections for persons who are incapable of self-determination can be justified in any way other than by the principle of beneficence. If not, so the criticism goes, then the National Commission adopted an incoherent position in thinking that respect for persons and beneficence are independent principles. Robert Veatch seems to both criticize and defend the National Commission for this apparent confusion:

The Belmont Report offers a three-principle theory that uses the Kantian term: "respect for persons." It subsumes autonomy under this broader notion, but in a strange way it also subsumes the welfare of the incompetent under respect for persons. This is hard to defend. Autonomy may be an element of a more fundamental notion of respect for persons, but it seems that the duty to serve the welfare of the incompetent is straightforwardly a part of the duty of beneficence. Nevertheless, if respect for persons includes autonomy, it could include other elements as well. . . . [I myself include] principles other than autonomy as part of respect for persons. If respect for persons includes only respect for autonomy, then nonautonomous persons are left stranded. . . . Respecting persons must involve . . . Veracity . . . Fidelity to promises . . . [and] Avoidance of killing.[5]

Veatch is suggesting that although the National Commission erred in its explication of respect for persons, its general viewpoint could perhaps be reconstructed and rendered viable.

2. The National Commission was very concerned that using utilitarian justifications of research had become too easy in the biomedical world. The Nazi experiments, Tuskegee, and the Jewish Chronic Disease Hospital cases all seemed to have been driven by a very utilitarian view of (social) beneficence that justified using humans on grounds of benefit to the broader public. However, the National Commission itself has been accused of having inadequate internal controls in its moral framework to protect research participants against abuse when there is the promise of major benefit for society. Two Commission members, Robert Cooke and Robert Turtle, sternly criticized the Commission's report on children as endorsing an unjustifiable utilitarian justification of research that placed children at undue risk.[6,7]

Whatever the merits of this criticism, the Belmont Report was written, in part, to ensure that we appropriately balance appeals to social utility in the justification of research. That is, a major purpose of the report was to properly balance the interests of research participants with those of science and society. Considerations of autonomy, justice, and risk control were set out to limit utilitarian overbalancing and investigator discretion. However, it is doubtful that the question of how best to control utilitarian balancing was ever resolved by the Commission.

3. Paradoxically, the Belmont Report and the National Commission more generally can be criticized for being overly protective of research participants—and consequently insufficiently utilitarian to meet the needs of certain classes of persons. The National Commission's emphasis was on the protection of humans from research injury. Research participation was conceived as a burden that individuals accepted in order to advance the public good and that should be distributed equitably. It is unclear why this assumption was so deep in the Commission's work, but it can likely be explained by the atmosphere of scandal that had emerged at the time. The nature and acceptability of the public's interest in research and the goals of research were little-explored matters in the Belmont Report. The notion that research is not always viewed by participants as burdensome was underexamined.

The AIDS epidemic altered this mind-set, perhaps forever. Whereas the Belmont Report sought to protect research participants, AIDS activists sought not protection from but inclusion in the research process. They wanted justice and respect for their autonomy, but not along the lines staked out in the Belmont Report. They wanted to be able to choose unapproved drugs; considerations of justice, they thought, should be used to allow them access to clinical trials. To them, the Belmont principles could be interpreted as protectionist to the point of excluding those who might benefit from research and from access to potentially beneficial drugs. In the end, this push for inclusion in research and broader access to the potential benefits of research altered the course of research ethics. Whether this development constitutes an expansion in the scope and use of the Belmont principles or a confrontation with these principles is debatable, but it certainly reconfigured research ethics[4,8] (see Chapters 9 and 23).

4. The Belmont Report has also been criticized for its abstractness and inability to resolve or otherwise treat practical moral problems. The report anticipated this criticism and cautioned that its principles "cannot always be applied so as to resolve beyond dispute particular ethical problems. The objective is [only] to provide an analytical framework that will guide the resolution of ethical problems arising from research involving human subjects." The National Commission thus warned readers that they should not expect to use Belmont principles as a checklist of federal regulations or as guidelines like recipes in cooking. Nonetheless, several critics have asked whether these principles are in any meaningful respect practical, or even useful. The concern is that norms as general as the Belmont principles underdetermine almost all moral judgments because there is too little content in abstract principles to determine concrete judgments.

Danner Clouser and Bernard Gert have objected to the Belmont principles, and all related analytical frameworks, contending that "principles" function more like chapter headings in a book than as directive rules and theories. Therefore, receiving no directive guidance from the principle, anyone who is working on a problem in bioethics is left free to deal with that principle in his or her own way and may give it whatever meaning and significance he or she wishes. Consider justice. The Belmont principle of justice (in the selection of research participants) instructs a moral agent to be alert to various matters of justice; but does such a general principle actually guide conduct? Other moral considerations besides the principle(s) of justice, such as moral intuitions and ethical theories, may be needed to do the real work of ethical reflection.[9–11]

This criticism merits careful attention, but can any system of principles, rules, or general guidelines escape this problem? Clouser and Gert maintain that some general moral rules can provide deep and directive substance, but these authors have had difficulty in clarifying and justifying this claim. Their point is no doubt correct for unspecified principles, but all abstract principles and rules will need some sort of specification-in-context to become directive. The National Commission anticipated this problem. It did not advance the Belmont principles as sufficient for resolving problems, but only as a starting point. The Commission noted that "other principles may be relevant" and that its principles should be able to "serve as a basic justification" for more "particular prescriptions and evaluations."

5. The Belmont Report has also been faulted for another, closely related reason: It gave no indication of how to prioritize or weigh its principles. Several commentators assert that the National Commission should have argued that one or more of its principles has priority—for example, that considerations of respect for persons and justice take priority over considerations of social benefit.[5,7,12] These critics support a model of basic moral principles and protections that cannot be violated under any circumstances, even if there is a clear and substantial benefit for society. Such restrictions—often said to be deontological in contrast to

utilitarian—are analogous to constitutional rights that constrain conduct and prohibit balancing of interests in various political and social matters. Some who propose such an ordinal or priority ranking of principles argue that it is the morally correct view; others are more concerned to show that the National Commission has not found a way out of situations in which its own principles come into conflict. Some critics also point out that a priority ranking of the sort they propose (to mitigate conflict between beneficence and either autonomy or social justice) would allow the National Commission to escape the accusation that its schema too readily invites utilitarian justifications of research protocols.

Other commentators have argued that the National Commission was correct in its assumption that the principles are more or less weighty depending upon the particular circumstances in which they are to be applied. These accounts are often referred to as balancing theories. They do not allow any principle in the basic analytical framework to have an ordered (or a priori) priority over any other principle. Thus, when principles conflict, the balance of right over wrong must be determined by assessing the weight of competing considerations as they emerge in the circumstance. What agents ought to do is determined by what they ought to do, all things considered. This appears to be the view presumed in the Belmont Report, and it seems also to be the view currently accepted in federal regulations for protocol review, waivers of consent, and the like.[13–15]

6. One former National Commission member, Albert Jonsen, and one staff member, Stephen Toulmin, have jointly questioned whether the National Commission actually used its framework of Belmont principles to support or defend its own bioethical conclusions.[16,17] They have argued that the Commission members believed and published as principlists, but actually worked as casuists. This thesis is not a criticism of the National Commission's substantive work, but rather a methodological comment on the use and limits of its principles. These authors hold that the National Commission's actual moral deliberations proceeded by the consideration of influential cases rather than by appeal to universal principles; and they think, more generally, that this paradigm of reasoning is the best method in bioethics. Jonsen and Toulmin present this understanding of the National Commission's work as follows:

> The one thing [individual Commissioners] could not agree on was why they agreed. . . . Instead of securely established universal principles . . . giving them intellectual grounding for particular judgments about specific kinds of cases, it was the other way around. . . . The locus of certitude in the Commissioners' discussions . . . lay in a shared perception of what was specifically at stake in particular kinds of human situations. . . . That could never have been derived from the supposed theoretical certainty of the principles to which individual Commissioners appealed in their personal accounts.[16]

The point is that National Commission members reasoned by appeal to particular cases and families of cases, and reached consensus through agreement on cases and generalization from cases. Principles were therefore of lesser importance than readers might suppose when they read the Belmont Report. Although the Belmont principles are important guiding ideals, they are overrated if revered for their practicality. Although Jonsen has supported the moral principles delineated in the Belmont Report, he has also maintained that in practical ethics, these principles must be interpreted and specified by the force of examples and counterexamples that emerge from experience with cases.[18] From this perspective, the National Commission should be thought of as using principles primarily as very general guiding ideals.

Enduring Legacy and Influence

The Belmont Report is one of the few documents that has influenced almost every sphere of activity in bioethics: moral theory and general standards of research ethics, government regulatory activity, bioethics consultation, and even medical practice. Its influence has arguably been as extensive in practice as in theory.

Many interested in the role of moral theory and principles in bioethics have honored Belmont for its framework of principles, even if those principles have not been widely analyzed in this literature. As Dan Brock has observed, "The Belmont Report . . . had great impact on bioethics because it addressed the *moral principles* that underlay the various reports on particular aspects of research."[19] Brock is noting the influence of the idea that a body of principles can be used to frame and discuss a wide range of practical moral problems.

In federal regulatory oversight and law, the Belmont Report has at times assumed a near canonical role. The Advisory Committee on Human Radiation Experiments noted in 1995 that

> Many conditions coalesced [historically] into the framework for the regulation of the use of human subjects in federally funded research that is the basis for today's system. . . . [T]his framework is undergirded by the three Belmont principles. The federal regulations and the conceptual framework built on the Belmont principles became so widely adopted and cited that it might be argued that their establishment marked the end of serious shortcomings in federal research ethics policies.[20]

Similarly, an Institute of Medicine report, issued by its Committee on Assessing the System for Protecting Human Research Participants, stated in 2002 that "The ethical foundations of research protections in the United States can be found in the three tenets identified in the Belmont Report."[21] Moreover, the Belmont principles found their way into every document the National Commission published, and these became the backbone of federal law. From this perspective, as Christine Grady has observed, "probably the single most influential body in the United States involved with the protection of human research subjects was the National Commission."[22]

The legacy of Belmont may be most enduring in areas of practice. Federal regulations require that all institutions receiving federal funds for research espouse a statement of principles for the protection of human research participants. Virtually all such institutions have subscribed to the Belmont principles as the basis of their efforts to assess research protocols from an ethical point of view. Professional associations, too, have widely recognized the authority and historical significance of the Belmont principles.[23] Eric Cassell has also argued that the Belmont principles have "permeated clinical medicine" as extensively as they have medical research.[24] His claim is that the Belmont principles were a significant force in a broad cultural shift in medicine toward a reworking of the relationship between doctor and patient.

Whatever the influence and enduring legacy of Belmont, it is not clear that scientists who today are involved in research with humans are any more familiar with the Belmont principles than their predecessors of several decades ago were familiar with documents such as the Nuremberg Code. When the National Commission deliberated, it seemed to some observers that the general system of protecting human research participants in the United States was in need of serious repair, that research investigators were not educated about research ethics, and that participants were not adequately protected. To some observers, the system seems today caught in a notably similar state of disrepair. From 1997 to 2002 a large number of hearings, bills, and reports by official, prestigious government bodies and government-mandated bodies in the United States concluded that the system of IRB review and the practice of informed consent—the core of research ethics established by the National Commission—are seriously defective.[8,21]

The National Commission and its Belmont Report may have succeeded both in "resolving" some major problems of research ethics and in bringing "oversight" to the research context, as historian David Rothman has claimed;[25] but this may have been a temporary, time-bound fix. Today the Belmont principles may be more revered than they are understood and practiced.

References

1. The National Commission for the Protection of Human Subjects of Biomedical and Behavioral Research. *The Belmont Report: Ethical Principles and Guidelines for the Protection of Human Subjects of Research.* Washington, D.C.: Department of Health, Education and Welfare; DHEW Publication OS 78-0012 1978. Available: http://www.hhs.gov/ohrp/humansubjects/guidance/belmont.htm.
2. Department of Health and Human Services, National Institutes of Health, and Office for Human Research Protections. The Common Rule, Title 45 (Public Welfare), Code of Federal Regulations, Part 46 (Protection of Human Subjects). [Online] June 23, 2005. Available: http://www.hhs.gov/ohrp/humansubjects/guidance/45cfr46.htm.
3. Jones JH. *Bad Blood,* 2nd ed. New York, N.Y.: The Free Press; 1993 [1981].
4. Levine C. Changing views of justice after Belmont: AIDS and the inclusion of "vulnerable" subjects. In: Vanderpool HY, ed. *The Ethics of Research Involving Human Subjects: Facing the 21st Century.* Frederick, Md.: University Publishing Group; 1996:105–26.
5. Veatch RM. Resolving conflicts among principles: Ranking, balancing, and specifying. *Kennedy Institute of Ethics Journal* 1995;5:199–218.
6. National Commission for the Protection of Human Subjects of Biomedical and Behavioral Research. Archived Materials 1974–78. Transcript of the Meeting Proceedings (for discussion of the Belmont Paper at the following meetings: February 11–13, 1977; July 8–9, 1977; April 14–15, 1978; and June 9–10, 1978), Kennedy Institute Library, storage facility, Georgetown University, Washington, D.C.
7. Marshall E. Does the moral philosophy of the Belmont Report rest on a mistake? *IRB: A Review of Human Subjects Research* 1986;8(6):5–6.
8. Moreno JD. Goodbye to all that: The end of moderate protectionism in human subjects research. *Hastings Center Report* 2001;31(3):9–17.
9. Clouser KD, Gert B. Morality vs. principlism. In: Gillon R, Lloyd A, eds. *Principles of Health Care Ethics.* London, England: John Wiley and Sons; 1994:251–66.

10. Gert B, Culver CM, Clouser KD. *Bioethics: A Return to Fundamentals.* New York, N.Y.: Oxford University Press; 1997:72–5.

11. Clouser KD, Gert B. A critique of principlism. *Journal of Medicine and Philosophy* 1990;15:219–36.

12. Veatch RM. From Nuremberg through the 1990s: The priority of autonomy. In: Vanderpool HY, ed. *The Ethics of Research Involving Human Subjects: Facing the 21st Century.* Frederick, Md.: University Publishing Group; 1996:45–58.

13. Ackerman TF. Choosing between Nuremberg and the National Commission: The balancing of moral principles in clinical research. In: Vanderpool HY, ed. *The Ethics of Research Involving Human Subjects: Facing the 21st Century.* Frederick, Md.: University Publishing Group; 1996:83–104.

14. Beauchamp TL, Childress JF. *Principles of Biomedical Ethics,* 6th ed. New York, N.Y.: Oxford University Press; 2008:chapters 1, 10.

15. Jonsen AR. The weight and weighing of ethical principles. In: Vanderpool HY. *The Ethics of Research Involving Human Subjects: Facing the 21st Century.* Frederick, Md.: University Publishing Group; 1996:64–5.

16. Jonsen AR, Toulmin S. *The Abuse of Casuistry.* Berkeley, Calif.: University of California Press; 1988:16–9.

17. Toulmin S. The National Commission on human experimentation: Procedures and outcomes. In: Engelhardt HT Jr., Caplan A, eds. *Scientific Controversies: Case Studies in the Resolution and Closure of Disputes in Science and Technology.* New York, N.Y.: Cambridge University Press; 1987:599–613.

18. Jonsen AR. Casuistry. In: Sugarman J, Sulmasy DP, eds. *Methods of Bioethics.* Washington, D.C.: Georgetown University Press; 2001: 112–3.

19. Brock D. Public policy and bioethics. In: Reich WT, ed. *Encyclopedia of Bioethics,* 2nd ed. New York, N.Y.: Macmillan Reference; 1995: 2181–8.

20. Advisory Committee on Human Radiation Experiments. *Final Report of the Advisory Committee on Human Radiation Experiments.* New York, N.Y.: Oxford University Press; 1996.

21. Institute of Medicine, Committee on Assessing the System for Protecting Human Research Participants (Federman DF, Hanna KE, Rodriguez LL, eds.). *Responsible Research: A Systems Approach to Protecting Research Participants.* Washington, D.C.: National Academies Press; 2002.

22. Grady C. *The Search for an AIDS Vaccine: Ethical Issues in the Development and Testing of a Preventive HIV Vaccine.* Bloomington, Ind.: Indiana University Press; 1995:42.

23. Pincus HA, Lieberman JA, Ferris S. *Ethics in Psychiatric Research.* Washington, D.C.: American Psychiatric Publishing, Inc.; 1999.

24. Cassell EJ. The principles of the Belmont Report revisited: How have respect for persons, beneficence, and justice been applied to clinical medicine? *Hastings Center Report* 2000;30(4):12–21.

25. Rothman DJ. Research, human: Historical aspects. In: Reich WT, ed. *Encyclopedia of Bioethics,* 2nd ed. New York, N.Y.: Macmillan Reference; 1995:2256.

Joan P. Porter   Greg Koski

Regulations for the Protection of Humans in Research in the United States

The Common Rule

Ethics and regulation of research with humans have coexisted in a somewhat uneasy relationship in the United States for the past 60 years. Wartime atrocities committed by Nazi doctors and scientists under the guise of "medical experimentation" set the stage for increasing awareness in the United States of ethical issues raised by experimentation on humans, even though few U.S. scientists at the time viewed their own work as "unethical." During the 1950s and 1960s, concerns about ethics and human research continued to spread within the U.S. scientific community and among the public as reports of abuses of human subjects in research, including children, became increasingly frequent. The monumental work by Jay Katz[1] provides a scholarly account and analysis of several troubling cases of human experimentation in the United States prior to revelation of the so-called Tuskegee Syphilis Study conducted by the U.S. Public Health Service from 1932 to 1972 (see Chapter 8). Similarly, the 1996 final report of the Advisory Committee on Human Radiation Experiments provides a detailed and sometimes chilling account of studies conducted by U.S. physicians and scientists with the support of the U.S. government during the years of the Cold War.[2]

Policies requiring informed consent and peer review of proposed research, intended to protect the interests of subjects and promote ethical conduct, were not enthusiastically embraced by much of the research community, even after adoption of federal regulations. Today, the research community readily, even if sometimes begrudgingly, acknowledges the need for an appropriate mechanism for ethical review of research and for protection of human research subjects, who now are often called research participants. In recent years, the view that protection of human subjects should be a primary goal of all responsible members of the

research community has become much more widely accepted and enthusiastically endorsed by scientists, the government, and the public than ever before. Still, imposition of federal regulations to achieve these goals is not considered necessary or appropriate by some in the research community, who argue that self-regulation ought to be sufficient. The enthusiasm for these processes is dampened by the logistical, administrative, and regulatory burdens they necessarily entail, rather than by lack of concern for ethical conduct or well-being of research subjects.

The notion that ethical conduct can be "enforced" by law is not well supported, and many scientists still resent mandatory review and modification of their proposals by review committees that, from the scientists' viewpoint, may not have sufficient expertise to properly carry out these tasks. Conversely, institutional review boards (IRBs), the bodies charged with review, approval, and oversight of human research in the United States, often believe that scientists are not well trained in research ethics. Not surprisingly, tensions remain among scientists, ethicists, patient advocates, and regulators, as well as among institutions and federal agencies that fund and conduct research with humans.

Passage of the National Research Act and the establishment of the National Commission for the Protection of Human Subjects in Biomedical and Behavioral Research (National Commission) in 1974 laid the foundation for formal adoption of federal regulations for protection of human subjects by the Department of Health, Education, and Welfare (DHEW), now the Department of Health and Human Services (DHHS). Prior to adoption of the regulations in 1981, similar practices had been implemented through policies instituted in the mid-1970s by the agencies of the Public Health Service for funding of its grants and contracts. The regulations were intended to implement an effective process for review, approval, and continuing oversight of research with humans within the framework of ethical principles identified in the National Commission's Belmont Report—namely, respect for persons, beneficence, and justice[3] (see Chapter 14).

The regulations themselves are process-oriented. They define what human subjects research is and what types of research are subject to regulation and review. They define the minimum requirements for composition of IRBs and the required elements of informed consent; more precisely, they spell out the elements and statements that must be included in a written consent form. They define an assurance process through which an institution wishing to receive federal funds for research makes a legally binding commitment to establish and maintain a program for the protection of human research participants, including providing resources and space for a duly constituted IRB. In doing so, they also create a mechanism for enforcement of the regulations through review and approval of an institution's assurance by the Office for Human Research Protections (OHRP) within the DHHS, formerly the Office for Protection from Research Risks (OPRR) within the National Institutes of Health (NIH).

The processes established in these regulations are intended to apply, in an operational sense, the ethical principles and practices set forth by the National Commission. The National Commission understood that regulations could not be expected to delineate on a case-by-case basis whether or not a given proposal was safe, ethical, or scientifically sound. Rather, the National Commission explained how these principles could be conscientiously applied during a review process that draws upon the collective knowledge and expertise of a committed panel of IRB members responsibly exercising good judgment in the interests of human research participants. The procedures cannot, in and of themselves, protect humans enrolled in research. A signature on a consent form does not mean that appropriately informed consent has been obtained, nor does approval by a quorum of an IRB ensure that a proposed study is ethical, safe, or will provide meaningful scientific data. These goals can be achieved only when all responsible parties do more than merely go through the process in compliance with minimal regulatory requirements.

This chapter discusses that portion of the federal regulations known as the Common Rule. The story of the Common Rule is one of trying to overcome government bureaucracy and statutory impediments to simplify the processes intended to promote responsible conduct, ethical study design, and safety of research subjects. Why did the creation of the Common Rule for federal departments and agencies, a project with noble intentions that ought to benefit everyone, take more than a decade to achieve? Even more perplexing is that having achieved the goal through great effort, many still view the Common Rule as ineffective and even as an impediment to progress and much needed reform. We will examine the historical context of the Common Rule, discuss its provisions and applications, and offer some thoughts about revisions that are still needed and associated reforms to the system for protection of humans in research.

Background and History of the Common Rule

The United States was among the first of a small but growing number of countries to adopt a formal, statute-based regulatory framework for protection of humans in research. The legislation passed by Congress in response to abuses of humans by government and private researchers was intended to prevent future abuses of the rights and welfare of research participants by establishing a system for review, approval, and oversight of all human research supported, conducted, or otherwise regulated by the U.S. government. This includes private research that is conducted to meet Food and Drug Administration (FDA) requirements but excludes some types of privately funded research for which there is no other mechanism to invoke federal jurisdiction.

The regulations promulgated by DHEW in 1974 under the statutory authority of the National Research Act (Pub. L. 93–348) replaced or augmented policies previously adopted by the agencies of the Public Health Service. Several years later, when the Department of Education was created and DHEW became DHHS, the regulations were transferred to DHHS, where they are incorporated in the Code of Federal Regulations (CFR), Title 45, Part 46, also referred to as 45 CFR 46.[4]

These regulations represented the government's efforts to respond to the National Commission's Belmont Report. The Belmont Report established an ethical framework for responsible conduct of research with humans and in so doing, laid a foundation of principles upon which a workable set of rules could be established to ensure that all human studies would be conducted ethically. As originally promulgated, the regulations broadly addressed research in the biomedical and behavioral sciences and set forth requirements for review and approval of proposed research by IRBs and a process of informed consent. Compliance with the regulatory requirements was to be enforced through an assurance process linked to the receipt of federal research support. Institutions receiving support from DHEW were required to give written assurance of compliance that the provisions of the regulations would be fulfilled. Failure to provide such an assurance would result in denial of DHEW support to institutions for research involving humans. To the core of those regulations, commonly referred to as Subpart A, were later added subparts pertaining to special groups of potential research participants deemed to warrant additional specific protections, among them pregnant women and fetuses (Subpart B), prisoners (Subpart C), and children (Subpart D). Originally, these additional provisions were deemed necessary to protect these "vulnerable" populations. Today, the view that women are vulnerable simply because they are pregnant is considered overtly paternalistic, so that terminology is less commonly used in this context. At the same time, the view that all research participants are vulnerable to exploitation has gained greater acceptance in view of widespread concern over the effectiveness of the existing system for protection of humans in research.

In this chapter, we will focus on 45 CFR 46, Subpart A, which is the DHHS's codification of the Common Rule. By now, other federal departments and agencies have codified the same rule at other sections of the code specific to each. When the regulations were first issued by DHEW, however they were not binding on other federal agencies, even though the need for comparable regulations for other agencies engaged in or supporting human research was evident. Nor were they acceptable to the FDA, which maintained its own process for regulation of clinical studies and approval of test articles under the Food, Drug, and Cosmetic Act. As an agency of DHHS, FDA does use the Common Rule when it conducts intramural research, however, and has its own internal IRB.

Table 15.1

Timeline of the Evolution of the Common Rule

Date	Event
May 1974	Basic Regulations Governing the Protection of Human Subjects Involved in Research issued by Office of the Secretary, Department of Health, Education and Welfare (30 FR 18914).
Nov. 1978	The President's Commission for the Study of Ethical Problems in Medicine and Biomedical and Behavioral Research is established by Pub. L. 95-622.
Jan. 1981	Public Health Service issues Final Regulation Amending Basic Department of Health and Human Services (DHHS) policy for the protection of human research subjects 45CFR46, Vol. 46, No. 16 (46 FR 8366).
Dec. 1981	The President's Commission issues its First Biennial Report on the Adequacy and Uniformity of Federal Rules and Policies, and their Implementation for the Protection of Human Subjects in Biomedical and Behavioral Research, "Protecting Human Subjects."
May 1982	Federal Coordinating Committee on Science, Engineering, and Technology (FCCSET) appoints an Ad Hoc Committee for the Protection of Human Subjects in Research, chaired by the Assistant Secretary for Health of DHHS.
Mar. 1983	Office of the Secretary, DHHS, issues Children Involved as Subjects in Research, Additional Protections, Final Rule, Vol. 48, No. 46 (48 FR 9814).
Oct. 1983	Interagency Human Subjects Coordinating Committee is chartered under FCCSET, chaired by Director, Office for Protection from Research Risks.
June 1986	Office of Science and Technology Policy (OSTP) issues Proposed Model Federal Policy for Protection of Human Subjects, Response to the First Biennial Report of the President's Commission for the Study of Ethical Problems in Medicine and Biomedical and Behavioral Research, Office of Science and Technology Policy, Vol. 51, No. 106 (51 FR 106).
Nov. 1988	OSTP issues a refined version of proposed Federal Policy for the Protection of Human Subjects; Notice and Proposed Rules, Vol. 53, No. 218 (53 FR 45661), launching three more years of debate and negotiation over the details of a Common Rule.
June 1991	OSTP publishes the Common Rule as Federal Policy for the Protection of Human Subjects; Notice and Rules, Vol. 56, No. 117 (56 FR 28003). Upon promulgation of the Common Rule, the Interagency Committee becomes a temporary subcommittee of FCCSET.
1994	Human Subjects Research Subcommittee placed under the auspices of the Committee on Health, Safety, and Food of the National Science and Technology Council (NSTC).
Oct. 1995	President Bill Clinton issues Executive Order 1295, Protection of Human Subjects and Creation of the National Bioethics Advisory Commission. Executive Order requires each department and agency that conducts, supports, or regulates research involving human subjects to review the protections of the rights and welfare of human subjects that are afforded by the department's or agency's existing policies and procedures and report to the Commission.
1997	NSTC is reorganized; Human Subjects Research Subcommittee becomes a subcommittee of the NSTC Committee on Science.

Not surprisingly, not all of the federal agencies shared a common view of which research projects ought to be subject to IRB review and approval, or, for that matter, what activities properly constituted research involving human subjects. At times, the policies and practices of some agencies actually conflicted with requirements of the regulations adopted by DHEW, a situation that caused great confusion at institutions engaged in research activities under the auspices of more than one funding agency, as well as some confusion and contentiousness among the agencies themselves. Therein lay the rationale and inspiration for a uniform regulatory framework afforded by a common rule.

Content of the Common Rule

The Common Rule is focused primarily on the processes of review, approval, and oversight of research with humans generally, rather than on being a substantive document specific to any one kind of research. These processes are based on three fundamental ethical principles found in the Belmont Report: (1) respect for persons, (2) beneficence, and (3) justice. Respect for persons requires that individuals be treated as autonomous agents and that persons with diminished autonomy are afforded additional protection. Informed consent is a requirement that derives from this principle, as is the consideration of special protections for vulnerable subjects who may not be able to consent fully to participation in research. Beneficence translates to (1) do no harm, and (2) maximize possible benefits and minimize possible harms. These concepts are reflected in the deliberations an IRB must make in its systematic assessment of risks and benefits. The third principle, justice, addresses who ought to receive the benefits of research and bear its burdens. The principle of justice requires that there be fair procedures and outcomes in the selection of research subjects. Each of these principles is embodied in the regulatory requirements.

The Common Rule applies to all research involving humans conducted, supported, or otherwise subject to regulation by any federal department or agency that takes appropriate administrative action to make the policy applicable to such research. Not all federal agencies and departments have adopted the Common Rule through regulation. In some cases, the departments and agencies may not see their activities as being research as defined by the regulations, or more specifically, may not consider that they are doing research with human subjects. Under the Common Rule, department and agency heads may determine how the rule will be applied, or not, to activities conducted or supported by their agencies. This flexibility was probably an important factor in acceptance of the rule by several federal agencies with widely varying interests and scope of research activities. The applicability section also describes six categories of exemptions from the Common Rule. It states, however, that research that takes place in foreign countries must follow the Common Rule or follow at least equivalent procedures determined and published by the department or agency head.

The Common Rule defines several terms that are used precisely in its application, particularly when compliance with its provisions is assessed. These include "research," "human subject," "minimal risk," "IRB approval," and many others. Many of these terms are further clarified in formal guidance issued by the departments and agencies, and their application may not always be entirely consistent from one agency to another. Even today, controversy exists over whether certain activities are rightfully considered "research," "human subjects research," or "research subject to regulation," and there are similar disputes over the definitions of "equivalent in protections to that in other countries" and "minimal risk." These controversies have been a source of continuing discussion, and sometimes confusion, among members of the research community as well as those who regulate it.

The written "assurance" that is required from institutions must describe how compliance with the rule will be achieved, including specification of principles that govern the conduct of the research, a description of the IRB(s) to be involved, written procedures that must be in place, and institutional responsibilities, including provision of adequate resources, space, and personnel to support the process.

Many of the Common Rule provisions deal with the IRB, including its membership, functions, operations, responsibilities, and authority. Among the basic responsibilities of IRBs, they must determine the following:

- Risks to research participants are minimized.
- Risks to participants are reasonable in relation to anticipated benefits, if any, to participants, and in relation to the importance of the knowledge that may reasonably be expected to result.
- Selection of participants is equitable, and special problems arising in research involving vulnerable populations, such as children, prisoners, pregnant women, and mentally, economically, or educationally disadvantaged people, have been considered.
- Informed consent is properly sought and documented.
- Appropriate monitoring is in place.
- Adequate provisions will be made to protect the privacy of research participants and to maintain the confidentiality of data.

The Common Rule also describes an expedited review procedure for certain kinds of research involving no more than minimal risk and for minor changes in approved research. In addition, DHHS publishes and regularly updates in the *Federal Register* a list of review categories that IRBs can use to expedite review of minimal risk research. The IRB chairperson or one or more experienced reviewers designated by the chairperson from among members of the IRB may carry out the expedited review. The list of expedited categories was last modified in November 1998 to clarify and expand the types of research for which IRB review could be expedited if the research were minimal risk.[5]

Importantly, the Common Rule details the criteria for IRB approval of research, suspension or termination of IRB approval, and arrangements by which cooperative research might be reviewed. It also covers IRB record-keeping requirements, required and additional elements of the consent form, criteria for waiving informed consent or documentation of informed consent, and other conditions that must be met when applications and proposals for IRB review lack specific plans for involvement of humans in research. Additional sections cover other conditions for administrative requirements and timing of reviews before research may begin.

In summary, the Common Rule lays out the process and specific requirements for review, approval, and oversight of research involving humans, but grants institutions and IRBs broad powers and flexibility with respect to the details of their implementation. This is considered by many to be the greatest

strength of the rule, and by others to be its greatest weakness. Some complain that the procedural requirements of the Common Rule impose unnecessarily rigid administrative impediments to the initiation of research, whereas others call for even more detailed and directive guidance for following its provisions, as will be discussed later in this chapter.

Development of the Common Rule

The creation and adoption by multiple agencies of a single rule for protection of humans in research was itself a major exercise in compromise, interagency diplomacy, and leadership. The President's Commission for the Study of Ethical Problems in Medicine and Biomedical and Behavioral Research (President's Commission) was established on November 9, 1978, by Pub. L. 95–622. One of the charges to the President's Commission was to report biennially to the president, Congress, and appropriate federal departments and agencies on the protection of humans involved in biomedical and behavioral research. The President's Commission was directed to conduct a review of the adequacy and uniformity of (1) the rules, policies, guidelines, and regulations of all federal departments and agencies regarding the protection of humans in biomedical or behavioral research that such departments and agencies conduct or support, and (2) the implementation of such rules, policies, guidelines, and regulations by such agencies, including appropriate recommendations for legislation and administrative action.

In December 1981, the President's Commission issued its first biennial report, entitled *First Biennial Report on the Adequacy and Uniformity of Federal Rules and Policies, and Their Implementation, for the Protection of Human Subjects.*[6] Morris B. Abram, chairman of the President's Commission, noted in his transmittal to the president:

> The Commission does not propose any major changes in the substance of the rules on human research, although a number of adjustments are recommended to recognize the flexibility needed by research institutions, particularly in responding to allegations of wrongdoing or other problems. We also propose a simple improvement in the reports filed by researchers, to provide information on the number of subjects and on any that are adversely affected by participation in a research project.
>
> The Commission does recommend one major organization change, namely that a uniform core of regulations be adopted, based upon the present rules of the Department of Health and Human Services, and that HHS become the lead agency in this field. This consolidation would eliminate needless duplication in the rules of the 23 other Federal entities that support or regulate research, thereby simplifying both local compliance with the rules and Federal oversight of the system. Copies of this report are being sent to all affected Federal agencies, with a request for action, pursuant to the Commission's enabling legislation.[6]

The Commission's report specified which departments and agencies it thought were involved. Barbara Mishkin of the President's Commission staff worked with Charles McCarthy, director of OPRR, to identify federal departments and agencies that conduct or support research involving human subjects, and it was here that this idea for a core policy was really begun. Ultimately, some of the agencies declared that that they did not do human subjects research, reducing the field to 16 or 17 agencies. In fact those agencies that indicated they were not doing any research may have been doing so, given that the definition of research is so broad.

The law that created the President's Commission required that each federal department or agency that received recommendations from the Commission with respect to its rules, policies, guidelines, or regulations, should publish the recommendations in the *Federal Register* and provide an opportunity for interested persons to submit written data, views, and arguments with respect to adoption of the recommendations. A decade of work to carry out the President's Commission's recommendations thus began.

From the outset it was clear that a coordinating mechanism would be necessary. For each federal department and agency to respond individually to the recommendations would be laborious and time consuming, if not unwieldy and impractical. Recent efforts to coordinate gathering and sharing of intelligence information among federal agencies, and even the need to create a new cabinet-level Department of Homeland Security to deal with a matter as essential and critical as defense against terrorism, dramatically underscore the complexity encountered when undertaking an interagency initiative of any kind, even when the rationale is sound and the need great. An interdepartmental or interagency initiative to achieve this type of coordination would prove challenging, especially because there were few clear-cut precedents for jointly publishing policies or regulations in common on issues of this scope.

OPRR Director McCarthy took the initiative with officials from the Office of Science and Technology Policy (OSTP), the Office of Management and Budget (OMB), and DHHS leadership to discuss how coordination could be accomplished with OPRR as the lead agency. On March 29, 1982, DHHS Secretary Richard S. Schweiker published the President's Commission's first biennial report on behalf of all the departments and agencies affected by the recommendations.[7]

In May 1982 the chairman of the Federal Coordinating Council for Science, Engineering and Technology (FCCSET) appointed an Ad Hoc Committee for the Protection of Human Research Subjects under the auspices of the FCCSET. This committee, chaired by Edward N. Brandt Jr., DHHS assistant secretary for health, was composed of representatives of affected departments and agencies. In consultation with OSTP and OMB, the Ad Hoc Committee was charged with developing responses to the recommendations of the President's Commission. An Interagency Human Subjects Coordinating Committee was chartered in October 1983 under the auspices of the FCCSET to provide continued interagency cooperation in the protection of humans in research after the Ad Hoc Committee had completed its assignment. It was chaired by the director of OPRR and had basically the same membership as the Ad Hoc Committee.

The Ad Hoc, and later standing, Committee met over many months to respond to the first recommendation in the President's Commission's First Biennial Report:

The President should, through appropriate action, require that all federal departments and agencies adopt as a common core the regulations governing research with human subjects issued by the Department of Health and Human Services (codified at 45 CFR 46), as periodically amended or revised, while permitting additions needed by any department or agency that are not inconsistent with these core provisions.[6]

The Committee produced a Model Policy to apply to research involving humans that is conducted, supported, or regulated by federal departments and agencies. The Model Policy encompassed only what was equivalent in scope to Subpart A of 45 CFR 46. Clearly OMB wished to have as much uniformity as possible and required several modifications and compromises in the Committee's draft that would minimize the "departures" from the core policy that had been added by various departments and agencies. After considerable discussion and negotiation, the department or agency heads, or their designees, concurred in the Model Policy in March 1985. It was not until June 3, 1986, however, that the Proposed Model Federal Policy was published in the *Federal Register* on behalf of 16 federal departments and agencies.[8]

During the intervening 14 months, OMB and OSTP acted to diminish the number of "departures" from the core policy through which many of the participating federal departments and agencies sought to accommodate their own organizational structures, procedures, and philosophies, and possibly to protect their own interests when deemed necessary. The position of the OMB was that there should be no departures unless there were statutory requirements for them in department and agency legislation, as was the case for the FDA. This position was not met with enthusiastic acceptance by the agencies, some of which may not have had specific legislative exceptions to substantiate their desired departures.

Despite the considerable efforts expended to promote uniformity among the agency positions, when the Model Policy was finally published there were still several departures indicated. Twelve agencies had no departures; the Department of Education had one; DHHS had two; FDA had two; and the Veterans Administration, now the Department of Veterans Affairs (VA), had many. To meet the concerns of the President's Commission that unnecessary and confusing regulations would impose burdens on institutions conducting research, the policy was drafted to have the following: uniform procedures for assurance and certification; consistency in IRB roles, responsibilities, and composition; provisions to assure compliance; procedures for expedited review; and provisions for obtaining and documenting informed consent. The specific intention was that departments and agencies could have their own implementing directives and procedures to supplement the Model Policy. The Model Policy was drafted in the form of a policy statement rather than in the form of a regulation so that departments and agencies could reference it within a reasonable time and in a manner that each department or agency was accustomed to using.

The President's Commission also recommended that the president authorize and direct the secretary of DHHS to designate an office with government-wide jurisdiction to coordinate, monitor, and evaluate the implementation of all federal regulations governing research with humans. The Ad Hoc Committee recommended that OPRR, then housed within the NIH, serve in the coordinating role. The OPRR director became the head of a standing committee of the FCCSET, the Interagency Human Subjects Coordinating Committee, which was chartered in 1983, and the Ad Hoc Committee was integrated into the new one. The new committee, composed of representatives of federal departments and agencies that conduct, support, or regulate research involving humans, was to evaluate the implementation of the Model Policy and recommend changes as necessary.

An Addition to the 1981 DHHS Regulations

On March 4, 1982, DHHS issued a "Notice of Waiver" in the *Federal Register.*[9] DHHS had been faced with a lawsuit raising the issue whether demonstration projects in the Social Security Administration constituted research under 45 CFR 46. The waiver was issued under 45 CFR 46(e). It pertained to demonstration projects approved under section 1115 of the Social Security Act, which test the use of cost-sharing, such as deductibles, copayment and coinsurance, in the Medicaid program. The rationale for the waiver was that it would facilitate the timely and efficient operation of demonstration projects that are likely to assist in promoting the objectives of the Medicaid program. Demonstration projects are pilot programs designed to determine if a particular practice or policy is effective in the setting(s) in which it is ultimately intended to be used. These projects are intended to provide evidence or proof that the practice or policy is valid or sound. The waiver was effected immediately with the publication of the Notice in the *Federal Register.* The Notice of Waiver was followed on March 22, 1982, with a "Notice of Proposed Rulemaking,"[10] whereby DHHS proposed to include among the types of research specifically exempt from the application of the regulatory requirement of 45 CFR 46, research and demonstration projects conducted under the Social Security Act and other federal statutory authority and designed to study certain public benefit or service programs, the procedures for obtaining benefits or services under those programs, and possible changes or alternative to those programs or procedures, including changes in methods or levels of payment. The argument was that these demonstration and service projects were already subject to procedures that provide for extensive review by high-level officials in the department and that IRB review would be duplicative and burdensome to state and local agencies and to other entities participating in demonstration projects. The proposed exemption would have added item (6) to the list in 46.101(b) as follows:

> Unless specifically required by statute, research and demonstration projects which are conducted by or subject to the approval of the Department of Health and Human Services, and which are designed to study, evaluate, or otherwise examine: (i) Programs under the Social Security Act, or other public benefit or service programs; (ii) procedures for obtaining benefits or services under those programs; (iii) possible changes in or alternatives to those programs or procedures; or (iv) possible changes in methods or levels of payment for benefits or services under those programs.[10]

Among the commentators on this provision was the President's Commission itself. The Commission proposed alternative language that would not have exempted research that reduced benefits to some recipients, whereas others in similar circumstances continued to receive a higher level of benefits. The Commission proposed that research projects in any way limiting or reducing the benefits to which recipients would otherwise be entitled would continue to be subject to IRB review. DHHS did not adopt the Commission's alternative, however.

The Final Rule was published on March 4, 1983, with language modified in response to public comment.[11] To ensure the continued protection of human research participants, DHHS added a specific requirement for written informed consent even if the research was exempt. In the Final Rule, DHHS modified the proposed exemption in 45 CFR 46 to indicate in part (i) of section 101 the following:

> If, following review of proposed research activities that are exempt from these regulations under paragraph (b)(6), the Secretary determines that a research or demonstration project presents a danger to the physical, mental, or emotional well-being of a participant or subject of the research or demonstration project, then federal funds may not be expended for such a project without the written, informed consent of each participant or subject.[11]

Section 116 was further modified by the addition of part (c), which provided that the IRB could approve a consent procedure that does not include or that alters some or all of the elements of informed consent; or it could waive consent altogether if the research or demonstration project is to be conducted by, or subject to, the approval of state or local government officials and is designed to study, evaluate, or otherwise assess the areas listed in 101(b)(6), and the research could not practicably be carried out without the waiver or alteration.

The drafting committee for the Model Policy now had an addition to DHHS regulations to consider for incorporation into the Model Federal Policy. The proposed Model Federal Policy published in 1986 changed the "public benefits exemption" only slightly in Section 101(b)(5) to drop the reference to programs under the Social Security Act and to change DHHS as the approving authority and to substitute in its place the department or agency head. Section 116(c) was similarly modified. The exemption remains as perhaps one of the most misunderstood and misused of the Common Rule exemptions.

Highlights of the Proposed Model Policy

The Model Policy was based on the 1981 version of 45 CFR 46, but there were some modifications. The Model Policy contained a definition of regulated research and identified which sections of the policy were applicable to regulated research. Some drafting had to be done to exclude FDA from the provision requiring assurances in advance of the conduct of research; this was considered to be inconsistent with the operating provisions of FDA's new drug approval (NDA) process.

Under then existing DHHS regulations, which had been adopted in 1981, certain classes of research were exempt from IRB review and approval. Changes in these exemptions were arguably the most significant modifications under the newly proposed Model Policy. The Model Policy revised certain exemptions to make them clearer. For example, in the 1981 version of Subpart A of the DHHS regulations, the exemption at 46.101(b)(2) read: "Research involving the use of educational tests (cognitive, diagnostic, aptitude, achievement), if information taken from these sources is recorded in such a manner that subjects cannot be identified, directly or through identifiers linked to the subjects."[12]

The exemption at 46.101(b)(3) read as follows:

Research involving survey or interview procedures, except where *all* of the following conditions exist: (i) Responses are recorded in a manner that the human subjects can be identified, directly or through identifiers linked to the subjects, (ii) the subject's responses, if they became known outside the research, could reasonably place the subject at risk of criminal or civil liability or be damaging to the subject's financial standing or employability, *and* (iii) the research deals with sensitive aspects of the subject's own behavior, such as illegal conduct, drug use, sexual behavior, or use of alcohol. All research involving survey or interview procedures is exempt, without exception, when the respondents are elected or appointed public officials or candidates for public office [emphasis added].[12]

And the exemption at 46.101(b)(4) read as follows:

Research involving the observation (including observation by participants) of public behavior, except where *all* of the following conditions exist: (i) Observations are recorded in such a manner that the human subjects can be identified, directly or through identifiers linked to the subjects, (ii) the observations recorded about the individual, if they became known outside the research, could reasonably place the subject at risk of criminal or civil liability or be damaging to the subject's financial standing or employability, and (iii) the research deals with sensitive aspects of the subject's own behavior such as illegal conduct, drug use, sexual behavior, or use of alcohol [emphasis added].[12]

The Model Policy, however, combined these three exemptions into two at sections 101(b)(2) and (3). These were as follows:

(2) Research involving the use of educational tests (cognitive, diagnostic, aptitude, achievement) survey procedures, interview procedures or observation of public behavior, *unless:*

(i) information obtained is recorded in such a manner that human subjects can be identified, directly or through identifiers linked to the subjects; *and*

(ii) any disclosure of the human subjects' responses outside the research could reasonably place the subjects at risk of criminal or civil liability or be damaging to the subjects' financial standing or employability [emphasis added].[8]

And,

(3) Research involving the use of educational tests (cognitive, diagnostic, aptitude, achievement), survey procedures, interview procedures or observation of public behavior that is exempt under paragraph (2), if:

(i) the human subjects are elected or appointed public officials or candidates for public office; or

(ii) federal statute(s) require(s) without exception that the confidentiality of the personally identifiable information will be maintained through the research and thereafter.[8]

In 1981, three requirements had to be in place if the research could not be exempted. In the Model Policy, only two criteria had to be met before the research could not be exempted.

To accommodate the Department of Justice and the Department of Education, a clause was added to the exemption at section 101(b)(3)(ii) that would permit research involving the use of

educational tests, survey procedures, interview procedures, or observation of public behavior to be exempt even if identifiers were recorded and a disclosure of the research participants' responses outside the research could place them at risk of criminal or civil liability or be damaging to their financial standing or employability. Under this provision, the research also could still be exempt if "federal statutes(s) require(s) without exception that the confidentiality of the personally identifiable information will be maintained throughout the research and thereafter."[8]

In this process, a new exemption was created that had to be negotiated with the FDA, the Environmental Protection Agency, and the Department of Agriculture to harmonize the terms with existing regulations and policies; this is known as the "taste and food quality evaluation study exemption." Each organization had its own terms in legislation or regulation that had to be carefully woven into the exemption to accomplish what all wanted to do to permit an exemption for taste and food quality evaluation studies where other safeguards were in place.

The Model Policy incorporated a new section, 101(g), to state what was only implicit in the DHHS regulation, namely, that the Model Policy does not affect any foreign laws or regulations that may otherwise be applicable and that provide additional protections for humans in research.[8] Furthermore, in section 101(h), it allows department and agency heads discretion in accepting equivalent procedures for research carried out in foreign countries, although it offers no definition or guidance as to what policies and procedures might be considered to provide "equivalent protections."[8] Departments and agencies are still struggling with how exactly to determine equivalency. For example, is another country's requirement to have an IRB-like body sufficient, or must that body have exactly the same kinds of functions and membership composition requirements as those under the Common Rule? To date, few departments or agencies have issued announcements of what would be equivalent protections in the method prescribed by section 101(h), although in 2002 the OHRP impaneled a DHHS working group to develop guidelines for making such a determination of equivalent protections. The report of that working group was published in July 2003 for public comments without further action at the time of this writing.[13]

A long period of negotiation was required with OMB and the Department of Justice regarding the language concerned with IRB membership. Section 107 of the Model Policy replaced the requirement in the DHHS regulations that if an IRB regularly reviews research that involves a special or "vulnerable" category of participants, the IRB must include one or more individuals who are primarily concerned with the welfare of those individuals. In the Model Policy, the inclusion of such an individual is left to the institution establishing the IRB. This was done in the spirit of deregulation. Although the 1981 DHHS regulations also indicated that no IRB may consist entirely of men or entirely of women, or entirely of members of one profession, OMB representatives in consultation with Department of Justice wanted the language to indicate the following:

Every nondiscriminatory effort will be made to ensure that no IRB consists entirely of men or entirely of women, including the institution's consideration of qualified persons of both sexes, so long as no selection is made to the IRB on the basis of gender. No IRB may consist entirely of members of one profession.[8] [finally incorporated as Section 107(b)]

This modification was requested in the spirit of moving away from any appearance of quotas.

By far the largest concern from public commentators concerned section 103(a) of the Model Policy and the "grace period." The 1981 regulations required certification of IRB review and approval by the institution receiving funds when the research is supported by a federal department or agency and not exempt. Along with the submission of an application or proposal for approval or support, an institution with an approved assurance covering the research was to certify that the application or proposal had been reviewed and approved by the IRB within 60 days of submission of the application or proposal. These were the institutions holding so-called Multiple Project Assurances, generally institutions with a large volume of research activity and well-established infrastructures for human research administration and oversight. Institutions without an approved assurance covering the research had to certify within 30 days after receipt of a request for such a certification from DHHS that the application or proposal had been approved by the IRB.

The Model Policy stated, however, that if the certification is not submitted with the application or proposal (or within 30 days after request for the institutions with no assurances covering the research), the application or proposal may be returned to the institution. The preamble to the Model Policy announced that there would be no grace period incorporated into the policy, whereas the 1981 DHHS regulations had explicitly permitted institutions that held an approved assurance to delay submission of certification of IRB review and approval until 60 days after submission of an application or proposal for financial support.

Most of the groups that represented the colleges and universities responded with concern that they couldn't work under this provision. They were used to turning in the certifications of IRB review long after the applications and proposals had been submitted to DHHS. Although the grace period was not explicitly noted in the Model Policy, this did not mean that there would be no grace period allowed. The idea was that each department and agency would need to decide what grace period it would permit and make that known through an information process other than incorporation explicitly into the Model Policy. When institutions and professional groups understood that the grace period was not being taken away in DHHS procedures simply by removing reference to it explicitly in the regulation, the swell of concern abated. DHHS had in the departure section of the published policy a comment that it would evaluate whether ending the grace period was an appropriate step before the next iteration of the policy could be published.

Two Years Later

The Model Policy next surfaced in the *Federal Register* on November 10, 1988.[14] The OSTP again published the proposed policy on behalf of the participating departments and agencies. Each time a proposed or final document was published in the *Federal Register,* the long bureaucratic process of department and agency clearance to the topmost echelons of the organizations had to occur. When administrations changed, new officials had to be briefed and convinced that the Model Policy or common regulations were important to issue.

The 1988 publication in the *Federal Register* served both as a notice that a final Model Policy was forthcoming and as a formal Notice of Proposed Rulemaking in compliance with the requirements of the Administrative Procedure Act. Over the course of the 2 years since its previous publication, there continued to be concerns on the part of the Interagency Committee and the OMB that too many departures could be made from the core policy.

As noted, over 200 public comments came in concerning the 1986 proposed Model Policy; most requested continuation of a grace period. The comments came primarily from medical schools and other academic institutions, some from professional associations, industry, IRBs, and research administrators. Almost unanimously, the respondents enthusiastically supported the concept of a Model Federal Policy, provided a grace period was retained. The Interagency Committee did revise the Final Model Policy to indicate that the certification of IRB review and approval must accompany the application or proposal unless the department or agency specified a later date for submission of the certification. DHHS announced in the preamble to the 1988 Model Policy/ Proposed Rule that it intended to retain the "grace period" administratively. Other departments and agencies would have to advise institutions of appropriate timing of certification through their information dissemination mechanisms.

Because the departments and agencies were not required to use the Model Policy, the burdens of redundant and confusing policies on institutions carrying out research involving humans could continue if inconsistencies in federal policies and procedures persisted. Further, DHHS, the Department of Energy, and some other departments and agencies had regulations that did not conform to the Model Policy and would have to be formally updated: The Model Policy itself was not binding. Clearly, regulations were in order.

The Interagency Committee, with the help of OMB, made several other changes in response to public comments on the 1986 proposed Model Policy. For example, one of the exemptions was modified so that the effect of disclosure of identifiable information on the "reputation" of an individual was to be taken into consideration. The taste and food quality evaluation exemption was clarified, a definition of IRB was included, and some further clarifications on reporting requirements were added.

One area of discussion in the preamble of the Final Model Policy/Notice of Proposed Rulemaking was that the Veterans Administration (VA), which had proposed many departures from the Common Rule, indicated that it did not intend to have assurances under Section 103 for its Medical Centers that participated in research. That policy changed dramatically in 1988. VA, which became a cabinet-level Department of Veterans Affairs the following year, indicated that it would withdraw all of its departures, but would narrowly construe exemptions and the informed consent provision to be consistent with other statutory requirements on it. VA recognized that it could, by internal policies that applied to its intramural research program, address many concerns about adequate protections for veterans and others in VA research.

The Department of Education now had two proposed departures from the Common Rule language. That department proposed that one of the exemptions relating to research involving the use of educational tests, survey procedures, interview procedures, or observations of public behavior could be used if the research was under a program subject to the General Education Provisions Act. In addition, the Department of Education now proposed another departure concerning membership on IRBs. This departure resulted from the special concern about providing additional safeguards for mentally disabled persons and handicapped children who are involved in research. Thus, the Department of Education proposed a rewording of language in section 107 of the Common Rule to apply to research under Department of Education auspices providing the following:

> When an IRB reviews research that deals with handicapped children or mentally disabled persons, the IRB shall include at least one person primarily concerned with the welfare of the research subjects. If an IRB regularly reviews research that involves other vulnerable categories of subjects, such as non-handicapped children, prisoners, or pregnant women, consideration shall be given to one or more individuals who are knowledgeable about and experienced in working with these subjects.[15]

FDA had two departures from the proposed Model Policy. First, FDA indicated that it must diverge from the proposal with regard to research that takes place in foreign countries. For clinical investigations that take place in a foreign country and are conducted under research permits granted by FDA, FDA must follow provisions of the Food, Drug, and Cosmetic Act; in other words, FDA does not have the authority to accept the procedures followed in a foreign country in lieu of the procedure required by FDA's authorizing legislation. The second departure was in the area of informed consent requirements. The Food, Drug, and Cosmetic Act requires that informed consent be obtained from all those enrolled in clinical investigations except in limited circumstances. Therefore, the FDA could not use the waiver provision offered in the proposed Model Policy.

Three More Years

Three years, and another round of public comments were to pass before publication of a final rule in 1991. Of course, during those years, there would be yet another change of administrations, another team of new players, and a new thrust to miniize regulations. The majority of public comments made on the 1988 "Notice of Proposed Rulemaking" were in three categories. First, some commentators were concerned because Sec.103(b)(5) of the Common Rule required institutions holding assurances to report unanticipated problems or scientific misconduct to department and agency heads. "Scientific misconduct" reporting appeared to expand the role of the IRB into areas covered by other regulations and policies and handled through channels other than the IRB in many institutions.

Additional concerns were raised about which kinds of suspensions of research made by the IRB had to be reported to department and agency heads—for example, whether suspensions simply for tardiness in submission of materials had to be treated the same way as suspensions for some substantive reason relating to the research. In response to concerns, the Interagency Human Subjects Coordinating Committee dropped from the Common Rule the requirement to report scientific misconduct. Further, the Preamble to the Common Rule clarified that reports did not have to be made to the heads of departments or agencies, but that they would be made to whomever in those organizations was delegated authority. Agencies had the flexibility to establish channels of reporting to meet their own individual requirements.

Another major concern involved the composition of IRBs. The majority of the comments were directed to the departure from the proposed Common Rule requested by the Department of Education in 1988. As noted, the department proposed that when an IRB reviews research that deals with handicapped children or mentally disabled persons, the IRB should include at least one person primarily concerned with the welfare of the research participants. The majority of the 21 commentators on this matter thought that the proposed departure was unnecessary and that there were many other groups that might need special representation on the IRB.

Negotiations in the OSTP and the OMB took place over many months so that a suitable arrangement could be worked out and all of the participating departments and agencies could move on to promulgate the Common Rule. The Department of Education withdrew its proposed departure regarding the Sec.101(b)(3) exemption and accepted the language we have today. The secretary of the Department of Education decided, however, to address the concerns outlined in the 1988 proposed departure concerning IRB composition by amending other regulations concerning the department's National Institute on Disability and Rehabilitation Research (34 CFR parts 350 and 356). In addition, the word *handicapped* was added to the examples of potentially vulnerable populations found in Sec.107 of the Common Rule.

A further set of comments involved the proposed exemptions. Some expressed concern that some of the exemptions would allow sensitive data to be used in such a way that subjects would be at risk. The regulations at 45 CFR 46 Subpart D, the so-called Children's Regulations promulgated by DHHS in 1983,[17] do not permit research involving survey or interview procedures, or observation of public behavior, except when the investigator(s) do not participate in the activities being observed.

The proposed Final Rule introduced a footnote to indicate that the exemptions could not be used for children. A provision of DHHS regulations was thus added with virtually no public input as an additional protection to children as a class of vulnerable individuals.

The area that had previously caused so much comment, the "grace" period, was again the area most addressed by the public in comments on the Notice of Proposed Rulemaking. Again, commentators wanted 60 days after submission of a research application or proposal to provide certification of IRB review and approval, as had been customary in DHHS policy. The Preamble to the Common Rule indicated that many federal departments and agencies do not have application review schedules that correspond to those of DHHS. A 60-day grace period is without relevance to their review systems. The proposed Final Rule made no reference to such a grace period, but rather indicated that certification must be submitted with the application or proposal or by such later date as may be prescribed by the department of agency to which the application or proposal is submitted. Thus, the timing was left to an administrative level of decision in each department or agency.

Finally, on June 18, 1991, OSTP published the Federal Policy for the Protection of Human Subjects as a Final Rule.[18] Upon promulgation of the final rule, the Interagency Committee became a temporary subcommittee of the FCCSET Committee on Life Science and Health (CLSH) and was redesignated as the CLSH Human Subjects Research Subcommittee. Sixteen federal departments and agencies had signed on, and the Central Intelligence Agency, which was required by Executive Order to follow DHHS rules, was also included. At last, after a decade of incubation and nurturing, the Common Rule, as it has come to be known, was born.

Now that the Common Rule has been in effect for more than a decade, its strengths and weaknesses have been probed and are better understood. Although the adoption of the Common Rule was itself a major milestone and accomplishment, its promise has never been fully realized, and perhaps never will be. Many have suggested that major and more fundamental reform may be necessary to achieve a more effective and efficient human research process. The DHHS Inspector General, the National Bioethics Advisory Commission (NBAC), the Government Accountability Office, and the Congress have questioned whether such reforms can be accomplished under the regulatory framework of the Common Rule. Understanding the basis for these concerns is critical for continuing progress.

The Following Years

In 1994, the Human Subject Research Subcommittee (HSRS) was rechartered under the auspices of the Committee on Health, Safety and Food of the National Science and Technology Council (NSTC), the successor to FCCSET. A restructuring of NSTC committees resulted in the redesignation of HSRS as a subcommittee of the NSTC Committee on Science (COS) in 1997.

On October 3, 1995, President Clinton issued Executive Order 12975, Protection of Human Subjects and Creation of National Bioethics Advisory Commission, requiring, among other provisions, each department and agency that conducts, supports, or regulates research involving humans to review the protections of the rights and welfare of humans in research that are afforded by the department's or agency's policies and procedures and report to NBAC. Furthermore, the Executive Order required that, to the extent practicable and appropriate, each affected department and agency develop professional and public education programs to enhance activities related to the protection of humans involved in research.

The Human Subject Research Subcommittee still exists as of 2007, and retains a coordinating role in interpreting policies and exchanging information about human research participant protection issues, but it had not attempted major harmonization efforts to streamline the federal regulatory and oversight processes for human research. Shortly after the creation of OHRP in June 2000, the charter for the subcommittee was revised to include other departments and agencies that were not part of the original group that promulgated the Common Rule or participated in its development. Additions included the Smithsonian Institution, the Appalachian Regional Commission, the National Foundation on the Arts and the Humanities, the Nuclear Regulatory Commission, the Social Security Administration, and the Small Business Administration.

Originally chaired by the director of OHRP, the Human Subject Research Subcommittee is now chaired by designees from both OHRP and the National Science Foundation. This structure essentially reflects the shared chairmanship of the parent Committee on Science, without a specific cochair from OSTP. The emphasis on behavioral and social science research relative to biomedical research is perhaps now more prominent given the change in leadership for the subcommittee. Organizationally and administratively, the Human Subject Research Subcommittee is

hierarchically placed so as to report to the NSTC Committee on Science, and it has limited autonomy and no policy-making authority.

Under its new charter and operating procedures, the subcommittee is charged with coordinating interpretation of policies and procedures for protections of humans involved in research across federal agencies, but it has made only modest progress in this area relative to the magnitude of the task at hand. The subcommittee also attempts to integrate interdepartmental approaches for the protection of human subjects, thereby supporting the department and agency heads who promulgated the Common Rule and other departments and agencies to which Executive Order 12975 applies. In so doing, the subcommittee provides a source of advice and a mechanism for development of a consistent approach to implementation of the final Common Rule, as well as a clear and uniform interpretation of the Common Rule and related federal policies.

The major strength of the subcommittee at this point in time is that it serves as a consistent and responsible forum for networking and exchange of information comparing and contrasting implementation practices. It also serves as a body from which federal liaisons and experts can be drawn to support work of such groups as the DHHS Secretary's Advisory Committee on Human Research Protections. Members of the subcommittee represent the interests and views of their own departments and agencies, and major regulatory or policy change requires agreement of all departments and agencies at the highest level before change can occur. Leadership of OMB and OSTP, or some other authority above the departments and agencies, is required now as it was in the past when the Common Rule was created. This makes changing the Common Rule difficult, even when change is consistent with the subcommittee's charge.

An example is the initiative to secure adoption of a unified assurance mechanism for use by all Common Rule agencies. Prior to December 2000, there had been a proliferation of several types of assurance mechanisms, both within DHHS and among the federal agencies. The assurance process had become an arcane paper-laden exercise in bureaucracy that utilized much of the resources and personnel of OPRR, focusing more on the assurance document itself than on substantive efforts to protect human subjects. The formal adoption in 2005 of a dramatically streamlined, uniform, federalwide assurance mechanism for the protection of humans in research—an effort spearheaded by OHRP, and endorsed by the Human Subject Research Subcommittee (or at least, not opposed by it)—was a significant accomplishment. That it took 5 years of discussions at the interagency level after approval by the Human Subject Research Subcommittee to secure final approval by OMB suggests that even when the agency representatives to HSRS may be in agreement, there is no assurance that others at the agency level will support a given change. Furthermore, changes are often subject to other procedural requirements, such as the Paperwork Reduction Act and the Administrative Procedure Act, compliance with which are necessary for OMB approval.

This example underscores the enormity of the achievement that we now call the Common Rule. It also demonstrates that without a central committee or office with appropriate authority to effect such changes, future efforts to simplify and harmonize policies and procedures across the federal departments and agencies for protection of human research participants established within the framework of the Common Rule will not be easy or timely, even if greatly desired. In fact, in its 1998 report on the status of the national human subjects protection process,[19] the DHHS Office of Inspector General concluded that the Common Rule might actually be an impediment to reform of the system because of the need to secure clearance and approval of any substantive changes from all of the signatory agencies.

The NBAC echoed this view and proposed the creation of an independent National Office for Human Research Oversight (NOHRO) to assume overall responsibility for federal human participant protection policies and their enforcement.[20] Over the past several years, legislation to strengthen and streamline the system for protection of humans in research has been introduced in both the House of Representatives and the Senate, but to date, none has advanced out of committee for votes on the floor, and few believe that much progress is likely until there is another tragedy resulting in harm to human subjects.

In the interim, several areas for action have been identified. Perhaps foremost among these is the need to harmonize provisions for additional protections beyond Subpart A for special populations of research subjects, including women and fetuses, prisoners, children, persons with impaired decision-making capacity, and those who participate in classified research. Such protections are currently provided for DHHS-supported or DHHS-conducted studies under Subparts B, C, and D, but these subparts have not been adopted by all of the signatories to the Common Rule. Within the past year, the DHHS Secretary's Advisory Committee on Human Research Protections, which replaced the National Human Research Protections Advisory Committee in 2002, continued to focus on the issues related to special protections, with participation by ex-officio members from departments and agencies other than DHHS. All recognize that making changes in the Common Rule through a regulatory change process will likely be a long and arduous path as all of the departments and agencies are tied together. This is unfortunate and somewhat ironic, because most major research institutions receiving federal support, under the terms of their institutional assurances, already apply the provisions of Subparts B, C, and D to all research conducted under those assurances regardless of the source of funding.

One of the greatest strengths of the Common Rule, ironically, is also one of its greatest weaknesses in practice. Because the Common Rule was intentionally stated in general terms, essentially providing guidelines and some requirements to implement the recommendations of the National Commission, its application permits a great deal of flexibility, but also requires a large measure of interpretation and good judgment. In an era when many institutions are still primarily concerned about the potential consequences of compliance failures, there is great hesitation to stray far from the well-beaten path.

Guidance on many of the provisions of the Common Rule has been offered by the federal agencies, but these are not always entirely consistent, leaving research institutions and their review boards in a difficult position. In some cases, the activity in question may be viewed by some agencies as research that is subject to regulation, whereas another agency may classify the very same activity as an educational exercise or a program evaluation that is not subject to regulation. Health services research, quality improvement activities, oral histories, and evaluation of education programs or public health programs are not discussed in detail in either the Belmont Report or the regulations, and agency guidance

has sometimes been insufficient or nonspecific. Additional guidance, in and of itself, may be useful on the one hand, but it can create even greater confusion when unusual cases arise that do not fit neatly within the analytical or practical framework used to formulate the guidance.

Many IRBs find it confusing, impractical, illogical, or even unethical to apply different regulations and standards for protection of humans in research simply on the basis of the source of support, particularly when the rules are supposedly based upon fundamental ethical principles for responsible conduct of research with humans, principles that ought to command widespread support. Indeed, the original intent behind promulgation of a true common rule, as envisioned by the President's Commission nearly a quarter century ago, was to avoid such confusion and its attendant inconsistencies and inefficiencies. Reconciliation of the outstanding differences in interpretation and application of the provisions of the Common Rule, and adoption of harmonized provisions for protection of those in need of protections in addition to those currently afforded under the Common Rule, ought to be a high priority for the federal government, not only for protecting the interests, rights, and well-being of research participants, but for promoting and facilitating the responsible conduct of high quality biomedical, social, and behavioral research in the interest of all. Many dedicated people are still striving to make it happen.

Disclaimer

The opinions presented in this paper are solely those of the authors. They do not represent the official policy or opinion of the Department of Veterans Affairs or of the Office of Research Oversight.

References

1. Katz J, with Capron AM, Glass ES. *Experimentation With Human Beings.* New York, N.Y.: Russell Sage Foundation; 1972.
2. Advisory Committee on Human Radiation Experiments. *Final Report of the Advisory Committee on Human Radiation Experiments.* New York: Oxford University Press; 1996.
3. The National Commission for the Protection of Human Subjects of Biomedical and Behavioral Research. *The Belmont Report: Ethical Principles and Guidelines for the Protection of Human Subjects of Research.* Washington, D.C.: Department of Health, Education and Welfare; DHEW Publication OS 78-0012 1978. [Online] Available: http://www.hhs.gov/ohrp/humansubjects/guidance/belmont.htm.
4. Department of Health and Human Services, National Institutes of Health, and Office for Human Research Protections. The Common Rule, Title 45 (Public Welfare), Code of Federal Regulations, Part 46 (Protection of Human Subjects). [Online] June 23, 2005. Available: http://www.hhs.gov/ohrp/humansubjects/guidance/45cfr46.htm.
5. Office for Protection from Research Risks, National Institutes of Health, Department of Health and Human Services. Protection of Human Subjects: Categories of Research That May Be Reviewed by the Institutional Review Board (IRB) Through an Expedited Review Procedure; Notice. *Federal Register* 1998;63(216):60364–7.
6. President's Commission for the Study of Ethical Problems in Medicine and Biomedical and Behavioral Research. *Protecting Human Subjects: First Biennial Report on the Adequacy and Uniformity of Federal Rules and Policies, and of Their Implementation, for the Protection of Human Subjects.* Washington, D.C.: U.S. Government Printing Office; 1981.

7. Department of Health and Human Services. Protection of Human Subjects: First Biennial Report on the Adequacy and Uniformity of Federal Rules and Policies, and Their Implementation for the Protection of Human Subjects in Biomedical and Behavioral Research; Report of the President's Commission for the Study of Ethical Problems in Medicine and Biomedical and Behavioral Research; Notice of Report for Public Comment. *Federal Register* 1982;47(60):13272–305.

8. Office of Science and Technology Policy, Executive Office of the President. Proposed Model Federal Policy for Protection of Human Subjects; Response to the First Biennial Report of the President's Commission for the Study of Ethical Problems in Medicine and Biomedical and Behavioral Research. *Federal Register* 1986;51(106):20204–17.

9. Office of the Secretary, Department of Health and Human Services. Waiver of Requirement as Applied to Medicaid Demonstration Projects Involving Cost-Sharing (Copayments, Deductibles, Coinsurance); Notice of Waiver. *Federal Register* 1982;47(43):9208.

10. Office of the Secretary, Department of Health and Human Services. Exemption of Certain Research and Demonstration Projects From Regulations for Protection of Human Research Subjects; Notice of Proposed Rulemaking. *Federal Register* 1982;47(55):12276–7.

11. Office of the Secretary, Department of Health and Human Services. Exemption of Certain Research and Demonstration Projects From Regulations for Protection of Human Research Subjects; Final Rule. *Federal Register* 1983;48(44):9266–70.

12. Office of the Secretary, Department of Health and Human Services. 45 CFR Part 46: Final Regulations Amending Basic HHS Policy for the Protection of Human Research Subjects; Final Rule. *Federal Register* 1981;465(16)8366–91.

13. Department of Health and Human Services. Report of the Equivalent Protections Working Group. [Online] July 17, 2003. Available: http://www.hhs.gov/ohrp/international/EPWG Report2003.pdf.

14. Office of Science and Technology Policy, Executive Office of the President. Federal Policy for the Protection of Human Subjects; Notice of Federal Policy for Protection of Human Subjects. *Federal Register* 1988;53(218):45660–82.

15. Secretary, Department of Education. 34 CFR Part 97. *Federal Register* 1988;53(218):45670.

16. Secretary, Department of Education. 34 CFR Parts 350 and 356. Protection of Human Subjects—Disability and Rehabilitation Research: General Provisions, Disability and Rehabilitation Research: Research Fellowships; Interim Final Regulations With an Opportunity to Comment. *Federal Register* 1991;56(117):28029–32.

17. Office of the Secretary, Department of Health and Human Services. 45 CFR Part 46: Additional Protections for Children Involved as Subjects in Research; Final Rule. *Federal Register* 1983;48(46):9814–20.

18. Office of Science and Technology Policy. Federal Policy for the Protection of Human Subjects; Final Rule. *Federal Register* 1991;56(117):28003–18.

19. Office of Inspector General, Department of Health and Human Services. *Institutional Review Boards: A Time for Reform.* OEI-01-97-00193. Washington, D.C.: DHHS; 1998. [Online] June, 1998. Available: http://oig.hhs.gov/oei/reports/oei-01-97-00193.pdf.

20. National Bioethics Advisory Commission. *Ethical and Policy Issues in Research Involving Human Participants, Vol. I.* Bethesda, Md.: NBAC; 2001. [Online] August 2001. Available: http://www.georgetown.edu/research/nrcbl/nbac/human/overv011.pdf

Juhana E. Idänpään-Heikkilä   Sev S. Fluss

International Ethical Guidance From the Council for International Organizations of Medical Sciences

The Council for International Organizations of Medical Sciences (CIOMS) was formally constituted by the World Health Organization (WHO) and the United Nations Educational, Scientific, and Cultural Organization (UNESCO) in 1949, and it still remains under the aegis of these two specialized UN agencies. Today, CIOMS has more than 70 international and national members, representing a significant proportion of the world's biomedical scientific community. Much of its work in the field of bioethics has been undertaken in close cooperation with WHO. In particular, its 1982 Proposed International Guidelines for Biomedical Research Involving Human Subjects—its first effort to generate guidance in this field—was the outcome of a joint project between CIOMS and WHO. The purpose of these proposed guidelines was to indicate how the ethical principles that were set forth in the 1975 version of the World Medical Association's Declaration of Helsinki[1] could be effectively applied, particularly in developing countries, given their socioeconomic circumstances, laws and regulations, and executive and administrative arrangements.

Just over a decade elapsed before the 1982 proposed guidelines were revised and, following very extensive consultation, the 1993 International Ethical Guidelines for Biomedical Research Involving Human Subjects were formulated and promulgated. Numerous innovative developments in biomedicine and new public health, ethical, and social challenges regarding research with humans in the 1990s required CIOMS to initiate, at the end of 1998, a process to update and revise its 1993 guidelines to respond to these new and often difficult questions. The revised version of the CIOMS Guidelines appeared in 2002.[2]

New Ethical Challenges for Biomedical Research

Research on the effectiveness and safety of disease treatment, diagnosis, and prevention has increased in developing countries, where the application of ethical principles formulated in industrialized countries requires careful consideration and adaptation. However, HIV/AIDS, malaria, tuberculosis, diarrhea, respiratory infections, and many neglected diseases are most prevalent in developing countries, and their control requires local research. Yet traditions of scientific research and the infrastructure for it are limited in many of these poorer locales.

Several new issues and questions have recently arisen in the context of multinational research. For example, low-income developing countries and countries in transition with many untreated patients have become attractive partners for multinational clinical trials. In these circumstances, the use of comparators other than the "best current therapeutic method" by the external sponsor have prompted lively discussion in the scholarly literature.[3–13] The rationale behind the departure from the "best current therapeutic method" standard is that there is a need to test low-cost and technologically appropriate public health solutions that poorer countries can afford, even if this means that comparators in such trials are not the best current interventions. Among the questions raised are the following: Is it not exploitative to conduct a clinical trial of a new product in a population that could not afford to buy it, making the benefits available only to the rich who live elsewhere? How has the study in question affected the research participants, their communities, or health care in their own country? Was there any prior agreement to make the new treatments available in the country concerned after termination of the study? If so, for how long will the new treatment be available? Is the new treatment affordable and sustainable there? (See Chapters 64–67.)

The revised 2002 CIOMS guidelines attempt to respond to questions of this kind, although consensus proved difficult to achieve during the revision process. The guidelines were designed to be of use, particularly in developing countries, in the following areas:

- Defining national policies on the ethics of biomedical research
- Applying ethical standards in local circumstances
- Establishing mechanisms for ethical review of clinical research, taking into account the 2000 revision of the Declaration of Helsinki[14] (see Chapter 13)

The Revision Process

The revision process elicited strong support from both WHO and the Joint United Nations Programme on HIV/AIDS (UNAIDS), involved expertise from both developed and developing countries, and consisted of a series of steps over a period of nearly four years. The revision process is summarized in Table 16.1.

Structure and Content of the 2002 Guidelines

The 21 guidelines are preceded by a detailed description of the background, an introductory discussion, a brief account of other

Table 16.1

CIOMS Guidelines Revision Timeline

Date	Event
Dec. 1998	First draft prepared by a consultant
May 1999	Steering Committee reviews draft, recommends papers to be commissioned
Mar. 2000	International consultation (report published in November 2000)[3]
Jan.–Mar. 2001	Five-day meeting of multinational drafting group; draft placed on the CIOMS website
July–Oct. 2001	Comments solicited from a wide range of institutions and individual experts
Oct. 2001	Multinational editorial group established
Jan. 2002	New draft placed on the CIOMS website
Feb. 2002	Draft text considered and endorsed by CIOMS Conference
Aug. 2002	Final text endorsed by CIOMS Executive Committee
Sept. 2002	Final text placed on the CIOMS website
Oct. 2002	Printed version of International Ethical Guidelines for Biomedical Research Involving Human Subjects published by CIOMS
Oct. 2002–2003	Procedures initiated to produce translations in as many languages as possible, notably WHO's official languages

international research ethics instruments and guidelines, an outline of the general ethical principles governing research ethics (based on the Belmont Report,[15] described in Chapter 14), and a preamble that discusses the nature and significance of research involving humans.

General Guidance for Clinical Research

Any clinical study involving humans, including placebo-controlled trials, must be scientifically sound and justified, and ethically acceptable. These prerequisites are outlined in the following terms in Guideline 1:

> The ethical justification of biomedical research involving human subjects is the prospect of discovering new ways of benefiting people's health. Such research can be ethically justifiable only if it is carried out in ways that respect and protect, and are fair to, the subjects of that research and are morally acceptable within the communities in which the research is carried out. Moreover, because scientifically invalid research is unethical in that it exposes research subjects to risks without possible benefit, investigators and sponsors must ensure that proposed studies involving human subjects conform to generally accepted scientific principles and are based on adequate knowledge of the pertinent scientific literature.[2]

The commentary on this guideline indicates that the methods used should be appropriate to the objectives of the research and that these considerations should be adequately reflected in the research protocol submitted for review to independent scientific and ethical review committees. These principles were widely accepted during the revision process; they have also been affirmed in a number of other recent documents providing guidance on ethical aspects of clinical research.[16–19]

Ethical Review Committees and Sanctions

Guideline 2 outlines the responsibilities of ethical review committees, stresses the need for sufficient resources, and suggests that review of protocols could be supported by payments. Ethical review committees should be independent of the research team, and any direct financial or other material benefit they may derive from the research should not be contingent on the outcome of their review. The CIOMS Guidelines are in agreement with paragraph 13 of the Declaration of Helsinki, which states that the ethical review committee should conduct further reviews as necessary in the course of the research, including monitoring of the progress of the latter.[14]

Guideline 2 goes beyond the Declaration of Helsinki, however, by recommending that ethical review committees may withdraw their approval if this is deemed necessary, and must report to the health authorities any serious noncompliance with ethical standards. Governmental, institutional, professional, or other authorities may then impose sanctions as a last resort.

There is general agreement that the ethical review committee is to verify that the safety, integrity, and human rights of the research participants are protected, thereby providing public reassurance about the soundness of research. However, mechanisms and procedures for local ethical review in some nonindustrialized countries are not well developed.[7–10,19,20]

Externally Sponsored Research

This topic has inspired lively discussion in recent years.[7–11,19,20] In Guideline 3, "externally sponsored research" means research undertaken in a host country but sponsored, financed, and sometimes wholly or partly carried out by an external international or national organization or pharmaceutical company with the collaboration or agreement of the appropriate authorities, institutions, and personnel of the host country.

The guideline states that the investigator should submit the research protocol for ethical and scientific review not only in the country of the sponsor but also to the health authorities of the host country, as well as a national or local ethical review committee. The investigator should also ensure that the proposed research is responsive to the health needs and priorities of the host country and meets this country's requisite ethical standards. Moreover, review of the protocol by the local ethical review committee is necessary to ensure that the means of obtaining informed consent are appropriate to local customs and traditions, as well as to assess the competence of the research team and the suitability of the proposed research site in the host country.

Research in Communities With Limited Resources

Guideline 10 states that research in populations or communities with limited resources should be responsive to the health needs and the priorities of the population or community and that any intervention or product developed, or knowledge generated, should be made reasonably available for the benefit of that population or community.

Prior to the trial, the sponsor and investigator should undertake negotiations with the representatives of stakeholders in the host country (such as the national government, the health ministry, local health authorities, and concerned scientific and ethical groups, as well as representatives of the communities and relevant nongovernmental organizations) to determine the practical implications of "responsiveness" to local health needs. In particular, they should discuss the reasonable availability of any potential intervention or product that the trial might develop.

The negotiations should cover the health-care infrastructure required for safe and rational use of the intervention or product, the likelihood of authorization for distribution, and decisions regarding payments, royalties, subsidies, technology and intellectual property, as well as distribution costs. Ideally, there should be an agreement in advance spelling out for whom, for how long, by whom, and at what cost a potential intervention or product resulting from a trial should be provided to the population with limited resources. These principles have also been adopted as a condition of externally sponsored research in certain other guidance documents.[16,19,20]

For research studies such as Phase I or early Phase II studies with pharmaceuticals or candidate vaccines, and when the outcome is scientific knowledge rather than a commercial product, such complex planning or negotiation is rarely, if ever, needed.

Informed Consent

Guidelines 4–6 provide comprehensive guidance on informed consent. The consent process, the use of comprehensible language and information, documentation of consent, requirements for waiver of consent, renewal of consent, cultural considerations, and consent to use biological materials, biological specimens, and medical records for research purposes are all covered. A total of 26 categories of information that must be communicated to prospective research subjects are listed in Guideline 5.

"Informed consent" is interpreted to mean a decision to participate in research, taken by a competent individual who has received the necessary information; who has adequately understood the information; and who, after considering the information, has arrived at a decision without having been subjected to coercion, undue influence or inducement, or intimidation.

The design and methods of placebo-controlled studies are often rather complicated. To explain research designs such as randomization and double-blinding using simple language, and to assure full comprehension by the prospective research participant, requires time and effort on the part of the investigator; but there must also be an opportunity for the individual to seek clarifications and ask questions. These principles are necessary in order to assure full comprehension of the study design and to make it clear that a prospective participant could be randomized to a placebo arm of the study.

As a rule, the prospective participants of placebo-controlled studies should be volunteers. If an individual is not capable of giving informed consent, a placebo-controlled study can rarely be considered appropriate and must in all cases be approved by an independent ethical review committee.

Vulnerable Persons, Children, and Pregnant Women

The term "vulnerable persons" is interpreted in Guideline 13 to mean those who are relatively (or absolutely) incapable of protecting their own interests because they may have insufficient power, intelligence, education, resources, strength, or other needed attributes to protect these interests. In all instances, research with persons thought to be vulnerable requires "special justification" and the means of protecting their rights and welfare must be "strictly applied."

Research with children is addressed in Guideline 14. The participation of children is indispensable for research into diseases of childhood as well as for clinical trials of drugs or vaccines that are intended for children. A sponsor of any new therapeutic, diagnostic, or preventive product that is likely to be indicated for use in children is obliged to evaluate its safety and efficacy for children before it is released for general distribution. Guideline 15 deals with research involving individuals who by reason of mental or behavioral disorders are not capable of giving adequately informed consent.

Guidelines 14 and 15 have a parallel structure and very similar content. In order to undertake research with children or those unable to consent by reason of mental or behavioral disorder, the following conditions must be satisfied: (1) the research question cannot be answered by research carried out with a less vulnerable population (e.g., competent adults); (2) the research must address an issue that is relevant to the particular study population (children and those unable to consent, respectively); (3) agreement to participate has been obtained to the extent of the individual's capabilities; (4) permission to enroll the individual in research has been granted by the appropriate authority (parent, family member or legally authorized representative); and (5) refusal to participate in the research should (almost always) be respected.

Guideline 16 provides guidance on the research participation of women. It states that investigators, sponsors, or ethical review committees should not exclude women of reproductive age from biomedical research, because the potential to become pregnant is not a sufficient ground for such exclusion. The guideline stresses the need for a thorough discussion of risks to the pregnant woman and to her fetus as a prerequisite for the woman's ability to make a rational decision to enroll in a clinical study. It further discusses the need for pregnancy tests and access to effective contraceptive methods.

According to Guideline 17, research with pregnant women should be performed only if it is relevant to the particular health needs of a pregnant woman or her fetus, or to the health needs of pregnant women in general. Reliable evidence from animal experiments, particularly regarding the risks of teratogenicity and mutagenicity, provides invaluable support for such studies.

Best Current Method, Active Comparator, and the Use of Placebos

There has been extensive discussion on the ethics of using placebo in comparative trials when a known therapy for the condition exists.[3–6,8,19,20] Much of this discussion was prompted by the 2000 version of the Declaration of Helsinki, in particular, its paragraph 29. Paragraph 29 states that the benefits, risks, burdens, and effectiveness of a new method should be tested against those of "the best current methods" but that this does not exclude the use of placebo, or no treatment, in studies in which no proven method exists.[14] When drafts of the revised CIOMS Guidelines were considered, interpretation of this paragraph became especially contentious as commentators raised the question of the standard of care to be provided to a control group.

When a method of treatment existed, those in favor of placebo use suggested that if the condition being studied was mild—such as baldness, smoking cessation, overweight, headache, allergic reactions, cough, or mild elevation of cholesterol or blood pressure—the use of placebo in comparative studies would be appropriate and ethical. However, they noted that proper surveillance of research participants should be assured, the duration of placebo use should be minimized, escape or reserve treatment should be available, and there should be valid informed consent from participants.

Furthermore, those favoring the use of placebos argued that the use of active comparators instead of placebos in controlled trials might produce unreliable results. The assay sensitivity in many conditions remains weak, the clinical symptoms and treatment response in some conditions may vary, or the spontaneous improvement rate may be high. Treatment response for certain conditions can also be modest and almost the same as with placebo. In these circumstances, a comparative study without a placebo arm may yield no reliable scientific results.

In fact, such clinical studies conducted without a placebo arm might be considered unethical because they may expose partici-

pants to unnecessary burdens and risks and also cause a waste of resources. In their discussion of a hypothetical comparative trial, Ezekiel Emanuel and Franklin Miller contend that the use of placebos instead of an active comparator may dramatically reduce the number of participants required to demonstrate a certain therapeutic response rate.[6] Failure to use placebos in such comparative trials could be considered unethical. Similarly, Robert Temple and Susan Ellenberg argue that the acceptability of placebo-controlled trials is determined by whether research participants will be harmed by deferral of therapy.[4] If they are not harmed, such trials can ethically be carried out.

The main argument against placebo use in comparative clinical trials includes the fact that, for a patient and a practicing physician, the comparison of a new therapy with existing therapies is the objective, rather than the comparison with placebo. An additional argument voiced against placebo use is that placebos may be harmful even in mild conditions, because as symptoms continue, the disease may worsen and may result in irreversible changes or even in death.

Many drug regulatory authorities, including the European Agency for the Evaluation of Medicinal Products[21] and the U.S. Food and Drug Administration (at 21 CFR 314.126),[22] however, have pointed out that they require placebo-controlled trials to demonstrate the efficacy and safety of new therapies, even in cases in which there is an existing therapy.

"Established Effective Intervention"

The CIOMS Guidelines depart in one respect from the terminology of the Declaration of Helsinki. "Best current method," the term used in the Declaration, is most commonly used to describe the active comparator that is ethically preferred in controlled clinical trials. For many conditions, however, there is more than one established "current" intervention, and expert clinicians do not necessarily agree on which is superior. In some cases in which there are several established "current" interventions, some expert clinicians recognize one as superior to the rest; some commonly prescribe another because the superior intervention may be locally unavailable, or prohibitively expensive, or unsuited to the capability of a particular patient to adhere to a complex and rigorous regimen.

In contrast to the Declaration of Helsinki's "best current method" terminology, the CIOMS Guidelines use the term "established effective intervention," which refers to all such interventions, including the best and various alternatives to the best. One could also hypothesize that this term may not exclude even placebo or no treatment as an intervention in some conditions. It is well known that placebo can be effective and is commonly used in some mild conditions and that application of no treatment is the best "therapeutic" intervention in some situations.

The CIOMS Guidelines suggest that in some cases, an ethical review committee may determine that it is ethically acceptable to use an established effective intervention as a comparator, even in cases in which such an intervention is not considered the best current intervention.

Appendices

There are a series of Appendices to the Guidelines. Appendix 1 consists of a list of 48 items to be included (when relevant to the study) in a protocol (or associated documents) for biomedical research involving human subjects. Appendix 2 reproduces the 2000 version of the Declaration of Helsinki—including the Note of Clarification on paragraph 29, adopted in 2002, which approved the use of placebo even when a current therapy is available, if necessary "for compelling and scientifically sound methodological reasons" and if it does not pose serious risk. The phases of clinical trials of vaccines and drugs are elucidated in Appendix 3. The remaining three Appendices deal with nonsubstantive matters.

Conclusions

The 2002 CIOMS Guidelines described in this chapter provide guidance for the ethical conduct of clinical research, taking into account discussions prompted by the 2000 version of the Declaration of Helsinki and considerations related to externally sponsored research in resource-poor countries. Standard of care, availability after a trial of an intervention or product developed as a result of the trial, and the use of placebos as comparators aroused lengthy debate during the revision process. CIOMS considers that the individual guidelines and the commentaries thereon offer useful and practical solutions. They emphasize the need to involve experts and ethical review committees from resource-poor countries in negotiations prior to the conduct of clinical trials in these countries.

Epilogue

In 1991, CIOMS, in cooperation with WHO, formulated International Guidelines for Ethical Review of Epidemiological Studies. Again in cooperation with WHO, these guidelines are currently being revised, with input from a number of distinguished experts in the fields of ethics and epidemiology, as well as relevant scientific institutions, associations, and other entities. It is hoped that the revision process will be completed by the end of 2007. It is anticipated that the final Guidelines will closely resemble, in terms of structure and format, the 2002 International Ethical Guidelines for Biomedical Research Involving Human Subjects.

References

1. World Medical Association. *Declaration of Helsinki: Recommendations Guiding Medical Doctors in Biomedical Research Involving Human Subjects.* Tokyo, Japan: WMA; October 1975. *Medical Journal of Australia* 1976;1:206–7.
2. Council for International Organizations of Medical Sciences, in collaboration with the World Health Organization. *International Ethical Guidelines for Biomedical Research Involving Human Subjects.* Geneva, Switzerland: CIOMS and WHO; 2002. [Online] November 2002. Available: http://www.cioms.ch/frame_guidelines_nov_2002.htm.
3. Levine RJ, Gorovitz S, Gallagher J, editors. *Biomedical Research Ethics: Updating International Guidelines: A Consultation.* Geneva, Switzerland: CIOMS; 2000.
4. Temple R, Ellenberg SS. Placebo-controlled trials and active controlled trials in the evaluation of new treatments. Part 1. Ethical and scientific issues. *Annals of Internal Medicine* 2000;133:455–63.
5. Idänpään-Heikkilä JE. Ethical principles for the guidance of physicians in medical research—The Declaration of Helsinki. *Bulletin of the World Health Organization* 2001;79:279.
6. Emanuel EJ, Miller FG. The ethics of placebo-controlled trials—A middle ground. *New England Journal of Medicine* 2001;345:915–9.
7. Benatar SR, Singer PA. A new look at international research ethics. *British Medical Journal* 2000;321:824–6.
8. Macklin R. After Helsinki: Unresolved issues in international research. *Kennedy Institute of Ethics Journal* 2001;11:17–36.
9. Angell M. Investigators' responsibilities for human subjects in developing countries. *New England Journal of Medicine* 2000;342:967–9.
10. Weijer C, Emanuel EJ. Protecting communities in biomedical research. *Science* 2000;289:1142–4.
11. Rothman KJ, Michels KB, Baum M. For and against: Declaration of Helsinki should be strengthened. *British Medical Journal* 2000;321:442–5.
12. Riis P. Perspectives on the fifth revision of the Declaration of Helsinki. *JAMA* 2000;284:3035–6.
13. Shapiro HT, Meslin EM. Ethical issues in the design and conduct of clinical trials in developing countries. *New England Journal of Medicine* 2001;345:139–42.
14. World Medical Association. *Declaration of Helsinki: Ethical Principles for Medical Research Involving Human Subjects.* Tokyo, Japan: WMA; October 2004. [Online] 2004. Available: http://www.wma.net/e/policy/b3.htm.
15. The National Commission for the Protection of Human Subjects of Biomedical and Behavioral Research. *The Belmont Report: Ethical Principles and Guidelines for the Protection of Human Subjects of Research.* Washington, D.C.: Department of Health, Education and Welfare; DHEW Publication OS 78–0012 1978. [Online] Available: http://www.hhs.gov/ohrp/humansubjects/guidance/belmont.htm.
16. World Health Organization. Guidelines for good clinical practice (GCP) for trials on pharmaceutical products. WHO Technical Report Series, No. 850, Annex 3. Geneva, Switzerland: WHO; 1995:97–137. [Online] Available: http://whqlibdoc.who.int/trs/WHO_TRS_850.pdf.
17. International Conference on Harmonisation of Technical Requirements for Registration of Pharmaceuticals for Human Use. *The ICH Harmonised Tripartite Guideline—Guideline for Good Clinical Practice.* Geneva, Switzerland: ICH; 1996. [Online] Available: http://www.ich.org/LOB/media/MEDIA482.pdf.
18. European Parliament and the Council of the European Union. Directive 2001/20/EC of the European Parliament and of the Council of 4 April 2001 on the approximation of the laws, regulations and administrative provisions of the Member States relating to the implementation of good clinical practice in the conduct of clinical trials on medicinal products for human use. *Official Journal of the European Communities* 2001;L121:34–44. [Online] Available: http://europa.eu.int/eur-lex/lex/LexUriServ/LexUriServ.do?uri=CELEX:32001L0020:EN:HTML.
19. European Group on Ethics in Science and New Technologies. *Opinion No. 17 to the European Commission: Ethical Aspects of Clinical Research in Developing Countries.* Brussels, Belgium: EGE; 2003. [Online] February 4, 2003. Available: http://ec.europa.eu/european_group_ethics/docs/avis17_en.pdf.
20. Nuffield Council on Bioethics. *The Ethics of Research Related to Healthcare in Developing Countries.* London, England: Nuffield Council on Bioethics; 2002. [Online] Available: http://nuffieldbioethics.org/fileLibrary/pdf/errhdc_fullreport001.pdf.
21. European Agency for the Evaluation of Medicinal Products. EMEA/CPMP Position Statement on the Use of Placebo in Clinical Trials With Regard to the Revised Declaration of Helsinki, EMEA/17424/01. [Online] June 28, 2001. Available: http://www.emea.eu.int/pdfs/human/press/pos/1742401en.pdf.

22. Food and Drug Administration, Department of Health and Human Services. Title 21 (Food and Drugs), Code of Federal Regulations, Part 314 (Applications for FDA Approval to Market a New Drug). [Online] April 1, 2006. Available: http://www.access.gpo.gov/nara/cfr/waisidx_06/21cfr314_06.html.

23. Council for International Organizations of Medical Sciences, in collaboration with the World Health Organization. *International Guidelines for Ethical Review of Epidemiological Studies.* Geneva, Switzerland: CIOMS; 1991. [Online] Available: http://www.cioms.ch/frame_1991_texts_of_guidelines.htm.

Pēteris Zilgalvis

The Council of Europe

The Council of Europe and Its Involvement in Bioethics

Founded in 1949, the Council of Europe is an intergovernmental organization with a pan-European mandate to foster political, legal, and cultural cooperation between its 46 member countries. Its Convention and the protocols that have been negotiated under its aegis form a set of legally binding treaties addressing a wide variety of topics at the international level. The Council is distinct from the 25-nation European Union (EU), although all EU member countries are also members of the Council of Europe. Its aims, as specified by its Statute, are to protect human rights and strengthen pluralist democracy, to enhance European cultural identity, and to seek solutions to the major problems of our time such as the bioethical problems addressed by the Convention on Human Rights and Biomedicine.

The most tangible results of intergovernmental cooperation in the Council are European conventions, drawn up as contracts between signatory nations. Each nation accepts a number of obligations in return for acceptance of the same obligations by other nations. These treaties are not legal instruments of the Council of Europe as such, but owe their existence to the member nations that sign and ratify them. Even though the treaties have a life of their own, they are in many cases followed by expert committees set up within the Council of Europe.[1] The Council of Europe has drawn up more than 200 multilateral conventions.[2]

Bioethics Instruments of the Council of Europe Relevant to Clinical Research Ethics

The Convention on Human Rights and Biomedicine

The Convention on Human Rights and Biomedicine is the first international agreement on the new biomedical technologies. Its full title is the Convention for the Protection of Human Rights and Dignity of the Human Being with regard to the Application of Biology and Medicine. It was opened for signature on April 4, 1997, in Oviedo, Spain, and by 2006, 34 countries had signed and 19 had ratified it, putting it into effect in those countries (see Tables 17.1 and 17.2). In addition to member countries, the following countries that took part in the preparation of the Convention may sign: Australia, Canada, the Holy See, Japan, and the United States. Mexico has requested permission to sign, and this has been granted by the Committee of Ministers.

The Convention on Human Rights and Medicine was prepared in order to establish a common, minimum level of protections for patients and human participants in research throughout Europe. Finding a consensus on such a minimum level was not a simple task. The traditions and approaches of some countries favored stringent prohibitions in some spheres. Others believed that some prohibitions could be seen as paternalistic and could deprive individuals of the choice, as well as the opportunity, to receive

Table 17.1

Signatories to the Convention on Human Rights
and Biomedicine as of 2006

Bosnia and Herzegovina	Iceland	San Marino
Bulgaria	Italy	Serbia
Croatia	Latvia	Slovakia
Cyprus	Lithuania	Slovenia
Czech Republic	Luxembourg	Spain
Denmark	Moldova	Sweden
Estonia	Montenegro	Switzerland
Finland	Netherlands	Turkey
France	Norway	Ukraine
Georgia	Poland	The former
Greece	Portugal	Yugoslav Republic
Hungary	Romania	of Macedonia

Table 17.2

Countries That Have Ratified the Convention on Human
Rights and Biomedicine as of 2006

Bulgaria	Greece	San Marino
Croatia	Hungary	Slovakia
Cyprus	Iceland	Slovenia
Czech Republic	Lithuania	Spain
Denmark	Moldova	Turkey
Estonia	Portugal	
Georgia	Romania	

some of the benefits from biomedicine. A balance also needed to be found between the freedom of research and the regulation of research to protect research participants.

Now or in the future, some countries may wish to offer a yet higher standard of protection; the Convention was drafted with such a possibility in mind. Article 27 (Wider Protection) states that none of the provisions shall be interpreted as limiting or otherwise affecting the ability of a party to grant a wider measure of protection with regard to the application of biology and medicine than is stipulated in the Convention.

The Convention first came into force on December 1, 1999. It is up to the countries that have signed and ratified it to implement its provisions in their national legislation. This process is followed by the Secretariat, specifically by the Bioethics Department and the Steering Committee on Bioethics (CDBI, Comité Directeur pour la Bioéthique) at the Council of Europe. These bodies also provide assistance, if needed, to signatories to adapt their institutions and legislation to the requirements of the Convention.

The Convention gives precedence to the human being over the sole interest of science or society. Its aim is to protect human rights and dignity, and all of its articles must be interpreted in this light. The term "human rights" as used in the title and text of the Convention refers to the principles enunciated in the European Convention for the Protection of Human Rights and Fundamental Freedoms of November 4, 1950, which guarantees the protection of such rights. The Convention on Human Rights and Biomedicine shares the same underlying approach as the 1950 pact as well as many ethical principles and legal concepts, and also elaborates on some of the principles found in that Convention.

Provisions of the Convention

Two types of provisions are contained in the Convention. Its first part is a codification of the principles of modern medical law in regard to informed consent and the protection of those unable to consent. Its second part addresses biomedical research and the new biomedical technologies, and provides that newly arising issues can be addressed in additional protocols. Thus, the Convention and its protocols are a system that can respond to new (and sometimes threatening) developments in biomedicine. An example of such a response was the rapid preparation of a protocol prohibiting human cloning after the disclosure of the birth of Dolly, the first cloned mammal, in late 1997. Another example is the provision of the draft Protocol on Biomedical Research addressing research in nonparty States (Article 29), which was developed in response to allegations of exploitation by Western researchers of research subjects from developing countries and central and eastern Europe.

Five additional protocols were originally proposed to supplement the Convention on Human Rights and Biomedicine. In order to address the ethical and legal issues raised by present or future scientific advances, protocols on the prohibition of cloning human beings and on transplantation of organs and tissues of human origin already have been opened for signature. In 2005, a draft protocol on human genetics was being written by a working party of high-level experts nominated by Council member states with the assistance of the Secretariat.

The so-called Additional Protocol on Biomedical Research was approved by the CDBI in June 2003. The Committee of Ministers of the Council of Europe, following its usual procedure, decided to send the draft Protocol to the Council of Europe's Parliamentary Assembly for an opinion in September 2003. It was opened for signature in January 2005, and by late that year had been signed by a dozen countries.

The Convention's purpose and object are set out in its Article 1: protecting the dignity and identity of all human beings and guaranteeing, without discrimination, respect for the integrity, other rights, and fundamental freedoms of every person. The Convention clearly states that an intervention in the health field may be carried out only after the patient has given free and informed consent (Article 5). It also provides safeguards for people who are unable to consent (Article 6); these include a requirement that the intervention be only be for that person's direct benefit, that when a minor is involved, the person or body responsible for that minor by law must authorize any intervention, and that the opinion of a minor must be taken into consideration as an increasingly determining factor in proportion to his or her age and degree of maturity.

Requirements for research to be undertaken on persons in the fields of biology and medicine are set out in the Convention in the chapter on scientific research as well as in other chapters, in particular, in the 2005 Additional Protocol Concerning Biomedical Research. The general rule for scientific research is set out in Article 15. It states that scientific research in biomedicine shall be carried out freely, subject to the provisions of the Convention and the other legal provisions ensuring the protection of the human being. The freedom of scientific research is a constitutionally protected right in some of the member states. For example, Article 20 ("Freedom of Science") of Switzerland's Constitution states: "The freedom of scientific research and teaching is guaranteed."[3]

The protection of persons who are unable to consent to research and of embryos in vitro are both specifically addressed in the Convention itself. Article 17 states that research on a person not able to consent to research may be undertaken only if the Convention's protective conditions are met, and it sets stringent conditions for permitting research that does not have the potential to produce results of direct benefit to the health of a person who is unable to consent. Such research may be approved if it has the aim of ultimately benefiting persons in the same age category, or afflicted with the same disease or disorder, or having the same condition, through significant improvement in scientific understanding of the condition, disease, or disorder. In addition, the research must entail only minimal risk and minimal burden for the individual concerned.

Article 18 of the Convention prohibits the creation of human embryos for research purposes and states that where the law allows research on embryos in vitro, that research must ensure adequate protection of the embryo. However, it does not prohibit research on excess embryos created for purposes of in vitro fertilization.

The Additional Protocol on Biomedical Research

The Additional Protocol on Biomedical Research will be the first legally binding international instrument to address the whole field of biomedical research, and it is not confined to pharmaceuticals.[4,5] The provisions of Articles 1 to 32 of this Protocol will be regarded as additional articles to the Convention on Human Rights and Biomedicine for the parties, and all the provisions of the Convention will apply accordingly.

The scope of the Protocol is set out in Article 2. The full range of research activities in the health field involving interventions on human beings are covered. This includes all phases of a research project, including selection and recruitment of participants. Paragraph 3 of this article states that, for the purposes of the Protocol, the term "intervention" covers physical interventions. It includes other interventions insofar as they involve a risk to the psychological health of the participant. The term "intervention" must be understood here in a broad sense; in the context of this Protocol it covers all medical acts and interactions relating to the health or well being of persons in the framework of health-care systems or any other setting for scientific research purposes. Questionnaires, interviews, and observational research taking place in the context of biomedicine constitute interventions if they involve a risk to the psychological health of the person concerned. One ramification of defining such research as coming within the scope of this Protocol is that review by an ethics committee would be required. The ethics committee could point out any potential problems in the research project to those submitting it for review. The Protocol does not address established medical interventions independent of a research project, even if they result in biological materials or personal data that might later be used in biomedical research. However, research interventions designed to procure biological materials or data are within the scope of the Protocol.

Research on archived biological materials and data is not covered by the Protocol. This is a point on which it differs from the 2000 version of the World Medical Association's Declaration of Helsinki, which includes "research on identifiable human material or identifiable data."[6,7] As noted above, an "instrument" on research on archived biological materials has been prepared by a working party of the CDBI. The instrument contains a chapter addressing biobanks, such as those recently developed in Estonia, Latvia, and the United Kingdom.[8] The CDBI has decided that this instrument should be a recommendation and not an additional protocol to the Convention. The Additional Protocol on Biomedical Research does not apply to research on embryos in vitro, but does apply to research on embryos in vivo.

The Protocol further states that research may only be undertaken if there is no alternative of comparable effectiveness. Comparable effectiveness refers to the foreseen results of the research, not to individual benefits for a participant. Invasive methods will not be authorized if other less invasive or non-invasive methods can be used with comparable effect. This does not imply that the Protocol authorizes or encourages using alternatives that are unethical. The Protocol does not evaluate the ethical acceptability of research on animals, using computer models, or other alternatives. These matters are addressed by other legal instruments, such as the Council of Europe Convention for the Protection of Vertebrate Animals used for Experimental and Other Scientific Purposes (1986) and relevant professional standards.

The Protocol specifies that research shall not involve risks to the human being disproportionate to its potential benefits. When medical research may be of direct benefit to the health of the person undergoing research, a higher degree of risk may be acceptable provided that it is in proportion to the possible benefit. For example, a higher degree of risk may be acceptable on a new treatment for advanced cancer, whereas the same risk would be quite unacceptable when the research is aimed at improving the treatment of a mild infection. A direct benefit to a person's health signifies not only treatment to cure the patient but also treatment that may alleviate suffering, thus improving quality of life.

Article 7 requires that research be undertaken only if the research project has been approved by the competent body after independent examination of its scientific merit and multidisciplinary review of its ethical acceptability. It is acknowledged that in some countries, the ethics committee could also act as the competent body, whereas in other cases or in other countries, the competent body might be a ministry or a regulatory agency (for pharmaceuticals, for instance), which would take the opinion of the ethics committee into account in formulating its decision. This provision is not intended to curtail the freedom of research. In fact, Article 4 of this Protocol states that biomedical research shall be carried out freely. However, this freedom is not absolute. It is qualified by the legal provisions ensuring the protection of the human being. Independent examination of the ethical acceptability of the research project by an ethics committee is one such protective provision. Allowing unethical research to utilize human beings would contravene their fundamental rights. It is the responsibility of parties to designate within the framework of their legal system the ethics committee or a different competent body that would act as the decision making organ in order to protect those taking part in the research.

Chapter III of the Protocol addresses ethics committees. Its Article 9 requires that research projects be submitted to independent examination in each country in which any research activity is to take place. This includes countries from which research subjects are to be recruited for research physically carried out in another country.

The article refers to "ethics committees." The drafters considered that this term covers ethics committees or other bodies authorized to review biomedical research involving interventions on human beings. In many countries this would refer to a multidisciplinary ethics committee, but review by a scientific committee might also be required. The article does not require a positive assessment by the ethics committee because the role of such bodies or committees may be solely advisory in some countries.

The purpose of the multidisciplinary examination, after the precondition of scientific quality has been met, is to protect the dignity, rights, safety, and well-being of research participants. Further, the article states that assessment of the ethical acceptability shall draw on an appropriate range of expertise and experience adequately reflecting professional and lay views. The existence of an independent ethics committee ensures that the interests and concerns of the community are represented, and the participation of laypersons is important in ensuring that the public can have confidence in the system for oversight of biomedical research. Such laypersons must not be health-care professionals and cannot have experience in carrying out biomedical research. However, expertise in an unrelated field, such as engineering or accountancy, does not preclude a person from being able to express lay views within the meaning of this article. Thus this article further details what is meant by the term "multidisciplinary." One may also conclude that it follows from this article that thought should be given to gender and cultural balance in the bodies carrying out the assessment. In creating an ethics committee, the nature of the projects that are likely to be presented for review should also be taken into account, and the committee may need to invite experts to assist it in evaluating a project in a specialized sphere of biomedicine. The ethics committee must produce an opinion containing reasons for its positive or negative conclusion. Whether the reasoning and conclusions are the final say on the project or are further considered by the competent body in granting or denying approval, the basis for the conclusion should be clearly comprehensible both to specialists in the field and to laypersons.

The independence of the ethics committee itself and of the individual members of the committee is addressed in Article 10. It states that parties to the protocol shall take measures to assure the independence of the ethics committees and that those committees shall not be subject to undue external influences. Members of the ethics committees must declare all circumstances that might lead to a conflict of interest. If such conflicts arise, those involved shall not participate in the review in question.

The fulfillment of the Convention's and the Protocol's requirement that multidisciplinary ethics committees review the acceptability of biomedical research projects has been particularly emphasized by the Council of Europe. Since 1997, the Council has been cooperating with its member countries on a program of multilateral and bilateral meetings, study visits, and informative materials on best practices in the ethical review of biomedical research—called the Demo droit Ethical review of Biomedical Research Activity (DEBRA). The independence of ethical review committees is paramount. As Senator Claude Huriet, who served as a *rapporteur* for a DEBRA meeting in Vilnius, wrote in the French Senate report on the protection of persons undergoing

biomedical research, the independence of the committees is the foundation of their credibility and legitimacy.[9]

Article 11 of the Protocol on Biomedical Research requires the researcher to submit all information necessary for the ethical assessment of the research project, in written form, to the ethics committee, and the Protocol's appendix lists items that are to be provided if they are relevant to the research project. These include details of all payments and rewards to be made in the context of the research project and of any potential further uses, including commercial uses, of the research results, data, or biological materials. Payments to research participants or to the researchers themselves are not prohibited, but the Protocol requires that the ethics committee be informed about the types and amounts, and the committee would have to consider their appropriateness.

Having received this information, the ethics committee might conclude, for example, that a payment to a research subject is excessive in relation to the inconvenience caused and is, in fact, an inducement to accept a higher level of risk. On the other hand, lucrative financial incentives for a doctor to enroll a large number of patients in a research project might call into question the physician's objectivity in explaining the positive and negative aspects of participation to his patients. Article 12 of the Protocol states that the ethics committee must be satisfied that "no undue influence, including that of a financial nature" has been exerted to persuade people to participate in research. If the ethics committee is not satisfied that no undue influence has been exerted, then the project should not receive a positive assessment unless changes are made to address the problem.

Neither the Convention nor the Protocol on Research takes a stand on patenting or on commercial use of research results, data, or biological materials. Rather, the fact that the motivation for participation in biomedical research for many persons may be out of solidarity is acknowledged. Information on foreseen commercial uses of their contribution to the research may be important to potential participants in making a decision on their participation. Again, in the interests of transparency, the ethics committee reviewing the research project and the potential research participant must be informed of such foreseen uses of the results, data, or biological materials.

Chapter IV of the Protocol addresses consent and information. Article 13 requires that people being asked to participate in a research project be given adequate information in a documented and comprehensible form, and it lists the items of information that they must receive. The same items of information must be furnished to those asked to provide authorization for the participation of a person in research (Article 16).

Consent to biomedical research is addressed by Article 14. Consent can be freely withdrawn at any phase of the research. Refusal to give consent or the withdrawal of consent shall not lead to any form of discrimination against the person concerned, in particular regarding the right to medical care. If the capacity of the person to give informed consent is in doubt, arrangements must be in place to verify whether or not the person has such capacity. Such persons may be those who have not been declared incapable of giving consent by a legal body, but whose capacity to give consent may be questionable due to an accident or due to a persistent or worsening condition, for instance. The aim of this requirement is not to set out any particular arrangement for verification but simply to require that such procedures exist. The arrangements would not necessarily be in the framework of the court system; they could be developed and implemented through professional standards in the medical sphere. The researcher is ultimately responsible for verifying that the participants from whom he obtains consent have the capacity to give the consent.

If the person in question is not able to give consent, then Chapter V ("Protection of Persons Not Able to Consent to Research") applies. Article 15 of this chapter is based on Article 17 of the Convention, which provides protection for those not able to consent to research. Both the Convention and the Protocol foresee the possibility of authorizing research in which there is no potential direct benefit to the research subject if additional conditions are fulfilled. One of these is that the research entails no more than minimal risk and minimal burden.

One of the critical comments made about the Convention was that it did not define "minimal risk" and "minimal burden." The draft Protocol now offers such a definition. It specifies that the research bears a minimal risk if, "having regard to the nature and scale of the intervention, it is to be expected that it will result, at the most, in a very slight and temporary negative impact on the health of the person concerned." It is deemed that research bears a minimal burden if it is to be expected that the discomfort will be, at the most, temporary and very slight for the person concerned. The Protocol adds that in assessing the burden for an individual, a person enjoying the special confidence of the person concerned shall assess the burden when appropriate. It might be said that this article is more explanatory than normative, but its political value in the very sensitive area of research on those not able to consent is unquestionable.

Chapter VI addresses specific situations, in particular those of persons in emergency clinical situations, pregnant or breastfeeding women, and persons deprived of their liberty. Research during pregnancy or breastfeeding is addressed by Article 18. The provision seeks to balance respect for the autonomy of the pregnant or breastfeeding woman with the need for special protection of the embryo, fetus, or child in the framework of any such research.

Safety and supervision are addressed by Chapter VII. Articles are included on minimization of risk and burden, assessment of health status, noninterference of research with necessary clinical interventions, and reexamination of ongoing research projects if relevant developments or events arise during the research. Article 23 ("Non-interference with Necessary Clinical Interventions") of this chapter states that the use of placebo is permissible when there are no methods of proven effectiveness or when withdrawal or withholding of such methods does not present unacceptable risk or burden.

Research in countries not party to this Protocol is addressed by Article 29. It specifies that sponsors and researchers within the jurisdiction of a party to the Protocol who plan to undertake or direct a research project in a country not party to the Protocol shall ensure that, without prejudice to the provisions applicable in that country, the research project complies with the principles on which the provisions of the Protocol are based. For example, if the nonparty country does not require independent ethical examination of research projects, then the project in question should be reviewed in the country that is a party to the Protocol. This does not imply that the country which is party to the Protocol can override the laws of the nonparty country state or authorize research that the nonparty country does not approve. Instead, it means that the researchers may be required to observe additional

conditions, over and above those of the nonparty country, if they choose to conduct research there.

Article 35 of the Protocol provides for its re-examination within the Committee referred to in Article 32 of the Convention on Human Rights and Biomedicine no later than five years from its entry into force, and thereafter at such intervals as the Committee may determine. Article 32 of the Convention identifies this Committee as the Steering Committee on Bioethics (CDBI), or any other Committee so designated by the Committee of Ministers.

Article 34 of the Protocol deals with wider protections. The text lays down common standards with which countries must comply, but it allows them to provide additional protections to human participants in biomedical research. A conflict may arise between the various rights established by the Protocol—for example, between a scientist's right of freedom of research and the rights of a research participant. However, the expression "wider protection" must be interpreted in the light of the purpose of the Protocol, as defined in Article 1, namely the protection of the human being with regard to any research in the field of biomedicine. In the example cited above, any additional statutory protection can only mean greater protection for a research participant.

Research on Biological Materials

The aforementioned work in the CDBI on research on biological materials was approved by its Steering Committee in October 2005 and submitted for adoption to the Committee of Ministers of the Council of Europe. The draft recommendation places a strong emphasis on consent to research on biological materials. When collecting samples, the initial consent for future use should be as specific as possible; materials collected for other purposes may only be used for research with appropriate consent or authorization. Exceptions are allowed if three conditions are fulfilled: (1) the research addresses an important scientific interest; (2) the aims could not be reached if one needs to obtain consent; and (3) there is no evidence that those who donated the tissue samples would object to such research use (Article 22). Those who have consented to tissue storage can withdraw their consent later or alter the scope of the consent. Tissue may not be removed after death without appropriate consent or authorization.

The recommendation also deals with transport of samples and discourages transfer to other countries that do not have an adequate level of protection (Article 16). Whenever samples are collected, clear conditions governing access and use of samples need to be established (Article 14).

Chapter V deals with biobanks, defined as collections of biological materials with a population basis that contain associated personal data, that will be used for multiple research projects, and that receive materials on a regular basis. The recommendation stipulates that such biobanks need to be subject to independent oversight and regular audits (Article 19), and that there should be a policy for access to the materials contained in them (Articles 19 and 20).

Conclusions

International cooperation is needed to extend the individual protections embodied in the Convention on Human Rights and Biomedicine beyond the member states of the Council of Europe. A number of observers have noted the tendency toward a certain homogenization of the law—in a positive sense—in the field of bioethics. Differences do remain between the approaches followed in the United Kingdom and on the Continent, and sometimes even more so between Europe and some other countries. However, the experience of the Convention, which is the first legally binding international instrument addressing the new biomedical technologies and has had tangible influence on national legislation, could be useful as the basis for a future, expanded discussion. The Standing Conference of European National Ethics Committees (COMETH) provides an opportunity for national ethics committees to come together biannually to discuss practical and ethical aspects of their work. Conferences such as the 1999 International Conference of the Council of Europe on ethical issues arising from the application of biotechnology will continue to be organized.

Disclaimer

The views expressed are personal and do not necessarily reflect any official position of the Council of Europe.

References

1. Polakiewicz J. *Treaty-Making in the Council of Europe.* Strasbourg, France: Council of Europe Publishing; 1999:10.
2. Council of Europe. Complete list of the Council of Europe's treaties. [Online] Available: http://conventions.coe.int/Treaty/Commun/Liste Traites.asp?CM=8&CL=ENG.
3. Federal Constitution of the Swiss Confederation. Adopted: April 18, 1999; in force: January 1, 2000. [Online] Available: http://www. admin.ch/ch/itl/rs/1/c101ENG.pdf.
4. Legal Affairs, Council of Europe. *Additional Protocol to the Convention on Human Rights and Biomedicine Concerning Biomedical Research.* European Treaty Series No. 195. Strasbourg, France: Council of Europe; 2005. [Online] January 25, 2005. Available: http://www.coe.int/t/e/legal_ affairs/legal_co-operation/bioethics/activities/biomedical_research/ 195%20Protocole%20recherche%20biomedicale%20e.pdf.
5. Directorate General I, Legal Affairs, Council of Europe. *Explanatory Report to the Additional Protocol to the Convention on Human Rights and Biomedicine Concerning Biomedical Research.* Strasbourg, France: Council of Europe; 2005. [Online] January 25, 2005. Available: http://www.coe .int/t/e/legal_affairs/legal_co-operation/bioethics/activities/biomed ical_research/195%20ER%20recherche%20biomedicale%20e.pdf.
6. World Medical Association. *Declaration of Helsinki: Ethical Principles for Medical Research Involving Human Subjects.* Tokyo, Japan: WMA; October 2004. [Online] 2004. Available: http://www.wma.net/e/policy/b3 .htm.
7. Zilgalvis P. The European Convention on Human Rights and Biomedicine: Competition for the Declaration of Helsinki? In: Deutsch E, Taupitz J, eds. *Forschungsfreiheit und Forschungskontrolle in der Medizin—Zur geplanten Revision der Deklaration von Helsinki [Freedom and Control of Biomedical Research: The Planned Revision of the Declaration of Helsinki].* Berlin, Germany: Springer-Verlag; 2000:261–71.
8. Raidla J, Nõmper A. The Estonian Genome Project and the Human Gene Research Act. In: Ziemele I, ed. *Baltic Yearbook of International Law, Volume 2.* The Hague, The Netherlands: Martinus Nijhoff Publishers; 2002:51–69.
9. Huriet C. Rapport d'information fait au nom de la commission des affaires sociales (1) sur le fonctionnement des comités consultatifs de protection des personnes dans la recherche biomédicale. *Les Rapports du Sénat* 2000–2001;267:2–173. [Online] April 6, 2001. Available: http://www.senat.fr/rap/r00–267/r00–2671.pdf.

Deryck Beyleveld   Sebastian Sethe

18

The European Community Directives on Data Protection and Clinical Trials

The two legislative instruments of the European Community (EC) with the greatest impact on medical research are Directive 95/46/EC, the "Data Protection Directive,"[1] and Directive 2001/20/EC on good clinical practice in clinical trials, the "Clinical Trials Directive."[2] Although Directive 95/46/EC had to be implemented by October 1998, there has as yet been no case law at the EC level on its requirements in relation to medical research. The deadline for implementation of Directive 2001/20/EC was May 2004, and, again, no case law about it has yet emerged. This renders it difficult to make definitive legal statements about many aspects of these directives. Consequently, our analysis is to a degree speculative and tentative, and some of the statements we make might be controversial.

Outline

After a brief explanation of the legal force of European Community directives, we outline the basic requirements of the Data Protection Directive and the Clinical Trials Directive, with emphasis on the rights of research participants. In the context of Directive 95/46/EC, which is older and in some ways more complex, we indicate the rights of data subjects and the duties of the data controller and assess the scope of the exemption for medical research. We also discuss specific points such as the requirement for consent, the further processing of data for purposes not initially envisaged, and some issues surrounding the anonymization of data. We conclude this section with a comment on the likely impact of the directive.

We discuss Directive 2001/20/EC in the second part of the chapter. We examine the role given to independent research ethics

committees (RECs) to protect the rights of research participants, the duties of research sponsors in relation to RECs, and the time limits for an REC to give an opinion. We also discuss some problematic aspects of the directive and evaluate its likely impact on medical research, in particular, highlighting the connection between the two directives regarding the role of RECs in ensuring data protection. We make brief reference to the Directive on Good Clinical Practice (2005/28/EC), which was to have been implemented nationally by January 29, 2006.[3]

The Legal Force of EC Directives

EC directives are legally binding on states of the European Economic Area (EEA), which comprises Iceland, Liechtenstein, and Norway in addition to the member states of the European Union. EC directives are directed in the first instance at member states, not individuals. Clinical researchers need to attend to their national law implementing an EC directive. However, as explained below, an EC directive informs the interpretation of national law and its provisions are applicable across countries. For these reasons, individuals will be assisted by some understanding of EC directives as well as of their national law.

EC directives have two parts: a preamble made up of recitals, and an operative part consisting of articles. Articles prescribe what must or may be achieved by implementation in national laws. Recitals, in addition to describing the legislative basis and context of the directive, provide reasons on which the directive is based and thus guidance on interpreting the articles. They are important because national authorities are required to interpret national law in the light of the purpose of the directive.[4] If a member state has failed to implement a directive, or if its implementing provisions are incompatible or not sufficiently precise, then any national provision must give way to EC law.[5] This holds *except* when the national law gives effect to an international obligation entered into before the member state became bound by the relevant Community treaty.[6]

Directive 95/46/EC—the Data Protection Directive

Aims of the Data Protection Directive

The aim of this directive is to enable the free flow of personal data while ensuring that fundamental rights and freedoms—in particular, but not limited to, privacy—are safeguarded (Article 1, Recitals 3 and 10). In so doing, the directive (see Recital 11) gives substance to the Council of Europe Convention for the Protection of Individuals with Regard to Automatic Processing of Personal Data of 1981.[7] It is therefore more accurate to view adequate safeguarding of fundamental rights and freedoms as a condition of the free flow of personal data, rather than as something merely to be weighed in the balance against having such a flow.

The directive has direct relevance for data collected and stored for research purposes. For example, there are specific rules for how long data can be stored, specific requirements for informed consent, and rules for future research use of stored data. Researchers and RECs need therefore be aware of the specific requirements of the Data Protection Directive, which may at times be more stringent than those required by research ethics regulations and guidelines.

Provisions and Definitions

At the risk of oversimplification, the directive lays down five principles of data protection (Article 6), specifies that data subjects have certain rights (Table 18.1), imposes certain duties on data controllers (Table 18.2), prohibits data controllers from processing sensitive personal data unless certain conditions are met (Table 18.3), and charts the official responsibilities of member states (Table 18.4).

There are some operative definitions: *Data controllers* are defined as any persons or institutions (private or public) that individually or jointly determine the purposes and means of processing (Article 2(d)). *Personal data*" is any information relating to an identified or identifiable natural person (*data subject*). Recital 26 specifies that data is personal if indirect identification is reasonably likely by the data controller or any other person. Although it may seem obvious that this means that data is personal if anyone is reasonably likely to be able to identify the data subject

Table 18.1
The Rights of Data Subjects

Data subjects have the right to the following:

- Access their personal data (Article 12)
- Object to processing of personal data on pressing legitimate grounds (Article 14(a))
- Object to the use of personal data for purposes of direct marketing (Article 14(b))
- Not be subjected to decisions that produce legal or other significant effects that are based solely on automated processing (Article 15)

Table 18.2
Duties of Data Controllers

Data controllers must do the following:

- Obtain data fairly by ensuring the individual is informed about the identity of the data controller, the persons or type of persons to whom the information will be disclosed, and the exact purpose the data is required for, including all secondary or future uses (Articles 10 and 11).
- Notify processing to the supervisory authority (Articles 19 and 28).
- Keep data only for the initially specified purpose and retain it no longer than necessary (Article 6.1(e)).
- Process data only in ways compatible with the initially specified purpose (Article 7.1(b)).
- Keep data safe and secure (Article 17).
- Keep data accurate, complete, and up-to-date, as well as adequate, relevant, and not excessive (Article 6.1© and (d)).
- Provide individuals with access to their personal data on request (Article 12).

Table 18.3
Conditions for Processing Data*

Personal data (Article 7)

Processing is legitimate only if there is unambiguous consent of the data subject; or if the processing meets one of the following criteria:

- Is necessary to perform or enter a contract to which the data subject is party
- Is necessary to comply with a legal obligation
- Is necessary to protect the vital interests of the data subject
- Is necessary in the public interest
- Is necessary in the exercise of official authority
- Is in the legitimate interests of the controller or recipients of the data and the protection of the fundamental rights and freedoms of the data subject is not overriding.

Sensitive personal data (Article 8, Recitals 33–36)

There is a blanket prohibition on processing sensitive personal data (Article 8(1)), which may be lifted under one of the following conditions:

- There is explicit consent of the data subject.
- Processing is necessary to protect the vital interests of the data subject (which, according to Recital 31 means "essential for the data subject's life") or of another person in cases in which the data subject physically or legally cannot give consent.
- The data has been manifestly made public by the data subject.
- Processing is necessary to establish, exercise, or defend a legal claim.
- Processing is in the substantial public interest (to be notified to the Commission, Recital 34, identifying scientific research and government statistics as an important reason of public interest that might justify processing).
- Processing is necessary for the purposes of preventive medicine, medical diagnosis, the provision of care or treatment, or the management of health-care services, and processing is by a health professional under the obligation of professional secrecy or by another person subject to an equivalent obligation of secrecy.

*It is important to note that these conditions are necessary but not in themselves sufficient. Just because a condition is met, it does not mean that all legal requirements are fulfilled.

Table 18.4

Official Responsibilities of Member States

Member states must, among other actions, do the following:

- Establish a public data protection authority (Article 28, Recitals 63 and 64).
- Require prior checking, by the authority or an independent data protection officer appointed by the data controller, of operations likely to pose specific risks to fundamental rights and freedoms (Article 20).
- Take measures to publicize all processing operations (Article 21).
- Provide judicial remedies for breaches of the specific rights (Article 22) and for the award of damages for violations (Article 23).
- Prohibit the transfer of personal data to countries outside the EEA unless certain conditions are satisfied (Article 26(1) and Recital 58), or the Commission has found that a country provides adequate protection. (This is of special relevance in the case of medical research, because this research is often sponsored by international companies. By 2007, only Argentina, Switzerland, and Canada had been recognized as providing "adequate protection.")

indirectly, the United Kingdom has apparently interpreted this differently. The U.K. Data Protection Act defines personal data, in effect, as data from which the data subject can be identified directly by anyone or indirectly by the data controller.[8] In the case of sensitive personal data, processing is prohibited unless certain conditions are satisfied. Data concerning health is in this category (Article 8(1), Recital 33).

The directive does not apply to anonymized personal data, but whether or not data can be considered anonymous is not always a straightforward decision. Anonymous data is sometimes confused and conflated with *reversibly anonymized* or *coded* data, in which personal data is encrypted so as to conceal a person's identity, but a key is being lodged with an overseer or custodian. However, it is evident from the directive's definition of personal data that coded data remains personal if the identity of the subject can be ascertained by anyone. Furthermore, if apparently anonymous health data can be combined with associated data, such as age of the person, and various locations and dates, it may be possible to deduce the identity of a patient reasonably easily, especially in the case of rare diseases.

Processing covers anything that can be done with personal data automatically or manually (Articles 2(b) and 3.1, Recital 27). However, the directive covers manual processing only if the data is part of, or intended to be part of, a *filing system* (Article 3, Recital 15), which is defined as a "structured set of personal data which are accessible according to specific criteria" (Article 2(c), Recitals 15 and 27). The directive does not cover processing of personal data for purposes that fall outside the scope of EC law or processing for purely personal or household purposes (Article 3.2; Recitals 12, 13, 16).

Most of the directive's provisions are subject to exemptions under specified conditions. Space precludes a detailed presentation, but the scope for exemption for medical research will be considered in more detail.

The Scope for Exemption of Medical Research

Directive 95/46/EC does not explicitly provide an exemption for medical research. The scope for exemption must be in-

ferred and collated from exemptions provided for research or statistics generally and for processing involving personal data on health.

For example, the prohibition against further processing (Article 6(1)(b)) provides that data must be collected for an explicit purpose, which according to Recital 28 must be determined at the time of collection, and must not be further processed in a way incompatible with that purpose. Regrettably, no guidance is provided about what would constitute compatible processing. This creates problems for interpreting the provision that further processing for historical, statistical, and scientific purposes is not to be considered incompatible, provided that states provide appropriate safeguards that "must, in particular, rule out the use of the data in support of measures or decisions regarding any particular individual" (Recital 29). Under the same conditions and for the same purposes, the prohibition against keeping personal data in a person-identifying form for longer than necessary may also be lifted (Article 6(1)(e)).

The prohibition on processing sensitive personal data (Article 8(1)), which includes data relating to a person's health, may be lifted when there are suitable specific safeguards (Recital 34), if specified by national law or the decision of the supervisory authority to be in the substantial public interest (see Article 8(4)). The prohibition may also be lifted for medical purposes, provided that data are processed by a health professional or another person under an obligation of professional secrecy (Article 8(3), see also Recital 33). Medical research is not expressly listed as a medical purpose in the directive. Nonetheless, some states—like the United Kingdom in schedule 3, paragraph 8 of the 1998 U.K. Data Protection Act[8]—treat it as such for the purpose of lifting the prohibition of Article 8(1).

The duty to provide information (Article 11(1)) when personal data was not obtained from the data subject does not apply for statistics or historical or scientific research, if the provision of information would be impossible or would involve disproportionate effort, or if recording or disclosure of data is expressly provided for by law (see also Recital 40). This exemption is not applicable when data was obtained from the data subject (except, possibly, when the processing for statistics or historical or scientific research was not anticipated at the time that the data was obtained; see Recitals 39 and 40 and further below).

The rights of access to personal data granted by Article 12 may be limited "when data are processed solely for the purposes of scientific research or are kept in personal form for a period that does not exceed the period necessary for the sole purpose of creating statistics," provided that the following criteria are met: the derogation is by a legislative measure; there is clearly no risk of breaching the privacy of the data subject; and adequate legal safeguards are provided—in particular, provided the data are not used to take measures or decisions regarding any particular individual (see Article 13(2).

In principle, Article 13(1) provides the widest scope for exemption. Member states may restrict the scope of the obligations and rights for specific purposes such as national security, inspection, and others. It is difficult to see the applicability of much of this for medical research. If Article 13 is invoked, Article 28(4) requires each national supervisory authority to hear "claims for checks on the lawfulness of data processing lodged by any person." At the very least, this suggests that member states may only appeal to Article 13 if they do so explicitly. Exemptions based on protecting "the rights and freedoms of others" (Article 13(g)) would need to be assessed on a case-by-case basis.

Finally, member states may permanently exempt data that has been held in manual filing systems since before Oct. 24, 1998 from Articles 6, 7, and 8, when the data is kept for the sole purpose of historical research.

Explicit Consent

There is some debate over the need to obtain explicit consent— which some member states have interpreted to be written consent, even though there is no compelling reason to do so—each time a patient's data is used in a new research project. The directive is not clear about whether the conditions for legitimate processing that are stated in Articles 7 and 8(2) are indiscriminate alternatives or whether consent must be sought wherever practicable and possible. If the jurisprudence of the European Court of Human Rights, which has persuasive force for EC law, is followed, then to process personal health data without explicit consent is to violate the right to private and personal life (Article 8(1) of the European Convention on Human Rights) and requires special justification to be permissible. This suggests that conditions other than explicit consent may be appealed to only if seeking explicit consent would be impracticable or disproportionate or would violate overriding values.[9]

Processing Data for Purposes Not Initially Declared

Article 10 applies to cases in which data was obtained from the data subject and requires the data subject to be informed about the purposes of the intended processing; Article 11(1) applies to cases in which data was not obtained from the data subject. However, the operative part of the directive does not cover the case in which data was obtained from the data subject, but the data controller now wishes to process the data for purposes not originally envisaged. It is arguable that, when data was obtained from the data subject for purposes not intended or envisaged at the time, such processing may proceed only if the data subject is contacted and informed. However, Recital 39, read with Recital 40, suggests that in relation to "unanticipated" disclosures to third parties, the data subject need be informed only if this would not be impossible or involve disproportionate effort.

In other words, where data was obtained from the data subject, the duty to inform the subject of unanticipated disclosures to third parties may be exempted (parallel to an Article 11(2) exemption to the duty under Article 11(1)). Thus, a purposive construction may permit extension to processing for purposes not "anticipated" at the time the data was obtained from the subject.[10]

Obtaining Data That Will Be Anonymized

It is not entirely clear whether the principles of protection apply to processing that will occur after personal data are rendered anonymous. For example, if researcher A collects data from data subject B, intending to render the data anonymous and process it for purpose P (or intends to pass nonpersonal data abstracted from the personal data to researcher C, and envisages that C will wish to process it for P), must A inform B of the envisaged processing and

its purpose? Because it is clear that anonymization is itself a process performed on personal data, and Article 10 requires the data subject to be informed of the purposes of processing, it is arguable that B must be informed at least of the intention to anonymize and the purposes of so doing. Whether this is indeed the case still requires authoritative clarification.[11]

Likely Impact of the Data Protection Directive

The pharmaceutical industry and medical researchers, epidemiological researchers in particular, have been antagonistic toward the directive, and some have called for medical research to be exempted altogether.[12] However, such calls are probably premature and even misplaced. They are premature because the impact of the directive is difficult to assess without authoritative guidance on uncertainties about what is personal data, when data is rendered anonymous, and so on. They appear misplaced in that they do not discriminate among different kinds of medical research (not all of which is an unqualified good) and they ignore the principle that a fundamental right or freedom cannot be set aside unless there is an unavoidable direct conflict with another more important fundamental right or freedom.

As it is, the directive creates a good deal of scope for research to continue. It does, however, require the value of medical research to be weighed against fundamental rights and freedoms— in particular, privacy—in the way that Article 8(2) of the European Convention on Human Rights permits derogation from the right to private life, and it does not create a presumption that the needs, let alone the mere convenience, of medical researchers in pursuing their research objectives take precedence.

Much will depend on the attitude of the supervisory authorities and their willingness to take action. However, if the directive is to be effective, RECs must play a central role in judging whether the directive is being complied with. If this role is marginalized, or if there is insufficient attention to the need for RECs to be independent (bearing in mind that RECs traditionally are dominated by medical researchers, and the researchers' involvement is essential for the value of medical research to be assessed expertly) or at least to be truly representative of opinion relevant to the public interest, then the directive will fail to achieve the objective stated in Article 1(1) in relation to medical research. Perhaps above all, the attitudes of medical researchers will be crucial. If they resist the directive's aims, then there is a good chance that the directive will not be effective, no matter what else is done.

Directive 2001/20/EC—"Clinical Trials Directive"

The Clinical Trials Directive must be viewed in the context of Directive 65/65/EEC,[13] the "Medicines Directive," which requires medicinal products for human use to have been subjected to clinical trials before they can be licensed and placed on the market (see Recital 1). Article 1(1) of the Clinical Trials Directive requires member states to impose requirements of good clinical practice on clinical trials conducted on human subjects when these investigate medicinal products for human use as defined in Article 1 of the Medicines Directive. The Commission has issued some further technical guidance[14] and recently, the Clinical Trials Directive has been supplemented by Directive 2005/28/EC on good clinical practice.

The initial impetus for the Clinical Trials Directive came from the pharmaceutical industry, which desires a harmonized process and set of standards for the granting of REC approval for clinical trials. Large parts of Directive 2001/20/EC are thus devoted to the role of RECs, and in this section we will focus on this aspect of good clinical practice management.

The Role of Ethics Committees

Article 2(k) of the directive defines an "ethics committee" as follows:

> an independent body in a Member State, consisting of healthcare professionals and non-medical members, whose responsibility it is to protect the rights, safety and wellbeing of human subjects [see also Recital 2] involved in a trial and to provide public assurance of that protection, by, among other things, expressing an opinion on the trial protocol, the suitability of the investigators and the adequacy of facilities, and on the methods and documents to be used to inform trial subjects and obtain their informed consent.

A clinical trial may begin only if the REC and/or the competent authority consider that the anticipated therapeutic and public health benefits justify the risks. Compliance with this requirement must be permanently monitored (Article 3(2)(a)). Clinical trials on minors and on adults incapable of giving their consent may not proceed without the endorsement of a specialist REC or one that has obtained specialist advice (Articles 4(h) and 5(g)).

Article 6, among other things, does the following:

- Provides a list of matters that RECs must, in particular, consider when formulating their opinions.
- Permits member states to devolve consideration of some of these things to the competent authority that each state must set up under Article 9.
- Permits the REC to make one request only for supplementary information when examining an application.

There must be only one REC opinion in each member state (Article 7). The favorable opinion of an REC must be communicated to all member states via a European database to which access is restricted (Article 11(1)(d)), and which is to be treated as confidential (Article 11(3)).

The competent authority must inform the REC when it suspends or prohibits a clinical trial (Articles 12(1) and (2)). Member states may provide for inspection reports for the purposes of verifying compliance with good clinical practice to be made available to the REC (Article 15(2)). RECs must be given the power to obtain from the investigator additional information on any reported deaths of subjects (Article 16(3)).

Although the directive requires that the risk/benefit balance in a clinical trial be constantly monitored (Article 3(2)(g)), this is the only aspect that expressly needs monitoring, and there is no prescription that this aspect be monitored by RECs. Penalties for breach of the national laws implementing the directive are at the discretion of member states; the directive itself does not prescribe any penalties for failure to submit to an REC or to adhere to its decision. However, trials conducted in breach of the directive will not be able to obtain regulatory approval in the EU for the tested products. The responsibilities of research sponsors are presented in Table 18.5.

Table 18.5
Sponsors' Duties in Connection With RECs

Sponsors must do the following:

- Not begin trials without the favorable opinion of an REC (Article 9(1)); authorization may be implicit as well as explicit (Recital 11).
- Submit any substantial amendments to protocols to the REC (Article 10(a)).
- Inform the REC of any urgent safety measures in emergency situations (Article 10(b)).
- Report to the REC all relevant information about suspected serious unexpected adverse reactions as well as relevant follow-up information (Article 17(a),(b)).
- Inform the REC when a clinical trial has ended (see Article 10(c)).

REC Time Limits

Generally, the REC has 60 days from the date of receipt of a valid application to give its reasoned opinion to the applicant and the competent authority. The time limit is suspended during an ongoing request for supplementary information. In the case of trials involving gene therapy, somatic cell therapy, or medicinal products containing genetically modified organisms, an extension is permitted of a maximum of 30 days, and a further 90 days in the event of consultation with a committee. There is no time limit in the case of xenogenic cell therapy.

Data Protection and RECs

Article 3(2)(c) specifies that a clinical trial may be undertaken only if, among other conditions, the data protection rights of research subjects are safeguarded in accordance with Directive 95/46/EC (see also Recitals 2 and 17). Regarding this, Article 6(3) states that when RECs prepare their opinions they must consider, among other factors, the following:

> (g) the adequacy and completeness of the written information to be given and the procedure to be followed for the purpose of obtaining informed consent and the justification for the research on persons incapable of giving informed consent as regards the specific restrictions laid down in Article 3.

The question has arisen whether the competence to consider data protection can be taken away from an REC and delegated to another agency. Reading Article 3(2)(c) with Articles 6(3)(g) and 6(4) seems to imply that RECs have a responsibility to safeguard subjects' data protection rights under Directive 95/46/EC that may not be devolved elsewhere.[15] This is reinforced by Article 6(1) of Directive 2005/28/EC,[3] according to which RECs must have procedures to handle the requirements of, in particular, Articles 6 and 7 of Directive 2001/20/EC.

Presumably to assist RECs to assess data protection matters, Article 8 of Directive 2001/20/EC requires the Commission to provide detailed guidance on "the application format and documentation to be submitted in an application for an ethics committee opinion, in particular regarding the information that is given to subjects, and on the appropriate safeguards for the protection of personal data."[16] The role that this gives to RECs in relation to data protection matters is surely appropriate. Research subjects are in a very weak position in relation to defending themselves from breaches of their data protection rights. They are usually not in a good position to find out that these rights have been violated. Even if they find out, they might be reluctant to complain, because they are in a vulnerable position in relation to their clinicians. In addition, they usually are not well placed to take legal action, through lack of knowledge and financial resources. Even if they do manage to take legal action, they might find the courts reluctant to award any meaningful redress unless there is some extrinsic harm. It is, therefore, altogether better for breaches to be prevented than for action to be taken only after a breach has occurred. RECs are in an excellent position to know of proposed breaches, and if they do not have responsibility to withhold approval from protocols that involve breaches of research subjects' data protection rights, a major means of protecting these rights will be absent.

Likely Impact of the Clinical Trials Directive

The Clinical Trials Directive is likely to have a positive impact in improving research subjects' rights in the area it covers, if only because it makes REC review a legal requirement for research to go ahead.

The interests of the pharmaceutical industry are clearly catered to in the time limits set for REC review and in the requirement for only one national opinion on the ethics of a clinical trial. Although implementation of these requirements will expedite ethical review, and that is a legitimate aim, the limits are arguably too tight and restrictive to be suitable in all cases if the safety and rights of research subjects are paramount.

The directive is restricted to clinical trials involving medicinal products for human use. From an ethical point of view, it is arguable that an opportunity has been missed to regulate clinical research generally. It must be noted that the directive's definition of good clinical practice has been complemented by the provisions of Directive 2005/28/EC. In Recital 8 of Directive 2005/28/EC, reference is made to the requirements of good clinical practice set by the International Conference on Harmonisation (ICH GCP),[17] and the 1996 version of the Declaration of Helsinki[18] is officially incorporated into Article 3 of Directive 2005/28/EC. This is significant because the Commission specifically chose to rely on the version in which the right of individual patients over the interest of science and society are framed in an especially strong manner. Nothing in either directive precludes member states from extending the requirements of good clinical practice in other areas, and many will choose to do so in order to simplify the structures of ethical review.

At the same time, cynics might suspect that the directive will serve to expedite research without necessarily giving greater protection to research subjects, because it will undoubtedly increase the appearance that such protection is improved. This has not stopped the pharmaceutical industry complaining that Directive 2001/20/EC will damage R&D (primarily on the grounds that a 60-day time limit for the REC to make a decision and a further 30 days for the competent authority to give approval is unacceptably long).[19] Whether this will be the case will depend very much (as with Directive 95/46/EC) on the independence, transparency, and accountability of REC review structures, and on the extent to which RECs are able to play a part in data protection. It will also depend on national laws in relation to who might be a legal representative for a minor or an incapacitated adult. On many of these matters, it will be possible to pass judgment only once member states have fully implemented the directive as well as its offspring, Directive 2005/28/EC.

References

1. Directive 95/46/EC of the European Parliament and of the Council of 24 October 1995 on the protection of individuals with regard to the processing of personal data and on the free movement of such data. *Official Journal of the European Communities* 1995;L281:31–50. [Online] Available: http://eur-lex.europa.eu/LexUriServ/LexUriServ. do?uri=CELEX:31995L0046:EN:HTML.

2. Directive 2001/20/EC of the European Parliament and of the Council of 4 April 2001 on the approximation of the laws, regulations and administrative provisions of the member states relating to the implementation of good clinical practice in the conduct of clinical trials on medicinal products for human use. *Official Journal of the European Communities* 2001;L121:34–44. [Online] Available: http://europa. eu/eur-lex/pri/en/oj/dat/2001/l _121/l _12120010501en 00340044.pdf.

3. Commission Directive 2005/28/EC of 8 April 2005 laying down principles and detailed guidelines for good clinical practice as regards investigational medicinal products for human use, as well as the requirements for authorisation of the manufacturing or importation of such products. *Official Journal of the European Union* 2005; L91:13–9. [Online] Available: http://eur-lex.europa.eu/LexUriServ/ site/en/oj/2005/l _091/l _09120050409en00130019.pdf.

4. *Von Colson and Kamann v. Nordrhein-Westfalen* (Case 14/83, Apr. 10, 1984, E.C.R. 01891).

5. *Amministrazione delle Finanze dello Stato v. Simmenthal SpA.* (Case 106/77, Mar. 9, 1978, E.C.R. 00629).

6. *Ministère public et Direction du travail et de l'emploi v. Jean-Claude Levy* (Case C-158/91, Aug. 2, 1993, E.C.R. I-04287).

7. Council of Europe. Convention for the Protection of Individuals with regard to Automatic Processing of Personal Data. Strasbourg, France: Council of Europe; 1981. [Online] January 28, 1981. Available: http://conventions.coe.int/Treaty/en/Treaties/Html/108.htm.

8. United Kingdom. Data Protection Act 1998. London, U.K.: Her Majesty's Stationary Office; 1998. [Online] Available: http://www. opsi.gov.uk/ACTS/acts1998/19980029.htm.

9. *M.S. v. Sweden* (28 EHRR 313, paragraphs 34–35, Aug. 27, 1997).

10. Beyleveld D. The duty to provide information to the data subject: Articles 10 and 11 of Directive 95/46/EC. In: Beyleveld D, Townend D, Rouillé-Mirza S, Wright J, eds. *The Data Protection Directive and Medical Research Across Europe.* Aldershot, U.K.: Ashgate Publishing Limited; 2005:69–88.

11. Beyleveld D, Townend D. When is personal data rendered anonymous? Interpreting Recital 26 of Directive 95/46/EC. *Medical Law International* 2004;6:73–86.

12. Cancer experts call for action on GMC's confidentiality rules. *Health Service Journal* (Nov. 2, 2000):4.

13. Council Directive 65/65/EEC of 26 January 1965 on the approximation of provisions laid down by law, regulation or administrative action relating to proprietary medicinal products. *Official Journal of the European Communities* 1965;22:0369–0373.

14. European Commission. Implementing texts for Directive 2001/20/EC. [Online] Available: http://ec.europa.eu/enterprise/ pharmaceuticals/pharmacos/dir200120ec.htm.

15. Beyleveld D, Townend D, Wright J, eds. *Research Ethics Committees, Data Protection and Medical Research in Europe.* Aldershot, England: Ashgate Publishing Limited; 2005.

16. Enterprise Directorate-General, European Commission. Detailed guidance on the application format and documentation to be

submitted in an application for an Ethics Committee opinion on the clinical trial on medicinal products for human use; ENTR/F2/BL D (2003). [Online] April 2003. Available: http://ec.europa.eu/enterprise/pharmaceuticals/pharmacos/docs/doc2003/april/cp-guidance-ec_23_0403.pdf.

17. International Conference on Harmonisation of Technical Requirements for Registration of Pharmaceuticals for Human Use. *The ICH Harmonised Tripartite Guideline—Guideline for Good Clinical Practice.*

Geneva: ICH; 1996. [Online] Available: http://www.ich.org/LOB/media/MEDIA482.pdf.

18. World Medical Association. *Declaration of Helsinki: Recommendations Guiding Physicians in Biomedical Research Involving Human Subjects.* Somerset West, Republic of South Africa: WMA; 1996. *JAMA* 1997;277:925–6.

19. Allen D. The EU Clinical Trials Directive could spell the end of UK R&D activity. *The Pharmaceutical Journal* 2003;271:364.

Eric M. Meslin   Summer Johnson

19

National Bioethics Commissions and Research Ethics

I. Introduction

One of the more visible features of the current bioethics and public policy landscape is the existence of national and transnational commissions of experts in science, law, bioethics, medicine, religion, and related disciplines. Unlike individual bioethicists, the credentials, expertise, and functions of whom have been the subject of considerable study and commentary,[1-4] these commissions are less well understood. They exist in many countries, tend to be established in response to particular events, cases, or problems, and are increasingly being referred to by governments, courts, professional organizations, and the media.[5-10]

Given the tremendous growth in biomedical research across the globe, it is not surprising that ethical, legal, and policy issues in research involving humans would be among the topics addressed by many of these bodies. Many countries are now facing similar issues: How should informed consent be obtained in clinical trials? What is the proper structure and function of ethics review bodies? How should the most vulnerable be protected in studies? Are there obligations to provide any ongoing treatment to patients at the conclusion of a clinical trial, and if so, on whose shoulders should these obligations fall? These topics, and others such as the conduct of human embryonic stem cell research, xenotransplantation, and genetic studies using human tissue samples, have been the focus of reports, studies, and recommendations by commissions appointed by governments and other nationally recognized organizations.

The aim of this chapter is to provide an overview of national commissions with particular attention to their activities related to research involving humans. The chapter is divided into three sections. In Section I, we set the stage by providing a brief history of the long-standing interactions between science, research, and government. In particular, we situate the existence and use of these commissions within a larger and richer context of the way advice can be provided on important social issues.

In Section II, we provide some working definitions of bioethics commissions gleaned both from the literature and from descriptive data obtained from a number of such commissions around the world. In providing a stipulative definition, we are able to examine these commissions and their work products, and we illustrate some of the ways that national commissions function in the area of research ethics.

In Section III, we discuss some of the implications for research ethics resulting from the existence of national commissions. In particular, we comment on the challenges that arise from trying to assess the potential impact that such commissions may have, both for their own countries and, given the growing number of these bodies, for research ethics issues that arise internationally.

II. A Brief History of the Interaction Between Science, Research, and Government

The gathering of scholars and experts to inquire into matters of social and political importance is a phenomenon that has been occurring for over 2,000 years. For example, the Great Library at Alexandria proved both politically and socially useful in its promotion of intellectual debate, scientific inquiry, and discovery through scholarly societies.[11] Scholars in various disciplines had met throughout early modern history in groups like the Compagnie du Gai Sçavoir (established in 1323);[12] the Academia Platonica

(1462–1522) founded by Cosimo de Medici to study Plato;[13] and the Barber Surgeons of Edinburgh, later called the Royal College of Surgeons of Edinburgh.[14] However, it was not until the 17th century that academies of science and medicine gained prominence throughout Western Europe. In the late 17th century, scholarly societies like the British Royal Society and the French Academy of Sciences began to conduct inquiries as a service for their governments. Later, as the relationship between science and government grew stronger, government-commissioned advisory bodies began to supplement (if not replace) the advice provided by independent scholarly societies. These temporary, specialized bodies became more common throughout the 18th and 19th centuries and were appointed for the sole purpose of reporting on topics of importance to the monarchy.

The use of royal commissions by governments established the precedent for using what in the United States are sometimes called "blue ribbon commissions"—groups of nationally and internationally renowned experts assembled to conduct inquiries and issue advice. One such blue ribbon commission, the Commission Charged by the King with the Examination of Animal Magnetism, led by Benjamin Franklin, investigated physician/scientist Anton Mesmer's claims about the healing power of animal magnetism. Franklin's commission rejected animal magnetism on both scientific and moral grounds;[15] but more importantly, the commission was one of the first to concern itself with issues in research ethics: the use and selection of human participants in research, the ethics of using unscientific medical treatments, and the "influence of the imagination" (the placebo effect) upon patients.[16] In the United States, the scientific establishment initially resisted the intermingling of science with politics. Scientists wanted to maintain a certain level of independence from government control and resisted the development of any state-sponsored institutions for research.[17] Despite this early independence, the U.S. government eventually gave great weight to the utility of science for government and society.

By the middle of the 20th century, commissions ceased to consist solely of politicians and political advisors, and began to include civilians from a variety of academic disciplines and backgrounds. This democratization of science and research, particularly in the post–World War II era marked a significant change for science policy making, particularly in the United States. This change in the interaction between government, science, and society would have repercussions not only in the basic sciences but would extend to medical, social, and behavioral research. Just as medical research entered a golden era of unprecedented expansion at this time, the increasing use of humans in medical experimentation raised profound questions about the ethical issues arising from the involvement of humans in medical studies. Henry Beecher's 1966 exposé of unethical conduct of research with humans published in well-respected research journals[18] and the extensive discussions by Pappworth[19] and Katz[20] contributed to a literature on medical research ethics that influenced both the public's perception of the value of science and the trust that government had in the ability of science to regulate itself.

In 1974, the U.S. Congress established the National Commission for the Protection of Human Subjects of Biomedical and Behavioral Research (the National Commission) "to identify the ethical principles of human subjects research and to recommend federal policy for research."[21] This was the first national bioethics commission in the United States, and it addressed important issues in research with humans, profoundly influencing both political and public opinion on medical practice and research in the process. In 1979, after preparing nine reports on topics such as research on the fetus, psychosurgery, and individuals who were institutionalized as mentally infirm, the National Commission published its most influential work, the *Belmont Report*, defining the ethical principles that ought to inform research involving humans,[22] a document that still has an impact on medical research three decades later[23] (see Chapter 14). Since that time, six time-limited national bioethics commissions of one form or another have been established in the United States.[24]

By the end of the 1980s, national bioethics commissions had been established in many other countries including Australia, Canada, Denmark, France, Hungary, Luxembourg, Malta, the Philippines, Sweden, the United Kingdom, and Zimbabwe. In 2005, national bioethics commissions existed in at least 85 countries, on every continent of the globe except Antarctica.[25]

III. National Bioethics Commissions: Definitions and Characteristics

Although definitional matters seem less important than normative ones, it is helpful to set out what national commissions are before examining what they do. No definition of a national bioethics commission has been formally adopted, but a consensus is gradually emerging, one that largely is based on the literature describing the history of public advisory commissions generally;[26–30] the history of bioethics commissions in particular;[5–10,31] the experiences of commission members and staff about the role, function, and effectiveness of commissions;[24,32–36] and the impact of these commissions.[37] Supplementing this scholarly work are the reports produced by the commissions themselves. To understand how commissions define themselves, we obtained reports from many who attended the Fourth Global Summit for National Bioethics Advisory Bodies in Brasilia (2003) and supplemented this material with information about commissions from the UNESCO[38] and the World Health Organization web sites.[25]

Definitions

We reviewed reports of more than 50 commissions and found that they tended to have the following characteristics:

- They were national-level advisory bodies. By "national-level," we mean that the commission aims to address bioethical issues deemed to be of importance to the country as a whole.
- They addressed issues in public bioethics. This characteristic is closely related to the one above, because issues of national importance can also be described as involving a notion of *public bioethics*—a term proposed more than a decade ago by John Fletcher who defined it as "[a] process . . . by which 'society' supports ethical inquiry prior to developing directions for public policy."[39] This definition is supported by the analytic literature on governmental, particularly executive, advisory bodies in the United States and some other countries. This characterization is also complementary to an emerging consensus in the political science literature about the role and function of executive advisory bodies.[26,29,40,41]
- They were established and funded either by a national government or other recognized national-level body. Although

most of the commissions that have contributed significantly to public discourse about research ethics were established by national governments or their agencies, a small minority were established by nongovernmental organizations (e.g., medical associations, foundations). Therefore, as in the first criterion, "national-level" also refers to a commission's location within the political system. Local or regional bioethics review boards or committees within a given country were omitted.

- Their members represented different disciplines, competencies, and perspectives. This means that a commission would typically include various academic, private, political, and public points of view. Among the more intriguing and persistent issues facing commissions is the way in which public representation or public engagement occurs. Some commissions, like those in the United States, are required by law to include opportunities for public input—whether by including members of the public or by convening open meetings accessible to members of the public. Other commissions have no such requirement.

Commission Characteristics

In addition, there are a number of characteristics that help to understand these bodies. These characteristics are important to understanding how these commissions function in diverse ways around the globe.

(i) Creation

Some commissions were created to address a particular topic; others were put in place to anticipate and address certain types of topics. A number of theories exist about why governments and or heads of state use commissions for various public policy problems. One theory suggests that governments use commissions as responses to crises, for policy analysis, as long-range educational projects, as issue avoidance or misdirection, or as "window dressing."[40] Bioethics commissions may emerge for several of these complementary reasons, but essentially they serve as a public response to particular controversial scientific or political events that present a public policy problem. As a general observation, bioethics commissions are often established in response to three primary cues: a scientific controversy, lack of knowledge, and lack of policy alternatives. In addition, when these three elements are satisfied, commissions can also be used as a means of resolving disagreement about which policy alternative is optimal.

In the area of ethical conduct of research with humans, commissions can be created as a means of generating research ethics guidance or providing oversight of human-participant research in a number of countries around the world. The U.S. National Commission arose from the establishment of a federal law, the *National Research Act*, which was itself the product of a series of prominent congressional hearings that highlighted concerns about research involving humans.[42] In contrast, the U.S. Advisory Committee on Human Radiation Experiments was established in 1995 in response to specific allegations about the conduct of radiation research on both military personnel and civilians.[43] The two most recent commissions—the National Bioethics Advisory Commission (NBAC) and the President's Council on Bioethics (PCB)—were established by a presidential Executive Order. However,

committees in other countries have had similar experiences in which public discourse and political attention to emerging issues in health care, science, technology, and research generated increased attention to the associated ethical, legal, and social issues and the need for policy analysis and education in these areas.[10,44,45–47]

(ii) Scope

Governmental bioethics commissions can address either a wide or a very narrow set of public bioethical issues. Although the majority of commissions are given a broad mandate to deal with research ethics topics in general or as needed, a few single-issue bodies also exist, usually influenced by governmental officials and government priorities. In our sample, these commissions dealt primarily with issues in assisted reproduction or biotechnology research. The Spanish National Commission on Assisted Human Reproduction is asked to "inform or advise in respect to assisted reproductive technologies and . . . the investigation or experimentation upon human fertility, gametes, and preembryos."[48] Alternatively, the Bioethics Advisory Commission of Singapore has included in its mandate "to protect the rights and welfare of individuals while allowing the biomedical sciences to develop and realize their full potential in Singapore, and for the benefit of humankind."[49] This kind of broad mandate allows commissions to address a variety of issues related to research with humans, either at the discretion of the commission members or based upon input from political leaders. This kind of "broad scope" advisory commission appears to be more common than the "narrow scope" commissions.

(iii) Accountability

Substantial variation exists in regard to accountability among bioethics commissions. We found that commissions tend to exist in a number of locations within governmental systems. Although the majority of governmental bioethics commissions are accountable to ministries or departments (e.g., health, education, science, culture), these bodies are also located under the auspices of research councils, heads of state and their cabinets, and funding agencies. Because no patterns are apparent in regard to particular types of commissions and their government location, it is likely that the development of bioethics commissions in various countries is largely dependent upon contingent factors including leadership interest in research with humans, funding availability, and other political factors.

(iv) Governance and Oversight

Commissions also differ with respect to specific governance issues such as the frequency of meetings, rules of procedure (e.g., voting, consensus), budgets, and staffing. These characteristics are often determined by a commission's terms of reference. These terms are usually written by the political authority to which the commission is accountable and vary according to the commission's function. For example, some protocol review commissions meet only on an "as-needed" basis, when protocols require review; other commissions meet monthly while they are generating policy recommendations for a report. The terms of reference can also govern other aspects of a commission including membership, topics to be addressed, and the powers given to the commission.

(v) Locus of Authority

Although the majority of national commissions described in this chapter trace their origins to the executive or legislative branches of their national governments, other "national" bioethics commissions trace their origins to nongovernmental sources. As with government bodies, these commissions are created to address issues considered to be of national importance by a particular group of leaders interested in bioethics and consist of members who represent a diversity of expertise, typically including various professional interests. One of the most influential and effective of these independent commissions is the United Kingdom's Nuffield Council on Bioethics. The Nuffield Council was established and is funded by a private foundation—the Nuffield Foundation—which is responsible for appointing the council's chair, whereas members are selected by the chairperson and currently sitting members. The Nuffield Council has been one of the most active and productive advisory commissions in the world, having produced more than a dozen major reports on bioethics topics, eight of which relate directly to research ethics.[50]

Other Bioethics Advisory Bodies

There are several countries whose primary public bioethics activity is not conducted through a national bioethics commission. These nongovernmental bioethics advisory bodies are of two different kinds: professional organization bodies and independent bioethics commissions. Often, economically developing countries conduct bioethics and public policy work in whatever institutions can support them and wherever interest in bioethics thrives. In some cases, these bodies can simply serve as nongovernmental sources of information and analysis. In other cases, these bodies may have an advantage over governmental commissions in that they are freer from political influence and limitations. On the other hand, the scope of authority and the influence of these bioethics advisory bodies may be much more limited than that of national bioethics commissions sponsored by governments.

A much smaller group of bioethics advisory bodies provide advice, recommendations, and information to professional associations and groups. Similar to national bioethics commissions, these professional bodies can serve a number of functions including policy recommendation, guidance generation, professional education, and protocol review. For example, the Cyprus Medical Association Bioethics Committee performed multiple functions including protocol review and policy recommendations on research ethics. It is one of three research ethics review bodies that have existed in Cyprus.[53] The most common location for these professional bioethics advisory bodies is in national-level medical societies or associations. Medical societies in the United States and the United Kingdom also serve similar policy, guidance, and educational functions.

IV. Commissions and Research Ethics

One hundred twelve national commissions have existed whose work has focused in whole or in part on issues arising from research involving humans. These commissions have addressed topics ranging from aging research to xenotransplan-

tation. Table 19.1 lists a range of topics addressed by these commissions.

Among national bioethics commissions, there is great variety in their functions with respect to research ethics. Below we describe a typology of various functions. These functions are not mutually exclusive, because a substantial number of commissions have served in more than one capacity. Moreover, a number of countries have or have had more than one national bioethics commission functioning at any one time. For example, Norway and Finland have a number of separate national-level research ethics commissions in areas such as medicine, the social sciences, and biotechnology. The presence of multiple bioethics commissions in a country often means that each commission serves a different role within the government.

Advice and Guidance

Advice is probably the most frequent service sought from national bioethics commissions. Commissions can be asked to provide advice on a wide range of bioethical issues or can be given a narrow mandate in just one area of public bioethics. Often these commissions are asked to conduct policy analysis and generate policy statements, as well as to provide general counsel to government officials or departments that require advice in regard to bioethical issues. Commissions can be given additional functions besides the provision of policy advice. Sometimes they can serve as protocol review bodies (usually serving as an appellate or specialized review body) or are given guidance or administrative powers. The first combination of duties has occurred in a number of countries including the Philippines, Slovenia, the United Kingdom, and China. Commissions combining policy advice and administrative duties are found in Mexico, Canada, Australia, and India. The United States has used national bioethics advisory commissions for three decades, with four commissions (the National Commission, the President's Commission, NBAC, and the current PCB) producing more than 20 advisory reports.

Some bodies, like the Central Ethics Committee on Human Research in India, are given the authority to produce guidance for research ethics in their country. This commission produced Ethical Guidelines for Biomedical Research on Human Subjects in 2000. Guidance commissions are also created with other functions included in their mandate. Commissions in Australia, Canada, Japan, India, and Mexico provide policy advice in addition to preparing guidance. Two other countries, Denmark and

Table 19.1

Selected Research Ethics Topics Addressed by National Commissions

Aging	Mental health
Children	Mental disorders
Cloning	Reproductive technologies
Genetics	Stem cell research
Genetic testing	Research on tissue samples
Informed consent	Vulnerable participants
International health research	Xenotransplantation
International clinical trials	

Thailand, combined guidance authority with the capacity for protocol review in their national bioethics commission.

Inquiry

Sometimes commissions are created to investigate an emerging policy issue about which there is insufficient information, policy alternatives, or consensus about which policy alternative is most justifiable. Commissions of this sort tend to have certain defined legal powers, such as subpoena power, that they exercise carefully. Internationally, a number of advisory bodies have been created to deal with such issues as human cloning and embryonic stem cell research, including commissions that rapidly emerged in response to public policy problems in countries such as Australia, Chile, France, the United States, and the United Kingdom.

Education and Training

A number of bioethics commissions have received the task of providing public and/or professional education on bioethical issues in their country. In particular, the Swedish National Council on Medical Ethics was charged to "stimulate exchange of information and ideas and promote discussion on new medical research and applications."[51] Similarly, commissions in Australia, Canada, the Dominican Republic, Estonia, and Greece each specifically mention an educational goal in their terms of reference.

Administration

Other governmental bioethics commissions function as administrators in dealing with regulatory issues in research ethics. In particular, Canada's National Council on Ethics in Human Research (NCEHR) has a mandate to assist research ethics boards (REBs) in "interpreting and implementing guidelines," assisting in resolving contentious issues in REBs, and "providing assistance to REBs" in quality control in review and oversight of research.[52] Another such commission is Brazil's National Commission for Ethics in Research, which similarly aims to foster and monitor review boards in its country.

Protocol Review

Governmental bioethics commissions frequently engage in research protocol review, often combining this role with another function such as policy advice or policy construction. Commissions can serve in a number of different capacities—for example, as national-level appeal bodies for resolving local ethics review committee disputes or confusion over research regulations. Other commissions conduct only specialized reviews: They review certain types of research protocols, such as gene transfer research (e.g., the U.S. Recombinant DNA Advisory Committee) or assisted reproduction and embryo research (e.g., the U.K. Human Fertilisation and Embryology Authority, and New Zealand's National Ethics Committee on Assisted Human Reproduction). Particularly in countries with less extensive research infrastructures, commissions can also serve either as a national ethics review committee required to review all research in a given country or as an ethics review committee that reviews only research conducted in a national-level or government-sponsored organization. Examples of the latter occur in China, Cyprus, Gambia, Latvia, Slovenia, and Zimbabwe. National-level institutional research ethics review bodies existed in three countries: Estonia, Kenya, and Venezuela. Some countries use their national ethics commission in a capacity that is complementary to local or regional research review. Australia is an example in which such a system is used.[44]

Table 19.2 provides a list of the commissions and, where possible, their major functions.

V. Commission Impact and Influence

Assessing Impact

National bioethics commissions that address research ethics issues exist in many countries and carry out different functions. To date, little consideration has been given to assessing the impact of such advisory bodies on research ethics. This is due in part to the inherent difficulties in measuring the impact of a national bioethics commission. Elisa Eiseman recently assessed the impact of the U.S. National Bioethics Advisory Commission (NBAC) on public policy[37] using the following methods:

- Tracking and analyzing responses from government agencies and departments to commission reports and recommendations
- Tracking and analyzing responses from professional societies, organizations, and foundations to commission reports and recommendations
- Tracking legislation that was introduced or enacted abroad that was a result (direct or indirect) of reports and recommendations
- Tracking policies, statements, and other documents from national scientific, medical, and bioethics bodies and international organizations that refer to or are based on any of the commission's reports or recommendations
- Tracking the peer-reviewed literature to assess the scholarly responses to reports and recommendations
- Tracking the media (print, visual, web) to determine the coverage given to particular topics or discussions

Eiseman's assessment concluded with the following observation:

NBAC has increased the awareness of the U.S. and foreign governments, international groups, the research community, and the public about complex bioethical issues, providing a forum for their public debate, and making recommendations that have been incorporated into the system of oversight for the protection of human research participants.[37]

By each of these methods, any commission could be judged to have a greater or lesser impact, so it is important to acknowledge (as Eiseman did) the inherent difficulties in any such assessment. The difficulties included the following:

- The impact of any report will have both a short-term and a long-term effect, and only the former can be addressed at any point in time.
- Reports developed earlier in a commission's tenure have a greater likelihood of being considered in policy discussions than those released later in a commission's tenure because interested parties have had more time to respond to the earlier reports.

Table 19.2

Commissions by Country and Type

Country	Title	Type(s)
Albania	Albanian Committee on Bioethics	Advisory
Algeria	National Council of Ethics in Science and Health	Advisory
Argentina	National Commission of Biomedical Ethics of Argentina	Advisory
Australia	National Bioethics Consultative Committee	Advisory
Australia	Australian Health Ethics Committee	Advisory
Austria	Austrian Commission on Bioethics	Advisory
Belgium	Belgian Advisory Committee on Bioethics	Advisory, Education
Bolivia	National Ethics and Bioethics Steering Committee of the Bolivian Academy of Medicine	Advisory, Guidance
Bolivia	National Bioethics Committee of Bolivia	Advisory
Brazil	National Commission for Ethics in Research	Guidance, Protocol Review
Burkina Faso	National Ethics Committee for Health Research	Guidance, Protocol Review
Cameroon	National Ethics Committee for the Protection of Medical Research Participants	Protocol Review
Canada	Royal Commission on New Reproductive Technologies	Inquiry, Advisory
Canada	National Council on Ethics in Human Research	Administrative
Canada	Interagency Advisory Panel on Research Ethics	Advisory
Canada	CIHR Standing Committee on Ethics	Advisory
Canada	Tri-Council Working Group (Joint effort of Medical Research Council of Canada, Natural Sciences and Engineering Research Council of Canada, and the Social Sciences and Humanities Research Council of Canada)	Advisory
China	Ministry of Health Ethics Committee	Advisory, Protocol Review
Congo	National Bioethics Committee	Protocol Review
Côte d'Ivoire	Côte d'Ivoire National Bioethics Advisory Commission	Advisory
Cuba	Cuban National Bioethics Commission	Advisory
Cyprus	Cyprus National Bioethics Committee	Protocol Review, Advisory
Czech Republic	Central Ethics Committee of the Ministry of Health of the Czech Republic	Advisory
Czech Republic	Bioethical Commission Associated to the Research and Development Council of the Government of the Czech Republic	Advisory
Denmark	Central Scientific Ethical Committee	Guidance, Protocol Review
Denmark	Danish Council of Ethics	Advisory
Dominican Republic	National Bioethics Commission	Advisory
Ecuador	Ecuador National Commission for Bioethics	Unknown
Egypt	Egyptian National Committee for Bioethics	Advisory
Estonia	Estonian Council on Bioethics	Advisory, Protocol Review, Guidance
Estonia	Human Research Ethics Committee	Protocol Review
Estonia	Ethics Committee of the Estonian Human Genome Project	Advisory
Ethiopia	National Health Research Ethics Review Committee	Guidance, Protocol Review
Finland	National Advisory Board for Biotechnology	Advisory
Finland	National Advisory Board for Health Care Ethics/Subcommittee on Medical Research Ethics	Advisory, Protocol Review
Finland	National Advisory Board on Research Ethics	Advisory, Education
France	French National Ethics Committee for the Ethics of Experimentation on Human Subjects	Advisory
France	National Consultative Ethics Committee on Health and Life Science	Advisory
Gambia	Gambia/Medical Research Council Joint Ethical Committee	Protocol Review
Georgia	National Bioethics Council of Georgia	Advisory, Protocol Review, Guidance
Germany	National Ethics Council	Advisory
Greece	Hellenic National Bioethics Commission	Advisory

Table 19.2 *(Continued)*

Country	Title	Type(s)
Hungary	Scientific and Research Ethics Committee of the Medical Research Council	Advisory
Iceland	National Bioethics Committee of Iceland	Advisory, Protocol Review, Guidance
India	Central Ethics Committee on Human Research	Guidance
Iran	Committee of Bioethics, National Committee for Ethics in Science and Technology	Unknown
Ireland	Irish Council for Bioethics	Advisory, Education
Israel	Bioethics Advisory Committee	Advisory
Italy	Italian National Bioethics Committee	Inquiry, Advisory
Italy	National Research Council Bioethics Commission	Guidance
Japan	Bioethics Committee of the Council for Science and Technology of Japan	Guidance
Kenya	National Ethical Review Committee	Protocol Review
Latvia	Central Medical Ethics Committee	Protocol Review
Lebanon	Bioethics Committee of the National Scientific Research Council	Unknown
Lithuania	Lithuanian Bioethics Committee	Administrative, Advisory
Luxembourg	National Ethics Advisory Commission on the Life Sciences and Health	Advisory
Malta	Bioethics Consultative Committee	Advisory
Mauritius	National Bioethics Committee of Mauritius	Unknown
Mexico	National Commission of Bioethics	Guidance, Advisory
Nepal	Nepal Health Research Council	Guidance, Protocol Review
Netherlands	Health Council of the Netherlands	Advisory
Netherlands	Central Committee for Research Involving Human Subjects	Protocol Review, Administrative
Netherlands	The Rathenau Institute	Education, Advisory
New Zealand	National Ethics Committee on Assisted Reproductive Technology	Advisory
New Zealand	Health Research Council Ethics Committee	Administrative
New Zealand	National Ethics Advisory Committee—the National Advisory Committee on Health and Disability Support Services Ethics	Advisory
New Zealand	National Ethics Advisory Committee	Advisory
Nigeria	National Ethics Committee of Nigeria	Unknown
Norway	National Committee for Research Ethics in the Social Sciences and Humanities	Advisory
Norway	National Committee for Medical Research Ethics	Advisory
Peru	Peruvian Bioethics Commission	Advisory
Philippines	National Health Research Ethics Committee	Administrative
Philippines	National Ethics Committee	Advisory
Poland	Commission for Research Ethics	Advisory
Portugal	National Council of Ethics for the Life Sciences	Advisory
Russia	Russian National Committee on Bioethics	Advisory
Saudi Arabia	National Committee for Medical and Bioethics	Guidance, Protocol Review
Senegal	National Health Research Council, Ethics Committee	Protocol Review
Senegal	National Ethics Committee	Unknown
Singapore	Bioethics Advisory Committee	Advisory
Slovakia	Central Ethics Committee for the Ministry of Health	Advisory
Slovenia	National Medical Ethics Committee	Advisory, Protocol Review
South Africa	National Health Research Ethics Council	Advisory, Protocol Review
Spain	Committee on Ethics for Science and New Technologies	Advisory
Spain	National Commission on Assisted Human Reproduction	Advisory, Education
Spain	Catalonian Bioethics Committee	Advisory, Administrative

(continued)

Table 19.2   (*Continued*)

Country	Title	Type(s)
Spain	Advisory Committee on the Ethics of Scientific and Technical Research	Advisory
Sri Lanka	National Science and Technology Commission	Education, Advisory
Sweden	Swedish National Council on Medical Ethics	Advisory
Sweden	The Swedish Council on Technology Assessment in Health Care	Advisory
Switzerland	Swiss National Advisory Commission on Biomedical Ethics	Advisory
Syria	Syrian National Bioethics Committee	Advisory
Tanzania	National Ethics Review Committee	Guidance, Protocol Review
Thailand	Ethical Review Committee for Research in Human Subjects	Guidance, Protocol Review
Tunisia	National Medical Ethics Committee	Advisory
Uganda	National Bioethics Committee of Uganda	Unknown
Ukraine	National Bioethics Commission	Advisory
United Kingdom	Nuffield Council on Bioethics	Advisory
United Kingdom	Medical Ethics Committee of the British Medical Association	Advisory
United Kingdom	Ethics and Governance Interim Advisory Group, U.K. Biobank	Advisory
United Kingdom	Human Fertilisation and Embryology Authority	Administrative, Guidance
United Kingdom	Human Genetics Commission	Advisory
United Kingdom	Central Office for Research Ethics Committees	Administrative
United States	Bioethics Advisory Commission	Advisory
United States	The President's Council on Bioethics	Education, Advisory
United States	Recombinant DNA Advisory Committee	Protocol Review, Advisory
United States	President's Commission for the Study of Ethical Problems in Medicine and Biomedical and Behavioral Research	Advisory
United States	Advisory Committee on Human Radiation Experiments	Inquiry
United States	National Commission for the Protection of Human Subjects of Biomedical and Behavioral Research	Advisory
United States	National Bioethics Advisory Commission	Advisory
Venezuela	Bioethics Commission of the Venezuelan Institute of Scientific Research	Protocol Review
Zimbabwe	Medical Research Council of Zimbabwe Ethics Committee	Protocol Review, Administrative

- Issues differed in their immediate importance to policy makers. For example, NBAC's reports on cloning and stem cell research were of immediate concern to policy makers and received a lot of attention, whereas the report on clinical trials research in developing countries received far less attention.
- When a government agency, professional society, or international organization develops policy or adopts guidelines that make use of or refer to a commission's work, it does not necessarily mean that the commission should be credited with having had a direct influence on the decision to develop or adopt guidelines.
- Much of a commission's contribution to the policy-making process has been to inform public discussion and debate over some highly contentious and value-laden issues, a contribution that is not easily measured.

One immediately recognizes that these methods (alone or in combination) are but proxies for assessing the full impact of a commission. Many indicators of impact are much less easily measurable but may be more substantial, such as changes in public attitudes on bioethics issues, increased interest in the field

of bioethics, or heightened awareness of issues on the part of policy makers. We recognize that further work must be done in this area if policy makers, legislators, health-care providers, and others are to understand and appreciate the value of such commissions.

Implications of National Bioethics Commissions for Research With Humans

For many countries, their national commissions are often the first source of consultation for their respective governments on emerging issues in science and technology.[54] Assigning a commission to address an issue provides government with the opportunity to step back and reflect rather than to precipitously act/react. This was an effective method used by President Bill Clinton in 1997 and 1998 when he directed NBAC to examine the issues arising from the cloning of the sheep "Dolly"[55] and from researchers' isolation of human embryonic stem cells, respectively.[56] In a similar vein, national and international discussion of the ethical issues arising from the conduct of clinical trials in developing countries was stimulated, in part, by the attention given to it by NBAC[57] and the Nuffield Council.[58] The ethical acceptability of placebos, harmonization of guidelines, and the obligation to provide posttrial benefits at the completion of trials were actively discussed by these two commissions before achieving wider discussion in the international community.[59]

For some commissions, the impact of their work may be direct and obvious. For example, the Central Ethics Committee on Human Research in India created research ethics guidelines that in 2007 were pending regulatory approval.[60, 61] Similarly, for more than two decades, the comprehensive work of France's National Consultative Ethics Committee on Health and Life Science has had a direct impact on French health law, including the recent revisions to the Laws on the Protection of Persons in Biomedical Research, commonly known as the French Bioethics Laws.[62,63]

However, individual commission productivity is only one frame of reference. In recent years, commissions around the world have begun to work together, benefiting from each other's expertise. Since 1995, five "global summits" of national bioethics commissions have convened—in San Francisco, Tokyo, London, Brasilia, and Canberra. These summits were facilitated by the efforts of national bioethics bodies in the United States, France, the United Kingdom, and Australia, and by the World Health Organization and the International Association of Bioethics. They have been productive in certain ways. For example, the Tokyo Summit produced a communiqué, the content of which suggests a willingness to use the combined knowledge and expertise of national commissions to address important issues in research ethics.[64] The work of these commissions, in concert with transnational organizations, has the potential to have a significant impact on issues of global bioethics.

VI. Conclusion

We think the future is promising for national bioethics commissions. In particular, we are optimistic about the untapped potential that these groups can draw on to influence both domestic and international research ethics policy. If the history of national commissions is a guide, we expect more countries to develop committees, and countries with existing committees to expand their use. As with all capacity building, time will tell whether efforts like these will be instrumentally as well as symbolically important. Because the existence of a commission often means greater access to the bioethics literature, the sharing of bioethics scholarship and work, and greater openness by public, private, and nongovernmental organizations, it is likely that many of the more pressing topics in research ethics—such as access to clinical trials, informed consent, and assessment of risk and potential benefit—will enjoy the fruits of national as well as transnational deliberation. As efforts to harmonize international research ethics policies and protocols take on great force, national bioethics commissions may offer resources previously unavailable to their governments.

As both repositories and conveyors of information, national bioethics commissions carry on an important tradition of bridging medicine, science, and ethics, with the aim of improving public discourse and policy. Beginning with the Great Library at Alexandria, through the Royal Societies and Royal Commissions of the early 18th and 19th centuries, to the present day, countries have made use of organized committees to advise societies and political leaders. Given the expansion of research involving humans, we expect that these advisory bodies will continue to be an important political tool throughout the 21st century.

Acknowledgments

The authors gratefully acknowledge the assistance of all bioethics commissions and their staff that provided information, reports, and related materials. These commissions and staff members are not responsible for any unintended errors in our reporting of their work. We also thank Elizabeth Garman, who helped collect reports from national commissions and assisted with the initial analysis; Amy Hatfield, who continues to collect bioethics commission reports for our database; and both Reidar Lie and Robert A. Crouch for helpful comments on an earlier draft.

Financial Disclosure

The Indiana University Center for Bioethics is supported by the Indiana Genomics Initiative (INGEN), which is supported by the Lilly Endowment, Inc.

References

1. Aulisio M, Arnold R, Youngner S, for the Society for Health and Human Values-Society for Bioethics Consultation Task Force on Standards for Bioethics Consultation. Health care ethics consultation: Nature, goals, and competencies. A position paper from the Society for Health and Human Values-Society for Bioethics Consultation Task Force on Standards for Bioethics Consultation. *Annals of Internal Medicine* 2000;133:59–69.
2. Cummins D. The professional status of bioethics consultation. *Theoretical Medicine and Bioethics* 2002;23:19–43.
3. Churchill L. Are we professionals? A critical look at the social role of bioethicists. *Daedalus* 1999;128:253–74.
4. Andre J, Fleck L, Tomlinson T. Improving our aim. *Journal of Medicine and Philosophy* 1999;24:130–47.
5. Walters L. Commissions and bioethics. *Journal of Medicine and Philosophy* 1989;14:363–8.
6. Williams JR. Commissions and biomedical ethics: The Canadian experience. *Journal of Medicine and Philosophy* 1989;14:425–44.
7. Wikler D. Bioethics commissions abroad. *HEC Forum* 1994;6:290–304.
8. U.S. Congress, Office of Technology Assessment. *Biomedical Ethics in U.S. Public Policy—Background Paper.* OTA-BP-BBS-105. Washington, D.C.: U.S. Government Printing Office; June 1993.
9. McNeill PM. *The Ethics and Politics of Human Experimentation.* New York, N.Y.: Cambridge University Press; 1993.
10. Halila R. The role of national ethics commissions in Finland. *Bioethics* 2003;17:357–68.
11. Biblioteca Alexandrina. The foundation of the museum and the library. Biblioteca Alexandrina, 2003. [Online] Available: http://www.bibalex.org.
12. Compagnie du Gai Sçavoir. [Online] Available: http://www.scholarly-societies.org/history/1323cgs.html.
13. Field A. *The Origins of the Platonic Academy of Florence.* Princeton, N.J.: Princeton University Press; 1988.
14. The Royal College of Surgeons Edinburgh. About the College. [Online] Available: http://www.rcsed.ac.uk/site/297/default.aspx.
15. McConkey K, Perry C. Franklin and Mesmerism revisited. *International Journal of Clinical and Experimental Hypnosis* 2002;50:320–31.

16. Franklin B, et al. Report of the commissioners charged by the King with the examination of animal magnetism. *International Journal of Clinical and Experimental Hypnosis* 2002;50:332–63.

17. Greenberg D. *The Politics of Pure Science,* 2nd ed. Chicago, Ill.: University of Chicago Press; 1999 [1967].

18. Beecher HK. Ethics and clinical research. *New England Journal of Medicine* 1966;274:1354–60.

19. Pappworth M. *Human Guinea Pigs: Experimentation on Man.* Boston, Mass.: Beacon Press; 1967.

20. Katz J, with Capron AM, Glass ES. *Experimentation with Human Beings.* New York, N.Y.: Russell Sage Foundation; 1972.

21. U.S. Congress. National Research Act of 1974. 7–12–1974. Public Law 93–348, Title H, Part A.

22. The National Commission for the Protection of Human Subjects of Biomedical and Behavioral Research. *The Belmont Report: Ethical Principles and Guidelines for the Protection of Human Subjects of Research.* Washington, D.C.: Department of Health, Education and Welfare; 1979. DHEW Publication OS 78–0012 1978. [Online] Available: http://www.hhs.gov/ohrp/humansubjects/guidance/belmont.htm.

23. Childress JF, Meslin EM, Shapiro HT, eds. *Belmont Revisited: Ethical Principles for Research With Human Subjects.* Washington, D.C.: Georgetown University Press; 2005.

24. Meslin EM, Shapiro HT. Some initial reflections on NBAC. *Kennedy Institute of Ethics Journal* 2002;12:95–102.

25. World Health Organization, Department of Ethics, Trade, Human Rights and Health Law. Interactive bioethics commission map. [Online] Available: http://www.who.int/ethics/committees/en/index.html.

26. Bell D. Government by commission. In: Cronin TE, Greenberg SD, eds. *The Presidential Advisory System.* New York, N.Y.: Harper & Row; 1969:117–23.

27. Wolanin TR. *Presidential Advisory Commissions: Truman to Nixon.* Madison, Wis.: University of Wisconsin Press; 1975.

28. Graham HD. The ambiguous legacy of American presidential commissions. *The Public Historian* 1985;7(2):5–25.

29. Zegart AB. Blue ribbons, black boxes: Toward a better understanding of presidential commissions. *Presidential Studies Quarterly* 2004;34:366–93.

30. Flitner DJ. *The Politics of Presidential Commissions.* Dobbs Ferry, N.Y.: Transnational Publishers; 1985.

31. Schüklenk U, Lott JP. Bioethics and (public) policy advice. In: Thiele F, Ashcroft RE, editors. *Bioethics in a Small World.* Berlin, Germany: Springer-Verlag; 2004:129–138.

32. Meslin EM. Engaging the public in policy development: The National Bioethics Advisory Commission report on "Research Involving Persons with Mental Disorders That May Affect Decisionmaking Capacity." *Accountability in Research* 1999;7:227–39.

33. Faden RR. The Advisory Committee on Human Radiation Experiments: Reflections on a Presidential Commission. *Hastings Center Report* 1996;26(5):5–10.

34. Gray BH. Bioethics commissions: What can we learn from past successes and failures? In: Institute of Medicine (Bulger RE, Bobby EM, Fineberg HV, eds.). *Society's Choices: Social and Ethical Decision Making in Biomedicine.* Washington, D.C.: National Academy Press; 1995:261–306.

35. Toulmin SE. The National Commission on Human Experimentation: Procedures and outcomes. In: Engelhardt HT Jr, Caplan AL, eds. *Scientific Controversies: Case Studies in the Resolution and Closure of Disputes in Scientific and Technology.* New York, N.Y.: Cambridge University Press; 1987:599–613.

36. Wikler D. Federal bioethics: Methodology, expertise, and evaluation. *Politics and Life Sciences* 1994;13(1):100–1.

37. Eiseman E. *The National Bioethics Advisory Commission: Contributing to Public Policy.* Arlington, Va.: RAND; 2003. [Online] 2003. Available: http://www.rand.org/pubs/monograph_reports/MR1546/.

38. United Nations Educational, Scientific and Cultural Organization (UNESCO). Bioethics Database. [Online] Available: http://www.unesco.org.

39. Fletcher JC. On restoring public bioethics. *Politics and the Life Sciences* 1994;13(1):84–6.

40. Wolanin T. *Presidential Advisory Commissions: Truman to Nixon.* Madison, Wis.: University of Wisconsin Press; 1975.

41. Graham HD. The ambiguous legacy of American presidential commissions. *The Public Historian* 1985;7(2):5–25.

42. Jonsen AR. *The Birth of Bioethics.* New York, N.Y.: Oxford University Press; 1998:94–8.

43. Advisory Committee on Human Radiation Experiments. *Final Report of the Advisory Committee on Human Radiation Experiments.* New York, N.Y.: Oxford University Press; 1996.

44. Chalmers D. Research ethics in Australia. In: National Bioethics Advisory Commission. *Ethical and Policy Issues in Research Involving Human Participants, Vol. II.* Bethesda, Md.: NBAC; 2001:A1–A66. [Online] Available: http://www.georgetown.edu/research/nrcbl/nbac/human/overv012.pdf.

45. Glasa J, ed., for the Council of Europe. *Ethics Committees in Central and Eastern Europe.* Bratislava, Slovak Republic: Institute of Medical Ethics and Bioethics Foundation; 2000.

46. Gefenas E. A short information about the Lithuanian national committee on biomedical ethics. *Journal International de Bioéthiques* 2000;11(1):63.

47. Sass HM. Ethical decision making in committee: A view from Germany. *Notizie di Politeia* 2002;18(67):65–81.

48. National Commission on Assisted Human Reproduction (Spain). 2004.

49. Bioethics Advisory Committee of Singapore. [Online] Available: http://www.bioethics-singapore.org/.

50. Nuffield Council on Bioethics. "Our Work." [Online] Available: http://www.nuffieldbioethics.org/go/ourwork/default_1.html

51. Swedish National Council on Medical Ethics. About the Council. [Online] Available: http://www.smer.gov.se/index.htm?lang=en&index=0&url=intro.html.

52. National Council on Ethics in Human Research. Ottawa, Canada. [Online] Available: http://ncehr-cnerh.org.

53. Privacy in Research Ethics & Law. Cyprus: RECs and medical research. [Online] Available: http://www.privireal.org/content/rec/cyprus.php.

54. Shapiro HT, Meslin EM. Relating to history: The influence of the National Commission and Its *Belmont Report* on the National Bioethics Advisory Commission. In: Childress JF, Meslin EM, Shapiro HT, eds. *Belmont Revisited: Ethical Principles for Research With Human Subjects.* Washington, D.C.: Georgetown University Press; 2005:55–76.

55. National Bioethics Advisory Commission. *Cloning Human Beings, Vol. I. Report and Recommendations.* Rockville, Md.: NBAC; 1997. [Online] Available: http://www.georgetown.edu/research/nrcbl/nbac/pubs.html.

56. National Bioethics Advisory Commission. *Ethical Issues in Human Stem Cell Research, Vol. I. Report and Recommendations.* Rockville, Md.: NBAC; 1999. [Online] Available: http://www.georgetown.edu/research/nrcbl/nbac/pubs.html.

57. National Bioethics Advisory Commission. *Ethical and Policy Issues in International Research: Clinical Trials in Developing Countries, Vol. I. Report and Recommendations.* Rockville, Md.: NBAC; 2001. [Online] Available: http://www.georgetown.edu/research/nrcbl/nbac/pubs.html.

58. Nuffield Council on Bioethics. *The Ethics of Research Related to Healthcare in Developing Countries.* London, U.K.: Nuffield Council on Bioethics; 2002. [Online] 24 April, 2002. Available: http://www.nuffieldbioethics.org/fileLibrary/pdf/errhdc_fullreport001.pdf.

59. Macklin R. *Double Standards in Medical Research in Developing Countries.* New York, N.Y.: Cambridge University Press; 2004.

60. Bagla P. India: New guidelines promise stronger bioethics. *Science* 2000;290:919.
61. Verma IC. Indian Code on human genetics and reproductive technology. In: Okamoto M, Fujiki N, Macer DRJ, eds. *Bioethics and the Impact of Human Genome Research in the 21st Century*. Christchurch, New Zealand: Eubios Bioethics Institute; 2001:102–3.
62. Aussage P. Bioethics in France. In: Okamoto M, Fujiki N, Macer DRJ, editors. *Protection of the Human Genome and Scientific Responsibility*. Christchurch, New Zealand: Eubios Bioethics Institute; 1996:59–60.
63. French National Consultative Committee on Ethics. Opinion No. 67. Opinion on the preliminary draft revision of the laws on bioethics. Paris, France: CCNE; 2001. [Online] Available: http://www.ccne-ethique.fr/english/pdf/avis067.pdf.
64. Global Summit of Bioethics Advisory Bodies. Tokyo Communiqué. In: National Bioethics Advisory Commission. 1998–1999 Biennial Report. Bethesda, Md.: NBAC; 1999. [Online] 1999. Available: http://www.georgetown.edu/research/nrcbl/nbac/pubs/Biennia198–99.pdf.

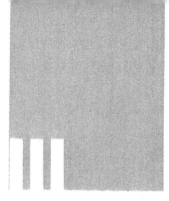

Context, Purpose, and Value
of Clinical Research

Alan Wertheimer

Exploitation in Clinical Research

Some writers on research ethics have argued that the principle "minimize exploitation" is a rationale—even *the* rationale—for many of the oft-mentioned principles of ethical research. The four canonical principles of bioethics (nonmaleficence, beneficence, respect for persons, and justice) do not invoke the language of exploitation, nor do some of the standard principles of research ethics, such as social value, scientific validity, fair participant selection, favorable risk-benefit ratio, and respect for human research participants. Still, it can be argued that many or all of these principles are based on a more general principle: minimize exploitation. For example, it can be argued that research that has no social value or is not scientifically valid is exploiting research participants because they are being "used" for no good end. Similar things can be said about research that involves unfair participant selection or that does not have a favorable risk-benefit ratio.

Yet despite the arguable breadth and power of the principle "minimize exploitation," the language of exploitation came to the fore only in the context of criticisms of research on vulnerable populations and, in particular, research in underdeveloped societies. This concern may have reached its apogee in response to the use of placebo-controlled trials that were designed to test the efficacy of a short course treatment of AZT in reducing maternal-fetal transmission of HIV when it was already known that a long-course treatment was effective. The trials were conducted in developing countries in which few could afford the long-course treatment and would probably not be able to afford the short-course treatment if it proved to be reasonably effective. Although the rationale for those trials was to find a less costly regimen that could be used in developing countries, the studies prompted an

outbreak of ethical outrage, much of it couched in terms of exploitation. Here are some representative examples:

- "Unless the interventions being tested will actually be made available to the impoverished populations that are being used as research subjects, developed countries are simply exploiting them in order to quickly use the knowledge gained from the clinical trials for the developed countries' own benefit."[1]
- " . . . the placebo-controlled trials are exploitative of poor people, who are being manipulated into serving the interests of those who live in wealthy nations."[2]
- " . . . there is always the nagging possibility that the assurances of such benefits may offer inordinate inducements to poor and impoverished populations and thus represent another form of exploitation."[3]
- "If the knowledge gained from the research in such a country is used primarily for the benefit of populations that can afford the tested product, the research may rightly be characterized as exploitative and, therefore, unethical."[4]
- "If the results of a clinical trial are not made reasonably available in a timely manner to study participants and other inhabitants of a host country, the researchers might be justly accused of exploiting poor, undereducated subjects for the benefit of more affluent populations of the sponsoring countries."[5]
- "Residents of impoverished, postcolonial countries, the majority of whom are people of color, must be protected from potential exploitation in research. Otherwise, the abominable

state of health care in these countries can be used to justify studies that could never pass ethical muster in the sponsoring country."[6]

- " . . . it is a fundamental ethical principle that those involved in research in developing countries . . . should not take advantage of the vulnerabilities created by poverty or a lack of infrastructure and resources."[7]

Yet despite the frequency with which commentators appeal to the language of exploitation, the term has been woefully under-analyzed in the bioethics literature. Indeed, the concept of exploitation has received relatively little attention from political and moral philosophers, who have been more concerned with liberty, equality, justice, and the like. There is little agreement on (or attention to) the defining characteristics of exploitative relations or transactions, and even less agreement as to why and whether exploitation is wrong.

In this chapter, I try to do the following. First, I illustrate the range of contexts in which the concept of exploitation is invoked. Second, I offer an account of the concept of exploitation and discuss several features and implications of this account. Third, I apply my account of exploitation to the sorts of charges that were raised in response to the maternal-fetal HIV trials. Although it will take some doing before we return to issues of exploitation in clinical research, rigorous analysis of these issues requires that we first step back from the immediate context and think in wider terms about the characteristics of exploitative transactions.

Examples of Alleged Exploitation

Consider the following examples, in which it often is or could be said that a practice is exploitative.

The Concept of Exploitation

The first task of any account of exploitation is to say when and why charges of exploitation are true. After all, people disagree as to whether the volunteer army is exploitative, whether universities do exploit student athletes, whether commercial surrogacy really does exploit surrogate mothers, and so on. We sometimes use the verb *exploit* in a morally neutral sense, in which we simply mean "to make use of." So we might say that the surgeon exploits his natural manual dexterity or that a baseball pitcher exploits the batter's inability to hit an inside curve ball. Those concerned with research ethics are interested in the morally charged sense of exploitation—the sort of exploitation in which it is thought that A wrongfully exploits B when A takes "unfair advantage" of B.

When is a practice or transaction exploitative? Although the concept of exploitation has not been central in the history of ethical theory, there are two traditions in which it has figured prominently. Karl Marx argued that capitalists exploit their workers when they do not pay workers the full value of their labor. Marx's view is consistent with the notion that exploitation involves taking unfair advantage of others, but is limited to the context of labor and relies on an almost universally rejected labor theory of value. Philosophers who have been inspired by Immanuel Kant have argued that one exploits another when one treats that person as a mere means to one's own ends, when one "uses" another person,

Table 20.1
Alleged Exploitation

Scenario	Description
Student athletes	It is often said that universities exploit their student athletes when they gain income, entertainment, and loyalty from alumni, whereas the athletes get little education and relatively few receive their degrees or go on to play professional sports.
Lumber	If there is a hurricane in Florida and lumber retailers were to raise their prices, we might say that they were exploiting their customers.
Strip club	It is often said that strip clubs exploit the women they employ or women as a group.
Volunteer army	It is sometimes claimed that the volunteer army exploits those citizens who lack decent civilian career opportunities: "A society as unjust as ours must draft its military to avoid unfair exploitation . . ."[8]
Rescue	Suppose that B's car slipped into a snowbank on a rural road late at night. A can pull B out by attaching a rope to his four-wheel drive pickup truck. A offers to help B for $200.
Nazis	Nazi doctors who performed hypothermia experiments on Jews were exploiting their victims.
Surrogacy	Commercial surrogacy involves the exploitation of the surrogate mothers.
Kidneys	The sale of bodily organs, such as kidneys, involves the exploitation of impoverished persons.
Interns	Hospitals exploit interns by requiring them to work long hours for relatively low pay.
Inducements	Medical researchers exploit people when they offer inducements to participate in research.
Embryonic stem cells	Embryonic stem cell research treats "nascent human life as raw material to be exploited as a mere natural resource."[9]
Unfair surgery	B needs life-saving surgery. A is the only surgeon available. A proposes to perform the surgery for $20,000 when the normal fee is $5,000. B agrees.

or when one "fails to respect the inherent value in that being."[10] The concepts of failing to respect or using are murky, and it is not clear when one treats another merely as a means.

Exploitation is best captured by the broader and simpler notion that one exploits another when one takes unfair advantage of that person.[11] As it stands, this definition is correct but not all that helpful. We must go a bit deeper. In what follows, I try to refine and amplify this definition.

1. *Exploitation requires the exploiter to benefit.* This distinguishes it from neglect or discrimination or paternalism. A cannot take unfair advantage of B unless A gets some *advantage* from B, unless A benefits from his use of B. A discriminates against B when A wrongly deprives B of some opportunity or benefit because of some characteristic of B that is not relevant to A's action. If clinical researchers discriminate against African Americans by excluding them from their study in violation of the principle of "fair participant selection,"

they would be doing something seriously unethical, but it would not be exploitation. A neglects B when A has an obligation to provide for B and fails to do so. For example, if a drug company chooses not to engage in research on drugs for malaria because it did not expect to make a profit on such drugs, it might be accused of neglecting the victims of malaria, but it could hardly be accused of exploiting them. A is wrongfully paternalistic to B if A acts so as to promote B's interests by interfering with B's liberty or autonomy. If a physician chooses not to disclose to his patient that she had cancer because he thought it would be in her interest not to know of her condition, the physician may have acted wrongly, but he did not exploit her, in part because he gains nothing from the failure to disclose and might even be putting himself at risk.

2. *Exploitation can involve benefit to those being exploited.* Some exploitative transactions or practices are clearly harmful to the exploitee and decidedly nonconsensual (see Table 20.1, "Nazis"). Importantly, in many cases exploitation can occur when the person seems to gain from the transaction and consents. Indeed, exploitation is of much less theoretical interest on a "no harm, no exploitation" rule. It is trivially true that it is wrong for A to gain from an action that unjustifiably harms or coerces B. By contrast, it is more difficult to explain when and why it might be wrong for A to gain from an action that also benefits B and to which B voluntarily consents.

For these reasons, it will be useful to make two sets of distinctions. First, we can distinguish between harmful exploitation and mutually advantageous exploitation. Mutually advantageous exploitation refers to those cases in which the exploitee and the exploiter gain from the transaction. In other words, it is the advantageousness of the transaction that is mutual. For instance, in Table 20.1 we might regard "unfair surgery" as exploitative even though B benefits greatly from the surgical procedure. In other words, "unfair surgery" is an example of mutually advantageous exploitation.

3. *Because exploitation can involve consent of the exploited, it is useful to distinguish between nonconsensual exploitation and consensual exploitation.* In cases of nonconsensual exploitation, the exploitee does not give consent at all or fails to give appropriately valid or voluntary consent, as when the consent is compromised by coercion, deception, or incompetence. By contrast, in cases of consensual exploitation, the exploitee makes a voluntary, informed, competent, and rational decision to agree to the transaction under the conditions in which she finds herself, even though she might not agree to it under better conditions or would prefer a more favorable transaction (see Table 20.1, "student athletes").

The two sets of distinctions (harmful/mutually advantageous and nonconsensual/consensual) are not equivalent. B could consent to being harmed by A, as when B agrees to sell a kidney for an unfair price. Nonetheless, the distinctions do overlap. Most cases of harmful exploitation are nonconsensual, and most cases of consensual exploitation are mutually advantageous. So for present purposes we can simplify things by distinguishing between harmful nonconsensual exploitation and mutually advantageous consensual exploitation.

4. *Exploitation mainly concerns unfair results rather than defective or unethical procedures.* Taking unfair advantage can be understood in two ways. First, it may refer to some dimension of the outcome of the exploitative act or transaction; that is, the transaction is substantively unfair. The benefit to A may be unfair because it is wrong for A to benefit at all by harming B or because A gains too much whereas B gains too little. Second, to say that A takes unfair advantage of B may imply that there is some sort of defect in the process by which the unfair outcome has come about, for example, that A has coerced B or deceived B or withheld information from B. Because A can exploit B, even when B consents voluntarily, exploitation does not necessarily involve a defect in process. It is, rather, mainly about unfair outcomes.

5. *To determine whether exploitation is harmful or mutually advantageous, use an "all things considered" analysis, rather than an analysis of each element of a transaction.* A engages in harmful exploitation of B when A gains by harming B. A engages in mutually advantageous exploitation when A gains wrongly or unfairly from a transaction with B that also benefits B. But how is it possible to distinguish between harmful and beneficial transactions? This is actually complicated. In asking how A's action affects B's interests, we must be careful to adopt an "all things considered" point of view. There are, after all, negative elements in virtually all uncontroversially beneficial transactions. Paying money for a good that is clearly worth the price is still a negative element in the transaction. It would be better to get it for free. Similarly, we do not say that a worker is harmed by employment merely because the worker prefers leisure to work. If the financial benefits to B from employment are greater than the cost of sacrificing leisure, then employment is beneficial to B, all things considered. So in deciding whether a case of alleged exploitation should be classified as harmful exploitation or mutually advantageous exploitation, we must look at its net effect on B. Even if the sale of a kidney has significant negative elements, it is possible that the value of the gains to the seller exceed the value of the costs, in which case it is a transaction that is beneficial to B.

6. *To determine whether exploitation is harmful or mutually advantageous, use an ex ante (before) rather than ex post (after) perspective in assessing the effects of a transaction on B.* Suppose that A enters into a type of business transaction with B, in which B expects, ex ante, to gain 80% of the time and lose 20% of the time. For example, A might sell B land on which B realistically hopes to find oil. We don't think that A has harmed B in those cases when the land produces no oil unless A knew that this would happen beforehand. To consider another example, if the sale of a kidney is advantageous to B ex ante, then even if B is harmed, ex post, by the sale of a kidney, it is a mutually advantageous transaction. Similarly, if B agreed to receive standard therapy for her medical condition, then this transaction is advantageous ex ante even if B doesn't benefit, or benefits less than her physician predicted, from the therapy. The general point is that one's assessment of the advantageousness of a transaction should not turn on the outcomes of that transaction; it should turn, instead, on an up-front and informed assessment of the possible outcomes and the probability that these outcomes will materialize.

7. *Vulnerability is not necessary or sufficient for exploitation.* It may be thought that a transaction is exploitative whenever A takes advantage of B's vulnerabilities or desperate situation to strike a deal. That is false. For if A makes a reasonable proposal that B has no alternative but to accept given B's desperate situation, it would be silly to say that A exploits B. If a doctor proposes to perform life-saving surgery for a reasonable fee, the patient is hardly exploited, even though the patient would not have agreed but for the fact that his or her life was in danger.

8. *Unequal benefits are also not necessary or sufficient for exploitation.* The most common view is that a transaction is unfair

when A gains much more than B. This view is also false. For if we measure the parties' gains by reference to the utility they receive, then the alleged exploitee may well gain more than the exploiter. If a doctor overcharges for life-saving surgery that only he can perform, the patient still gains much more than the doctor. The doctor gets some money; the patient gets his or her life. On closer inspection, the exploiter's power over the exploitee stems precisely from the fact that the exploiter does not stand to gain too much. The exploiter can easily walk away from the transaction, whereas the exploitee cannot. Unequal benefit is therefore a problematic criterion of exploitative transactions, for on that view, many paradigmatically exploitative transactions would turn out not to be exploitative at all.

9. *It is important to determine whether the exploitee's consent to a transaction is valid.* Let us assume that a transaction is mutually advantageous although unfair and hence exploitative. It is still important to distinguish between consensual and nonconsensual exploitation because there may be reason to prohibit nonconsensual exploitation, but to permit consensual exploitation. So when is a transaction consensual? There are many ways that consent can be invalidated, but I will discuss only two: coercion and seductive offers. Limited choice does not necessarily lead to coercion. Many people claim that B's consent is coerced when B has no reasonable alternative but to consent. This is wrong. Suppose that B will die unless his or her leg is amputated, and B therefore agrees to the amputation. B's consent is valid, even though B has no reasonable alternative but to agree. A coerces B to do X only when A proposes to violate B's rights if B refuses to do X.[12] And A certainly doesn't propose to violate B's rights if he or she doesn't agree to the amputation. People can and do give appropriately voluntary consent even when they make choices that they would not have made under more favorable circumstances or more just background conditions.

Coercion is often confused with a different defect in consent. Seductive offers, or what is often referred to as undue inducement, can also compromise the validity of consent. A makes a seductive offer when A's offer distorts B's ability to make a reasonable judgment about his or her long-term interests. This can occur when A's proposal contains such great short-term benefits that it causes B to excessively discount the long-term costs and to make a decision that does not serve his or her long-term interests. "Kidneys" is not a case of coercion, because A does not propose to make B worse off if B refuses to consent. But B's consent may not be valid if A's offer gets B to make an unreasonable judgment. If kidney donors systematically overestimate the economic benefits of donation and underestimate the long-term costs, then we would have reason to question the validity of their consent.

The main point is that there are numerous cases of alleged and actual exploitation in which B would not have agreed under better or perhaps more just background conditions, but in which B is fully informed as to the consequences of various choices and fully capable of making such choices. Such conditions may obtain in "kidneys," "surrogacy," "rescue," and "lumber." Precisely because B's objective situation is what it is, it may be reasonable for B to agree to proposals to which those who are better situated would not agree. Although it would not be rational for an affluent American to sell a kidney for $25,000, it does not follow that it is irrational for an impoverished Egyptian to do so.

10. *Unfairness is based on a normative standard.* If a transaction or interaction between A and B is mutually advantageous, B gains as well as A. A transaction is exploitative only if the outcome is unfair to B, even if B gains or benefits. When is a transaction unfair? This is the most difficult issue for an account of exploitation.

If we cannot evaluate the fairness of a transaction by comparing how much utility the parties receive, then we must measure the fairness of their gains against a normative standard as to how much the parties ought to gain. Unfortunately, that standard is notoriously difficult to specify. A promising but not unproblematic candidate is to measure the parties' gains against what they would have gained in a "hypothetical competitive market," in which there was relatively complete information.[11] On this view, there is no independent standard of a "just price" for goods or services such as lumber, kidneys, or labor. Furthermore, the just price is not whatever the actual market yields, because the market has many known imperfections. Rather, we evaluate the parties' gains by what they would have received under relatively perfect market conditions, just as we may try to determine the "fair market value" of a home by what the home would sell for under relatively perfect market conditions in that locale.

Acknowledging all of the difficulties, and granting that reasonable people may disagree about the appropriate standard, mutually advantageous transactions can be unfair by reference to an appropriate normative standard, and A exploits B when A gains more than A should or B gains less than B should from the transaction.

11. *Exploitation is distinct from background injustice.* Exploitation is transaction-specific. It does not follow that the transaction itself is unfair or exploitative just because a transaction may leave B worse off than background justice requires. Consider "surrogacy" in Table 20.1. If society should provide people with an adequate standard of living, then a woman might consider serving as a surrogate only because society has not fulfilled its obligations and her background conditions are therefore unjust. Still, it does not follow that A's transaction with B is exploitative or unjust if A bears no responsibility for causing B's unjust background condition, nor does A have an obligation to repair those conditions. To put the point slightly differently, we must distinguish between two claims: (1) A takes advantage of unfairness to B; and (2) A takes unfair advantage of B.

It is important to see that (1) does not entail (2). Other commentators disagree. They argue, "If we gain advantage from an interaction with another, and that advantage is due in part to an injustice he has suffered, we have failed to give him appropriate respect;"[10] in other words, we have taken unfair advantage of him. To see why this is mistaken, consider this case:

> *Unemployed Lawyer:* B has been unjustly fired from his position with a law firm, where he earned $150,000 per year. A local community college offers him a position teaching law courses for $35,000 per year.

Even if the community college is taking advantage of an injustice that has been done to B, it does not follow that it is exploiting B. If B has a complaint, it is with those who fired him, not with those who propose to hire him for a much lower salary.

This distinction between a transaction that is exploitative and background conditions that are unjust is important for clinical researchers. If clinical researchers take advantage of the unjust background conditions in which people in developing societies find themselves, it does not follow that they are taking unfair advantage of the people. They may or may not be doing so. To say that they are taking unfair advantage of the people, it must be shown that researchers have a specific—not general humanitarian—obligation to provide more to their research participants than they are actually providing.

Put somewhat differently, it is absolutely crucial to distinguish between moral defects in B's background situation and moral defects in the transactions that occur within that situation. Justice relates to background situations, whereas exploitation relates to transactions. People often focus on the wrong target. Although we often have moral reason to object to the background situation in which people find themselves, the relative invisibility of background situations compared with transactions, and our relative helplessness with respect to people's unfortunate or unjust background situations, may lead us to wrongly object to transactions that are themselves completely ethical.

Arguments for Intervention

It is always wrong to take unfair advantage of or to exploit another person. Interestingly, however, the force of that wrongness is much less clear. Many people believe we should prohibit or otherwise remedy all types of exploitation, be it harmful and nonconsensual exploitation or mutually advantageous and consensual exploitation. They justify their view with the following logic: (1) If a transaction is exploitative, it should not be permitted. (2) Transaction X is exploitative. (3) Therefore, X should not be permitted. This is not well argued. For even if it is true that some transactions are exploitative, it does not automatically follow that X should be prohibited. Although it is always wrong to exploit another person, it is sometimes ethically permissible, all things considered, to allow an unethical transaction to occur.

Now some people question whether a mutually advantageous and consensual transaction could be exploitative. It might be thought that there can be nothing seriously wrong about an agreement from which both parties benefit and in which A has no obligation to enter into any transaction with B. This is false. There can be transactions in which B consents and gains advantage, but which are wrong because A is treating B unfairly. Recall a paradigmatic example of exploitation, such as "rescue," in which B's car slips into a snowbank on a rural road late at night. A can pull B out by attaching a rope to his four-wheel drive pickup truck. A offers to help B for $200. Suppose that Table 20.2 represents the gains in utility from three hypothetical transactions in which scenario 2 is "rescue."

As noted above, a fair transaction does not necessarily yield equal utility gains. Because being rescued is important to B, she gets as much utility in the unfair transaction (scenario 2) as does A. And if B were rescued for only $20 (scenario 3), she would get

Table 20.2
"Rescue" and Its Alternatives

Scenario	Description	A's Benefit	B's Benefit
1	No transaction	0	0
2	Unfair transaction ($200)	5	5
3	Fair transaction ($20)	2	8

much more overall utility than A. Still, even if A is under absolutely no obligation to transact with B, we might still think A has moral reasons to be fair to B, especially because A benefits from the interaction with B. Charging $200 for a few minutes of work is arguably unfair, however much B benefits from that work.

Yet even if A's behavior is seriously wrong, it does not follow that we should prevent A and B from transacting on those terms. It is always important to distinguish between two claims: (1) A's action X is wrong; and (2) we should prevent A from doing X. I believe it would be seriously wrong for someone to give a speech in which he denies that the Holocaust happened. I believe that it might be wrong for a woman to abort her male fetus because she wanted a girl. It certainly does not follow, however, that it would be right to prevent the person from delivering that speech or to prevent the woman from having an abortion. Similarly, it does not follow that just because A is engaged in wrongful exploitation of B that we would be justified in preventing A from exploiting B. We might be so justified, but that must be determined independently, that is, on grounds other than that the transaction is exploitative.

What would justify interfering with a case of mutually advantageous consensual exploitation, a case in which B both gains and consents to the exploitation? We sometimes interfere with transactions on paternalistic grounds, in order to protect B from making a decision that does not advance her own interests. But a paternalistic argument for interference cannot apply to mutually advantageous exploitation. Paternalism is justifiable only when B's important interests are at serious risk of being harmed. Even if we think it legitimate to interfere with someone for her own good (as when we require people to wear seat belts), we cannot justify intervention on paternalistic grounds if the exploitative transaction is advantageous to the exploitee and if interference is not likely to result in a transaction that is more beneficial to B.

Obviously, we could justifiably interfere with mutually advantageous and consensual transactions if they give rise to harm to others. For example, even if allowing kidney sales were beneficial to the participants directly involved, such a policy might have diffuse negative effects on the way in which we think about persons and their bodies. Although averting harm to others may be an important reason to limit certain transactions, it is an empirical question—and often an extraordinarily complex empirical question—as to whether interfering with a practice would actually avert harm to others. Unfortunately, these sorts of claims are often made without any evidence or appreciation of the need for evidence. Moreover, this line of argument for intervention actually has nothing to do with exploitation per se. The point is not to protect the exploitee, but to protect others.

The strongest argument for intervention in mutually beneficial and consensual exploitative transactions is that a policy of disallowing unfair transactions makes it more likely that a fairer transaction will occur than that no transaction will occur. Reconsider the matrix of the benefits in "rescue." Suppose A proposes that he gets $200. B counters that they should agree on $20. A rejects B's proposal and replies that it is either $200 or no transaction. Given these options, B is prepared to pay $200. At first glance it seems that society is not justified in preventing B from paying the unfair $200, for given the choice between being exploited and not rescued, B would rather be exploited. Nonetheless, if we prohibit A from entering into an unfair transaction with B, it is possible that A will propose a fair transaction rather than refusing to transact with B. After all, A benefits from a fair transaction with B and so has no reason to refuse to transact with B if the unfair transaction is prohibited. It is important to recognize that this is a strategic argument for prohibiting exploitation rather than one about inherent evils of exploitation.

However, there are problems with prohibiting exploitation if the strategic argument does not apply. Suppose that A is under no obligation to transact with B on any terms. Then A proposes terms that are unfair to B. If we prevented A from transacting with B on unfair terms, then A would choose not to transact with B at all. In this case, prohibiting A from exploiting B is actually worse for B than allowing A to exploit B. In the context of research, this may raise the following question: Can the state or the writers of a code of ethics or an institutional review board justifiably prevent a transaction that is good for the parties involved, is worse for no one else, and to which the parties give perfectly rational consent under the nonideal conditions in which they find themselves?

Some would argue, "No." By claiming that some exploitation may be "permissible," I do not mean that it is ethically permissible for A to exploit B. A acts wrongly in exploiting B. Permissible exploitation means that society should permit A to exploit B and that it would be wrong for society to prevent A from exploiting B. There is a very strong presumption in favor of accepting this principle. Although I do not think it incoherent to claim that there might be deontological reasons to reject such a principle, such a view is difficult to justify. Moreover, because permitting this kind of exploitation precludes intervention only when the parties consent to the transaction, one cannot easily reject the principle on the Kantian ground that it allows A to use B as a mere means to his own ends. For it is at least plausible to maintain that A does not treat B as a mere means if B's valid consent is a necessary condition of any transaction between A and B.

Although I lack a knockdown argument for contending that we should permit exploitative transactions when doing so is better for all concerned, I suspect that this is a plausible principle of nonideal ethical theory as contrasted with ideal ethical theory. Whereas ideal moral theory aims to provide the principles for a just society and a just world, nonideal moral theory aims to provide the principles by which individuals, the state, and organizations should act under unjust or nonideal moral conditions. Although ethics must ask how things should be, ethics must also ask what we should do given that things are not as they should be.

The ethics of clinical research in developing countries is a problem of nonideal moral theory. In a more just world, these nations would not be so underdeveloped. But just because a transaction would not occur under ideal or just conditions, it does not follow that it is wrong for it to occur under nonideal conditions. Given the nonideal background conditions under which people find themselves, there should be a very strong presumption in favor of principles that would allow people to improve their situations if they give appropriately robust consent, and if doing so has no negative effects on others, even if the transaction is unfair, unjust, or exploitative.

Exploitation in Clinical Research

How does this analysis of exploitation in general apply to exploitation in clinical research? There are many famous examples of research that involved harmful or nonconsensual exploitation: the Nazi doctors, the Jewish Chronic Disease Hospital, and Tuskegee are a few examples (see Chapters 2, 6, and 8). These cases are important examples of exploitation. However, we are obviously justified in seeking to prevent harmful or nonconsensual exploitation. Mutually advantageous consensual exploitation may be less serious, but it poses more complex ethical challenges. Consider the following case:

> Pharma, a large American pharmaceutical company, wants to test a new antibiotic, Q, for meningitis. There is a standard treatment, T, for meningitis, but Pharma believes Q may be more effective or have fewer side effects than T. Pharma could run an active-controlled trial in the United States, in which it tests Q against T, but it prefers to run a placebo-controlled trial in Ecuador, because a placebo-controlled trial requires a smaller sample size, produces cleaner statistical results, and will save Pharma money. Because virtually no one in Ecuador can afford T, people are willing to enroll in a trial for which they have a 50% chance of receiving Q. If Q proves successful, it will not be generally affordable by the citizens in Ecuador even if it obtains regulatory approval.

Many will charge that such a study is a paradigmatic case of exploitation. They would argue something like the following.

1. If a practice is exploitative, it should not be permitted.
2. Randomized placebo-controlled trials such as Pharma's proposed trial of Q in Ecuador are exploitative.
3. Therefore, we should prohibit a randomized placebo-controlled trial of Q in Ecuador.

As it stands, this argument moves much too quickly. First, it is not clear just who is regarded as the victim of exploitation. Some statements suggest that the participants in this study would be exploited, that researchers would be taking advantage of the participants' vulnerabilities to get them to participate in studies from which half can expect not to benefit at all because a known treatment is withheld from them. Other statements imply that it is the nation or its citizens who are exploited. In this view, it is not so much that the participants are treated unfairly. After all, they stand to gain and they do consent to participate in the research. Rather, it is the nation of Ecuador that is exploited because its citizens are used to test drugs that won't be available there even if the research is successful..

Second, despite the confidence with which these charges of exploitation are often advanced, to say that the proposed trial is exploitative requires an account of an unfair transaction. We cannot just assume that the terms of these transactions are unfair. All the critics seem to implicitly or explicitly accept that Pharma would not be acting unfairly toward the citizens of Ecuador or potential research participants if it chose to do its research in the United States, in which case it would do nothing for people in Ecuador. How much does the company owe research participants or the nation of Ecuador if it chooses to do research there?

Many discussions of exploitation in clinical research implicitly accept something like the following argument.

1. A researcher does not act wrongly by choosing not to do research with B.
2. If the researcher profits from a mutually advantageous and consensual transaction with B, the researcher acquires special obligations toward B, including obligations of fairness.

3. It is worse for researchers to treat B unfairly than to fail to interact with B, even though B benefits from the research and consents to it.

Assume that the benefits in utility for Pharma and its research participants would be something like those in Table 20.3. Many seem to believe, in effect, that Pharma acts more wrongly in (B) than in (A) with respect to Ecuadorians, even though Ecuadorian research participants are better off in (B) than in (A). According to this analysis, once Pharma conducts research in Ecuador, it acquires obligations toward research participants or other Ecuadorians that it would not have if it neglected them—that is, if it had chosen to do its research in the United States. Perhaps the company must make Q available to all those who participated in the trial or provide other benefits to Ecuador. On this view, the wrongness of Pharma's behavior does not correspond to its effect on the well-being of Ecuadorians. Before we decide that *Pharma* would be exploitative, we have to think long and hard as to how much the Pharmas of this world owe research participants (or their nations) when they interact with them.

Third, let us assume for the sake of argument that Pharma does exploit Ecuadorian research participants, that it would be treating them unfairly. It is still not clear whether we should accept the premise that if research is exploitative, then it should not be permitted. If we believe that we should permit some cases of mutually advantageous consensual exploitation, then it is arguable that we should permit Pharma to conduct its trial. Let us assume that all participants receive care that is at least as good as, and probably better than, if the trial had not been conducted at all. After all, even those who receive the placebo may be receiving better (and certainly no worse) than normal care in Ecuador. Moreover, all the research participants stand to gain ex ante (they have a 50% chance of receiving beneficial treatment) even though they do not all gain ex post. Second, if Pharma is not permitted to conduct a placebo-controlled trial in Ecuador, it is possible that the company will either abandon the study or go elsewhere. I do not mean that Pharma would merely threaten to abandon the investigation as a bargaining tactic to secure what it regards as a better arrangement. Rather, I mean that Pharma might in fact abandon the investigation or go elsewhere if it is not allowed to conduct a placebo-controlled trial in Ecuador. It would, for example, prefer (A) to (C). With these assumptions in mind, let us now consider the various claims and prescriptions that are frequently linked to the claim that this sort of research is exploitative.

Table 20.3
Expected Utilities of Three Research Scenarios

Scenario	Description	Pharma's Utility	Ecuadorian Research Participant's Utility
A	Active-controlled trial in U.S.	900	0
B	Placebo-controlled trial in Ecuador	1,000	1
C	Active-controlled trial in Ecuador	800	2

The Declaration of Helsinki states, "The benefits, risks, burdens and effectiveness of a new method should be tested against those of the best current prophylactic, diagnostic, and therapeutic methods"[13] (see Chapter 13). The Pharma trial seems to be incompatible with this principle, unless one fudges with the notion of the "best current . . . methods" by arguing that we should adopt a "local" standard, under which the best current method is no treatment at all. But the real question is not whether Pharma's trial is compatible with the principles of the Declaration of Helsinki or other similar documents, but whether we should accept the principles articulated in the Declaration of Helsinki or other comparable documents. If Pharma proposed to run an active-controlled trial in the United States, thereby providing no care to anyone in Ecuador, it would not violate the principles of the Declaration of Helsinki. So if Pharma Pharmaceuticals is not required to provide any care at all to Ecuadorians, why should we insist that it provide the best current method of care to all participants in the study?

We can consider the Declaration of Helsinki's "best current . . . methods" principle in terms of the strategic argument for intervention. In the developed world, if we insist that active-controlled trials be used whenever a standard therapy exists and whenever there are no very strong scientific reasons for preferring a placebo-controlled trial, there is little risk that the research will simply go away. Although the drug companies might prefer placebo-controlled trials because they are cheaper, quicker, and provide better data, the potential participants in the developed world are helped by rules that force researchers to treat patients better than they otherwise might. After all, if patients are assured of the best current methods of care, there is no reason why they should consent to participate in a placebo-controlled trial.

By contrast, the strategic argument may or may not work so easily in the developing world. On the one hand, a developing nation may fear that the researchers will go elsewhere if too many constraints are placed on research. Precisely for that reason, it is possible that such constraints will prevent a "race to the bottom" among developing nations that are competing for the inadequate benefits of being used for such research. On the other hand, it is also possible that—given such constraints—the researchers will decide that they might as well use active-controlled trials in their own nations. There may be little reason for Pharma to run an active-controlled trial in Ecuador when it could run such a trial in the United States, especially if it needs to invest in upgrading the Ecuadorian health-care system to ensure adequate diagnostic tests and therapeutic interventions to conduct the trial. If that is right, prohibiting Pharma from conducting a placebo-controlled trial in Ecuador cannot be justified as the best strategy for improving the lot of potential research participants in Ecuador or other developing nations. In any case, it is an empirical question as to whether disallowing such trials will work to the advantage of potential participants or increase the welfare of persons in developing nations. This will not be solved by calling some study exploitative or by ethical discussion.

We must also ask how much moral weight we should place on the benefits that accrue to the researchers or to the citizens of the developed society as contrasted with the effects of the trials on the participants. First, there is the issue of commercial profit. Although seeking profit is not itself unethical, it might be thought that Pharma cannot justify running placebo-controlled trials if its primary motivation is simply to save money and fatten its coffers.

Interestingly, however, the standard arguments cited previously do not appeal to worries about commercial profits. After all, such studies could easily be conducted by nonprofit organizations such as the National Institutes of Health. Rather, the main claim is that it is wrong for citizens in developed societies to gain large benefits from trials conducted on citizens of developing societies who may not benefit at all. Recall the statement from the Council for International Organizations of Medical Sciences (CIOMS): "If the knowledge gained from the research in such a country is used primarily for the benefit of populations that can afford the tested product, the research may rightly be characterized as exploitative and therefore, unethical."[4]

Should we accept this argument? I'm not sure. First, this argument does not claim that the research participants are exploited. Rather, it implies that the society or nation is exploited. Second, the country may or may not be exploited, but even if it is, we have to ask whether that is sufficient reason to block such research if three conditions are all fulfilled: (1) the research participants give informed consent; (2) the individual research participants stand to benefit from such research; and (3) their participation in such research does not render their fellow citizens worse off. In addition, it should be noted that the benefit that accrues to citizens of the affluent nations is not something trivial, like cheaper running shoes made in sweatshops in Thailand. Rather they may be getting life-saving medications. The CIOMS statement raises difficult moral questions, and I do not propose to try to resolve them here. I suggest only that the moral truth of the matter is much more complex than the statement suggests.

Some argue that there is something particularly morally obnoxious about a practice in which the affluent entice the poor to provide a service that will primarily benefit the rich. Why should the burden of clinical research be borne by the poor? The answer might be, It is not a burden for anyone, and not a burden for the poor. This is not like asking the poor to take the radioactive and other toxic waste produced by the rich. Moreover it is very unclear that medical research is qualitatively different from a wide variety of practices in which the affluent directly or indirectly hire the less affluent to provide goods or services, as when they work as nannies, gardeners, and domestics. Nor is it acceptable to argue that these occupations are not life-threatening; the affluent also effectively hire others to engage in dangerous jobs such as coal mining, construction work, or volunteer (professional) soldiering. Some bioethicists often assume without argument that there is something morally special about hiring others to serve as participants for medical trials that distinguishes such "hirings" from other sorts of hirings. It is not clear just why that is so.

Of course, this assumes that the participants in studies such as Pharma actually give valid informed consent. There are two questions that we might ask here: (1) Do the participants give valid consent? (2) If not, is it possible that this sort of research could be conducted with valid informed consent? Clearly, the answer to both questions will turn on our criteria for valid consent. Although we cannot resolve that here, it is possible that the answer to (1) is often "no." It is possible that many people do not understand that they are consenting to participate in a placebo-controlled clinical trial as opposed to consenting to medical treatment. They may suffer from the "therapeutic misconception." But the current available data do not substantiate this claim, at least when compared with participants in developed countries.

We should distinguish between these sorts of cognitive deficiencies in a participant's consent and worries that are often advanced about the voluntariness of the consent. It is often argued that a research participant's consent is not voluntary when he or she has "no acceptable alternative." And it is argued that impoverished potential participants who would ordinarily have no medical care available have no choice but to participate in a study in which they have a chance of obtaining medical care and that their consent is consequently invalid on grounds of coercion. But this line of argument is incorrect. A's proposal is coercive only if A proposes to violate B's rights if B rejects the proposal. The central fact is that Pharma did not propose to violate a potential participant's rights should a potential participant decide not to participate.

It might be noted in this connection that many bioethicists have expressed worries about providing inducements to research participants. CIOMS worries that the offer of monetary payments may "induce prospective subjects to consent to participate in the research against their better judgment."[4] And there may be similar worries about the inducement of therapeutic treatment. We must be careful to properly interpret the phrase "against their better judgment." It is important to distinguish between two claims:

1. The inducements constitute a seductive offer that motivates people to consent to participate when doing so does not advance their interests.
2. Given the people's objective circumstances, the inducements make it rational for them to participate.

Note that in (2), the inducements are large enough to render participation compatible with the participants' better judgment given the objective conditions in which they find themselves, although participation might have been against their better judgment in the absence of those inducements or under different conditions. The real tragedy of poverty is not that (1) is often true, but that (2) is often true. David Rothman writes that "abject poverty is harsh enough without people having to bear the additional burdens of serving as research subjects."[14] But the point could easily go the other way. We might say, after all, that abject poverty is harsh enough without denying people the opportunity to make their lives somewhat less miserable by participating in biomedical research and receiving benefits that they would not otherwise receive. The British Marxist economist Joan Robinson once remarked that for people in many poor countries, "the misery of being exploited by capitalists is nothing compared to the misery of not being exploited at all."[15] Whether a similar view might be correct with regard to clinical research is one of the questions that must be raised and answered.

Worries about exploitation in clinical research often focus not just on the treatment of the experimental participants but on the benefits to the community when the study is over. Recall these two statements: "Unless the interventions being tested will actually be made available to the impoverished populations that are being used as research subjects, developed countries are simply exploiting them in order to quickly use the knowledge gained from the clinical trials for the developed countries' own benefit;"[1] and "If the results of a clinical trial are not made reasonably available in a timely manner to study participants and other inhabitants of a host country, the researchers might be justly accused of exploiting poor, undereducated subjects for the benefit of more affluent populations of the sponsoring countries."[5]

Although the commentators have not been precise about this, they may be arguing that the research would not be exploitative if the products that result from such studies were to be made available to present or future citizens of the host country (so-called reasonable availability). Why should the benefit to future citizens render it permissible to exploit present research participants? They might be arguing that the exploitation of the research participants inherent in the research would be counterbalanced and outweighed by the benefit to other citizens. But this view would seem to violate some of the standard principles for ethical clinical research. We don't say that the exploitation of research participants is justified by gains to other persons.

Consider the following statement: "If the intervention being tested is not likely to be affordable in the host country or if the health care infrastructure cannot support its proper distribution and use, it is unethical to ask persons in that country to participate in the research, since *they* will not enjoy any of its potential benefits [emphasis added]."[16] But who is the "they" to whom Shapiro and Meslin refer? After all, it is often true that the persons who participate in research will not, themselves, enjoy any of its potential benefits. If it is wrong to ask B to participate in research from which B will not benefit, then it is not clear why it becomes permissible just because B's fellow citizens may benefit. And if it is not wrong to ask B to participate in such research, then I do not see why it should be necessary that B's fellow citizens will also benefit.

Moreover, if it is morally crucial that benefits of doing research with impoverished persons be made available to other impoverished persons, it is not clear to me why the nation is the relevant moral unit here. Suppose that the Pharma trial was a success and that Pharma had to choose between making the results of research available to citizens of Ecuador or Uganda and that it would do more good to do so in Uganda. Do the citizens of Ecuador have a claim on those treatments just because other Ecuadorians participated in the research? Perhaps, but why?

To the extent that the principle of reasonable availability—the principle that a successful result of a clinical trial should be made available in the host country—is motivated by principles of distributive justice, we must be careful not to conflate valid concerns about the distribution of medical resources in the world with concerns about the relationship among the participants or the nations involved in particular studies. It is possible that insisting upon reasonable availability, when feasible, will generate a shift of resources from the more affluent persons of the world (through their governments) to the less affluent. But if reasonable availability is not feasible, then insisting on reasonable availability as a precondition for a trial will result in no study at all, and will result in less redistribution, not more.

In this connection, it is also important to distinguish between the claim that the distribution of resources in the world is unjust and the claim that a sponsoring nation (or the home country of the sponsors) is causally responsible for the injustice. Crouch and Arras argue that the misery of people in underdeveloped societies "must be due in no small measure to the flagrantly unjust behavior of the former colonial powers, which plundered their natural resources and subjugated their peoples."[5] Certainly, this is sometimes right, but equally often this is false. The poorest societies of the world are those that have had the least economic contact with the highly industrialized nations. They have suffered not because imperialism has made them worse off, but because the affluent nations have found too little there to be exploited. Of course, even if the industrialized nations have not caused the poverty of the underdeveloped society, they may still have an obligation to ameliorate that poverty. The question is whether insisting on reasonable availability is the best way to do that and why the burden of ameliorating background injustice should be placed on clinical researchers.

Many commentators have argued, in effect, that to allow a placebo-controlled trial in a developing nation that would not be permitted in a developed society is to countenance moral relativism or a double ethical standard. If the Pharma trial would not be permitted in the United States, then it should not be permitted in Ecuador: "Residents of impoverished, postcolonial countries, the majority of whom are people of color, must be protected from potential exploitation in research. Otherwise, the abominable state of health care in these countries can be used to justify studies that could never pass ethical muster in the sponsoring country."[6]

Or, as Marcia Angell puts it, "Acceptance of this ethical relativism could result in widespread exploitation of vulnerable Third World populations for research programs that could not be carried out in the sponsoring countries."[17]

This is much too quick. Those who would defend trials such as Pharma in Ecuador but who would oppose such trials in the United States are not necessarily guilty of ethical relativism or applying double standards. Rather, an argument for allowing clinical trials to which the parties give voluntary informed consent maintains that this principle of informed consent should be universally applied. More importantly, all things are not equal between the United States and Ecuador. If, for example, it would be irrational for Americans to consent to participate in a placebo-controlled trial because they can assure themselves of a standard treatment, but it would not be irrational for Ecuadorians to do so because no treatment is available to them, then insisting that rational consent can be taken as valid will have different implications in the two societies, but there is no relativism or double standard here.

The most important point is this: We will not resolve questions as to the justifiability of studies such as the Pharma trial simply by invoking the derisive language of exploitation. This is just demagoguery. We will resolve them by the rigorous examination of ethical arguments and by the painstaking empirical study of the relevant data as to the effects of various policies on people's lives.

Empirical study is crucial. The principles of research ethics are not just high-minded ideals. They are regulations that affect what happens. Without endorsing any particular method of doing cost/benefit analysis, it would be highly unethical to ignore the consequences of imposing regulations in the world as we find it, however well intentioned. It's not just that regulations can be costly. Some regulations are actually self-defeating in their own terms. The FAA once considered a proposal that would have required young children to be placed in a child restraint on an airplane rather than allowing them to be held by an adult. The goal was to reduce infant deaths, and it was demonstrable that there would be (a few) fewer deaths on airplanes if infants were so restrained. Good idea? Probably not. The regulation would have saved relatively few lives at great cost because virtually everyone dies in most airplane accidents. More importantly, there is good reason to think that this regulation would actually have led to more infant deaths because the extra cost of buying a ticket for one's child would motivate some parents to drive rather than fly, and being a passenger in a car is less safe than being held by an adult in a plane.

Similarly, it is possible that however well intentioned the principles designed to minimize exploitation in clinical research, the consequences of adopting those principles might well be worse for the people that they are designed to help. I do not claim that this is so. I suggest only that we must study the effects of such regulations on the people that they are designed to help and we should not assume that good intentions will be matched by good results. Interested parties should withdraw some of their heavy rhetorical artillery and begin the hard work of deliberating about the best ethical principles for the decidedly nonideal conditions that we encounter.

References

1. Annas GJ, Grodin M. Human rights and maternal-fetal HIV transmission prevention trials in Africa. *American Journal of Public Health* 1998;88:560–3.
2. Bayer R. The debate over maternal-fetal HIV transmission prevention trials in Africa, Asia, and the Caribbean: Racist exploitation or exploitation of racism? *American Journal of Public Health* 1998;88: 567–70.
3. Bhutta ZA. Ethics in international health research: A perspective from the developing world. *Bulletin of the World Health Organization* 2002;80:114–20.
4. Council for International Organizations of Medical Sciences, in collaboration with the World Health Organization. *International Ethical Guidelines for Biomedical Research Involving Human Subjects.* Geneva, Switzerland: CIOMS and WHO; 2002. [Online] November 2002. Available: http://www.cioms.ch/frame_guidelines_nov_2002.htm.
5. Crouch RA, Arras JD. AZT trials and tribulations. *Hastings Center Report* 1998;28(6):26–34.
6. Lurie P, Wolfe SM. Unethical trials of interventions to reduce perinatal transmission of the human immunodeficiency virus in developing countries. *New England Journal of Medicine* 1997;337:853–6.
7. Nuffield Council on Bioethics. *The Ethics of Research Related to Healthcare in Developing Countries.* London, England: Nuffield Council on Bioethics; 2002. [Online] April 24, 2002. Available: http://www.nuffieldbioethics.org/fileLibrary/pdf/errhdc_fullreport001.pdf.
8. Wasserman D. Enlistment and exploitation. *Report from the Institute for Philosophy and Public Policy* 1991;11(2):6–7.
9. Kass L. *Life, Liberty and the Defense of Dignity.* San Francisco, Calif.: Encounter Books; 2002.
10. Sample RJ. *Exploitation: What It Is and Why It's Wrong.* Lanham, Md.: Rowman and Littlefield; 2003.
11. Wertheimer A. *Exploitation.* Princeton, N.J.: Princeton University Press; 1997.
12. Wertheimer A. *Coercion.* Princeton, N.J.: Princeton University Press; 1986.
13. World Medical Association. *Declaration of Helsinki: Ethical Principles for Medical Research Involving Human Subjects.* Tokyo, Japan: WMA; October 2004. [Online] 2004. Available: http://www.wma.net/e/policy/b3.htm.
14. Rothman DJ. The shame of medical research. *The New York Review of Books* 2000;47(19):60–4.
15. Robinson J. *Economic Philosophy.* Chicago, Ill.: Aldine; 1962.
16. Shapiro HT, Meslin EM. Ethical issues in the design and conduct of clinical trials in developing countries. *New England Journal of Medicine* 2001;345:139–42.
17. Angell M. The ethics of clinical research in the third world. *New England Journal of Medicine* 1997;337:847–9.

Robert J. Levine

The Nature, Scope, and Justification
of Clinical Research

What Is Research? Who Is a Subject?

This chapter begins with an examination of the nature and scope of medical practice. As we shall see, there are several alternative visions of the nature and scope of medical practice. *Clinical research* is a subset of a larger category called *biomedical research*, which has as its purpose the enhancement or improvement of medical practice. We cannot begin to consider the nature, scope, and justification of clinical research until we have a clear understanding of the enterprise it is intended to serve. This chapter also includes a review of the definitions of *research* and *human subject* that have been developed in the context of developing policy to safeguard the rights and welfare of human research subjects.

Definitions

The term *clinical* is derived from the Greek *klinikos* meaning "of or pertaining to a bed."[1] Its original usage in the context of medical practice referred to a physician who attends bedridden patients, a clinician. It has since developed multiple meanings. A *clinic* commonly means a place where ambulatory (not bedridden) patients go to receive advice and treatment from health-care professionals. (It is also worth noticing, perhaps with some alarm, that we now have legal clinics and tennis clinics.)

In this chapter, the term *clinical research* means research involving human subjects that is designed to advance the goals of medicine (and other health-care professions). Some clinical research contributes directly to enhancing the professional capabilities of physicians and other health-care professionals through the development of new therapeutic (including diagnostic and preventive) interventions or procedures. Some other clinical research is de-

signed to contribute to the fund of knowledge in those sciences that are traditionally considered "basic" in the medical setting, such as biochemistry, physiology, pathology, pharmacology, epidemiology, molecular biology, and the cognate behavioral sciences; some, but not all, such research contributes indirectly to enhancing the professional capabilities of health-care professionals by adding to or refining the fund of knowledge that provides the basis for future research aimed at the development of new therapeutic modalities.

Biomedical research, which has the same purpose as clinical research, includes research that does not involve humans as subjects. The terms *clinical research* and *biomedical research* are, in common parlance, often used interchangeably. Much of the research carried out in medical school departments of medicine or surgery is biomedical research, which does not involve humans as subjects; those who do this research are commonly called clinical investigators, and the reports of their research findings are published in such vehicles such as the *Journal of Clinical Investigation. Investigation,* in this sense, means "research."

The Domain of Medicine

In the introduction to his monumental work on the history of medicine, Henry Sigerist states:

> The scope of medicine is so broad that it includes, under any circumstances, infinitely more than the physician's actions. The task of medicine may be outlined under the following four headings: 1. Promotion of health; 2. Prevention of illness; 3. Restoration of health; and 4. Rehabilitation.[2]

In the traditional medical model, the focus is on the last two functions and their extensions. A person who feels ill initiates contact with a physician with the hope—and increasingly since the mid-20th century, the expectation—that he or she will be treated and consequently rendered healthy. The physician first makes a diagnosis, naming the disease that is causing the patient to feel ill. Based upon the diagnosis the physician can perform the other functions expected of him or her.[3] The physician can provide (1) a prognosis, predicting what will become of the patient, and (2) therapy designed to cure the disease, to delay the progress of or compensate for its disabling manifestations, or to relieve symptoms. Finally, the physician is expected to care for the patient, with all that the word *care* implies.[4]

The principal focus of the medical profession and of biomedical research is on disease. In the modern concept of a disease, it is a distinct entity, the presence of which is verifiable objectively; it has a cause, and if we can identify the cause the physician can either cure or prevent it, or the means for its cure or prevention inevitably will be developed by the biomedical researcher. This view of disease presupposes that it is something distinct from the person who contracts it and that if rid of it, the person will be normal (healthy).

The doctrine that each disease is a distinct entity, the presence of which is verifiable objectively, was established firmly in the closing years of the 18th century by a group of Parisian physicians whose intellectual leader was Xavier Bichat.[5] Their philosophical perspective was largely that of the French *ideologues* who accepted the philosophical empiricism of Locke; their concentration was on the careful observation of phenomena and their correlations and an avoidance of speculation and theory. Under their influence, two major traditions of medical science—each of which had yielded a classification of disease—were fused: (1) careful and systematic observation of the living sick person (clinical observation), and (2) systematic dissection of the dead person (necropsy), which yielded a body of knowledge known as morbid anatomy (forerunner of pathology, the study of diseases).

Morbid anatomy became the dominant science of clinical medicine because at the time, it was the only science of the human body that could provide objective evidence of concrete abnormalities. Most diseases were named after the abnormality found at necropsy. Thus, if a disease produced inflammation of the liver, it was named hepatitis (*hepar* = liver; *itis* = inflammation). During the late 18th and most of the 19th centuries, most maneuvers now recognized as the modern physical examination were developed. The ultimate test of a diagnostic maneuver was that it could predict what would be found at necropsy, and the ultimate test of a physician was that he or she could predict what would be found at necropsy.[3] Through the remainder of the 19th and into the 20th century, other natural sciences were applied with increasing success to the description of normal and abnormal structure and function, to the identification of the causes of diseases, and to the mechanisms through which they produce malfunction and disability. With time, names began to be assigned to diseases according to their causative agents, for example, streptococcal sore throat (named for the bacteria that cause it); or by the physiological (e.g., high blood pressure) or biochemical (e.g., phenylketonuria) aberrations through which they might be identified.

Although the scientific disciplines used to identify and explain disease have evolved, the necessity of objective verification remained constant. Lack of objective verification may cast doubt on the legitimacy of a discipline, on a proposed disease entity, or on the credibility of a patient. Thus, the specialty of dynamic psychiatry was admitted very slowly and grudgingly into the traditional medical profession. Early acceptance of organic psychiatry into departments of neurology was based on the fact that anatomical abnormalities, if any, were found in the brain and that some mental illnesses were caused by infection (e.g., syphilis), vitamin deficiency (e.g., pellagra), or hormonal imbalances (e.g., hypothyroidism).[5] Full acceptance of dynamic psychiatry was delayed until the mid-20th century, when it was demonstrated that some severe behavioral disorders responded favorably to either surgery (e.g., frontal lobotomy), electroconvulsive therapy, or drugs (e.g., tranquilizers).

The modern examination of a patient by a physician evolved in the same philosophical tradition. A patient must receive an "adequate" examination consisting first of a complete "history" including a systematic quest for complaints that the patient may have neglected to mention and for diseases that may either be familial or related to environment or habits. After the initial examination the physician formulates an "impression" (equivalent to a hypothesis) as to what might be wrong. Evidence of the possible presence of various diseases is pursued with further diagnostic testing. When all the necessary data are available, the physician makes a diagnosis (equivalent to a theory). At this point, the other functions of the physician begin. If there is objective evidence of disease, a diagnosis is made; if not, a problem is presented to both physician and patient.

Until recently, a dichotomy was made between organic and functional illness. The former classification was assigned to patients having validated diseases, whereas the latter was a suspect set. Patients with functional illness were informed that there was nothing wrong and that they should stop complaining, or else the physician delicately suggested that they might see a psychiatrist—a suggestion that until recently patients usually resisted and frequently rejected.[6] Talcott Parsons vividly described the sick role as one in which an individual might be excused from his or her usual obligations only on the conditions that (1) the sick role was legitimized by a physician and (2) the sick person was obligated to cooperate with the physician's healing efforts.[7] The paradigmatic experience is when a doctor's note is required to permit return to school or work after an alleged illness. Consider the plight of the person with a functional illness.

Since the Second World War, several things have happened to change the composition of medicine. Three have had a profound impact on the orientation of biomedical research. First, the concept of disease began to expand. Disease, always recognized as a type of abnormality, gradually came to be equated with any deviance from accepted norms.[8] But now the deviations increasingly derived their objective verification through the devices of the social and behavioral as well as the natural sciences. The identification of some sorts of children with learning disabilities as diseased or sick led to the development of therapies that often enhance their abilities; however, it reversed the model presented earlier. In some cases such children are "diagnosed" by school authorities and sent home with a note *to* the doctor. Illegitimate classification of a group may be associated with the social stigmatization of being sick without any possibility of therapy. As we label as diseases such things as alcohol abuse and drug abuse, inappropriate aggression and deviant sexual behavior, we begin to blur the distinctions between sin, crime, and disease. One who deviates from accepted norms may now be offered the choice between the criminal role and the sick role. The physician, accustomed to playing legitimizer, may now be called upon to function as illegitimizer.[7]

As a consequence of the success of the struggle against infectious diseases—until the early 20th century the perennial greatest killers of people—a new constellation of diseases has emerged to dominate the lists of causes of death. These include the familiar triad of heart disease, cancer, and stroke. Treatment of these diseases is most effective if begun before they become manifest as illness. For example, high blood pressure, by producing relentless destruction of arteries over a period of many years, eventually produces heart attacks, strokes, and kidney failure, which, in turn, cause disability and death. Treatments of high blood pressure, begun before the patient feels ill, will greatly reduce the incidence of disabling and lethal complications. The physician, who is accustomed to dealing with patients who feel ill, is increasingly called upon to work with people who, although they may have diseases, feel well.[5]

As a consequence of these and other factors, strong forces have developed within and without the medical profession to change its primary orientation toward the maintenance of health rather than the treatment of disease. There has been an increasing emphasis on the approaches of public health and preventive medicine, and both of these disciplines have influenced the practice of medicine. The World Health Organization provides the following definition in its constitution: "Health is a state of complete physical, mental and social well-being and not merely the absence of disease or infirmity."[9] Unlike disease, the presence of health is not objectively verifiable. Thus, the researcher has difficulty focusing on health as a definitive objective.

Public health, which is concerned with maintaining the health of populations, had its origins in the development of sanitation techniques for purposes of preventing contagious diseases. A story of one of its early successes (probably apocryphal, but often rehearsed) demonstrates the characteristic nature of its approaches and emphasizes that it is not always necessary to know the exact cause of a disease in order to prevent it.[10] During an epidemic of cholera in London in 1854, John Snow observed that most fatally infected people seemed to have used the water pump at Broad Street. He persuaded the city authorities to remove the handle from the pump; almost immediately thereafter the epidemic disappeared.

In the 20th century the domain of public health has been extended to manipulations of the environment generally so as to maintain physical, mental, and social health. Among its concerns are improvement of working conditions (to prevent occupational diseases), urban planning (to reduce mental illness, drug abuse), clean air and water, highway safety, and so on.

Preventive medicine, which is concerned with doing something to or for an individual person in order to prevent future disease, also had its origins in the combat against infectious diseases.[10] One of its notable early triumphs was the finding in the 18th century that persons could be protected from severe cases of smallpox (variola) by deliberately infecting them with material from persons with mild cases (variolation); subsequently, it was found that even more satisfactory protection could be afforded by deliberate infection with a closely related and much milder disease, cowpox (vaccination). The latter finding was based on Edward Jenner's observation that milkmaids who contracted cowpox (vaccinia) retained a permanent immunity to smallpox.

In the late 19th and early 20th centuries, vaccines were developed that produced lasting protection against many of the major infectious diseases. Further, it was discovered that many severe diseases were due to nutritional deficiencies that could be prevented by appropriate diets, and the probability of acquiring some other diseases, for example, emphysema and venereal diseases, could be minimized through modification of personal habits. The approaches of preventive medicine have been extended into preventive therapy with a current emphasis on early detection of such diseases as high blood pressure and glaucoma so that they might be treated before disabling or lethal complications ensue.

For the purpose of discussing clinical research, I shall assume that the domain of medicine includes preventive medicine and public health. For the reason I mentioned earlier, I shall further assume that it does not embrace the additional component covered in the WHO definition of health. Biomedical research is concerned with physical and mental but not necessarily with social well-being.

Biomedical Research in Relation to Medicine

A revolution in medical education was launched in 1910 by Abraham Flexner, who proposed in his report to the Carnegie Foundation that U.S. medical schools should be reconstructed to emulate the highly successful European (particularly German) university-based model. He suggested that all medical schools should have full-time faculties, that the teachers of medicine should be actively engaged in research, and that medical students should be educated in what he called the laboratory sciences.[11] By the late 1930s, all U.S. medical schools conformed to the Flexnerian model.

The disciplines that came to be known as the biomedical sciences are those that Flexner identified as the laboratory sciences. In general, they have comprised most of the first two years of the medical school curriculum; they are commonly referred to as the basic sciences to distinguish them from the primary focus of the second two years, the clinical studies. There is a general tendency to refer to research in these disciplines as biomedical research, whether or not it conforms to the definition used here.[12]

These basic sciences include anatomy (the study of bodily structure), physiology (the study of bodily function), biochemistry, pathology, pharmacology (the study of drugs), and microbiology (the study of microorganisms, many of which can cause disease). With the addition of statistics, behavioral sciences, molecular biology, immunology, and genetics, this model remains generally intact. In the 20th century, biochemistry, defined by Joseph S. Fruton as "efforts to explain biological phenomena in terms of the specific properties of chemical substances present in living organisms," emerged as the natural science having the greatest power to provide an explanatory theory for the nature of health and disease as well as the development of remedies.[12] The approaches of biochemistry and molecular biology now dominate most research and explanatory theory in the aforementioned sciences.

If we accept the definition of medicine developed in the preceding section, it becomes apparent that biomedical research includes parts of almost all the natural, behavioral, and social sciences as well as many aspects of engineering. For example, although it is absurd to say that sociology is a biomedical science, it is clear that its research approaches are being applied to the development of explanatory theories for health and diseases and, further, that social science research may suggest approaches to the improvement of public health and to the development of improved medical facilities. Although the researcher is more attracted to the study of disease than of health, this does not mean that he or she eschews the study of normal processes. The concept of a normal process presents no problem to the researcher; rather, it is the totality of the concept of health that defies scientific validation. The researcher knows that an understanding of disease—deviation from normal—is contingent upon a thorough understanding of the normal. As stated earlier, a disease is conceived as a distinct entity that has a cause; if we can identify the cause, the physician can either cure or prevent it, or the means for its cure or prevention inevitably will be developed by the biomedical researcher. The last part of this statement may be recognized as an article of faith that forms the basis for the mainstream of modern biomedical research.[13]

The foundations for this article of faith were established by the proof of the germ theory of disease and the consequent successes of immunization and chemotherapy.[5] In 1876, Robert Koch first demonstrated beyond doubt that a specific disease (anthrax) was caused by specific bacteria. He developed a set of tests (Koch's postulates), which must be satisfied if an organism is to be accepted as the cause of a disease. Within a short period of time, bacteria that caused many diseases were identified. Aside from firmly fixing the concept of "one disease, one cause" in the tradition of biomedical research, this event had three other important practical consequences.

First, it was possible to isolate these bacteria and grow large numbers of them in pure culture. These cultured bacteria could be treated in various ways so as to render them less virulent. The less virulent bacteria could be administered to normal persons causing little or no illness but conferring a lasting immunity to the disease (immunization). Subsequently, very similar techniques have been applied to the isolation of other microbes and the development of immunizations (vaccines) against them.

Second, it was found that some dyes selectively stained certain cells—either bacteria or the cells of animal tissues—but not others. Presumably, their affinity for specific cells was based upon their chemical properties. It occurred to Paul Ehrlich that some poisonous chemicals might be developed that would have an affinity for bacteria but not other cells. Such chemicals would be "magic bullets" in that they would kill the cause of the disease without killing the other cells of those who were diseased. Among the chemotherapeutic agents (chemical therapies) found by this approach are sulfa drugs (derivatives of the original aniline dyes with which Ehrlich worked) and antibiotics.

Third, it was possible to inject disease-causing bacteria into animals and to produce in the animals the same diseases the bacteria caused in humans (animal models). Thus it became possible to perform increasingly sophisticated studies on the nature of disease. Further, it became possible to test the new vaccines and chemotherapeutic agents to see if they truly effected prevention or cure without seriously damaging the animal.

The expression *biomedical research* ordinarily calls to mind research on human subjects. Yet the vast majority of biomedical research activity is conducted on animals or their tissues, cells, or even parts of cells.[14] Some is done on plants, and some uses nothing derived from living sources, for example, developmental engineering designed to improve devices such as cardiac pace-makers. Because a need for prior animal experimentation is emphasized in such documents as the Nuremberg Code and the Declaration of Helsinki, it is often thought that its purpose is to try something out on animals to see if it is sufficiently safe to be tried in humans. However, much biomedical research is devoted to the development of animal models of human disease. The purposes of developing animal models are essentially those established in the development of the germ theory. The models provide efficient systems for the studies of mechanisms of disease, providing the basis for the development of more effective therapeutic technologies. Additionally, the availability of animal models greatly facilitates searches for causes, cures, and preventions.

Increasingly, the public tries to ensure the achievement of its research objectives through priority funding of "mission-oriented" or "targeted research."[14] The researcher, perplexed by this, argues that one cannot commission discoveries; these are nearly always accidents. One cannot legislate that a scientist, such as Wilhelm Roentgen, while exploring a fundamental problem in physics, will accidentally discover the X-ray. Rather, through legislation one can create environments in which young prospective scientists will learn how to do research and how to deal with discoveries, their validation and their application to the solution of problems. Comroe and Dripps identified the 10 most important advances in the treatment of cardiovascular and pulmonary diseases—which currently account for more than half the deaths in the United States—and analyzed the sorts of research upon which they were based. Research was defined as "clinically oriented" (analogous to "mission-oriented"), even if performed entirely on animals, tissues, cells, or fragments of cells, if the author mentioned even briefly an interest in a medical problem. By these criteria, 41% of key articles leading to the development of the 10 most important advances were not clinically oriented. Thus, they conclude, if the public chooses to fund only clinically oriented research, it will sacrifice such advances as the development of antibiotics, polio vaccine, and so on.[14]

Conflicts Between Medical Practice and Research

There are important conflicts between the traditions and motivations of physicians and researchers. As much as we have attempted to fuse science with medicine, much of the practice of medicine is not scientifically based. Much of what the physician does in practice is dictated by authority.[15] For centuries the authority was Hippocrates (5th century B.C.) as updated by Galen (2nd century A.D.); no physician dared challenge the teachings of Galen until the Renaissance was well established. Subsequently, although some authority (or the statements of some authorities) has been established through the scientific method, the vast majority of physicians' activities—particularly the caring functions—have no scientific validation. Further, the average physician, who has not participated in what scientific validation there is, must accept the statements of the new authorities with faith that the science upon which they are based is sound and accurately reported.

The researcher, by contrast, challenges authority. If there is one overriding ethic in research, it is to learn and to tell the truth. Authority, as established in the Hippocratic Corpus, instructs physicians to use treatment to help the sick according to *their* ability or judgment but never to injure or wrong them. Put another way, to help, or at least to do no harm.[16] Truth is dispensed to the patient as cautiously and judiciously as any powerful remedy, with a clear weighing of the potential adverse consequences. For thousands of years, the physician has known that a sick person who is convinced that he or she will feel better as a consequence of taking some remedy almost always will.[17] Thus, while administering remedies, some of which were fantastic and nearly all of which were inert, the ancient physician uttered some mystical or magical incantation. The post-Renaissance physician was admonished by authorities to label a prescription with something in Latin that had no meaning to the patient (and often no meaning at all), for example, tincture of Condurango; the modern physician finds that labeling a drug with a long chemical name has similar effects. At times, the modern physician knowingly prescribes an inert substance called a placebo—from the Latin: "I shall please"—usually to produce relief of symptoms.

Similarly, it is in the tradition of the physician not to tell the patient the truth about diagnosis or prognosis unless the physician is reasonably certain that on balance the consequences of doing so will produce more benefit than harm.[18] There are several other important conflicts. Physicians, by virtue of both the immediacy of contact with patients and the expectations of patients, are impelled to do something. Scientists, who can select their problems, are impelled to learn something. Physicians, whose "problems" select them, are constrained by their oath to conduct their practices with utmost confidentiality, and until recently were required by modern medical ethics to shun advertising. Scientists, whatever their primary motivations, can ordinarily achieve their rewards only through publication.

The conflicting motivations of the physician and the researcher produce the most dramatic tensions when both functions are being performed simultaneously by the same individual.[19] Some authors have argued that these conflicts are essentially irreconcilable and—in the interests of protecting the patient who might also be asked to play the role of subject—that the roles of physician and researcher should always be played by different individuals.[20,21] Others argue that the roles should not be separated because in the final analysis the best assurance that the welfare of research subjects will be protected derives from the motivations, or "conscience," of the physician.[22]

The tensions between the motivations and value systems of the researcher and physician are exemplified well in the widely used research design known as the randomized clinical trial (RCT). The problems associated with the RCT have been discussed extensively.[21,23] Although the RCT was designed primarily to test new drugs,[24] it has since been applied to the evaluation of old drugs, vaccinations, surgical interventions, social policy interventions, and even intercessory prayer.[23]

The RCT is a controlled study. That is to say, the therapy that is to be evaluated is administered to part of the subject population while another part—as similar as possible in all important respects—receives either another therapy or no therapy. The purpose of having simultaneous controls is to avoid the fallacy of *post hoc ergo propter hoc* reasoning, the mistaken belief that because B occurs after A, A must be the cause of B.

The significance of the results of the RCT is established through statistical analysis. Frequently, in order to generate sufficiently large numbers for statistical analysis in a reasonably short period of time, it is necessary to involve several medical centers in the study; thus, the design of the protocol and the evaluation of the results may be conducted in a center remote from that in which any particular patient-subject is being studied.

Controlled experimentation and statistical analysis are not recent innovations. The credibility of the former was established firmly in the 18th century when James Lind applied it to demonstrate that scurvy could be treated successfully by feeding citrus fruits to afflicted people. The power of statistical analysis to resolve otherwise irreconcilable conflicts over the relative merits of a particular form of therapy was established in the 19th century. One of its first triumphs was to demonstrate that bloodletting—in the early part of that century, the most popular form of therapy for all fevers—was much more dangerous than no therapy at all.[5]

In the 20th century additional features were introduced to the RCT. First, the suggestibility of patients, known and used to advantage by physicians for centuries, was acknowledged as a cause of some apparent drug-induced results. This is overcome by "blinding" the subjects (not letting them know which therapy they are receiving).[23] When the therapy is designed to produce relief of symptoms, the control group often receives a placebo.[25] It was then acknowledged that the biases of investigators might also influence results. Random assignment of patient-subjects to treatment and control groups is done to minimize these and other biases. Similarly, biases in the interpretation of results are eliminated through use of the "double-blind" technique; that is, neither the investigator nor the subject knows until the conclusion of the study who is in which group, treatment or control.[23]

One can easily see how—in the negotiations for informed consent for participation in an RCT—nearly all the traditions and motivations of the physician must be suspended. Similarly, the effects on expectations and wishes of many patients may be devastating. There are those who argue that the entire process is so technological and dehumanizing that its use should be sharply curtailed.[21] On the other hand, there are scientists[24] and physicians[26] who hold that the power of the RCT to develop sound information on the relative merits of therapies is so great that it would be unethical to introduce a new therapy without this sort of validation.

Ethical Justification of Biomedical Research

Biomedical research as a field of human activity is justified in terms of the good it can and often does produce. It has as its purpose the advancement of goals that are greatly valued by our society—enhancing the capabilities of physicians (and other health-care professionals) to serve the health interests of people. Some biomedical research projects do this directly and others indirectly by adding to or refining the fund of knowledge that provides the basis for future therapeutic innovations and improvements. The value of biomedical research is such that many commentators believe that society has a strong obligation to conduct, support, or otherwise encourage it. I have argued that society does have such an obligation but that this is not society's strongest obligation.[27] As an obligation of society, biomedical research's priority is not as high as, for example, the obligation to protect its members from harm and to secure the conditions of its preservation. Hans Jonas helps us put the nature of this obligation in perspective:

Unless the present state [conditions of life in our society] is intolerable, the melioristic goal [of biomedical research] is in a sense gratuitous, and this is not only from the vantage point of the present. Our descendants have a right to be left an un-plundered planet; they do not have a right to new miracle cures. We have sinned against them if by our doing, we have destroyed their inheritance . . . not . . . if by the time they come around arthritis has not yet been conquered (unless by sheer neglect).[28]

In the ethical justification of any particular research project, the first consideration is also an appraisal of the value and validity of the anticipated consequences.[29] The scientific design of the research must be adequate; otherwise one cannot anticipate accurate results (validity). Inaccurate results are of no value to society. Moreover, the anticipated results must be of sufficient value to justify the exposure of human subjects to the risks of harm presented by the project (value).

In addition to these beneficence-related requirements, the ethical justification of particular projects requires responsiveness to rules or norms related to the ethical principles of respect for persons and justice. As stated in Guideline 1 of the International Ethical Guidelines for Biomedical Research Involving Human Subjects, promulgated by the Council for International Organizations of Medical Sciences (CIOMS),

> The ethical justification of biomedical research involving human subjects is the prospect of discovering new ways of benefiting people's health. Such research can be ethically justifiable only if it is carried out in ways that respect and protect, and are fair to, the subjects of that research and are morally acceptable within the communities in which the research is carried out. Moreover, because scientifically invalid research is unethical in that it exposes research subjects to risks without possible benefit, investigators and sponsors must ensure that proposed studies involving human subjects conform to generally accepted scientific principles and are based on adequate knowledge of the pertinent scientific literature.[30]

Regulatory Definition of Research

The definition of research contained in the U.S. federal regulations for the protection of human subjects is, at the time of this writing, a topic of serious controversy. In this section, I shall review the origins of this definition with the aim of providing insight into its intended meaning and then survey briefly the controversy over its meaning. The definition in the U.S. regulations, codified at 45 CFR 46.102(d), is as follows:

> *Research* means a systematic investigation, including research, development, testing and evaluation, designed to develop or contribute to generalizable knowledge. Activities which meet this definition constitute research for purposes of this policy, whether or not they are conducted or supported under a program which is considered research for other purposes. For example, some demonstration and service programs may include research activities.[31]

This definition was derived from that recommended by the National Commission for the Protection of Human Subjects of Biomedical and Behavioral Research (hereafter, the National Commission) and published in its Belmont Report[32] (see Chapter 14). It is worth noting in passing that the entire body of federal regulations that came to be known as the Common Rule is based on the recommendations of the National Commission.

The National Commission's definition is in the following paragraph:

> For the most part, the term "practice" [of medicine or behavioral therapy] refers to interventions that are designed solely to enhance the well-being of an individual patient or client and that have a reasonable expectation of success. The purpose of medical or behavioral practice is to provide diagnosis, preventive treatment or therapy to particular individuals. By contrast, the term "research" designates an activity designed to test a hypothesis, permit conclusions to be drawn, and thereby to develop or contribute to generalizable knowledge (expressed, for example, in theories, principles, and statements of relationships). Research is usually described in a formal protocol that sets forth an objective and a set of procedures designed to reach that objective.[32]

The National Commission, knowing the danger of stipulated definitions in policy documents,[33] adhered closely to the definition provided in *Webster's Third New International Dictionary:* "Studious inquiry or examination; especially: critical and exhaustive investigation or experimentation having for its aim the discovery of new facts and their correct interpretation, the revision of accepted conclusions, theories, or laws in the light of newly discovered facts, or the practical applications of such new or revised conclusions, theories or laws."[34]

The first thing we notice about the National Commission's definition is that it was developed in contrast to a vaguely defined activity called *practice.* Why was the definition of practice so equivocal? Because the National Commission wanted to focus its attention on the relationship between the individual practitioner (medical or behavioral) and patient (or client). There are other types of practices including, for example, public health and "practice for the benefit of others" (a class of activities in which interventions or procedures are applied to one individual with the expectation that they will enhance the well-being or convenience of one or many others).[33] Such practices include, for example, organ donation, vaccination, quarantine, and heavy tranquilization of disruptive patients in a mental institution.

The National Research Act (Pub. L. 93–348), which established the National Commission, directed it to "consider . . . the boundaries between biomedical or behavioral research and the accepted and routine practice of medicine."[35] It did this because several prominent physicians regarded this as a very important and exceedingly difficult task.[36] Jay Katz identified "drawing the line between research and accepted practice . . . [as] the most difficult and complex problem facing the Commission."[36] Thomas Chalmers stated, "It is extremely hard to distinguish between clinical research and the practice of good medicine. Because episodes of illness and individual people are so variable, every physician is carrying out a small research project when he diagnoses and treats a patient."[36]

Chalmers, of course, was only echoing the views of many distinguished physicians who had spoken on this issue earlier. For example, in the classic volume, *Experimentation with Human Subjects,* Herrman Blumgart asserted: "Every time a physician administers a drug to a patient, he is in a sense performing an experiment."[18] Francis Moore added, "every (surgical) operation of any type contains certain aspects of experimental work."[37] In 1975 the National Commission assigned me the task of writing a paper on this topic to inform the Commission's considerations of the boundaries. In that paper I wrote: "It is fortunate that sharp definitions of the boundaries are not required. Even a superficial examination of this problem (contained in this paper) will reveal the impossibility of describing mutually exclusive subsets (one called research and one called practice) of the universe of activities in which health care professionals may be engaged."[38] I revised this position later after I identified the barriers to defining research and practice as mutually exclusive sets.[33,39]

In the 1970s, when the National Commission was doing its work, there were two major types of barriers to distinguishing medical practice from research. One was the fact that much of medical practice entails experimentation. The other was the widespread use of poorly defined terms to describe the use of innovative therapies. I will discuss these below.

Experimentation in Clinical Practice

Blumgart and Moore were right: The practice of medicine is characterized by experimentation. Chalmers illustrates the source of confusion by using the terms *research* and *experimentation* interchangeably. But these words are not synonyms. According to *Webster's Third New International Dictionary,* experiment means: "1a: A test or a trial; b (1) A tentative procedure or policy—especially: One adopted in uncertainty as to whether it will answer the desired purpose or bring about the desired result. . . ."[34] A consideration of the treatment of a patient with antihypertensive drugs will illustrate the experimental nature of clinical practice. The physician usually prescribes a relatively low dose of a drug that is likely to be both safe and effective. At the next office visit, the physician may discover that the patient's blood pressure remains high, in which case he or she will ordinarily increase the dose of the drug. This process is repeated until either the blood pressure decreases to the desired level or the maximum recommended dose is attained. In the latter case, the physician will ordinarily prescribe another drug—one that is known to have effects that are additive to or synergistic with the first drug. Again, the dose is escalated as needed. If there is an unacceptable side effect of the drug, it is discontinued and replaced by another drug. All of this experimentation is intended "solely to enhance the well-being of an individual patient" and not "to develop or contribute to generalizable knowledge." In other words, it is clinical practice and not research.

One of the ethical problems presented by much research, particularly the RCT, is that the patient-subject is deprived of the therapeutic experimentation that characterizes clinical practice. For the duration of most RCTs, the subject receives a fixed dose of either the drug being evaluated or the comparator.

Terminological Inexactitude

An important barrier to the development of a satisfactory definition of research was the use of language that implied that the use of "nonvalidated therapies" was research. The Food and Drug Administration (FDA) referred to drugs that had not been approved for commercial distribution as "investigational." Physicians seeking informed consent to the use of investigational drugs are required by FDA, as codified at 21 CFR 50.25(a)(1), to tell patients that "the study involves research" even when there is no research, as in the case of "compassionate use."[40] (*Compassionate use* means the use of an investigational drug for the treatment of patients who do not satisfy the eligibility criteria for drug trials that may be in progress. The FDA permits the use of some investigational drugs in situations in which no alternative drug is available or the treating physician believes that available alternatives would be clearly inferior for the patient. For example, the patient's disease may be refractory to approved alternatives or the patient may have experienced unacceptable side effects to all known approved alternatives. The FDA does not endorse use of the term *compassionate*.)

The FDA has the authority to regulate interstate commerce in drugs (among other things), and its regulations forbid sending across state lines drugs it had not approved for commercial distribution. Sponsors of new drugs who wish to ship drugs across state lines for the purpose of conducting research to evaluate their safety and efficacy are required to file a document called "Notice of Claimed Investigational Exemption for a New Drug." Although the adjective *investigational* is intended to apply to the exemption, with the passage of time, the shorthand expression *investigational new drug* (IND) became commonly used.[41] This confusing usage persists to this day.

Another linguistic infelicity was the use of the term *therapeutic research* to identify research involving the use of interventions or procedures intended to provide direct health benefit for the individual patient-subject. Therapeutic research was distinguished from *nontherapeutic research*, in which there was no possibility of direct health benefit for the individual subject. It is not clear to me when the use of this distinction began to be made in discussions of the ethics and regulation of clinical research. The original Declaration of Helsinki (1964) distinguished nontherapeutic clinical research from clinical research combined with professional care. In the 1975 revision of the Declaration, "medical research combined with professional care" is designated "clinical research," and "nontherapeutic biomedical research" is also called "non-clinical biomedical research." The National Commission recognized that this terminology contributed to the problem in defining *research*. More importantly, it recognized that all policy documents and all discussions that rely on this distinction contain serious errors. Accordingly, it rejected this distinction and replaced it with more suitable terms. A full discussion of this topic is beyond the scope of this discussion; interested readers are referred to the cited publications.[25,33,42]

Conceptual Clarification

The National Commission also addressed the problem of how to deal with clinical interventions that did not conform to what Congress called "the accepted and routine practice of medicine." In the words of the National Commission,

> When a clinician departs in a significant way from standard or accepted practice, the innovation does not, in and of itself, constitute research. The fact that a procedure is "experimental," in the sense of new, untested or different, does not automatically place it in the category of research. Radically new procedures of this description should, however, be made the object of formal research at an early stage in order to determine whether they are safe and effective. Thus, it is the responsibility of medical practice committees, for example, to

insist that a major innovation be incorporated into a formal research project.

Research and practice may be carried on together when research is designed to evaluate the safety and efficacy of a therapy. This need not cause any confusion regarding whether or not the activity requires review; the general rule is that if there is any element of research in an activity, that activity should undergo review for the protection of human subjects.[32]

This class of activities is most commonly called *innovative therapy;* I proposed that it should be called *nonvalidated practice* because the defining attribute was not novelty; it was lack of validation (demonstration of safety and efficacy), and the Commission's reasoning about how to deal with such practices applies to diagnostic and preventive measures, not only therapies.[33]

As already noted, the National Commission rejected the concepts of therapeutic and nontherapeutic research. Instead of *nontherapeutic research,* the National Commission simply refers to *research* which is, by definition, something other than therapeutic. More cumbersome language is employed by the National Commission to convey the meaning intended most commonly by those who had used the expression *therapeutic research.* For example, in the Commission's report *Research Involving Prisoners,*[43] recommendation 2 states in part: "Research on practices, both innovative and accepted, which have the intent and reasonable probability of improving the health or well-being of the individual may be conducted. . . . " The same concept is reflected in recommendation 3 of the report *Research Involving Children.*[44] It is made clear that the risks and benefits of therapeutic maneuvers are to be analyzed similarly notwithstanding the status of the maneuver as either nonvalidated or standard (accepted). "The relationship of benefits to risks . . . (should be) at least as favorable to the subject as that presented by any" available alternative. The risks of research maneuvers designed to benefit the community at large are justified differently. If the risks are greater than minimal, special substantive and procedural protections are required.

The concept rejected by the National Commission is that entire research projects could (or should) be classified as therapeutic. All research projects include some components that are nontherapeutic. The Commission recommended that the separate components of the research be classified as either "beneficial" or "nonbeneficial" and each justified accordingly. The language recommended by the National Commission in *Research Involving Children* is in the federal regulations at 45 CFR 46.405: "intervention or procedure that holds out the prospect of direct benefit for the individual subject, or by a monitoring procedure that is likely to contribute to the subject's well-being."[31] The process of sorting out the procedures and interventions according to whether they hold out, or do not hold out, the prospect of direct benefit for the purpose of justification of their risks is called *component analysis.*[33,45,46]

Controversy Over the Definition of Research

Controversy over the definition of research began even before the promulgation in 1981 of the revision of the federal regulations that contained it. Although some said that the definition was not inclusive enough, most commentators who challenged the definition asserted that it was overly inclusive. In general, the complaints

about the definition were, and continue to be, complaints about the consequences of the definition: Anything that was included within the definition would be covered by the federal regulations for the protection of human subjects. Anxiety was provoked by the National Commission's statement in the Belmont Report of the reason for defining research: "It is important to distinguish between biomedical and behavioral research, on the one hand, and the practice of accepted therapy on the other, in order to know what activities ought to undergo review for the protection of human subjects of research."[32]

Some social and behavioral researchers who testified at hearings held by the National Commission claimed that all they did in their research activities was to talk with their subjects. Therefore, they argued, any attempt to regulate this activity would be unconstitutional, an infringement of their first amendment right to freedom of speech. Institutional review board (IRB) review, they argued, would be a "prior restraint" on speech, and this is forbidden by constitutional law.[33] Social and behavioral scientists complained, and continue to complain,[47] that the definition created a forced fit of their activities into the medical model. Those who protested did not succeed in getting the definition changed; their protests, however, did succeed in getting the regulation writers to create exemptions from coverage by the federal regulations—exemptions that had not been recommended by the National Commission.

The level of complaint appeared to subside during the 1980s and early 1990s only to return forcefully since the mid-1990s. The crescendo in the level of complaint coincided with the increasingly aggressive enforcement of regulatory compliance by the federal Office for Protection from Research Risks and its successor, the Office for Human Research Protections (OHRP). In response to threats of regulatory sanctions, IRBs and other parts of the institutional human subjects protection system have become increasingly attentive to the bureaucratic details of their review and approval activities. Researchers have always considered the IRB review process burdensome,[48] and many find it intolerable.[49] Several groups of researchers have proposed that the definition of research should be changed; in general, they are proposing to change the definition so that most or all of their activities would not be considered research. I believe their motivation is to escape from the increasingly burdensome experience of regulatory compliance.

Examples of the fields in which researchers are striving to redefine research are public health,[50] quality improvement,[51] social and behavioral research,[47] and health policy research.[52] Their proposed revisions, each carefully gerrymandered to reduce their own compliance burdens, are not consistent with each other's. I have recommended to each of them that they discontinue their efforts to revise the definition of research. Instead, they should appeal for revisions of the list of exemptions from coverage by the Common Rule. For example, public health officials should appeal for exemptions for their outbreak investigations rather than quibble over whether such investigations are research or public health practice. There is nothing in an outbreak investigation that presents to the subjects risks as great as those presented by research on public benefit or service programs (particularly "possible changes in or alternatives to those programs"), a category that is already exempted at 45 CFR 46.101(b)(5) of the U.S. federal regulations.[31] Further discussion of this topic is beyond the scope of this chapter.

Definition of "Human Subject"

The U.S. federal regulations define *human subject* and further terms contained within this definition as follows:

> 45 CFR 46.102 (f) *Human subject* means a living individual about whom an investigator (whether professional or student) conducting research obtains (1) data through intervention or interaction with the individual, or (2) identifiable private information.
>
> *Intervention* includes both physical procedures by which data are gathered (for example, venipuncture) and manipulations of the subject or the subject's environment that are performed for research purposes. *Interaction* includes communication or interpersonal contact between investigator and subject. *Private information* includes information about behavior that occurs in a context in which an individual can reasonably expect that no observation or recording is taking place, and information which has been provided for specific purposes by an individual and which the individual can reasonably expect will not be made public (for example, a medical record). Private information must be individually identifiable (i.e., the identity of the subject is or may readily be ascertained by the investigator or associated with the information) in order for obtaining the information to constitute research involving human subjects.[31]

When the foregoing definition made its debut in the revised federal regulations promulgated in 1981 (it had not been recommended by the National Commission), it attracted little or no attention. It became the subject of considerable controversy in 1999 shortly after the occurrence of what came to be known as the Virginia Commonwealth University incident.[53–55] Researchers sent a copy of a questionnaire by mail to the home of one of their adult research subjects. When it arrived, her father opened the envelope and found that the information solicited in the survey instrument included some aspects of the medical history of the subject and other members of her family. Some of the information was of a highly personal and sensitive nature. He protested to various officials at the university and in the government that he and his family were involved in this study as research subjects without their informed consent. The matter was referred to OHRP, which ruled that he was right; he was a research subject and, because the solicited information was both private and sensitive, consent from the family members should have been obtained.

The ensuing challenges to the definition of *human subject* focused nearly exclusively on whether it was reasonable to require consent from the individuals (variously referred to in the debates as *secondary subjects* or *third parties*) about whom private and sensitive information was solicited. I do not intend to discuss here the merits of the arguments for or against the reasonableness of this requirement; such analysis is beyond the scope of this chapter. These debates have much in common with the efforts of some professionals to alter the definition of research so that they might be spared the burdens of regulatory compliance. The issue is not the definition; the issue is whether or not there should be a requirement for consent of the "secondary subjects." Those who believe that consent should not be required should focus their attention on revising (or negotiating the interpretation of) the regulatory justifications for "waivers and alterations" of the elements of informed consent at 45 CFR 46.116(d),[31] and not on the definition of *human subject*.

Participants or Subjects?

In recent years some commentators have attempted to replace the word *subject* with *participant*. The motivation for this appears to be a concern with egalitarianism. To some, the word *subject* implies subjugation, as in "the King and his subjects;" the parallel would then be "the researcher and his or her subjects." The word *participant,* by contrast, implies a moral equality between the researcher and the participant; they are each participants in the program known as research. We have seen similar egalitarian gestures in the past. In the 1970s, for example, such distinguished scholars as Jay Katz and Paul Ramsey attempted to replace the word *subject* with *co-adventurer* or *joint venturer*. Clearly these efforts had no lasting effect. The word *subject* in this context was never intended in the sense of *subordinate*. It was introduced into the lexicon of medicine around the beginning of the 19th century in the sense of "the subject matter of an art or science," or "that which forms or is chosen as a matter of thought, consideration or inquiry, a topic, a theme."[1] The patients who were presented to senior clinicians or professors for teaching purposes or for clinical consultations were called subjects. In the early 19th century, one definition of *subject* was "a person who presents himself for or who undergoes medical or surgical treatment."

Undoubtedly, the researcher and the subject should be regarded as moral equals. There is nothing about the word *subject,* properly understood, that is inconsistent with that. They are, however, moral equals who are performing in differing roles. If the day comes that all persons engaged in research are called participants, it will be necessary to invent new language to designate which of the participants is responsible for negotiating informed consent, which will be eligible to share in the Nobel Prize, and which are entitled to compensation in case of research-induced injury.

Summary

Clinical research is defined as that subset of biomedical research in which the subjects of research are human beings. Biomedical research is defined as research having as its ultimate aim the advancement of the goals of medicine. The domain of medicine is defined most narrowly in the traditional medical model, which focuses the attention of the physician on a patient who either feels ill or has a disease, the presence of which is subject to objective verification. The broadest view of the domain of medicine holds that the primary concern of the profession is the maintenance of health, a state of complete physical, mental, and social well-being, not merely the absence of disease. Thus, biomedical research may be seen—according to the traditional medical model—primarily as the application of the natural sciences. In relation to a broader view of the domain of medicine, which includes preventive medicine and public health, biomedical research is extended to include some aspects of virtually all natural, behavioral, and social sciences.

Since early in the 19th century there has been a systematic effort to blend the scientific method into the practice of medicine.

And yet there are important conflicts between the traditions, assumptions, and motivations of physicians and researchers. As a consequence of these conflicts, serious problems may be presented to patients, subjects, physicians, and investigators. These problems are exemplified well in the peculiarly 20th-century device known as the randomized clinical trial.

The definitions of *research* and *human subject* contained in the U.S. federal regulations are each the focus of current controversy. The cause of these controversies is not the definitions themselves. It is the regulatory actions that are contingent on the definitions and their interpretation. The controversies would likely be abated if appropriate additions were made to the list of activities that are exempt from coverage by the regulations and if the regulatory criteria for waiver or alteration of the elements of informed consent were interpreted differently.

Acknowledgments

This work was funded in part by grant number 1 P30 MH 62294 01A1 from the National Institute of Mental Health and a grant from The Patrick and Catherine Weldon Donaghue Medical Research Foundation. Portions of this paper were adapted or abridged from previous publications of the author, particularly, *Ethics and Regulation of Clinical Research,* 2nd ed. New Haven, Conn.: Yale University Press, 1988; and Biomedical research. In: Reich WT, ed. *Encyclopedia of Bioethics.* New York, N.Y.: The Free Press; 1978.

References

1. *Oxford English Dictionary,* 2nd ed. New York, N.Y.: Oxford University Press; 2004.
2. Sigerist HE. *A History of Medicine. Vol. 1: Primitive and Archaic Medicine.* New York, N.Y.: Oxford University Press; 1951:7.
3. Feinstein AR. *Clinical Judgment.* Baltimore, Md.: Williams & Wilkins Co.; 1967:385.
4. Reich WT. Historical dimensions of an ethic of care in healthcare. In: SG Post, ed. *Encyclopedia of Bioethics,* 3rd ed. New York, N.Y.: Macmillan Reference; 2004:361–7.
5. Shryock RH. *The Development of Modern Medicine,* rev. ed. New York, N.Y.: Alfred A. Knopf; 1947:129ff.
6. Cassell EJ. Illness and disease. *Hastings Center Report* 1976;6(2):27–37.
7. Parsons T. *The Social System.* Glencoe, Ill.: The Free Press; 1951.
8. Freidson E. *Profession of Medicine: A Study of the Sociology of Applied Knowledge.* New York, N.Y.: Dodd, Mead & Co.; 1970.
9. World Health Organization. *Constitution of the World Health Organization.* Geneva, Switzerland: WHO, 1994 [1948]. [Online] Available: http://www.who.int/about/en/.
10. Burton LE, Smith HH. *Public Health and Community Medicine for the Allied Medical Professions,* 2nd ed. Baltimore, Md.: Williams & Wilkins Co.; 1975.
11. Flexner A. *Medical Education: A Comparative Study.* New York, N.Y.: Macmillan Co.; 1925.
12. Fruton JS. The emergence of biochemistry. *Science* 1976;192:327–34.
13. Thomas L. The future impact of science and technology on medicine. *Bioscience* 1974;24:99–105.
14. Comroe JH, Dripps RD. Scientific basis for the support of biomedical science. *Science* 1976;192:105–11.
15. Green FHK. The clinical evaluation of remedies. *Lancet* 1954;264:1085–91.
16. Jonsen AR. Do no harm. *Annals of Internal Medicine* 1978;88:827–32.
17. Shapiro AK. A contribution to the history of the placebo effect. *Behavioral Science* 1960;5:109–35.
18. Blumgart HL. The medical framework for viewing the problem of human experimentation. In: Freund PA, ed. *Experimentation With Human Subjects.* New York, N.Y.: George Braziller; 1970:39–65.
19. Katz J. The regulation of human research: Reflections and proposals. *Clinical Research* 1973;21:785–91.
20. Beecher HK. *Research and the Individual: Human Studies.* Boston, Mass.: Little, Brown & Co.; 1970:289–92.
21. Fried C. *Medical Experimentation: Personal Integrity and Social Policy.* New York, N.Y.: American Elsevier Co.; 1974.
22. Levine RJ. Uncertainty in clinical research. *Law, Medicine and Health Care* 1988;16:174–82.
23. Levine RJ. Randomized clinical trials: Ethical considerations. In: Edwards RB, editor. *Advances in Bioethics, Vol. 5.* Stamford, Conn.: JAI Press; 1999:113–45.
24. Hill AB. Medical ethics and controlled trials. *British Medical Journal* 1963;1:1043–9.
25. Levine RJ. Placebo controls in clinical trials of new therapies for conditions for which there are known effective treatments. In: Guess HA, Kleinman A, Kusek JW, Engel LW, eds. *The Science of the Placebo: Toward an Interdisciplinary Research Agenda.* London, England: BMJ Books; 2002:264–80.
26. Chalmers TC, Block JB, Lee S. Controlled studies in clinical cancer research. *New England Journal of Medicine* 1972;287:75–8.
27. Levine RJ. An ethical perspective. In: Spilker B, ed. *Quality of Life and Pharmacoeconomics in Clinical Trials,* 2nd ed. Philadelphia, Pa.: Lippincott-Raven; 1996:489–95.
28. Jonas H. Philosophical reflections on experimenting with human subjects. In: Freund PA. *Experimentation With Human Subjects.* New York, N.Y.: George Braziller; 1970:358–78.
29. Freedman B. Scientific value and validity as ethical requirements for research: A proposed explication. *IRB: A Review of Human Subjects Research* 1987;9(6):7–10.
30. Council for International Organizations of Medical Sciences, in collaboration with the World Health Organization. *International Ethical Guidelines for Biomedical Research Involving Human Subjects.* Geneva, Switzerland: CIOMS and WHO; 2002. [Online] November 2002. Available: http://www.cioms.ch/frame_guidelines_nov_2002.htm.
31. Department of Health and Human Services, National Institutes of Health, and Office for Human Research Protections. The Common Rule, Title 45 (Public Welfare), Code of Federal Regulations, Part 46 (Protection of Human Subjects). [Online] June 23, 2005. Available: http://www.hhs.gov/ohrp/humansubjects/guidance/45cfr46.htm.
32. The National Commission for the Protection of Human Subjects of Biomedical and Behavioral Research. *The Belmont Report: Ethical Principles and Guidelines for the Protection of Human Subjects of Research.* Washington, D.C.: Department of Health, Education and Welfare; DHEW Publication OS 78–0012 1978. [Online] Available: http://www.hhs.gov/ohrp/humansubjects/guidance/belmont.htm.
33. Levine RJ. *Ethics and Regulation of Clinical Research,* 2nd ed. New Haven, Conn.: Yale University Press; 1988.
34. Gove PB, ed. *Webster's Third New International Dictionary.* Springfield, Mass.: G.C. Merriam Co.; 1971.
35. National Research Service Award Act of 1974. Public Law 93–348; Title II.
36. Kay EM. Legislative history of title II—protection of human subjects of biomedical and behavioral research—of the National Research Act: PL 93–348. Unpublished manuscript prepared for the National Commission, 1975.
37. Moore FD. Therapeutic innovation: Ethical boundaries in the initial clinical trials of new drugs and surgical procedures. In: Freund PA, ed. *Experimentation With Human Subjects.* New York, N.Y.: George Braziller; 1970:358–78.

38. Levine RJ. The boundaries between biomedical or behavioral research and the accepted and routine practice of medicine. In: National Commission for the Protection of Human Subjects of Biomedical and Behavioral Research. *The Belmont Report: Ethical Principles and Guidelines for the Protection of Human Subjects of Research, Appendix I.* DHEW Publication No. (OS) 78–0013. Washington, D.C.: DHEW; 1978:1.1–1.44.

39. Levine RJ. Clarifying the concepts of research ethics. *Hastings Center Report* 1979;9(3):21–6.

40. Department of Health and Human Services, Food and Drug Administration. Title 21 (Food and Drugs), Code of Federal Regulations, Part 50 (Protection of Human Subjects). [Online] April 1, 2006. Available: http://www.gpo.gov/nara/cfr/waisidx_06/21cfr50_06.html.

41. Levine RJ. Commentary on E. Howe's and E. Martin's "Treating the Troops." *Hastings Center Report* 1991;21(2):27–9.

42. Levine RJ. The need to revise the Declaration of Helsinki. *New England Journal of Medicine* 1999;341:531–4.

43. National Commission for the Protection of Human Subjects of Biomedical and Behavioral Research. *Research Involving Prisoners: Report and Recommendations.* DHEW Publication No. (OS) 76–131. Washington, D.C.: DHEW; 1976. [Online] Available: http://www.bioethics.gov/reports/past_commissions/Research_involving_prisoners.pdf.

44. National Commission for the Protection of Human Subjects of Biomedical and Behavioral Research. *Research Involving Children: Report and Recommendations.* DHEW Publication No. (OS) 77–0004. Washington, D.C.: DHEW; 1977. [Online] Available: http://www.bioethics.gov/reports/past_commissions/Research_involving_children.pdf.

45. Levine RJ. The National Commission's ethical principles with special attention to beneficence. In: Childress JF, Meslin EM, Shapiro HT, eds. *Belmont Revisited: Ethical Principles for Research with Human Subjects.* Washington, D.C.: Georgetown University Press; 2005:126–35.

46. Weijer C. The ethical analysis of risk. *Journal of Law, Medicine and Ethics* 2000;28:344–61.

47. Center for Advanced Study, University of Illinois. *The Illinois Whitepaper. Improving the System for Protecting Human Subjects: Counteracting IRB "Mission Creep."* [Online] 2005. Available: http://www.law.uiuc.edu/conferences/whitepaper.

48. Kavanagh C, Matthews D, Sorenson JR, Swazey JP. We shall overcome: Multi-institutional review of a genetic counseling study. *IRB: A Review of Human Subjects Research* 1979;1(2):1–3,12.

49. Levine RJ. Institutional review boards: A crisis in confidence. *Annals of Internal Medicine* 2001;134:161–3.

50. Secretary's Advisory Committee on Human Research Protections. Minutes of the meeting of October 4 and 5, 2004. [Online] Available: http://www.hhs.gov/ohrp/sachrp/mtgings/mtg10–04/min10–04.html.

51. Baily MA, Bottrell M, Lynn J, Jennings B. The ethics of using QI methods to improve health care quality and safety: A Hastings Center Special Report. *Hastings Center Report* 2006;36(4):S1–S40. [Online] Available: http://www.thehastingscenter.org/pdf/using_qi_methods_to_improve_health_care_quality_safety.pdf.

52. Lynn J, Johnson J, Levine RJ. The ethical conduct of health services research: A case study of 55 institutions' applications to the SUPPORT project. *Clinical Research* 1994;42:3–10.

53. Botkin J. Protecting the privacy of family members in survey and pedigree research. *JAMA* 2001;285:207–11.

54. National Institutes of Health Behavioral and Social Sciences Research Coordinating Committee. Minutes of the Meeting of April 13, 2001. [Online] Available: http://obssr.od.nih.gov/BSSRCC/Minutes/April2001.pdf.

55. Rubin R. Whose medical history is it, anyway? *USA Today* Apr. 8, 2001.

Ezekiel J. Emanuel   Christine Grady

Four Paradigms of Clinical Research and Research Oversight

The understanding of appropriate ethical protections for participants of biomedical research has not been static. It has developed over time, with the evolution of biomedical research as well as social values. Since World War II, four major paradigms of research and research oversight have been operative in the United States. These paradigms incorporate different values and provide different approaches to research oversight and the protection of research participants.

For hundreds of years, research to test interventions had been sporadic.[1,2] Little distinction was made between experimentation and therapy. Evidence of the effectiveness, and even safety, of medical interventions was rare.[3] Until the late 19th century, most therapies could properly be considered experimental in the sense that they lacked empirical evidence for their effectiveness. Researchers were usually physicians, motivated to do what they thought best for their patients, and trusted to do the right thing.[4] There were no specific codes of ethics, laws, or regulations governing the conduct of researchers, but peer judgment and influence served to contain fraud and abuse.[5] For instance, in 1897 Giuseppe Sanarelli, an Italian researcher working on yellow fever, declared he had produced yellow fever by injecting a bacillus into five people.[1,6,7] At a 1898 medical meeting, William Osler condemned Sanarelli saying: "To deliberately inject a poison of known high degree of virulency into a human being, unless you obtain that man's sanction, is not ridiculous, it is criminal."[6]

Systematic biomedical research began to grow as an enterprise after the development of penicillin and the passage in 1938 of the U.S. Food, Drug, and Cosmetic Act, which required evidence of safety before a product was marketed.[8] Just before World War II, there was dramatic growth in research as an enterprise. Large pharmaceutical companies were starting up; both public and private money was devoted to research; and research became increasingly centralized, coordinated, standardized in method, and publicly supported.

Since the beginning of World War II, understanding of the ethics and oversight of human subjects research has proceeded through four distinct periods or paradigms. Each period embodied different perspectives on research and its dangers and different conceptualizations of the goals of oversight. Each period also advanced a different underlying ethical principle guiding the protections of research participants; each empowered different institutions to implement the protections, and each had its own way of balancing protection of research participants against other important values in biomedical research. At least in the United States, the change from one period to another was frequently catalyzed by crises or scandals. To some degree the periods represent "swings of the regulatory pendulum"[9] but, as will become clear, these swings were not along just one dimension.

Importantly, these periods or paradigms should not be thought of as Kuhnian paradigms with radical, instantaneous paradigm shifts.[10] The transition between paradigms evolved over time, usually due to crises or scandals that forced a reexamination of the existing research oversight paradigm. The ideas that evolved, and were subsequently espoused, had antecedents in the prior paradigm. Furthermore, the dominant ideas and values of a prior paradigm often remained operative and influential in subsequent paradigms. Indeed, distinct paradigms can coexist, and it might be argued that none of the paradigms has been entirely supplanted. Nevertheless, although precise dates cannot be given for each period, there are important changes between periods symbolized and encapsulated in the values of research oversight that become dominant.

Because the different paradigms overlap, controversies about the oversight system and the ethics of research are frequently disagreements over what values and which paradigms should be dominant. There may also be disagreements over what types of research studies the particular protections apply to. That is, one paradigm and its protections may clearly apply to intervention studies, but there might be controversy over whether they apply to epidemiology, pharmacokinetic, or normal physiology studies. Indeed, some of the more recent paradigms probably apply only to some types of studies. Table 22.1 summarizes the four paradigms and their important features.

Period 1: Researcher Paternalism

World War II had a profound impact on Western society, emphasizing the need for people to contribute to the social good. The importance of individual sacrifice for society's benefit was palpable. Indeed, in Britain it was thought that society's very survival depended upon such sacrifice, and in the United States there was a strong sense that if not survival, then certainly the country's winning of the war depended upon such sacrifice. Obviously this belief was manifest directly in fighting the war, but it also influenced related activities, such as biomedical research. Beginning with the war and extending for nearly three decades, the dominant view was that biomedical research was important for society's benefit and progress against diseases.[4] Individual sacrifice was necessary for research and was justified by the tremendous good it would produce for all of society.[11] The war analogy was vivid, visceral, and, with the victory, validated by experience. Frequently, it was implicitly and explicitly invoked to justify clinical research.

Biomedical research during this period has been described as "unashamedly utilitarian."[12] The federal government and the pharmaceutical industry supported intensive research efforts to develop vaccines and antibiotics to help soldiers at risk from infectious diseases. This research frequently involved available and captive populations in prisons, orphanages, homes for the emotionally or developmentally disturbed and other institutions.[13] Research was justified as a way for such groups to make their contribution to society. Biomedical research was clearly seen as distinct from therapy; participants who were not necessarily in need of therapy were accepting a personal burden in order to make a contribution to society.

Although utilitarianism is not the only philosophical approach that can justify individual sacrifice for the greater good of society, it is the best developed and accepted rationale. During this period, utilitarianism implicitly or explicitly became the dominant justification for research; and the dominant ethical principle guiding research and research oversight was social value. The ratio of risks to benefits for individual research participants might have been unfavorable—with high risks for the individual. But risks to the individual were thought to be outweighed by the emphasis on social value, the value of the knowledge to be gained for society.

By the late 1960s, clinical research was under attack and researchers found it necessary to articulate the philosophical justification for research, specifying the benefits of biomedical research for society and the need for individual sacrifice to achieve those benefits. For instance, Hans Jonas attacked the underlying paradigm when he attacked the war image, specifically the idea that research with humans was necessary for society's survival.[14] He also rejected the utilitarian philosophy underlying the research paradigm:

> We may observe that averting a disaster always carries greater weight than promoting a good. Extraordinary danger excuses extraordinary means. . . . Much weaker is the case where it is a matter not of saving but of improving society. Much of medical research falls into this category. As stated before, a permanent death rate from heart failure or cancer does not threaten society. . . . The destination of research is essentially melioristic. It does not serve the preservation of the existing good from which I profit myself and to which I am obligated. Unless the present state is intolerable, the melioristic goal is in a sense gratuitous. . . . [Consequently, t]he surrender of one's body to medical experimentation is entirely outside the enforceable "social contract."[14]

Probably no one was more explicit in defending clinical research against Jonas's view than Walsh McDermott, one of the leading figures in postwar American medicine. In 1967, when addressing a colloquium on clinical research, McDermott argued:

> When the needs of society come in head-on conflict with the rights of an individual, someone has to play God. We can avoid this responsibility so long as the power to decide the particular case-in-point is clearly vested in someone else, for example, a duly elected government official. But in clinical investigation, the power to determine this issue of "the individual versus society" is clearly vested in the physician. . . . [A]s a society we enforce the social good over the individual good across a whole spectrum of non-medical activities every day, and many of these activities ultimately affect the health or the life of an individual. . . . I submit that the core of this ethical issue as it arises in clinical investigation lies in [that] to ensure the rights of society, an arbitrary judgment must be made against an individual. . . . [W]e have seen large social payoffs from certain experiments in humans . . . we could no longer maintain, in strict honesty, that in the study of disease the interests of the individual are invariably paramount. . . . To be sure, by careful attention we can cut down the number of instances in which the problem presents itself to us in its starkest form. But there is no escape from the fact that, if the future good of society is to be served, there will be times when the clinical investigator must make an arbitrary judgment with respect to an individual.[15]

Louis Lasagna, chair of Department of Pharmacology and Toxicology at the University of Rochester, agreed that individuals could be sacrificed for the greater social good and noted that the best protection for research participants was the ethical researcher:

> Society frequently tramples on the rights of individuals in the "greater interest." . . . [T]he good of the individual and the good of society are often not identical and sometimes mutually exclusive. I submit that the successful development of such an ethical conscience, combined with professional skill, will protect the patient or experimental subject much more effectively than any laws or regulations. . . . I believe it is

Table 22.1
Four Periods and Paradigms of Research Oversight

Period/Paradigm	Dates	Triggering Event	Key Protection	Conception of Clinical Trial Participant	Roles of Research and Health Care	Underlying Philosophy	Highlighted Ethical Principle
Researcher paternalism	1940–early 1970s	World War II	Researchers' judgment	A passive subject of research	Sharp distinction between care and research	Utilitarianism	Social value
Regulatory protectionism	Early 1970s–late 1980s	Jewish Chronic Disease Hospital Scandal; Tuskegee Syphilis Study; Beecher's revelations	IRB review and individual informed consent	A vulnerable patient	Research priorities seen as threat to clinical care	Principlism	Independent review
Participant access	Late 1980s–mid-1990s	AIDS epidemic; breast cancer movement	Individual autonomy	An informed consumer	Clinical trials viewed as best, cutting-edge clinical care	Individual rights–based theory	Informed consent
Community partnership	Mid-1990s	Genetic research among Ashkenazi Jews and aboriginal communities; international HIV/AIDS research	Host community collaboration	An active "participant" in the research enterprise	Research and clinical practice go hand in hand	Communitarianism	Collaborative partnership

inevitable that the many will continue to benefit on occasion from the contributions—sometimes involuntary—of the few. The problem is to know when to say "Halt!"[16]

During this period, the main protections for research participants were the integrity of the researcher and the researcher's judgment. Informed consent was seen as a lesser protection. At the end of the 19th century, Walter Reed had obtained consent for his yellow fever experiments. Over the next 70 years, researchers typically obtained informed consent to research from healthy volunteers. However, consent to research from patients receiving experimental treatments was much more inconsistent. More important than informed consent, it was argued, was the caring, compassionate researcher. Researchers were seen as concerned with the participants' well-being and wanting to protect them. The judgment of researchers regarding the types of research projects they thought were reasonable, as well as what risks and risk-benefit ratios were reasonable, was deemed an appropriate and acceptable safeguard. Individual researchers' judgments about what was reasonable were influenced by what the wider research community deemed acceptable, and that remained an important protection. Nonetheless, the main protection was really researcher paternalism.[4,15,16]

This view was widespread. One of the persons most responsible for ending this paradigm—although he did not intend to end it—was Henry Beecher. Through his 1966 article in the *New England Journal of Medicine* delineating 22 cases of abuse of research participants, he catalyzed a transformation that changed the paradigm of research and research oversight.[17] Yet throughout his career he maintained that the care and integrity of the researcher, rather than informed consent, was the best way to protect research participants. In this sense, he very much supported a kind of researcher paternalism paradigm, although his aim was to emphasize that researchers had to have the right goals in mind:

> The ethical approach to experimentation in man has several components; two are more important than the others, the first being informed consent. The difficulty of obtaining this is discussed in detail. . . . Secondly, there is the more reliable safeguard [for the research participant] provided by the presence of *an intelligent, informed, conscientious, compassionate, responsible investigator* [emphasis added].[17]

Importantly, the researcher paternalism paradigm for protecting research participants was not an isolated phenomenon; the social values that informed it influenced other areas of medicine. Paternalism cohered with both the prevailing ethics of clinical care and the legal standards of informed consent for clinical care at that time. During this period, almost everyone agreed that physicians should influence treatment decisions for patients. Although it was accepted that physicians should obtain patients' consent for medical procedures, the amount of information the physician disclosed was based on what the physician community determined was reasonable to tell the patient, the so-called professional standard. For instance, in the landmark *Natanson* v. *Kline* case, the Kansas Supreme Court held: "The duty of the physician to disclose . . . is limited to those disclosures which a reasonable medical practitioner would make under the same or similar circumstances."[18]

It also was accepted that physicians might not tell patients about their cancer or other serious, life-threatening illness out of

concern for their best interests.[19] Indeed, the physician was frequently entrusted with deciding what was best for the very sick patient without gaining the patient's informed consent.[20]

Period 2: Regulatory Protectionism

The period of researcher paternalism came to an end in the early 1970s after a series of scandals. The Jewish Chronic Disease Hospital case, Henry Beecher's revelation of many unethical practices in clinical research at leading medical centers, and the Tuskegee Syphilis Study, among others, discredited researchers as concerned protectors of participants' well-being and interests[17,21,22] (see Chapters 6, 7, and 8).

What became clear through many of these cases was that researchers were not always judiciously weighing social value over individual risk-benefit assessments when they were in tension. Rather, researcher paternalism was sometimes a cover for blatantly unethical practices with few social benefits. In both the Jewish Chronic Disease Hospital case and the Tuskegee Syphilis Study, pervasive deception was used to enroll and retain relatively powerless participants.[17,21,22] Although deception might not have had an adverse physical impact in the former case, it certainly prevented many African Americans from getting curative therapy in the Tuskegee case. Furthermore, in some cases, including Tuskegee, the social value of the research was highly questionable.[21,22] Beecher summarized the problem: "Undoubtedly all sound work has [the good of society] as its ultimate aim, but such high flown expressions are not necessary and have been used within recent memory as cover for outrageous ends."[23]

The cumulative effect of these scandals was to repudiate researchers as effective overseers of the interests of participants and the ethics of research, and to question the underlying utilitarian justification for research ethics. The scandals led to a period of intense debate about the scope and limitations of research involving human subjects. Passage of the National Research Act in 1974 and the creation of the National Commission for the Protection of Human Subjects of Biomedical and Behavioral Research led to a comprehensive reassessment of the ethics of research and the appropriate oversight system.[24] The result was a regulatory system for federally funded research, codified in 1981 as Title 45, Code of Federal Regulations, Part 46, entitled "Protection of Human Subjects,"[26] which a decade later became the Common Rule (see Chapter 15).

The underlying view informing this oversight system was that biomedical research, although valuable and in some sense necessary, was inherently dangerous and a threat to the well-being of participants. The goals of therapy and research were distinct. The goal of the oversight system was protectionism—to protect participants from researchers and the inherent risks that they and their research posed. Institutional review board (IRB) review and individual informed consent were thought to be the best mechanisms to protect research participants from the risks and burdens of research. In addition, special protections were built into the regulations for various groups deemed especially vulnerable to the threat and harms posed by research—prisoners, pregnant women, and children.[27-30]

A critical aspect of the protections put into place during this period was that decision-making authority about research was partially taken away from physician researchers and put it into the hands of independent review groups, government regulators, and research participants themselves.[31] IRB review and informed consent did not come out of nowhere. As noted, informed consent for research studies from healthy volunteers had increasingly been standard practice since the turn of the century and was performed consistently with patients at certain institutions. Research review committees had been established at various institutions, such as the Clinical Center of the National Institutes of Health (NIH).[32] Nevertheless, before adoption of the federal regulations, there were no uniform rules regarding the content of informed consent or the composition and operation of the independent review committees. Furthermore, under the researcher paternalism paradigm, neither informed consent nor independent review was seen as mandatory, especially in research with patients. As in the case of the Jewish Chronic Disease Hospital, researchers felt that obtaining consent might upset the participants and that therefore it could be suspended. And much research was conducted without any independent review. Thus, a major element of the change in paradigm was to formalize informed consent by requiring written, signed informed consent documents, formalizing the review process and, at least for federally funded research, making both informed consent and independent review mandatory.[24,27] The underlying ethical philosophy was one of principlism formalized by Tom Beauchamp and James Childress in their book *Principles of Biomedical Ethics*[33] and the National Commission's Belmont Report,[34] which Beauchamp took a leading role in writing (see Chapter 14). This approach eschews comprehensive ethical theories in favor of mid-level principles that are shared and can be justified by a variety of ethical theories, particularly utilitarianism and deontology. Three ethical principles—respect for persons, beneficence, and justice—became linked to and justified specific requirements for regulating research: informed consent, determination of a favorable risk-benefit ratio, and fair selection of subjects.[33]

Ironically, although these protections emphasized informed consent and were justified in part by appeals to the principle of respect for persons, they remained somewhat paternalistic, although in a manner different from the research paternalism of the previous paradigm. For example, the new federal regulations prohibited most research with prisoners.[27,29] This restriction clearly limited prisoner autonomy but was believed to be justified because of the coercive circumstances of prison. Similarly, research with pregnant women was limited. The constraint on the autonomy of women was justified by the need to protect their fetuses.[28]

Once again, the oversight of clinical research was not being reassessed in isolation. At the same time there was a pervasive social reassessment of the ethical norms governing medical practice as well as a reevaluation of informed consent. The claim that professional ethics, codes, and oaths established by physicians should serve as normative standards was being attacked. Physician-generated rules for physicians were viewed as inadequate and suspect.[20,35] Instead, universal ethical principles that were independent of the profession, such as beneficence and autonomy, became the basis for ethical medical practice. As Robert Veatch argued in his book, *A Theory of Medical Ethics,*

What is being questioned is the authority of a professional group to set its own ethical standards and to adjudicate disputes about the conduct of its members. . . . Our conclusion is that a professional ethics grounded in nothing more than

agreement, custom, or vote by a group's members can have no ethical bite. No one outside the group would have any reason for conforming to the professional ethical judgments.[36]

Veatch argued for a social contract to replace the profession's ethics. Regardless of his specific alternative, the key point was that general ethical norms should be controlling, not norms specified by the profession for itself. This clearly mirrored the change from research oversight based upon professional judgment to oversight that was imposed from outside and derived from independent ethical principles.

Similarly, in 1972, the *Canterbury* v. *Spence* ruling by a federal appellate court delineated a different standard for assessing the amount of information that should be disclosed to patients as part of the informed consent process for medical interventions.[34,37] The court rejected a professional standard and articulated a patient-centered standard in which the goal was to give patients the power to decide what was in their interest rather than entrusting their interests to physicians.[34,36]

Mortimer Lipsett of the NIH explicitly recognized in 1982 that a utilitarian justification of individual sacrifice for the good of society was no longer tenable. In his defense of Phase I oncology studies, he recognized the centrality of individual autonomy in research:

The larger questions about the ethics of phase I clinical trials of cancer chemotherapies have not been discussed in depth. . . . [I]s this phase I trial an example of the sacrifice of the individual for the good of society? . . . The question is philosophical in nature, and the answers are conditioned by the prevailing morals of society. It is clear that in certain circumstances we mandate individual sacrifice for the good of society. For example, the citizen drafted into the armed services may have to risk his life without prospect of immediate personal gain, although, even here, remote personal gain, such as preservation of home, family, and way of life can be invoked. Although this social contract has been generally accepted . . . considerations change. A foundation stone of our moral and legal framework is autonomy—the right to personal inviolability, control of one's person, and the exercise of free will in taking risks. . . . In medical research, the imperative for sacrifice is not present, nor is it part of the social contract today. One need only recall the horrors of medical experimentation during World War II to appreciate the brutal extension of the utilitarian philosophy of sacrifice of the individual for a societal purpose.[38]

Period 3: Participant Access

Beginning in the late 1980s, the oversight system built around protecting potential research participants from researchers and the risks of research began to be attacked. Although the change was heralded by heated emotion and protests, the cause was not a scandal in which people were being harmed by research but a new health crisis, the AIDS crisis. The fatal nature of the disease and the paucity of effective treatments induced a demand for more research. People with HIV faced the prospect of dying inevitably and quickly. To them, trying a therapy that was unproven, potentially risky but also potentially beneficial, seemed reasonable. They argued that participation in clinical research was a benefit that individuals should not be denied, rather than a harm to be protected against. They assailed federal regulations aimed at protecting research participants as obstacles rather than safety measures.[13] They viewed protectionism as discriminatory in that it prevented them from getting experimental interventions that they wanted. Rather than protecting them from potential exploitation, they considered exclusion or limited access to trials as harmful and unjust. HIV patients rejected regulatory protections from researchers and research interventions and demanded access to experimental interventions. Activists asserted an autonomous right to try risky but potentially beneficial treatments—a right that they claimed should trump regulatory protectionism and paternalism. Martin Delaney of Project Inform said, "People with life-threatening illnesses have rights that supersede those of society to control their behavior."[39]

To the AIDS activists, regulations that forced them to die without trying something were more dangerous than researchers with unproven experimental interventions. Just as relying on researcher paternalism often exposed people to excessive risks, HIV activists argued that regulatory protections exposed people to the excessive risk of doing nothing. The justification for regulatory protections in research was challenged as the regulations' consequences and costs were exposed.[40] Delaney recounts,

> The epidemic will not pause for the traditional modes of science; AIDS has forced the acceleration of the procedures and processes of clinical investigation, as well as the mechanisms of regulations. . . . The basic concept of human experimentation has been radically altered—from protecting individuals from research to attempting to ensure individuals access.[39]

The regulatory pendulum began to move.

This period marked not only another major reassessment of research but also substantive changes in the way federal research agencies did business. Research was now perceived not as necessarily harmful but as a societal good—and as an opportunity for treatment. Concomitantly, researchers were not to be feared as enemies but to be seen as allies. Moving away from an emphasis on protection against research, laypeople and patient advocates began demanding access to research. Many advocates and patients argued that more efficient and equitable studies could be done, with better patient compliance, if community physicians participated in clinical trials. A number of programs were established to allow clinical providers in the community to participate in conducting research, such as the Community Consortium in San Francisco, the American Foundation for AIDS Research's (AmFAR) community coalition, and the Community Programs for Clinical Research in AIDS (CPCRA) formed by the National Institute of Allergy and Infectious Diseases (NIAID).[13] The line between research and treatment was blurred as participation in research was seen as the best, and sometimes only, way to obtain needed treatment, and was being offered by community physicians in community clinics. And, it was argued, the best protection against harm and exploitation was the judgment of individuals about what was in their own best interests, not government regulations or bureaucrats deciding what risks were excessive. Delaney writes,

> [R]egulators contend that desperate patients don't know what's good for them, that access to experimental treatments must be controlled by those with the proper scientific train-

ing . . . many feel this argument smacks of "big brother." . . . No one disputes that the multiphase steps of clinical research are a proven way to quantify the effects of a drug. The question is whether those steps should be equally required when seeking to restrain a contagious, world-wide epidemic as when judging a new cold tablet or pain remedy. AIDS is the medical equivalent of war. . . . The question should be, "who gets to decide what risks are acceptable: the bureaucracy in Washington or the patient whose life is on the line?"[39]

Although this trend began with HIV, it was subsequently reinforced by activists associated with other serious diseases for which there also were few effective interventions or cures. Thus, advocates for people with breast cancer, diabetes, Alzheimer's, and other diseases adopted similar pleas for access to clinical trials. Additionally, critics charged that certain groups who were traditionally underrepresented in research were being denied not only the possible benefits of participation but also the benefits of the application of knowledge gained through research. In the early 1990s, the NIH began to require that federally funded researchers enroll more people from traditionally underrepresented groups such as women and ethnic minorities, and later children.[41,42]

Interestingly, this view also began to be supported by organized medicine. Beginning in 1995, the American Medical Association's Council on Ethical and Judicial Affairs began considering equitable access to research trials across different groups, including sociodemographic groups. The Council even explored whether researchers had an obligation to secure funding for participation for those too poor to pay for the various medical interventions required by a trial. Ultimately, the Council rendered a much less innovative opinion. It recognized that "ethical considerations in clinical research have traditionally focused on protecting research subjects" and urged that under the rubric of protectionism groups should not be "categorically excluded, or discouraged, from research protocols."[43] However, the Council fell short of demanding access for participants from these groups.

The underlying ethical principle emphasized in this period was the right to autonomy. According to this view, individuals did not need to be protected by regulation; rather, they should be entrusted to know their own good and their own best interests, and they should be free to pursue them. After all, as Mill said, the individual knows best what is in his or her best interest and is in the best position to pursue it. Autonomy was invoked as overriding the protections provided by the federal regulations. Activists demanded changes in the oversight system. They succeeded in getting a faster Food and Drug Administration (FDA) approval process for therapies aimed at life-threatening diseases as well as a change in the clinical outcomes used to determine effectiveness.

Importantly, this new paradigm directed at access to trials had limited applicability. It was most relevant to intervention trials, but not to other types of medical research such as physiology studies or studies recruiting healthy volunteers.

Again, this perspective did not arise in isolation from the wider society. It was during Ronald Reagan's presidency that individualism and the free market were championed and government regulation was strongly attacked as interfering with individual freedom. The arguments by the AIDS activists can be seen, at least in part, as an adaptation of this libertarian, individual autonomy view to the domain of research ethics. The words of activists could have come from libertarians: "If public and individual good are not clearly harmed, then government should not stand in the way. That is the American way."[39]

The pendulum swing to emphasizing the benefits of research and the preeminence of individual choice over societal restraints also occurred against the sociopolitical backdrop of a strong and visible gay rights movement, patients' rights movements, and patient and public skepticism about medical and scientific authority.

Period 4: Collaborative Partnership

Beginning in the mid-1990s, the limitations and potential drawbacks of the participant-access model began to become apparent in three areas: genetic research, research in developing countries, and increased patient demands for participation in planning research.

With dramatic growth in understanding of the human genome and how genes function, families and communities were increasingly being enrolled in research attempting to identify genes that cause disease. Such research implicated not just individuals but extended families and entire communities. Research involving Ashkenazi Jews, for example, especially research to identify genes related to mental disorders, and research that involved aboriginal populations prompted calls for extra protections for communities and for new involvement of communities in the planning, conduct, and dissemination of research.[44,45] Involvement of communities, it was argued, was the best way to protect them from stigma and other potential harms from genetics research. It was observed that the existing federal research regulations focused on individuals and did not mention communities. This seemed to leave communities vulnerable.

Another development that stimulated reevaluation of benefits and risks was the growth of research in developing countries sponsored by developed countries—which some critics viewed as scandalous. Research on perinatal HIV transmission conducted in developing countries and sponsored by the NIH and the Centers for Disease Control and Prevention (CDC) in the late 1990s was attacked for using placebo controls in the trials and for succumbing to what many saw as an ethical double standard.[46,47] Much debate and commentary ensued, especially about the possibility of exploitation of people in developing countries by researchers from rich, developed countries[48–55] (see Chapters 64–67). One frequently recommended response to the possibility of exploitation was to develop partnerships with the community in which the research was being conducted.[56]

At home, activist demands for easier access to clinical trials eventually led to demands for a greater role in research decision making. HIV and breast cancer activists fought for inclusion at the research table, and gradually but increasingly were consulted on the establishment of research priorities, review of protocols, lobbying for funding, and even recruiting clinical trial participants. Ultimately, several groups became less concerned with individual autonomy in deciding about enrollment in a particular study and more focused on community participation in the entire research process, from funding priorities to protocol development to dissemination of results.[39]

In 2005, the United States was in the midst of this trend toward collaborative partnership in the research enterprise. The idea was far from widely endorsed and solidified. Nevertheless

important attempts were being made to realize this paradigm. For instance, the FDA regulations guiding emergency research promulgated in 1996 require community consultation[57] (see Chapter 27). Although the purpose and process of community consultation was not well delineated in the regulations, the inclusion of this requirement was a clear recognition of the need for community partnership, even if the mechanism for achieving it remained somewhat undeveloped.

This paradigm may well apply only to a segment of research, such as epidemiology and intervention studies. Nevertheless, collaborative partnership constitutes a new paradigm of research and research oversight. This paradigm is based on the recognition that clinical research does not occur in isolation; clinical research is a collaborative, social enterprise. This is obviously true in that it involves a community of scientists. But, more important, at least for certain types of research, especially disease-specific studies, it also involves a community of participants, medical practitioners, as well as the larger society required to fund the research and also assimilate the results into the health delivery system. The community is a necessary partner for successful research.

In the past, this collaborative partnership was implicit, even hidden. In the current paradigm, it is more explicit, more formalized, and more extensive. Community involvement is an important part of the process of establishing research priorities through public advocacy as well as participation on advisory boards and funding organizations. The community is involved in oversight of research through growing participation on IRBs and on monitoring boards. Community participation may extend to negotiating benefits from the research, assistance with recruitment, and then integrating results into guidelines, reimbursement policies, and other aspects of the delivery system.

The community partnership paradigm rejects professional paternalism as a protection because the responsibilities and privileges of the researcher occur only within a wider social framework. It recognizes that risks and benefits both during and after research are best evaluated by involved communities. In addition, this paradigm lessens the emphasis on individual autonomy and the protections of individual informed consent. Importantly, it does not reject these protections, but places them into a wider context of protections that need to be satisfied prior to seeking the consent of individuals. In this way, community partnership is based more on a communitarian model and less on an individual rights model.

Future

Over the past 70 years or so, the paradigm governing ethical treatment of participants in clinical research has evolved though several stages: from a model based on the social value of research and trust in investigators to one of stringent protections against the dangers posed by researchers and research itself; then to a paradigm that rejected protectionism and demanded wide opportunity to participate in research; and finally to a model that recognizes the importance of the community in ensuring the relevance and integrity of research practices. At least in terms of the involvement of ordinary citizens in the clinical research enterprise, there has been great progress and expansion. The early period of research paternalism minimized the involvement of participants and the public; the currently operative collaborative partnership paradigm has integrated them as key participants in the entire research enterprise.

Each of these transitions has been catalyzed by scandals, crises, and/or changes in the nature of research practices. Although one paradigm was dominant at any particular historical moment, there has certainly been overlap. Strains of argument and reasoning from prior paradigms persist. The shift between paradigms is evolutionary rather than one of radical breaks, so there is continuity between prior and future paradigms, as well as change in emphases and in dominant values.

How the understanding of clinical research and ethical oversight may evolve in the future is unclear. Greater engagement of research participants throughout the process—from the development of research agendas and protocols to the conduct and dissemination of research and the altering of health policies in response to research results—is certain to shift the paradigm again. Currently, there is an enormous need for greater focus on how that participation can occur most efficiently and effectively in order to promote societal good through valuable research while respecting and attending to the rights and well-being of individuals and communities.

Acknowledgment

An earlier version of this chapter was published as a journal article in 2006. Emanuel E, Grady C. Four paradigms of clinical research and research oversight. *Cambridge Quarterly of Health Care Ethics* 2006; 16(1):82–96.

References

1. Lilienfeld AM. Ceteris paribus: The evolution of the clinical trial. *Bulletin of the History of Medicine* 1982;56:1–18.

2. Bull JP. The historical development of clinical therapeutic trials. *Journal of Chronic Diseases* 1959;10:218–48.

3. Rothman DJ. Ethical and social issues in the development of new drugs and vaccines. *Bulletin of the New York Academy of Medicine* 1987;63:557–68.

4. Halpern SA. *Lesser Harms: The Morality of Risk in Medical Research.* Chicago, Ill.: University of Chicago Press; 2004.

5. Howard-Jones N. *Human Experimentation and Medical Ethics.* Geneva, Switzerland: World Health Organization; 1982.

6. Bean WB. Walter Reed and the ordeal of human experiments. *Bulletin of the History of Medicine* 1977;51:75–92.

7. Lederer SE. *Subjected to Science: Human Experimentation in America Before the Second World War.* Baltimore, Md.: The Johns Hopkins University Press; 1994.

8. U.S. Food and Drug Administration. History of the FDA: The 1938 Food, Drug, and Cosmetic Act. [Online] Available: http://www.fda.gov/oc/history/historyoffda/section2.html.

9. Edgar H, Rothman DJ. New rules for new drugs: The challenge of AIDS to the regulatory process. *Milbank Quarterly* 1990;68(Suppl.1):111–42.

10. Kuhn TS. *The Structure of Scientific Revolutions,* 2nd ed. Chicago, Ill.: University of Chicago Press; 1970.

11. Altman LK. *Who Goes First? The Story of Self-Experimentation in Medicine.* Berkeley, Calif.: University of California Press; 1998 [1987].

12. Rothman DJ. Ethics and human experimentation—Henry Beecher revisited. *New England Journal of Medicine* 1987;317:1195–9.

13. Arno P, Feiden K. *Against the Odds: The Story of AIDS Drug Development, Politics, and Profits.* New York, N.Y.: Harper-Collins Publishers; 1992.

14. Jonas H. Philosophical reflections on experimenting with human subjects. *Daedalus* 1969;98:219–47.

15. McDermott W. The changing mores of biomedical research. II. Challenge and discussion: Opening comments. *Annals of Internal Medicine* 1967;67(Suppl.7):39–42.

16. Lasagna L. Some ethical problems in clinical research. In: Mendelsohn E, Swazey JP, Taviss I, eds. *Human Aspects of Biomedical Innovation.* Cambridge, Mass.: Harvard University Press; 1971:98–110.

17. Beecher HK. Ethics and clinical research. *New England Journal of Medicine* 1966;274:1354–60.

18. *Natanson v. Kline,* 350 P.2d 1093 (Kan. 1960).

19. Oken D. What to tell cancer patients: A study of medical attitudes. *JAMA* 1961;175:1120–8.

20. Katz J. *The Silent World of Doctor and Patient.* New York, N.Y.: The Free Press; 1984.

21. Jones JH. *Bad Blood: The Tuskegee Syphilis Experiment,* 2nd ed. New York, N.Y.: The Free Press, 1993 [1981].

22. Brandt A. Racism and research: The case of the Tuskegee Syphilis Study. *Hastings Center Report* 1978;8(6):21–9.

23. Beecher HK. Experimentation in man. *JAMA* 1959;169:461–78.

24. U.S. Congress. National Research Act of 1974. Pub. L. No. 93–348, 93rd Congress, 2nd Session, July 12, 1974.

25. Advisory Committee on Human Radiation Experiments. *Final Report of the Advisory Committee on Human Radiation Experiments.* New York, N.Y.: Oxford University Press; 1996.

26. Office of the Secretary, Department of Health and Human Services. 45 CFR Part 46: Final Regulations Amending Basic HHS Policy for the Protection of Human Research Subjects; Final Rule. *Federal Register* 1981;465(16):8366–91.

27. Department of Health and Human Services, National Institutes of Health, and Office for Human Research Protections. The Common Rule, Title 45 (Public Welfare), Code of Federal Regulations, Part 46 (Protection of Human Subjects). [Online] June 23, 2005. Available: http://www.hhs.gov/ohrp/humansubjects/guidance/45cfr46.htm.

28. The National Commission for the Protection of Human Subjects of Biomedical and Behavioral Research. *Research on the Fetus: Report and Recommendations.* DHEW publication No. (OS) 76–127. Washington, D.C.: DHEW; 1975. [Online] Available: http://www.bioethics.gov/reports/past_commissions/research_fetus.pdf.

29. The National Commission for the Protection of Human Subjects of Biomedical and Behavioral Research. *Research Involving Prisoners: Report and Recommendations.* DHEW Publication No. (OS) 76–131. Washington, D.C.: DHEW; 1976. [Online] Available: http://www.bioethics.gov/reports/past_commissions/Research_involving_prisoners.pdf.

30. The National Commission for the Protection of Human Subjects of Biomedical and Behavioral Research. *Research Involving Children: Report and Recommendations.* Washington D.C.: U.S. Government Printing Office; 1977. [Online] Available: http://www.bioethics.gov/reports/past_commissions/Research_involving_children.pdf.

31. The National Commission for the Protection of Human Subjects of Biomedical and Behavioral Research. *Institutional Review Boards: Report and Recommendations.* Washington, D.C.: U.S. Government Printing Office; 1978.

32. Fletcher J. The evolution of the ethics of informed consent. In: Berg K, Tranoy K, eds. *Research Ethics.* New York, N.Y.: Alan Liss, Inc.; 1983:187–228.

33. Beauchamp TL, Childress JF. *Principles of Biomedical Ethics.* New York, N.Y.: Oxford University Press; 1979.

34. The National Commission for the Protection of Human Subjects of Biomedical and Behavioral Research. *The Belmont Report: Ethical Principles and Guidelines for the Protection of Human Subjects of Research.*

Washington, D.C.: Department of Health, Education and Welfare; 1979. DHEW Publication OS 78–0012 1978. [Online] Available: http://www.hhs.gov/ohrp/humansubjects/guidance/belmont .htm.

35. Berg JW, Appelbaum PS, Lidz CW, Parker LS. *Informed Consent: Legal Theory and Clinical Practice,* 2nd ed. New York, N.Y.: Oxford University Press; 2001.

36. Veatch R. *A Theory of Medical Ethics.* New York, N.Y.: Basic Books; 1981.

37. *Canterbury v. Spence,* 464 F.2d 772 (D.C. Cir. 1972).

38. Lipsett M. On the nature and ethics of phase 1 oncology trials of cancer chemotherapy. *JAMA* 1982;248:941–2.

39. Delaney M. The case for patient access to experimental therapy. *Journal of Infectious Diseases* 1989;159:416–9.

40. National Research Council. *The Social Impact of AIDS in the United States.* Washington, D.C.: National Academy Press; 1993.

41. National Institutes of Health. Guidelines for the inclusion of women and ethnic minorities in research. *NIH Guide to Grants and Contracts* March 18, 1994; 23(11).

42. National Institutes of Health. NIH Policy and guidelines on the inclusion of children as participants in research involving human subjects. *NIH Guide to Grants and Contracts* March 6, 1998; 1998. [Online] Available: http://grants.nih.gov/grants/guide/notice-files/not98–024.html.

43. Council on Ethical and Judicial Affairs, American Medical Association. Subject selection for clinical trials. *IRB: A Review of Human Subjects Research* 1998;20(2–3):12–5.

44. Weijer C, Goldsand G, Emanuel EJ. Protecting communities in research: Current guidelines and limits of extrapolation. *Nature Genetics* 1999;23:275–80.

45. Weijer C, Emanuel EJ. Protecting communities in biomedical research. *Science* 2000;289:1142–4.

46. Lurie P, Wolfe SM. Unethical trials of interventions to reduce perinatal transmission of the human immunodeficiency virus in developing countries. *New England Journal of Medicine* 1997;337: 853–6.

47. Angell M. The ethics of clinical research in the third world. *New England Journal of Medicine* 1997;337:847–9.

48. Levine RJ. The "best proven therapeutic method" standard in clinical trials in technologically developing countries. *IRB: A Review of Human Subjects Research* 1998;20(1):5–9.

49. Crouch RA, Arras JD. AZT trials and tribulations. *Hastings Center Report* 1998;28(6):26–34.

50. Grady C. Science in the service of healing. *Hastings Center Report* 1998;28(6):34–8.

51. Cleaton-Jones PE. An ethical dilemma: Availability of anti-retroviral therapy after clinical trials with HIV infected patients are ended. *British Medical Journal* 1997;314:887–8.

52. Wilmshurst P. Scientific imperialism: If they won't benefit from the findings, poor people in the developing world shouldn't be used in research. *British Medical Journal* 1997;314:840–1.

53. Glantz LH, Annas GJ, Grodin MA, Mariner WK. Research in developing countries: Taking "benefit" seriously. *Hastings Center Report* 1998;28(6):38–42.

54. Annas GJ, Grodin MA. Human rights and maternal-fetal HIV transmission prevention trials in Africa. *American Journal of Public Health* 1998;88:560–2.

55. Shapiro H, Meslin E. Ethical issues in the design and conduct of clinical trials in developing countries. *New England Journal of Medicine* 2001;345:139–42.

56. Emanuel E, Wendler D, Killen J, Grady C. What makes clinical research in developing countries ethical? The benchmarks of ethical research. *Journal of Infectious Diseases* 2004;189:930–7.

57. U.S. Food and Drug Administration. Guidance for Institutional Review Boards, Clinical Investigators, and Sponsors: Exception from Informed Consent Requirements for Emergency Research; Draft Guidance. [Online] March 30, 2000. Available: http://www .fda.gov/ora/compliance_ref/bimo/err_guide.htm.

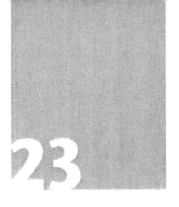

Rebecca Dresser

The Role of Patient Advocates and Public Representatives in Research

During the 1980s and 1990s, patient advocates became vocal participants in debates over biomedical research. Patient advocates helped persuade government officials to change rules governing access to clinical trials and unapproved medications. They joined scientific teams designing, conducting, and reviewing research. They lobbied for more government funds for research that could help their constituents, as well.

These developments occurred around the world. For example, the United Kingdom's National Health Service enlisted patient advocates to evaluate research priorities and help in planning health studies.[1] Developed nations sponsoring studies in developing countries worked with community representatives to plan and carry out the research.[2]

Advocates' insistence on participating in research decision making has changed the politics of biomedical research. Not everyone embraces the changes, however. Scientists worry that advocates focus too much on cures and treatments, without recognizing the importance of basic research. Researchers also fear that good science is threatened by the desire of seriously ill people to "try anything" after conventional therapies have failed. Public officials are unsettled by the apparent competition among patient advocacy organizations seeking government research dollars.

The contemporary patient advocacy movement offers many potential benefits. Advocacy could contribute to a biomedical research enterprise more in tune with the needs of the people the enterprise is designed to assist. It could prevent researchers' personal and professional aims from exerting too much control over research priorities. It could make the potential harms and benefits of research participation less mysterious to people enrolling in studies. It offers fresh opportunities for communication and exchange

between scientists and the society they serve, which could give researchers valuable insights into the human side of the problems they study, and at the same time give members of the public a more realistic picture of how research works and what it can achieve.

Yet these positive outcomes cannot be guaranteed. Genuine communication between scientists and the public is all too rare. Bridging the gap between the two worlds requires mutual willingness to learn and to value the other's knowledge. Shared decision making also costs money. Some will challenge the use of scarce resources to increase public involvement, and others will try to add public involvement cheaply, primarily for public relations purposes.

Advocates and other public participants confront these challenges from a variety of perspectives. Many advocates act as paid or unpaid representatives of specific disease interest groups. Other advocates fill a different role, that of general lay or public representative—sometimes without affiliation with a specific health organization. A third category of advocates comprises those representing communities and ethnic groups with particular interests in health research.

In the United States, the general public and patient advocates entered the biomedical research arena by two different routes. Public participation began with the emergence of the U.S. research oversight system. During the 1960s, as people became aware that research participants had been exposed to serious risks without their awareness or consent, scientists and government officials faced growing demands for safeguards to prevent similar violations in the future. Once officials and their advisers went to work on an oversight system to protect research participants, public representation surfaced as a key component of ethics review.

Designers of the oversight system thought that scientists and physicians too easily lost sight of their duty to put participants' interests above other research aims. They believed that "outsiders" could add an essential moral perspective to judgments about the ethics of proposed studies. Through this process, public oversight became an integral and enduring feature of U.S. research policy. By the early 1980s, federal government policy required ethics review committees to include individuals lacking employment or other personal ties to the institution in which the research would be conducted.

In the ethics review context, it was primarily government officials, professionals, and scholars who argued for a public role in research decision making. The strongest demand for public involvement came not from grass roots activists, but from "experts" designing the oversight system. By contrast, patient advocates became involved in research on their own initiative. Responding to personal and family health threats, advocates undertook a variety of activities in the research arena.

Patient advocates got their start battling restrictive regulations controlling access to promising experimental interventions. Beginning in the 1980s, activists sought to expand patients' opportunities to benefit from biomedical research. Advocates thought research policies focused too much on avoiding risks to research participants and the public, and too little on promoting research benefits. The rules seemed to impede unnecessarily the development of new treatments to aid people in desperate need.

The U.S. pioneers in this form of advocacy were HIV/AIDS and breast cancer activists. By the 1990s, practically every disease or injury had its advocacy organization; many celebrities and public officials had also become involved in activities to raise awareness about research needs in specific areas.

Contemporary research advocates engage in many different activities. Much of their work focuses on three areas. First, advocates representing many disease constituencies help to plan, conduct, and evaluate research. Second, advocates promote policies allowing more people to participate in disease-related research. Third, advocates engage in extensive fund-raising, in both public and private sectors. This includes lobbying the government for more funds and participating in priority setting at health research agencies.

The remainder of this chapter examines these activities in detail. The first three sections focus on patient advocacy activities, and the fourth section examines public participation in research ethics oversight. The chapter concludes with ideas for enhancing the contributions that advocates and other public representatives make to research practices and policies.

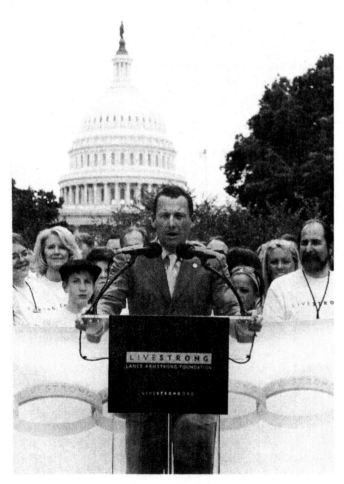

Figure 23.1. Lance Armstrong, champion cyclist and founder of the Lance Armstrong Foundation, a nonprofit education and advocacy group, addresses an audience with the U.S. Capitol Building in the background. Source: © Lance Armstrong Foundation, 2006. Reproduced with permission.

Advocates on the Research Team

Many advocates seek to exert influence over the way biomedical research is conducted. This goal is shared by patient and community activists worldwide. Advocates representing numerous constituencies want to help researchers decide what problems to study, how to study them, and how to apply study results.

U.S. and International Origins

During the 1980s, as gay men in the United States sought to cope with the growing HIV/AIDS epidemic, they looked to medicine for assistance. Activists initially campaigned for more funding and a heightened national commitment to study the condition. Once an intensified research program was under way, however, advocates discovered that they had many disagreements with traditional research methods.

The focus of activist discontent was the randomized clinical trial (RCT). The RCT is commonly regarded as the gold standard for determining whether an experimental drug or other intervention is good enough to enter the realm of accepted therapy. Participants in an RCT are randomly assigned to different groups. Often one group in an RCT is assigned to receive a placebo, an agent believed to have no direct effect on the condition being studied. Adding a placebo group allows scientists to separate the improvements produced by the experimental and other active agents under study from any improvements caused by the placebo effect.[3]

To the HIV/AIDS activists, many of the RCT conventions seemed shockingly inhumane. In their eyes, it was unethical to give people with a life-threatening disease an inactive agent instead of a promising new experimental drug. They criticized other aspects of the RCT, as well. For example, people with HIV/AIDS were often told that during trial participation, they would have to refrain from taking other medications, including drugs designed to relieve symptoms unrelated to the study. Some people also were excluded from trials because their past medication use might improperly influence study findings. Activists eventually persuaded researchers that some restrictive RCT demands could be relaxed without reducing the scientific value of the findings.[4]

Quick to learn from their counterparts in the HIV/AIDS community, breast cancer activists began in the early 1990s to demand a greater role in the research process. At first, their influence was most visible in the U.S. Department of Defense (DoD) Program for Breast Cancer Research.[5] In 1993, advocates persuaded the U.S. Congress to set aside $210 million of the DoD budget for breast cancer research. Because DoD was not a traditional biomedical research sponsor, the agency lacked established conventions for determining which studies it would fund. Activists saw this as an opportunity for a fresh approach to research decision making.[6] The system that emerged gave advocates a role in determining the overall goals of the DoD program, as well as in selecting the proposals that received funding.

Breast cancer activists also created a training program to give advocates the scientific knowledge that would enable them to gain the respect of biomedical researchers.[7] And at the international level, the U.S.-based National Breast Cancer Coalition organized conferences to promote and strengthen advocacy efforts worldwide.[8]

Separately, the participatory research movement—which supports community involvement in planning and conducting health research—has been applied to health research in many Asian, African, and Latin American nations. Participatory research holds that members of the study population possess knowledge that is as essential to a project's success as is the scientific and

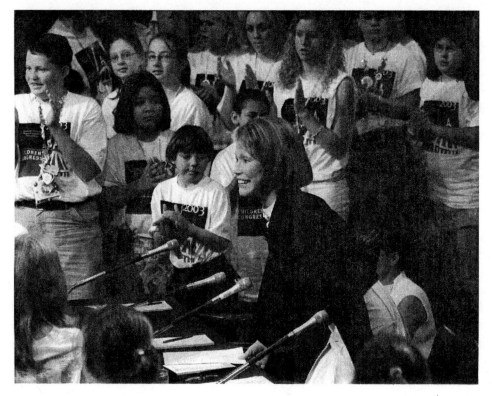

Figure 23.2. Mary Tyler Moore, International Chairman of the Juvenile Diabetes Research Foundation, testifies at a 2003 Senate hearing on behalf of increased NIH funding for diabetes research. Moore and the children pictured all have Type 1 diabetes. Photo credit: Camera One, NYC. © Juvenile Diabetes Research Foundation. Reproduced with permission.

medical knowledge researchers contribute. Fully realized, participatory research contemplates "researchers and local people work[ing] together as colleagues with different skills to offer, in a process of mutual learning where local people have control over the process."[9]

Participatory researchers and the early HIV/AIDS and breast cancer activists shared similar aims. By the mid-1990s, these aims had been accepted in mainstream research settings, as well. For example, a 1995 *British Medical Journal* editorial declared that "patients should help to decide which research is conducted, help to plan the research and interpret the data, and hear the results before anyone else."[10]

Strengths and Weaknesses of Advocate Involvement

Enlisting representatives of the study population as members of the research team highlights the moral and social dimensions of the biomedical research enterprise. The approach recognizes that this form of research is conducted not simply to answer abstract questions, but to provide health benefits to society. Once one accepts this concept of biomedical research, it is not difficult to envision the contributions affected people can make to improved research quality.

First, members of the community can provide information about which health problems, and which aspects of particular health problems, are most important for scientists to study. As one health researcher put it, "[g]reater lay involvement in setting the research agenda would almost certainly lead to greater open mindedness about which questions are worth addressing. . . ."[11]

Second, representatives of affected groups can provide guidance on study design. For instance, a British researcher reported that when women were told of a proposed study of aspirin to reduce hypertension in pregnant women, they "asked why there were no plans to follow up the babies of women participating in the trial—[given that] for decades women had been warned not to take aspirin during pregnancy because it might harm their babies."[11]

Third, community representatives can help decide whether research results should change clinical practice. For example, after a study showed that large doses of antimalarial drugs during pregnancy could increase infants' birth weights, New Guinea women "living in mud floored huts" pointed out that in their circumstances, bigger babies could make childbirth more risky for both mothers and children.[11]

Fourth, community representatives can contribute to decisions on research merit. Lay representatives can be as qualified as researchers to evaluate the social value of research. They can also remind scientists and other review panelists "that we don't want simply jewel-like studies that will stay on library shelves but studies that will actually make a difference."[12]

Fifth, community representation can promote ethical research. Consulting with members of the study population "ensures both that their interests are central to the project or study, and that they will not be treated simply as objects."[12] Community members are in a position to know what prospective participants should understand before deciding whether to enroll in a study.[10] As HIV/AIDS activists demonstrated, advocates can also supply a participant-centered perspective on the potential benefits and harms accompanying study participation. Patient and community

advocates can foster justice in the choice of research participants, as well, by evaluating whether research will impose disproportionate burdens on a community or a community's access to research benefits will be unfairly limited. And involving representatives can protect the community from further contact with researchers who "'parachuted' in, took samples, and disappeared with nothing of value resulting in the community."[13]

Community involvement can be useful at the practical level, too. For example, researchers in Uganda reported that community representatives addressed potential difficulties involving local politics that would have presented "a quagmire for the unwitting outsider."[14] Recruitment approaches attuned to local concerns can increase study enrollment. Although the process of involving representatives will add to a project's expense, "in the long run the net result will be an improvement in efficiency as a consequence of increased community support, more rapid recruitment, and enhanced cooperation on the part of subjects."[15]

In sum, more community involvement could improve research in a variety of ways. But the endeavor is far from risk-free. Though many scientists and clinicians are enthusiastic about community participation, others remain unpersuaded.

Among scientists, there is continuing controversy over whether laypersons should participate in merit review of research proposals. Some researchers contend that community representatives on peer review panels are unqualified to judge the caliber of competing proposals. The controversy over merit review reflects divergent perceptions of research merit. Those who perceive a threat to scientific quality see merit in its more narrow technical sense, whereas their opponents see merit as a broader concept that includes social value.

Another threat arises when affected communities seek control over research data and publication of results. Disadvantaged communities most frequently seek this authority, citing past exploitation in research or other social contexts. For the community representatives and researchers supporting them, local control is a reasonable response to prior injustices and to an unfair convention giving researchers nearly absolute control over data and results.[13]

On the other side are scholars and researchers worried about threats to academic freedom and research integrity. An agreement giving a community substantial control over the written products of research "opens up the possibility of serious restrictions on [the researcher's] academic freedom, and encroachment on the academic authority of his . . . university."[16] Censorship of results could also impede development of health benefits for the public.

Community involvement creates new issues for advocates, as well. When representatives of the affected community work with investigators to plan, conduct, implement, and evaluate research, they become part of the research enterprise. In the process, they may experience difficulties in maintaining their independence and legitimacy as community representatives. Moreover, some researchers may seek community input primarily for its symbolic or public relations value. In this situation, researchers may pretend to consider community views, but proceed to do what they would have done anyway. If the community opposes what researchers do, or a study has a negative community impact, representatives will be seen as complicit in the objectionable activity.[14]

Other challenges are related to community representation. Personal experience cannot in itself confer knowledge of "what it is like" for others in similar situations. Thus, the diversity of individuals within a community adds complexity to the task of representation. At minimum, direct and ongoing communication with a reasonable number of other community members is essential to legitimate representation.

To succeed in this endeavor, researchers and patient advocates will need additional education, as well as reflection on the best ways to address the new challenges they face. The conclusion of this chapter offers ideas for responses to some of these challenges.

Expanded Access Activities

Patient advocates in the United States are enthusiastic proponents of government policies promoting expanded access to experimental interventions. Advocates contend that investigational agents and procedures offer people fighting serious illness renewed hope when standard therapies have failed. They also contend that involving more people in research is essential to delivering better therapies to the patients of tomorrow.

Contributions to Policy Revisions

During the 1980s, advocates for people with HIV/AIDS mounted a vigorous attack on the rules governing access to unproven interventions. Faced with a lethal epidemic and no effective treatments, activists were intensely committed to the search for new drugs to reduce death and suffering. As they embarked on this mission, they collided with a drug development system that was slow, inflexible, and highly risk-averse.

Displaying banners proclaiming "Red Tape Is Killing Us,"[17] HIV/AIDS activists protested the U.S. Food and Drug Administration (FDA) rules on drug testing. They joined drug manufacturers and conservative policy groups in lobbying for policy changes.[4] By becoming part of this unusual coalition, activists helped set in motion revisions that made experimental agents more available to seriously ill people.[18]

Although the driving force for FDA action was the HIV/AIDS emergency, the new policy measures had a much broader impact. They produced, for example, wider and quicker access to investigational agents targeted at cancer, Alzheimer's disease, Parkinson's disease, multiple sclerosis,[18] and heart disease.[19] Because of these revisions, seriously ill individuals unable to benefit from available treatments now enjoy increased liberty to seek help from promising but unproven interventions.

Activists were also key figures in producing a second set of policy changes affecting clinical research. In this development, women's health organizations joined community health advocates in supporting policies aimed at increasing the participation of women and underrepresented ethnic groups in clinical trials.

This move led to two major policy changes. In 1993, the FDA abandoned its rule against including "women of childbearing potential" as participants in early phases of drug testing. Officials said studying a new agent's effects in both genders was needed so that any gender-related differences could be identified early and adequately studied in later phases of clinical trials.[20]

The same year, the U.S. Congress directed officials at the National Institutes of Health (NIH) to ensure that women and members of minority groups were included in government-funded studies. Officials then established guidelines to promote gender and ethnic diversity in study populations. The guidelines instructed researchers to collect data that would allow valid analyses of possible gender and ethnic differences in response to experimental interventions.[21]

With the encouragement of patient advocates, Congress and agency officials then turned to two remaining barriers to research participation. To make patients more aware of their opportunities to enroll in clinical trials, Congress directed health officials to establish a public database with information about government and privately sponsored trials of "experimental treatments for serious and life-threatening diseases and conditions."[22]

Financial barriers to research participation were the second target of government action. Research grants ordinarily do not include money to cover hospitalization and other costs of routine patient care for people enrolled in studies. Some insurers were unwilling to pay for such care on grounds that trial participants received interventions not established as safe and effective.[23] At the behest of advocacy groups and researchers, officials sought to expand reimbursement for heath-care services to trial participants.[24] Some states enacted laws requiring coverage[25] and in 2000, President Clinton directed the Medicare program to cover routine patient care costs for beneficiaries enrolled in clinical trials.[24]

Activists were enthusiastic partners in the campaign to expand patients' access to clinical trials and investigational interventions. These programs were consistent with the advocacy view that clinical trials "are the best means of finding the cause, cure, and prevention" of serious diseases.[26] The consequences of expanded access might not be all good, however.

Ethics of Expanded Access

In campaigning for expanded access, advocates could cite three established research ethics principles to support their position.[27] The first was respect for individual autonomy in choices about experimental interventions. Advocates argued that restrictive drug testing policies improperly interfered with constituents' freedom to accept possible harm from exposure to unapproved agents in exchange for a chance to improve or extend their lives.

Advocates for women and ethnic minorities also stressed the value of free choice. Exclusionary policies and practices denied women the freedom to decide for themselves whether to enter trials that could improve health care for others and, possibly, their own care. Advocates supporting the two remaining government efforts to expand access invoked patients' freedom of choice, too. The government-sponsored clinical trials database would give patients coping with illness a wider array of alternatives. Insurance coverage for trial participants would remove financial constraints on patient choice.

Activists calling for expanded access appealed to the ethical principle of beneficence, as well. Activists representing people with HIV/AIDS and other serious conditions stressed the benefits patients could gain through participating in clinical trials or using investigational agents outside a trial. Trying experimental interventions offered people with terminal illness a chance of benefit and presented insignificant risk, in light of their dire situations.

Advocates for underrepresented groups also invoked the beneficence principle in arguing that the failure to collect adequate data deprived women and ethnic minorities of medical benefits. Advocacy support for government efforts to publicize research enrollment opportunities and secure insurance coverage for clinical trials rested on the beneficence principle, too. If more of today's patients enrolled in research, future patients would gain more health benefits.

Justice was the third ethical concept advocates cited to support expanded access. Restrictive approaches were a reaction to past cases in which scientists imposed unconscionable burdens on historically disadvantaged groups. But protecting disadvantaged groups from an unfair share of research burdens kept them out of clinical trials that could improve or extend their lives. Members of disadvantaged groups also received possibly inappropriate medical advice and treatment based on narrowly focused research.[28]

Although expanded access can advance a number of ethical objectives, access alone cannot produce a more ethical research policy. To achieve this broader goal, additional ethical considerations must be taken into account. Moreover, the costs of expanded access must be acknowledged and reduced as much as possible.

A person can make an autonomous decision to enroll in a study or try an unproven agent only when the decision is adequately informed. The need for adequate understanding underlies the informed consent requirement. Yet empirical evidence suggests that many research participants fail to comprehend important information about the studies they join.[29] True freedom is not advanced when people choose investigational agents or procedures because they have inflated hopes of therapeutic benefit. If informed decision making fails to accompany expanded access, individual autonomy will be diminished, rather than enhanced.

Another major ethical justification for expanded access is its potential to increase the benefits available through biomedical research. There is no question that expanded access can produce benefits for participants, such as extended life, reduced discomfort, satisfaction from actively fighting one's disease, and solace in contributing to better care for others. At the same time, one should not underestimate the risks presented by investigational agents and procedures. Such interventions can produce physical, psychological, and financial burdens.

Although justice is also cited as an ethical basis for expanded access, financial and social inequalities limit this impact. Expanded access to research and unproven interventions must not be confused with expanded access to health care. Increased opportunities to enroll in clinical trials can do little to meet the needs of those unable to afford adequate health-care coverage. Any personal health benefits people gain through study participation often end with the study. Similarly, the campaign to secure insurance reimbursement for trial participants' patient care costs overlooks people with no insurance at all.

At the same time, expanded access policies require researchers to recruit more members of disadvantaged groups for study participation. Recruitment programs aimed at such groups frequently offer reimbursement for travel, child care, meal, and other expenses associated with study participation.[30] However, such incentives can induce people to join studies they would refuse if they were financially better off. The outcome could be that members of disadvantaged groups end up bearing an undue share of research burdens and lacking a fair share of the health benefits produced through such research.[31]

Thus, expanded access can have both good and bad consequences. At its best, expanded access can increase individual freedom, enhance research benefits, and produce a more just allocation of research benefits and harms. At its worst, expanded access can foster uninformed decisions to try unproven interventions and lead low-income people to join studies in hopes of obtaining a fraction of the health services they need.

Advocates can play an important role in determining how expanded access turns out. Prospective research participants are not well served when advocates downplay the risks of trying unproven interventions or imply that access to research is equivalent to access to proven treatment. When advocates represent constituents in the policy arena, they assume a responsibility to assess access realistically. The final part of this chapter describes ways of meeting this responsibility.

Research Funding Activities

During the 1990s, U.S. officials faced heightened pressure from patient advocates seeking government dollars for health research. Advocates said the intensified congressional lobbying stemmed in part from their dissatisfaction with NIH funding decisions. They claimed that though NIH officials gave lip service to the importance of public participation in research priority setting, scientists actually controlled the agency's funding agenda. Advocates also charged that the agency played favorites, granting certain disease-specific interest groups overly generous amounts for studies on their constituents' health problems.

In response to these developments, NIH officials created more opportunities for advocates to help set funding priorities. But officials and patient advocates confront difficult ethical and policy issues as they seek to achieve the goal of increased public participation.

Advocacy's Potential Contributions

It is not surprising that people affected by disease and injury seek increased government funding for research on their particular conditions. In this sense, advocacy for research funding is simply an instance of the interest group politics shaping U.S. policy in all areas. Supporters say that patient advocates could help produce: (1) a research budget more consistent with public preferences and interests; (2) better-informed government officials and scientists; and (3) valuable health benefits.

Those favoring the changes say that scientific dominance has led to allocation choices that deviate from public preferences and the overall public good. They also suspect that scientists have been overly responsive to certain interest groups, and they contend that creating a more open and inclusive system could yield allocation decisions more consistent with the needs and values of the people whose tax dollars pay for federal research.[32]

Besides producing a more democratic research budget, patient advocates supply valuable information to government officials. A graphic account of living with a serious illness or caring for an injured family member conveys personal knowledge missing from the facts and figures officials ordinarily rely on to make allocation decisions. Moreover, although channeling money to particular areas cannot in itself ensure scientific progress, financial resources are a necessary foundation for such progress. Funds enable scientists to conduct exploratory research, obtain training in previously neglected areas, share ideas, and formulate new avenues for investigation.

Advocacy also raises public awareness of a condition. Increased awareness can lead to higher rates of state and local funding, as well as charitable giving by the general public, wealthy individuals, private foundations, and industry.

Advocacy's Risks

A major concern is that advocacy for research funds could encourage unfair and inequitable allocations of limited public dollars. The problems arise because groups with the most effective presentations and best access to officials can gain disproportionate advantage over others. For example, one explanation offered for the lack of research on improving end-of-life care is that "dying patients do not form an energetic, ongoing constituency to advocate for more research," nor do "their survivors [who] tend to be exhausted and grieving."[33]

Partisan research lobbying could also lead to inefficient resource allocation. This would occur if powerful interest groups persuaded officials to award funds for research on particular conditions without proper regard for the quality of proposed studies.[34] Poor-quality studies are unlikely to make any contribution to improved health care.

Research advocacy also consumes resources. When organizations spend substantial amounts to lobby for research funding, rather than for improvements in health-care delivery, housing, and other social needs, they arguably compromise their constituents' interests. When organizations focus on increasing funds for research on one condition, they ignore the fact that many of their constituents could be vulnerable to harm from other diseases or injuries.

New Roles for Advocates

With advocates' increased abilities to influence priority setting come changed roles and responsibilities. In many situations, decision makers may expect advocates to represent interests beyond those of their customary constituents. Advocates thus could be asked to express perspectives and values on behalf of the general public, or of a large subset of the population, such as elderly persons, medically underserved communities, or those at risk for genetic diseases. Accompanying this new role are new obligations, obligations that for the most part remain to be defined.

Advocates should recognize that a single-disease focus could be detrimental to their constituents' interests. Many constituents have multiple health needs over the course of their lives; thus, federally funded studies on different health problems could benefit them. Nearly all constituents have loved ones whose health care could be improved by research in a variety of areas. Constituents could also benefit from government support for social programs, such as health care and housing assistance. Advocates exploring these issues with constituents may find that narrowly targeted lobbying for research funding is inconsistent with constituents' actual preferences.

A single-interest approach to research advocacy raises more general moral concerns, as well. When advocates lobby to obtain the maximum possible research support for their specific constituents, they overlook the compelling needs of persons with other health problems.

By putting the spotlight on priority setting, advocates have created an opportunity to develop a more thoughtful approach to allocating biomedical research funds. According to a government report on priority setting, there is "no right amount of money, percentage of the budget, or percentage of projects for any disease."[34] But this claim is only partly correct. The "right" amount or percentage is a function of choices regarding which conditions merit more research attention than others, together with scientific and practical judgments on where it is realistic to expect progress. Increased public participation could produce a clearer picture of the relevant values and their relative importance.

There is reason for hope that advocates can contribute to fairness in research funding allocation. Although advocates have different ideas on how funds would be best allocated, most share a common desire to reduce the suffering and death inflicted by illness and injury. Though their constituents' interests affect their preferences on funding, most participants begin with altruistic intentions, too. In the concluding section, I offer principles to guide advocates in funding allocation activities.

Research Oversight Activities

The practice of appointing members of the public to committees reviewing studies involving human participants has long-standing public support. In the United States and worldwide, many policies require committees to include one or more public members. For example, guidelines issued by the Council for International Organizations of Medical Sciences and the World Health Organization advise that committees should include "lay persons qualified to represent the cultural and moral values of the community and to ensure that the rights of the research subjects will be respected."

Government officials, commentators, and review committee members point to five general justifications for including public members. First, public members add a common sense, "ordinary person" worldview that is often missing when professionals discuss research proposals.[36] The presence of public members can "transform the committees from closed associations of like-minded professionals who 'understand' one another into a more open forum of community responsibility."

Second, the public member's presence increases the chance that decisions will be consistent with local community attitudes and values. Situating ethics review in the setting in which research is conducted means that ethical judgments will be sensitive to actual conditions in the community.[38] Members of the general public are likely to be aware of particular religious, cultural, or economic factors that could affect local reactions to specific research projects.[39]

Third, the public members help to apply specific ethical and regulatory standards. Public members delineate the real-world meanings of basic ethical concepts. For instance, public members are highly qualified to evaluate whether a proposed consent form and process will give individuals the information they need to decide about study participation.[40]

Fourth, public members make research more transparent to the broader community. If ordinary people know that studies will be scrutinized by someone like them, they will be less worried about the possibility of hidden research improprieties. When they press investigators and researchers on the committee to describe study goals, procedures, and risks in plain language, public members remind scientists of their responsibilities to communicate with ordinary people.

The public member's fifth contribution is representation. Many assume that unaffiliated institutional review board (IRB) members have a special responsibility to represent research participants. Thus, they are instructed "to see through the eyes of the patient and imagine what he or she is being asked to go through."[41] At the same time, public members receive conflicting messages about their representation responsibilities. Public members are portrayed as representing the general public, poor people and other vulnerable groups, and most expansively, "patient-subjects, future patients, and the research profession all at once."[42] Public members' activities on the IRB could vary substantially depending on which group they decide to represent.[43]

Advocates in Ethics Oversight

Critics claim that the public member does little to disrupt "business as usual" in the research enterprise. For example, a 1998 government report declared that few research ethics review committees "seem to seek or be able, on a constant basis, to recruit and maintain lay and/or nonaffiliated members who play an active, effective role in helping the [committees] stay focused on their mission of protecting subjects."[44] Critics cite three problems with the current situation. First, public participants lack the technical knowledge and independent perspective that would enable them to participate fully in research ethics deliberations. Second, they operate in a system that minimizes their power and impact. Third, they lack a definite constituency to guide their contributions to research ethics deliberations.

Reformers dissatisfied with the current situation propose a number of remedies, such as increasing the proportion of public members on oversight committees[45] and improving training opportunities for public members.[46] Another potential remedy is to enlist more patient advocates to participate in ethics review.

To date, patient advocacy groups have devoted relatively little attention to research ethics oversight. Most of their energy has gone into promoting research through activities such as fundraising and lobbying for increased access to clinical trials. Although there are a few notable exceptions,[47] advocates have generally stayed away from research ethics review committees and debates over whether the rights and interests of research participants are adequately protected.

Yet there are good reasons for advocates to join research ethics oversight. Advocates familiar with clinical research issues would be much better equipped than most public members to evaluate investigators' proposed disclosure procedures, data collection methods, and other matters affecting study participants. Advocates could also bring personal knowledge to research oversight. Because of their close connections to patients, they are more likely than other committee members to appreciate the psychological, familial, and economic conditions affecting research participants. This is a perspective that can rarely be supplied by the attorneys, ethicists, chaplains, and other nonscientists serving on ethics review panels.

Advocates could bring passion, commitment, and energy to ethics deliberations, too. Many advocates are accustomed to negotiating with clinicians and researchers. This experience makes advocates less likely than other laypersons to be intimidated by professionals participating in ethics review. Advocates skilled in communicating with both expert and lay audiences would also be highly qualified to express participants' concerns in ethics oversight activities.

At the same time, advocates themselves could benefit from such participation. Participating in protocol review would give advocates a deeper understanding of the research process and could be an effective antidote to unrealistic expectations about what research can deliver. The experience could sensitize advocates to the problems of patients outside their ordinary constituencies, which could have a beneficial impact in other advocacy work.

Not all patient advocates would be suited to oversight work. Yet their performance in other areas suggests that many could do an excellent job. Enlisting more advocates for ethics oversight would also be relatively easy to do. This proposal thus has the advantage of being simpler to implement than other suggestions for ethics oversight reform.[43] It would require no formal policy revisions; instead, all that would be needed is cooperation among advocacy organizations, review committees, and oversight officials.

Conclusions

By the end of the 20th century, patient advocates were an undeniable presence in biomedical research. Advocates made individual studies more responsive to the patients and communities that the research was intended to benefit. They persuaded U.S. agencies to adopt requirements for gender and ethnic diversity in study populations. They helped make experimental innovations more widely available to seriously ill people. They convinced government agencies to boost funding for biomedical research.

In many respects, the emergence of research advocacy is a welcome development. At the foundation of modern research ethics is the belief that research practice and policy ought not be decided by scientists alone. Rather, the values and preferences of the broader community must guide the conduct of research.

For the most part, however, the broader community has been excluded from the research world. Advocates are capable of changing this situation. The most effective advocates combine an intimate awareness of illness and caregiving with medical knowledge. This mixed expertise equips them to apply abstract ethical principles to specific study situations. Many advocates are vocal and articulate, and have strong ties to people who must live with the consequences of research decisions. At this point in time, advocates are better prepared than anyone else to represent the community in research decision making.

The emergence of patient advocacy also makes it possible to explore research ethics from the bottom up. Not enough has been done to discover what participants value, resent, and would change about the research experience. Advocates have knowledge to fill these gaps. Advocates could help scientists and professional ethicists to see research from the point of view of research participants and patients in the community.

At the same time, advocacy raises a multitude of unrecognized and unresolved ethical issues, and the time is ripe for systematic inquiry into these issues. Advocates are a trusted and powerful force in the research arena. Their choices and actions have a significant impact on constituents and others. To preserve their influence, and use it wisely, advocates must confront the moral dimensions of their work.

Ethical Principles for Research Advocacy

A review of advocacy's influence on research points to three ethical principles for advocates. First, advocates should be truthful when communicating with others about research. In much of their work, advocates convey tidings of hope to constituents and the public. The optimism undoubtedly provides solace to patients and families and is effective in fund-raising. The problem is that optimism can create unfounded expectations about research prospects. Biomedical research over the past 50 years has produced a few sudden and significant advances, many incremental improvements, and numerous advances in knowledge that have not yet produced actual health benefits.[48] Thus, talk of imminent cures is almost always disingenuous.

Advocates have a responsibility to be realistic when they speak and write about research. Conveying inflated optimism about what research can deliver deprives patients and families of the facts they need to make research, health-care, and other personal decisions. Such optimism can foster public support for research policies and funding allocations that rest on implausible beliefs. It can damage advocates' credibility, as well.

Research advocacy should also be guided by a second ethical principle: appreciation for the diversity of constituents. Like advocates, constituents are a heterogeneous group. Some constituents have the necessary self-assurance, education, and economic wherewithal to be savvy research consumers. Others, however, do not. As a result, a "one-size-fits-all" approach to advocacy risks compromising the interests of certain constituents.

The challenge for advocates is to take into account constituents' different interests and situations. It is fine to promote the liberty of constituents prepared to exercise it, but safeguards are needed for those lacking the ability to protect themselves. Advocacy efforts to date seem most tailored to confident, well-educated patients able to take full advantage of their expanded research opportunities. Advocates should supplement this approach with programs to assist constituents who are not in this situation.

The third ethical principle is to reject parochialism in research advocacy. Advocates applying this principle will support policies and funding allocations to expand constituents' access not only to promising experimental interventions, but also to established health care. These advocates will not concentrate solely on research if significant numbers of constituents lack access to standard treatments of proven benefit. In campaigning to secure insurance coverage for patients in clinical trials, they will endorse measures to make both trials and established treatments more accessible to uninsured patients.

Advocates applying this principle will take into account patients outside their immediate constituencies, too. On first glance, such an approach may appear to conflict with advocates' responsibilities to pursue the most advantageous outcomes for their constituents. Yet often there is no real conflict. Constituents themselves are vulnerable to other health problems, and most have family and friends at risk for or affected by a wide range of diseases. Thus, constituents have interests in maintaining research and other programs designed to assist people with a variety of conditions.

At a broader level, advocates should support measures that promote fair representation for all affected groups in research deliberations. Advocates should also consider collaborating to devise a comprehensive plan for meeting the nation's health needs. A collaborative approach would reduce unseemly and self-defeating competition among interest groups. Moreover, an alliance of advocacy organizations would be a powerful force in shaping government, industry, and charitable support for research, health care, and other social services.

Preparing for Advocacy's Next Phase

In the next decade, advocates will confront a multitude of questions. At least three broad topics are likely to demand their attention. One is whether HIV/AIDS activism should continue as the model for research advocacy. As the first modern disease activists, HIV/AIDS advocates set the tone for those who followed. The success of HIV/AIDS advocacy prompted other disease interest groups to adopt similar goals and strategies. Now it is time for advocates to examine the virtues and pitfalls of the HIV/AIDS advocacy approach.

Several features of HIV/AIDS advocacy remain worthy of imitation. Most prominent is an emphasis on acquiring scientific and medical knowledge. Traditional patient advocacy organizations were content to leave research decisions to the scientific community. But HIV/AIDS activists proved that patient advocates could be valuable participants in such decision making. The grass roots character of HIV/AIDS advocacy is another feature with persistent appeal. Close involvement with local groups enables advocates to stay in touch with constituents' individual concerns.

Other features of HIV/AIDS activism seem less suited to future research advocacy. Certain deviations from the HIV/AIDS advocacy model might be in order for organizations representing people with cancer, heart disease, chronic obstructive lung disease, dementia, and other common serious conditions. In this context, emphasizing the search for a cure could diminish the attention given to patients' basic needs for health care and appropriate living situations. Cures for degenerative and chronic conditions arising later in life also are less likely to emerge than are cures for infectious diseases like HIV. Another lesson comes from the HIV/AIDS activists who eagerly embraced disease theories and interventions that were later discredited.[4] These advocates learned the hard way that assertions and anecdotes cannot substitute for rigorous research, and that initially exciting interventions often fail to live up to their promise.

Private sector advocacy is another area demanding attention. To date, advocacy has focused on government research policies. But with industry controlling a growing percentage of biomedical research, advocacy belongs in the private sector, too. Advocates could offer assistance to industry sponsors seeking to meet ethical standards. They could also address research priority setting in the private sector by encouraging firms to develop medications and other innovations that would fill significant gaps in existing therapy.

The increased commercialization of biomedical research confronts advocacy organizations with internal issues, for industry sponsors sometimes seek to enlist advocates as partners in various endeavors. To avoid ethical and legal problems, advocacy organizations should adopt conflict of interest policies. Such policies should define when disclosure of corporate support is sufficient to address ethical concerns, and when support must be rejected as incompatible with the advocacy mission.

In the future, research advocates will also encounter an array of novel biomedical technologies. Advocates already have begun to participate in policy discussions on xenotransplantation,[49] stem cell,[50] and gene transfer[51] research. Innovations in biomedical research require advocates to develop new kinds of scientific expertise. Acquiring such knowledge is a necessary step in developing defensible positions on the ethical and policy issues raised by these research innovations. As in the case of human embryo research, novel technologies may also produce contentious debate over the extent to which patients' interests ought to trump other social concerns.

Everyday research advocacy will generate plenty of future challenges, too. Advocates may have difficulty sustaining constituent and public enthusiasm if research fails to deliver dramatic treatment improvements. Researchers and officials in various settings may regard advocates primarily as public relations tools and turn a cold shoulder to patient-centered reforms. Politicians and entrepreneurs may attempt to manipulate research advocacy to advance their own agendas.

Biomedical research both reflects and influences the values of the society in which it occurs. Advocates have fiercely campaigned to put patients' interests at the forefront of research deliberations. Now they face pressure to refine their approach to constituent representation, cultivate alliances with other advocacy groups, and acknowledge the limits of research as a means to advance patients' interests.

Acknowledgment

This chapter is based on my book *When Science Offers Salvation: Patient Advocacy and Research Ethics*. New York, N.Y.: Oxford University Press; 2001.

References

1. Hope T. Medical research needs lay involvement. *Journal of Medical Ethics* 1998;24:291–2.
2. Edejer TT. North-south partnerships: The ethics of carrying out research in developing countries. *British Medical Journal* 1999;319:438–41.
3. Rothman KJ, Michels KB. The continuing unethical use of placebo controls. *New England Journal of Medicine* 1994;331:394–8.
4. Epstein S. *Impure Science: AIDS, Activism, and the Politics of Knowledge*. Berkeley, Calif.: University of California Press; 1996.
5. Institute of Medicine. *A Review of the Department of Defense's Program for Breast Cancer Research*. Washington, D.C.: National Academy Press; 1997.
6. Rich IM, et al. Perspective from the Department of Defense Breast Cancer Research Program. *Breast Disease* 1998;10:33–45.
7. National Breast Cancer Coalition. Education and Training. [Online] 2002. Available: http://www.natlbcc.org.
8. National Breast Cancer Coalition. NBCC's International Initiative. [Online] 2002. Available: http://www.natlbcc.org.
9. Cornwall A, Jewkes R. What is participatory research? *Social Science and Medicine* 1995;41:1667–76.
10. Goodare H, Smith R. The rights of patients in research. *British Medical Journal* 1995;310:1277–8.
11. Chalmers I. What do I want from health research and researchers when I am a patient? *British Medical Journal* 1995;310:1315–8.

12. In Quotes: NIMH's Hyman on mental health research. *Science and Government Report* Aug. 15, 1998.
13. Herbert CP. Community-based research as a tool for empowerment: The Haida Gwaii Diabetes Project example. *Canadian Journal of Public Health* 1996;87:109–12.
14. Seeley JA, Kenegeya-Kayonda JF, Mulder DW. Community-based HIV/AIDS research—Whither community participation? Unsolved problems in a research programme in rural Uganda. *Social Science and Medicine* 1992;34:1089–95.
15. Levine C, Dubler NN, Levine RJ. Building a new consensus: Ethical principles and policies for clinical research on HIV/AIDS. *IRB: A Review of Human Subjects Research* 1991;13(1–2): 1–17.
16. Fox RC. Contract and covenant in ethnographic research. In: King NMP, Henderson G, Stein J, eds. *Beyond Regulations: Ethics in Human Subjects Research*. Chapel Hill, N.C.: University of North Carolina Press; 1999:67–71.
17. Spiers H. Community consultation and AIDS clinical trials: Part II. *IRB: A Review of Human Subjects Research* 1991;13(4):1–6.
18. Shulman S, Brown J. The Food and Drug Administration's early access and fast-track approval initiatives: How have they worked? *Food and Drug Law Journal* 1995;50:503–31.
19. Temple R. Are surrogate markers adequate to assess cardiovascular disease drugs? *JAMA* 1999;282:790–5.
20. Food and Drug Administration. Guideline for the Study and Evaluation of Gender Differences in the Clinical Evaluation of Drugs; Notice. *Federal Register* 1993;58(139):39405–16.
21. National Institutes of Health. NIH Policy and Guidelines on the Inclusion of Women and Minorities as Subjects in Clinical Research—Amended, October 2001. [Online] October 2001. Available: http://grants.nih.gov/grants/funding/women_min/guidelines_amende_10_2001.htm.
22. U.S. Congress. Food and Drug Modernization Act, U.S. Code, Vol. 42, §282 (j) (1999 Supplement).
23. Stapleton S. Is best cancer care available? *American Medical News* 1998;41(Aug. 3).
24. National Cancer Institute. Clinical trials and insurance coverage. [Online] 2002. Available: http://cancertrials.nci.nih.gov.
25. Hoffman S. A proposal for federal legislation to address health insurance coverage for experimental and investigational treatments. *Oregon Law Review* 1999;78:203–73.
26. National Breast Cancer Coalition. Legislative Accomplishments. [Online] 2002. Available: http://www.natlbcc.org.
27. The National Commission for the Protection of Human Subjects of Biomedical and Behavioral Research. The Belmont Report: Ethical Principles and Guidelines for the Protection of Human Subjects of Research. Washington, D.C.: Department of Health, Education and Welfare; 1979. [Online] April 18, 1979. Available: http://www.hhs.gov/ohrp/humansubjects/guidance/belmont.htm.
28. Dresser R. Wanted: Single, white male for medical research. *Hastings Center Report* 1992;22(1):24–9.
29. Advisory Committee on Human Radiation Experiments. *Final Report of the Advisory Committee on Human Radiation Experiments*. New York, N.Y.: Oxford University Press; 1996.
30. Swanson GM, Ward AJ. Recruiting minorities into clinical trials: Toward a participant-friendly system. *Journal of the National Cancer Institute* 1995;87:1747–59.
31. Institute of Medicine. Women and Health Research. Washington, D.C.: National Academy Press; 1994.
32. Sarewitz D. Social change and science policy. *Issues in Science and Technology* 1997;14:29–32.
33. Institute of Medicine. *Approaching Death: Improving Care at the End of Life*. Washington, D.C.: National Academy Press; 1997.
34. NIH Working Group on Priority Setting. *Setting Research Priorities at the National Institutes of Health*. NIH Pub. No. 97-4265. Washington,

D.C.: NIH; 1997. [Online] Available: http://www.nih.gov/about/researchpriorities.htm.

35. Council for International Organizations of Medical Sciences, in collaboration with the World Health Organization. International Ethical Guidelines for Biomedical Research Involving Human Subjects. Geneva, Switzerland: CIOMS and WHO; 2002. [Online] November 2002. Available: http://www.cioms.ch/frame_guidelines_nov_2002.htm.

36. Veatch R. Human experimentation committees: Professional or representative? *Hastings Center Report* 1975;5(5):31–40.

37. Curran WJ. Government regulation of the use of human subjects in medical research: The approach of two federal agencies. *Daedalus* 1969;98:542–94.

38. The National Commission for the Protection of Human Subjects of Biomedical and Behavioral Research. *Institutional Review Boards: Report and Recommendations.* DHEW Publication No. (OS) 78–0008. Washington, D.C.: Government Printing Office; 1978.

39. Davis AM. Exception from informed consent for emergency research: Drawing on existing skills and experience. *IRB: A Review of Human Subjects Research* 1998;20(5):1–8.

40. President's Commission for the Study of Ethical Problems in Medicine and Biomedical and Behavioral Research. *Implementing Human Research Regulations.* Washington, D.C.: Government Printing Office; 1983.

41. Porter JP. What are the ideal characteristics of unaffiliated/nonscientist IRB members? *IRB: A Review of Human Subjects Research* 1986;8(3):1–6.

42. Porter JP. How unaffiliated/nonscientist members of institutional review boards see their roles. *IRB: A Review of Human Subjects Research* 1987;9(6):1–6.

43. McNeill PM. *The Ethics and Politics of Human Experimentation.* New York, N.Y.: Cambridge University Press; 1993.

44. Office of Inspector General, Department of Health and Human Services. *Institutional Review Boards: A Time for Reform.* OEI-01-97-00193. Washington, D.C.: DHHS; 1998. [Online] June 1998. Available: http://oig.hhs.gov/oei/reports/oei-01-97-00193.pdf.

45. Institute of Medicine. *Responsible Research: A Systems Approach to Protecting Research Participants.* Washington, D.C.: National Academies Press, 2003.

46. Edgar H, Rothman DJ. The institutional review board and beyond: Future challenges to the ethics of human experimentation. *Milbank Quarterly* 1995;73:489–506.

47. Merton V. Community-based AIDS research. *Evaluation Review* 1990;14:502–37.

48. Klaidman S. *Saving the Heart.* New York, N.Y.: Oxford University Press; 2000.

49. Institute of Medicine. *Xenotransplantation: Science, Ethics, and Public Policy.* Washington, D.C.: National Academy Press; 1996.

50. Perry D. Patients' voices: The powerful sound in the stem cell debate. *Science* 2000;287:1423.

51. Foubister V. Intense scrutiny confronts gene therapy. *American Medical News* 2000;43(Feb. 28).

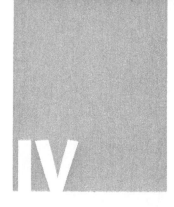

IV

Scientific Design

Steven Joffe   Robert D. Truog

24

Equipoise and Randomization

Most observers believe that randomized controlled trials (RCTs) offer the highest standard of evidence about the safety and efficacy of proposed new treatments.[1] When a new therapy's benefits are dramatic, nonrandomized studies may suffice to show its advantages. However, therapeutic advances more often involve small to moderate incremental benefits. Such benefits may be of substantial public health importance, particularly for common conditions.[2] Without the ability to conduct RCTs, efforts to evaluate such benefits are fraught with potential for error.

However, RCTs raise ethical challenges. In particular, randomizing patients to receive the experimental therapy, or a conventional therapy, or perhaps placebo, creates a dilemma. Clinicians are ethically required to offer patients the best available therapy. But researchers may propose to offer some participants in the trial an intervention that does not meet this "best available" standard.

Randomization is controversial in part because it draws attention to the uneasy coexistence of experimentation and therapy that exists in most clinical research. Notions of equipoise, which invoke some form of indifference between the interventions offered in a trial, have played a central role in efforts to reconcile the tensions between the roles of clinician and experimenter inherent in RCTs, and have found a place in the U.S. Department of Health and Human Services guidance regarding research design.[3]

However, equipoise is not universally accepted as the solution to the problems raised by RCTs. Definitions of equipoise vary, many authors doubt that it succeeds in reconciling the obligations of science and care, and more radically, some recent critics deny any need for such reconciliation. The epistemological assumptions underlying the notion of equipoise are also debated.[4] Finally, even

if the argument for equipoise is correct, it ignores many of the ethical questions that RCTs pose.

In what follows, we outline the rationale for and methodological basis of RCTs, review the history of equipoise, discuss the different conceptions and critiques of equipoise, attempt to situate the challenges associated with RCTs within a systematic framework for ethical research, and suggest scientific and policy implications of these challenges. We also review the relevant empirical data in order to tie normative discussions of equipoise and other ethical concerns to the real-world practice of RCTs.

Before beginning, another word about terminology is in order. Because there are numerous competing notions of equipoise, and the word itself is so unfamiliar in ordinary discourse, in this chapter we will favor a neutral term—*indifference*—unless we are discussing specific conceptions of equipoise advocated by particular authors.

Randomized Trials: Core Conception and Methodological Rationale

All clinical research that aims to inform choices about prophylactic, diagnostic, or therapeutic interventions involves comparing the relative merits of two or more possibilities. Consider a hypothetical single-arm study that appears to show improved outcomes among individuals exposed to a new intervention, compared with outcomes among a historical control group of patients exposed to a standard intervention. There are at least five potential explanations for this apparent benefit. It may result from between-group differences in demographic or other characteristics independently associated with the outcome under study—that is, from confounding due to selection bias. For example, individuals receiving the new intervention may be younger or healthier than the historical controls. Or, the benefit may result from differences in investigators' interactions with or observations of subjects—that is, from better supportive care, more intensive diagnostic testing, or reduced loss to follow-up. The improvement could be a placebo effect related to expectations about the new therapy. It might simply be due to chance. Finally, it may represent a true difference in treatment efficacy. These alternative explanations for the observed data must be considered whether or not results favor one of the treatments.

RCTs employ three or more devices to minimize the likelihood of false-positive and false-negative errors (see Table 24.1). First, they use concurrent controls, thereby permitting direct comparison between groups[5] and eliminating confounding by temporal trends. Second, they divide participants into groups using some method of random allocation, thereby increasing the likelihood that the groups will be comparable at baseline.[6] This is important because, though methods to adjust for known covariates are available, these methods are both imperfect and unable to control for unmeasured or unrecognized confounding variables. Third, RCTs employ statistical tests and sample size calculations to quantify and control the chances of false-positive and false-negative results. In addition, many trials conceal treatment allocation from subjects and/or investigators (a technique known as single- or double-blinding) to reduce the chance that investigators or subjects will tilt the trial by unconsciously favoring one group over the other. Finally, some trials use placebos to facilitate blinding. Such rigorous methodology helps maximize the scientific validity that is among the primary requirements for ethical research.[7]

Of these five error-minimizing devices, use of concurrent controls and statistical tests present no special ethical problems,

Table 24.1
Error-Minimizing Features of Randomized Trials

Feature	Purpose
Concurrent controls	• Eliminate between-group differences due to temporal trends • Enable direct comparisons
Randomization	• Reduce likelihood that groups will differ at study entry
Statistical tests, sample size calculations	• Control chances of false-positive and false-negative results
Blinding*	• Reduce likelihood that investigators will interact with or observe study participants in ways that differ systematically between groups • Reduce chance that participants will behave or report symptoms in ways that differ systematically between groups • Distinguish physiologic from placebo effects
Placebo administration**	• Facilitate blinding when interventions differ in observable ways between groups

*Not all randomized trials involve blinding or placebo controls.

**In a subset of trials involving placebos, participants in the control arm may be asked to forgo treatment that is available in the context of standard care.

though the choice of statistical approaches may have ethical implications,[8] as discussed below. Randomization, however, has been debated for at least 40 years. Blinding, though less scrutinized, also raises ethical challenges. Special concerns related to placebos arise when control participants are asked to forgo therapy that is otherwise available[5,9–12] (see Chapter 25).

There are two general statistical approaches to designing and analyzing RCTs. The most prevalent method, called frequentist, begins with a null hypothesis: that there is no difference in outcome between Treatment A and Treatment B. Before the trial begins, investigators define a probability threshold, called an alpha error, beyond which they will reject the null hypothesis as statistically improbable. The experiment proceeds, and the data are used to calculate the conditional probability, assuming the null hypothesis is true, of "observing a result equal to or more extreme than what was actually observed."[13] If this conditional probability (or P value) is smaller than the predefined alpha error, the null hypothesis is rejected and the alternative hypothesis—that there is a difference in outcome between Treatment A and Treatment B—is accepted by default. It is critical to note the common misconception that the P value describes the probability that the observed difference reflects a false positive. The P value represents the probability of the observed data given no true difference, not—as often assumed—the probability of no true difference given the observed data.[14]

An alternative analytic approach, called Bayesian, eschews null hypotheses and hypothesis tests. Instead, it starts with an assumption (which may be either subjective or evidence-based) about the true difference in outcome between Treatment A and Treatment B. This assumption takes the form of a prior probability distribution. The experiment is conducted, and the data are used to calculate a measure of the weight of the evidence (known as the Bayes factor or likelihood ratio). This measure is then combined mathematically with the prior distribution to generate a posterior probability distribution. The posterior distribution represents an updated estimate, taking into account information learned from the experiment, of the true difference between A and B.[15–17]

Historical Perspective

Most discussions of the ethics of RCTs have revolved around the possibility of conflict between research and treatment. The felt need to defend RCTs as consistent with physicians' therapeutic obligations was evident by 1949, when Walker and Barnwell cited the lack of "genuine ignorance or doubt that the drug in question has any therapeutic value" to justify their decision against randomizing in an early U.S. Veterans Administration study of streptomycin for pulmonary tuberculosis.[18] Fisher, who developed the statistical theory underlying randomization, wrote in 1958 that RCTs are acceptable "so long as no body of medical opinion can say with confidence that one [new drug] is better than the other." (Interestingly, in the same article he criticized the mounting but nonrandomized evidence of an association between cigarette smoking and lung cancer as insufficient to prove causation.)[19] Hill, who helped design the earliest published RCT, the British streptomycin trial, wrote in 1963: "Only if, in his state of ignorance, [the doctor] believes the treatment given to be a matter of indifference can he accept a random distribution of the patients to the different groups."[20] Importantly, Hill did not invoke indifference in defending the decision to randomize tuberculosis patients to streptomycin versus observation. Rather, because insufficient streptomycin was available to treat all eligible patients, he viewed a random lottery as a fair way to ration the drug while facilitating collection of valuable data[21] (see Chapter 4).

Charles Fried's 1974 treatise systematized the theoretical case for the indifference requirement, pointed to the clinician-investigator at the bedside as the primary locus of the moral dilemma, and suggested ways to resolve or lessen the quandary, including emphasis on informed consent and greater openness to nonrandomized designs.[22] Fried's essay opened the modern history of the notion of equipoise.

The Ethics of Randomization

Ethical concerns about randomization, the most striking feature of RCTs, focus on two related but separable aspects of trial conduct. First, some critics object that participants must forgo their right to "personal care."[22,23] Put differently, physicians have a duty, grounded in the fiduciary nature of the patient-doctor relationship, to make individualized treatment recommendations in the context of patients' particular values and circumstances. When physicians also act as investigators, randomization seems to force them to violate this duty. Second, commentators raise the more consequentialist concern that randomization may require assignment of some participants to therapy that is likely to be inferior, even though the preliminary evidence supporting that judgment falls short of conventional standards of methodological rigor. Emerging data during the course of a trial that appear to favor either treatment exacerbate these problems. Reviews of ethical aspects of RCTs are available.[24,25]

The most common defense of RCTs is to claim a state of indifference between the two treatments—that is, that they are "an equal bet in prospect."[25] Many versions of this requirement have been proposed. Mostly they vary along two dimensions—whether indifference is for physician-investigators or patient-subjects to determine, and whether it should operate at the individual or community level. (Table 24.2 attempts to clarify the nomenclature.) Although these views of indifference vary, they share the intuition that it is ethical to conduct a trial or enroll a patient when there are no strong reasons to favor one treatment over the other. Thus, under indifference, clinician-investigators can fulfill their commitments to personal care while avoiding charges of giving patients predictably inferior therapy.

Table 24.2
Four Conceptions of Equipoise

	Clinician-Investigator	Patient-Subject
Individual*	Individual equipoise**	Patient equipoise
Community	Clinical equipoise†	Community equipoise

*The *uncertainty principle* invokes individual preferences among both clinician-investigators and patient-subjects.

**Sometimes called *theoretical equipoise* or *Fried's equipoise*.

†To complicate matters, Gifford has used *community equipoise* to refer to Freedman's notion of clinical equipoise.[30]

Fried's view, which others have termed *individual* or *theoretical* equipoise, established the benchmark for subsequent authors.[22] (Table 24.3 catalogs the key positions in the debate.) Concerned mainly about randomization's challenge to personal care, Fried held that it is ethically problematic for a physician who favors either treatment to offer enrollment in a trial if his or her preferred treatment is available outside the trial. Furthermore, personal care requires that physicians consider patients as individuals with unique values and circumstances, not as generic exemplars of a given condition. Fried contended that when physicians take such individual factors into account, instances of genuine indifference between treatments for particular patients will be rare. For Fried, physicians' fiduciary obligations require that they share their beliefs with their patients and recommend their preferred treatment when it is available. Variations of this position continue to appear.[23,25–33]

The difficulties of conducting RCTs within the constraints of the requirement that individual physicians be indifferent are obvious. Physicians will usually have at least weak treatment preferences, which would impose moral obligations at a minimum to share their preferences with patients and perhaps even to recommend against or decline involvement with the trial. Also, the physicians who conduct a trial are often the same individuals who have led the clinical development of the intervention; they are naturally motivated because they believe the intervention may be superior to standard therapy. Demanding that those who developed the experimental treatment be indifferent about its merits in comparison with standard therapy might seem an unreasonable constraint. Furthermore, even if physicians are indifferent at the start of the trial, they will often develop preferences as it progresses. And they cannot ethically agree to the withholding of interim results to avoid this problem, because doing so violates their obligations of advocacy and fidelity. Though Fried did not wish to create an insurmountable barrier to RCTs, it is difficult to imagine beginning a trial or bringing it to completion in the moral universe he describes. As Hellman and Hellman have argued, "even if randomized clinical trials were much better than any alternative . . . the ethical dilemmas they present may put their use at variance with the primary obligations of the physician. . . . We must develop and use alternative methods for acquiring clinical knowledge."[23]

Before discussing responses to Fried, an aside about the problem of personal care is in order. Because randomization spotlights the fact of experimentation, it sometimes seems like a methodological streetlamp under which we search for our lost ethical keys. In fact, virtually all intervention studies—not just RCTs—challenge obligations of personal care.[34] Consider a single-arm trial that has enrolled 18 subjects, none of whom responded to the experimental agent.[35] The protocol specifies closing the trial and declaring the drug ineffective if none of the first 19 subjects responds. Is it ethical to enroll the next eligible patient if alternatives are available? Or consider the more pedestrian example of a chemotherapy research protocol that specifies a white blood cell (WBC) count of 1500/uL before beginning each cycle. Adherence to the protocol would require that the subject who arrives in clinic with a WBC of 1450/uL be sent home, even if proceeding with therapy would be clinically reasonable. Thus, if the argument from personal care holds, RCTs are hardly unique in presenting ethical challenges to the conduct of clinical research.

An alternative view holds that standards within the clinical community, rather than individual physicians' inclinations,

Table 24.3

Equipoise and Other Responses to the Problem of Treatment Preferences in Randomized Trials

Position	Core Argument	Representative Citations
Arguments From Equipoise		
Individual equipoise	Physicians must view the treatments offered in an RCT as "equal bets in prospect" in order to enroll patients. Some advocates of this position argue that this condition is unlikely ever to be met and would therefore discard RCTs on ethical grounds.	Fried[22]; Hellman & Hellman[23]; Markman[31]; Royall[28]; Hellman[26]; Gifford[30]; Edwards et al.[25]
Equipoise among expert clinicians	An RCT is ethical if there is uncertainty or disagreement within the expert clinical community about the relative merits of the two therapies.	Freedman[36] ; Miller & Weijer[40]; Weijer et al.[188]; Weijer[37]
Standards of evidence	An RCT is ethical if there is no scientifically validated reason to favor either treatment in the trial.	Levine[1]
Patient equipoise and informed consent	Patients, rather than clinicians, must be indifferent among the various treatment options when enrolling in a trial. Closely related to the view that the patient-subject's informed consent, not the objective state of knowledge or physicians' beliefs, is the primary ethical precondition for RCT participation.	Angell[41]; Marquis[42]; Lilford[43]; Ashcroft[44]; Veatch[45]; Menikoff[46]; Gifford[39]
Community equipoise	The locus of uncertainty or disagreement includes not just expert clinicians, but also patients and their representatives.	Karlawish & Lantos[47]
Uncertainty	The ethical precondition for enrolling a patient in a trial is a state of uncertainty—not necessarily of equal prior probabilities—on the part of clinician and patient about which of two or more treatments is preferred. Combines features of individual and patient equipoise.	Peto et al.[2]; Peto & Baigent[49]; Sackett[48]; Enkin[51]
Alternatives to Equipoise		
Altruism	Patients' desires to assist in learning something of value justifies their participation in RCTs.	Meier[53]; Royall[54]
Social contract	By virtue of the benefits they receive from prior research, persons have correlative obligations to participate in trials, even at some limited cost to themselves.	Wikler[57]; Gifford[56]
Consequentialism	Experimentation in RCTs cannot be reconciled with patients' rights to optimum personal care. Only an ethic that looks to the greatest good for the greatest number can justify such trials.	Marquis[62]
Debate rests on false premises	Notions of equipoise are based on a misconception about the relationship between research and therapy in RCTs. It ought to be discarded in favor of a conception that is specific to research.	Miller & Brody[66]

should determine whether RCT participation is acceptable. Freedman's 1987 description of *clinical equipoise,* which took this approach, was perhaps the most influential response to Fried's challenge.[36] Freedman argued that physicians' knowledge—and therefore the scope of their therapeutic obligations—is collective and professional rather than individual in nature. If so, he argued, clinicians who offer participation in RCTs are behaving ethically so long as there exists "an honest, professional disagreement among expert clinicians about the preferred treatment."[36] In Freedman's view, absent professional consensus, a clinician's hunches or preferences pose no moral barrier to trial recruitment.

In a recent extension of Freedman's work, Weijer noted that clinical research often includes some procedures "administered with therapeutic intent and others that answer the research question" (presumably, the experimental treatment under study in an RCT is among the procedures "administered with therapeutic intent").[37,38] He argued that the equipoise requirement applies specifically to these "therapeutic" procedures. Based on the work

of the U.S. National Commission for the Protection of Human Subjects of Biomedical and Behavioral Research, he advocated a "components approach" in which each element of a trial would be judged according to standards appropriate to its intent. Thus, a biopsy undertaken exclusively to address a scientific hypothesis would be acceptable if risks were minimized and were reasonable in relation to the knowledge gained (i.e., a research-specific evaluation standard). In contrast, administration of a promising new agent with therapeutic expectations in the context of a randomized trial would be acceptable if it met Freedman's test of clinical equipoise.

Levine has argued that a trial is ethical if "there is no scientifically validated reason to predict that Therapy A will be superior to Therapy B. Further, there must be no Therapy C known to be superior to either A or B."[1] This position bears a fundamental kinship with Freedman's statement of clinical equipoise, because what constitutes a "scientifically validated reason" depends on community standards.

Although individual and clinical equipoise differ in a number of ways,[39] the contrast in moral locus of decision making is among the most salient. Recently, Miller and Weijer have suggested that the choice between equipoise at the individual or clinical community level represents a false dilemma; both may be ethically necessary.[40] They argue that clinical equipoise is a social condition that legitimates the initiation or continuation of a trial, whereas individual equipoise justifies the clinician-investigator's decision to offer or recommend trial enrollment to a patient. In practice, sorting through these conditions is often difficult. In Box 24.1, we describe a case in which, to the clinicians involved, neither level of equipoise seemed sufficient by itself to justify a trial.

A third important conception of the indifference requirement, hinted at by Fried and developed more fully by others, emphasizes the views of the patient-subject rather than the clinician-investigator.[41–46] The acceptability of trial participation depends crucially on how the subject values the various probabilities and outcomes associated with trial enrollment, because it is the subject who will experience the consequences. Thus the subject, not the clinician-investigator, must be reasonably indifferent between the treatments offered in the trial.

Two features of the patient indifference perspective bear mention. First, because only the subject can provide ethical justification for trial participation, the argument rests entirely on valid informed consent. Proponents have not considered this principle's implications for RCTs, such as trials involving young children or occurring in emergency situations, in which autonomous consent is not possible. Second, this view highlights the need to think broadly about what endpoints we have in mind when we speak of being indifferent between two treatments. Clinician-investigators might be indifferent with respect to the trial's "hard" endpoints—mortality or major morbidity—but prospective trial participants are likely to consider factors such as quality of life and practical burdens as well.[39] Mastectomy and local resection with radiation may result in similar survival for most women with limited-stage breast cancer, but many women will have strong preferences depending on how they value such factors as disfigurement and the possibility of local recurrence. Lilford and Jackson have shown how one might model such tradeoffs to arrive at "effective" equipoise.[27]

Just as Freedman highlighted the role that lack of consensus within the expert clinical community plays in legitimizing an RCT, others have emphasized the importance of disagreement or indifference within the patient community.[47] According to this position, for a trial to be ethical, the community that must be in equipoise includes representatives of those who would be eligible for the trial. As with clinicians, individual patients and communities of patients may have complementary roles in legitimizing a trial.

A final group of authors argues that uncertainty, not equipoise, best articulates the ethical basis for RCTs.[2,48–51] According to Peto and Baigent,

> A patient can be entered if, and only if, the responsible clinician is substantially uncertain which of the trial treatments would be most appropriate for that particular patient. A patient should not be entered if the responsible clinician or the patient are for any medical or non-medical reasons reasonably certain that one of the treatments that might be allocated would be inappropriate for this particular individual (in comparison with either no treatment or some other treatment that could be offered to the patient in or outside the trial).[49]

At first blush, it is not entirely evident how this "uncertainty principle" differs from some conceptions of equipoise. (Compare it with Levine's formulation above.) One important difference, however, is that, against Freedman, advocates of the uncertainty principle wish to place the moral onus back on the individual physician and patient who must decide about trial participation, rather than on the community of experts.[52] Proponents of the uncertainty principle also reject the "etymological connotation of an equal balance between . . . the alternatives to be tested" inherent in the word *equipoise*.[51] They insist instead that, for an RCT to be ethical, the metaphorical "confidence intervals" around one's hunches of benefit must include the possibility of no effect or of harm. This is a much less fragile conception than the individual equipoise described by Fried.[51] Nevertheless, the uncertainty principle qualifies rather than radically revises the notion of equipoise.

Reconciling Clinical and Scientific Obligations in Randomized Trials

The justifications for RCTs reviewed above all invoke some version of the indifference requirement. However, some authors suggest that indifference may be neither necessary nor sufficient to justify trials. These commentators offer frameworks that—either alone or in combination with arguments from indifference—might provide alternative ethical foundations for RCTs.

One defense of RCTs appeals to patients' altruism to justify a limited loss of benefit associated with the possibility of randomization to inferior therapy.[53,54] In Meier's words, "most of us would be quite willing to forgo a modest expected gain in the general interest of learning something of value."[53] Like the patient indifference approach, invoking altruism as a defense of trials rests heavily on valid consent and raises problems for trials involving those who lack capacity to consent.[54] It is also amenable to empirical investigation of participants' reasons for enrolling in trials.[55]

A second justification appeals to the notion of social contract. Gifford, in a promising account, explored such an approach to

---

Box 24.1
A Case Involving Different Conceptions of Equipoise

In 2004, clinicians at Boston Children's Hospital discussed an RCT involving assignment of critically ill children to groups that would receive red blood cell transfusions at threshold hematocrits of either 21% or 27%. Though the current local practice was to transfuse at about 21%, no data existed to support this cutoff and practices varied across institutions. On the basis of this broader disagreement, a few clinicians argued for an ethical obligation to support the trial in order to help resolve this important question. Most, however, insisted that unless there was personal uncertainty, or at least disagreement within the local group, it would not be ethical to enroll patients. Thus three versions of the equipoise position were in play in this debate: (1) clinical equipoise, as described by Freedman; (2) equipoise within the *local* expert community; and (3) individual equipoise, as described by Fried.

reconciling patients' self-interests and right to personal care with efforts to advance the common good. He suggested that "morality and political institutions are conceptualized as . . . cooperative ventures for mutual advantage, and each person can see that it is in his interest to have such an institution."[56] RCTs might be among the institutions that invite justification in this way. Wikler took a similar line, asking us to imagine a choice of "citizenship in one of two societies. In the first, doctors always give their patients the best care they can, whereas in the second, patients are sometimes slighted in the interest of medical progress. The state of the art of medicine, however, is more advanced in the second than in the first."[57] Many people, he argued, would choose citizenship in the second society. Several authors have considered the broader but related question, based on considerations of fair play and free ridership, of whether persons have prima facie obligations to participate in clinical research.[58–61]

A third option invokes the consequentialist notion that the social benefits of trials outweigh their costs to individuals. For example, Marquis reluctantly suggested that an ethics of conscription, defended on consequentialist grounds, might be necessary to justify the conduct of these trials.[62] Others have discussed the broader role of consequentialism in the ethics of medical research.[50,63–65]

Finally, in 2003 Franklin Miller and Howard Brody posed a radical challenge to the central question underlying the equipoise debate. They argued that concerns about equipoise derive from the widely held but (they believe) incoherent "similarity position," which holds that "the ethics of clinical trials rest on the same moral considerations that underlie the ethics of clinical medicine."[66] In their view, this position contradicts the fundamental assumption of research ethics, as articulated in the Belmont Report of the National Commission for the Protection of Human Subjects of Biomedical and Behavioral Research: "The ethics of clinical trials must start with the realization that medical research and medical treatment are two distinct forms of activity, governed by different ethical principles"[67] (see Chapter 14). According to the Belmont Report, clinical care involves activities "that are designed solely to enhance the well being of an individual patient or client and that have a reasonable expectation of success," whereas research denotes "an activity designed to test an hypothesis, permit conclusions to be drawn, and thereby to develop or contribute to generalizable knowledge."[67] To suggest that equipoise can unite the ethical conditions for these two activities represents a category mistake.

Rather than ask whether an RCT satisfies clinical equipoise, Miller and Brody would assess it against principles appropriate to the evaluation of research.[7] The key question is not, as proponents of clinical equipoise argue, how the interventions offered in a trial compare with competent medical practice. Rather, investigators and reviewers must ensure that the study does not exploit subjects. This condition requires that the question is worth asking, the methods are sufficient to answer the question at hand, the risk-benefit ratio—integrating risks and benefits to individual participants with benefits to the community of future patients—is favorable, and subjects give valid informed consent. The most important implication of this view is that, to estimate the risk-benefit ratio of any study involving human subjects, one must incorporate considerations of societal benefit.[67,68] The confusion at the heart of the various arguments from indifference lies in their denial that this is as true for RCTs as it is for other research designs.

Miller and Brody's framework is particularly helpful for analyzing and justifying studies, such as certain placebo trials, that offer some subjects less expectation of benefit than they might receive under standard care. However, conceptual questions and practical problems remain, and though the authors attempt to address these, it is not clear how their proposal will play out in the clinic.[69] For example, can we realistically ask individuals to trade the status of patient for that of subject when they enter a trial, or must we articulate a coherent vision of them simultaneously as patients and subjects? If patients, particularly those with serious illnesses, come to physicians with expectations of receiving optimum therapy, how will the explicit denial of therapeutic obligations affect subject recruitment and trust in research?[70,71] On what normative grounds do we proceed when studying persons who cannot provide informed consent, such as children or patients involved in emergency exception research? Given these considerations, Weijer and Paul Miller counter that the components approach discussed above, which assesses research and therapeutic elements of a trial according to different criteria, better reflects the insights of the National Commission.[72]

Practical Responses to the Problem of Reconciling Clinical and Scientific Obligations

As noted previously, various formulations of the indifference requirement offer potential solutions both to the problem of personal care and to the concern that some patients might be randomized to predictably inferior therapy. Conceptual debates focus mainly on the deontological issues related to personal care, and secondarily on the more consequentialist problem of assignment to inferior therapy. In contrast, discussions about practical ways to ameliorate these problems seek primarily to minimize the number of subjects who receive inferior therapy.

A historically important suggestion for ensuring indifference is to randomize beginning with the first person exposed to a drug.[73] This argument recognizes that preliminary, usually uncontrolled data available prior to the first RCT tend to disturb indifference sufficiently to make subsequent studies ethically and logistically challenging. Although theoretically plausible, in the real world there are valid reasons that new therapies do not reach the point of evaluation in an RCT until after they have been evaluated (sometimes extensively) in early-phase research.[74] By this time, evidence for their efficacy already exists. Nor does this suggestion resolve the practical problem caused by trends that emerge during the course of the study. Knowledge of such trends could lead to treatment preferences among clinician-investigators and potential subjects that could threaten study completion.

The practical challenge posed by interim data has led to the standard but controversial practice of withholding the information from investigators, referring physicians, and enrolled and potential subjects.[75] Veatch has written that withholding such information may sometimes be acceptable when subjects are aware of and consent to it in advance, but that "where the information really is crucial such consent to ignorance will be morally unacceptable."[76] Levine held that it is acceptable to "ask the subject to consent to . . . acceptance of the standards of proof agreed upon within the community of professionals" regarding emerging efficacy trends.[1] Freedman suggested that clinical equipoise alleviates the ethical difficulties caused by emerging trends, because until the evidence is sufficient to convince the expert clinical community, clinical equipoise is maintained.[36] He further argued that, if clinical equipoise suffices to justify a trial, then withholding interim data should be unnecessary. (The routine concealment of such data suggests that, though investigators may endorse the abstract notion of clinical equipoise, they are unwilling to bet their own trials on it.) Finally, Lilford et al. argued against the withholding of interim results.[75]

In concert with the practice of withholding interim results, data monitoring committees (DMCs)—also known as data safety and monitoring boards (DSMBs)—are widely used to deal with the problem of emerging trends[50] (see Chapter 53). DMCs, which should be independent of the sponsor and principal investigator, review interim data regarding toxicity and efficacy. They are charged with deciding when the accumulated evidence justifies closing the trial. Ideally, the decision to close a trial respects protocol-specified stopping guidelines that function to preserve both the scientific validity and the ethical integrity of the trial. DMCs may close trials early for several reasons, including poor accrual or other logistical problems, unanticipated toxicity in one or both arms, lack of an emerging difference between arms (futility), or unexpectedly strong evidence for a difference between arms (efficacy). In the context of the present discussion, their major role is to close a trial when the data are sufficient to answer the research question. The possibility of stopping early minimizes the number of subjects assigned to the less effective treatment, while permitting the better therapy to be offered sooner and to larger numbers of patients outside the trial. Decisions about early stopping, which are the subject of considerable statistical discussion, are among the most ethically charged in all of clinical research[53,77–79] and will always generate controversy.[80,81] In our view, they require greater attention from the research ethics community than they have heretofore received.

Decisions about when to stop an individual trial are obviously connected to judgments about when to declare uncertainty resolved and a particular line of inquiry closed. This critical issue has received only limited attention in the research ethics literature.[82] Despite the concerns that they raise,[1] it has been customary to conduct confirmatory trials in many circumstances. Guidance from the U.S. Food and Drug Administration (FDA) states that "the usual requirement for more than one adequate and well-controlled investigation reflects the need for *independent substantiation* of experimental results. A single clinical experimental finding of efficacy, unsupported by other independent evidence, has not usually been considered adequate scientific support for a conclusion of effectiveness."[83] Parmar has described Bayesian methods for making explicit decisions about when residual uncertainty justifies confirmatory trials.[84]

A second strategy for minimizing the number of subjects exposed to the inferior intervention involves unbalanced randomization, with a ratio favoring the preferred arm.[85,86] A more complicated approach has been called *adaptive randomization*, or "play-the-winner."[86,87] In this design, subjects are initially assigned to the experimental or standard treatment in a fixed ratio. However, as the data begin to favor one treatment or the other, the allocation ratio tilts toward the preferred arm. When there are large differences between treatments and results are available in the short run, such a design can be completed successfully.[88,89] However, when differences are smaller or primary outcomes require long-term follow-up, adaptive randomization may not be feasible.

Although unbalanced randomization and play-the-winner strategies may reduce the number of subjects exposed to the inferior intervention, this advantage may be more than offset by the problem of justifying to those assigned to the nonpreferred arm why it is ethical for them to be recruited into the trial. Adaptive designs are also subject to methodological challenge, as changes in participants' prognostic profiles over the course of the trial (e.g., lesser severity of illness late in the trial) might lead to differences between groups and confound the interpretation of treatment effects.[90]

Yet another way to minimize suboptimal treatment for individual participants, as implemented by Kadane in a cardiac anesthesia trial,[91] involves Bayesian strategies for assigning study participants to treatment arms. Before the start of the trial, a group of experts made treatment recommendations for hypothetical patients with various prognostic profiles. These predictions were used to develop computer models that could provide treatment recommendations for individuals meeting the trial's eligibility criteria. Data that emerged over the course of the trial were used to update these models continually. If the experts' (computer-modeled) recommendations for a particular eligible patient unanimously favored one arm, the patient was assigned to that arm. In contrast, if there was any disagreement among the recommendations, clinical equipoise was said to exist and the patient underwent random allocation. This method has the virtue of individualization and might reduce assignment of patients to predictably inferior therapy, but is labor intensive and has not found widespread acceptance.

Two other proposals for reducing the tension between experimental validity and personal care merit consideration. First, Peto et al.[2] have advocated the use of "large simple trials," rather than the more typical and highly regimented "explanatory" designs.[92] Such trials are distinguished by their broad eligibility criteria, reduced data collection requirements, and limited specification of treatments in the study beyond the particular intervention under evaluation.[49] From the point of view of reconciling research and treatment imperatives, such trials have the virtue of minimizing the experimental constraints and practical burdens that protocols place upon patients and physicians. As a result, they have many scientific advantages, including facilitating very large sample sizes, decreasing complexity and cost, enhancing the generalizability (external validity) of the study findings, and reducing the gap between the efficacy as measured in controlled settings and effectiveness as seen in ordinary practice.[93–96] They also reduce the gap between personal and protocol care. Thus, for compelling ethical as well as scientific reasons, they merit serious consideration.

Finally, Veatch[76] and Silverman[97] have advocated "semi-randomized" or "comprehensive cohort" trials on both ethical and methodological grounds. In such studies, patients are offered the choice of Treatment A, Treatment B, or random assignment. Analytically, the primary comparison involves only the randomized subjects. However, subjects who choose direct assignment to Treatment A or Treatment B constitute useful observational cohorts. In particular, outcomes within these groups can shed light on whether the results of the primary comparison are generalizable to the population of persons who would not accept randomization (and who might differ in systematic ways from those willing to be randomized). This approach offers randomization as a genuine choice, reducing the need for physicians to choose between fidelity to patients as unique individuals and allegiance to the experimental method. Although one might worry that few patients offered participation in such a trial would accept random assignment, such unwillingness might cast doubt on the ethical justification for randomization in the first place. Several comprehensive cohort trials have been successfully conducted.[98–100]

Empirical Data

Though the relationship of normative to descriptive ethics is an uneasy one, some questions about the ethics of RCTs lend themselves to empirical answers.

How often do RCTs comparing experimental with standard therapies find the new treatment to be better? The observation that trials favor the experimental treatment most of the time would suggest the absence of systematic indifference within the institution of clinical trials. Knowledge of the proportion of past trials favoring the experimental treatment would also inform estimates of prior probabilities associated with future trials.[101] Most such studies have not found strong advantages to experimental treatment. Reviewing surgery and anesthesia trials, Gilbert et al. found reasonable symmetry between studies favoring the experimental treatment and those favoring the standard.[60] Colditz et al. came to similar conclusions in trials of medical therapies.[102] Chlebowski and Lillington observed that 16% of meeting abstracts describing RCTs of adjuvant therapy for localized breast cancer and only 2% of abstracts describing RCTs for metastatic breast cancer favored experimental treatment.[103] Machin et al. noted that 28% of published RCTs for solid tumors from the British Medical Research Council favored the experimental treatment.[104] Djulbegovic et al. reported that 44% of published RCTs for multiple myeloma favored the standard treatment, whereas 56% favored the innovation.[105] They also found that industry-sponsored and placebo-controlled trials were more likely than other trials to favor the innovation, raising concerns about systematic departure from indifference. Joffe et al. observed that 29% of adult cancer trials sponsored by a publicly funded U.S. cooperative group favored the experimental treatment, whereas only 3% favored the standard treatment; on average, experimental treatment was associated with a 20% improvement in anticancer efficacy when compared with standard treatment.[106] Finally, Soares et al. found no evidence that trials sponsored by a radiation oncology cooperative group favored the experimental treatment.[107]

Do RCTs proceed despite compelling prior evidence that one treatment is better? Lau et al. used cumulative meta-analysis to evaluate the strength of evidence over time for or against 15 interventions for myocardial infarction.[108] For some interventions, trials continued years after benefits had been shown with high confidence. For example, 15 RCTs of intravenous streptokinase (SK) were reported and 32,095 subjects enrolled after 1977, by which time SK had been proven superior to control with Cumulative $P < 0.001$. Similar results have been seen in other settings.[109,110] Such continuation of trials long after differences have been convincingly shown is difficult to defend on scientific or ethical grounds.

Do physicians have preferences for treatment arms, and do they affect recruitment? Though surprisingly few data are available, treatment preferences appear both to be common among physicians and to reduce their willingness to enroll patients. For example, Taylor et al. surveyed surgeons participating in a slow-accruing trial comparing mastectomy with local excision for breast cancer.[111] About 20% believed that one or the other treatment was inappropriate for patients. Other work has shown that many physicians are uncomfortable with randomization, either because of treatment preferences or because it seems to violate the norms of the patient-doctor relationship.[112,113] Alderson found that few health-care professionals thought indifference was possible for breast cancer trials.[114] Cheng et al. described how prior beliefs led investigators to reject an RCT of a promising new therapy for melioidosis, a life-threatening infectious disease, despite considerable uncertainty about the new therapy's effectiveness.[115] Finally, Clark et al. applied the term "jumping-the-gun" to refer to physicians' tendencies to treat patients off-protocol with interventions that have not yet been proven in RCTs, a phenomenon that probably reflects early loss of indifference among individual physicians.[116]

Do patients have preferences for treatment arms, and do those preferences affect their enrollment decisions? Few data characterize preferences among patients considering or enrolled in RCTs. Jenkins and Fallowfield asked approximately 200 cancer patients considering participation in RCTs about their reasons for accepting or declining trial entry.[55] Three-quarters of those interviewed decided to participate in the RCT. Approximately 80% of those who accepted the trial, versus 14% who declined, agreed that "either treatment in the trial would be suitable," suggesting that treatment preferences explain at least some patients' decisions not to enter the trial. Jack et al. observed similar effects.[117] A review of the literature on trial accrual concluded that "patient preferences for one of the study treatments . . . appear to limit their willingness to take part in randomized trials."[118] Finally, in a recent trial of a molecularly targeted agent for chronic myeloid leukemia, 18% of those assigned to the standard arm—versus only 2% of those assigned to the experimental arm—either withdrew consent or crossed over to the alternative treatment before meeting the study endpoint, indicating both strong preferences and a willingness to act on them.[119]

Beyond Equipoise: A Systematic Overview of Ethical Issues in RCTs

Although notions of equipoise have dominated debates over the ethics of RCTs, these trials raise many other challenging questions. A comprehensive discussion is beyond the scope of this chapter. Here, we attempt to identify issues of particular salience to RCTs, locate them within a general framework for judging the ethics of clinical research,[7] and briefly review the relevant literature. Table 24.4 provides an overview.

Social or Scientific Value

In general, whether a research question is worth asking is independent of the study design, and therefore the requirement for social value has no special implications for RCTs. However, as discussed above, new trials sometimes begin long after any reasonable uncertainty about the preferred intervention is re-

Table 24.4

Randomized Trials and the Criteria for Ethical Research

Criterion	Issues and Questions Relevant to Randomized TrialsTCH
Social or scientific value	Has the study question previously been answered? • Confirmatory trials • Cumulative meta-analyses • Objective of answering unresolved questions versus changing clinical practice
Scientific validity	How much incremental validity does the RCT offer, compared with alternate designs? What problems compromise the validity of RCTs in practice? • Subversion of randomization • Underpowered trials • Publication bias • Concerns about generalizability
Fair selection of participants	(No special problems related to randomized designs)
Favorable risk-benefit ratio	Do the study treatments satisfy the indifference requirement? • Loss of personal care • Loss of expected utility for some subjects Is there a generic benefit (trial effect) from RCT participation? When should a study be stopped? What should the control treatment be when there is no standard of care?
Independent review	(No special problems related to randomized designs)
Informed consent	Is informed consent always necessary? • Randomized consent (Zelen) design • Minimal-risk RCTs • Emergency exception research
Respect for potential and enrolled participants	Is withholding of information from trial participants acceptable? • Study arm assignment (blinding) • Interim results

solved.[108–110] The question of when to conduct a confirmatory trial is controversial,[1,84,120] and requires further normative exploration. The history of neonatal extracorporeal membrane oxygenation (ECMO) provides an illustrative example (see Box 24.2). Finally, performing a trial in hopes of influencing slow-to-change practice patterns, despite the fact that the study question has previously been answered, is ethically problematic.[120]

Scientific Validity

The primary justification for randomization is its ability to minimize bias compared with alternative allocation strategies. Few deny that RCTs offer scientific benefits, but their exact magnitude is a matter of contention.[121] Early reports suggested that studies using historical or concurrent nonrandomized controls overestimated benefits from experimental therapies, compared with RCTs, primarily because controls in RCTs often had better

outcomes than controls in other designs.[102,122,123] Recent meta-analyses comparing randomized with nonrandomized studies, however, offer a more complicated picture. Concato et al.[124] and Benson and Hartz[125] found that effects observed in well-conducted nonrandomized controlled trials were similar to those seen in RCTs. In contrast, Ioannidis et al. found that discrepancies between randomized and nonrandomized trials were common, even when the latter were restricted to prospective comparisons.[126] Thus, in our view, further empirical work is needed to quantify the magnitude of the scientific benefits from RCTs.

Even assuming substantial incremental validity, several practical problems threaten RCTs' claim to methodological priority. First, inadequate allocation concealment raises questions about the assumption of baseline comparability.[127,128] Furthermore,

---

Box 24.2
Trials of Neonatal ECMO

By the early 1980s, uncontrolled case series suggested that certain critically ill neonates who were expected to die with conventional treatment could survive if treated with extracorporeal membrane oxygenation (ECMO), a complex, expensive, and risky new therapy. A group of investigators began an RCT to compare outcomes among infants treated with ECMO or conventional treatment.[88] Because the investigators' prior expectations strongly favored ECMO (before initiating the trial, the investigators expected a 90% chance of survival with ECMO and 10% chance of survival with conventional treatment), they adopted several unusual design features to "soften the ethical dilemma."[88] First, they employed single-consent prerandomization, whereby only parents of those infants assigned to experimental treatment (ECMO) were asked for permission to enroll their child.[158] Second, they used adaptive randomization (i.e., allocation probabilities increasingly favored the treatment that had been more successful among prior subjects).[87] When the study ended, 1 child had been assigned to conventional treatment and died, whereas 11 children had been assigned to ECMO and survived. This difference was statistically significant.

In 1986, investigators at Harvard initiated a second RCT of ECMO versus conventional treatment.[159] They justified another trial because "the disparity in group size [in the first RCT] provided little concurrent experience concerning the relative efficacy of the two therapies," and because they were concerned that rapidly decreasing mortality rates with conventional treatment made using historical controls problematic. This trial also used single-consent prerandomization. In addition, it employed a different form of adaptive randomization whereby all infants were randomized to either ECMO or conventional treatment until there were four deaths in one arm, after which all subsequent infants were directly assigned to the favored treatment. In this trial, 6 out of 10 infants treated with conventional treatment, versus 19 out of 20 infants treated with ECMO, survived ($p < 0.05$).

Though ECMO subsequently entered standard practice in the United States, it was not accepted in the United Kingdom at the time. Thus U.K. physicians, dissatisfied with the methods employed in the trials described above, initiated a conventional RCT in 1993.[90] By the fifth interim analysis three years later, mortality was 54/92 (59%) in the conventional arm and 30/93 (32%) in the ECMO arm ($p = 0.0005$). Upon the recommendation of the DMC, the trial was closed. The appropriateness of conducting this trial, giving the prior evidence favoring ECMO, has been hotly debated.[120]

participants in some blinded trials may make informed guesses about their treatment assignments, raising the possibility of un-acknowledged postrandomization biases.[129,130] Second, many RCTs are underpowered, increasing the prevalence of false-negative results.[131] Third, evidence of publication bias (i.e., lower publication rates among negative than among positive RCTs) suggests that the literature systematically overstates the effectiveness of new treatments.[132–138] Fourth, participants in RCTs are often unrepresentative of the populations to which inferences are made, raising concerns that study results may not generalize to nontrial practice.[94,95,139–143] Fifth, despite RCTs' methodological rigor, bias may creep into authors' qualitative conclusions.[144]

Finally, Wikler argues that the standard P value cutoff of 0.05 for declaring statistical significance is "not a medical or statistical truth, but a clinician's convention."[57] It reflects a value-laden tradeoff between expected risks and benefits for present subjects and the degree of confidence desired before adopting new therapies. Also, as noted previously, because the P value fails to take into account the prior probability that the new treatment is superior to the standard, it can encourage misleading conclusions about the likelihood that an observed difference is a false positive.[14,16] Various strategies to deal with the practical and inferential problems of the P value, including relaxing the traditional 0.05 cutoff for rare diseases or low-risk/low-cost interventions and using Bayesian or mixed frequentist-Bayesian analytic techniques, have been proposed.[13,14,16,145–147]

Favorable Risk-Benefit Ratio

The Belmont Report enjoins us to consider risks and benefits to study participants, together with societal benefits from the knowledge gained, in evaluating the risk-benefit ratio of a particular study.[67] As Miller and Brody point out, the societal advantages of rigorous research design strengthen the ethical argument for RCTs, even when the indifference claim is weak.[66] On the other hand, RCTs open up the possibility that some participants may be disadvantaged by assignment to a predictably inferior therapy.[25] As we noted previously, the various conceptions of indifference in part represent efforts to resolve this conundrum. DMCs and early stopping rules are further efforts to walk the tightrope between advantages to society and costs to present patients.

It is difficult to estimate how much benefit, if any, subjects forgo by taking part in RCTs. Scant data indicate that experimental therapies in RCTs offer at best a small advantage over standard therapies.[60,103–106] However, some claim the existence of a benefit from trial participation itself,[25,148–150] though one of us has questioned the methodological basis for this conclusion.[151] In any case, the weight of evidence suggests that in most cases one sacrifices little or nothing in terms of disease outcome by agreeing to participate in an RCT.

Recently, controversy has erupted over whether RCTs with mortality or major morbidity endpoints must include standard-care control arms.[152–155] This debate, inspired by a trial involving patients with acute respiratory distress syndrome (ARDS), raises important questions of social value, scientific validity and risk-benefit ratio[156] (see Box 24.3).

In the ARDS trial, subjects were randomized to receive either large or small tidal volumes delivered by a mechanical ventilator,

in which either option was judged at the start of the trial to be within the range of acceptable care. This design presented at least three questions at the interface of ethics and scientific methodology: (1) In the absence of a routine-care control arm (that is, a third arm of the trial in which tidal volumes would have been determined by the bedside clinicians), could the trial determine whether either treatment under study was preferable to current practice? (2) Were subjects randomized to either arm put at unnecessary risk compared with routine care? (3) Did the absence of a routine-care arm hinder the DMC's ability to evaluate whether participants were experiencing adverse outcomes using interim data?[152,157] Answering these questions is complex. Some have argued, for example, that a routine-care arm would not have been helpful in this trial, because routine care was not defined and was known to vary across a wide spectrum of practice. This lack of definition might have rendered any comparisons between the experimental arms and the routine-care control arm uninterpretable. At a minimum, the debate highlights the critical question

---

Box 24.3
The ARDSNet Controversy

In 1996, the Acute Respiratory Distress Syndrome Network (ARDSNet) initiated a multicenter randomized trial comparing mortality among critically ill patients treated with "traditional" high-volume mechanical ventilator breaths versus those treated with low-volume breaths.[156] At the start of the trial, practice varied considerably across intensive care units, with some preferring lower-volume and others higher-volume approaches. In addition, physicians generally adjusted their approach to mechanical ventilation based on the patient's clinical state. There was no consensus about the preferred ventilator strategy.

Against this background, trial participants were randomized to receive either high-volume or low-volume mechanical ventilation, with subsequent adjustments based on prespecified physiologic criteria. The high-volume strategy reflected approximately the 80th percentile of common practice, whereas the low-volume strategy reflected approximately the 3rd percentile.[153] About 860 subjects enrolled. In 1999, upon the recommendation of the Data Monitoring Committee (DMC), the trial closed early when convincing evidence for reduced mortality in the lower-volume arm emerged.

In July 2002, two critical-care physicians and two statisticians raised concerns about the trial, as well as about a second ARDSNet trial that was under way, with the Office for Human Research Protections (OHRP), which has regulatory jurisdiction over most U.S. human subjects research.[153] They argued that the absence of a routine-care control arm (either individualized ventilator management or volumes reflecting approximately the median in routine practice) potentially put subjects at increased risk. The additional risk could derive from the assignment of some participants to an inappropriate "control" arm, or from the inability of the DMC to monitor directly whether the participants in the two arms were experiencing poorer outcomes than they would have if they had received routine care. In response to this and other complaints, OHRP launched an investigation of the completed trial and requested that a second ARDSNet trial raising similar issues be suspended. Though ultimately it exonerated both trials and permitted the second trial to proceed, OHRP called for further debate about whether trials should be required on ethical grounds to include a routine-care control arm.[157]

of what role research ethics should play with regard to considerations of scientific design.[155]

Informed Consent

In general, informed consent to RCTs does not raise qualitatively different concerns from consent to other forms of intervention research. As with other designs, consent to RCTs is viewed by most as central to individuals' acceptance of the role of subject in addition to (or instead of) that of patient. However, several issues specific to RCTs have arisen.

Discomfort among physician-investigators with the mandate to obtain written informed consent has contributed to recruitment problems and even threatened the completion of some trials.[111] One response to this problem, advocated by Zelen, is to randomize eligible patients before requesting consent.[158] Investigators could then request consent only from those assigned to the experimental arm (single-consent design), or from those assigned to both arms (double-consent design). In either case, the trial would be analyzed on the basis of initial group assignment rather than treatment received (i.e., intent to treat). The single-consent approach, which withholds material information from some subjects, was deemed unethical by the U.S. National Institutes of Health when used in the Harvard Neonatal ECMO Trial.[89,159] The double-consent strategy is more palatable, though it too has been challenged on both ethical and methodological grounds. For example, Ellenberg[160] and Altman et al.[161] have argued that because of subject refusal and the need for intention-to-treat analyses, prerandomized trials may underestimate treatment effects and have reduced power when compared with conventional RCTs. Prerandomization is also inapplicable to blinded trials. Furthermore, it is possible that unbalanced presentations by investigators[162] (i.e., emphasizing benefits to those assigned to experimental therapy and uncertainty or risks to those assigned to standard therapy) or investigators' glossing over the difficult issue of randomization itself might lead subjects to consent who would have refused under the conventional design. On the basis of these arguments, Marquis has condemned prerandomization as "either unnecessary or unethical."[163]

Truog et al. have argued that informed consent to RCT participation may be ethically optional under limited circumstances, including (1) availability of all treatments outside the trial without the requirement for consent, (2) minimal incremental risk, (3) "genuine clinical equipoise," and (4) no basis for treatment preference among reasonable persons.[164] Middle-ground alternatives, such as opt-out consent designs,[165] are also available.

Trialists, ethicists, and regulators have recognized the impossibility of obtaining informed consent or proxy permission in some emergency trials, such as those for cardiac arrest[166] (see Chapter 27). In the United States, regulators have waived the requirement for informed consent to such trials if certain stipulations, including advance community consultation and notification, are met.[167] This emergency exception, although controversial, suggests that informed consent is not seen as ethically mandatory for all RCTs.

Empirical data on participants' or proxies' understanding of randomization are conflicting.[25] Several studies demonstrate problems with recognition of the method of treatment allocation or the underlying rationale for its use.[168–174] Other studies, however, paint a less pessimistic picture.[175–178]

Respect for Potential and Enrolled Participants

Emanuel et al. suggest that respect for subjects includes permitting withdrawal, protecting privacy, informing subjects of newly discovered risks or benefits, sharing results, and maintaining subject welfare.[7] For the most part, respect for subjects in RCTs raises no unique issues. One major difference, however, is that withholding information about treatment assignment and interim results is more common in RCTs than in other study designs.

Despite the fact that blinding challenges obligations of personal care as much as randomization (indeed, its methodological rationale is in part to preclude personal care),[179] it has received far less attention in the ethics literature. Clinicians who take part in blinded trials cannot easily make individualized dose adjustments, have difficulty interpreting adverse events, and may struggle with drug interactions. Although well-designed protocols will help investigators minimize risks to subjects as they navigate most situations, unanticipated circumstances can arise. Most commentators accept blinding if prospective subjects are aware of and agree to the fact that neither they nor the investigator will know their treatment assignment.[1,180] Nevertheless, this reliance on consent raises problems for pediatric and other research that relies on proxy permission. In such trials, blinding (a clearly nontherapeutic procedure) might be ethically justified if it was both scientifically necessary and involved at most a minor increment over minimal risk.[37,181]

Finally, respect for subjects would ordinarily include access to interim findings. The common practice of withholding interim results in RCTs further impairs personal care and increases the likelihood that subjects will receive a less effective treatment despite mounting evidence for its inferiority. At the same time, it may be practically necessary for trials to reach completion. As discussed above, withholding results is usually justified by reference to subjects' prior consent.[1,76,180] Some commentators, however, argue that such "consent" to ignorance is invalid, at least in certain circumstances, and that trial results should be freely available.[75,76] As with blinding, an alternate defense of the practice of withholding interim results might invoke methodological necessity and limited incremental risk.[37,181]

Study Design and Policy Implications

The appropriate methodological and policy response to the debates over RCTs depends largely on whether one agrees with Freedman and his followers that clinical equipoise succeeds in reconciling perfectly clinicians' obligations to help advance medical science and to care for individual patients. The main practical effect of adopting this position is to prohibit trials, especially involving placebo controls, in which equipoise does not obtain.[10–12] If, however, one believes as we do that RCTs (along with virtually all clinical research) may require accommodation between clinical and scientific commitments, the policy implications are more profound. At the extreme, viewing obligations to patients as absolute may require abandoning RCTs entirely.[23] Less radically, one can seek to reduce inconsistencies between the clinical and scientific objectives of providing care within RCTs and to justify any compromises that remain. Several design and policy options merit consideration.

1. *Allocating treatments in ways that minimize losses to current patients:* Adaptive randomization and Bayesian allocation techniques might enhance expected utility for prospective subjects. Nevertheless, they do not entirely negate the charge that RCTs may require sacrificing the interests of some patients in pursuit of medical progress.[28,57]

2. *Expanding the range of choices available to patients:* When experimental treatments are available outside trials, patients could be offered the choice of randomization or direct assignment to standard or experimental therapy.[76] This would diminish concerns that the withholding of patients' (or their physicians') preferred treatment compels enrollment in RCTs. However, few data indicate whether participation in the primary analytic (i.e., randomized) groups would be sufficient to make this design feasible in practice.

3. *Conducting pragmatic trials:* In some circumstances, pragmatic trials, including large simple trials, may help reconcile the competing aims of RCTs without compromising scientific rigor.[2,49,93,182] In such trials, deviations from standard care are kept to the minimum necessary for experimental validity. In addition to the ethical advantages, proponents make scientific (enhanced generalizability) and logistical (lower cost, easier recruitment) arguments for such trials. Taken together, they form a compelling case for conducting a pragmatic trial when it can successfully answer the study question.

4. *Exploring Bayesian analytic techniques:* The implications of Bayesian statistical analysis for ethical conceptions of RCTs have received little attention. On the one hand, they might result in continuing trials beyond their stopping point under the frequentist paradigm, thus straining the indifference requirement past the point required by the $P = 0.05$ convention.[14,16] At the same time, by reminding us that both patients and physicians generally hold prior probabilities, Bayesian approaches could force greater emphasis on disclosure of preferences and on patient choice than is currently the norm.[43]

5. *Maximizing the return on investment from every RCT:* If the pursuit of scientific rigor through RCTs involves some concessions by present patients, then practical problems that compromise the quality of the information gained are especially troubling. Regarding publication bias, for example, one response envisions mandatory prospective registration of every RCT in a publicly accessible database.[183–184] Efforts to ensure that trials are adequately powered and to assess their generalizability to the populations of interest are also warranted.

6. *Weighing alternate designs:* Fried argued that proponents of RCTs wrongly characterize their advantages over other designs as "a gulf as sharp as that between the kosher and the non-kosher."[22] Nonrandomized concurrent controls, historical controls, or continuous quality improvement may occasionally offer feasible alternatives when RCTs prove ethically or practically untenable.[28,89,115,185] Shatz has written that "researchers ought to utilize alternative designs when they seem scientifically appropriate, and perhaps even when loss of scientific accuracy—which translates into possible losses for future patients—can be justified by reference to the interests of present patients."[24] At the same time, recent trials of high-dose chemotherapy for metastatic breast cancer[186] and of hormone replacement therapy for postmenopausal women[187] illustrate the dangers of relying on nonrandomized evidence. In our view, to avoid RCT orthodoxy investigators should consider alternative designs in each controversial case and provide specific justification for the decision to proceed with a randomized design.

Unresolved Ethical Issues and Data Requirements

Our review of the literature demonstrates four major areas that require additional data or greater conceptual clarity.

First, limited empirical evidence about the methodological or practical consequences of alternative designs exists. For example, how would comprehensive cohort designs affect trial enrollment and interpretation? How often do the restrictive eligibility criteria and tightly controlled conditions of many RCTs lead to answers that are internally valid but poorly generalizable to the population of interest?[189] How much bias is introduced by using concurrent but nonrandomized controls together with statistical adjustment techniques?[124,125] Answers to these questions are crucially important to informed policy decisions about clinical research.

Second, the views of prospective participants about the tradeoffs inherent in RCTs are poorly understood. For example, we know little about how individuals who enroll in trials view their status as both patient and subject, how often they have preferences for standard or experimental therapy, what reasons they hold for accepting randomization, or how they view the relationship between their own medical care and contributing to medical progress.

Third, the choices we make when defining the boundaries of uncertainty require explicit justification in full view of their consequences for patients and subjects.[82] Because they attempt to estimate treatment effects and their attendant uncertainties directly, Bayesian methods may prove especially fruitful here.[16]

Finally, despite the extensive debates over the past half-century, there is as yet no agreement on the fundamental justification for or appropriate use of randomized trials. Thus there is an overarching need for conversation among patients, methodologists, clinicians, and ethicists about the moral basis of RCTs. Existing writings, although rich and professionally diverse, do not always demonstrate the kind of interdisciplinarity or empirical grounding required to advance the debate. Because randomization largely highlights rather than fundamentally alters the dilemmas that are integral to most intervention studies, such conversation should transcend the narrow context of RCTs and aspire to articulate a solid ethical foundation for all clinical research.

References

1. Levine RJ. *Ethics and Regulation of Clinical Research,* 2nd ed. New Haven, Conn.: Yale University Press; 1986.

2. Peto R, Collins R, Gray R. Large-scale randomized evidence: Large, simple trials and overviews of trials. *Journal of Clinical Epidemiology* 1995;48:23–40.

3. Department of Health and Human Services, Office for Human Research Protections. *Protecting Human Research Subjects: Institutional Review Board Guidebook.* Rockville, Md.: OHRP; 1993. [Online] Available: http://www.hhs.gov/ohrp/irb/irb_guidebook.htm.

4. Ashcroft R. Equipoise, knowledge and ethics in clinical research and practice. *Bioethics* 1999;13:314–26.
5. Temple R, Ellenberg SS. Placebo-controlled trials and active-control trials in the evaluation of new treatments. Part 1: Ethical and scientific issues. *Annals of Internal Medicine* 2000;133:455–63.
6. Harrington DP. The randomized clinical trial. *Journal of the American Statistical Association* 2000;95:312–5.
7. Emanuel EJ, Wendler D, Grady C. What makes clinical research ethical? *JAMA* 2000;283:2701–11.
8. Palmer CR. Ethics and statistical methodology in clinical trials. *Journal of Medical Ethics* 1993;19:219–22.
9. Ellenberg SS, Temple R. Placebo-controlled trials and active-control trials in the evaluation of new treatments. Part 2: Practical issues and specific cases. *Annals of Internal Medicine* 2000;133:464–70.
10. Rothman KJ, Michels KB. The continuing unethical use of placebo controls. *New England Journal of Medicine* 1994;331:394–8.
11. Freedman B, Weijer C, Glass KC. Placebo orthodoxy in clinical research. I: Empirical and methodological myths. *Journal of Law, Medicine, and Ethics* 1996;24:243–51.
12. Freedman B, Glass KC, Weijer C. Placebo orthodoxy in clinical research. II: Ethical, legal, and regulatory myths. *Journal of Law, Medicine, and Ethics* 1996;24:252–9.
13. Goodman SN. Toward evidence-based medical statistics. 1: The P value fallacy. *Annals of Internal Medicine* 1999;130:995–1004.
14. Lee SJ, Zelen M. Clinical trials and sample size considerations: Another perspective. *Statistical Science* 2000;15:95–110.
15. Spiegelhalter DJ, Freedman LS. Bayesian approaches to randomized trials. *Journal of the Royal Statistical Society A* 1994;157:357–416.
16. Goodman SN. Toward evidence-based medical statistics. 2: The Bayes factor. *Annals of Internal Medicine* 1999;130:1005–13.
17. Lewis RJ, Wears RL. An introduction to the Bayesian analysis of clinical trials. *Annals of Emergency Medicine* 1993;22:1328–36.
18. Walker AM, Barnwell JB. Clinical evaluation of chemotherapeutic drugs in tuberculosis. *Annals of the New York Academy of Sciences* 1949;52:742–9.
19. Fisher RA. Cigarettes, cancer and statistics. *Centennial Review* 1958;2:151–66.
20. Hill AB. Medical ethics and controlled trials. *British Medical Journal* 1963:1043–9.
21. Doll R. Controlled trials: The 1948 watershed. *British Medical Journal* 1998;317:1217–20.
22. Fried C. *Medical Experimentation: Personal Integrity and Social Policy.* New York, N.Y.: American Elsevier Publishing Co., Inc.; 1974.
23. Hellman S, Hellman DS. Of mice but not men: Problems of the randomized clinical trial. *New England Journal of Medicine* 1991;324:1585–9.
24. Shatz D. Randomized clinical trials and the problem of suboptimal care: An overview of the controversy. *Cancer Investigation* 1990;8:191–205.
25. Edwards SJ, Lilford RJ, Braunholtz DA, et al. Ethical issues in the design and conduct of randomised controlled trials: A review. *Health Technology Assessment* 1998;2(15):1–132.
26. Hellman S. The patient and the public good. *Nature Medicine* 1995;1:400–2.
27. Lilford RJ, Jackson J. Equipoise and the ethics of randomization. *Journal of the Royal Society of Medicine* 1995;88:552–9.
28. Royall RM. Ethics and statistics in randomized clinical trials. *Statistical Science* 1991;6:52–62.
29. Hellman D. Evidence, belief, and action: The failure of equipoise to resolve the ethical tension in the randomized clinical trial. *Journal of Law, Medicine, and Ethics* 2002;30:375–80.
30. Gifford F. Community-equipoise and the ethics of randomized clinical trials. *Bioethics* 1995;9:127–48.
31. Markman M. Ethical difficulties with randomized clinical trials involving cancer patients: Examples from the field of gynecologic oncology. *Journal of Clinical Ethics* 1992;3:193–5.
32. Menikoff J. The hidden alternative: Getting investigational treatments off-study. *Lancet* 2003;361:63–7.
33. Menikoff J. Full disclosure: Telling patients when not being a research subject is a good choice. *Perspectives in Biology and Medicine* 2005;48(Suppl.):S139–S149.
34. Appelbaum PS, Roth LH, Lidz CW, Benson P, Winslade W. False hopes and best data: Consent to research and the therapeutic misconception. *Hastings Center Report* 1987;17(2):20–4.
35. Sordillo PP, Schaffner KF. The last patient in a drug trial. *Hastings Center Report* 1981;11(6):21–3.
36. Freedman B. Equipoise and the ethics of clinical research. *New England Journal of Medicine* 1987;317:141–5.
37. Weijer C. The ethical analysis of risk. *Journal of Law, Medicine, and Ethics* 2000;28:344–61.
38. Weijer C, Miller PB. When are research risks reasonable in relation to anticipated benefits? *Nature Medicine* 2004;10:570–3.
39. Gifford F. Freedman's "clinical equipoise" and "sliding-scale all-dimensions-considered equipoise." *Journal of Medicine and Philosophy* 2000;25:399–426.
40. Miller PB, Weijer C. Rehabilitating equipoise. *Kennedy Institute of Ethics Journal* 2003;13:93–118.
41. Angell M. Patients' preferences in randomized clinical trials. *New England Journal of Medicine* 1984;310:1385–7.
42. Marquis D. How to resolve an ethical dilemma concerning randomized clinical trials. *New England Journal of Medicine* 1999;341:691–3.
43. Lilford RJ. Ethics of clinical trials from a Bayesian and decision analytic perspective: Whose equipoise is it anyway? *British Medical Journal* 2003;326:980–1.
44. Ashcroft R. Giving medicine a fair trial: Trials should not second guess what patients want. *British Medical Journal* 2000;320:1686.
45. Veatch RM. Indifference of subjects: An alternative to equipoise in randomized clinical trials. *Social Philosophy and Policy* 2002;19:295–323.
46. Menikoff J. Equipoise: Beyond rehabilitation? *Kennedy Institute of Ethics Journal* 2003;13:347–51.
47. Karlawish JH, Lantos J. Community equipoise and the architecture of clinical research. *Cambridge Quarterly of Healthcare Ethics* 1997;6:385–96.
48. Sackett DL. Why randomized controlled trials fail but needn't: 1. Failure to gain "coal-face" commitment and to use the uncertainty principle. *Canadian Medical Association Journal* 2000;162:1311–4.
49. Peto R, Baigent C. Trials: The next 50 years. Large scale randomised evidence of moderate benefits. *British Medical Journal* 1998;317:1170–1.
50. Pocock SJ. When to stop a clinical trial. *British Medical Journal* 1992;305:235–40.
51. Enkin MW. Clinical equipoise and not the uncertainty principle is the moral underpinning of the randomised controlled trial: Against. *British Medical Journal* 2000;321:757–8.
52. Sackett DL. Equipoise, a term whose time (if it ever came) has surely gone. *Canadian Medical Association Journal* 2000;163:835–6.
53. Meier P. Terminating a trial—The ethical problem. *Clinical Pharmacology and Therapeutics* 1979;25:633–40.
54. Royall RM. Ignorance and altruism. *Journal of Clinical Ethics* 1992;3:229–30.
55. Jenkins V, Fallowfield L. Reasons for accepting or declining to participate in randomized clinical trials for cancer therapy. *British Journal of Cancer* 2000;82:1783–8.
56. Gifford F. The conflict between randomized clinical trials and the therapeutic obligation. *Journal of Medicine and Philosophy* 1986;11:347–66.

57. Wikler D. Ethical considerations in randomized clinical trials. *Seminars in Oncology* 1981;8:437–41.

58. Caplan AL. Is there a duty to serve as a subject in biomedical research? In: Caplan AL. *If I Were a Rich Man Could I Buy a Pancreas?* Bloomington, Ind.: Indiana University Press; 1992:85–99.

59. Almy TP. Meditation on a forest path. *New England Journal of Medicine* 1977;297:165–7.

60. Gilbert JP, McPeek B, Mosteller F. Statistics and ethics in surgery and anesthesia. *Science* 1977;198:684–9.

61. Mosteller F. Innovation and evaluation. *Science* 1981;211:881–6.

62. Marquis D. Leaving therapy to chance. *Hastings Center Report* 1983;13(4):40–7.

63. McDermott W. The changing mores of biomedical research. II. Challenge and discussion: Opening comments. *Annals of Internal Medicine* 1967;67(Suppl.7):39–42.

64. Eisenberg L. The social imperatives of medical research. *Science* 1977;198:1105–10.

65. Lasagna L. Some ethical problems in clinical investigation. In: Mendelsohn E, Swazey JP, Taviss I, eds. *Human Aspects of Biological Innovations.* Cambridge, Mass.: Harvard University Press; 1971:98–110.

66. Miller FG, Brody H. A critique of clinical equipoise: Therapeutic misconception in the ethics of clinical trials. *Hastings Center Report* 2003;33(3):19–28.

67. The National Commission for the Protection of Human Subjects of Biomedical and Behavioral Research. *The Belmont Report: Ethical Principles and Guidelines for the Protection of Human Subjects of Research.* Washington, D.C.: Department of Health, Education and Welfare; DHEW Publication OS 78-0012 1978. [Online] April 18, 1979. Available: http://www.hhs.gov/ohrp/humansubjects/guidance/belmont.htm.

68. Miller FG. Research ethics and misguided moral intuition. *Journal of Law, Medicine, and Ethics* 2004;32:111–6.

69. Brody H, Miller FG. The clinician-investigator: Unavoidable but manageable tension. *Kennedy Institute of Ethics Journal* 2003;13:329–46.

70. Miller FG, Rosenstein DL. The therapeutic orientation to clinical trials. *New England Journal of Medicine* 2003;348:1383–6.

71. Grunberg SM, Cefalu WT. The integral role of clinical research in clinical care. *New England Journal of Medicine* 2003;348:1386–8.

72. Weijer C, Miller PB. Therapeutic obligation in clinical research. *Hastings Center Report* 2003;33(3):3.

73. Chalmers TC, Block JB, Lee S. Controlled studies in clinical cancer research. *New England Journal of Medicine* 1972;287:75–8.

74. Brody BA. *The Ethics of Biomedical Research: An International Perspective.* New York, N.Y.: Oxford University Press; 1998.

75. Lilford RJ, Braunholtz D, Edwards S, Stevens A. Monitoring clinical trials—Interim data should be publicly available. *British Medical Journal* 2001;323:441–2.

76. Veatch RM. *The Patient as Partner: A Theory of Human-Experimentation Ethics.* Bloomington, Ind.: Indiana University Press; 1987.

77. Baum M, Houghton J, Abrams K. Early stopping rules—Clinical perspectives and ethical considerations. *Statistics in Medicine* 1994;13:1459–69.

78. DeMets DL, Pocock SJ, Julian DG. The agonising negative trend in monitoring of clinical trials. *Lancet* 1999;354:1983–8.

79. Parmar MK, Griffiths GO, Spiegelhalter DJ, Souhami RL, Altman DG, van der Scheuren E. Monitoring of large randomised clinical trials: A new approach with Bayesian methods. *Lancet* 2001;358:375–81.

80. Bryant J, Wolmark N. Letrozole after tamoxifen for breast cancer—What is the price of success? *New England Journal of Medicine* 2003;349:1855–7.

81. National Breast Cancer Coalition. NBCC Raises Concerns About Halting of Letrozole Clinical Trial. [Online] 2003. Available: http://www.natlbcc.org/bin/index.asp?strid=627&btnid=1&depid=20.

82. Lantos JD, Frader J. Extracorporeal membrane oxygenation and the ethics of clinical research in pediatrics. *New England Journal of Medicine* 1990;323:409–13.

83. Food and Drug Administration. *Guidance for Industry: Providing Clinical Evidence of Effectiveness for Human Drug and Biologic Products.* Rockville, Md.: FDA; 1998. [Online] May, 1998. Available: http://www.fda.gov/cder/guidance/1397fnl.pdf.

84. Parmar MK, Ungerleider RS, Simon R. Assessing whether to perform a confirmatory randomized clinical trial. *Journal of the National Cancer Institute* 1996;88:1645–51.

85. Avins AL. Can unequal be more fair? Ethics, subject allocation, and randomised clinical trials. *Journal of Medical Ethics* 1998;24:401–8.

86. Palmer CR, Rosenberger WF. Ethics and practice: Alternative designs for phase III randomized clinical trials. *Controlled Clinical Trials* 1999;20:172–86.

87. Zelen M. Play-the-winner rule and the controlled clinical trial. *Journal of the American Statistical Association* 1969;64:131–46.

88. Bartlett RH, Roloff DW, Cornell RG, Andrews AF, Dillon PW, Zwischenberger JB. Extracorporeal circulation in neonatal respiratory failure: A prospective randomized study. *Pediatrics* 1985;76:479–87.

89. Truog RD. Randomized controlled trials: Lessons from ECMO. *Clinical Research* 1992;40:519–27.

90. UK Collaborative ECMO Trial Group. UK collaborative randomised trial of neonatal extracorporeal membrane oxygenation. *Lancet* 1996;348:75–82.

91. Kadane JB, ed. *Bayesian Methods and Ethics in a Clinical Trial Design.* New York, N.Y.: John Wiley and Sons, Inc.; 1996.

92. Sackett DL, Gent M. Controversy in counting and attributing events in clinical trials. *New England Journal of Medicine* 1979;301:1410–2.

93. Tunis SR, Stryer DB, Clancy CM. Practical clinical trials: Increasing the value of clinical research for decision making in clinical and health policy. *JAMA* 2003;290:1624–32.

94. George SL. Reducing patient eligibility criteria in cancer clinical trials. *Journal of Clinical Oncology* 1996;14:1364–70.

95. Fuks A, Weijer C, Freedman B, Shapiro S, Skrutkowska M, Riaz A. A study in contrasts: Eligibility criteria in a twenty-year sample of NSABP and POG clinical trials. *Journal of Clinical Epidemiology* 1998;51:69–79.

96. Cochrane AL. *Effectiveness and Efficiency: Random Reflections on Health Services.* London, U.K.: Nuffield Provincial Hospitals Trust; 1972.

97. Silverman WA. Patient preferences and randomised trials. *Lancet* 1994;344:1023.

98. Link MP, Goorin AM, Miser AW, Green AA, Pratt CB, Belasco JB, et al. The effect of adjuvant chemotherapy on relapse-free survival in patients with osteosarcoma of the extremity. *New England Journal of Medicine* 1986;314:1600–6.

99. Schmoor C, Olschewski M, Schumacher M. Randomized and non-randomized patients in clinical trials: Experiences with comprehensive cohort studies. *Statistics in Medicine* 1996;15:263–71.

100. Henshaw RC, Naji SA, Russell IT, Templeton AA. Comparison of medical abortion with surgical vacuum aspiration: Women's preferences and acceptability of treatment. *British Medical Journal* 1993;307:714–7.

101. Chalmers I. What is the prior probability of a proposed new treatment being superior to established treatments? *British Medical Journal* 1997;314:74–5.

102. Colditz GA, Miller JN, Mosteller F. How study design affects outcomes in comparisons of therapy. I: Medical. *Statistics in Medicine* 1989;8:441–54.

103. Chlebowski RT, Lillington LM. A decade of breast cancer clinical investigation: Results as reported in the Program/Proceedings of the American Society of Clinical Oncology. *Journal of Clinical Oncology* 1994;12:1789–95.

104. Machin D, Stenning SP, Parmar MK, et al. Thirty years of Medical Research Council randomized trials in solid tumours. *Clinical Oncology* 1997;9:100–14.

105. Djulbegovic B, Lacevic M, Cantor A, Fields KK, Bennett CL, Adams JR, et al. The uncertainty principle and industry-sponsored research. *Lancet* 2000;356:635–8.

106. Joffe S, Harrington DP, George SL, Emanuel EJ, Budzinski LA, Weeks JC. Satisfaction of the uncertainty principle in cancer clinical trials: Retrospective cohort analysis. *British Medical Journal* 2004; 328:1463–7.

107. Soares HP, Kumar A, Daniels S, et al. Evaluation of new treatments in radiation oncology: Are they better than standard treatments? *JAMA* 2005;293:970–8.

108. Lau J, Antman EM, Jimenez-Silva J, et al. Cumulative meta-analysis of therapeutic trials for myocardial infarction. *New England Journal of Medicine* 1992;327:248–54.

109. Clark O, Adams JR, Bennett CL, Djulbegovic B. Erythropoietin, uncertainty principle and cancer related anaemia. *BMC Cancer* 2002;2:23.

110. Antman EM, Lau J, Kupelnick B, Mosteller F, Chalmers TC. A comparison of results of meta-analyses of randomized control trials and recommendations of clinical experts: Treatments for myocardial infarction. *JAMA* 1992;268:240–8.

111. Taylor KM, Margolese RG, Soskolne CL. Physicians' reasons for not entering eligible patients in a randomized clinical trial of surgery for breast cancer. *New England Journal of Medicine* 1984;310:1363–7.

112. Taylor KM, Feldstein ML, Skeel RT, Pandya KJ, Ng P, Carbone PP. Fundamental dilemmas of the randomized clinical trial process: Results of a survey of the 1,737 Eastern Cooperative Oncology Group investigators. *Journal of Clinical Oncology* 1994;12:1796–805.

113. Taylor KM. Physician participation in a randomized clinical trial for ocular melanoma. *Annals of Ophthalmology* 1992;24:337–44.

114. Alderson P. Equipoise as a means of managing uncertainty: Personal, communal and proxy. *Journal of Medical Ethics* 1996;22:135–9.

115. Cheng AC, Lowe M, Stephens DP, Currie BJ. Ethical problems of evaluating a new treatment for melioidosis. *British Medical Journal* 2003;327:1280–2.

116. Clark WF, Garg AX, Blake PG, Rock GA, Heidenheim AP, Sackett DL. Effect of awareness of a randomized controlled trial on use of experimental therapy. *JAMA* 2003;290:1351–5.

117. Jack WJ, Chetty U, Rodger A. Recruitment to a prospective breast conservation trial: Why are so few patients randomised? *British Medical Journal* 1990;301:83–5.

118. Gotay CC. Accrual to cancer clinical trials: Directions from the research literature. *Social Science and Medicine* 1991;33:569–77.

119. O'Brien SG, Guilhot F, Larson RA, Gathmann I, Baccarani M, Cervantes F, et al. Imatinib compared with interferon and low-dose cytarabine for newly diagnosed chronic-phase chronic myeloid leukemia. *New England Journal of Medicine* 2003;348:994–1004.

120. Lantos JD. Was the UK collaborative ECMO trial ethical? *Paediatric and Perinatal Epidemiology* 1997;11:264–8.

121. Gehan EA, Freireich EJ. Non-randomized controls in cancer clinical trials. *New England Journal of Medicine* 1974;290:198–203.

122. Sacks H, Chalmers TC, Smith H, Jr. Randomized versus historical controls for clinical trials. *American Journal of Medicine* 1982;72: 233–40.

123. Miller JN, Colditz GA, Mosteller F. How study design affects outcomes in comparisons of therapy. II: Surgical. *Statistics in Medicine* 1989;8:455–66.

124. Concato J, Shah N, Horwitz RI. Randomized, controlled trials, observational studies, and the hierarchy of research designs. *New England Journal of Medicine* 2000;342:1887–92.

125. Benson K, Hartz AJ. A comparison of observational studies and randomized, controlled trials. *New England Journal of Medicine* 2000;342:1878–86.

126. Ioannidis JP, Haidich AB, Pappa M, et al. Comparison of evidence of treatment effects in randomized and nonrandomized studies. *JAMA* 2001;286:821–30.

127. Schulz KF, Chalmers I, Hayes RJ, Altman DG. Empirical evidence of bias: Dimensions of methodological quality associated with estimates of treatment effects in controlled trials. *JAMA* 1995;273:408–12.

128. Schulz KF. Subverting randomization in controlled trials. *JAMA* 1995;274:1456–8.

129. Byington RP, Curb JD, Mattson ME. Assessment of double-blindness at the conclusion of the beta-Blocker Heart Attack Trial. *JAMA* 1985;253:1733–6.

130. Howard J, Whittemore AS, Hoover JJ, Panos M. How blind was the patient blind in AMIS? *Clinical Pharmacology and Therapeutic* 1982;32:543–53.

131. Freiman JA, Chalmers TC, Smith H, Kuebler RR. The importance of beta, the type II error and sample size in the design and interpretation of the randomized control trial: Survey of 71 "negative" trials. *New England Journal of Medicine* 1978;299:690–4.

132. Sterling TD. Publication decisions and their possible effects on inferences drawn from tests of significance—Or vice versa. *Journal of the American Statistical Association* 1959;54:30–4.

133. Rosenthal R. The "file drawer problem" and tolerance for null results. *Psychological Bulletin* 1979;86:638–41.

134. Dickersin K, Chan S, Chalmers TC, Sacks HS, Smith H. Publication bias and clinical trials. *Controlled Clinical Trials* 1987;8:343–53.

135. Dickersin K, Min YI. Publication bias: The problem that won't go away. *Annals of the New York Academy of Sciences* 1993;703:135–46.

136. Stern JM, Simes RJ. Publication bias: Evidence of delayed publication in a cohort study of clinical research projects. *British Medical Journal* 1997;315:640–5.

137. Ioannidis JP. Effect of the statistical significance of results on the time to completion and publication of randomized efficacy trials. *JAMA* 1998;279:281–6.

138. Krzyzanowska MK, Pintilie M, Tannock IF. Factors associated with failure to publish large randomized trials presented at an oncology meeting. *JAMA* 2003;290:495–501.

139. Antman K, Amato D, Wood W, Carson J, Suit H, Proppe K, et al. Selection bias in clinical trials. *Journal of Clinical Oncology* 1985;3:1142–7.

140. Winger MJ, Macdonald DR, Schold SC, Jr., Cairncross JG. Selection bias in clinical trials of anaplastic glioma. *Annals of Neurology* 1989;26:531–4.

141. Cottin V, Arpin D, Lasset C, Cordier JF, Brune J, Chauvin F, et al. Small-cell lung cancer: Patients included in clinical trials are not representative of the patient population as a whole. *Annals of Oncology* 1999;10:809–15.

142. Bertelsen K. Protocol allocation and exclusion in two Danish randomised trials in ovarian cancer. *British Journal of Cancer* 1991;64:1172–6.

143. Ward LC, Fielding JW, Dunn JA, Kelly KA, for the British Stomach Cancer Group. The selection of cases for randomised trials: A registry survey of concurrent trial and non-trial patients. *British Journal of Cancer* 1992;66:943–50.

144. Als-Nielsen B, Chen W, Gluud C, Kjaergard LL. Association of funding and conclusions in randomized drug trials: A reflection of treatment effect or adverse events? *JAMA* 2003;290:921–8.

145. Tan SB, Dear KB, Bruzzi P, Machin D. Strategy for randomised clinical trials in rare cancers. *British Medical Journal* 2003;327:47–9.

146. Lagakos SW. Clinical trials and rare diseases. *New England Journal of Medicine* 2003;348:2455–6.

147. Slutsky AS. Prone positioning of patients with acute respiratory failure: The editorialist replies. *New England Journal of Medicine* 2002;346:297.

148. Lantos JD. The "inclusion benefit" in clinical trials. *Journal of Pediatrics* 1999;134:130–1.

149. Braunholtz DA, Edwards SJ, Lilford RJ. Are randomized clinical trials good for us (in the short term)? Evidence for a "trial effect." *Journal of Clinical Epidemiology* 2001;54:217–24.

150. Stiller CA. Centralised treatment, entry to trials and survival. *British Journal of Cancer* 1994;70:352–62.

151. Peppercorn JM, Weeks JC, Cook EF, Joffe S. Comparison of outcomes in cancer patients treated within and outside clinical trials: Conceptual framework and structured review. *Lancet* 2004;363:263–70.

152. Miller FG, Silverman HJ. The ethical relevance of the standard of care in the design of clinical trials. *American Journal of Respiratory and Critical Care Medicine* 2004;169:562–4.

153. Steinbrook R. How best to ventilate? Trial design and patient safety in studies of the acute respiratory distress syndrome. *New England Journal of Medicine* 2003;348:1393–401.

154. Steinbrook R. Trial design and patient safety—The debate continues. *New England Journal of Medicine* 2003;349:629–30.

155. Drazen JM. Controlling research trials. *New England Journal of Medicine* 2003;348:1377–80.

156. Acute Respiratory Distress Syndrome Network. Ventilation with lower tidal volumes as compared with traditional tidal volumes for acute lung injury and the acute respiratory distress syndrome. *New England Journal of Medicine* 2000;342:1301–8.

157. Office for Human Research Protections. Letter to Lee E. Limbird, Associate Vice Chancellor for Research, Vanderbilt University, July 25, 2003. [Online] Available: http://www.hhs.gov/ohrp/detrm_letrs/YR03/jul03af.pdf.

158. Zelen M. A new design for randomized clinical trials. *New England Journal of Medicine* 1979;300:1242–5.

159. O'Rourke PP, Crone RK, Vacanti JP, et al. Extracorporeal membrane oxygenation and conventional medical therapy in neonates with persistent pulmonary hypertension of the newborn: A prospective randomized study. *Pediatrics* 1989;84:957–63.

160. Ellenberg SS. Randomization designs in comparative clinical trials. *New England Journal of Medicine* 1984;310:1404–8.

161. Altman DG, Whitehead J, Parmar MK, Stenning SP, Fayers PM, Machin D. Randomised consent designs in cancer clinical trials. *European Journal of Cancer* 1995;31A:1934–44.

162. Snowdon C, Elbourne D, Garcia J. Zelen randomization: Attitudes of parents participating in a neonatal clinical trial. *Controlled Clinical Trials* 1999;20:149–71.

163. Marquis D. An argument that all prerandomized clinical trials are unethical. *Journal of Medicine and Philosophy* 1986;11:367–83.

164. Truog RD, Robinson W, Randolph A, Morris A. Is informed consent always necessary for randomized, controlled trials? *New England Journal of Medicine* 1999;340:804–7.

165. Rogers CG, Tyson JE, Kennedy KA, Broyles RS, Hickman JF. Conventional consent with opting in versus simplified consent with opting out: An exploratory trial for studies that do not increase patient risk. *Journal of Pediatrics* 1998;132:606–11.

166. Biros MH, Lewis RJ, Olson CM, Runge JW, Cummins RO, Fost N. Informed consent in emergency research: Consensus Statement from the Coalition Conference of Acute Resuscitation and Critical Care Researchers. *JAMA* 1995;273:1283–7.

167. Department of Health and Human Services. Waiver of Informed Consent Requirements in Certain Emergency Research; Waiver. *Federal Register* 1996;61(192):51531–3. [Online] Available: http://www.hhs.gov/ohrp/humansubjects/guidance/hsdc97–01.htm.

168. Kodish E, Eder M, Noll RB, Ruccione K, Lange B, Angiolillo A, et al. Communication of randomization in childhood leukemia trials. *JAMA* 2004;291:470–5.

169. van Stuijvenberg M, Suur MH, de Vos S, et al. Informed consent, parental awareness, and reasons for participating in a randomised controlled study. *Archives of Disease in Childhood* 1998;79:120–5.

170. Snowdon C, Garcia J, Elbourne D. Making sense of randomization: Responses of parents of critically ill babies to random allocation of treatment in a clinical trial. *Social Science and Medicine* 1997;45:1337–55.

171. Benson PR, Roth LH, Appelbaum PS, Lidz CW, Winslade WJ. Information disclosure, subject understanding, and informed consent in psychiatric research. *Law and Human Behavior* 1988;12:455–75.

172. Aaronson NK, Visser-Pol E, Leenhouts GH, et al. Telephone-based nursing intervention improves the effectiveness of the informed consent process in cancer clinical trials. *Journal of Clinical Oncology* 1996;14:984–96.

173. Simes RJ, Tattersall MH, Coates AS, Raghavan D, Solomon HJ, Smartt H. Randomised comparison of procedures for obtaining informed consent in clinical trials of treatment for cancer. *British Medical Journal* 1986;293:1065–8.

174. Davis SW, Nealon EO, Stone JC. Evaluation of the National Cancer Institute's clinical trials booklet. *Journal of the National Cancer Institute Monographs* 1993;14:139–45.

175. Howard JM, DeMets D. How informed is informed consent? The BHAT experience. *Controlled Clinical Trials* 1981;2:287–303.

176. Joffe S, Cook EF, Cleary PD, Clark JW, Weeks JC. Quality of informed consent in cancer clinical trials: A cross-sectional survey. *Lancet* 2001;358:1772–7.

177. DCCT Research Group. Implementation of a multicomponent process to obtain informed consent in the Diabetes Control and Complications Trial. *Controlled Clinical Trials* 1989;10:83–96.

178. Coyne CA, Xu R, Raich P, et al. Randomized, controlled trial of an easy-to-read informed consent statement for clinical trial participation: A study of the Eastern Cooperative Oncology Group. *Journal of Clinical Oncology* 2003;21:836–42.

179. Vickers AJ, de Craen AJ. Why use placebos in clinical trials? A narrative review of the methodological literature. *Journal of Clinical Epidemiology* 2000;53:157–61.

180. Lantos J. Ethics, randomization, and technology assessment. *Cancer* 1994;74:2653–6.

181. Department of Health and Human Services, National Institutes of Health, and Office for Human Research Protections. The Common Rule, Title 45 (Public Welfare), Code of Federal Regulations, Part 46 (Protection of Human Subjects); Subpart D—Additional Protections for Children Involved as Subjects in Research. [Online] June 23, 2005. Available: http://www.hhs.gov/ohrp/humansubjects/guidance/45cfr46.htm#subpartd.

182. Crouch RA. Eligibility, extrapolation and equipoise: Unlearned lessons in the ethical analysis of clinical research. *IRB: Ethics and Human Research* 2001;23(4):6–9.

183. Simes RJ. Publication bias: The case for an international registry of clinical trials. *Journal of Clinical Oncology* 1986;4:1529–41.

184. Dickersin K, Rennie D. Registering clinical trials. *JAMA* 2003; 290:516–23.

185. Berwick DM. Harvesting knowledge from improvement. *JAMA* 1996;275:877–8.

186. Stadtmauer EA, et al., for the Philadelphia Bone Marrow Transplant Group. Conventional-dose chemotherapy compared with high-dose chemotherapy plus autologous hematopoietic stem-cell transplantation for metastatic breast cancer. *New England Journal of Medicine* 2000;342:1069–76.

187. Rossouw JE, Anderson GL, Prentice RL, LaCroix AZ, Kooperberg C, Stefanick ML, et al. Risks and benefits of estrogen plus progestin in healthy postmenopausal women: Principal results from the Women's Health Initiative randomized controlled trial. *JAMA* 2002;288:321–3.

188. Weijer C, Shapiro SH, Glass KC. Clinical equipoise and not the uncertainty principle is the moral underpinning of the randomised controlled trial—for and against—education and debate. *British Medical Journal* 2000;321:756–8.

189. Vist GE, Hagen KB, Devereaux PJ, Bryant D, Kristoffersen DT, Oxman AD. Systematic review to determine whether participation in a trial influences outcome. *British Medical Journal* 2005;330:1175.

Franklin G. Miller

The Ethics of Placebo-Controlled Trials

Randomized clinical trials test the efficacy of experimental or existing treatments by comparing them with a control intervention. The control group may receive a placebo disguised to appear indistinguishable from the treatment under investigation or standard treatment. Placebo-controlled trials have generated considerable ethical controversy and debate when they are used to evaluate treatments for patients with particular disorders despite the availability of proven effective treatment. Critics of placebo-controlled trials in these circumstances have argued that the use of placebos in the control group rather than proven effective treatment is unethical.[1,2] It is alleged to violate the therapeutic obligation of physicians, by randomizing patients to an intervention known to be inferior to standard treatment. These placebo-controlled trials contravene the principle of "clinical equipoise," which is widely held to be an ethical foundation for the design and conduct of randomized clinical trials.[3,4] Defenders of such placebo-controlled trials have contended that placebo controls are ethically justifiable in these circumstances provided that sound methodological reasons support their use and that they do not expose research participants to excessive risks of harm.[5–7] At the heart of the debate are fundamental issues concerning the nature and ethical justification of clinical research.

The ethics of clinical research has two objectives: promoting valuable and rigorous science in the service of human health and safeguarding the rights and well-being of research subjects.[8] Because these objectives can conflict, ethical analysis of many difficult issues, including placebo-controlled trials, involves the careful weighing and balancing of competing considerations of scientific methodology and subject protection. Whether placebo-controlled trials can be ethically justified in research on disorders with proven effective treatments depends on an understanding of the strength and weakness of alternative scientific methods for evaluating treatments. After introducing the rationale for placebo-controlled trials as a rigorous method of testing treatment efficacy, this chapter examines the methodological difficulties associated with active-controlled trials, especially those designed to test equivalence or "noninferiority." It then reviews leading regulatory standards and codes of ethics relating to the use of placebo controls and undertakes a critique of clinical equipoise. This critique paves the way for developing an ethical framework for determining when placebo-controlled trials are justified despite the existence of proven effective treatment. Finally, the chapter discusses the difficult ethical issues concerning the use of placebo-controlled trials for "vulnerable" populations: children and cognitively impaired adults.

The "Gold Standard"

The history of the placebo-controlled trial has been traced to an experiment to evaluate the therapeutic efficacy of "animal magnetism" or "mesmerism" conducted in 1784 by a French royal commission headed by Benjamin Franklin.[9,10] The randomized, double-blind, placebo-controlled trial, however, did not become a common method of clinical research until the mid-20th century.[9] It is widely regarded as the most rigorous method for testing treatment efficacy.[11] A basic understanding of the rationale for testing treatments in placebo-controlled trials is necessary to appreciate the ethical debate.

Two distinctions are useful at the outset: (1) the distinction between absolute and relative efficacy and (2) that between superiority and equivalence trials. Absolute efficacy is indicated by credible evidence that a treatment for a given disorder produces improvement in a relevant clinical outcome. It is typically measured by demonstrating a statistically significant and clinically important superiority of the treatment over a placebo control in a double-blind randomized trial. Relative efficacy is indicated by credible evidence that a treatment under investigation is better (or no worse) than a standard treatment with respect to a relevant clinical outcome, as measured by an active-controlled randomized trial. Thus, the primary purpose of the placebo-controlled trial is to ascertain whether a treatment under investigation for a defined group of patients with a given disorder has absolute efficacy. This is determined by observing specified clinical outcomes of patients randomly assigned to an investigational treatment or a placebo control. Placebo-controlled trials are typically conducted under double-blind conditions, with the aim of making it impossible for either patient-subjects or investigators rating trial outcomes to know whether the experimental treatment or placebo was received.

Superiority trials are designed to show that an investigational treatment is better than a suitable control treatment with respect to a relevant clinical outcome. Equivalence (or noninferiority) trials are designed to demonstrate that an investigational treatment is not inferior to a standard treatment. Placebo-controlled trials, which test absolute efficacy, are superiority trials. Active-controlled trials comparing two or more treatments may be designed either as superiority trials or equivalence trials. As discussed below, equivalence trials pose distinctive methodological problems.

The scientific merit of placebo-controlled trials can be illustrated by comparing them with "open label" trials—single-arm clinical trials without randomization, control groups, or masking of the treatment under investigation. Consider an eight-week open label trial of an experimental treatment T in patients diagnosed with major depression. Suppose that this trial demonstrates that 70% of the patients experienced a 50% or greater reduction of depressive symptoms, as compared with baseline measurement, using a standard rating scale. Does it follow that T is an effective treatment for depression? The patients improved, but did their reduction in symptoms result from taking T? This is a question of causation, the answer to which requires guarding against the fallacy of post hoc ergo propter hoc (after that, therefore because of that).

In the case of such an open label trial, the temporal sequence of an observed improvement following the administration of treatment does not imply that the treatment caused the improvement. The patients might have improved without T, owing to spontaneous remissions or the fact that depression has a characteristic pattern of waxing and waning symptoms. Alternatively, they may have improved because they hoped and expected relief from taking a new treatment, thereby manifesting a placebo effect. Similarly, the clinical attention of investigators from an esteemed research institution, involving diagnostic assessment and measurement of study outcomes, may also have contributed to improved mood reported by these patients. The fact that both the patients and the investigators knew that all trial participants received T may have biased the mood ratings in the direction of symptomatic improvement. Perhaps the patients reported feeling better because they wanted to please the investigators or thought that they ought to feel better after taking an antidepressant.[12] All these factors can confound judgments of treatment efficacy. The purpose of the placebo-controlled trial is to conduct a rigorous experiment that controls for these confounding factors in order to make valid causal inferences about treatment efficacy.

A placebo-controlled trial of T would randomize patients with major depression to T or a suitable placebo control (PT). Ideally, the placebo-controlled trial administers test conditions that vary only in the fact that half the patients receive T (an agent with certain pharmacologic properties) and half receive an identically appearing "inert" placebo (for example, a sugar pill) without any known pharmacologic properties. If the patients receiving T are observed to have a significantly greater reduction in symptoms of depression than those receiving PT, then it is inferred that the pharmacologic properties of T are responsible for this result. For example, if half of the trial participants receiving T experience a 50% symptom reduction, as compared with one-quarter of those on placebo, and this difference is statistically significant, then T has therapeutic efficacy.

The placebo-controlled trial is not a perfect tool for testing absolute therapeutic efficacy. Most importantly, inferences about treatment efficacy may not be valid if the double-blind conditions of a trial are unsuccessful, such that trial participants or investigators are able to discern whether the investigational treatment or placebo has been administered. Nonetheless, there is no more rigorous method that is feasible for testing treatment efficacy with respect to disorders that lack treatment, or when existing treatments have not been proven effective.

Active-Controlled Trials

When proven effective treatment already exists for a given disorder, it is natural to think that any new treatment should be tested exclusively against the standard treatment. Apart from ethical concerns of protecting research participants, the use of placebo-controlled trials in this circumstance would seem to lack scientific or clinical value. Clinicians want to know whether an experimental treatment is as good or better than existing treatment, not whether it is better than "nothing."[1] From this point of view, although first generation investigational treatments should be tested against placebo, second and subsequent generation treatments should be evaluated exclusively in comparison with existing treatments in active-controlled trials.[2] This perspective, however, can be challenged on methodological grounds.

Three methodological reasons support the use of placebo-controlled trials despite the existence of proven effective treatment. First, assessing the absolute efficacy of experimental treatments remains desirable, as distinct from evaluating relative efficacy in comparison with standard treatment. The new treatment may or may not be more effective than the standard treatment. However, the difference in efficacy between the experimental and standard treatments is likely to be smaller than the difference between the experimental treatment and placebo. Therefore, in order to have adequate statistical power to evaluate efficacy, a placebo-controlled trial would require fewer subjects than an active-controlled superiority trial, because the sample size needed to detect a difference between experimental and control interventions varies inversely with the anticipated magnitude of this difference. Indeed, if the anticipated difference between the experimental treatment and placebo is twice as large as that between the former and standard treatment, then approximately four times as many subjects would be required for the active-controlled superiority trial.[13] Accordingly, placebo-controlled trials are more efficient. Because they require fewer subjects, they can be completed more quickly and at less cost. This makes it advantageous to demonstrate the absolute efficacy of experimental treatments in placebo-controlled trials before planning larger scale active-controlled trials.

Second, as compared with active-controlled trials, placebo-controlled trials afford a more accurate determination of whether adverse events observed during a trial are caused by the pharmacologic properties of the investigational drug or reflect the symptomatic expression of the disorder.[14] The lack of a control group not receiving pharmacologic treatment makes active-controlled trials less advantageous in this respect. To be sure, this assessment is complicated by the fact that placebo controls are often associated with reported adverse effects that mirror those of the investigational treatment; however, a higher incidence of adverse effects in the treatment arm as compared with the placebo arm can be attributed to the pharmacologic properties of the treatment.

Third, active-controlled superiority trials may not be feasible for testing new drugs, especially when they are not expected to be substantially more effective than existing treatment. Nonetheless, these new drugs may offer considerable clinical value if they have a more favorable side-effect profile. Furthermore, when existing treatment is only partially effective, providing measurable relief of symptoms for some but not all patients, the availability of new treatments can expand the range of therapeutic options, even though they are no better on the whole than standard treatment.[6] Under these conditions, it is possible to conduct active-controlled trials designed to test the equivalence or noninferiority of an experimental and a standard treatment.

Active-controlled equivalence trials, however, are subject to serious methodological difficulties.[5,6,15] A finding of no significant difference between the two treatments does not imply that the new treatment is effective. It is possible that in this particular trial neither the experimental drug nor active comparator was effective. Many standard, proven effective drugs are not uniformly effective in clinical trials. Without a placebo control to validate absolute efficacy, active-controlled equivalence trials may not be capable of discriminating between apparent and real equivalence. This difficulty can be surmounted when standard drugs are consistently and robustly effective, making it probable that the lack of observed difference amounts to equivalence. Otherwise, active-controlled equivalence trials, in contrast to superiority trials, do not permit valid inferences about treatment efficacy; that is, they lack "assay sensitivity."[5] This methodological limitation of the active-controlled equivalence trial is analogous to the more obvious inability of open label treatment trials to discriminate between true and apparent treatment efficacy. In both cases, the difficulty derives, in large part, from the use of a trial method that is not designed to determine the *superiority* of an experimental treatment to an appropriate control group.

These methodological considerations are ethically significant. The greater efficiency of placebo-controlled trials means that rigorous initial tests of efficacy can be conducted without exposing large numbers of subjects to potentially ineffective agents.[16] These trials also provide clinically useful information on the side effects of new treatments as compared with an untreated control group. Moreover, serious problems can arise when active-controlled

equivalence trials are used as evidence for licensing or validating treatments in cases where active-controlled *superiority* trials would not be feasible. These equivalence studies could lead to licensing new treatments, or validating available treatments that previously have not been proven effective for a given disorder, when these treatments in fact are no better than a placebo intervention. Because most drugs cause unwanted and potentially harmful side effects, drugs that lack specific pharmacologic efficacy—therapeutic benefit beyond a placebo response—do not have an acceptable risk-benefit ratio.

Nevertheless, these methodological considerations, though ethically relevant, are not sufficient to justify the use of placebo-controlled trials to test treatments for a disorder when proven effective therapy exists. Further ethical analysis is necessary to evaluate whether placebo controls that withhold proven effective treatment are acceptable, and whether the risks from placebo assignment are not excessive and are justifiable by the value of the knowledge to be gained from the research. Though related, these are logically distinct issues. Some prominent critics of placebo-controlled trials have argued that use of placebo controls in these circumstances is morally wrong regardless of whether they are harmful.[2] Before undertaking a critical examination of these ethical issues, I review the guidance available from existing regulatory standards and codes of ethics.

Regulatory Standards and Codes of Ethics

Regulatory standards and codes of ethics differ in their guidance concerning placebo-controlled trials when standard, effective treatments exist. United States federal regulations governing research with humans contain no explicit prohibition or restriction of the use of placebo controls in clinical trials.[17] Research involving humans can be approved by institutional review boards (IRBs) provided that several conditions are met, including the following: (a) "Risks to subjects are minimized . . . by using procedures which are consistent with sound research design and which do not unnecessarily expose subjects to risk"; (b) "[r]isks to subjects are reasonable in relationship to anticipated benefits, if any, to subjects, and the importance of the knowledge that may reasonably be expected to result"; and (c) "[i]nformed consent will be sought from each prospective subject or the subject's legally authorized representative."[17]

However, the *Institutional Review Board Guidebook* prepared by the Office for Protection from Research Risks (now the Office for Human Research Protections), which oversees research with humans, states, "A design involving a placebo control should not be used where there is a standard treatment that has been shown to be superior to placebo by convincing evidence."[18] Regulations and guidelines of the U.S. Food and Drug Administration (FDA) require "adequate and well-controlled" studies to demonstrate the effectiveness of drugs as a condition of approving their clinical use.[19] Although the FDA does not require placebo controls, its policy gives a decided preference to placebo-controlled trials when such trials do not pose risks of death or serious harm. FDA regulations define an "adequate and well-controlled study" as one that "uses a design that permits a valid comparison with a control to provide a quantitative assessment of drug effect."[19] Among the variety of control conditions considered, the regulations mention placebo controls first. Concerning active treatment controls the regulations state: "The test drug is compared with known effective therapy; for example, where the condition treated is such that administration of placebo or no treatment would be contrary to the interest of the patient."[19]

It might be thought that FDA regulations should favor active-controlled trials whenever standard, effective treatment exists, because use of placebo controls in such cases is "contrary to the interest of the patient." However, in a supplementary advisory on placebo-controlled and active-controlled study designs, the FDA points out the methodological limitations of active-controlled designs: "For certain drug classes, such as analgesics, antidepressants or antianxiety drugs, failure to show superiority to placebo in a given study is common. . . . In those situations active control trials showing no difference between the new drug and control are of little value as primary evidence of effectiveness and the active control design, the study design most often proposed as an alternative to use of a placebo, is not credible."[20]

The FDA position on the issue of placebo-controlled trials has been developed in detail by Robert Temple and Susan Ellenberg.[5,6] They argue that in view of the methodological considerations favoring placebo-controlled trials, placebo controls are justifiable as long as patients randomized to placebo are not exposed to known risks of irreversible harm, such as death, disease progression, or permanent functional disability. This stance is also reflected in the guidelines for control group selection adopted by the International Conference on Harmonisation of Technical Requirements for Registration of Pharmaceuticals for Human Use, which formulates recommended regulatory policy for the United States, the European Union, and Japan.[21]

The Declaration of Helsinki, endorsed by the World Medical Association, is the leading international code of ethics for clinical research. In an influential article entitled, "The Continued Unethical Use of Placebo Controls," Kenneth Rothman and Karin Michels appealed to the Declaration to support their position that placebo-controlled trials are unethical in disorders for which treatments of proven efficacy exist.[1] The relevant principle of the Declaration cited in favor of this ethical stance was the following: "In any medical study, every patient—including those of a control group, if any—should be assured of the best proven diagnostic and therapeutic method."[22] Critics of this ethical position have responded that the cited language would also appear to rule out any randomized clinical trial comparing a standard with an experimental treatment.[23,24] The point of these trials is to determine if the experimental treatment is at least as effective as standard treatment. Patients randomized to experimental treatment are not assured "the best proven" treatment, because the efficacy of the experimental treatment has yet to be determined, and is the very issue under investigation in the trial.

The Declaration of Helsinki was extensively revised in 2000. Its prohibition of placebo-controlled trials when proven effective therapy exists was made unambiguous: "The benefits, risks, burden and effectiveness of a new method should be tested against those of the best current prophylactic, diagnostic and therapeutic methods. This does not exclude the use of placebo, or no treatment, in studies where no proven prophylactic, diagnostic or therapeutic method exists."[22] Nevertheless, a year later, the World Medical Association issued a Note of Clarification concerning the stance of the Declaration on the use of placebo-controlled trials, which states that placebo controls may be ethically justifiable despite the availability of proven effective treatment in two cir-

cumstances: "(1) [w]here for compelling and scientifically sound methodological reasons its use is necessary to determine the efficacy or safety of a prophylactic, diagnostic or therapeutic method, or (2) [w]here a prophylactic, diagnostic or therapeutic method is being investigated for a minor condition and the patients who receive placebo will not be subject to any additional risk of serious or irreversible harm."[22] The Declaration of Helsinki now appears internally inconsistent, containing a provision that prohibits placebo-controlled trials when proven effective treatment exists and a Note of Clarification that permits them under two conditions (see Chapter 13).

The latest version (2002) of the International Ethical Guidelines for Biomedical Research Involving Human Subjects promulgated by the Council for International Organizations of Medical Sciences (CIOMS) permits the use of placebo controls despite the existence of "an established effective intervention" under two conditions: "when withholding an established effective intervention would expose subjects to, at most, temporary discomfort or delay in relief of symptom;" or "when use of an established effective intervention as comparator would not yield scientifically reliable results and use of placebo would not add any risk of serious or irreversible harm to the subjects."[25] This second condition provides more sound guidance than the comparable first condition in the Note of Clarification of the Declaration of Helsinki, because it limits the use of placebo controls when methodologically indicated to situations that do not pose serious or irreversible harm (see Chapter 16). The CIOMS guidelines also address the use of placebo controls to test interventions for use in less developed countries when an established effective intervention is not available. This controversial aspect of the debate over placebo-controlled trials is outside the scope of this chapter (see Chapters 64–67).

The lack of consistent guidance on the use of placebo-controlled trials in the extant regulations and codes of ethics reflects the unresolved ethical controversy over this issue. In any case, these documents have limited utility for ethical analysis, because they typically do not provide any systematic ethical rationale for the positions they adopt. The next section assesses critically the leading ethical argument against the use of placebo-controlled trials when proven effective treatment exists.

Clinical Equipoise

The principle or doctrine of *clinical equipoise,* first articulated by Benjamin Freedman, is widely regarded as central to the ethical justification of randomized clinical trials (RCTs)[3,26] (see Chapter 24). To understand this principle and its bearing on the ethics of placebo-controlled trials, it is useful to place it within the context of philosophical inquiry concerning "the RCT dilemma." During the 1980s, philosophers interested in research ethics recognized a tension between the obligation of physicians to offer optimal care to their patients ("the therapeutic obligation") and the limitations on medical treatment provided in the context of randomized clinical trials. Don Marquis addressed this problem in a 1983 essay, "Leaving Therapy to Chance."[27] The title is significant, suggesting that the randomized clinical trial is a form of therapy rather than an activity of clinical research ethically distinct from therapeutic medicine. Marquis began his essay, "Consider this dilemma: according to an argument that is hard to refute, the procedure for conducting randomized clinical trials of anticancer drugs is incompatible with the ethics of the physician-patient relationship. If this problem is to be resolved, then either a key procedure for achieving scientific knowledge in medicine must be given up or unethical behavior by physicians must be tolerated."[27]

Fred Gifford, following the lead of Marquis, examined the RCT dilemma in greater depth. He described the problem as follows: "The central dilemma concerning randomized clinical trials (RCTs) arises out of some simple facts about causal methodology (RCTs are the best way to generate the reliable causal knowledge necessary for optimally-informed action) and a prima facie plausible principle concerning how physicians should treat their patients (always do what it is most reasonable to believe will be best for the patient)."[28] Neither Marquis nor Gifford found what they regarded as a satisfactory solution, and neither considered the possibility that the ethical norms governing the therapeutic relationship between physician and patient may not be appropriate for guiding the ethics of clinical trials.

Freedman offered a solution to the RCT dilemma that gained widespread acceptance within bioethics and the medical world. In a landmark article published in 1987, he argued that in clinical trials, the tension between scientific experimentation and the therapeutic obligation of physicians could be overcome by means of the principle of "clinical equipoise."[3] The term *equipoise* had been coined by Charles Fried to describe an ethically necessary condition for conducting a randomized clinical trial: physician-investigators must be indifferent between the therapeutic value of the experimental and control treatments evaluated in the study.[29] Physician-investigators not in a state of equipoise would be inviting patients to enroll in a trial allocating up to half of them to treatment they believed to be inferior.

Freedman argued that Fried's formulation of equipoise was unduly constraining and failed to reflect the nature of medicine as a social practice according to a professional standard of care. He labeled Fried's original concept of equipoise *theoretical equipoise* (sometimes called *individual equipoise*) and contrasted it with his favored concept of *clinical equipoise* (sometimes called *collective equipoise*). In the latter sense of equipoise, any individual investigator or physician might believe that one arm of the randomized clinical trial offers a therapeutic benefit over the other arm, but the medical profession as a whole remains divided as to which arm is the better treatment. According to Freedman, the trial would be ethical so long as the professional community has not yet reached consensus, which recognizes that "medicine is social rather than individual in nature."[3] What makes clinical equipoise an ethical requirement of randomized clinical trials is that only when it is satisfied will patients be assured that they will not be randomized to treatment known to be inferior. In a later article, Freedman and his colleagues described clinical equipoise, and its implications for placebo-controlled trials, in the following way:

That principle can be put into normative or scientific language. As a normative matter, it defines ethical trial design as prohibiting any compromise of a patient's right to medical treatment by enrolling in a study. The same concern is often stated scientifically when we assert that a study must start with an honest null hypothesis, genuine medical uncertainty concerning the relative merits of the various treatment arms included in the trial's design. These principles allow for testing new agents when sufficient information has accu-

mulated to create a state of clinical equipoise vis-à-vis established methods of treatment. At the same time they foreclose the use of placebos in the face of established treatment, because enrolling in a trial would imply that a proportion of enrollees will receive medical attention currently considered inferior by the expert community.[2]

To evaluate critically the principle of clinical equipoise, it is important to appreciate the ethically significant differences between clinical research and medical care.[30,31] In routine medical care, physicians are obligated to offer individualized therapy to particular patients consistent with the professional standard of care. Risks of diagnostic and treatment interventions are justified exclusively by the prospect of medical benefits to the patient. In contrast, clinical trials differ from medical care in their purpose, characteristic methods, and justification of risks. The randomized clinical trial is an experiment designed to answer a scientific question, not a form of personal therapy. Clinical trials aim at developing knowledge that can lead to improving the medical care of future patients, not at promoting the medical best interests of those enrolled in research. Unlike routine medical care, randomized clinical trials assign patient-participants to treatment (or placebo) by a random method; they are often conducted under double-blind conditions; and they typically restrict the dosing of experimental and control treatments and the use of concomitant treatments in accordance with the study protocol. These trials often contain a drug "washout" phase prior to randomization, designed to avoid confounding the evaluation of the investigational treatment with the effects of medication that patients were receiving prior to trial participation. Additionally, clinical trials include procedures designed to measure trial outcomes, such as blood draws, biopsies, lumbar punctures, and imaging procedures, which carry some degree of risk of harm or discomfort to participants without offering them compensating benefits. Similarly, outside the context of clinical trials, studies of patients designed to improve understanding of pathophysiology administer research procedures that pose risks without holding out the prospect of medical benefits to them. These risks of clinical research are justified by the value of knowledge to be generated. In sum, clinical research routinely incorporates features of study design that are not justifiable within the ethical framework of medical care.

These key differences between medical care and clinical research are ethically significant. In view of these differences, the ethical principles that guide medical care are not the same as those that guide clinical research. To be sure, in the abstract, the leading principles of beneficence and nonmaleficence (as well as autonomy and justice) apply to both activities.[26] However, the meaning of these principles differs importantly in the case of clinical research and medical care. Beneficence and nonmaleficence in medical care are patient-centered norms that guide physicians in the treatment of their particular patients. Together, they prescribe optimal medical attention, or, at least, conformity to the professional standard of care. In clinical research, beneficence concerns promoting the social good of improving health by means of producing generalizable knowledge; and nonmaleficence limits the risks to which research participants can be exposed for the sake of this goal. The investigator in conducting clinical research typically does not function primarily as the personal physician of enrolled patient-participants, and therefore is not subject to the same therapeutic obligations that govern medical care.

Although intuitively appealing, clinical equipoise is fundamentally mistaken. This principle conflates the ethics of clinical research with the ethics of medical care. The RCT dilemma, for which clinical equipoise was proposed as a solution, is a false dilemma. Clinical equipoise, and all other forms of equipoise, make sense as a normative requirement for clinical trials only on the presumption that physician-investigators who conduct these trials have a therapeutic obligation to the research participants enrolled in them. The "therapeutic obligation" of investigators, forming one horn of "the RCT dilemma," constitutes a misconception about the ethics of clinical trials. The presumption that randomized clinical trials must be compatible with the ethics of the physician-patient relationship assumes erroneously that the randomized clinical trial is a form of therapy, thus misapplying the principles of therapeutic beneficence and nonmaleficence that govern clinical medicine to the fundamentally different practice of clinical research. It is impossible to maintain strict fidelity to doing what is best medically for individual patients in the context of ethical randomized clinical trials, because they are not designed for, and may conflict with, personalized care. The project of bridging the gap between therapy and research via the doctrine of clinical equipoise is doomed to fail.

Accordingly, clinical equipoise provides mistaken guidance about the ethics of placebo-controlled trials. Control groups in clinical trials that depart from a validated standard of medical care require justification but they are not inherently unethical. Placebo controls should be understood as no different in principle from any research procedures that pose risks to participants without a prospect of compensating medical benefit.[30] Placebo controls are unethical if they are not necessary to answer a clinically valuable scientific question, or if they pose excessive risks. However, the normative assumptions behind clinical equipoise—which evaluate clinical trials with respect to the prevailing medical standard of care—are ethically irrelevant to the situation of clinical research.

Clinical equipoise is also misguided because it confuses a valid methodological principle with a dubious stance on the ethics of selecting appropriate control groups for randomized clinical trials. Freedman and his colleagues have equated the methodological, and ethical, requirement that clinical studies have "an honest null hypothesis" and the ethical norm that physician-investigators have a therapeutic obligation to patient-participants, so that it is unethical to randomize them to known inferior treatment.[2,3] These two components of clinical equipoise, however, are not equivalent. To have scientific and potential clinical value, all clinical trials require an honest null hypothesis. There must be sufficient uncertainty about the hypothesis being tested in a clinical trial to make it worth conducting. Randomized clinical trials comparing an experimental treatment with placebo typically are instituted to test an honest null hypothesis. It is not known whether the experimental treatment being evaluated would be superior to a placebo control with respect to study outcomes. Yet when proven effective treatment exists for the disorder under investigation, these placebo-controlled trials violate clinical equipoise because randomization to placebo involves treatment that is known to be inferior to available therapy.[2,4] The critical assessment of clinical equipoise must detach the sound principle of scientific merit enjoining an honest null hypothesis from the erroneous ethical principle that control groups must always conform to the scientifically validated standard of medical care.

Charles Weijer, a leading advocate of clinical equipoise, has recently claimed that "[p]lacebo-controlled trials in the context of

serious illnesses such as depression or schizophrenia are ethically egregious precisely because no competent physician would fail to offer therapy to a patient with the condition."[32] But given the differences between the ethics of clinical research and the ethics of medical care, appealing to what competent physicians would do in medical practice has no inherent ethical bearing on what is justifiable in the context of clinical research. Instead, we should be concerned about the methodological rationale for use of placebo controls and the consequences to patient-participants of placebo assignment.

Ethical Framework for Placebo-Controlled Trials

Ethical evaluation of placebo controls as a scientific tool for testing treatment efficacy requires attention to five issues: (1) methodological rationale, (2) fair selection of participants, (3) assessment of risks from placebo assignment, (4) safeguards to minimize risks, and (5) informed consent.[7,33] Participant selection is addressed briefly in the final section of this chapter devoted to placebo-controlled trials in children and cognitively impaired adults.

Methodological Rationale

The use of placebo controls must be methodologically necessary or desirable to achieve valid trial results. For the reasons indicated above, initial efficacy evaluation of experimental treatments in comparison with placebo controls is desirable, notwithstanding the fact that proven effective treatment exists, provided that the risks from receiving placebo are not excessive. Additionally, in comparing new treatments with standard treatments, placebo controls will often be necessary to assure the internal validity of trials designed to evaluate equivalence. Without a placebo control, it often would be difficult, if not impossible, to determine whether apparent equivalence reflected the efficacy of both treatments or the fact that neither was effective. This holds for chronic disorders with waxing and waning symptoms when existing treatments often are only partially effective, such as depression and anxiety, migraine headaches, multiple sclerosis, and stable angina. Randomized trials of these disorders evaluate treatments on subjective outcomes of symptom relief and have high rates of placebo response. Without placebo controls, trials showing lack of significant differences between experimental and standard treatments will not permit valid inferences regarding treatment efficacy.

When placebo controls are not methodologically indicated, they should not be used.[34] Two asthma clinical trials demonstrate the unnecessary, and therefore unethical, use of placebo controls. These two studies compared combination therapy with monotherapy as well as placebo.

The first study enrolled patients with "a history of at least 1yr of intermittent or persistent asthma symptoms treated with inhaled corticosteroids for at least 6 wks before the prestudy visit."[35] Patients were randomized to receive either the inhaled corticosteroid beclomethasone combined with the leukotriene antagonist montelukast (193 subjects), bechlomethasone monotherapy (200 subjects), montelukast monotherapy (201 subjects), or placebo (48 subjects). The trial lasted 16 weeks.

The second study enrolled patients who "had a medical history of asthma . . . of at least 6 months' duration that required pharmacotherapy over the 6 months preceding the study."[36] For this 12-week trial, patients were randomized to receive one of three treatments or placebo: the combination of the inhaled corticosteroid fluticasone propionate and the long-acting beta-agonist salmeterol (92 subjects), either of these alone as monotherapy (92 and 90 subjects each), and placebo (82 subjects).

Both studies were powered to detect significant differences between combination therapies and monotherapies. The statistical analysis section of the first study stated: "This sample size allowed detection, with 95% power (at alpha = 0.05; two-sided test), of a 6.0 percentage point difference in FEV1 (percent change from baseline) and a 10.0% difference in daytime symptoms score (change from baseline) between the additivity and beclomethasone treatment groups."[35]

In these trials, there was no clear or compelling scientific or clinical rationale for placebo controls. Because both employed sample sizes powered to detect significant treatment differences between combination and monotherapy, placebo controls were methodologically unnecessary. They could, and should, have been designed as active-controlled superiority trials without placebo controls, thus avoiding the exposure of asthmatic patients in need of maintenance treatment to placebo for up to 12 or 16 weeks. In the article reporting the results of the first study, the authors stated, "The placebo group was included to validate the clinical benefit from inhaled corticosteroid treatment."[35] However, demonstrating the *superiority* of the combination therapy to monotherapy would provide all the validation needed for this clinical trial. Moreover, because all the active treatments were approved medications that had been shown to be superior to placebo in previous clinical trials, comparison to placebo did not add valuable scientific information.

Demonstrating that the combination therapies were superior to placebo also lacks clinical value. Combination therapy should be administered in clinical practice only if it is likely to be more effective than monotherapy. In fact, both studies showed that combination therapy was superior to monotherapy—outcomes that could be demonstrated without comparison with placebo.

Why were placebo controls thought to be needed in these two studies evaluating combination therapy? One reason might be the belief that the FDA requires placebo controls for asthma clinical trials. This is suggested by the fact that the first study, which enrolled patients in 18 countries, included placebo controls only at U.S. sites. (The second study was conducted exclusively in the United States.) Although FDA guidelines appear to favor placebo controls whenever studies do not pose risks of serious, irreversible harm, they do not question the credibility of active-controlled superiority trials, in contrast to active-controlled equivalence trials.[5,6,19] Hence, use of placebo in these two studies, which could have been executed as active-controlled superiority trials, without placebo controls, would not find any support in this appeal to FDA requirements.

Patients randomized to placebo in these two studies fared worse with respect to primary and secondary outcome measures including forced expiratory volume in 1 second at the end of the study compared with baseline, asthma symptom scores, withdrawal owing to asthma exacerbations, and use of albuterol. These results do not suggest that those receiving placebo were irreversibly harmed; however, they were placed at some risk of harm from asthma exacerbation and experienced symptoms associated with discomfort, which may have caused temporary functional disability. Without a solid methodological rationale for placebo controls, it is impossible to justify exposing patient volunteers to the risks and discomforts of withholding or withdrawing effective treatment.

Assessment of Risks

The risks of placebo controls derive from the placebo intervention itself and from the risks of withholding proven effective treatment. When placebos consist of inert substances, ingested by mouth, the risks of the placebo itself generally are nonexistent or minor. Placebo injections and more invasive placebos, such as "sham surgery," carry risks from the invasiveness of the placebo procedure and accompanying treatment such as anesthesia.[37,38] Risk assessment here will focus on pill placebos, for which the risks of concern stem from lack of effective treatment.

It is important to recognize that a wide range of therapeutic benefits falls within the category of "proven effective" treatment. Therapeutic benefits include complete cures, more or less effective prophylaxis or symptom control, slowing progression of disease, and varying extent of symptom relief. Treatments may work in these ways for varying proportions of patients. Accordingly, the risks from withholding effective treatment will depend on the degree and probability of efficacy for patients receiving treatment and the severity of consequences for the health and well-being of patients in the placebo arm from lack of standard treatment during the course of trial participation. When existing treatments are only partially effective, or the benefit-risk ratio of standard treatment is marginal owing to relatively severe side effects, patients may not be disadvantaged by receiving placebo.

Assessing the risks of harm from receiving placebo in clinical trials requires attention to three dimensions of risk: (1) severity, (2) probability, and (3) duration of harm. At one end of the severity spectrum is the experience of mild symptoms with minimal threats to health, resulting from receiving placebo in trials of new treatments for conditions such as allergic rhinitis, heartburn, or headaches. At the other end of the spectrum, such as trials of cancer chemotherapy and antibiotics for a life-threatening infection, the use of a placebo control would pose substantial risks of serious irreversible harm, in view of illness severity and effectiveness of standard treatment. The use of placebo controls at the mild end of the severity spectrum is unlikely to evoke ethical concern, except for those who take a categorical stance that placebo controls are unethical whenever proven effective treatments exist. These studies are consistent with the Declaration of Helsinki's permission for placebo-controlled trials in "minor" disorders in its recent Note of Clarification described above. On the other hand, everyone agrees that placebo controls are unethical if withholding available treatment would be likely to expose research subjects to death or irreversible morbidity. The more difficult cases lie in the middle range between the two ends of the severity spectrum.

Some commentators have taken the position that the only risks that raise concern about placebo assignment are death or irreversible morbidity.[5,6] Yet discomfort or distress and temporary functional disability may reach a level of severity that makes them serious harms, to which research participants should not be exposed.[7] An example is placebo-controlled trials of drugs administered to prevent nausea and vomiting caused by highly emetogenic chemotherapy to treat various cancers. In 1981, research demonstrated robust and statistically significant differences between metoclopramide and placebo for the treatment of nausea and vomiting induced by cisplatin.[39] In the early 1990s, the new antiemetic agent ondansetron was tested in placebo-controlled trials for patients naïve to previous chemotherapy who were receiving cisplatin.[40] Because it was known that lack of prophylactic antiemetic treatment was likely to result in repeated vomiting in patients receiving cisplatin, and that an effective antiemetic agent was available, these trials were arguably unethical.[7,8] Indeed, the need for placebo controls was doubtful, as a contemporaneous active-controlled trial demonstrated that ondansetron was superior to metoclopramide in reducing the incidence of nausea and vomiting in connection with cisplatin therapy.[41] Although vomiting induced by chemotherapy is not life-threatening and does not cause irreversible disability, it represents serious, avoidable harm that is more than a minor discomfort. Nausea and vomiting induced by chemotherapy can be sufficiently severe to cause patients to refuse subsequent chemotherapy, or it may increase the risk of nausea and vomiting for those who undergo further chemotherapy.

The ethical concern over severe discomfort produced by trials that withhold antiemetic treatment was evidenced by a 1996 article written by seven investigators, including the lead authors of the previous placebo-controlled studies, entitled "Are More Antiemetic Trials With a Placebo Necessary?"[42] They compiled the results of placebo-controlled trials of three antiemetic agents evaluated in connection with cisplatin chemotherapy. The article contained a table presenting the individual results for all 48 patients randomized to placebo in these trials. According to the pooled results, 98% of those receiving placebo experienced vomiting (median of six emetic episodes), as compared with 49% of those pretreated with one of the three antiemetic drugs. The authors concluded that "[c]andidate antiemetic agents should only be tested against active comparators."[42]

Accordingly, risks of concern for placebo-controlled trials should include short-lived but severe discomfort and temporary disability, as well as death and irreversible damage. What, then, counts as excessive risk? And who decides? There is no reasonable way to formulate exactly the probability, severity, and duration of potential harm that would make the risks of placebo controls excessive. The question calls for careful investigation and judgment. Such risk-benefit assessments are made by research sponsors, investigators, and most importantly by ethics review boards (ERBs) and research participants.

ERBs, charged with prospective approval of research protocols, must carefully assess the risks from placebo assignment when this involves withholding proven effective treatment. The review boards must determine that the risks have been minimized, that they are not intolerable or excessive, and that they are justifiable by the value of the knowledge to be gained by the study. Once placebo-controlled trials have been reviewed and approved by ERBs, patients make their own judgments about whether they are prepared to accept the risks of trial participation. In the case of chronic conditions for which placebo-controlled trials are common, patients are familiar with the symptoms of their disorder: For example, they know what it is like to experience symptoms of depression, anxiety, multiple sclerosis, or migraine attacks. Therefore, they are well placed to decide whether the risks of nontreatment, or less than standard treatment, are acceptable to them.

Some systematic data are available to inform risk assessments of placebo-controlled trials. A comprehensive review of placebo-controlled trials of chronic, stable angina showed that the risks of adverse events did not differ significantly between the drug and placebo groups.[43] A meta-analysis of antidepressant trials in the FDA database, encompassing thousands of patients, found that those depressed patients receiving placebo were not at significantly greater risk of suicide or attempted suicide.[44] In addition, the patients receiving placebo experienced a mean 31% symptom reduction during trial participation, as compared with 41% symptom reduction for patients who received investigational or active comparator drugs. Thus it appears that, in the aggregate, depressed patients receiving placebo controls in short-term trials are not made worse off or disproportionately disadvantaged as compared with those receiving pharmacologic treatment. A study of placebo-controlled studies in schizophrenia registered with the pharmaceutical regulatory authority of the Netherlands over a 10-year period ending on December 31, 2002, including more than 7,000 patients, also found no significant differences in suicide or attempted suicide between those patients receiving active drugs and those receiving placebo.[45] In contrast, there is some evidence from placebo-controlled asthma trials that patients maintained on inhaled corticosteroid treatment prior to trial entry who have treatment withdrawn by virtue of being randomized to placebo are more likely than trial participants receiving maintenance treatment to experience symptomatic worsening and to be withdrawn from research owing to asthma exacerbation.[33,46] More systematic research is needed on the consequences of placebo assignment across the spectrum of placebo-controlled trials in disorders with proven effective treatment.

Safeguards to Minimize Risks

Careful screening of prospective patient volunteers for placebo-controlled trials is required to minimize risks. Severely ill patients at heightened risk of deterioration or of severe suffering from lack of treatment should be excluded. Prospective patient volunteers should be encouraged to consult with their physicians prior to deciding whether or not to enroll in a placebo-controlled trial.[47,48] For those who lack a physician, consultation with a clinician not involved in the research project is desirable.

The duration of the placebo period should be limited to the shortest time required for adequate efficacy testing. During the conduct of the clinical trial, monitoring procedures are necessary to protect patient volunteers.[49] For severely ill patients, consideration should be given to limiting placebo-controlled trials to inpatient settings with constant monitoring and the ready availability of "rescue" medications in case of significant deterioration. In outpatient trials, investigators should maintain frequent contact with patient volunteers to assess symptomatic worsening and intervene appropriately. Consideration should be given to requiring research protocols to specify criteria for removing patient volunteers from clinical trials owing to symptom severity or other adverse consequences. In any case, clinical judgment will be necessary, and investigators should err on the side of patient safety.

Informed Consent

Elements of informed consent do not differ essentially in placebo-controlled trials from other forms of clinical research. Some points, however, deserve emphasis. It is imperative that patient volunteers understand the nature of the study under consideration, how it differs from standard clinical practice, the meaning of *placebo*, the rationale for placebo use, random assignment, the probability of receiving a placebo, blinding of patient volunteers and investigators, alternatives for potentially effective treatment outside the research setting, and other pertinent aspects of study design. Among the risks that must be disclosed and understood are lack of improvement that patient volunteers randomized to placebo might have experienced if they had received standard treatment and the chance of symptomatic worsening during the placebo phase.

A variety of evidence indicates that many patients enrolled in randomized clinical trials are confused about, or fail to appreciate, the differences between routine therapy in medical practice and trial participation.[50] The invitation to enroll in treatment studies at medical institutions may foster "therapeutic misconceptions" that lead patients to believe that in clinical trials they are being assigned treatment according to clinical judgments about what is in their best medical interests.[51] Consequently, special efforts are desirable to educate patient volunteers about the differences between clinical trials and personalized medical care. Educational aids may be helpful prior to the informed consent process for a particular study, such as computerized tutorials that explain the key elements of randomized, placebo-controlled trials.

Vulnerable Populations

Children and incompetent adults are vulnerable research subjects because they are not able to give informed consent. Children either lack or have not fully developed the capacities of understanding, reasoning, and making choices necessary for giving informed consent to research participation, or they have not reached the age of consent. Adults with various severe cognitive impairments have lost these capacities or may have never achieved them.

Placebo-controlled trials that would be unethical in the case of adults capable of giving informed consent obviously would also be unethical for children and incompetent adults. However, placebo-controlled trials that are ethical for adults may be unethical for individuals from these vulnerable populations. Two key ethical questions need to be addressed in determining whether it is justifiable to enroll children or incompetent adults in placebo-controlled trials. First, is it fair to enroll those unable to give informed consent? Second, should there be stricter limits on the risks of receiving placebo for trials enrolling children or incompetent adults than for competent adults? It is agreed that enrollment of children and cognitively incapacitated adults in research requires safeguards such as authorization by parents in the case of children and appropriate surrogate decision makers in the case of incompetent adults. Assent within the capabilities of the subject should also be obtained. Because these are generic safeguards for clinical research they will not be discussed here.

Children

As a general rule, it is unfair to enroll children in research when their participation is not necessary to answer the scientific question posed by the research.[52] Some disorders occur solely or predominantly in children, such that clinical trials testing treatments for these conditions will require the enrollment of children.

Whenever possible, initial safety and efficacy testing should involve adults before proceeding to appropriate trials in children. However, just as unnecessary inclusion of children is unethical, excluding children from clinical trials may be morally problematic. Rigorous scientific knowledge about the safety and efficacy of treatment of adults with a given disorder is not adequate for guiding the care of children with the same condition, owing to biological differences between children and adults.[53] Excluding children from clinical trials on grounds of protecting the vulnerable can produce clinical vulnerability of children who must be treated by physicians without adequate evidence concerning the safety and efficacy of drugs tested only in adults.

Placebo-controlled trials of experimental treatments when no treatment is clinically available for a given disorder, or when existing treatments have not been rigorously evaluated, are just as acceptable in children as in adults, provided that the rule of initial testing in adults, when possible, has been followed. Can placebo-controlled trials testing experimental drugs enroll children when pharmacologic treatment that is proven effective in children exists? It might be argued that withholding proven effective treatment from a control group of children is unethical, because they cannot consent to forgo potentially effective treatment. The lack of informed consent makes these studies problematic in the case of children, as it does for all research with children that carries risks without the prospect of compensating medical benefits. Nonetheless, we should focus on the potential harm from receiving placebo rather than the fact of withholding treatment. If deviation from standard medical care is not inherently unethical for adults, it is not clear that it should necessarily be unethical for children.

Consider a placebo-controlled trial to evaluate a new treatment for allergic rhinitis. With children who regularly experience mild to moderate symptoms, the harms of forgoing treatment are likely to be minimal, provided that the trial is short term, the investigators have specified reasonable criteria for stopping trial participation in case of symptom worsening, and trial participants are carefully monitored. Accordingly, if placebo-controlled trials are methodologically necessary to test the absolute or relative efficacy of new treatments for childhood disorders, such as depression or anxiety, categorical exclusion of children is unreasonable.

Should there be a more stringent limitation of allowable risks in children from receiving a placebo control than for competent adults? As discussed above, the issue of where to set a risk threshold in adults is a matter of judgment. In the case of children, it is desirable to put some constraints on the upper limit of allowable risk. The U.S. federal regulations concerning research with children may be helpful in this regard. Placebo controls should be understood as "an intervention or procedure that does not hold out the prospect of direct benefit for the individual subject."[54] So understood, subpart D of the regulations permits placebo-controlled trials in children when the risks of placebo assignment are more than minimal under three key conditions: "(a) the risks represent a minor increase over minimal risk; (b) the intervention or procedure presents experiences to subjects that are reasonably commensurate with those inherent in their actual or expected medical, dental, psychological, social, or educational situations; and (c) the intervention or procedure is likely to yield generalizable knowledge about the subjects' disorder or condition that is of vital importance for the understanding and amelioration of the subjects' disorder or condition."[17] Minimal risks are defined as those that children are likely to experience in daily life, making a minor increase over minimal a small increment of additional risk.

The use of placebo controls to evaluate antidepressants in children with depression might fall within an acceptable risk threshold.[54] The justification of placebo, however, would depend on a reasonable determination that children are not exposed to more than a minor increase over minimal risk from the lack of pharmacologic treatment during short-term placebo-controlled trials. Placebo-controlled trials that exclude children suspected to be at higher risk of suicide, limit trial duration to the shortest period necessary to demonstrate acute efficacy, employ reasonable criteria for stopping trial participation in the event of serious clinical deterioration, and implement careful monitoring might qualify as providing placebo interventions that fall within a minor increase over minimal risk.

Additionally, to approve such a trial, an IRB would need to judge that the use of the placebo control would lead to generalizable knowledge of "vital importance." Several considerations support such a judgment. Depression is a serious disorder of relatively high prevalence in children.[55] Comparatively few antidepressant trials have been conducted in children.[56] Treatments that are effective in adults are not necessarily effective in children, as trials evaluating tricyclic antidepressants have demonstrated.[55] High rates of placebo response, coupled with lack of strong and consistent efficacy of currently available treatments for childhood depression,[55,56] provide the rationale for including placebo controls to generate valid efficacy data.[7] Without a placebo control, the validity of antidepressant trials is open to question. The use of placebo controls in childhood depression appears consistent with criteria promulgated by the American Academy of Pediatrics, which permit placebo controls "when the disease process is characterized by frequent, spontaneous exacerbations and remissions."[57]

Incompetent Adults

The ethical considerations relating to appropriate enrollment of children in clinical trials and setting allowable risk limits are also pertinent to research with incompetent adults. Incompetent adults should not be enrolled in placebo-controlled trials unless their participation is scientifically necessary to test hypotheses about treatment efficacy. A major difference between children and incompetent adults is that children as a class are incapable of giving informed consent, whereas adults with disorders that put them at risk of lacking decisional capacity may or may not be capable of giving informed consent for research. In other words, diagnostic categories generally are not indicative of incompetence.[58] Because incompetent adults should not be enrolled in placebo-controlled trials when others who can give informed consent are available, some process of assessing capability to give informed consent is needed to determine whether or not cognitively impaired adults lack competence. For example, patients with schizophrenia on the whole score below normal controls on standard evaluations of capacity to give informed consent.[59] However, most, but not all, are capable of giving informed consent to research participation, especially when intensive educational efforts are employed.[60] The National Bioethics Advisory Commission recommended assessment of the capacity to give informed consent by professionals independent of the research team for all more than minimal risk research involving individuals with mental disorders that affect decision-making capacity.[61]

Placebo-controlled trials, however, may evaluate treatment appropriately targeted at severely ill patients who lack the capacity to give informed consent. Whether enrollment of incompetent adult patients is ethically acceptable will depend, in part, on the level of risks posed by the placebo control. The threshold of a minor increase over minimal risk might also be reasonable for incompetent adults. It is conceivable that higher risks from placebo assignment might be acceptable if those enrolled have formulated clear research advance directives authorizing their participation in greater than minimal risk research.[62] In this case, the potential clinical value of the research and the methodological rationale for use of placebo would need to be compelling.

Conclusion

Over the past decade, the conduct of placebo-controlled trials in the face of proven effective treatment has generated intense controversy and debate. The points in contention are complex, including disputed methodological issues and competing ethical perspectives. Categorical rejection of such placebo-controlled trials, which invokes the concept of clinical equipoise, is subject to serious theoretical and practical problems. This chapter has presented an ethical framework for assessing the design and conduct of placebo-controlled trials that includes criteria for a sound methodological rationale, acceptable level of risks, informed consent or authorization by appropriate surrogate decision makers, and safeguards to protect enrolled participants. In permitting placebo-controlled trials despite the existence of proven effective treatment, provided that the trials satisfy suitable ethical criteria, this ethical framework aims at appropriately balancing the twin objectives of clinical research ethics: promoting rigorous research aimed at improving health and medical care, and protecting research participants from harm and exploitation.

Acknowledgments

In writing this chapter, I have incorporated ideas and/or text from the following articles: Miller FG. Placebo-controlled trials in psychiatric research: an ethical perspective. *Biological Psychiatry* 2000;47:707–16; Emanuel EJ, Miller FG. The ethics of placebo-controlled trials—A middle ground. *New England Journal of Medicine* 2001;345:915–9; Miller FG, Shorr AF. Unnecessary use of placebo controls. *Archives of Internal Medicine* 2002;162:1673–7; Miller FG, Brody H. What makes placebo-controlled trials unethical? *American Journal of Bioethics* 2002;2(2):3–9; Miller FG, Brody H. A critique of clinical equipoise: Therapeutic misconception in the ethics of clinical trials. *Hastings Center Report* 2003; 33(3):19–28; and Miller FG, Wendler D, Wilfond B. When do the federal regulations allow placebo-controlled trials in children? *Journal of Pediatrics* 2003;42:102–7. I am indebted to my coauthors for their contributions to collaborative research on the ethics of placebo-controlled trials.

Disclaimer

The views expressed here are the author's own and do not represent any positions or policies of the National Institutes of Health, the Public Health Service, or the Department of Health and Human Services.

References

1. Rothman KJ, Michels B. The continuing unethical use of placebo controls. *New England Journal of Medicine* 1994;331:394–8.
2. Freedman B, Glass KC, Weijer C. Placebo orthodoxy in clinical research. II: Ethical, legal, and regulatory myths. *Journal of Law, Medicine, and Ethics* 1996;24:252–9.
3. Freedman B. Equipoise and the ethics of clinical research. *New England Journal of Medicine* 1987;317:141–5.
4. Freedman B. Placebo-controlled trials and the logic of clinical purpose. *IRB: A Review of Human Subjects Research* 1990;12(6):1–6.
5. Temple R, Ellenberg SE. Placebo-controlled trials and active-control trials in the evaluation of new treatments. Part 1: Ethical and scientific issues. *Annals of Internal Medicine* 2000;133:455–63.
6. Ellenberg SE, Temple R. Placebo-controlled trials and active-control trials in the evaluation of new treatments. Part 2: Practical issues and specific cases. *Annals of Internal Medicine* 2000;133:464–70.
7. Emanuel EJ, Miller FG. The ethics of placebo-controlled trials—A middle ground. *New England Journal of Medicine* 2001;345:915–9.
8. Emanuel EJ, Wendler D, Grady C. What makes clinical research ethical? *JAMA* 2000;283:2701–11.
9. Kaptchuk TJ. Intentional ignorance: A history of blind assessment and placebo controls in medicine. *Bulletin of the History of Medicine* 1998;72:389–433.
10. Green SA. The origins of modern clinical research. *Clinical Orthopaedics and Related Research* 2002;405:311–9.
11. Clark PI, Leaverton PE. Scientific and ethical issues in the use of placebo controls in clinical trials. *Annual Review of Public Health* 1994;15:19–38.
12. Kienle GS, Kiene H. The powerful placebo effect: Fact or fiction? *Journal of Clinical Epidemiology* 1997;12:1311–8.
13. Sackett DL. Why randomized controlled trials fail but needn't: 2. Failure to employ physiological statistics, or the only formula a clinician-trialist is ever likely to need (or understand!). *Canadian Medical Association Journal* 2001;165:1226–37.
14. Spilker B. *Guide to Clinical Trials.* Philadelphia, Penn.: Lippincott, Williams, and Wilkins; 1991.
15. Makuch RW, Johnson MF. Dilemmas in the use of active control groups in clinical research. *IRB: A Review of Human Subjects Research* 1989;11(1):1–5.
16. Leon AC. Placebo protects subjects from nonresponse: A paradox of power. *Archives of General Psychiatry* 2000;57:329–30.
17. Department of Health and Human Services, National Institutes of Health, and Office for Human Research Protections. The Common Rule, Title 45 (Public Welfare), Code of Federal Regulations, Part 46 (Protection of Human Subjects). [Online] June 23, 2005. Available: http://www.hhs.gov/ohrp/humansubjects/guidance/45cfr46.htm.
18. Department of Health and Human Services, Office for Human Research Protections. *Protecting Human Research Subjects: Institutional Review Board Guidebook.* Rockville, Md.: OHRP; 1993. [Online] Available: http://www.hhs.gov/ohrp/irb/irb_guidebook.htm.
19. Department of Health and Human Services, Food and Drug Administration. Title 21 (Food and Drugs), Code of Federal Regulations, Part 314 (Applications for FDA Approval to Market a New Drug). [Online] April 1, 2006. Available: http://www.access.gpo.gov/nara/cfr/waisidx_06/21cfr314_06.html.
20. Food and Drug Administration. Supplementary Advisory: Placebo-controlled and active-controlled drug study designs, 1989. In: Brody B. *The Ethics of Biomedical Research: An International Perspective.* New York, N.Y.: Oxford University Press; 1998.
21. International Conference on Harmonisation of Technical Requirements for Registration of Pharmaceuticals for Human Use. E10: Choice of Control Group and Related Issues in Clinical Trials. [Online] July 20, 2000. Available: http://www.ich.org/LOB/media/MEDIA486.pdf.
22. World Medical Association. Declaration of Helsinki: Ethical Principles for Medical Research Involving Human Subjects. Tokyo, Japan: WMA; October 2004. [Online] 2004. Available: http://www.wma.net/e/policy/b3.htm.
23. Lasagna L. The Helsinki Declaration: Timeless guide or irrelevant anachronism? *Journal of Clinical Psychopharmacology* 1995;15:96–8.
24. Levine RJ. The need to revise the Declaration of Helsinki. *New England Journal of Medicine* 1999;341:531–4.
25. Council for International Organizations of Medical Sciences in collaboration with the World Health Organization. *International Ethical Guidelines for Biomedical Research Involving Human Subjects.* Geneva, Switzerland: CIOMS and WHO, 2002. [Online] November 2002. Available: http://www.cioms.ch/frame_guidelines_nov_2002.htm.
26. Beauchamp TL, Childress JF. *Principles of Biomedical Ethics,* 5th ed. New York, N.Y.: Oxford University Press; 2001.
27. Marquis D. Leaving therapy to chance. *Hastings Center Report* 1983;13(4):40–7.
28. Gifford F. The conflict between randomized clinical trials and the therapeutic obligation. *Journal of Medicine and Philosophy* 1986;11:347–66.
29. Fried C. *Medical Experimentation: Personal Integrity and Social Policy.* New York, N.Y.: American Elsevier; 1974.
30. Miller FG, Brody H. What makes placebo-controlled trials unethical? *American Journal of Bioethics* 2002;2(2):3–9.
31. Miller FG, Brody H. A critique of clinical equipoise: Therapeutic misconception in the ethics of clinical trials. *Hastings Center Report* 2003;33(3):19–28.
32. Weijer C. When argument fails. *American Journal of Bioethics* 2002;2(2):10.
33. Miller FG. Placebo-controlled trials in psychiatric research: An ethical perspective. *Biological Psychiatry* 2000;47:707–16.
34. Miller FG, Shorr AF. Unnecessary use of placebo controls. *Archives of Internal Medicine* 2002;162:1673–7.
35. Laviolette M, Malmstrom K, Lu S, Chervinsky P, Pujet J-C, Peszek I, Zhang J, Reiss TF. Montelukast added to inhaled beclomethasone in treatment of asthma. *American Journal of Respiratory and Critical Care Medicine* 1999;160:1862–8.
36. Kavuru M, Melamed J, Gross G, LaForce C, House K, Prillaman B, Baitinger L, Woodring A, Shah T. Salmeterol and fluticasone propionate combined in a new powder inhalation device for the treatment of asthma: a randomized, double-blind, placebo-controlled trial. *Journal of Allergy and Clinical Immunology* 2000;105:1108–16.
37. Horng S, Miller FG. Is placebo surgery unethical? *New England Journal of Medicine* 2002;347:137–9.
38. Horng S, Miller FG. Ethical framework for the use of sham procedures in clinical trials. *Critical Care Medicine* 2003;31(Suppl.):S126–S130.
39. Gralla RJ, Itri LM, Pisko SE, Squillante AE, Kelsen DP, Braun DW, Bordin LA, Braun TJ, Young CW. Antiemetic efficacy of high-dose metoclopramide: randomized trials with placebo and prochlorperazine in patients with chemotherapy-induced nausea and vomiting. *New England Journal of Medicine* 1981;305:905–9.
40. Cubeddu LX, Hoffman IS, Fuenmayor NT, Finn AI. Efficacy of ondansetron (GR 38032f) and the role of serotonin in cisplatin-induced nausea and vomiting. *New England Journal of Medicine* 1990;322:810–6.
41. Marty M, Pouillart P, Scholi S, Drox J P, Azab M, Brion N, Pujade-Lauraine E, Paule B, Paes D, Bons J. Comparison of the 5-hydroxytryptamine3 (serotonin) antagonist ondansetron (GR

38032 7f) with high-dose metoclopramide in the control of cisplatin-induced emesis. *New England Journal of Medicine* 1990;322:816–21.

42. Kris MG, Cubeddu LX, Gralla RJ, Cupissol D, Tyson LB, Venkat-raman E, Homesley HD. Are more antiemetic trials with placebo necessary? Report of patient data from randomized trials of placebo antiemetics with cisplatin. *Cancer* 1996;78:2193–8.

43. Glasser SP, Clark PI, Lipicky RJ, Hubbard JM, Yusuf S. Exposing patients with chronic, stable, exertional angina to placebo periods in drug trials. *JAMA* 1991;265:1550–4.

44. Khan A, Warner HA, Brown WA. Symptom reduction and suicide risk in patients treated with placebo in antidepressant clinical trials: An analysis of the Food and Drug Administration database. *Archives of General Psychiatry* 2000;57:311–7.

45. Storosum JG, van Zweiten BJ, Wohlfarth, et al. Suicide risk in placebo vs. active treatment in placebo-controlled trials for schizophrenia. *Archives of General Psychiatry* 2003;60:365–8.

46. Miller FG, Shorr. Ethical assessment of industry-sponsored clinical trials: A case analysis. *Chest* 2002;121:1337–42.

47. Levine RJ. *Ethics and Regulation of Clinical Research*, 2nd edition. New Haven, Conn.: Yale University Press; 1986:111–2.

48. Chen DT, Miller FG, Rosenstein DL. Clinical research and the physician-patient relationship. *Annals of Internal Medicine* 2003; 138:669–72.

49. Quitkin FM. Placebos, drug effects, and study design: A clinician's guide. *American Journal of Psychiatry* 1999;156:829–36.

50. Lidz CW, Appelbaum PS. The therapeutic misconception: Problems and solutions. *Medical Care* 2002;40(supplement):V55–V63.

51. Appelbaum PS, Roth LH, Lidz CW, Benson P, Winslade W. False hopes and best data: Consent to research and the therapeutic misconception. *Hastings Center Report* 1987;17(2):20–4.

52. Wendler D. Informed consent, exploitation and whether it is possible to conduct human subjects research without either one. *Bioethics* 2000;14:310–39.

53. Wiznitzer M, Findling RL. Why do psychiatric drug research in children? *Lancet* 2003;361:1147–8.

54. Miller FG, Wendler D, Wilfond B. When do the federal regulations allow placebo-controlled trials in children? *Journal of Pediatrics* 2003;42:102–7.

55. Wagner KD, Ambrosnin PJ. Childhood depression: Pharmacological therapy/treatment. *Journal of Clinical Child Psychology* 2001;30:88–97.

56. Ambrosini PJ. A review of pharmacotherapy of major depression in children and adolescents. *Psychiatric Services* 2000;51:627–33.

57. American Academy of Pediatrics. Guidelines for the ethical conduct of studies to evaluate drugs in pediatric populations. *Pediatrics* 1995; 95:286–94.

58. Chen DT, Miller FG, Rosenstein DL. Enrolling decisionally impaired adults in clinical research. *Medical Care* 2002;40(Supplement): V20–V29.

59. Grisso T, Appelbaum PS. *Assessing Competence to Consent to Treatment.* New York, N.Y.: Oxford University Press; 1998.

60. Carpenter WT, Jr., Gold JM, Lahti AC, et al. Decisional capacity for informed consent for schizophrenia research. *Archives of General Psychiatry* 2001;158:712–7.

61. National Bioethics Advisory Commission. *Research Involving Persons With Mental Disorders That May Affect Decisionmaking Capacity, Vol. I.* Rockville, Md.: NBAC; 1998. [Online] December 1998. Available: http://www.georgetown.edu/research/nrcbl/nbac/capacity/TOC.htm.

62. Wendler D, Prasad BS. Core safeguards for clinical research with adults who are unable to consent. *Annals of Internal Medicine* 2001; 135:514–23.

Franklin G. Miller   Donald L. Rosenstein

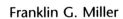

Challenge Experiments

Challenge experiments are among the most controversial forms of clinical research. They involve experimental interventions aimed at perturbing the biological or psychological functioning of human beings for the purpose of developing scientific knowledge about diseases and their treatment. Challenge agents include drugs, inhaled or ingested substances, physical or psychological stimuli, and pathogens. No precise definition of challenge experiments has been developed, such that it is not always clear whether a particular investigation falls into this category. These studies characteristically offer no prospect of medical benefit for the enrolled participants. In this chapter we concentrate on two types of challenge studies: symptom-provoking experiments with psychiatric patients and infection-inducing experiments with healthy volunteers. Psychiatric symptom-provoking studies include administering challenge procedures known to evoke panic attacks, depressive symptoms, obsessions, and psychotic experiences.[1] Infection challenge experiments have induced diseases such as cholera, malaria, influenza, shigella, and E. coli.[2]

Psychiatric symptom-provoking studies have received considerable public and professional attention, owing to ethical concerns about research involving mentally ill patients that emerged in the mid-1990s. This prompted a report on this area of research by the National Bioethics Advisory Commission, *Research Involving Persons With Mental Disorders That May Affect Decisionmaking Capacity*.[3] In contrast, relatively little attention has been devoted to the ethics of infection-inducing challenge experiments in the news media or in the medical or bioethics literature.[4] Assessing these two forms of challenge experiments together offers a fruitful opportunity for reflecting on ethical issues presented by clinical research that exposes volunteers to risks without the prospect of medical benefits.

Framing the Ethical Assessment of Challenge Experiments

Clinical research is typically designed and supervised by physicians with the use of medical equipment and procedures, and conducted in clinical settings. It is therefore commonly presumed that clinical research should be compatible with the ethical principles of therapeutic medicine, or that clinical investigation is morally problematic if it departs significantly from the ethics of medical care. In this light, challenge experiments appear morally shocking. How can it possibly be ethical for physicians to provoke symptoms of mental illness in psychiatric patients or induce infectious diseases in healthy individuals for the sake of scientific investigation? Isn't this the sort of abusive experimentation carried out by Nazi physicians? To be sure, the participants are volunteers, rather than concentration camp prisoners. Nonetheless, these challenge experiments involve physicians deliberately exposing humans to interventions that induce pathological conditions associated with physical or psychic distress and with the potential for lasting harm. The duties of physicians to care for the sick and avoid harm that is not compensated by medical benefit appear to be flagrantly violated by this form of clinical research.

Although understandable, this moral perspective on challenge studies is mistaken. It transports moral intuitions appropriate to evaluating medical care to the fundamentally different context of clinical research.[5] Medical care is devoted to producing therapeutic benefit to particular patients by means of diagnostic and treatment interventions. Clinical research, on the other hand, is devoted to producing scientific knowledge for the benefit of society that can aid in the understanding and treatment of disease. Whereas in clinical care, the risks of medical interventions to which patients are exposed must be justified by the potential for therapeutic benefit to them, in clinical research the risks of experimental procedures are typically justified, entirely or in part, by the value of the knowledge to be gained from the investigation. It follows that the ethical principles of beneficence and nonmaleficence applicable to both medical care and clinical research must be understood as having different implications for these two domains. In medical care, these principles are understood as having an individualized, patient-centered focus. In clinical research, by contrast, beneficence concerns the social value of scientific knowledge; and nonmaleficence places constraints on the level of risks to which it is ethical to expose research subjects for the sake of this social goal.

Nontherapeutic challenge procedures aimed at scientific knowledge would be morally egregious in the context of medical care. However, their use in clinical research must be assessed in accordance with the ethical requirements appropriate to this endeavor. The departure from, or symbolic violation of, the moral ethos of medical care posed by challenge experiments is, in itself, ethically irrelevant. What makes challenge studies morally problematic is their potential to exploit research participants for the good of society. As in the case of all clinical research, this form of experimentation stands in need of ethical justification in accordance with standard ethical requirements. To be ethical, challenge experiments must have scientific or social value; employ valid methods of investigation; select participants fairly; minimize risks and justify them by the potential knowledge to be gained from the research; be reviewed and approved by a research ethics committee; enroll participants who have given informed consent or with ethically appropriate surrogate authorization; and they must be conducted in a way that adequately protects the rights and well-being of research participants.[6]

In an ethical assessment of challenge experiments it is important to distinguish the use of challenge procedures as diagnostic tools in therapeutic medicine from their use as research probes in clinical research. Challenge procedures are commonly administered in the context of medical care for purposes such as determining sensitivity to allergens, airway reactivity, and as evidence of cardiac abnormalities. The purpose is to diagnose disease or dysfunction for the sake of guiding treatment. Challenge experiments in clinical research lack this patient-centered therapeutic purpose; they are administered to develop scientific knowledge about groups of patients with particular disorders.

Social Value

The first ethical consideration in assessing clinical investigation is the potential value of the knowledge it can yield. Valueless clinical research exploits human participants by exposing them to risks without the prospect of producing scientific knowledge. To be ethically justified, experiments that impose substantial risks or burdens must offer commensurate potential knowledge value.

Psychiatric symptom-provoking studies administer challenge procedures to patients and healthy volunteers to investigate the pathophysiology of psychiatric disorders, with the ultimate aim of improving the diagnosis and treatment of mental illness. The study of evoked symptoms and associated neurobiological phenomena under experimental conditions has contributed to elucidating the role of neural circuitry and the functioning of neural transmitters in psychiatric disorders.[7-8] For example, the roles of dopamine and glutamate in the symptomatic expression of schizophrenia have been explored by challenge experiments that have administered amphetamines and ketamine to schizophrenic patients. Tryptophan depletion experiments and the administration of alpha-methylparatyrosine (AMPT) have contributed to our understanding of the role of the serotonergic and noradrenergic neural systems in depression, respectively. It is hoped that this valuable method of scientific investigation, employed over the past 40 years, might eventually lead to diagnostic tests for psychiatric disorders, reliable indicators of optimal treatment selection, or new targets for treatment interventions. Whether or not such clinically relevant developments accrue directly from psychiatric symptom-provoking studies, improved knowledge of pathophysiology and response to treatment is likely to be produced by combining these experiments with brain imaging techniques and genetic tests associated with predisposition to psychiatric illness.

The social value of clinical research may extend beyond specific scientific knowledge. Psychiatric symptom-provoking studies have contributed to the social understanding of mental illness as biologically mediated brain disorders, bringing psychiatry squarely within the domain of somatic medicine. By identifying psychiatric disorders as "real" disturbances in biological functioning rather than purely mental or neurotic phenomena, this understanding has led to a decline in the social stigma of mental illness and the more widespread acceptance of pharmacological treatment. It has also helped absolve parents from misplaced guilt about causing severe mental illness, such as schizophrenia, in their children by means of childrearing practices. Although relevant to the historical assessment of symptom-provoking studies, the social value deriving from improved understanding of mental illness cannot justify any specific prospective experiment. This requires a judgment of potential scientific value relating to the hypotheses to be tested by the study in question.

By virtue of their role in vaccine development, infection-inducing challenge studies offer the prospect of contributing substantially to generating clinically relevant scientific knowledge.[2] These challenge experiments, which involve deliberate exposure of healthy volunteers to infectious diseases, have been used especially to evaluate initial efficacy of experimental vaccines before conducting large-scale field trials. Once human challenge models are developed, such that they can reliably and safely transmit infectious disease, they are typically used in experiments comparing those who receive candidate vaccines with unvaccinated controls. Preliminary indications of efficacy are determined by the differential responses of vaccinated and unvaccinated research participants to the infection challenge.

Expeditious development of effective vaccines can help spare many people from morbidity or death associated with infectious diseases. Pilot data on the efficacy of an experimental vaccine obtained by means of infection challenge experiments can limit the exposure of thousands of humans in field trials to only the most promising vaccine candidates. By weeding out candidate vaccines that do not demonstrate the ability to protect challenged participants, the use of a challenge model can significantly increase the efficiency of vaccine development by reducing the time and cost of testing candidate vaccines. Accordingly, infection-inducing challenge experiments can contribute substantially to public health. In addition to their role in initial efficacy testing of vaccines, infection challenge experiments have been used to elucidate the pathogenicity of microbes and to understand factors contributing to protective immunity, disease acquisition, and disease severity.[2,4]

Participant Selection

Both psychiatric symptom-provoking and infection challenge experiments raise issues of fairness in selecting research participants. By virtue of aiming to improve the understanding of the pathophysiology of psychiatric disorders, symptom-provoking studies must necessarily recruit patients with mental illness. However, targeting severely ill patients who may have compromised capacity to give informed consent is unethical if the research questions that symptom-provoking experiments are designed to address can be answered by studying fully capacitated patients.[9] Nonetheless, some valuable research questions can be answered only by recruiting those who are incapable of giving informed consent. Ethics review boards must determine whether the potential scientific value and the risk-benefit ratio of proposed experiments justify enrolling incompetent individuals with informed authorization by family members. Similar issues of participant selection are raised by psychiatric or infection challenge experiments designed to enroll children.

Infection-inducing challenge experiments recruit healthy volunteers who are financially compensated for research participation. No systematic data are available on the volunteer population for these experiments. To the extent that these studies are more likely to recruit economically disadvantaged individuals, concerns may be raised about the fairness of participant selection. However, a blanket policy of excluding such individuals would arguably be discriminatory.

Risks of Challenge Experiments

A key ethical issue in the assessment of challenge experiments is whether the risks to participants can be justified by the value of the knowledge to be gained from the research. The risk of greatest concern is death, which might arise from the unexpected adverse consequences of the challenge agent, from suicide provoked by exacerbated psychiatric symptoms, or by the complications of induced infectious disease. For example, in the famous yellow fever experiments in 1900, supervised by Walter Reed, the first volunteers were members of the research team.[10] Volunteers were deliberately exposed to the challenge of mosquito bites in Cuba with the aim of establishing the transmission of yellow fever. One of the researchers died and another recovered after a serious bout of yellow fever. Over the past 30 years during the era of prior review of clinical research in the United States by Institutional Review Boards (IRBs), there had been no reports of death or lasting harm from either psychiatric symptom-provoking or infection challenge experiments. However, an asthma challenge experiment conducted at Johns Hopkins University resulted in the death of a young, healthy volunteer in 2001.[11]

Contemporary infection challenge experiments are almost always limited to those diseases that resolve on their own without adverse consequences or that can be fully eradicated by treatment. According to a retrospective review of 18 challenge experiments involving the infection of 128 healthy volunteers with malaria via mosquito challenge, no participants had lasting sequelae.[12] However, 97% of participants experienced one or more symptoms. The most common symptoms were arthralgia or myalgias (79%), headache (77%), chills (68%), and fever exceeding 38° C with a median duration of two days (61%). With adequate procedures for monitoring and treatment, the risks to volunteers from infection challenge experiments are mainly physical discomfort, which may be severe. For example, in a study administering cholera bacteria to determine an optimal challenge model for future efficacy testing of candidate vaccines, 34 of 40 volunteers developed diarrhea, which was classified as "severe" in ten participants.[13]

Short-lived discomfort, rather than lasting harm, is also the major risk of psychiatric symptom-provoking studies. In these experiments, the discomfort takes the form of psychic distress. For most symptom-provoking studies the symptoms that they produce are typically of brief duration and of mild to moderate intensity: for example, a panic attack lasting a few minutes, temporary increase in anxiety and obsessive thoughts in patients with obsessive-compulsive disorder (OCD), or short-lived depressive symptoms; however, some participants experience more pronounced symptomatic responses. Articles presenting the results of symptom-provoking experiments usually report only aggregate data describing the mean degree of change in symptom rating scales produced by a challenge stimulus as compared with a placebo control. These data do not indicate symptom severity of individual participants or the level of distress experienced by those with provoked symptoms. Systematic investigation of psychic distress produced by various psychiatric challenge paradigms would aid in risk-benefit assessment of prospective studies. Some articles, however, include narrative descriptions of more intense reactions, which illustrate the potential of these studies to cause psychic distress. Three examples are presented below.

Metergoline Administered to OCD Patients[14]
The magnitude of the change during the metergoline study period was within the subclinical category as assessed by the NIMH Global Anxiety Scale (4 to 6) for all but two patients. Over the four-day metergoline period, one patient (patient 5) developed gradually mounting anxiety, which remained unabated for three days, after the study was terminated. Another patient (patient 7) who was well-controlled on clomipramine, reported a similar experience peaking in the evening of day 3 of metergoline administration. She reported being "frantic," "agitated," and very fearful and noted a dramatic increase in compulsive checking. On the evening of day 3, she reported three hours of moving repeatedly in and out of her house during a severe thunderstorm to check on a specific item in her backyard. This sudden attack of anxiety and compulsive behavior was very unusual and distressing for her, as she had not experienced similar symptoms for months.

Tryptophan Depletion Following Treatment for Depression[15]
She began to cry inconsolably and described her emotions as being "out of control." She said that she did not know why she was crying but could not stop. She also described psychic

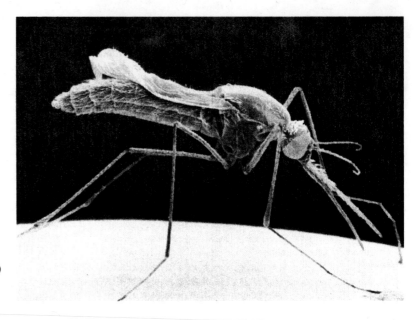

Figure 26.1. Scanning Electron Micrograph (SEM) of *Anopheles stephensi*. Source: BSIP/Photo Researchers, Inc. Reproduced with permission.

anxiety, difficulty concentrating, loss of energy, loss of self-confidence, and a sense that nothing was worthwhile. She felt as if all the gains she had made over the past few weeks had "evaporated," and her HDRS [Hamilton Depression Rating Score] increased to 34. . . . By the following morning she said that she felt "back to herself," with an HDRS score of 9. She commented that the previous day had been a "nightmare" but that she had learned that the depression was not her "fault." She also noted that, although she would not want to repeat the test, it had been worthwhile because of what she learned about her illness.

Lactate Infusion in Vietnam Veterans With Posttraumatic Stress Disorder[16]
Except for patient 6, all the men became depressed and felt guilty during flashbacks. . . . Patient 7 burst into tears during a lactate flashback as he saw his best friend blown up by a booby-trapped grenade.

One potential indicator of severity of distress caused by psychiatric challenge studies is the need for treatment to manage symptoms caused by the experimental provocation. Whether or not counteractive treatment was administered is not typically reported in research articles. One article describing an amphetamine challenge of 16 patients with borderline personality disorder reported, "Two patients had a significant psychotic experience following amphetamine on the first day and were treated with neuroleptic."[17]

Studies addressing the safety of psychiatric symptom-provoking studies have seldom been conducted. A recent report of the outcome of 30 schizophrenic patients receiving 90 ketamine challenge infusions is encouraging.[18] The patients in the aggregate experienced a 30% increase in psychotic symptoms, with a return to baseline 90 minutes after the infusion. No serious adverse events occurred following any of the ketamine challenges. Outcomes for 25 of these patients were matched to a comparable group of 25 patients who did not receive ketamine, over an average

follow-up period of 265 days. No differences were observed in measures of psychopathology, psychiatric care, or amount of antipsychotic medication.

Minimizing Risks

Achieving an acceptable risk-benefit ratio requires that research risks are minimized to the extent possible. The requirement to minimize risks does not mean that risks must be eliminated, for that would make almost all clinical research impossible to conduct. Risks are to be minimized with respect to the task of answering valuable scientific questions by means of scientifically valid methods. Study designs should be evaluated to determine if they can be modified to pose less risk to participants without compromising or undermining the scientific validity of data to be generated by the study.

Challenge procedures must be sufficiently potent to answer research questions without placing participants at excessive risks of harm. Multiple dimensions of the design and conduct of challenge experiments are relevant to the requirement of minimizing risks. For pharmacologic challenge studies, careful attention must be given to the dose of the challenge agent, its route of administration (for example, intravenous versus oral), the frequency of administration, and invasiveness of the challenge procedure. For a scientifically successful and ethically appropriate symptom-provoking experiment, the challenge procedure must be potent enough to elicit characteristic symptoms but not so strongly provocative as to cause severe or long-lasting distress. Generally, infection challenge studies should be limited to inducing infections that are self-limiting or can be fully eradicated by treatment without lasting adverse consequences. Supportive care, such as adequate hydration, is required to protect participants from avoidable complications. Review of the literature and communication with other investigators may help determine safe challenge procedures. The investigator who supervised the asthma challenge experiment that led to the death of a volunteer was criticized for not undertaking a thorough literature review of the risks of administering hexamethonium, a ganglionic blocker that was not licensed for clinical use.[11]

Risks are also minimized by careful determination of eligibility criteria aimed at excluding those who might be at higher risk of harm from the challenge experiment. In the case of psychiatric symptom-provoking studies, avoiding the provocation of suicidal behavior is of paramount importance, which calls for screening to exclude those with known risk factors for suicide. For infection challenge experiments, eligible subjects must be determined to be in good health and without any compromise to their ability to fight infection.

To protect participants during the course of challenge experiments, adequate procedures for monitoring their condition are required. Whenever risks of challenge procedures are substantial, these studies should usually be conducted in in-patient settings staffed with competent clinicians and equipped with the medical resources required to respond to any adverse events.

Infection-inducing challenge experiments may pose risks to individuals who are not research participants, because volunteers may transmit infectious disease to others with whom they come into contact. Careful screening of prospective volunteers can reduce the risk of disease transmission to those most vulnerable to infection: for example, by excluding pregnant women and volunteers who live in households with infants. Volunteers, furthermore, must practice adequate contraception while capable of transmitting infection. Infection control procedures for research and clinical staff who come into contact with volunteers and isolation of volunteers while they remain infectious may be indicated for some challenge experiments.

Justifying the Risks of Challenge Experiments

Should there be any limit to the level of risks that are justifiable in challenge experiments? The question is most pertinent to high-risk infection challenge studies that would form an integral part of a vaccine development program that has a compelling public health rationale. Consider the prospect of challenge experiments inducing infectious diseases for which treatment is nonexistent or not effective in fully eradicating disease, symptoms are severe, and/or serious morbidity or mortality is likely to result: for example, smallpox, SARS, HIV, or hepatitis C. Although the U.S. federal regulations governing research with humans do not place any upper limit on allowable research risks,[19] it is unlikely that any public funding agency or ethics review board would endorse such an experiment. However, it is worth pondering whether the famous experiments with healthy volunteers conducted by Walter Reed on the transmission of yellow fever—then a potentially lethal disease without treatment—would be considered ethical by our contemporary standards.

The Nuremberg Code, developed in the wake of the brutal Nazi concentration camp experiments, states the following: "No experiment should be conducted where there is an *a priori* reason to believe that death or disabling injury will occur; except, perhaps, in those experiments where the experimental physicians also serve as subjects."[20] The qualification of an *a priori* reason is critical. Because a research participant dies as a result of a medical experiment, it does not follow that the research was unethical. For example, one's ethical conclusions about the asthma challenge

experiment at Johns Hopkins—in which a healthy volunteer died—will depend on what was antecedently known or knowable about the risks of the challenge procedures proposed for use in the study.

The Nuremberg Code's suggestion of an exception to the upper limit for justifiable risk in the case of self-experimentation by investigators raises an interesting question. It is doubtful that inclusion of self-experimentation would, by itself, make a high risk study ethical that would otherwise be judged unethical. Nonetheless, self-experimentation deserves ethical attention. In justifiable, higher risk studies involving healthy volunteers, such as some infection challenge studies, should members of the research team be prepared to volunteer to demonstrate their willingness to assume the same risks and discomforts that they ask of healthy volunteers?

Most commentators would probably take the position that the risks of lasting harm from some possible challenge experiments are so great that they cannot be justified regardless of the potential social value of the research. Whether there should be any upper limits on temporary discomfort not associated with lasting harm is more questionable. Some would argue that there should be no limit on how much discomfort is allowed in such research, because competent adults presented with adequate information about an infection-inducing challenge study have the right to decide how much discomfort or inconvenience they are willing to accept. Others, including the authors, would contend that some studies might be likely to produce such a magnitude of discomfort that it would be unethical to recruit volunteers.

How can it be determined whether the potential value of knowledge to be gained from a given study can justify the risks posed to healthy volunteers? There are no formulas available. The assessment calls for carefully considered and deliberated judgments by research sponsors, investigators, and ethics review boards. Ethics review boards must assess each protocol for challenge experiments on its own merits, weighing the benefits of potential scientific knowledge and possible future clinical applications against the severity of risks of lasting harm and temporary discomfort that the challenge procedures are likely to produce.

Informed Consent

Challenge experiments do not raise unique issues relating to informed consent. As in other forms of psychiatric investigation, psychiatric symptom-provoking studies prompt concerns about the ability of various groups of psychiatric patients to give informed consent for research participation. Clinical experience and the research literature do not support the view that, as a class, psychiatric patients have compromised decision-making capacity.[21] On the whole, diagnostic categories are not reliable indicators of the capability of individual patients to give informed consent. Paul Appelbaum and his colleagues found that a group of 26 female outpatients with major depression performed well on the MacArthur Competence Assessment Tool—Clinical Research (MacCAT-CR), which evaluated their capacity to give informed consent to a study of maintenance psychotherapy.[22] William Carpenter and his research team used this same capacity assessment instrument to evaluate the decisional capacity of 30 patients with schizophrenia with respect to a hypothetical randomized trial of a novel antipsychotic medication.[23] A comparison group of normal volunteers was assessed with the MacCAT-CR for a comparable clinical trial. Those with schizophrenia performed significantly worse on the Understanding, Reasoning, and Appreciation scales of the instrument. However, following an educational intervention, those with schizophrenia performed as well as the normal volunteers.

For patients considered at risk of compromised decision-making capacity, adequate safeguards should be implemented to assure that they give informed consent to participation in challenge experiments. The National Bioethics Advisory Commission[3] has recommended capacity assessment by independent professionals for all research studies involving those with mental disorders that may affect decision-making capacity that present greater than "minimal risk"—defined in terms of the type of risks "ordinarily encountered in daily life or during the performance of routine physical or psychological examinations or tests." The alternative requirement that prospective participants pass a test of comprehension of symptom-provoking studies may be no less effective and more efficient.[24]

The context and timing of informed consent for some symptom-provoking studies deserves attention. In a number of studies, amphetamine and methylphenidate challenges have been administered to patients with schizophrenia shortly after psychiatric hospitalization, during a period when they were acutely psychotic and before they received treatment.[1] This linkage between treatment and symptom-provoking studies has the potential to interfere with informed consent. Acutely ill patients in need of treatment for psychotic disorder may lack the capacity to give informed consent at the time of hospitalization and prior to antipsychotic treatment. Additionally, patients who are seeking treatment may not fully appreciate the nontherapeutic nature of the symptom-provoking experiment. They may believe that its purpose is to obtain clinically relevant information about their condition. Finally, they may view research participation as a condition of receiving treatment, thus compromising the voluntariness of their choice to enroll in the challenge experiment. Compelling reasons must justify symptom-provoking studies under these circumstances. If an ethics review board approves such research, tests of comprehension and perhaps an independent capacity assessment would be indicated.

In our experience as members of an IRB reviewing mental health research, we have found that informed consent documents prepared by investigators for IRB review have often failed to be explicit about the purpose of symptom-provoking studies. It is especially misleading to describe symptoms produced by these challenge experiments as "side effects." The aim of eliciting characteristic symptoms to study psychiatric disorders should be clearly articulated at the beginning of consent forms. It is also necessary that these documents describe the symptoms anticipated to be provoked and the fact that the experiment is being used solely for research and not to generate information relevant to the diagnosis or treatment of individual patient-participants.

Infection challenge experiments enroll healthy volunteers who are not at risk of impaired decision-making capacity. In view of the burdens imposed on those participating in these studies, a thorough process of information disclosure prior to research enrollment is critical to assure that prospective volunteers understand the purpose of challenge experiments; the procedures involved, including isolation if relevant; the risks of the induced infection and measures taken to minimize these risks; the type, level, and duration of discomfort likely to be experienced; what can or will be done to alleviate discomfort; and the fact that there are no individual health-related benefits from research participation.

The major ethical concern relating to informed consent for these studies is the potential adverse effects of payment as an inducement to participate. Sometimes a high level of payment is characterized as "coercive," but this confuses threatened penalties for not participating with an incentive to volunteer. The term "undue inducement," often used to describe incentive payments for research thought to be excessive, is also problematic. Because it is not clear what counts as due inducement to participate in research, determinations of undue inducement are apt to be arbitrary. Ezekiel Emanuel has persuasively argued that when the necessary ethical requirements for clinical research are satisfied, then there are no grounds for assessing any level of inducement as undue.[25]

Nevertheless, when substantial payment is offered to volunteer for an infection challenge experiment, safeguards need to be in place to protect individuals from the prospect that the payment might impair their judgment about research participation. Two issues are of concern in this context. First, the offer of payment may cause people to lie about risk factors that would exclude them from study participation. To the extent possible, objective tests should be used to determine study eligibility. When risk factors can be identified only from history-taking, careful assessment is required and confirmatory medical evidence is desirable. Prospective participants must be counseled about the personal importance of truthful communication and informed about the specific health risks of participation if they possess various risk factors. Second, the offer of payment may prompt prospective participants to discount the risks of the challenge experiment.[26] This problem can be counteracted by requiring that individuals pass a test of comprehension, including the major risks of study participation, prior to permitting research enrollment. A similar requirement is appropriate for psychiatric symptom-provoking studies when treatment is offered as an inducement to participate.

Patients typically have not been paid as an inducement to, or compensation for, research participation. Consideration should be given to providing modest payment for participating in psychiatric symptom-provoking studies as a way of signifying the difference between research participation and medical care.[26] This could help dispel any confusion that the research is being conducted to generate diagnostic information for the benefit of patients.

Right to Withdraw From Research

In some infection challenge studies, volunteers are isolated for a period of time following the induced infection in order to prevent transmitting the infection to others. Such restriction on the freedom of research volunteers should not be permitted unless it is judged by investigators and IRBs to be necessary to protect the public health. Isolation or constraints on the ability to leave the research facility conflicts with the norm of research ethics that volunteers are able to withdraw from research participation at any time without interference or penalty. However, restrictions on freedom to withdraw from research participation or a research facility are not unique to infection-inducing challenge experiments. For example, psychiatric patients in studies that withdraw their medication may not be free to leave the research facility if they are judged to be a danger to themselves or to others.

Challenge experiments using isolation should limit the time volunteers spend in isolation to that necessary to eliminate the risk of infecting others. The need for isolation places an added burden on the process of informed consent. All volunteers must be fully cognizant of and agree voluntarily to the isolation requirements. Although participants may not be allowed to leave the research facility for a specified period, this does not preclude their right to withdraw from further exposure to infectious agents and/or other unwanted research procedures.

Conclusion

Challenge experiments constitute a valuable form of clinical investigation. They are perceived as ethically objectionable, in large part, because of misguided moral intuitions that evaluate these studies in the light of ethical norms appropriate to medical care. As in the case of all clinical research, challenge experiments must be carefully planned, prospectively reviewed, and conducted with the aim of promoting valuable research and protecting participants from harm and exploitation.

References

1. Miller FG, Rosenstein DL. Psychiatric symptom-provoking studies: an ethical appraisal. *Biological Psychiatry* 1997;42:403–9.
2. Kotloff KL. Human challenge studies with infectious agents. *Journal of Investigative Medicine* 2003; 51(Suppl.1):S6–S11.
3. National Bioethics Advisory Commission. *Research Involving Persons With Mental Disorders That May Affect Decisionmaking Capacity, Volume I.* Rockville, Md.: NBAC; 1998. [Online] December 1998. Available: http://www.georgetown.edu/research/nrcbl/nbac/capacity/TOC .htm.
4. Miller FG, Grady C. The ethical challenge of infection-inducing challenge experiments. *Clinical Infectious Diseases* 2001;33:1028–33.
5. Miller FG. Research ethics and misguided moral intuition. *Journal of Law, Medicine and Ethics* 2004;32:111–6.
6. Emanuel EJ, Wendler D, Grady C. What makes clinical research ethical? *JAMA* 2000;283:2701–11.
7. D'Souza DC, Berman RM, Krystal JH, Charney DS. Symptom provocation studies in psychiatric disorders: scientific value, risks, and future. *Biological Psychiatry* 1999;46:1060–80.
8. Bremner JD, Vythilingam M, Ng CK, et al. Regional brain metabolic correlates of alpha-methylparatyrosine-induced depressive symptoms: implications for the neural circuitry of depression. *JAMA* 2003;289:3125–34.
9. Wendler D. Informed consent, exploitation and whether it is possible to conduct human subjects research without either one. *Bioethics* 2000;14:310–39.
10. Lederer SE. *Subjects to Science: Human Experimentation in America Before the Second World War.* Baltimore, Md.: The Johns Hopkins University Press; 1995.
11. Steinbrook R. Protecting research subjects—the crisis at Johns Hopkins. *New England Journal of Medicine* 2002;346:716–20.
12. Preston Church LW, Lee TP, Bryan JP, et al. Clinical manifestations of plasmodium falciparum malaria experimentally induced by mosquito challenge. *Journal of Infectious Diseases* 1997;175:915–20.
13. Sack DA, Tacket CO, Cohen MB, et al. Validation of a volunteer model of cholera with frozen bacteria as the challenge. *Infection and Immunity* 1998;66:1968–72.
14. Benkelfat C, Murphy DL, Zohar J, et al. Clomipramine in obsessive-compulsive disorder. *Archives of General Psychiatry* 1989;46:23–8.
15. Delgado PL, Charney DS, Price LH, et al. Serotonin function and the mechanism of antidepressant action: reversal of antidepressant induced remission by rapid depletion of plasma tryptophan. *Archives of General Psychiatry* 1990;47:411–8.
16. Rainey JM, Aleem A, OrtizA, et al. A laboratory procedure for the induction of flashbacks. *American Journal of Psychiatry* 1987;144: 1317–9.
17. Schulz SC, Cornelius J, Jarret DB, et al. Pharmacodynamic probes in personality disorders. *Psychopharmacology Bulletin* 1987;23:337–41.
18. Lahti AC, Warfel D, Michaelidis T, et al. Long-term outcome of patients who receive ketamine during research. *Biological Psychiatry* 2001;49:869–75.
19. Department of Health and Human Services, National Institutes of Health, and Office for Human Research Protections. The Common Rule, Title 45 (Public Welfare), Code of Federal Regulations, Part 46 (Protection of Human Subjects). [Online] June 23, 2005. Available: http://www.hhs.gov/ohrp/humansubjects/guidance/45cfr46.htm.
20. Annas GJ, Grodin MA, eds. *The Nazi Doctors and the Nuremberg Code.* New York, N.Y.: Oxford University Press; 1992.
21. Chen DT, Miller FG, Rosenstein DL. Enrolling decisionally-impaired adults in clinical research. *Medical Care* 2002;40(Suppl.):V20–V29.
22. Appelbaum PS, Grisso T, Frank E, et al. Competence of depressed patients for consent to research. *American Journal of Psychiatry* 1999;156:1380–4.
23. Carpenter WT, Gold JM, Lahti AC, et al. Decisional capacity for informed consent in schizophrenia research. *Archives of General Psychiatry* 2000;57:533–8.
24. Wendler D. Can we ensure that all research subjects give valid consent? *Archives of Internal Medicine* 2004;164:2201–4.
25. Emanuel EJ. Ending concerns about undue inducement. *Journal of Law, Medicine and Ethics* 2004;32:100–5.
26. Dickert N, Grady C. What's the price of a research subject? Approaches to payment for research participation. *New England Journal of Medicine* 1999;341:198–203.

Jason H. T. Karlawish

Emergency Research

History

Research that enrolls people with acute, serious, and life-threatening illnesses without their informed consent, referred to as emergency research, presents substantial ethical challenges. These challenges focus on how to justify enrolling critically ill persons when the investigator cannot obtain informed consent from either the participants or their proxies. Many Western nations have struggled to define the appropriate regulations to guide this kind of research. Perhaps the most illustrative of these efforts occurred in the United States during the 1990s.[1] The controversy over appropriate regulations became so contentious that for three years there was a moratorium on the research while researchers, institutional review boards (IRBs), and research regulators debated whether the principles of research ethics were adequate to justify a waiver of informed consent, and if they were, how such a waiver should be implemented.[2,3]

Ultimately, the U.S. Food and Drug Administration (FDA), an arm of the Department of Health and Human Services (DHHS), issued a set of regulations in 1996 that outlined conditions for the waiver of informed consent in emergency research, after which clinical trials resumed.[4] Although the policy arguments were waged in nuanced debates over the precise wording and intent of the government's basic clinical research regulations, known as the Common Rule,[5] the controversy and its resolution are an excellent case study in issues that transcend the particulars of regulatory language. The issues include the openness of IRB review, who should participate in research review, the justification of research risks, and the role of proxy informed consent.

Clinical trials involving emergently ill persons who are unable to provide informed consent themselves are a relatively recent event in the history of research with humans. The scientific and clinical infrastructure to launch large trials studying important questions in the care of the acutely ill were not capable of facilitating research until the late 1970s—when researchers in cardiology, neurology, emergency medicine, and critical care began to discover the mechanisms of acute, serious, and life-threatening conditions such as myocardial infarction and head injury. Motivated by data that suggested plausible hypotheses for interventions, these investigators and the emergency medical system established an infrastructure for clinical trials to test potential treatments for emergently ill patients.

Some of this research produced dramatic successes. The randomized controlled trials of drugs that opened up clotted coronary arteries demonstrated a reduction in mortality from heart attacks.[6] These "clot buster" drugs rapidly became the standard of care for acute myocardial infarction. In contrast, other trials demonstrated that some initially promising interventions, such as hypothermia for acute head injury, were not effective.[7] In these studies, informed consent was often impossible to obtain from research participants, but the research continued nonetheless, under a variety of rationales for waiving consent.

In the mid-1990s, the U.S. clinical research infrastructure and the DHHS agencies charged with human participant protections came into sharp conflict. The problem was the ethical appropriateness of enrolling people with emergent illness who could not provide informed consent and who had no legally authorized representative available to do so. Clinical investigators and research regulators disagreed over the adequacy of human participant protections for the waiver of both patient and proxy informed consent. The judgment of research regulators in the DHHS that there existed no regulatory guidance for the waiver of informed consent placed a moratorium in 1993 on all emergency research involving a waiver of informed consent unless it was approved by the Secretary of the DHHS.[8]

Prior to this moratorium, how did investigators justify emergency research? They relied on at least one of three justifications: (1) deferred consent; (2) a waiver granted by the FDA for testing an emergency investigational new drug (IND); or (3) a waiver based upon a series of requirements in the Common Rule anchored to the construct of minimal risk. Individually, each of these solutions was ethically inadequate, but collectively they contained many of the elements of the ethical principles used to permit emergency research with a waiver of informed consent.

Deferred consent meant obtaining consent from participants or their proxies to remain in a research protocol after the investigator had already enrolled them in the research.[9] Although researchers who used deferred consent argued that it fulfilled the requirement for informed consent,[10,11] the practice only gave the participant (or proxy) an opportunity to withdraw after enrollment. Hence, it lacked one of informed consent's key components—the ability to choose prior to enrollment. Although deferred consent arguably respected a person's autonomous choice to continue participating in a study, it did not substitute for an informed prospective consent.

A second justification researchers used to waive informed consent in the late 1970s and 1980s was the repeated application of the FDA's rule for the use of an intervention in an unplanned, emergency situation for the benefit of a patient, known as an IND waiver.[12] Investigators argued that they could invoke the IND waiver multiple times for each eligible patient and that it thereby constituted a legitimate mechanism for waiving informed consent. Although this repeated practice of the IND waiver does capture the investigator's judgment that the intervention is potentially beneficial, the waiver refers specifically to a treatment situation. Research may contain components that are given with therapeutic intent, but it inherently includes components to generate knowledge about the efficacy and safety of the intervention. Hence, a waiver of informed consent for treatment purposes cannot be extended to justify exposing a person to research procedures such as randomization.

The third rationale that investigators used was the Common Rule's guidelines for the waiver and modification of informed consent when, as is the case in emergency research, the research could not occur without the waiver.[11] These guidelines required that the research risks were minimal, the waiver would not adversely affect the participants' rights and welfare, steps would be taken to inform the participants of the research, and the research could not be practicably carried out without the waiver.[5] But the Common Rule, first promulgated in 1981, did not clearly articulate what risks *minimal risk* applied to and how to interpret the definition of minimal risk. Substantial disagreement over these issues meant that a waiver on the basis of minimal risk could not settle the controversy.

For three years, emergency research in the United States was halted because federal research regulators argued that no adequate participant protections existed for the waiver of informed consent in emergency research. Until regulations were written that could justify it, all such research was prohibited unless the secretary of the DHHS authorized it. Although the secretary's permission may have granted an investigator legal authority, it did not address any of the unresolved ethical issues. These issues were finally addressed and the moratorium ceased in October 1996 when the DHHS issued regulations that established conditions to permit research with the waiver of an informed consent, the so-called emergency research regulations.[4] These regulations established criteria for the review and approval of emergency research done under a waiver of informed consent (see Table 27.1).

The 1996 emergency research regulations describe a process that engages the investigator, study sponsor, IRB, and general public and that affects the spectrum of activities in the design and conduct of research. This process includes (1) consultation with the leaders of the community about the research design and plans; (2) informing the community about the research; (3) preparing three kinds of informed consent forms—a standard informed consent form for the participant, a form for the family or legally authorized representative to provide proxy informed consent, and a form for consent to continue in the research; and (4) informing the community of the study's results.

These requirements included substantial innovations. Although the new regulations made no effort to clarify the minimal risk controversy, they introduced a novel risk-benefit assessment, namely, that research had to be "potentially beneficial" to the participants. The process of informed consent was expanded to include a role for family rather than the narrowly defined "legally authorized representative." Finally, the process of research review and approval was extended beyond the usual institutional structures. The

Table 27.1

Requirements for Waiver of Informed Consent in U.S. Emergency Research

Necessity: Evidence supports the need to do the research, and the proposed participants are the only population that could reasonably participate in the research.

1. Informed consent from the participant or the participant's legally authorized representative is not practical.

2. Risk-benefit assessment: The research is "potentially beneficial" to the participants.

3. Engagement of the community of potential participants at the beginning and close of the research: The community of potential participants has input into the research design and conduct to determine its social worth and learns about the research results.

4. IRB-to-IRB communication: If one IRB fails to approve the research, the sponsor should inform the remaining IRBs of this fact.

5. Ongoing review of the research: A data safety and monitoring board is in place.

6. Due diligence to obtain consent from participants or their proxy is exercised.

7. Respect for proxy or participant assent and dissent after enrollment.

8. Regulatory review: The FDA and investigator meet to discuss study design and whether the research could be conducted without a waiver of informed consent, and, if the research could not be practicably done without a waiver, how to apply the regulations to the proposed study design.

regulations required consultation with leaders of the community from which research participants would be drawn and required that the community be informed of the proposed research and its results. "Community consultation" was probably the most innovative and controversial of the new regulations' requirements.

The emergency research controversy was a unique opportunity in the ethics of research with humans. By removing the usual protection of informed consent from the participant or a proxy, the research community had to engage a core issue: What are adequate protections for research with humans when the core protection of informed consent is absent? The controversy that brought emergency research to a halt in the United States was resolved by a set of regulations specific to emergency research. Although the problem was solved and the research resumed, this resolution missed an opportunity to settle the general issue of the responsible conduct of research that involves noncompetent adults.

Core Conception and Methodological Rationale

The core concept of emergency research is based on two attributes: (1) the characteristics of enrolled participants; and (2) the impact of the timing of the intervention on the ability to obtain informed consent from either the participants or their proxies. A research project is emergency research when the participants have an acute, serious, and life-threatening condition; the investigator must administer the intervention to the participants within a limited amount of time; and this time limit prevents the research team from obtaining informed consent from either the participants or their proxies.

This definition is conceptually sensible, and investigators can usually apply it. Assume that the first criterion is fulfilled, namely, that the potential participants have an acute, serious, and life-threatening condition. An investigator can generally obtain informed consent for a study whose intervention can be given over the course of days after the acute event. Participants have days to consider the option of enrolling and, in the event a person is not competent to consent, the investigator has time to locate a proxy. Such a study is not emergency research. At the other extreme, an investigator generally cannot obtain informed consent for a study from the patient or the patient's proxy when the intervention must be delivered within minutes of an acute and entirely unexpected event. Such a study is emergency research. But in between these extremes, when does the timing of an intervention transform the research from nonemergency research to emergency research?

Much of the controversy over this question has to do with how one interprets the judgment that it is not practical to obtain informed consent from either the participant or the participant's proxy.[13,14] For example, a study of diaspirin cross-linked hemoglobin for traumatic hemorrhagic shock had a 30-minute window of intervention to randomly administer either the study intervention or blood to patients with acute hemorrhage.[15] Even under these conditions, the investigators enrolled 6% of the participants with prospective informed consent. Hence, informed consent is *possible* with as little as a 30-minute window. But how should an investigator and IRB decide whether this is practicable?

An assessment of the practicality of obtaining prospective informed consent from the participant or the participant's proxy requires a consideration of at least four factors: (1) whether the onset of becoming eligible for a research study can be anticipated

in advance; (2) the proximity of the participant or a proxy to the study site; (3) the financial and personnel resources needed to obtain informed consent from either the participant or a proxy; and (4) the impact of different consent methods on the scientific value of the study. The following two cases illustrate how these factors interact to determine the economic and scientific costs of a requirement for informed consent from either the person prior to illness (advance informed consent) or from a proxy after the person is ill.

In both cases, the studies proposed to recruit persons who were admitted to hospital and then suffered acute cardiac arrest. Under these conditions, advance informed consent from the person is possible. That is, at the time of admission to the hospital, the patients grant consent to be enrolled if they should become eligible for the study. In the first case, the study compared manual chest compressions to a new device to perform chest compressions during cardiopulmonary resuscitation.[16] The study used advance informed consent from the participants who were admitted to hospital.[16] This informed consent practice enrolled 18 participants out of 2,131 prospectively consented patients screened from 7,100 patients. Thus, among participants who granted advance informed consent, approximately 1% were enrolled. With this enrollment rate, the investigators estimated that the study would take 16 years to complete.

In the second case, the study proposed to compare two drugs for cardiac resuscitation.[14] In planning the practicality of advance consent, the investigators identified 85 patients out of 8,000 patients admitted to telemetry units who might have been included over a 14-month enrollment period.[14] As in the other case, the ratio of people granting advance consent to enrolled participants would be approximately 1%. These two cases demonstrate that it is possible to obtain informed consent, but the costs can be substantial. These costs include the number of study staff and sites needed to screen and discuss the study with potentially eligible participants, and the time needed to enroll participants.

Another cost of informed consent is scientific. Specifically, the requirement for informed consent can selectively reduce the enrollment of certain subpopulations. This in turn limits the generalizability of the results because underrepresented populations are excluded from the study, thereby diminishing the social worth of the research. For example, investigators conducting a study of hypothermia for persons with acute brain injury initially used prospective informed consent and then changed to a waiver of informed consent after it became lawful to do so in 1996.[13] The time during which the intervention could be administered was eight hours. During the period of prospective informed consent, the study enrolled 7.2 participants per month. In contrast, during the period when enrollment occurred under a waiver of informed consent, the study enrolled 10.6 participants per month. Whereas the other studies cited above reported enrollment rates of 1% to 6% using informed consent, in this study, a reasonable proportion of participants could be enrolled with prospective informed consent. From the perspective of cost, a requirement for informed consent increased study costs, but not prohibitively.

But the investigators noted differences in the characteristics of the persons enrolled under the requirement for informed consent versus those enrolled under the waiver of informed consent. During the period of prospective informed consent, minority groups were underrepresented by 30%. This gap was closed when the requirement for informed consent was waived. Hence, the informed consent requirement had an impact on the generalizability of the results because the study could say nothing about populations similar to those who were excluded under the informed consent requirement. The requirement for informed consent diminished the social worth of the research.

The economic and scientific costs of informed consent are also interdependent. Even if the financial resources did exist to conduct a 16-year study, the results of such a study might not be valid. The added sites might not be qualified to do the research, and as the duration of a study grew, the administration at study sites would change and interest might wane. Collectively, these factors could compromise the quality of the data collected. In addition, a 16-year study would substantially delay production of useful data and publication of potentially valuable knowledge to the clinical community.

Emergency research is controversial because it suggests that society is willing to trade off a core research participant protection—informed consent—in the pursuit of efficiency and the interests of society. The claim that a project counts as an instance of emergency research is a judgment that must be made through negotiation with all interested parties. In fact, the finding that a protocol is emergency research may vary from site to site. At one site, the consensus may be that a project is not emergency research because prospective informed consent is practical. For example, an urban medical center may find that families are likely to be available in time for an informed consent discussion and thus a waiver of informed consent is not necessary. In contrast, a rural medical center may find that the distance between the families and the hospital is so great that the costs of enrolling only those whose families or proxies can provide informed consent are not acceptable. At that site, the same project would be thought of as emergency research.

Ethical Issues

The voluntary choice of the competent person to enroll in research is a core protection that fulfills the requirement of respect for persons.[17] But is this protection an absolute requirement for the responsible conduct of research? During the 1970s in the United States, the National Commission for the Protection of Human Subjects of Biomedical and Behavioral Research (National Commission) addressed whether it was possible to ethically conduct research in which the participant's signature on an informed consent form is either impossible or unnecessary. The National Commission addressed the ethics of research that involves selected populations and its recommendations were subsequently written into federal regulations for research that involves the following groups: children who are by law not competent to consent,[5(subpart D)] prisoners whose captive environment substantially restricts their voluntary choice,[5(subpart C)] and persons with mental illness severe enough to warrant institutionalization.[18] The National Commission also developed guidelines that resulted in federal regulations for research in which written informed consent from the participant was either infeasible,[5(46.116(d)(1–4))] such as research involving deception, or seemed excessively protective, such as a study that used existing samples initially gathered for clinical purposes without written informed consent.[5(46.117(c)(2))]

The conceptual framework the National Commission developed to address research that involves vulnerable persons or research in which written informed consent from the participant

was infeasible or seemed excessively protective was a substantial step away from the strict requirement of informed consent. By relaxing informed consent as an absolute requirement for all research with humans, while at the same time preserving core protections, the National Commission established a new standard that recognized that the social worth of research could outweigh a strict adherence to the informed consent requirement. In sum, vulnerable persons should have access to research and its potential benefits, and many kinds of valuable research not otherwise practicable without a waiver or modification of informed consent were permissible.

The conceptual framework relied on nuanced applications of the principles of beneficence and justice.[19] Waivers and modifications of written informed consent from the participant are permissible if the research risks and potential benefits fulfilled specific criteria. Parental, prisoner, or proxy consent was appropriate if the research presented no more than minimal risk, or in the case of greater than minimal risk research, if the research either had a reasonable prospect of potential benefit to the participant, could produce results relevant to the class of participants, or had been reviewed and approved by a national panel. The National Commission also articulated the *necessity requirement*. This term described the finding that the research was relevant to the vulnerable population and could not be otherwise done with a nonvulnerable population. The National Commission was thus developing a framework that justified research risks based on balancing study risks against either the potential benefits to the participants or against the importance of the knowledge that could reasonably be expected to result from the research.

This conceptual framework was consistent with two of the National Commission's recommendations in its general guidelines for research with humans. First, its guidelines for IRB review of research required that the IRB judge risks reasonable in relation to the potential benefits to participants and to the importance of the knowledge that could reasonably result from the research. Second, the framework was consistent with the guidelines for waivers and modifications of informed consent in the general conduct of research. An IRB could modify the elements of informed consent, such as the requirement for the participant's signature, or even waive informed consent entirely, if the research risks were minimal, if the waiver or modification would not adversely affect the participants' rights and welfare, and if the research could not practicably be carried out without the waiver or modification.

This model suggests that although the National Commission never specifically addressed the waiver of informed consent in research that involves persons with critical illness, it articulated many of the elements that might justify waiving informed consent in emergency research. But the model is incomplete. Specifically, the National Commission never addressed two shortcomings. These shortcomings remain the source of substantial disagreement in the ethics of research that involves noncompetent adults.[1,19,20] First, although the National Commission rejected the distinction between therapeutic and nontherapeutic research, it never clarified what risks should be balanced against the potential benefits to participants and what risks should be balanced against the importance of the knowledge to be gained from the research. Second, the National Commission did not clearly articulate how to interpret its own definition of minimal risk that was subsequently adopted by federal regulators when they wrote the Common Rule: "*Minimal risk* means that the probability and magnitude of harm or discomfort anticipated in the research are not greater in and of themselves than those ordinarily encountered in daily life or during the performance of routine physical or psychological examinations or tests."[5(46.102(i))] A clear limitation in this definition is the absence of a comparison group to which an IRB could refer when answering the question of to whose daily life the risks of research should be compared. Should the IRB compare the risks of the research to the risks encountered in the daily lives of the potential participants of the research or in the daily lives of healthy persons? A previous version of the regulations stated healthy persons but this was edited out to yield the unanchored definition in the Common Rule.[21] The commentary to the Common Rule stated that the edited definition referred to the risks faced by the potential participants of research.[21]

The authors of the Common Rule would later explain that this edit to the minimal risk definition was intended to permit a waiver of informed consent for research that involved persons with head injury, that is, emergency research.[22] Unfortunately, this was a quick fix without the necessary public discussion of a substantial modification in the nature and intent of the rules for waiver and modification of informed consent. Both politically and ethically, it was ambitious but naive to think that a single word modification in the definition of minimal risk, with an explanation in the commentary section, would settle the issue of when it is appropriate to waive informed consent. Such limited treatment of the issue by the federal officials who wrote the regulations was insufficient when the National Commission had never tackled the general issues of research that involves persons who are cognitively impaired as a result of either physical or mental illness, or the waiver of informed consent in research that involves these participants. In the end, the National Commission's particular recommendations for research that involves the institutionalized mentally ill were never adopted into regulations.

As a result of these shortcomings, investigators and IRBs had little if any explicit guidance for the conduct of emergency research. The Common Rule required that an investigator obtain informed consent from participants or their legally authorized representatives,[5(46.116)] and it directed that when a research project enrolled "vulnerable subjects," the IRB should ensure that additional safeguards are included.[5(46.111(b))] But no detailed procedures existed for obtaining consent from a legally authorized representative, or what to do if such a representative is not available, or what additional protections IRBs and investigators should consider. This limited guidance and the shortcomings in the standard for assessment of research risks precipitated much of the emergency research controversy, the moratorium, and the need for further regulations.

Despite these limitations, the National Commission's conceptual framework was significant for establishing that informed consent was not an absolute requirement and that it could be relaxed when other protections were adequate. The strategies IRBs and investigators did take to justify emergency research—deferred consent, treatment IND waiver, and waived informed consent on the basis of minimal risk—were arguably insufficient. But collectively they suggested that the National Commission's conceptual model could be adapted along with other considerations to create adequate participant protections to permit the waiver of informed consent. The emergency research controversy was a chance to pick up where the National Commission and the authors of the 1981 Common Rule left off. Unfortunately, the emergency research regulations that were issued in 1996 did not do that. Specifically, the regulations did not address the shortcomings in the application of the minimal risk definition and the justification of research risks.

The 1996 regulations focused on four elements: (1) risk-benefit assessment based on the necessity requirement and potential benefit; (2) a process to assess risks and benefits that emphasizes open, public, and ongoing review; (3) a continued role for informed consent; and (4) the ability to opt out of research.

Risk-Benefit Assessment Based on the Necessity Requirement and Potential Benefit

A core defense of the waiver of informed consent was the principle of beneficence. Investigators consistently asserted that there was legitimate uncertainty in the expert community as to the correct approach to manage emergently ill patients. They designed their research projects to settle this uncertainty and determine the benefits of promising interventions for participants who suffered substantial morbidity and mortality even after receiving standard care. Investigators noted a common framework in the provisions of the Common Rule for research that involved children and in the Commission's draft regulations and proposed guidelines for research that involved noncompetent adults that permitted proxy consent in the case of research risks that were minimal or research that was potentially beneficial. However, these regulations and guidelines set out standards for when it is permissible to obtain the informed consent from a parent or proxy, not the waiver of informed consent.

The 1996 emergency research regulations created a novel category of permissible research risk and benefit called a "potential . . . to provide a direct benefit to the individual subjects."[4] The regulations instructed IRBs to judge whether a study met this standard based on a tripartite risk benefit assessment: "risks associated with the investigation are reasonable in relation to (1) what is known about the medical condition of the potential class of participants, (2) the risks and benefits of standard therapy, if any, and (3) what is known about the risks and benefits of the proposed intervention or activity."[4]

The standard suggests three risk assessments. Risks are to be compared to the severity of the medical condition, the risks and benefits of standard therapy, and the risks and benefits of the proposed intervention. There are a number of shortcomings in this tripartite standard.[20] First, it does not articulate which risks are to be used in each of these assessments. Research includes risks that are part of interventions that may help participants (so-called therapeutic components, such as the proposed intervention), and it also includes risks that are part of the intervention but done solely to generate generalizable knowledge (so-called nontherapeutic components, such as additional blood draws and randomization). Second, the first assessment—risks compared to the severity of the medical condition—suggests that the sicker the participant population is, the more justifiable are increased research risks. Although this is accepted in clinical care, it is not at all appropriate that increasing vulnerability justifies increasing research risks, in particular risks that are associated with nontherapeutic components. Third, the balancing of "risks associated with the investigation" with "risks and benefit for the proposed intervention" is at least vague and even incoherent. What risks of the investigation are distinct from the risks of the proposed intervention? Fourth, the balance between risk and the importance of the knowledge that may reasonably result is entirely absent. In summary, although the spirit of the requirement reflects the principle of beneficence, the requirement is vague in instructing an IRB how it should assess the research risks and potential benefits in order to arrive at the judgment that the research has a "potential . . . to provide a direct benefit to the individual subjects."

This is a substantial shortcoming in the regulations and a missed opportunity to settle the loose ends of the National Commission's work. It resurfaced in 1998 when the National Bioethics Advisory Commission (NBAC) proposed regulations for research that involves adults with impaired decision-making capacity.[23] Those regulations, like the 1996 emergency research regulations, should have stipulated clearly what kinds of research risks could be justified by potential benefits to the participants and what research risks were justified by the importance of the research questions. A model to guide this assessment is "component analysis" and was developed by Charles Weijer[19] and adopted by NBAC in 2001 in its summary recommendations for the revision of U.S. human participant research regulations.[24]

Component analysis recognizes that clinical trials characteristically include activities intended to benefit the participants and procedures to evaluate such activities. In other words, research has therapeutic and nontherapeutic components. Dividing research into these respective components assists in justifying research risks. In the case of therapeutic components, the essential consideration is whether legitimate uncertainty exists over which approach to manage emergently ill patients is the preferred one. This epistemological condition, called equipoise,[25] describes a consensus that the available evidence suggests, but is not sufficient to support the claim, that an intervention is at least as effective and safe as existing treatments. A clinical trial is necessary to gather that evidence.

In contrast, the nontherapeutic components of research are the procedures that are done to assure that the study fulfills the requirements of generalizable knowledge. Such procedures include techniques such as randomization, blinding, and tests and questionnaires that are not normally included in standard care of persons with the condition under study. The risks of these components are justified by the value or importance of the knowledge that the research is expected to produce.

How much risk in nontherapeutic components is appropriate in research that enrolls participants without participant or proxy informed consent? The risks justified by nontherapeutic components should be no more than minimal risk, or to avoid the contentious definition, an increment of *acceptable risk*. In accord with the principle of justice, this increment of risk should not be based on the severity of the participant's illness because that would effectively mean that sicker participants could be exposed to greater risks because they are sick. It should be based on the standard of a reasonable person.

A Process to Assess Risks and Benefits That Emphasizes Open, Public, and Ongoing Review

In addition to creating a new conceptual model of research risk and benefit assessment, the 1996 regulations created a process for assessing research risks and benefits. The regulations require the study sponsor and investigator to consult with representatives of the communities from which participants will be drawn and, prior to the start of the research, to publicize to these communities plans for the research and its risks and expected benefits. In the event an IRB at one proposed study site does not approve a study, the regulations require the IRB to document its refusal and require the sponsor to disseminate this report to investigators and IRBs at other sites. During the course of the research, a data safety and monitoring board (DSMB) should review the conduct of the study. Finally, at the close of the research, the sponsor should disclose the results to the community in which the research was conducted. The general theme of this process is an open and public discussion of the risks, potential benefits, and social worth of research.

Among these requirements, the most innovative are the requirements for community consultation, public disclosure, and sharing the determinations of other IRBs. This model of democratic deliberation is novel to the social structure of research review, approval, and monitoring. Typically, in nonemergency research, studies are designed by the expert medical community based on its consensus that equipoise exists. The IRB at each study site reviews the research risks and potential benefits and determines whether they are appropriate. IRB membership includes a representative of the community and the IRB is empowered to bring in additional members as necessary to assist in reviewing a study. The IRB does not routinely seek the input of the participant community. The results of IRB review are not routinely shared with other IRBs reviewing the same protocol. Public disclosure of results is not expected, and in the case of some research, especially research done for advancing corporate interests, disclosure may not occur.

The requirements for community consultation, public disclosure and the sharing of IRB determinations alter this social structure. The requirement that the sponsor and the investigator consult with representatives of the community from which participants will be drawn include suggestions for public meetings to discuss the protocol, the creation of a panel of community members as consultants to the IRB, and the addition to the IRB of community members who are not affiliated with the institution. The goal of these efforts is to promote the public's comprehension of the study and the proposed waiver of informed consent and to elicit community opinions and input. Although there is no formal requirement that the community approve the research, the acts of consultation and disclosure provide the community the opportunity to weigh in on what are permissible risks in the pursuit of research to develop new therapies. Sharing the results of an IRB's deliberations with other IRBs opens up the scope of IRB deliberations to other IRBs. The net effect of all of these requirements is a more public discussion of the research.

In principle, these proposals have substantial merit and conceptual sense. The history of AIDS research suggests that there is good reason to proactively involve the community of potential participants in the process of research review.[26,27] In AIDS research, patients with the disease sharply and vocally disagreed with the standard approach that investigators proposed to determine whether a drug should be used to treat a person with AIDS; in early trials, the proposed endpoints to establish an intervention's efficacy included reducing the number of deaths. Although such an endpoint provides solid proof of efficacy according to the expert medical community, people with AIDS argued that it meant clinical trials exposed them to unnecessary risks in the pursuit of generalizable knowledge and slowed the process of developing effective therapies. Instead, they successfully argued that trials should measure intermediate endpoints that were used in clinical decision making, such as CD4 cell count. Such involvement expands the community that assesses the therapeutic components from an expert medical community to a more democratic community that includes potential participants. In other words, clinical equipoise becomes community equipoise.[27] One could imagine a similar dialogue occurring in a discussion of an emergency research protocol. For example, the community might have input into the judgment that death is the appropriate endpoint to assess an intervention's efficacy or whether the waiver of informed consent was necessary on the basis of the costs and social worth of the research.

Some of the rhetoric to justify community consultation was that it was the "consent of the community."[28] However, the use of the term *consent* in this context does not mean that community consultation replaces the individualized ethic of informed consent. Informed consent is designed to respect an individual's autonomy. A group consultation simply cannot do that. Instead, the ethical issue raised by the requirement for community consultation and disclosure in the emergency research regulations relates to the principle of justice and whether the social structure of research is sufficient to assure that the rights and interests of participants are adequately protected. In the case of AIDS research, patient advocacy groups proactively sought a place at the table and as a result revised the social structure of AIDS research. But the emergency research controversy did not start with public outcry, and the requirement for community consultation did not come from the public asking for a role in research review. This may reflect the fact that the community did not know about the issues, and even when the community did know, that it did not care. The limited coverage in the popular press of the emergency research controversy and the lack of public engagement in spite of the press reports suggests this. But it is also possible that the failure of the public to demand a place in the social structure of research reflected the lack of an organized community to make that demand. In other words, community consultation and public disclosure at the start and end of a study were meritorious proposals but without a clear social structure to support them.

This lack of a social structure was revealed when investigators attempted to fulfill the requirement of community consultation. They struggled with identifying who is the community, and who are its representatives, and who can legitimately speak about the social worth of research. Investigators were faced with the unusual exercise of looking closely at how their eligibility criteria defined who they would recruit, how they would identify leaders who could speak for the community, and what the dialogue with those leaders would involve. In some kinds of studies, the eligibility criteria define a well-circumscribed group, such as narcotics addicts who would be recruited for an intervention for acute overdose. This is a group that can be reached through addiction counseling centers, the courts, and even popular venues for drug trade. But who are their leaders? Other kinds of studies defined increasingly heterogeneous groups such as persons at risk for a heart attack or persons at risk for an automobile accident. Are the leaders of these communities persons who provide health care, politicians, or those who speak up when suitably informed? Finally, the press and other media showed that they were not accustomed to playing a role in the social structure of research.

Poststudy disclosure of studies that were halted on the basis of safety took the form of sensational stories about the waiver of informed consent rather than balanced presentations of the study results.[29]

A Continued Role for Informed Consent

The core of the emergency research controversy was the claim that obtaining informed consent—whether from the participant or from the participant's legally authorized representative—was not practicable. But this is a judgment based upon scientific and economic factors. In some cases, informed consent may not be practicable, but it is possible. The 1996 regulations require that investigators and IRBs address this possibility. The investigator should have IRB-approved informed consent forms in place for the participant and the participant's legally authorized representative in the event informed consent might be obtained at either the time of enrollment or even prior to eligibility using the mechanism of advance informed consent.

This requirement sends a mixed message about the adequacy of the other participant protections. The regulations require that although the balance of the risks and potential benefits and the process to assess them support a waiver of informed consent, the investigators should still make an effort to get informed consent. But if the original judgment was that informed consent is not practicable and its waiver is justified on the basis of a public finding of permissible risks and social worth, why is informed consent thought necessary? This requirement illustrates the unresolved tension in the very definition of emergency research: whether it is appropriate to say that informed consent is not practical, and if it is appropriate, what considerations should enter into the judgment?

Because the regulations require procedures to obtain informed consent when it is possible, they raise the question of what counts as a reasonable effort to secure consent. This suggests that sites should set benchmarks for the expected proportion of participants who will provide informed consent. This benchmark would be informed by previous studies and pilot studies of the proportion of eligible participants who are either themselves capable of informed consent or who will have proxies available to provide informed consent.

The Ability to Opt Out

The regulations require that the investigator locate the legally authorized representative or family of the participants who are enrolled under a waiver of informed consent to disclose that the patient is in the study and obtain "consent to continue in the study." Although this is not informed consent, it does permit a participant the opportunity to withdraw from the study. It is a sensible protection for those who find participation in research objectionable in principle and therefore wish to withdraw their data or cease receiving ongoing study interventions.

Empirical Data

The public's reaction to the emergency research regulations was largely quiet. This may in part reflect the lack of a clear group that represents persons with an emergent illness. It may also indicate that the public did not have the same concerns as researchers and regulators. The few studies of public attitudes that have been conducted suggest that the waiver of informed consent in emergency research does not elicit substantial public concern.[30] More than half of people questioned are willing to participate in such research, and most are willing to allow a family member to serve as a proxy. The experience with actual emergency research protocols suggests that people are typically willing to remain in the research and do not feel that the failure to obtain informed consent is an indignity.[15] What people do express concern over is focused more often on the fairness of selecting their community as the study population, the risks of the intervention, and who will profit from the research.[31]

The Process of Public Disclosure and Community Consultation

Experience with the process of community consultation and public disclosure generally shows that investigators do not regard it as a valuable part of the design and review of their research. Instead, they regard it as a hassle[14] and have difficulty in delineating the requirements and responsibilities for implementing the rule.[32] Most of the communication with the public is informing the public without discussion or exchange of information, so-called one-way communication.[33] One-way communication to announce discussions generally results in limited attendance at public forums. For example, advertisements in a newspaper with a daily circulation of 250,000 to a metropolitan area of 1.5 million people resulted in 12 calls, 20 preregistrations, and 25 attendees at a community consultation meeting.[16] Experience suggests that there may be a vocal minority who want the option to prospectively state their dissent to enrollment using medic alert bracelets or notations on a driver's license similar to the indication for organ donation.[31] The experience with two-way communication suggests that the investigators and IRBs should ask the community the following questions: Does the community recognize the problem the research is designed to address? Are the research risks reasonable with respect to the potential benefits and the importance of the research problem? Finally, given previously voiced concerns about who will profit from the research, investigators should have a clear answer to this question when meeting with members of the public.

The Role and Function of the DSMB

One of the requirements for an emergency research protocol is a DSMB. As important as this board is for the ongoing monitoring of study risks and benefits, there is limited data on how well DSMBs function to protect participants. The case of an emergency research protocol shut down by its DSMB because of substantial numbers of deaths in the intervention group[29] raised two issues that are common to the design and conduct of DSMBs but for which limited data or standards exist to guide investigators.[34] The first issue is DSMB membership. Specifically, what proportion, if any, of the membership of the DSMB should include representatives of the community? A plausible case can be made that just as community consultation is necessary at the start of the trial, it is necessary over the course of the trial. Hence, community repre-

sentation on the DSMB may be appropriate. However, who should serve in this role and what expertise should be required are not evident. The second issue is how the DSMB should balance protecting the interests of the participants with preserving the credibility and integrity of the research. Although unplanned subgroup analyses to assess interim risks, benefits, and results are potentially informative, they may lack sufficient credibility on which to base decisions about whether to stop a trial. One potentially useful strategy to help a DSMB work through the balance between participants' interests and study credibility is an upfront discussion among the members about how they would respond to various kinds of scenarios over the course of the trial.[35] Such a group exercise would force members to express their views on what counts as credible evidence and the degree of risk to which they are willing to expose participants in order to get these data.

Policy Implications

The inability to obtain informed consent to research from emergently ill persons challenges nations to address whether they will relax a core protection for participants in the interests of other patients and society. Although the regulations developed in the United States make such research possible, they present investigators, IRBs, study sponsors, and research regulatory agencies with a number of requirements that researchers generally regard as burdensome. A retrospective review of the number of cardiac arrest trials published during the period of 1992 to 2002 documents a temporal decline in the proportion of studies conducted in the United States compared with all other countries that corresponds to the issuance of the 1996 regulations.[36] This decline suggests that the regulations present a burden to sponsors and researchers, especially researchers who wish to conduct small, single site studies that typically lack the resources to fulfill the requirements for a waiver of informed consent under the 1996 regulations. Or it may reflect that sponsors are taking their research overseas to countries that do not have similar regulatory requirements. Although fewer small and single-site studies may increase the quality of emergency research studies, it does limit the opportunity for innovation and rapid development and testing of new treatments which can occur as a result of small and single-site studies.

The second policy implication is a potential weakening of trial sponsors' ability to protect proprietary data. The regulations' requirements for public disclosure, community consultation, and informing other IRBs if one institution's IRB rejects a project potentially open up the largely private world of research to wider scrutiny of preclinical data, intellectual property ownership, and research results. Such scrutiny might inhibit a private sponsor from supporting an emergency research project.

Study Design Implications

An inability to waive informed consent for research that involves emergently ill persons would have substantial impact on the design of studies to develop interventions to improve the care of these patients. In many cases, the research simply would not be done. Instead, evidence would be gathered by case reports, animal models, and inferences from interventions for related conditions in persons who can provide informed consent or prospective non-randomized cohort studies that examine the outcomes of variations in the standard of care (assuming such variations exist). Each of these kinds of studies has substantial limitations when compared with the randomized controlled trial.

If informed consent is an absolute requirement, there would be some cases when a small portion of the participant population could either provide prospective consent or have a legally authorized representative available to do so on their behalf. In these studies, participant recruitment would be slow and costly. At the close of such studies, the data would be difficult to interpret because of changes over time in the standard of care and legitimate concerns regarding the quality of the data that arise because study sites that enroll participants infrequently are likely to have mistakes in data gathering and the training of study personnel.

The 1996 regulations allowed investigators to avoid these problems. The implications of these rules on study design include allowing investigators to use techniques such as randomization, control groups, and blinding.

Conclusion

The U.S. controversy over emergency research was dramatic, contentious, and resolved with a set of regulations that many researchers regard as cumbersome and an impediment to valuable research and some ethicists regard as a weakening of the structure of human participant protections.

European Union countries have regulations suggesting that a waiver of informed consent would be illegal unless the "direct benefit to the patient outweighs the risks."[37] But this position is ethically questionable. It mistakenly applies to *research* a set of conditions that justify the waiver of informed consent for *treatment*. This approach cannot, however, ethically justify research because study protocols have components that are not intended to benefit participants.

Addressing three unresolved ethical issues might close this disquieting gap between scientific practice and ethical norms. First, there is a need for a coherent conceptual framework to assess research risks and benefits. A framework based on component analysis that separately examines the risks of therapeutic and nontherapeutic procedures seems the most sensible framework. Second, there is a need for a conceptual framework to guide the judgment that informed consent is not practicable. Particular attention is needed to examine cases when informed consent is possible but costly and a threat to scientific value and validity. The third issue arises at the intersection of ethics and political science. The requirement for community consultation suggests that existing local and national structures may not adequately represent the interests of potential participants in the design and review of research. But community consultation is a vague construct without clear institutional structures to support it.

Empirical studies can inform the discussion of these ethical issues. Studies of both researchers and the public should explain how people perceive the moral harm of waiving informed consent in the conduct of research that involves nontherapeutic research risks, the acceptability of waiving informed consent on the basis of considerations of science and costs, and the consequences of changes to the institutional structures for the design and review of research that are intended to expand community input.

References

1. Karlawish JHT, Hall JB. The controversy over emergency research: A review of the issues and suggestions for a resolution. *American Journal of Respiratory and Critical Care Medicine* 1996;153:499–506.
2. Spivey WH, Abramson NS, Iserson KV, MacKay CR, Cohen MP. Informed consent for biomedical research in acute care medicine. *Annals of Emergency Medicine* 1991;20:1251–65.
3. Biros MH, Lewis RJ, Olson CM, Runge JW, Cummins RO, Fost N. Informed consent in emergency research: Consensus statement from the Coalition Conference of Acute Resuscitation and Critical Care Researchers. *JAMA* 1995;273:1283–7.
4. Food and Drug Administration, Department of Health and Human Services. Title 21 (Food and Drugs), Code of Federal Regulation, Part 50.24: Exception from informed consent requirements for emergency research. [Online] April 1, 2006. Available: http://a257.g.akamaitech.net/7/257/2422/10apr20061500/edocket.access.gpo.gov/cfr_2006/aprqtr/21cfr50.24.htm.
5. Department of Health and Human Services, National Institutes of Health, and Office for Human Research Protections. The Common Rule, Title 45 (Public Welfare), Code of Federal Regulations, Part 46 (Protection of Human Subjects). [Online] June 23, 2005. Available: http://www.hhs.gov/ohrp/humansubjects/guidance/45cfr46.htm.
6. Brody BA. *Ethical Issues in Drug Testing, Approval, and Pricing.* New York, N.Y.: Oxford University Press; 1995:5–98.
7. Clifton GL, Miller ER, Choi SC, et al. Lack of effect of induction of hypothermia after acute brain injury. *New England Journal of Medicine* 2001;344:556–63.
8. Ellis G. Informed consent: Legally effective and prospectively obtained: Office for Protection from Research Risks. *OPRR Reports* 1993:93.
9. Levine RJ. Research in emergency situations: The role of deferred consent. *JAMA* 1995;273:1300–2.
10. Abramson NS, Meisel A, Safar P. Deferred consent: A new approach for resuscitation research on comatose patients. *JAMA* 1986;255:2466–71.
11. Prentice ED, Antonson DL, Leibrock LG, Kelso TK, Sears TD. IRB review of a Phase II randomized clinical trial involving incompetent patients suffering from severe closed head injury. *IRB: A Review of Human Subjects Research* 1993;15(5):1–7.
12. Food and Drug Administration, Department of Health and Human Services. Title 21 (Food and Drugs), Code of Federal Regulations, Part 50 (Protection of Human Subjects). [Online] April 1, 2006. Available: http://www.access.gpo.gov/nara/cfr/waisidx_06/21cfr50_06.html.
13. Clifton GL, Knudson P, McDonald M. Waiver of consent in studies of acute brain injury. *Journal of Neurotrauma* 2002;19:1121–6.
14. Kowey P, Ornato J. Resuscitation research and emergency waiver of informed consent. *Resuscitation* 2000;47:307–10.
15. Sloan EP, Koenigsberg M, Houghton J, et al. for the DCLHb Traumatic Hemorrhagic Shock study group. The informed consent process and the use of the exception to informed consent in the clinical trial of diaspirin cross-linked hemoglobin (DCLHb) in severe traumatic hemorrhagic shock. *Academic Emergency Medicine* 1999;6:1203–9.
16. Kremers MS, Whisnant DR, Lowder LS, Gregg L. Initial experience using the Food and Drug administration guidelines for emergency research without consent. *Annals of Emergency Medicine* 1999;33:224–9.
17. National Commission for the Protection of Human Subjects of Biomedical and Behavioral Research. The Belmont Report: Ethical principles and guidelines for the protection of human subjects of research. Washington, D.C.: Department of Health, Education and Welfare; DHEW Publication OS 78-0012 1978. [Online] Available: http://www.hhs.gov/ohrp/humansubjects/guidance/belmont.htm.
18. Office of the Secretary, Department of Health, Education, and Welfare. 45 CFR Part 46: Protection of Human Subjects. Proposed Regulations

on Research Involving Those Institutionalized as Mentally Disabled; Proposed Rule. *Federal Register* 1978;43(223):53950–6.

19. Weijer C. The ethical analysis of risk. *Journal of Law, Medicine, and Ethics* 2000;28:344–61.

20. McRae AD, Weijer C. Lessons from everyday lives: A moral justification for acute care research. *Critical Care Medicine* 2002;30:1146–51.

21. Office of the Secretary, Department of Health, Education, and Welfare. 45 CFR Part 46: Proposed Regulations Amending Basic HEW Policy for the Protection of Human Research Subjects; Proposed Rule. *Federal Register* 1979;44(158):47688–98.

22. McCarthy CR. To be or not to be: Waiving informed consent in emergency research. *Kennedy Institute of Ethics Journal* 1995;5: 155–62.

23. National Bioethics Advisory Commission. *Research Involving Persons With Mental Disorders That May Affect Decisionmaking Capacity, Vol. I.* Rockville, Md.: NBAC; 1998. [Online] December 1998. Available: http://www.georgetown.edu/research/nrcbl/nbac/capacity/ TOC.htm.

24. National Bioethics Advisory Commission. Assessing risks and potential benefits and evaluating vulnerability. In: NBAC. *Ethical and Policy Issues in Research Involving Human Participants, Vol. I.* Bethesda, Md.: NBAC; 2001:69–96. [Online] August 2001. Available: http:// www.georgetown.edu/research/nrcbl/nbac/human/overv011 .pdf.

25. Freedman B. Equipoise and the ethics of clinical research. *New England Journal of Medicine* 1987;317:141–5.

26. Epstein S. *Impure Science: AIDS, Activism, and the Politics of Knowledge.* Berkeley, Calif.: University of California Press; 1996:181–354.

27. Karlawish JHT, Lantos J. Community equipoise and the architecture of clinical research. *Cambridge Quarterly of Healthcare Ethics* 1997;6: 385–96.

28. Ellis G. Perspectives from OPRR. PRIM&R Annual Meeting—IRBs: Encountering the Special Problems of this Decade. Boston, Mass., October 19, 1995.

29. Lewis RJ, Berry DA, Cryer H III, et al. Monitoring a clinical trial conducted under the Food and Drug Administration regulations allowing a waiver of prospective informed consent: The diaspirin cross-linked hemoglobin traumatic hemorrhagic shock efficacy trial. *Annals of Emergency Medicine* 2001;38:397–404.

30. Smithline HA, Gerstle ML. Waiver of informed consent: A survey of emergency medicine patients. *American Journal of Emergency Medicine* 1998;16:90–1.

31. Santora TA, Cowell V, Trooskin SZ. Working through the public disclosure process mandated by use of 21 CFR 50.24 (exception to informed consent): Guidelines for success. *Journal of Trauma* 1998;45:907–13.

32. Biros MH, Fish SS, Lewis RJ. Implementing the Food and Drug Administration's final rule for waiver of informed consent in certain emergency research circumstances. *Academic Emergency Medicine* 1999;6:1272–82.

33. Shah AN, Sugarman J. Protecting research subjects under the waiver of informed consent for emergency research: Experiences with efforts to inform the community. *Annals of Emergency Medicine* 2003;41:72–8.

34. Ellenberg SS, Fleming TR, DeMets D. *Data Monitoring Committees in Clinical Trials: A Practical Perspective.* Chichester, England: John Wiley & Sons Ltd.; 2002.

35. Freedman L, Anderson G, Kipnis V, et al. Approaches to monitoring the results of long-term disease prevention trials: Examples from the Women's Health Initiative. *Controlled Clinical Trials* 1996;17:509–25.

36. Nichol G, Huszti E, Rokosh J, Dumbrell A, McGowan J, Becker L. Impact of informed consent requirements on cardiac arrest research in the United States: Exception from consent or from research? *Resuscitation* 2004;62:3–23.

37. European Parliament and the Council of the European Union. Directive 2001/20/EC of the European Parliament and of the Council of 4 April 2001 on the approximation of the laws, regulations and administrative provisions of the Member States relating to the implementation of good clinical practice in the conduct of clinical trials on medicinal products for human use. *Official Journal of the European Communities* 2001;L121:34–44. [Online] Available: http://europa .eu.int/eur-lex/lex/LexUriServ/LexUriServ.do?uri=CELEX: 32001L0020:EN:HTML

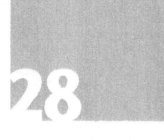

David Wendler

Research With Biological Samples

The collection and storage of human biological samples has become integral to health research. The number of stored samples, estimated to be in the hundreds of millions, if not billions, increases daily as researchers and clinicians routinely obtain samples and store them for research purposes.[1] To identify an appropriate consent process for research with human biological samples, commentators have relied largely on theoretical considerations. Not surprisingly, this approach has led to divergent practices[2] and conflicting recommendations.[3–13]

Some commentators endorse prospective consent, whereas others argue that individuals should provide consent for each new study at the time the study is proposed. There is also disagreement among those who endorse prospective consent. Some advocate asking individuals to authorize future research on the disease being studied, and to separately authorize research on other diseases.[14] Others propose to offer individuals even more choices, including how the samples will be stored, which investigators may use the samples, and what types of research may be performed on them.[15,16] Finally, some hold that consent is not needed at all for research with biological samples that poses minimal risk.[17]

Reliance on different consent practices has the potential to undermine the scientific value of human biological samples and greatly increase the costs of conducting such research. Divergent consent practices require investigators to track the various types of consent obtained for different samples and may preclude the pooling of samples. One way to avoid these problems is to consider whether data on individuals' views support an ethically appropriate and uniform consent process that could be adopted across institutions and around the world.

Relevance of Empirical Data on Individuals' Views

Empirical research has yielded substantial data on individuals' views regarding consent for research with human biological samples,[18] yet few studies have considered the implications of these data for consent practices. This paucity of analysis may trace in part to concerns over the so-called "is-ought" gap between empirical data and moral conclusions. Briefly, the is-ought gap refers to the view that empirical data concern the way the world is, whereas moral conclusions concern the way the world ought to be. Hence, it is unclear to what extent empirical data can shed light on moral controversies and debates. To address this concern, it is important to understand the ethical relevance of empirical data on individuals' views for consent practices.

Any consent process must respect individuals' autonomy and values, and protect them from serious risks. If only one kind of consent process for research with human biological samples were consistent with these ethical goals, appeal to empirical data would be unnecessary. Institutions, investigators, and institutional review boards/research ethics committees (IRBs/RECs) could simply adopt the ethically preferred approach.

Analysis reveals, however, that these ethical considerations are consistent with a number of consent practices. For example, respect for autonomy implies that individuals should be allowed to make their own life decisions. Yet, respect for autonomy does not clearly favor a single kind of consent process. It does not, for example, clearly support prospective consent for unspecified future studies versus asking individuals for consent at the time each new study

Figure 28.1. Stored Tissue Repository. Source: Guido Sauter, University Medical Center Hamburg-Eppendorf. Reproduced with permission.

is proposed. When theoretical considerations alone do not identify a unique approach, data on individuals' views can be useful, in several ways, to identifying a best practice among the ethically acceptable options.

First, empirical data on individuals' views can be vital to determining which of the ethically acceptable approaches are supported by the so-called reasonable person standard. The reasonable person standard can be understood as a response to the fact that even straightforward research studies involve more information and more choices than any single person could possibly absorb and understand. This fact raises the question of what information and which choices should be offered to individuals as part of the informed consent process. According to the widely held reasonable person standard, investigators should make these decisions based on the preferences of the reasonable person: What information does the reasonable person want to make this decision, and which choices does the reasonable person want to be offered? Empirical data can be useful for helping to estimate the views of the reasonable person. In particular, by identifying areas of general consensus, empirical data can provide insight into the views of the reasonable person.

Second, moral analysis implies that investigators should respect individuals' fundamental values. Empirical data can be useful in this regard by identifying fundamental values as they pertain to research with biological samples. For example, empirical data might reveal that the collection of certain types of biological samples, such as semen or ova, conflict with the values of some groups but not others.

Third, respect for persons provides a reason to respect their preferences. All things being equal, investigators should respect the preferences of research participants, even when the preferences

in question do not rise to the level of fundamental values. This is also true when the preferences are not widely shared, in which case they may not be addressed by considerations related to the reasonable person standard, which focuses on preferences that apply to most individuals. Empirical research provides an important mechanism for identifying even relatively uncommon preferences regarding research with biological samples. For example, empirical data might reveal that a certain group of individuals does not want to contribute samples for research purposes, even though the majority of individuals are willing to have their samples so used. This finding could alert investigators to restrict the use of samples obtained from individuals who belong to this group.

To assess the policy implications of empirical data on individuals' views, it is important to recognize that all empirical studies have limitations. The results of survey research in particular can be sensitive to numerous aspects of a given study, including which groups were surveyed, framing effects of the questions, current events at the time the survey was administered, and the possibility that individuals may not have understood some questions or may simply have provided the answers they thought the interviewers wanted to hear. To address these limitations, it is vital to determine the extent to which the data are consistent across studies that surveyed different groups, and whether different questions and methodologies were used.

Literature Search

A comprehensive search was conducted using PubMed for studies published in English that report data on individuals' views regarding consent for research with biological samples (see Appendix 28.1 for details). Studies about individuals' views on research with embryos, as well as studies about the use of biological samples for clinical purposes, were excluded. This search identified 2,483 articles. The titles of all the identified articles were reviewed by the author for any terms related to individuals' views regarding consent for research with biological samples. The abstracts of articles with any relevant terms or phrases were retrieved and reviewed, and the full texts of all potentially eligible articles were reviewed to determine whether they included quantitative or qualitative data on individuals' views regarding consent for research with biological samples. This process yielded 29 unique articles. Finally, references and bibliographies of the 29 articles were reviewed using the same method. This search yielded 2 additional articles.

Empirical Findings

The literature search identified 31 studies that provide empirical data on the views of more than 33,000 individuals regarding consent for research with human biological samples. A summary of these studies is presented in Table 28.1. Most of the studies were quantitative, with a few qualitative studies, hearings, and focus groups. The studies, conducted in the United Kingdom, France, India, Japan, Singapore, Sweden, Uganda, and the United States, assessed the views of employees, religious leaders, patients, current research participants, past research participants, parents of research participants, relatives of deceased individuals, and the general public. Fourteen studies assessed the views of research

Table 28.1

Individuals' Views on Consent for Research With Biological Samples

Respondent Type; Donor/Nondonor	Author, Year	Population; Response Rate	Willing to Provide Sample for Research	Willing to Allow Study of Other Diseases	Comments
Subject; donor	Matsui, 2005[19]	5,361 Japanese; 98.0%	> 90.0%	N/A	Willingness to provide sample for genetic research 5–9% lower
	Hoeyer, 2005[20]	1,200 Swedes; 80.9%	N/A	N/A	48.5% want results; 35.5% not aware they gave a sample
	Chen, 2005[21]§	1,670 U.S.; 100%	90.8%	87.1%	6.7% refused all research
	Wendler, 2005[22]§§	347 Ugandans; 98%	95%	85.0%	54% want results; 4% think may be used for nonresearch
	McQuillan, 2003[23]#	3,680 U.S.; 79.7%	85.3%	85.3%	84% agree to genetic research; minorities slightly less willing
	Stegmayr, 2002[24]	1,409 Swedes; 95.2%	93.0%	N/A	3% oppose industrial research; 22.3% recontact for new projects
	Malone, 2002[25]	7,565 U.S.; 100%	93.7%	86.9%	4% lower consent rate for less detailed consent form
	Wendler, 2002[26]##	814 U.S.; 94% / 47%	N/A	91.9%	88% want results; consent more important for clinically derived samples
	Nakayama, 1999[27]	120 Japanese; 88%	98.5%*	N/A	92% remembered donating; 61% thought it was for clinical care
Patient; donor	Pentz, 2005[28]	315 U.S.; 70%	95%	95%	76% prefer consent once; 14% state consent is unnecessary
	Jack, 2003[29]	3,140 English; 100%	98.8%	N/A	Only 2 individuals concerned about commercial research
	Moutel, 2001[30]	170 French; 30%	100%	N/A	None thought that DNA "storage duration should be limited"
	Hamajima, 1998[31]	583 Japanese; 95.7%	95%	N/A	Some decliners concerned about spreading their disease
Public; donors	Womack, 2003	106 U.K.; 71.0%	100%	N/A	5% stated family or deceased opposed tissue donation
	Kozlowski, 2002[33]	3,383 U.S.; 70%	18%	N/A	Study solicited genetic samples by mail from random individuals
Patient; nondonors	Start, 1996[34]	450 U.K.; 91.0%	83%†	N/A	Some concerned with spreading their disease
	Goodson, 2004[35]	100 English; 100%	82.0%††	N/A	35% want results; 75% "not happy" to contribute to cloning
Public; nondonors	Roberts, 2005[36]	63 U.S.; N/A	N/A	N/A	Support genetic research; concern about children/prisoners
	DeCosta, 2004[37]	59 Indians; 96.6%	86.0%	N/A	14% fewer willing to provide sample of child's blood
	Hoeyer, 2004[38]	1,000 Swedes; 59.6%	N/A	N/A	48% "feel respected" if get results
	Wong, 2004[39]	708 Singaporeans; 70.3%	49.3%	N/A	38.1% unwilling to donate due to fear of needles/injections
	Ashcroft, 2003[40]	155 U.K.+; N/A	100%	N/A	Want control; oppose cloning; want new consent for new tests
	PSP, 2002[41]++	16 U.K. focus groups; N/A	N/A	N/A	Support research; willing to contribute biological samples
	Stolt, 2002[42]	21 Swedes; N/A	N/A	N/A	Support research on other diseases; some want results
	Asai, 2002[43]	21 Japanese; N/A	N/A	N/A	Support research; concerned about risks; some want results
	Schwartz, 2001[44]	1,383 U.S. Jewish Am.; 20%	> 80.0%	> 80.0%	Want consent for each study, but not offered general consent
	Wang, 2001[45]	3130 U.S.; 84%	79%	79%	21% not willing to donate nor store blood for genetic research

Table 28.1 (*Continued*)

Respondent Type; Donor/Nondonor	Author, Year	Population; Response Rate	Willing to Provide Sample for Research	Willing to Allow Study of Other Diseases	Comments
	Welcome Trust, 2000[46]	16 U.K. focus groups; N/A	N/A	N/A	Most would provide sample; prefer disease-specific research
	NBAC, 2000[47]	7 U.S. hearings; N/A	N/A	N/A	Support research, including for profit; endorse one-time consent; concerned about confidentiality
	Merz, 1996[48]	99 U.S.; 0–20%	60%	87%	26% want results; 30% would restrict drug company access
	Phan, 1995[49]	21 U.S.+++; 48.8%	N/A	N/A	90.5% support genetic research; concerned about confidentiality

N/A = Indicates that the study does not provide quantitative data on the relevant question. § Denominator varies for different questions. §§ Respondents were guardians who donated children's blood samples. # Using year 2000 data. ## Most respondents were subject donors; the remainder were public nondonors. * Of the 96 respondents who participated in the follow-up survey. ** Donated deceased family members' tissue. † Percentage who would agree to their left over tissue being used for *medical research*; †† Percentage who were "happy" for tissue to be used for *cancer research*. + 35 individuals in focus groups; 120 in individual interviews. ++ Also interviewed clinicians, patients, community leaders and organization spokespersons. +++ Respondents were religious leaders from the Midwest.

participants, patients or members of the general public who had donated samples for research purposes; 17 studies assessed the views of patients or members of the general public who had not donated a sample for research.

Taken together, the studies yield consistent findings, despite being conducted around the world, over a 10-year period, in different groups, using different methods. The studies reveal that the vast majority of individuals want to decide whether their biological samples are used for research purposes. When given a choice, 80–95% of individuals are willing and 5–10% are not willing to contribute a biological sample for research purposes.

Most objections to providing samples are due to factors other than their use in research. For example, some individuals expressed concern regarding the method of obtaining samples. Only 50% of respondents in one study were willing to provide a sample for research, but 38% of those who were unwilling cited a fear of needles or injections as their reason.[39] Similarly, in another study, most respondents who declined even to consider the possibility of providing a sample of their deceased relative's tissue cited the time required for the discussion.[32] Only 18% of the respondents in yet another study provided a genetic sample for research.[33] However, these individuals were contacted through random digit dialing by investigators unknown to them. In addition, respondents were required to complete a telephone interview, agree to receive a kit for obtaining genetic samples, follow the instructions in order to use the kit themselves, and mail the sample back to the investigators. The low rate of donation in this study likely traces, at least in large measure, to the fact that respondents were contacted by strangers and providing a sample would be time consuming and difficult.

Consistent with the finding that most objections trace to factors related to obtaining the samples, rather than the actual research use of the samples, all six studies that focused exclusively on leftover samples found extremely low opposition to samples being used for research purposes. More than 90% of the respondents in five of the six studies were willing to donate their leftover samples for research purposes.[24,25,28,29,31] In the remaining study, 83% of patients were willing to donate their leftover tissue for

research and only 2% were unwilling.[34] The other patients skipped the relevant question in the survey or were unsure of their views regarding donation. Furthermore, many of those who were unsure or unwilling to donate expressed concern over the possibility of spreading their disease to others.

Studies that investigated different consent options found that the vast majority of individuals who are willing to provide samples for research are willing to provide samples for research in general, without restriction regarding the type of research for which their samples would be used. Even the five studies that assessed research on potentially stigmatizing diseases found that most individuals are willing to provide their samples for such research. Two studies found that individuals are equally or slightly more willing to provide samples for research on potentially stigmatizing conditions (Alzheimer's;[28] HIV[22]); two others found that individuals are slightly less willing (Down syndrome;[35] Alzheimer's[25]); and one study found mixed results (mental illness, equally willing; homosexuality, slightly less willing).[44] The only proposal that elicited consistent opposition in the four studies that assessed the issue was the use of samples in research aimed at cloning human beings.

In seven studies that explicitly addressed the issue, the majority of individuals were willing to provide one-time general consent and rely on IRBs/RECs to determine when their samples would be used in future research projects.[20,22–25,28,38] The apparent exception to this acceptance of one-time general consent found that approximately 70% of respondents thought consent was needed for each project. However, as the authors note, these respondents were not offered the option of one-time consent.[44]

Three studies assessed commercial research, finding that individuals are only slightly less willing to provide a sample for commercial compared to academic research.[24,29,48] Finally, nine studies assessed whether individuals want information on the studies for which their samples will be used. A significant percentage, ranging from 26%[48] to 88%,[26] want such information. Because the studies tend to ask about information in general, it is unclear whether individuals want information on the goals of the studies, their own results, grouped results, or some combination of these types of information.

Implications for Informed Consent

Contemporary commentators, following the philosopher David Hume, often cite a gap, the so-called is-ought gap, between empirical data and ethical conclusions.[50,51] Empirical data concern the way the world is; ethical conclusions concern the way the world ought to be. To assess the implications of empirical data on individuals' views, it is important to recognize the is-ought gap, yet not overstate its significance. The is-ought gap does not imply that empirical data are irrelevant to ethics. Instead, this gap implies that it is impossible to derive moral conclusions about what we ought to do or which policy we ought to adopt from empirical data alone. To derive ethical conclusions, empirical data must always be supplemented by and analyzed in the context of the relevant moral considerations.

Moral analysis establishes that any consent process should respect individuals' autonomy and values and that it should protect them from unwarranted risks. However, these considerations are consistent with a number of consent processes for research with biological samples. In this context, empirical data on individuals' views provides a way to identify which consent process is best supported by the reasonable person standard and best respects individuals' fundamental values.

The data reveal consistent and strong evidence that individuals around the world want to control whether their biological samples are used for research purposes. When given a choice, the vast majority of individuals choose to provide a sample, whereas a small minority of individuals do not want their samples used for research purposes. The data also reveal that the vast majority of individuals endorse one-time general consent and are willing to rely on IRBs/RECs to determine when their samples will be used in future research projects.

Because these data are so consistent across surveys and survey populations, they provide an estimate for the consent process best supported by the reasonable person standard. Specifically, these data suggest that the reasonable person standard supports a default practice of offering individuals a simple, binary choice of whether their samples may be used for research, with the stipulation that future decisions regarding research uses will be made by an IRB/REC.[52,53] In addition to respecting individuals' autonomy by allowing them to decide whether their samples are used for research, this approach respects the small minority who do not want their samples used for research by allowing them to keep their samples out of the research pool. This approach also protects individuals by ensuring their samples are used for future research only when the reviewing IRB/REC finds that the research project poses no more than minimal risk, including any risk of group harms.

Although this consent process should be suitable for most studies, there may be compelling reasons to modify it in some cases, either by waiving consent or soliciting more detailed consent. The consistency of the data implies that the default of offering a simple, binary choice should be modified only in rare cases. Specifically, the fact that individuals want to control whether their samples are used for research implies that consent typically should be obtained even when samples will be anonymized. Conversely, the fact that individuals are willing to have their samples used for research on all conditions—including potentially stigmatizing conditions and conditions from which they do not suffer—implies that only rarely will there be a need to detail the different kinds of research for which their samples might be used.

Implementation

To implement this approach, the consent form and process should include at least the following five elements: (1) request to obtain samples for future research; (2) risks, if any; (3) absence of direct benefits; (4) information, if any, to be provided to individuals; and (5) reliance on IRB/REC to review and approve future research provided it poses no greater than minimal risk (see Box 28.1).

Several studies found that individuals often assume samples obtained for research will be used for their own clinical care.[27] To address this confusion, the consent process should inform individuals that the research will not benefit them. The finding that many individuals would like information regarding future research studies implies, at a minimum, that individuals should be told what information will be provided to them regarding future studies.

The consent process should also include additional elements as appropriate (see Box 28.1). In cases in which individuals retain the right to remove their samples from the research pool, they should be so informed. When samples are obtained as part of clinical care or other research, individuals should be told whether their decision regarding samples will have any impact on their clinical care or research participation.

Box 28.1.
Suggested Wording of Consent Forms

A. Possible Wording

"We would like to use your blood (tissue) sample in future studies to learn how to improve people's health. The researchers conducting these studies will not contact you for more information. Your sample will be used only when an independent group, called an institutional review board [research ethics committee], determines that the research is important and ethical, and poses no more than minimal risk to you. These future research projects will not benefit you personally, and are not part of your medical care. All information you provide will be kept confidential as far as possible. However, there is always a very small chance that some information may be released."

B. Possible Additions When Relevant

Optional provision: "No matter what you decide, it will not affect how we treat you."

Individual information: "We will provide you with any information from future studies that may have an impact on your health."

Study information: "Information on the nature [findings] of future research projects will be posted on our website [provided in some other way]."

Future removal: "If you decide in the future that you no longer want to allow your sample to be used for research, please contact the study doctors and any remaining sample will be removed."

The data reveal that many individuals want information about the studies for which their samples are used. The data do not indicate whether individuals want information on the research goals of the studies, pooled results, individual results, or some combination of these types of information. These data also do not address why individuals want this information, for instance, whether they are curious or think the information might be relevant to their clinical care; nor do the data address how individuals might balance receiving information with protecting their confidentiality, and the possibility that some information might cause them anxiety. Recommendation of a uniform approach to this issue will require further research and analysis.

IRBs/RECs should not approve research projects that involve using individuals' samples for purposes that conflict with the individuals' fundamental values. The several studies that assessed the issue reveal that many individuals are opposed to their samples being used for research dedicated to cloning human beings. Hence, investigators should not be allowed to use samples for this type of research without first obtaining specific informed consent. Finally, the vast majority of studies focused on blood and tissue samples. Individuals may be more willing to provide some types of samples, such as hair or sweat, and less willing to provide other types of samples, such as semen or placenta.[54]

Implications for Ethics Review

Most commentators argue that research with human biological samples should be subject to ethical review and approval. Most guidelines agree with this approach. In 2004, however, the U.S. Office for Health Research Protections ruled that if the samples were not obtained specifically for the research project in question, and if an arrangement was in place to keep investigators from obtaining the identities of the donors, then the samples are considered not identifiable—and therefore are not subject to U.S. regulations or IRB review.[55]

The existing data indicate that the vast majority of individuals are willing to provide biological samples for research purposes and to rely on IRBs/RECs to protect them from risks. The data do not indicate, however, whether individuals would be willing to rely on investigators to decide when their samples are used for research purposes in the absence of IRB/REC review and approval. Until future research is conducted on individuals' views, and on whether investigators would provide sufficient protections without IRB/REC oversight, the existing data support requiring IRB/REC review and approval. Hence, in the absence of compelling considerations to the contrary, it seems reasonable to argue that ethics review should be required.

Conclusion

Many proposed approaches to consent for research with biological samples are consistent with the moral considerations of respecting individuals' autonomy and values, and protecting them from untoward risks. In this context, empirical data can help to identify the preferred approach by estimating the views of the reasonable person and identifying individuals' relevant values and preferences.

The existing empirical data reveal that the vast majority of individuals want to control whether their samples are used for

Appendix 28.1

Articles Found in PubMed by Type and Number

Search Terms	Number Found
Limits: All Fields, in English, Humans	1,770
views and stored samples	4
attitudes and stored samples	8
perceptions and stored samples	4
opinions and stored samples	1
public and stored samples	177
views and biological samples	23
attitudes and biological samples	22
perceptions and biological samples	0
opinions and biological samples	3
public and biological samples	652
views and biospecimens	0
attitudes and biospecimens	0
perceptions and biospecimens	0
opinions and biospecimens	0
public and biospecimens	1
views and biobanks	1
attitudes and biobanks	3
perceptions and biobanks	1
opinions and biobanks	1
public and biobanks	11
views and genetic research	20
attitudes and genetic research	158
perceptions and genetic research	22
opinions and genetic research	5
public and genetic research	664
Limits: Title/Abstract, in English, Humans	713
consent and stored samples	40
consent and biological samples	37
consent and biospecimens	0
consent and biobanks	9
consent and genetic research	180
empirical data and stored samples	1
empirical data and biological samples	11
empirical data and biospecimens	0
empirical data and biobanks	0
empirical data and genetic research	31
survey and stored samples	72
survey and biological samples	106
survey and biospecimens	0
survey and biobanks	0
survey and genetic research	202
donate and stored samples	1
donate and biological samples	10
donate and biospecimens	0
donate and biobanks	1
donate and genetic research	12

research purposes. The vast majority of individuals also endorse one-time general consent. These data support offering individuals a simple binary choice of whether their samples may be used for research purposes, with the stipulation that an IRB/REC will decide when their samples are used. This approach respects individuals' autonomy and is supported by the reasonable person standard for informed consent. In particular, this approach allows all individuals to control whether their samples are used for research, and allows the minority who do not want their samples used to keep them out of the research pool. This approach has the additional virtues of not burdening individuals with unwanted choices, and avoiding unnecessarily burdening institutions with the need to track the specific choices that attach to individual samples under other approaches to consent.

Acknowledgments

Thanks to Bernice Elger, Benjamin Wilfond, Rebecca Pentz, and Ezekiel Emanuel for their helpful comments on earlier versions of the manuscript. The opinions expressed are the author's own. They do not represent any position or policy of the National Institutes of Health, Public Health Service, or Department of Health and Human Services.

References

1. Azarow KS, Olmstead FL, Hume RF, Myers J, Calhoun BC, Martin LS. Ethical use of tissue samples in genetic research. *Military Medicine* 2003;168:437–41.
2. White TH, Gamm J. Informed consent for research on stored blood and tissue samples: A survey of institutional review board practices. *Accountability in Research* 2002;9:1–16.
3. Clayton EW, Steinberg KK, Khoury MJ, Thomson E, Andrews L, Kahn MJ, Kopelman LM, Weiss JO. Informed consent for genetic research on stored tissue samples. *JAMA* 1995;274:1786–92.
4. Stephenson J. Pathologists enter debate on consent for genetic research on stored tissue. *JAMA* 1996;275:7.
5. Reilly PR, Boshar MF, Holtzman SH. Ethical issues in genetic research: Disclosure and informed consent. *Nature Genetics* 1997;15:16–20.
6. Association of American Medical Colleges. *Health Data Security, Patient Privacy, and the Use of Archival Patient Materials in Research.* AAMC Policy Statement. Approved: AAMC Executive Council, February 27, 1997.
7. Knoppers BM, Laberge C. Research and stored tissues: Persons as sources, samples as persons? *JAMA* 1995;274:1807.
8. Rothstein MA. Expanding the ethical analysis of biobanks. *Journal of Law Medicine and Ethics* 2005;33:89–101.
9. Mashcke KJ, Murray TH. Ethical issues in tissue banking for research: The prospect and pitfalls of setting international standards. *Theoretical Medicine and Bioethics* 2004;25:143–55.
10. Winickoff DE, Winickoff RN. The charitable trust as a model for genomic biobanks. *New England Journal of Medicine* 2003;349:1180–4.
11. Hakimian R, Korn D. Ownership and use of tissue specimens for research. *JAMA* 2004;292:2500–5.
12. Van Diest PJ, Savulescu J. No consent should be needed for using leftover body material for scientific purposes: For and against. *British Medical Journal* 2002;325:648–51.
13. Lo B, Chou V, Cedars MI, Gates E, Taylor RN, Wagner RM, Wolf L, Yamamoto KR. Consent from donors for embryo and stem cell research. *Science* 2003;301:921.
14. National Action Plan on Breast Cancer. Model Consent Form for Biological Tissue Banking: Focus Group Report. [Online] 1998.

Available: http://www.4woman.gov/napbc/catalog.wci/napbc/model_consent.htm.
15. Council of Europe, Steering Committee on Bioethics. *Draft Explanatory Report to the Proposal for an Instrument on the Use of Archived Human Biological Materials in Biomedical Research.* Strasbourg, Council of Europe, 2002. [Online] October 14, 2002. Available: http://www.coe.int/t/e/legal_affairs/legal_co-operation/bioethics/activities/biomedical_research/cdbi-inf%282002%296e.pdf.
16. National Bioethics Advisory Commission. *Research Involving Human Biological Materials: Ethical Issues and Policy Guidance, Vol. I.* Rockville, Md.: NBAC; 1999. [Online] August 1999. Available: http://www.georgetown.edu/research/nrcbl/nbac/hbm.pdf.
17. The American Society of Human Genetics. Statement on informed consent for genetic research. *American Journal of Human Genetics* 1996;59:471–4.
18. Ring L, Lindblad AK. Public and patient perception of biobanks and informed consent. In: Hansson MG, Levin M, ed. *Biobanks as Resources for Health.* Uppsala, Sweden: Uppsala University; 2003.
19. Matsui K, Kita Y, Ueshima H. Informed consent, participation in, and withdrawal from a population-based cohort study involving genetic analysis. *Journal of Medical Ethics* 2005;31:385–92.
20. Hoeyer K, Olofsson B, Mjorndal T, Lynoe N. The ethics of research using biobanks: Reason to question the importance attributed to informed consent. *Archives of Internal Medicine* 2005;165:97–100.
21. Chen DT, Rosenstein DL, Muthappan PG, Hilsenbeck SG, Miller FG, Emanuel EJ, Wendler D. Research with stored biological samples: What do research participants want? *Archives of Internal Medicine* 2005;165:652–5.
22. Wendler D, Pace C, Talisuna A, Maiso F, Grady C, Emanuel E. Research on stored biological samples: The views of Ugandans. *IRB: Ethics and Human Research* 2005;27(2):1–5.
23. McQuillan GM, Porter KS, Agelli M, Kington R. Consent for genetic research in a general population: The NHANES experience. *Genetics in Medicine* 2003;5:35–42.
24. Stegmayr B, Asplund K. Informed consent for genetic research on blood stored for more than a decade: A population based study. *British Medical Journal* 2002;325:634–5.
25. Malone T, Catalano PJ, O'Dwyer PJ, Giantonio B. High rate of consent to bank biologic samples for future research: The eastern cooperative oncology group experience. *Journal of the National Cancer Institute* 2002;94:769–71.
26. Wendler D, Emanuel E. The debate over research on stored biological samples: What do sources think? *Archives of Internal Medicine* 2002;162:1457–62.
27. Nakayama T, Muto K, Yoshiiike N, Yokoyama T. Awareness and motivation of Japanese donors of blood for research. *American Journal of Public Health* 1999;89:1433–4.
28. Pentz RD, Billot L, Wendler D. Research on stored biological samples: Views of African American and white American cancer patients. *American Journal of Medical Genetics* 2006;140;733–9.
29. Jack AL, Womack C. Why surgical patients do not donate tissue for commercial research: Review of records. *British Medical Journal* 2003;327:262.
30. Moutel G, Montgolfier S, Meningaud JP, Herve C. Bio Libraries and DNA storage: Assessment of patient perception and information. *Medicine and Law* 2001;20:193–204.
31. Hamajima N, Tajima K, Oya H, et al. Patients' views on residual blood use for research purposes. *Japanese Journal of Cancer Research* 1998;89:341–6.
32. Womack C, Jack AL. Family attitudes to research using samples taken at coroner's postmortem examinations: Review of records. *British Medical Journal* 2003;327:781–2.
33. Kozlowski LT, et al. Using a telephone survey to acquire genetic and behavioral data related to cigarette smoking in "made-anonymous"

and "registry" samples. *American Journal of Epidemiology* 2002;156: 68–77.

34. Start RD, Brown W, Bryant RJ, Reed MW, Cross SS, Kent G, Underwood JCE. Ownership and uses of human tissue: Does the Nuffield bioethics report accord with opinion of surgical inpatients? *British Medical Journal* 1996;313:1366–8.

35. Goodson ML, Vernon BG. A study of public opinion on the use of tissue samples from living subjects for clinical research. *Journal of Clinical Pathology* 2004;57:135–8.

36. Roberts LW, Warner TD, Geppert CM, Rogers M, Green Hammond KA. Employees' perspectives on ethically important aspects of genetic research participation: A pilot study. *Comprehensive Psychiatry* 2005;46:27–33.

37. DeCosta A, D'Souza N, Krishnan S, Chhabra MS, Shihaam I, Goswami K. Community based trials and informed consent in rural north India. *Journal of Medical Ethics* 2004;30:318–23.

38. Hoeyer K, Olofsson BO, Mjorndal T, Lynoe N. Informed consent and biobanks: A population-based study of attitudes towards tissue donation for genetic research. *Scandinavian Journal of Public Health* 2004;32:224–9.

39. Wong ML, Chia KS, Yam WM, Teodoro GR, Lau KW. Willingness to donate blood samples for genetic research: A survey from a community in Singapore. *Clinical Genetics* 2004;65:45–51.

40. Ashcroft R, Kent J, Williamson E, Goodenough T. *Ethical Protection in Epidemiological Genetic Research: Participants' Perspectives. Final Report.* November 2003.

41. People Science and Policy Ltd. *BioBank UK: A Question of Trust: A Consultation Exploring and Addressing Questions of Public Trust.* London, England: People Science & Policy Ltd.; 2002. [Online] March 2002. Available: http://www.mrc.ac.uk/pdf-biobank_public_consultation.pdf.

42. Stolt UG, Liss PE, Svensson T, Ludvigsson J. Attitudes to bioethical issues: A case study of a screening project. *Social Science and Medicine* 2002;54:1333–44.

43. Asai A, Ohnishi M, Nishigaki E, Sekimoto M, Fukuhara S, Fukui T. Attitudes of the Japanese public and doctors toward use of archived information and samples without informed consent: Preliminary findings based on focus group interviews. *BMC Medical Ethics* 2002;3:E1.

44. Schwartz MD, Rothenberg K, Joseph L, Benkendorf J, Lerman C. Consent to the use of stored DNA for genetics research: A survey of attitudes in the Jewish population. *American Journal of Medical Genetics* 2001;98:336–42.

45. Wang SS, Fridinger F, Sheedy KM, Khoury MJ. Public attitudes regarding the donation and storage of blood specimens for genetic research. *Community Genetics* 2001;4:18–26.

46. The Wellcome Trust and Medical Research Council. *Public Perceptions of the Collection of Human Biological Samples.* [Online] October 2002. Available: http://www.ukbiobank.ac.uk/docs/perceptions.pdf.

47. Wells JA, Karr D. Mini hearings on tissue samples and informed consent. In: National Bioethics Advisory Commission. *Research Involving Human Biological Materials: Ethical Issues and Policy Guidance, Vol. II.* Rockville, Md.: NBAC; 2000:G1–G53. [Online] January 2000. Available: http://www.georgetown.edu/research/nrcbl/nbac/hbmII.pdf.

48. Merz JF, Sankar P. DNA banking: An empirical study of a proposed consent form. In: Weir RF, ed. *Stored Tissue Samples: Ethical, Legal, and Public Policy Implications.* Iowa City, Iowa: University of Iowa Press; 1998:198–225.

49. Phan KL, Doukas DJ, Fetters MD. Religious leaders' attitudes and beliefs about genetics and the human genome project. *Journal of Clinical Ethics* 1995;6:237–46.

50. Hume D. *A Treatise of Human Nature.* Harmondsworth, England: Penguin Books; 1969 [1739].

51. Gewirth A. The "is-ought" problem resolved. *Proceedings and Addresses of the American Philosophical Association* 1973–1974;47:34–61.

52. Clayton EW. Informed consent and biobanks. *Journal of Law, Medicine, and Ethics* 2005;33:15–21.

53. Buchanan A. An ethical framework for biological samples policy. In: National Bioethics Advisory Commission. *Research Involving Human Biological Materials: Ethical Issues and Policy Guidance, Vol. II.* Rockville, Md.: NBAC; 2000:B1–B31. [Online] January 2000. Available: http://www.georgetown.edu/research/nrcbl/nbac/hbmII.pdf.

54. Jenkins GL, Sugarman J. The importance of cultural considerations in the promotion of ethical research with human biologic material. *Journal of Laboratory and Clinical Medicine* 2005;145:118–24.

55. Department of Health and Human Services, Office for Human Research Protections. Guidance on research involving coded private information or biological samples. [Online] August 10, 2004. Available: http://www.hhs.gov/ohrp/humansubjects/guidance/cdebiol.pdf

Eric T. Juengst   Aaron Goldenberg

29

Genetic Diagnostic, Pedigree, and Screening Research

Interest in genetic approaches to biomedical research problems has been high for almost 100 years, since Archibald Garrod used Gregor Mendel's rediscovered theory of inheritance to explain human "inborn errors of metabolism" in 1908.[1] From the point of view of clinical research ethics, sadly, many chapters of this history are viewed today as examples of how biomedical science can be exploited by social prejudices to the detriment of marginalized people. Borrowing from the successes of both stock breeding and the germ theory of disease, early human geneticists moved quickly from biased pedigree studies and racist anthropologies to draconian prescriptions for preventing hereditary disease and improving the public's health. In the United States, policy makers translated these *eugenic* conclusions into selective immigration restrictions and involuntary sterilization programs; Germany under fascism took them further, to coercive selective breeding programs and genocide.[2–8] By mid-century, the Nuremberg trials had transformed *eugenics* into an epithet and launched our contemporary concern with clinical research ethics on the lessons of the medical experiments undertaken in its name[9] (see Chapters 2 and 12).

Over this same period, biochemists, cell biologists, and geneticists working with animal and plant models were steadily illuminating the cellular and molecular mechanisms of genetic inheritance.[10] Since World War II, the resulting field of molecular genetics has inspired new waves of interest in research that might produce a *genetic medicine* for the future.[11] With the elaboration of the genetic code and the role of DNA mutations in *molecular disease,* a new discipline of medical genetics was able to use molecular markers to track and predict health problems in families and populations, and with the development of methods for manipu-

lating DNA, a new *biotechnology* made it possible to contemplate a comprehensive molecular analysis of the human genome. Today, in the wake of the Human Genome Project and the human genetic research it makes possible, clinical scientists whose specialties range from infectious disease to psychiatry are conducting family studies to isolate genetic variants, developing diagnostic tests based on those variations, and screening populations with those tests to assess the variants' prevalence and distribution.

With the widespread adoption of genetic approaches to biomedical research problems has also come new attention to the ethical issues that human genetic research can raise. Against the historical backdrop of eugenics, genetic researchers have reason to be sensitive to the potentially stigmatizing power of genetic information and acutely concerned to fulfill their obligations to respect the rights and interests of the individuals, families, and groups they study. Their challenge has been that, although genetic family studies, testing trials, and population screening surveys have been conducted for decades, there has been little consensus about how they should be designed and conducted from an ethical point of view.

As new research teams take up genetic approaches, investigators and institutional review boards (IRBs) alike quickly discover that both the federal research regulations and the research ethics literature are only beginning to explore this area. If anything, the prevailing standards seem to assume that cohorts of biomedical research subjects usually consist of individual strangers, rather than people who live with each other as families and communities. At the same time, a variety of homegrown practices and policies have evolved within the human genetics research community to address these challenges.[12] Unfortunately, these precedents can bewilder as easily as they illuminate. Although homegrown approaches to specific problems are often defended passionately by their advocates, almost all these approaches have their critics as well.

In 1993, the federal Office for Protection from Research Risks (OPRR; now the Office for Human Research Protections, OHRP) issued a second edition of its *Institutional Review Board Guidebook,* which included a new section addressing human genetic research. That section opens with the caveat: "Some of the areas described in this Section present issues for which no clear guidance can be given at this point, either because not enough is known about the risks presented by the research or because no consensus on the appropriate resolution of the problem yet exists."[13] In fact, 10 different open research policy questions can be found in that section, under two broad headings: issues in recruitment for and consent to genetic studies, and issues in information disclosure and control.[14] The *Institutional Review Board Guidebook* has never been updated, but many of the questions it raises have been the subject of research and policy discussion over the last decade. For some questions, a consensus has emerged that provides a way forward for researchers. Other questions have been substantially superseded by new ones. Still others remain hotly contested. Five topics warrant special consideration:

1. The status of research participants' relatives as "human subjects" in pedigree and genetic diagnostic studies
2. Protecting the voluntariness of research participation in pedigree and genetic diagnostic studies
3. Respecting the rights and interests of communities in population screening studies
4. Defining researcher obligations to disclose research findings to participants in both family and population-based genetic studies
5. Defining participant rights regarding the control of genetic materials and research results in both family and population-based genetic research

This chapter reviews each of these five topics with three aims in mind: (1) to identify further empirical research needs; (2) to draw out any public policy implications of its discussion to date; and (3) to suggest lessons for the design and conduct of genetic research studies. The next section begins by explaining the core conception and rationale for each of the three kinds of genetic research that raise these issues: genetic family studies, diagnostic genetic testing research, and population-based genetic screening studies. This will help display the common genetic etiology of the issues to be reviewed and the different ways they manifest themselves in different contexts.

Core Conception and Methodological Rationale

Genetic Family (Pedigree) Studies

The oldest form of genetic research is to observe the pattern of inheritance of a particular trait across multiple generations of a family. Today, these genealogical *pedigree* studies are used to help pinpoint the chromosomal location of the DNA coding regions, or *exons,* that seem most closely tied to an inherited trait, or *pheno-*

type, in order to seek clues into the phenotype's causes. By comparing the inheritance of a panel of known molecular markers in the DNA with the familial occurrence of a particular inherited trait, specific markers that have been transmitted through the family in the same pattern as the trait can be identified. This is a sign that the DNA markers and the exons most tightly correlated with the phenotype reside together on the same section of chromosomal DNA. Where a causal hypothesis can explain the relationship between the proteins prescribed by these exons and the phenotype, the coding regions can be collectively identified as the gene for the familial trait. Once *mapped* in this way, the causal gene can be isolated by even more fine-grained techniques and deciphered, or *sequenced,* at the molecular level, providing a key clue to the pathogenesis of the clinical problem.[15]

As higher resolution marker maps become available, such genetic *linkage studies* involving large families are becoming increasingly common across the biomedical research landscape. They are already being used in attempts to discover the etiology of health problems as diverse as deafness, heart disease, colon cancer, and schizophrenia.[16] They have become particularly important in the etiology of diseases such as breast cancer, which are understood to be predominantly environmentally caused, but which also seem to run in some families. In these cases, the hope is that if the inherited germ-line mutation can be isolated in families, it may shed light on the environmentally induced somatic cell mutations that are its sporadic counterparts. With the Human Genome Project's production of comprehensive, fine-grained genetic marker maps beginning in the 1990s, and the first complete sequencing of the human genome in 2003, the pace of these gene-identification studies has increased dramatically[17] (see Figure 29.1).

Genetic Diagnostic Testing Research

Genetic linkage studies produce a measure of the proximity between a trait's correlated markers and its causal gene known as a *lod score.*[18] Flanking markers that have lod scores indicating that they are 1,000 times more likely to be physically linked to the relevant coding regions are considered reliable indicators of the location of the causal gene. This means that they can also be used as clinically detectable surrogates for the gene long before tests can be developed that directly target the relevant DNA exons themselves. Then, if specific molecular mutations can be identified within the exons as necessary and sufficient conditions for the emergence of the clinical phenotype, molecular probes for these versions of the genes (or *alleles*) can be quickly developed as powerful prognostic tests for use within at-risk families.[19]

For individuals who have a familial risk of carrying alleles that are causally correlated with health problems for themselves or their children, the identification of these genes or their markers through clinical testing can provide the benefit of increased certainty about their personal genetic status. For those who are found not to carry the deleterious alleles, this benefit is reassurance and relief. For those who *test positive* for the targeted mutations, the benefit depends on how well they can use the knowledge of their carrier status to prevent or prepare for its ill effects. Genetic diagnostic research, usually involving pilot studies of clinical testing protocols with high risk families, attempts to optimize this process by gathering evidence on its dynamics and sequelae before the tests are introduced into general clinical practice.[20]

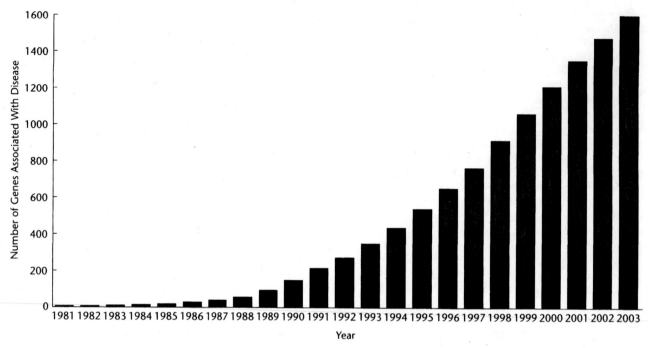

Figure 29.1. Cumulative Pace of Gene Discovery, 1981–2003. Minimum estimated values are represented. Source: National Human Genome Research Institute (http://www.genome.gov/Pages/News/PaceofDisease GeneDiscovery.pdf).

Population Screening Research

The rationale for identifying and tracking the inheritance of genetic variants in particular families also fuels research interest in studies of genetic variation at the level of human groups and populations. Since the beginning of the Human Genome Project, there have been calls to systematically map the genetic variation within our species.[21] The initial interest was primarily genealogical: Physical anthropologists and population geneticists would use comparative genotyping to produce the molecular clues they need to reconstruct more completely the global history of human migration and differentiation. But today interest in the ways in which human groups vary at different genetic loci is much broader within biomedicine, as scientists apply the fruits of genome research to their work in epidemiology,[22] molecular diagnostics,[23] pharmacogenetics,[24] and the analysis of complex genetic traits.[25] Much of this interest is driven by the prospect of a *genomic medicine*, in which diagnostic protocols, therapeutic interventions, and preventive measures could be tailored to each patient's genetic profile.[26]

Whatever its focus, all population genomic research involves collecting DNA samples from individual members of different human groups, genotyping them (through marker mapping or DNA sequencing) at one or more loci, and comparing the results. Almost by definition, a complicating feature of many population genomic studies is the fact that this research is increasingly cross-cultural and international. Large genetic variation studies like the Haplotype Mapping Project are increasingly collaborative efforts between scientists in different countries who collect and compare DNA from populations chosen for their phenotypic diversity. Even genetic studies that involve mainstream U.S. immigrant communities, such as African Americans or the Ashkenazim, can quickly

take investigators all across the globe. As a result, cultural, linguistic, and socioeconomic factors complicate population genetics research in much the same way they complicate international epidemiological research, raising questions about the collective interests of the human groups being studied, and their decision-making role in this context.

Ethical Issues

"Secondary Subjects" and Informational Privacy

Conceptually, family-based gene-hunting studies start with the identification of a person who expresses the inherited trait in question (a *proband*, or *index case*), and then reconstructs as much of the trait's pattern of inheritance within the proband's extended family as possible. This genetic pedigree is used to distinguish family members who carry the causal gene from those who do not. For most well-defined genetic conditions, linkage study subjects are recruited from clinical practice settings in which multiple family members have become involved in genetic evaluation and counseling, and the family pedigree for the condition is already at least partially established. As one researcher has noted,

> It takes an immense amount of time and detective work to construct a pedigree: to check the genetic relatedness of individuals, hunt down clinical information (such as clinical work-ups of living members and autopsy reports on those who have died) and obtain blood, tissue and other samples from family volunteers. Doing the genetic marker studies—

the laboratory work—is relatively expeditious compared to constructing the pedigree and getting the samples from family members.[27]

Ethical questions, however, arise even in the initial stages of this process. The proband can provide investigators access to his or her own clinical records, which may well include family medical histories compiled for clinical purposes. But does the provision of information by the proband about family members for research purposes involve them involuntarily in the research, potentially breaching their privacy? This issue came to the forefront in 1999 when the father of a participant in a genetic twin study being conducted by behavioral genetic researchers at Virginia Commonwealth University (VCU) protested the fact that personal and medical information about him had been solicited from his daughter in the course of the study. In its resulting investigation, OPRR suggested that the VCU IRB should have considered the probands' family members as "secondary" research subjects, and should have required the investigators to secure the family members' consent before collecting this information about them. Because the OPRR and the FDA used this rationale to temporarily suspend all human subjects research at the Virginia Commonwealth University, genetic researchers and IRBs around the country reacted to this ruling with considerable alarm. Scientists complain that the "reality is that restricting the ability of a researcher to collect family history data without obtaining informed consent from family members will result in many projects being abandoned for logistical and financial reasons."[28]

Appropriating clinical family history information to launch a new genetic family study is a practice so traditional that it was ethically invisible within the research community until this case raised the issue. But at stake is not only the privacy of the genetic information disclosed about other family members, but also the voluntariness of their involvement in the study.

Empirical Research

To date, there has been little systematic study of the relative consequences of constructing pedigrees with or without the consent of the family members involved. However, there is a good bit of data on the public's general attitudes toward the use of medical records for research purposes without consent. Coy summarizes a series of five public opinion polls conducted between 1993 and 2001, before the VCU case raised the profile of this issue. A significant majority of the public consistently expressed opposition to the prospect of researchers using their medical records without their consent, even when research confidentiality safeguards were emphasized.[29] On the other hand, one survey found that 64% of respondents would, if asked, consent to the use of their medical records by "researchers at a university conducting a study about a medical condition that had affected some of the respondent's family members."[30]

This data needs to be followed up with more specific studies in the genetic research context, but it does suggest that the public is interested in having control over the research uses of personal medical information, particularly as that use moves further away from direct clinical care for themselves or their family members.

Policy Implications

The federal regulations governing clinical research define *human subjects* as living individuals about whom investigators collect information that is both identifiable with the individuals and private (45 CFR 46.102(f)).[31] One early policy response to the VCU case was a statement from the American Society of Human Genetics, which argued that, although the family history information gathered in constructing pedigrees was identifiable, it was not private, because it was usually known to other family members.[32] But as Botkin notes, "there are different spheres of privacy and a decision to share information with close friends and family does not imply a willingness to share information more broadly."[33]

In 1993, although acknowledging that "no consensus on this issue has yet been reached," OPRR suggested that IRBs might "draw a distinction between information about others provided by a subject that is also available to the investigator through public sources (for example, family names and addresses) and other personal information that is not available through public sources (for example, information about medical conditions or adoptions)."[13] IRBs could then allow investigators to collect only the former, public facts about the family in the index case. This strategy has been promoted and expanded by several commentators in the wake of the VCU case.[33]

If the information gathered from family members is both identifying and private, thus categorizing them as human subjects, IRBs and investigators must determine whether informed consent can be waived. This process begins by asking if the research involves more than minimal risk to secondary subjects. Botkin argues that the collection of highly sensitive private information, such as psychiatric history or sexual orientation, may indicate that a study poses more than minimal risk. Botkin also recognizes how advances in genetic research may raise particular concerns regarding potential stigma or discrimination based on genetic risk information. This is especially true for studies in which new knowledge is generated that may indicate genetic risks for disease in healthy individuals.[33]

Study Design Implications

The recruitment strategy that flows most naturally from the "secondary subject" discussion is to have the proband provide a bare family tree (one that contains information already publicly available elsewhere), and for the investigators to convert this tree into a genetic pedigree by soliciting relevant health data from each relative directly. In order to pursue the linkage analysis further, investigators must request and collect DNA (usually from a blood sample) from as many members of the extended family as possible. This recruitment approach anticipates the fact that the relatives will all have to be contacted eventually anyway if the study is to proceed to the next stage. If the investigator's solicitation includes an invitation to contribute the preliminary genetic data as well as blood, the subjects' ability to control their own involvement in the study is enhanced.[34]

Other researchers take stronger measures to insulate prospective subjects from premature involvement. Some investigators do not construct family trees immediately, but have the probands carry letters to their relatives explaining the study and inviting them to contact the investigators if they want to become involved.[35] As a result, the researchers only receive pedigree information from those family members who actively volunteer for the study. Although this approach does the best job of giving the potential subjects control over the situation, it is important to note its imperfections. If enough family members volunteer for the study, even those who declined to participate may find themselves involved, as information about them is inferred from analyses of their offspring and forbears. This approach may also potentially decrease overall participation of family members in studies; however this effect has yet to be determined empirically.

This approach, moreover, highlights a second issue: In some cases it may be the proband's own privacy that the recruitment process puts at risk. This concern arises primarily for genetic studies of socially stigmatizing conditions like psychiatric disorders, the diagnosis of which may not be generally shared within an extended family.[36] To rely on a proband to contact and recruit members of his or her extended family is to assume that the proband's diagnosis is one that can be shared with relatives without prejudice; for this reason most psychiatric geneticists take the responsibility to contact the family themselves. Here, the imposition on the family is justified out of a concern to protect the proband's privacy.[37]

Unless it is handled adeptly, this strategy quickly meets limitations. Without a reference to the proband's diagnosis of, for example, schizophrenia, how do the investigators adequately explain to a proband's cousin why they are interested in her participation in their family linkage study of this disease? One approach to this problem involves discussing the importance of preserving confidentiality for every participant within a family study. This educational approach may also give the family member the chance to learn more about the illness being studied while both keeping the proband's diagnosis confidential and reducing the confusion of a family member concerning why this family was chosen for the study.[37]

Finally, a different kind of family privacy and consent question comes up at the conclusion of a genetic study when investigators are preparing to publish their results. To present their data, investigators must publish the pedigrees on which they based their work. It is easy enough to present the pedigrees anonymously, but the family trees they provide are readily decipherable by family members and those who know them. It is thus possible for family members to learn not only about the carrier status of other relatives, but also other facts relevant to the genetic analysis, such as adoptions, stillbirths, and instances of misidentified paternity.

One common practice within human genetics is to scramble pedigrees for publication by changing the gender and birth order of family members in order to disguise their identities, yet preserve the essential genetic story the pedigree tells.[35] The original data is then kept available for inspection only by other *bona fide* researchers. As linkage analysis spreads into other medical fields, this approach is meeting increased resistance: Although the traditional publication practice of placing bars across the eyes of patients obscured information irrelevant to the topic, this approach also modifies the scientific data in question. A National Institutes of Health (NIH) research team learned this lesson to its chagrin when it published a "disguised" pedigree of an Egyptian family that disclosed the existence of two children in which "paternal genotype inconsistencies" were identified.[38] The results of this disclosure within the immediate family were disastrous, and led to new guidance to the NIH IRBs that, when misidentified paternity is uncovered in a genetic family study,

if the disease is rare with few subjects available, and it is scientifically impractical to discard the pedigree, then the results of the data analysis could be published without publishing the pedigree itself, with the pedigree made available to bona fide investigators who request it. If the pedigree must be

included in the publication, the nuclear family in which the incompatibility occurs could be left out of the pedigree. If it is necessary to publish the complete pedigree, an approach could be made to the family to elicit admission of nonpaternity and to request permission to publish.[39]

This approach, in fact, is the one that would be most compatible with other existing guidelines for protecting the privacy of clinical research subjects in the medical literature.[40] But it challenges the time-honored convention of using pedigree diagrams as a convenient graphic summary of family study data, and it leaves open important ethical questions. From whom should the investigators solicit permission from within the family? Everyone represented in a pedigree? Only those who carry the mutation in question? Only family members with special interests at stake, like the two Egyptian children and their parents? Although each of these approaches has its advocates, none is entirely satisfactory. Moreover, they all give rise to an additional question: What should investigators do in the face of intrafamilial disagreements over permission to publish data about their family?

A recent empirical study attempted to assess how investigators and journals are addressing the various challenges of publishing pedigrees while attempting to protect the privacy of family members.[41] The three-part study examined the attitudes and experiences of human genetics researchers regarding privacy and confidentiality issues related to the publication of pedigrees. It also surveyed editors of biomedical journals concerning their policies and practices regarding pedigrees, and reviewed recent articles from a number of prominent journals that publish genetics research to assess the documentation of consent and information available to authors with respect to published pedigrees. The study found a wide array of practices among both journals and investigators with respect to the protection of privacy and confidentiality in the publication of pedigrees.

For example, 36% of investigators reported that family members were not informed that their pedigrees would be published and 78% did not obtain consent specifically for pedigree publication. Additionally, 19% of investigators reported that they had altered pedigrees to protect the privacy and confidentiality of family members; however, of those respondents, 45% did not disclose these alterations to journals. Of the 14 journal editors that responded to the survey, only three had specific policies for dealing with potential identifying information in pedigrees, and in the two-year review of journal articles, none had explicit documentation of informed consent for pedigree publication.

The results of this study demonstrate that practices by investigators and journals are not conforming to established recommendations regarding the protection of privacy and confidentiality of human subjects in pedigree research. The current practice of pedigree alteration may also affect the integrity of scientific communication. The authors involved with this study recommend more explicit policies for informed consent, documentation, and peer review regarding pedigree publication, including an active stand against pedigree alteration and better management of identifying information in published pedigrees.[41]

Recruitment Strategies

Enlisting research subjects to help recruit their relatives has been defended as a means to enhance family members' ability to make voluntary choices regarding participation in genetics research. However, families are not composed of equal peers. In many situations, the subject-recruiter or family facilitator is recruited from the charged atmosphere of the clinic. These subjects, who are motivated by their clinical need to find "their gene," usually proceed as advocates of the research. Thus the pressure of compelling family relationships may simply replace the researcher's influence in recruiting potential subjects.[42] This problem may be greater for cohesive, hierarchically organized families from cultural groups that have not yet been affected by the 20th century breakdown of the family, families whose size also tends to make them ideal subjects for linkage analysis.

One response to this problem is for researchers to approach families collectively by presenting their research projects at large gatherings like family reunions, and inviting all interested individuals to contact them to become involved.[37,43] Some teams of researchers also rely on lay organizations, like genetic disease support groups, to make the initial contact with families in the context of the community support they are providing.[44] However, these approaches also pose risks to the goal of achieving autonomous participation: Family members may actually feel less free to demur in large group settings, and lay-led support groups vary in expertise, understanding, and objectivity (particularly when they are helping to fund the research itself).

Empirical Research

There have been very few empirical studies of participant reactions to different recruitment approaches.[43] A study of proband and parental assistance in identifying relatives for cystic fibrosis carrier testing research found 30.1% of 203 eligible families declining to provide contact information for relatives,[45] and a focus group study of cancer genetic research participants reported reluctance to serve as an intermediary for the researcher.[46] On the other hand, the literature includes many calls by genetic health voluntary and advocacy organizations for participant-led recruitment efforts, and many family studies proceed in this fashion.[47]

Policy Implications

Some argue that because the family is the proper clinical unit of analysis (and allegiance) for geneticists who counsel patients, most questions about the disclosure of intrafamilial genetic information should not be regarded as problems about confidentiality in professional practice.[48] If that argument succeeds for genetic counseling, should it not also apply to genetic research? Similarly, others now argue that taking the family seriously means that IRBs or investigators should not attempt to police the inevitable psychosocial forces that come into play in familial decision making, any more than they would second-guess an individual volunteer's internal deliberations. Researchers would do better, they argue, to monitor their own influence and leave the family's internal dynamics intact.[49] Whether the family should be regarded as an entity that can justify these arguments that may discount the privacy and autonomy of individuals is, of course, the question.[50–52]

Study Design Implications

Whether individual family members or the family as a whole are considered the unit of analysis in a family linkage study, the recruitment of family members should be part of the original protocol and study design, and must involve thoughtful consideration regarding the confidentiality of both the proband and other participating family members. The nature of the particular study, recruitment goals, and family dynamics should also be taken into consideration when developing a recruitment strategy. It is important that these strategies balance the research quality and the need for adequate participant accrual to achieve scientific validity with potential harms to family participants such as invasion of privacy, unwanted disclosure of disease risk information, or familial pressure to participate. These issues should be highlighted during all stages of a recruitment process including identification, contacting, and actual recruitment of family members.

In 2004, a multidisciplinary ad hoc expert group was convened by the Cancer Genetics Network to explore the scientific and ethical issues surrounding the recruitment of participants for familial genetic research. This group reviewed the various recruitment methods used in family studies with regard to privacy, confidentiality, and participant accrual for each stage of the recruitment process (see Figure 29.2).[43] Initial contact with potential participants may be conducted by the study's investigators or by enrolled participants who may wish to contact family members themselves in order keep their identity confidential until they agree to be in the study. Although the latter approach may maximize privacy, it may also put undue burden on the participants and thus lower accrual. Alternatively, although investigator-initiated contact may raise accrual rates, some family members may feel that because an investigator has contact information, and possibly some health information, their privacy has already been invaded. A third, intermediary approach would be for enrolled participants to inform family members about the study and that an investigator will be contacting them to discuss participation. This approach takes the actual burden of recruitment off the shoulders of participants, but allows them to take the family's best interest into account.

Unfortunately, none of these approaches deals with the problem of unwanted disclosure of information to family members before an informed consent process can take place. In dealing with this issue, it is increasingly important that the researcher consider the family dynamics of potential participants. Kathleen Bonvicini claims that it is important to pay attention to "individual family roles, level of cohesiveness, levels of power/influence, and family interactions" when designing a recruitment strategy. For example, the recruitment of a family leader from an older generation may help in the recruitment of subsequent generations of family members. Bonvicini also explains that the informal communication between family members, such as the family "grapevine," can also help in the dissemination of information about the study and recruitment.[37]

Once initial contact is made and basic information concerning the study is given to potential participants, they are usually given the opportunity to be further contacted by the investigators regarding participation using either an *opt-out* or *opt-in* approach. In situations in which enrolled participants make the initial contact, family members must opt in by contacting the investigator in order to receive more information about the research. Alternatively, family members can also opt in by permitting their contact information to be given to the investigator. In situations in which the investigator makes the initial contact, family members may be asked to opt in by contacting the investigators directly if they would like further information about the research, or may only need to

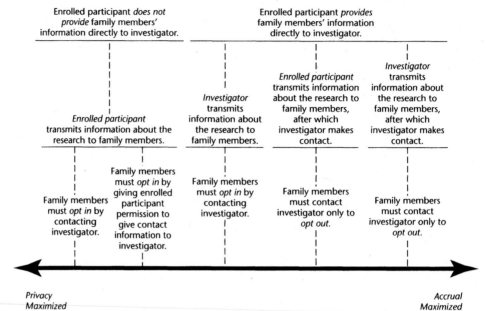

Figure 29.2. Overview of Family-Based Recruitment Methods. Source: Beskow LM et al. Ethical issues in identifying and recruiting participants for familial genetic research. *American Journal of Medical Genetics* 2004;130A:424–31. © 2004 Wiley-Liss, Inc. Reproduced with permission.

contact investigators to opt out if they do not wish to be further contacted. Although the opt-in approach maximizes the privacy of family members, an opt-out approach may increase accrual rates for a study. The decision to use either of these methods may depend on both the needs and goal of the study and the families involved in the research.[43]

Community Interests

Genetic research projects that are framed in terms of identified human groups can have repercussions for all the groups' members, even when not all are directly enrolled in the study.[53,54] In fact, it is only through their group identity that the harms of population genomic research can come back to haunt individual subjects.[55] As a result, some commentators have begun to argue that where genetic studies impose group-level risks, a decision to incur shared risks is most appropriately made at the level of the group as a whole. Some have proposed that this moral concern be translated into a fourth principle for clinical research ethics (in addition to the Belmont Report's respect for persons, beneficence and justice) called "respect for communities."[56]

The principle of respect for communities is often put into practice through a call for "community engagement" as a prerequisite for population-based genetic studies. Over the last decade, such calls have come from a wide range of potential research participant groups, communities, and research policy makers,[57] and there have been some anecdotal reports of participant attitudes and researcher experiences with community consultation exercises.[58–62] To date, however, there has been very little empirical research evaluating different approaches to community engagement or documenting its consequences for participating communities and groups.

The idea of community engagement has its origins in practices employed in a wide variety of research areas that recruit subjects because of their membership in a certain population, including public health research,[63] cultural anthropology,[64] research on

emergency medical procedures, and research with sovereign nations like Native American tribes.[65] Community engagement has been brought into discussions of population genetic studies relatively recently, however, largely in response to the collapse of one of the earliest proposed sequels to the Human Genome Project, the ill-fated Human Genome Diversity Project (HGDP).

In 1991, a group of population geneticists and physical anthropologists released a plan to sample DNA from the "world's most ancestrally representative" human populations, to create a global data and tissue bank for human genetic variation studies.[66] The proposal was originally framed as an attempt to preserve genetic material from "vulnerable" and "vanishing" human populations before assimilation and oppression drove them to extinction. When the planners released a list of 400 isolated ethnic, linguistic, and tribal groups they felt met this criterion, the project encountered a firestorm of critical reaction from advocates of indigenous peoples. The advocates pointed out that none of the listed groups had ever been approached about their willingness to be included in the research and, to the extent that the groups were vulnerable to extinction, the preservation of their DNA would not be their first concern.[67–69] The HGDP never survived this political controversy beyond its planning stages. However, a rear-guard attempt to redress the disaster by the North American advocates of the project did create the starting place for current discussion of community involvement in genetic variation research.

The North American Committee (NAmC) for the HGDP developed a "model protocol" for DNA sample collection that "requires that researchers participating in the HGDP show that they have obtained the informed consent of the population, through its culturally appropriate authorities where such authorities exist, before they begin sampling."[70] For the NAmC, this requirement essentially meant ratcheting up all the protections that are afforded to individual human subjects in biomedical research to the group level, on the ground that "the group—whether one family, a set of family, a genetic disease organization or an ethnic group—is really the research subject."[53]

The NAmC vision of group consent is a robust way to recognize the principle of respect for communities. The model protocol gives groups the rights to grant or deny investigators access to their members, to withdraw from research at any time, to have their group identity protected as a matter of confidentiality, and to negotiate the ways in which their DNA samples will be studied and used. It even instructs researchers to let refusals at the group level trump the informed consent of individual members who might otherwise volunteer.[70]

The NAmC concept of group consent is best exemplified by the kinds of negotiations that occur between researchers and self-governing groups like the American Indian nations. These were the "ancestral populations" of interest to the HGDP in North America, and many tribes already have formal legal mechanisms for vetting research proposals involving their communities. The Navajo, for example, not only review all biomedical research proposals at the tribal level before giving scientists access to their people, but insist on the right to censor all publications emanating from any research they approve.[71] On the other hand, the indigenous American Indian peoples are still sovereign nations in their own right, and can impose such requirements quite independently of whether or not researchers recognize a moral need for population-based consent. For these groups, in other words, the NAmC protocol works well, but is also largely irrelevant.

Unfortunately, for other kinds of populations, in which the group consent would be a new protection, the protocol is less apt. In fact, the committee recognizes that "researchers can only seek consent from a broader representative of a population if such a representative exists." For study populations larger than single families or the residents of a specific locale, it argues, the need for group consent "depends necessarily on two things: the population's view of its identity and the existence within the broader group of entities that the population itself recognizes as culturally appropriate authorities." Apart from Native American and Canadian peoples, the committee concludes, "most other ethnic groups in those two countries do not have those kinds of cultural identities or group-wide culturally appropriate authorities."[71]

Very few of the populations of interest for current genetic variation research have political structures that can claim to be their culturally appropriate authorities, and all of the populations of interest will be larger than the populations of specific families or sampling sites. Attempting to apply this full-blooded concept of group consent to nonsovereign genetic populations encounters major conceptual, ethical, and practical difficulties, which have been more extensively discussed elsewhere.[72] In brief, such an attempt would founder on two fronts: First, both our practice of nesting local groups within larger social communities and the global diasporas of most human populations mean that no socially identified group with the culturally appropriate authority to do so can have the reach to speak for all those in a given genetic population who might become research subjects.[73] No matter how careful researchers are to get permission from the right authorities in a local self-identified social group, as long as that group is nested within a larger genetic population, the group's ability to protect itself from the consequences of the research will be compromised by any other subpopulation's decision to participate, and its decision to participate will in turn put those other groups at risk. In response to this, some advocates argue that researchers must attempt to consult with the largest supervening group relevant to the research problem.[54] In doing so, of course, they will inevitably find themselves dealing with populations that transcend ethnic, national, and even continental borders.

Second, suggesting that any socially identified group could speak for such populations would reinforce (by tacitly endorsing) the view that there really is a biological justification for the social boundaries we draw around and between each other—a view population geneticists don't believe and expect to discredit.[74] Whatever moral standing the human superfamilies of interest to population genomics may have, in the modern world it will only very rarely be the moral standing of sovereign nations.

These concerns have convinced most advocates for group interests in genetic research that simply treating populations as if they were individual research subjects is naïve, and that more nuanced interpretations of what it means to respect communities in this context will be required.[54] Under various labels, two models of community engagement are beginning to appear in various official recommendations to genetic variation researchers. Although both models conform better to the realities of population genomic research, both also remain haunted by the same kinds of issues that limit the utility of the NAmC protocol for group consent.

Policy Implications

The first approach is to reframe the process of community interaction to retract the gatekeeping role of group consent. Because genetic populations are not the sorts of groups that can claim autonomy as moral communities, it makes no sense to hinge the recruitment of their members on some corporate permission. Thus, for example, the "Points to Consider for Population-based Genetic Research" developed by the NIH stresses that: "Community consultation is not the same as consent. In the majority of cases, communities in the United States are not required to give consent or approval for research in which its members participate, nor is it reasonable to attempt to obtain community consent or approval."[75]

Instead of consent or approval, the NIH guidelines explain that "community consultation is a vehicle for hearing about the community's interests and concerns, addressing ethical issues and communicating information about the research to the community."[75] The purpose of this interchange is to solicit the study population's help in identifying any "intracommunity" or "culturally specific" risks and potential benefits, so that the research can be designed in ways that best protect the group's interests.[65]

This interpretation of community engagement places much more emphasis on preserving the special values and cultural lifeways of a given population than on treating the population as a politically autonomous entity. The ethical emphasis has shifted from respecting the group to protecting its members as research participants vulnerable to group-related harms. Nevertheless, the ethical requirements continue to share with the group consent model the importance of identifying and interacting with consultants who can accurately and fairly represent the population's values.[64] As Marshall and Rotimi point out, this can be difficult:

> Despite the obvious benefits of community advisory boards, there are limits and constraints on their ability to represent the values of diverse community members. . . . In some cases community leaders on advisory boards may be politicians. Community activists represent another powerful group who might serve on such boards. Religious leaders or local celebrities also might be asked to participate on the boards. Investigators must be sensitive to the social and political agendas

of members on community advisory boards and try to minimize the potential for addressing priorities that may be relevant to only a minority of the local population.[64]

Of course, the increasing dispersion of human populations around the world means that in fact most human superfamilies no longer share common "culturally specific risks" and benefits. This leads even the staunchest advocates of community engagement to the counterintuitive point of arguing that, for study populations like "general ethnic, racial or national populations, e.g., Ashkenazi Jews, American Indians, Puerto Ricans, etc.," the lack of distinctive common interest and structured social interaction means that "community review may not be required and even for geographically dispersed populations that share distinctive beliefs and practices, like the Amish or the Hmong, limited social interactions between members of the study population make intra-community risks unlikely."[54]

Study Design Implications

Diverse, dispersed genetic superfamilies of the sort useful to genetic variation studies will not often enjoy the level of organization that can make representative consultations possible. For these cases, Sharp and Foster suggest that all that may be required is the form of community engagement they call "community dialogue": an effort to interact with the local communities and institutions at the specific site from which members of a given genetic population will be recruited, in order to acquaint them with the investigators' mission in advance of individual subject enrollment.[54] The key move in this interpretation is to acknowledge the complexity of human population structure by sacrificing the ambition to protect all members of a genetic population from the potential harms of the research, and to refocus on the particular families and locale from which investigators hope to solicit DNA samples.

Instead of attempting to respect the genetic population as a moral community, or attempting to protect all its individual members from potential harm, the practice of community engagement is reinterpreted by this approach to be simply a matter of establishing a viable political collaboration with the local community in which the recruitment of individuals for DNA sampling is to take place. Because this does not even require that the community representatives bring any special expertise to the research design, the language can shift from "consultation" and "review" to "dialogue" and "engagement"—terms more often used to describe attempts to teach than to learn. In fact, as the range of "local" risks and benefits widens for any specific genetic population across the global spectrum of cultural, political, and social environments, the utility of any specific advice becomes diluted to the vanishing point, until only the most generic biomedical design considerations become relevant to researchers.[75] As the NIH "Points to Consider" warn,

> Community-wide "buy-in" to the goals of the research project may improve the ability to recruit study participants. However, community consultation is not a substitute for careful, systematic preliminary studies that provide the foundation for choosing the study population, developing sampling or recruitment plans, designing protocols and measurement tools, and planning analytic strategies. A wide variety of social science methods and statistical data are available for assessing the characteristics of communities. Investigators must be

cautious about relying on anecdotal information gained in the course of community consultation to guide the development of their research plans.[75]

Narrowing the focus from broad study populations to localized communities does make the prospect of community engagement more plausible. Localized communities will be able to produce representatives authorized to speak for their membership more easily than unorganized populations. Local communities are more likely to face common intracommunity risks and needs that might be usefully communicated in designing the research at that site. And to build trust and negotiate access to community members, it will be much more effective to work at the local level.

Nevertheless, it remains important to appreciate the limits of this approach. The kinds of study populations that are of most interest to genetic variation researchers, the international human superfamilies whose genetic variations disclose the patterns of disease susceptibilities within the species, will be those least well served by the practice of community engagement. If the concern is to give those larger population groups some involvement in research that may affect them, even negotiating a full-blown "community partnership" with one localized subset of the population is as likely to be an example of the problem as it is a step toward justice: To the extent that the researcher does not confine his scientific claims to the local community at hand, that community's decisions about participation preempt the interests of the rest of the population.

Moreover, for these same reasons, investigators cannot honestly let local communities speak for the population, and cannot promise that local research designs will protect the communities from population-related harms incurred by studies at other locales. Thus, in this most attenuated model of community engagement, even the local communities to which the principle of respect for communities could apply cannot be afforded a robust interpretation of that ideal.

Reporting Research Findings to Participants

So far, the issues we have described all arise at the outset of a new genetic study, during the process of recruiting and enrolling subjects. As human genetic studies progress and begin to yield results, however, other questions emerge. These questions all concern the management of the information that investigators uncover about their subjects.

Most human genetic studies begin as basic research projects in molecular and human genetics, and often have relatively indirect connections with the kinds of clinical services that are relevant to the education and counseling of individuals regarding the results of genetic tests. Thus, one traditional approach to managing findings has been to condition subjects' participation on the understanding that no individual findings will be disclosed to subjects under the auspices of the study. This approach was justified, in part, by the slow pace of research that isolated disease genes, which allowed the clinical community to prepare for the translation of research findings into clinical practice further in advance. Even when researchers are confident that the information they have uncovered is reliable, they are often uncertain about their own obligations to provide the clinical services required to convey it back to their subjects. The traditional view has been that, clinical researchers may minimize potential harm to subjects by separating, as thoroughly as possible, their research role from clinical roles. If a genetic test reaches the level of reasonable medical certainty, and a subject wishes presymptomatic testing to learn the risk of carrying a particular defective gene, the subject can be referred to a qualified clinical genetic counselor for provision of such information (rather than obtaining genetic liability test results in the research setting).[36]

Hence, for example, the linkage studies that localized markers for the Huntington's disease gene established the policy of withholding preliminary research results from all subjects until the level of scientific confidence in the reliability of the markers justified the establishment of pilot clinical testing programs.[76]

Others, however, question whether the traditional separation of research and clinical roles is in the participant's/patient's best interest in these situations. Information transferred to regular medical records would become more widely accessible to insurance companies and employers, exposing the family members to increased socioeconomic risks as a result of their research participation.[77] Moreover, the pace of research to isolate genes is quickly putting pressure on this traditional approach. Many investigators now find themselves in possession of information that seems to be reliable enough to use clinically in the absence of a developed program for delivering the information. In addition, individuals and families sometimes request early results directly from the researchers, and their requests are supported by those who argue that subjects should have the right to information about themselves at all stages of the research, particularly when it could have a bearing on clinical decision making.[78] For example, one team reports that,

> We believe that the major responsibility of this type of investigation (to their subjects' welfare) is formal education of the affected individuals, particularly those newly diagnosed, their families and their physicians. . . . As part of the education component in our study, a detailed session is conducted during the study visit; all local subjects are afforded a clinical visit to review all data with the polycystic kidney disease (PKD) physician; and all patients and all doctors receive a detailed letter describing the data obtained.[79]

This position reflects a growing view that the relationship between genetic researchers and research participants should be one of collaboration and codiscovery, rather than simply one of scientific observer and participants observed. On the strongest version of this view, even the clinical significance of the research results is not particularly relevant: Research participants simply enjoy a basic right to know everything that the researcher knows about them. In fact, legal concerns have already been raised about "look-back liability" on the part of investigators who hold, but do not communicate, important findings.[80]

Policy Implications

Three different kinds of research results prove particularly troubling to researchers in defining the limits of their obligations to inform their participant partners: unanticipated findings that are potentially stigmatizing; findings that have clinical implications for health problems unconnected with the research topic; and

preliminary findings of possible clinical relevance that remain to be validated for clinical use.

Unanticipated findings.   One of the more common unanticipated consequences of tracing the inheritance of DNA markers within a family can be the inadvertent disclosure of misidentified paternity. This is not a new issue for clinical geneticists, who encounter it in the context of prenatal testing and carrier screening for recessive diseases.[81] However, for clinical researchers from other specialties interested in late onset diseases of adults like breast cancer, this risk is still underappreciated. Longstanding recommendations to address that risk up front in the informed consent process are rarely followed outside of traditional medical genetic settings.[82,33]

For many people, ancestral relationships are as important to their identities as their living relations. Despite our modern belief that individual human potential transcends genealogy, biological lineage continues to provide most people in many cultures with their names, their inheritances, and their connections to history.[83] This is why population genetic studies that promise to confirm, enrich, or extend the ancestral lineage stories of particular families are of such interest, and why the interpretation and communication of their results can be so controversial.[73] The seduction of genetic genealogies has already tempted governments and tribes to propose DNA-based tests to secure lineage-based membership in indigenous tribes for political purposes,[84, 85] and led religious communities to use genetic markers to adjudicate the orthodoxy of aspirants' claims to be coreligionists.[86] As often as not, those efforts will be inconclusive or exclusionary.

In both ancestry and paternity cases, genetic studies can exacerbate the problem of genealogical essentialism, in other words, "the view that the genealogical family is the 'real' one and that knowing blood kin is essential for establishing a stable personality and identity."[87] In challenging either our remote or immediate origin stories, genetics provokes the same question: What does it mean to be a "descendant," and what role should biology play in determining the rights and privileges that should attend the role?[88]

Plieotropy.   The second set of problematic results from genetic studies reflects the fact that some clinically significant alleles will be "plieotropic" in their expression, meaning that a single gene or allelic variation has multiple phenotypic effects. Plieotropic alleles may convey risks for very different health problems with different prospects for treatment. For example, consider the preliminary but highly public association of APOE genotypes with risk for Alzheimer's disease (AD). APOE genotyping is also under investigation by cardiologists as a risk factor for hyperlipidemia and its clinical sequelae, atherosclerosis and myocardial infarction. In fact, the same allele of the APOE gene, the 4 allele, seems to convey the highest risk for both coronary artery disease (CAD) and AD.[89,90] Presumably, the ethicolegal requirements of informed consent now require cardiologists to disclose to their research subjects that information on AD risk will be contained in the results of any APOE genotyping they perform.

Moreover, the researcher's commitment to candor and the patient's "right to know" would also seem to require that researchers divulge the AD risk results when patients ask for that information after testing has already been conducted as part of a study in cardiovascular genetics. And, of course, the researcher's professionalism means that all of those disclosures should be performed according to the professional standards of care established for that task. Unfortunately, if those standards follow the recommendations emerging from the neurologists' current discussions of APOE genotyping for AD risk, it will be difficult for other researchers, like cardiologists, to conduct APOE testing in the setting of their research without becoming professionally competent to counsel participants about the meaning of the test for their AD risks as well.

This difficulty arises because most of the new practice guidelines on APOE genotyping for AD risk take as their model the protocols developed to govern the clinical introduction of prognostic testing for Huntington's disease,[91,92] for which no effective treatment exists. This paradigm sets the ethical standards for APOE genotyping for AD risk quite a bit higher than they have been to date in cardiological research contexts, because the model's focus is on protecting the patient from the psychosocial risks of testing rather than on preventing the harms it predicts. Moreover, these psychosocial risks do not depend on either the subject's awareness of the information or its ultimate scientific validity. If parties outside the research relationship, including the patient's family and clinicians, labor under the belief that APOE gentoyping will predict AD risk, their reactions can still harm the patient. Thus, the most recent recommendations regarding APOE genotyping urge that "in deciding whether or not to carry out APOE genotyping for any purpose, physicians and patients should bear in mind that genotype disclosure can have adverse effects on insurability, employability, and the psychosocial status of patients and family members."[92] Thus, they conclude that "future clinical applications of genotyping should be offered only when pre-test and post-test counseling, education and support are available."[92]

In other words, to be consistent with the most relevant current recommended policies and practices regarding genetic testing, it appears that all research uses of a versatile genetic test like APOE genotyping will have to be governed by the protocols required by its most problematic use. This means that, in order to protect participants in cardiovascular research from the psychosocial sequelae of having their APOE genotype interpreted as a risk predictor for Alzheimer's disease, cardiologists must perform their testing according to the guidelines devised by neurologists for AD risk assessment—guidelines that the neurologists themselves are not yet ready to implement because of the scientific uncertainties that still haunt the association.[92] As genome research yields an increasing number and variety of such "spoiler associations," it will become important for biomedical researchers to coordinate their efforts across specialties, so that important research tools are not hamstrung by similarly contentious professional policy claims.

Preliminary findings. Finally, because gene-hunting has been an incremental affair, using maps and sequence data to triangulate our way to alleles of interest and then assessing the expression of those alleles in populations, it almost always generates tentative conclusions along the way. Where these findings seem to hold the promise of clinical relevance, bench scientists and epidemiologists find themselves concerned about their obligations to warn participants of these findings.

In part, this issue reflects the need for a better translational bridge between the laboratory and clinical practice, a need that has spurred the dramatic growth of genetic diagnostics research. In the absence of effective therapies, the promise of accessible genetic information lies in its ability to allow individuals and their families to identify, understand, and sometimes control their inherited health risks. That ability, in turn, depends on two conditions: the validity of the clinical risk predictions that the information provides and the patients' ability to assess that validity realistically. This means that the decision to declare a particular genetic test ready for use as a clinical decision-making tool depends on much more than guaranteeing the test's ability to reliably identify its target mutations. It also requires a professional judgment about the clinical significance of the test results and the concomitant risks of that information for patients and their families: the features that comprise what some call a test's "clinical validity."[93]

Assessing those features of the test, and developing testing protocols that can optimally address them, requires answering epidemiological, psychosocial, and health services research questions that go well beyond the usual purview of molecular genetics.[16,93] Over the last decade, at the recommendations of policy bodies like the National Academy of Sciences[16] and the Department of Health and Human Services Secretary's Advisory Committee on Genetic Testing, the field of genetic diagnostic research has emerged to provide the evidence needed to craft safe and effective protocols for the clinical delivery of genetic risk information.[94] Professional policy statements like those governing the disclosure of APOE4 risk information are often precautionary placeholders in the absence of such data.

Study Design Implications

Despite the development of policies and protocols for the careful translation of genetic research findings into clinical practice, however, bench scientists often feel obligated to disclose accidental or expected research results that they find clinically or socially important for participants to know. This has led to attempts to develop practical approaches to deciding when to disclose research results, even in advance of well-developed clinical protocols. Three types of approaches are increasingly common.

One approach is to establish decision-making guidelines by suggesting the variables that should be considered in each instance. For the most part, these algorithms track the risk/benefit calculus familiar in clinical medicine. For example, one early report recommended that investigators make their decision about the disclosure of early finding on the basis of the following three variables: (1) the magnitude of the threat posed to the subject, (2) the accuracy with which the data predict that the threat will be realized, and (3) the possibility that action can be taken to avoid or ameliorate the potential injury.[95] These are the principles that typically govern decisions to disclose information in clinical medicine, and routinely dominate medical ethical discussions of clinical truth-telling, the limits of confidentiality,[96] and professional obligations to offer unsolicited medical advice.[97] Most recent recommendations on the question of reporting research results to subjects simply elaborate on these consequentialist principles.[98–100] Thus, one reviewer concludes:

> Thus in the end perhaps genetics research is best served by the routine practices of disclosure utilized in the medical treatment area. Disclosure of results, which are material to a patient's decision-making in the areas of health and reproduction could become the standard of care so long as the information is reasonably believed to offer some clinical benefit to the subject. Disclosure to family members may also fall under a materiality standard, with disclosure becoming a duty if the genetic infirmity is susceptible to treatment or prevention. As the study of the human genome gives way to

the practice of genetic medicine, our sensibilities about disclosure may follow in its path.[101]

For all its strengths, this approach faces two major objections. The first is that it ignores the ideal of "partnership" to which many researchers and participants aspire. For those who view genetic research as a robustly "collaborative enterprise" between scientists and volunteers, titrating disclosures against a risk/benefit algorithm may not show enough respect to the participants' right "to know everything the investigator knows about them."[102] The second objection is that, in practice, the prerequisites imposed by applying clinical standards of care, such as the clinical validation of test results, the use of Clinical Laboratory Improvement Amendments (CLIA)–approved laboratories, and the observance of Health Insurance Portability and Accountability Act (HIPPA) privacy regulations, may, as in the case of APOE4 genotyping, make it inappropriate for researchers to disclose many of the findings that they feel compelled to report to their volunteers.[100] Applying clinical standards suitable to the therapeutic relationship, in other words, may mask or distort distinctive elements of the researcher/volunteer relationship that both parties would be loath to sacrifice.

A second, procedural approach to these issues is to recommend the creation and use of committees that would be comparable to the data safety and monitoring boards (DSMBs) used by clinical trials.[103] These committees (often misnamed as project ethics committees) are charged with deciding when study findings are clinically reliable and useful enough to disclose to the research subjects.[104] To the extent that they involve research subjects, family representatives, or community members from the study populations, these committees may potentially offer a useful middle ground between paternalistic and client-centered views. This approach has been particularly successful when researchers are working with organized communities and disease groups, although it faces many of the same challenges discussed above for other forms of community engagement at earlier stages in the research process.[64] Although these committees may utilize similar standards for clinical evaluation as other researchers or policy makers, they are in a unique position to help define the magnitude of potential threats to their communities, provide more accurate information on key social variables, and evaluate study criteria in light of their own values.

Finally, a third approach is to plan research communications in a stepwise fashion. In this model, participating families or communities are brought into the planning of research studies early on so that they can have as full as sense as the researchers of the potential information that might be generated, even before they agree to participate in the study. This process allows the study team both to alert the participants to the possibility of unexpected, uncertain, or unhappy findings, and at the same time to gain a sense of their expectations regarding information reporting and a more refined understanding of what results would be considered problematic by their volunteers.[54] Then, as data is collected and analyzed, the research team communicates aggregate results to the participants, via newsletters or reports, in progressively more refined and validated form. This approach shapes the disclosure in keeping with the volunteers' own values, but also shifts to them the responsibility for ascertaining their individual results.[105]

Increasingly, as tests for genetic factors in more complex diseases become available, the question will become less whether one has the mutation in question, but what that means for one's future.

To be able to use the results of genomic research intelligently, research participants will need to be able to think even more than they must today in terms of shifting ranges of probabilities that are influenced by both genes and environmental factors.[106] As they learn to do this, both subjects of research and investigators will find themselves swimming upstream against our culture's tendency to interpret genetic risk factors in a deterministic, even fatalistic fashion.[107] It is this willingness to read too much into genetic risk assessments that raises the stakes of the researcher's decision to disclose preliminary research results, because it both drives the interest of participants and exacerbates most of the ancillary psychosocial risks they might face. Part of the clinical researcher's job in optimizing the personal utility of genetic information will be finding ways to counter this misleading inclination.

Control and Benefit-Sharing

Returning research results to participants inevitably raises their expectation of being able to control the consequences of their participation, especially when communication is cloaked in the language of "partnership." Partnerships are usually characterized by shared decision making and mutual benefit. But this leads to a final set of issues for genetic researchers: How much control and what kinds of benefit-sharing can genetic researchers honestly promise?

For example, research participants are routinely told that they are free to withdraw from studies at any time. Yet in genetic family studies, their participation consists of their presence on a pedigree and their DNA in a freezer. Traditionally, most researchers have regarded DNA samples like other donated human biological material, as material over which the sample sources no longer hold a claim. For example, one group draws on the *Moore v. Regents of the University of California* case[108] to argue, "According to a 1990 California Supreme Court case, a cell line is 'factually and legally distinct' from the cells taken from a subject, and therefore cannot be considered the 'property' of that subject."[36] However, unlike most donated tissue, DNA samples in a family collection gain their research value precisely to the extent that they continue to represent their donors. Thus, when another group considered the issue, it determined the following:

> Participants at the conference agreed that subjects in pedigree studies have the right to refuse to participate any further in the research, and should be able to have their names removed from a pedigree. There was also a consensus that the subjects could withdraw their personal DNA sample or require that it not be used in any further research, assuming that they had not formally transferred ownership to the researchers. However, subjects were not considered to have any control over the information obtained by investigators from their DNA samples, and researchers are free to use such information for further analysis consistent with approved research protocols.[52]

For investigators contemplating publication, this consensus yields mixed advice. The "names" of family members who deny permission to publish data should not be included, but does this extend to the anonymous symbols that signify them in the chart as well? Or are those symbols, conveying gender, genotype, and family relationships, simply "information obtained by the investigators," over which family members have no further control?[44]

Part of the reason the "ownership" of research data and materials becomes a question in genomic studies is that the pedigree information and DNA samples collected in the course of particular gene-hunting projects can often be used to support subsequent projects. Traditionally, tissues and blood samples donated for research have been considered to be available for further study by researchers. Many consent forms for linkage studies make this assumption explicit to their subjects by having them provide blanket permission "for further research" with their samples. An increasingly common view today, however, is that "the day for informal donations of DNA samples is past,"[109] and that new molecular studies of collected samples should be subject to the same requirements as the original family study that generated the resource. The strongest view is that the participants should know and agree to any molecular studies conducted on their DNA samples that were not specifically discussed under the initial consent without a "blanket consent" option. One statement of this position appears in the institutional guidelines developed by the IRB of the Johns Hopkins University:

> A subject cannot give consent to participate in a future experiment of unknown risk. Prior to recontacting donors who have either agreed to future testing or whose samples are stored and with whom consent for future testing was not discussed, investigators must seek an opinion from the . . . IRB regarding the appropriateness of the risk:benefit ratio and possible impact of test results on the subjects. . . . If consent is given for genomic screening using a particular set of probes—identified as probes for a particular disease under study—probes identified with other diseases may not be used unless further consent is obtained for the study of the individual's DNA with those new probes.[79]

Of course, one category of research that has traditionally been exempt from the regulations that apply to research involving humans has been research with anonymous human tissue, and most of the human cell lines that are used for biomedical research are distributed through the genetic research community without any traditional personal identifiers attached.[110] As genetic mapping, DNA sequencing, and genotyping technologies progress, however, the adequacy of that practice will continue to be pressed by our increasing ability to retrospectively link samples to their human sources. Because DNA profiles are themselves remarkable personal identifiers, there may be no way to completely "anonymize" individual DNA sequence data. Foreseeing the day when it may become valuable to research to post complete "personal genome projects"[111] on the Internet as open source research resources, calls for "health information altruists" are already being made.[112]

In addition to questions about the limits of participant control of samples and information, there has been increasing discussion of the need for a variety of forms of "benefit sharing" with genetic research participants, at both family and group levels. Three different models of benefit-sharing are emerging, although they are not often well distinguished: (1) profit-sharing plans, in which the research participants negotiate intellectual property rights and financial stakes in any commercialized outcomes of the research; (2) health-care dividend plans, in which participants are provided with privileged access to any health-care products or services generated by the research; and (3) "reciprocity" agreements, in which participants are given benefits unrelated to the research itself, in recognition of their contribution to the research. Each of these approaches has strengths and weaknesses, and they are only just beginning to be evaluated empirically.

Policy Implications

Most genetic researchers strive to avoid profit-sharing approaches by having participants relinquish claims to any commercial benefits of a study. However, in recent years a number of the voluntary health organizations of families at risk for particular genetic conditions have begun experimenting with the profit-sharing approach.[113] Again, this trend has been galvanized by a dispute: In 1997, Miami Children's Hospital obtained a patent that covered all diagnostic and therapeutic uses of the gene for aspartoacylase and its mutations, which cause Canavan's disease. The research leading up to this discovery had been organized largely by families of children with Canavan's disease, who recruited the scientist Reuben Matalon, raised the funding, and participated as DNA donors in the research. The families sued Miami Children's Hospital, arguing that the use of the patent to sell genetic testing back to the community that made it possible was unfair and likely to restrict access to the test.[114] In the wake of that case, other organizations—like PXE International, devoted to another rare genetic disease, pseudoxanthoma elasticum—have taken care to negotiate material transfer agreements with researchers, retaining rights to patent ownership for discoveries related to "their genes."[115] The Genetic Alliance, an umbrella group for rare genetic disease organizations, has now launched a Biobank initiative modeled on the PXE International profit-sharing approach.

The rationale for the profit-sharing approach is two-fold. On one hand, disease groups argue that they make material contributions to the research, well beyond the DNA samples that their family members may contribute. They are often the ones who bring scientific attention to their disease, maintain the registries of families that are key to research recruitment, facilitate that recruitment, and sometimes even fund the research. Second, by preserving a financial stake in the research, these groups strive to protect access to any health-care services that result from the research for their constituents.

As a policy matter, however, the profit-sharing approach does raise some challenges. First, it risks imputing ownership of particular mutations or alleles to the participating group. Unlike populations, these genetic disease advocacy groups are "genetic communities" in the sense that their membership is defined by a genotype many members share. Unlike clans, the families that constitute them are not genealogically related. When such a group patents "its" gene after underwriting the gene's discovery, the group explicitly adopts the "ownership" paradigm, even when it does so defensively and on behalf of its constituency. But what obligations to that constituency flow from this move? Little attention has been given to how competing interests within such groups should be adjudicated by researchers in negotiating the disposition of this intellectual property, or whether the advocacy group itself acquires any different obligations of accountability to people carrying "its" genotype than scientific or corporate patent-holders would. What does it mean to be a loyal member of such a community, when different scientific research groups come courting, or when rival advocacy groups claim to be one's representative?

Because the main stated interest of disease groups in advocating profit-sharing approaches is to gain access to health-care benefits, another popular model has been to condition group participation on privileged access to research-related health care, regardless of ownership. For example, in 2000 the revised Declaration of Helsinki endorsed the view that "[a]t the conclusion of the study, every patient entered into the study should be assured of access to the best proven prophylactic, diagnostic and therapeutic methods identified by the study."[116]

The "health dividends" approach is defended as a realistic way to recognize a family's or community's role in assuming the risks of research, and of allowing researchers to do what is in their power to help redress the lack of health-care access that research participants from disadvantaged communities may face. It does, however, face two dangers that are familiar to investigators in other clinical research settings. The first is that by promising health-care benefits from basic genetic research studies, the researchers may foster unrealistic expectations among participants, encouraging the "therapeutic misconception" (see Chapter 58). Perhaps even more important, where there are foreseeable benefits, this approach can establish a forced choice dilemma for disadvantaged participants, compromising the voluntariness of their participation in any particular study.

One response to these challenges has been to attempt to disconnect the health benefits provided by researchers from the topic of the research itself. For example, in its policy statement on benefit sharing, the international Human Genome Organization says that, in addition to research-related health dividends, "immediate health benefits as determined by community needs could be provided . . . and that profit-making entities [should] dedicate a percentage (1–3% of their annual net profit) to healthcare infrastructure and/or to humanitarian efforts."[117] Often, such benefits are negotiated by communities during or after their participation in research as a gesture of "reciprocity" on the part of researchers.

The reciprocity approach has several important policy advantages. It does not impute "ownership" of particular genetic patterns or variants to the participants. It does not risk unrealistic expectations about the therapeutic outcomes of genetic research. It can provide collective benefits to both participating and nonparticipating segments of the group. And it can be better adapted to meet the highest priority local needs. On the other hand, it does raise some important questions. For example, is there a community that can benefit? Does the proposed reciprocity constitute extortion or bribery? Is the proposed reciprocity proportional to the group's contribution?

Although the first wave of contemporary literature on this topic portrayed genetic information as "the common heritage of humankind,"[1] and thus unsuited to ownership and exploitation by subsets of the species, the organization of genetic research in terms of community membership is shifting the tone of the ownership debate dramatically. Although the ownership framework continues to be debated in international policy circles,[118] as human communities have come to be (mistakenly) identified with unique human superfamilies, such communities seem to have begun to accept the idea that their genes are akin to the natural resources under their local control.[119] Complaints of "biopiracy," and pleas for "benefit-sharing" and "reciprocity" on behalf of communities under genetic study, as well as charges of unfairness and neglect by

those left out of genetic diversity research, all suggest a rising sense that, in fact, subsets of the species do have claims on the genetic information that distinguishes them and should be compensated appropriately for its use by others.[102]

Conclusion

Genes (and their variations) seem to have acquired the status that germs held in Archibald Garrod's day a century ago, as the most promising causal factors to investigate in addressing questions of human health and disease.[2] As these investigations gather momentum in the clinical research arena, they are provoking reassessments of the traditional conventions of human genetics research and pioneering new questions for research ethics. So far, the discussion of these issues has proceeded largely without the benefit of the evidence that might help their sound resolution. Fortunately, there is a growing interdisciplinary community of researchers devoted to gathering this evidence, and support from the scientific community for their efforts.[120] Our review suggests a four-part agenda for further empirical and policy research by this community, addressing four questions that cut across all the issues identified above.

What Does It Mean to Participate in Human Genetic Research?

As genomics makes possible increasingly fine-grained studies of human genetic variation, both globally and locally, it will become more important for genome researchers and science policy makers to become sophisticated students of human cultural, social, and political variation as well. Understanding research participants' beliefs and attitudes about themselves, their family relations, lineage, community, and ethnic identity will be critical to the success of this science. These beliefs and attitudes shape the participants' interpretation of the research experience and lay the foundation for any research risks or possible benefits that might emerge.

What Social Values Influence the Pace and Direction of Genomic Research?

Questions about the translation of new genetic knowledge into practical health benefits sometimes get relegated "downstream" from genetic research ethics, as issues in the clinical delivery or dissemination of genetic discoveries. However, studies of academic/industry relationships in genomics make it clear that entrepreneurial thinking about the prospect for application occurs quite early in the human genetic and genomic research process. The increasing interest in benefit-sharing arrangements with research participant communities is also encouraging basic scientists to design research with practical outcomes in mind. Finally, behind these incentives, most scientists are motivated by more or less well formed public health goals. Careful empirical and policy studies of benefit-sharing, the commercialization of cutting-edge science, the regulatory system that governs the translational pathway in the United States, and the public health goals of genetic medicine, will provide useful perspectives on regulatory regimes at the institutional, governmental, and international levels.

What Challenges Can We Anticipate From the Frontiers of Genetic Science?

New advances in genome-wide analysis will increase the speed and scope of genetic research exponentially over the next decade, making it possible for clinical investigators to take genomic approaches to complex traits and conditions that have been hitherto beyond their reach. New sequencing technologies promise to propel this work even further by dramatically lowering research costs, and their combination with improved gene transfer technology will open up new horizons for molecular medicine. Novel issues will be generated for clinical investigators and research participants when these tools begin to be used in human studies, challenging current conventions regarding individual informed consent, research participant privacy, research risks, and research aimed at "genetic enhancement." Anticipating and identifying these new issues in advance is the exercise of scientific moral imagination that can be informed by careful empirical forecasting of scientific progress.

What Are Responsible Policy Options in Designing and Conducting Human Genetic Research?

Experiments in policy making for genetic research ethics are proliferating, as investigators, bioethics scholars, professional societies, and regulatory bodies suggest and implement different approaches to the issues we have reviewed. Now the data from these experiments needs to be analyzed. Comparative assessments of genetic research projects with families, communities, and populations operating under different regimes can help provide empirical evidence of researchers' and participants' actual experience with them, and help inform more careful ethical and legal critiques of the alternatives.

It is not a coincidence that genetic research attracts special attention within clinical research ethics, even when its issues are common to other parts of biomedicine. In addition to the historical shadow under which it operates and the scientific excitement about its promise, the intrinsic subject matter of human genetics—our biological differences and relationships—will always provoke ethical issues. Genetics is a science that speaks to the very traits that animate our most profound and volatile human rights issues and it will challenge clinical researchers and the research participants who work with them as long as our genetic identities are important ingredients in human assessments of social standing.[121]

Acknowledgment

Support for this chapter comes through a grant (1P50HG003390–01) from the National Human Genome Research Institute of the U.S. National Institutes of Health.

References

1. Bearn AG, Miller ED. Archibald Garrod and the development of the concept of inborn errors of metabolism. *Bulletin of the History of Medicine* 1979;53(3):315–28.

2. Adams MB. *The Wellborn Science: Eugenics in Germany, France, Brazil and Russia*. New York, N.Y.: Oxford University Press; 1990.

3. Duster T. *Backdoor to Eugenics*, 2nd ed. New York, N.Y.: Routledge; 2003 [1990].

4. Kevles DJ. *In the Name of Eugenics: Genetics and the Uses of Human Heredity*. Cambridge, Mass.: Harvard University Press; 1985.

5. Ludmerer KM. *Genetics and American Society: A Historical Appraisal*. Baltimore, Md.: The Johns Hopkins University Press; 1972.

6. Rafter NH. *White Trash: The Eugenic Family Studies, 1877–1919*. Boston, Mass.: Northeastern University Press; 1988.

7. Müller-Hill B. *Murderous Science: Elimination by Scientific Selection of Jews, Gypsies and Others, Germany 1933–1945*. New York, N.Y.: Oxford University Press; 1988.

8. Paul DB. *Controlling Human Heredity: 1865 to the Present*. Amherst, N.Y.: Humanity Books; 1998.

9. Annas GJ, Grodin MA, eds. *The Nazi Doctors and the Nuremberg Code: Human Rights in Human Experimentation*. New York, N.Y.: Oxford University Press; 1992.

10. Keller EF. *The Century of the Gene*. Cambridge, Mass.: Harvard University Press; 2000.

11. Collins FS, Guttmacher AE, Drazen JM, eds. *Genomic Medicine*. Baltimore, Md.: The Johns Hopkins University Press; 2004.

12. Frankel MS, Teich AH, eds. *Ethical and Legal Issues in Pedigree Research*. Washington, D.C.: American Association for the Advancement of Science; 1993.

13. Department of Health and Human Services, Office for Health Research Protections. *Protecting Human Research Subjects: Institutional Review Board Guidebook*. Rockville, Md.: OHRP; 1993:5–42. [Online] Available: http://www.hhs.gov/ohrp/irb/irb_guidebook.htm.

14. Juengst ET. Respecting human subjects in genome research: A preliminary policy agenda. In: Vanderpool HY, ed. *The Ethics of Research Involving Human Subjects: Facing the 21st Century*. Frederick, Md.: University Publishing Group; 1996:401–29.

15. Green ED, Waterston RH. The Human Genome Project: Prospects and implications for clinical medicine. *JAMA* 1991;266:1966–75.

16. Andrews LB. *Assessing Genetic Risks: Implications for Health and Social Policy*. Washington, D.C.: National Academy Press; 1994.

17. National Human Genome Research Institute, National Institutes of Health. Cumulative Pace of Gene Discovery 1981–2003. [Online] Available: http://www.genome.gov/Pages/News/PaceofDiseaseGeneDiscovery.pdf.

18. Risch N. Linkage strategies for genetically complex traits. I. Multilocus models. *American Journal of Human Genetics* 1990;46:222–8.

19. Cooper DN, Schmidtke J. Molecular genetic approaches to the analysis and diagnosis of human inherited disease: An overview. *Annals of Medicine* 1992;24:29–42.

20. Wilfond BS, Nolan K. National policy development for the clinical application of genetic diagnostic technologies: Lessons from cystic fibrosis. *JAMA* 1993;270:2948–54.

21. Committee on Human Genome Diversity, Commission on Life Sciences, National Research Council. *Evaluating Human Genetic Diversity*. Washington, D.C.: National Academy Press; 1997.

22. Collins FS, Guyer MS, Charkravarti A. Variations on a theme: Cataloging human DNA sequence variation. *Science* 1997;278:1580–1.

23. Sutherland GR, Richards RI. DNA repeats—A treasury of human variation. *New England Journal of Medicine* 1994;331:191–3.

24. Weinshilboum R, Wang L. Pharmacogenomics: Bench to bedside. *Nature Reviews Drug Discovery* 2004;3:739–48.

25. Risch N, Merikangas K. The future of genetic studies of complex human diseases. *Science* 1996;273:1516–7.

26. Knoppers BM, ed. *Populations and Genetics: Legal and Socio-Ethical Perspectives*. Leiden, The Netherlands: Brill Academic Publishers; 2003.

27. Cook-Deegan RM. Privacy families and human subject protections: Some lessons from pedigree research. *Journal of Continuing Education in the Health Professions* 2001;21:224–37.

28. Renegar G, Rieser P, Manasco P. Family consent and the pursuit of better medicines through genetic research. *Journal of Continuing Education in the Health Professions* 2001;21:265–70.

29. Coy KL. The current privacy environment: Implications for third-party research. *Journal of Continuing Education in the Health Professions* 2001;21:203–14.

30. Princeton Survey Research Associates for the California Healthcare Foundation. *Medical Privacy and Confidentiality Survey.* [Online] January 1999. Available: http://www.chcf.org/documents/ihealth/topline.pdf.

31. Department of Health and Human Services, National Institutes of Health, and Office for Human Research Protections. The Common Rule, Title 45 (Public Welfare), Code of Federal Regulations, Part 46 (Protection of Human Subjects). [Online] June 23, 2005. Available: http://www.hhs.gov/ohrp/humansubjects/guidance/45cfr46.htm.

32. The American Society of Human Genetics Social Issues Subcommittee on Familial Disclosure. ASHG Statement: Professional disclosure of familial genetic information. *American Journal of Human Genetics* 1998;62:474–83.

33. Botkin J. Protecting the privacy of family members in survey and pedigree research. *JAMA* 2001;285:207–11.

34. Department of Health and Human Services, Office for Health Research Protections. *Protecting Human Research Subjects: Institutional Review Board Guidebook.* Rockville, Md.: OHRP; 1993, "Recruitment of Subjects," 4–20. [Online] Available: http://www.hhs.gov/ohrp/irb/irb_guidebook.htm.

35. Simpson SA. Case study on bipolar mood disorder: Ethical and legal issues. In: Frankel MS, Teich AH, eds. *Ethical and Legal Issues in Pedigree Research.* Washington, D.C.: American Association for the Advancement of Science; 1993:44–6.

36. Shore D, et al. Legal and ethical issues in psychiatric genetic research. *American Journal of Medical Genetics* 1993;48:17–21.

37. Bonvicini KA. The art of recruitment: The foundation of family and linkage studies of psychiatric illness. *Family Process* 1998;37:153–65.

38. Compton JG, et al. Linkage of epidermolytic hyperkeratosis to the type II keratin gene cluster on chromosome 12q. *Nature Genetics* 1992;1:301–5.

39. Austin HA, Kaiser M. Summary Report to the Human Subjects Research Advisory Committee on the Meetings of the Intramural Working Group on Human Genetics Research. Bethesda, Md.: NIH; 1993:2–3 (unpublished).

40. Powers M. Publication-related risks to privacy: Ethical implications of pedigree studies. *IRB: A Review of Human Subjects Research* 1993;15(4):7–11.

41. Botkin JR, et al. Privacy and confidentiality in the publication of pedigrees: A survey of investigators and biomedical journals. *JAMA* 1998;279:1808–12.

42. Leppert M. Case study on colon cancer. In: Frankel MS, Teich AH, eds. *Ethical and Legal Issues in Pedigree Research.* Washington, D.C.: American Association for the Advancement of Science; 1993:199.

43. Beskow LM, et al. Ethical issues in identifying and recruiting participants for familial genetic research. *American Journal of Medical Genetics* 2004;130A:424–31.

44. Gray J. Case study on Huntington's Disease. In: Frankel MS, Teich AH, eds. *Ethical and Legal Issues in Pedigree Research.* Washington, D.C.: American Association for the Advancement of Science; 1993:90–6.

45. Sorenson JR, et al. Proband and parent assistance in identifying relatives for cystic fibrosis carrier testing. *American Journal of Medical Genetics* 1996;63:419–25.

46. Kreiger N, et al. A qualitative study of subject recruitment for familial cancer research. *Annals of Epidemiology* 2001;11(4):219–24.

47. Glass KC, et al. Structuring the review of human genetics protocols: Gene localization and identification studies. *IRB: A Review of Human Subjects Research* 1996;18(4):1–9.

48. Wachbroit R. Rethinking medical confidentiality: The impact of genetics. *Suffolk University Law Review* 1993;27:1391–410.

49. Parker LS, Lidz CW. Familial coercion to participate in genetic family studies: Is there cause for IRB intervention? *IRB: A Review of Human Subjects Research* 1994;16(1–2):6–12.

50. Wachbroit R. Who is the patient? A moral problem. *Maryland Medical Journal* 1989;38:957–9.

51. Christie RJ, Hoffmaster CB. *Ethical Issues in Family Medicine.* New York, N.Y.: Oxford University Press; 1986.

52. Shinn R. Family relationships and social policy: An ethical inquiry. In: Frankel MS, Teich AH, eds. *Ethical and Legal Issues in Pedigree Research.* Washington, D.C.: American Association for the Advancement of Science; 1993:9–25.

53. Greely HT. The control of genetic research: Involving the "groups between." *Houston Law Review* 1997;33:1397–430.

54. Sharp RR, Foster MW. Involving study populations in the review of genetic research. *Journal of Law, Medicine, and Ethics* 2000;28:41–51, 53.

55. Foster MW, Eisenbraun AJ, Carter TH. Genetic screening of targeted subpopulations: The role of communal discourse in evaluating sociocultural implications. *Genetic Testing* 1997–1998;1:269–74.

56. Weijer C, Goldsand G, Emanuel EJ. Protecting communities in research: Current guidelines and limits of extrapolation. *Nature Genetics* 1999;23:275–80.

57. Juengst ET. Community engagement in genetic research: The "slow code" of research ethics? In: Knoppers BM, ed. *Populations and Genetics: Legal and Socio-Ethical Perspectives.* Leiden, The Netherlands: Brill Academic Publishers; 2003:181–98.

58. Schulz A, Caldwell C, Foster S. "What are they going to do with the information?" Latino/Latina and African American perspectives on the Human Genome Project. *Health, Education and Behavior* 2003;30:151–69.

59. Marshall PA, Rotimi C. Ethical challenges in community-based research. *American Journal of the Medical Sciences* 2001;322:241–5.

60. Haimes E, Whong-Barr M. Competing perspectives on reasons for participation and non-participation in the North Cumbria Community Genetics Project. In: Knoppers BM, ed. *Populations and Genetics: Legal and Socio-Ethical Perspectives.* Leiden, The Netherlands: Brill Academic Publishers; 2003:199–216.

61. Sharp RR, Foster MW. Community involvement in the ethical review of genetic research: Lessons from American Indian and Alaska Native populations. *Environmental Health Perspectives* 2002; 110(Suppl. 2):145–8.

62. Bowekaty MB. Perspectives on research in American Indian communities. *Jurimetrics* 2002;42:145–8.

63. Gostin L. Ethical principles for the conduct of human subject research: Population-based research and ethics. *Law, Medicine, and Health Care* 1991;19(3–4):191–201.

64. Marshall PA, Rotimi C. Ethical challenges in community-based research. *American Journal of the Medical Sciences* 2001;322:259–63.

65. Foster MW, et al. The role of community review in evaluating the risks of human genetic variation research. *American Journal of Human Genetics* 1999;64:1719–27.

66. Cavalli-Sforza LL, et al. Call for a worldwide survey of human genetic diversity: A vanishing opportunity for the Human Genome Project. *Genomics* 1991;11:490–1.

67. Dodson M, Williamson R. Indigenous peoples and the morality of the Human Genome Diversity Project. *Journal of Medical Ethics* 1999;25:204–8.

68. Lock M. Genetic diversity and the politics of difference. *Chicago/Kent Law Review* 1999;75:86–111.

69. Reardon J. *Race to the Finish: Identity and Governance in an Age of Genomics.* Princeton, N.J.: Princeton University Press; 2004.

70. Weiss KM, et al. North American Regional Committee of the Human Genome Diversity Project: Proposed model ethical protocol for collecting DNA samples. *Houston Law Review* 1997;33:1431–74.

71. Navajo Nation. Tribal Code, Title 13 (Health & Welfare), para. 10.

72. Juengst ET. Groups as gatekeepers to genomic research: Conceptually confusing, morally hazardous and practically useless. *Kennedy Institute of Ethics Journal* 1998;8:183–200.

73. Davis DS. Groups communities and contested identities in genetic research. *Hastings Center Report* 2000;30(6):38–45.

74. Lee SS, Mountain J, Koenig BA. The meanings of "race" in the new genomics: Implications for health disparities research. *Yale Journal of Health Policy, Law and Ethics* 2001;1:33–75.

75. National Institutes of Health. Points to Consider When Planning a Genetic Study That Involves Members of Named Populations. [Online] 2002. Available: www.nih.gov/sigs/bioethics/named_populations.html.

76. MacKay CR, Shea JM. Ethical considerations in research on Huntington's disease. *Clinical Research* 1977;25(4):241–7.

77. Biesecker BB, et al. Genetic counseling for families with inherited susceptibility to breast and ovarian cancer. *JAMA* 1993;269:1970–4.

78. Wertz DC, Fletcher JC. Communicating genetic risks. *Science, Technology and Human Values* 1987;12(3&4):60–6.

79. Folstein M. Report of the Clinical Genetic Research Guidelines Committee. Baltimore, Md.: Johns Hopkins University Hospital Joint Committee on Clinical Investigation; 1993.

80. Offit K, et al. The "duty to warn" a patient's family members about hereditary disease risks. *JAMA* 2004;292:1469–73.

81. Ross LF. Disclosing misattributed paternity. *Bioethics* 1996;10:114–30.

82. President's Commission for the Study of Ethical Problems in Medicine and Biomedical and Behavioral Research. *Screening and Counseling for Genetic Conditions.* Washington, D.C.: U.S. Government Printing Office; 1983:55.

83. Modell JS. *Kinship with Strangers: Adoption and Interpretations of Kinship in American Culture.* Berkeley, Calif.: University of California Press; 1994.

84. Elliott C, Brodwin P. Identity and genetic ancestry tracing. *British Medical Journal* 2002;325:1469–71.

85. Tallbear K. DNA blood and racializing the tribe. *Wicazo Sa Review* 2000;17:2–19.

86. Parfitt T. Genes, religion and history: The creation of a discourse of origin among a Judaizing African tribe. *Jurimetrics* 2002;42:209–19.

87. Post SG. Adoption theologically considered. *Journal of Religious Ethics* 1997;25:149–68.

88. Roberts DE. The genetic tie. *University of Chicago Law Review* 1995;62(1):209–73.

89. Davignon J, Gregg RE, Sing CF. Apolipoprotein E polymorphism and atherosclerosis. *Arteriosclerosis* 1988;8:1–21.

90. Kosunen O, et al. Relation of coronary atherosclerosis and apolipoprotein E genotypes in Alzheimer patients. *Stroke* 1995;26:743–8.

91. Lennox A, et al. Molecular genetic predictive testing for Alzheimer's disease: deliberations and preliminary recommendations. *Alzheimer Disease and Associated Disorders* 1994;8:126–47.

92. National Institute on Aging/Alzheimer's Association Working Group. Apolipoprotein E genotyping in Alzheimer's disease. *Lancet* 1996;347:1091–5.

93. Holtzman NA, et al. Predictive genetic testing: From basic research to clinical practice. *Science* 1997;278:602–5.

94. Secretary's Advisory Committee on Genetic Testing, National Institutes of Health. *Enhancing the Oversight of Genetic Tests: Recommendations of the SACGT.* [Online] July, 2000. Available: http://www4.0d.nih.gov/oba/sacgt/reports/oversight_report.pdf.

95. Reilly P. When should an investigator share raw data with the subjects? *IRB: A Review of Human Subjects Research* 1980;2(9):4–5.

96. Winter PR, et al. Notification of a family history of breast cancer: Issues of privacy and confidentiality. *American Journal of Medical Genetics* 1996;66:1–6.

97. Ratzan RM. Unsolicited medical opinion. *Journal of Medicine and Philosophy* 1985;10:147–62.

98. Quaid KA, Jessup NM, Meslin EM. Disclosure of genetic information obtained through research. *Genetic Testing* 2004;8:347–55.

99. National Bioethics Advisory Commission. *Ethical and Policy Issues in Research Involving Human Participants, Vol. I.* Bethesda, Md.: NBAC; 2001. [Online] Available: http://www.georgetown.edu/research/nrcbl/nbac/human/overv011.pdf.

100. Renegar G, et al. Returning genetic research results to individuals: Points-to-consider. *Bioethics* 2006;20:24–34.

101. Laidlaw SA, Raffel LJ, Daar DF. Genetic testing and human subjects in research. *Whittier Law Review* 2002;24(2):429–72.

102. Merz JF, et al. Protecting subjects' interests in genetics research. *American Journal of Human Genetics* 2002;70:965–71.

103. MacKay CR. Discussion points to consider in research related to the human genome. *Human Gene Therapy* 1993;4:477–95.

104. Kodish E, Murray TH, Shurin S. Cancer risk research: What should we tell subjects? *Clinical Research* 1994;42:396–402.

105. Beskow LM, et al. Informed consent for population-based research involving genetics. *JAMA* 2001;286:2315–21.

106. LeRoy B. Where theory meets practice: Challenges to the field of genetic counseling. In: Bartels DM, LeRoy B, Caplan AL, eds. *Prescribing Our Future: Ethical Challenges in Genetic Counseling.* New York, N.Y.: Aldine de Gruyter; 1993:39–54.

107. Holtzman NA. *Proceed with Caution: Predicting Genetic Risks in the Recombinant DNA Era.* Baltimore, Md.: The Johns Hopkins University Press; 1989.

108. Curran WJ. Scientific and commercial development of human cell lines: Issues of property ethics and conflict of interest. *New England Journal of Medicine* 1991;324:998–1000.

109. Hannig VL, Clayton EW, Edwards KM. Whose DNA is it anyway? Relationships between families and researchers. *American Journal of Medical Genetics* 1993;47:257–60.

110. Gey GO, Coffman WD, Kubicek MT. Tissue culture studies of the proliferative capacity of cervical carcinoma and normal epithelium. *Cancer Research* 1952;12:264–5.

111. Church GM. Genomes for all. *Scientific American* 2006;294(1):47–54.

112. Kohane IS, Altman RB. Health-information altruists—A potentially critical resource. *New England Journal of Medicine* 2005;353:2074–7.

113. Patrick T. PXE International: Harnessing intellectual property law for benefit-sharing. In: Knoppers BM, ed. *Populations and Genetics: Legal and Socio-Ethical Perspectives.* Leiden, The Netherlands: Brill Academic Publishers; 2003:377–95.

114. Marshall E. Genetic testing: Families sue hospital scientist for control of Canavan gene. *Science* 2000;290:1062.

115. Smaglik P. Tissue donors use their influence in deal over gene patent terms. *Nature* 2000;407:821.

116. World Medical Association. *Declaration of Helsinki: Ethical Principles for Medical Research Involving Human Subjects.* Tokyo, Japan: WMA; October 2004. [Online] 2004. Available: http://www.wma.net/e/policy/b3.htm.

117. Hugo Ethics Committee. Hugo Ethics Committee statement on benefit sharing: April 9, 2000. *Clinical Genetics* 2000;58:364–6.

118. Thorsteindottir H, et al. Do patents encourage or inhibit genomics as a global public good? In: Knoppers BM, ed. *Populations and Genetics: Legal and Socio-Ethical Perspectives.* Leiden, The Netherlands: Brill Academic Publishers; 2003:487–504.

119. Merz JF, McGee GE, Sankar P. "Iceland Inc."? On the ethics of commercial population genomics. *Social Science and Medicine* 2004;58:1201–9.

120. Juengst ET. Self-critical federal science? The ethics experiment within the U.S. Human Genome Project. *Social Philosophy and Policy* 1996;13(2):63–95.

121. Juengst ET. FACE facts: Why human genetics will always provoke bioethics. *Journal of Law, Medicine, and Ethics* 2004;32:267–75.

David Wendler   Franklin G. Miller

30

Deception in Clinical Research

Testing research hypotheses and answering scientific questions are sometimes accomplished by deceiving research participants. Deception is most commonly associated with psychological and social science research, in which data suggest that investigators often deceive participants. However, deception also occurs in a broad range of clinical research.[1] For example, clinical trials designed to assess the impact of expectancy on drug-craving and drug-taking behaviors sometimes deceive participants. One testing paradigm involves asking research participants to perform various manual tasks, for instance, responding to a red light on a computer screen, after receiving an injection of a drug such as cocaine. To distinguish drug effects from expectancy effects, this paradigm administers the drug in only half of the testing sessions and administers saline in the other sessions, but tells participants that they will receive the drug in all the sessions.

In some cases, clinical investigators may deceive research participants for what is perceived to be the good of the participants themselves, for instance, suggesting that an individual's disease has not progressed to the point that research testing reveals. Such deception raises obvious ethical concerns, but not issues that are unique to clinical research, and we will not address them here. We will instead focus on the question of whether and under what conditions it might be ethically acceptable to deceive research participants for scientific purposes.

Most commentators agree that deceiving research participants for scientific purposes is prima facie unacceptable. Most commentators also agree that the deception of research participants for scientific purposes can be justified in some cases—that is, that such deception is not, in practice, always ethically unacceptable. Much of the debate, then, focuses on the conditions under which

deception might be acceptable. Not surprisingly, the extent to which one finds deception in clinical research acceptable depends on how problematic one takes deception to be, which, in turn, depends in large measure on the extent to which one thinks that deception harms or wrongs research participants.

Many researchers assume that deception typically is relatively harmless and conclude that any restrictions on its use should be modest. These individuals would allow deceptive research for a broad range of studies, and would allow deception in cases in which nondeceptive methods are possible but would be more burdensome or onerous, perhaps requiring more participants or a longer study. Many commentators assume, in contrast, that deception is seriously unacceptable, and should be permitted only in extraordinary circumstances, if at all. These commentators often conclude that deception should be allowed for scientific purposes only when the research has very significant social value and would be impossible to conduct using nondeceptive methods.

Behind much of the debate over the ethical acceptability of deception in clinical research is the assumption that the use of deception necessarily conflicts with respect for participant autonomy. Either participants can provide valid informed consent, or investigators can rely on deception, but not both.[2-5] Against this assumption, some writers have argued that investigators can conduct deceptive studies while respecting the autonomy of the research participants by prospectively informing them that will be deceived, but not informing them of the nature of the deception. For example, in the deceptive studies of drug-craving and drug-taking behaviors, participants might be informed that the study has not been described accurately in all its details, without telling them which details have been misdescribed. Here too, as in a good deal of the deception debate, more data would be instructive, data on how deception and its alternatives affect participants and the validity of scientific findings.

The Nature of Deception

Deception occurs when investigators communicate—understood broadly to include written, spoken and behavioral communication—in ways that can reasonably be expected to result in some participants developing false beliefs. For example, investigators might tell participants that they will all receive active medication when only half of them will receive active medication and the other half will receive placebo. Deception in the clinical setting typically is intentional. That is, the investigator intends to deceive the participant and communicates in a way that is expected to lead to false beliefs on the part of participants. Moreover, the investigators rely on the fact that the participants are likely to develop false beliefs. It is the fact that the participants develop false beliefs in the drug testing paradigm mentioned previously that allows the investigators to distinguish expectancy effects from drug effects. Typically, we consider deception especially problematic when it involves the deceiver intentionally deceiving another person and then relying on the deception for the benefit of individuals other than those deceived.

Deception typically occurs as the result of investigators providing false information to participants. For example, in a study of continuous positive airway pressure (CPAP) versus placebo in sleep apnea, participants were told that the inert placebo pill was "intended to improve airway function."[6] The investigators used a misdescribed placebo pill as the control out of concern that those familiar with CPAP would have been able to distinguish CPAP from sham CPAP.

Investigators also may deceive participants by withholding pertinent information from them. In a study of chronic obstructive pulmonary disease (COPD), investigators attached a chronolog to participants' inhalers to measure whether they were "dumping" study medications.[7] To ensure accurate measurements, participants "were not informed of the chronolog's date- and time-recording capabilities."[7]

Whether a given instance of communication or failure to communicate constitutes deception depends upon what it is reasonable to expect individuals to conclude on the basis of the communication (or lack thereof). For this reason, reasonable people may disagree on whether a given instance of communication constitutes deception. To assess the impact of expectancy, one research design tells participants that a light will appear on their computer screen and then they will receive an injection of a drug. The design assesses expectancy by delaying the injection of drug for some time after the light appears. This design relies on the fact that participants expect to receive the injection just after the light appears. Is this design deceptive?

It is deceptive if it is reasonable to expect that participants, told that they will receive an injection of drug after the light appears, will conclude that they will receive an injection *immediately* after the light appears. If it is reasonable to expect that participants, told that they will receive an injection of drug after the light appears, will conclude that they will receive an injection at some time relatively soon but not necessarily immediately after the light appears, then the design may not be deceptive, depending upon how long the delay happens to be. Because our expectations re-

garding the beliefs reasonable individuals will develop may not be clear in this case, it may be unclear whether this design involves deception.

To consider a more prominent example, what does the present analysis imply about whether placebo-controlled studies are inherently deceptive? A typical blinded placebo trial randomly assigns some to receive drug and others to receive placebo, while withholding from participants information regarding which they are receiving. Furthermore, active steps are taken, such as double blinding and placing drug and placebo in identical capsules, to ensure that participants do not discern whether they have been assigned to receive drug or placebo. Clearly, then, placebo trials withhold important information from participants, and as a result participants often end up with false beliefs about what they are taking. Some end up with the belief that they are taking drug when, in fact, they are receiving a placebo. Are these trials therefore inherently deceptive? (Critics of placebo trials claim that participants typically are able to discern whether they are receiving active drug or placebo, allaying one's concerns regarding the potential for deception, but raising concerns regarding the scientific usefulness of placebo-controlled studies.)

Placebo-controlled trials in which all participants are told that they will receive an active drug clearly are deceptive. A trial that simply withheld any information regarding the contents of the research "tablets" would arguably be deceptive as well. In the absence of information to the contrary, one expects that tablets provided in the context of a clinical trial contain active medication. It is less clear that placebo-controlled trials are deceptive when participants are informed that placebos are being used, and that they will not be told whether they are receiving active medication or placebo. If participants are provided this information, it seems the reasonable response would be to remain agnostic over whether they are receiving medication or placebo, implying that standard placebo-controlled designs are not inherently deceptive.

Trials involving sham procedures, in contrast, sometimes involve an element of deception. In these trials, researchers manipulate the sham procedure, not so that participants will remain agnostic over whether they are receiving the real or the sham procedure, but in such a way as to engender the false belief in the participants that they are receiving the real procedure. Thus, even though participants are informed in advance that they will receive either a real or a sham intervention, active steps are taken to convince all the participants that they are receiving the real treatment.[8]

The Milgram Experiments

The contemporary debate about deception in clinical research was fueled by Stanley Milgram's experiments on obedience in the early 1960s.[9] In the wake of the disclosure of horrific acts during World War II, perpetrated by ostensibly ordinary Germans who claimed simply to be following orders, Milgram designed a series of experiments to assess the extent to which ordinary Americans would likewise obey authority figures.

Milgram recruited participants and paired them with a second individual who was identified as another participant, but in fact was working with Milgram. The "confederate" was placed in what was described as an electric chair and given a series of tasks to perform. This individual intentionally made a series of mistakes.

At each mistake, the participants were instructed by a researcher in a white coat to administer shocks of increasing severity to the individual. The accomplices in the chairs would feign increasing levels of agony as the participants were instructed to give, and often complied with giving, greater and greater shocks.

Milgram's widely criticized experiments were clearly deceptive. Participants were told that they were delivering actual shocks, and the actors strapped in the chair reacted in ways to reinforce this belief. Milgram's experiments led to widespread discussion on what precisely are the harms of deception in clinical research. Milgram responded to his critics on several occasions, and even conducted follow-up research on the participants to assess the extent to which they had been harmed.[10] Many of the participants reported to Milgram that they did not experience long-term harm as a result of their participation and were supportive of the research. Critics have questioned whether long-term harms are the relevant metric and whether participants can be trusted to report accurately whether they experienced serious trauma, especially when asked by the very individual who perpetrated the deception in the first place, raising further questions about the best methods for empirically assessing the possible harms of deception for scientific purposes.

What Makes Deception in Scientific Investigation Ethically Problematic?

At the outset, it is useful to appreciate the conflict between the ethos of science and the use of deceptive techniques. Science aims to discover and communicate the truth about the natural world and human conduct. There are sound methodological reasons for using deception to probe the truth about human attitudes and beliefs, and their effects on behavior. It follows, however, that when deception is used, a conflict between the means and ends of scientific investigation ensues: The end of discovering the truth is pursued by the means of deliberate untruth.

It might be argued that deception in scientific investigation is no more problematic than the pervasive and accepted use of deception in daily life and social contexts.[11] In a 2004 news article reporting advances in the design of computers to simulate human responsiveness, Clifford Nass, a professor of communication at Stanford University, is quoted as endorsing the use of deception in research: "We spend enormous amounts of time teaching children to deceive—it's called being polite or social. The history of all advertising is about deceiving. In education, it's often important to deceive people—sometimes you say, 'Boy you are really doing good,' not because you meant it but because you thought it would be helpful."[12]

Deception in ordinary life typically is justified on the grounds that it is for the benefit of the individual who is being deceived. For instance, the "polite" and "social" deception that Nass cites is justified on the ground that it is better to deceive someone slightly than criticize them or hurt their feelings. Notice, however, that this condition is not relevant to deceiving research participants for scientific purposes and the benefit of society in general, through the development of generalizable knowledge.

A major ethical concern with deception in research is its potential to violate legitimate trust. Individuals generally trust that the research in which they are invited to participate is worthwhile, that it will not expose them to undue risks of serious harm, and that they will be treated fairly. When participants discover that they have been deceived, which typically occurs during the process of debriefing at the end of study participation, they may lose trust in scientific investigation. As we argue below, the issue of trust is likely to be especially important for research involving patient subjects conducted in clinical settings.

Deception of research participants also clearly conflicts with the ethical norms governing clinical research.[1,13] First, it violates the principle of respect for persons by infringing the right of prospective research participants to choose whether to participate in research based on full disclosure of relevant information. Second, it may manipulate individuals to volunteer when they would otherwise not have chosen to do so had they been informed accurately about the nature of the research, including its use of deception. For these reasons, deception as it is currently practiced in many clinical research studies is incompatible with informed consent.

Finally, deception in research raises ethical concern because it can be corrupting for the professionals who practice it and for those who witness it. According to an ancient perspective in moral philosophy, moral character depends on habits of conduct.[14] The use of deception in research may interfere with the disposition not to lie or deceive persons. This problem is compounded when the study design requires deception at the initiation of the trial, as well as maintenance of the deception during the conduct of research. Those who witness deception, especially if performed or sanctioned by professionals in positions of authority, may develop skewed perceptions of the ethics of deception, which may have negative consequences for the development of moral character. For these reasons, deception in research is prima facie wrongful.

The Harms of Deception and the Value of Deceptive Studies

The previous section concludes, as most commentators assume, that deception in clinical research is prima facie unethical, but can be justified in some circumstances. Hence, much of the debate concerns the extent to which deceptive studies should be permitted: Should deceptive studies be allowed in a relatively broad range of cases, or in extraordinary circumstances only? This debate over balancing the costs of deception against the value of deceptive studies occurs for two general kinds of studies.

First, in some cases investigators must deceive research participants to answer the scientific questions posed by the study. Earlier, we considered some examples of drug expectancy studies that pose just this dilemma. Assuming that there is no way to assess the effects of expectancy without deceiving the research participants, institutional review boards (IRBs) must determine whether the value of answering these questions justifies the harms of the deception involved. This is a difficult calculation to make; it is an impossible calculation to make unless one has some estimate for the potential harms of deception. It is worth noting that this calculation is made all the more difficult by the fact that an individual study rarely, if ever, definitively answers any given scientific question on its own. Only a series of studies, including future studies that may or may not occur, and which are usually not under the purview of the reviewing IRB, can answer the scientific questions posed by most trials.

A second, less examined need to balance the potential harms of deception against the anticipated value of deceptive research arises with respect to studies in which the use of nondeceptive means is theoretically possible, but is to varying degrees difficult or impractical. For example, one experimental paradigm for studying aggression in humans challenges participants to accumulate points by typing into a computer that, they are told, is connected to another computer operated by someone who may steal some of their points. In fact, the participant's computer is programmed to occasionally, and arbitrarily, subtract points from the participant's accounts. The investigators measure aggression as a function of how participants respond to these "thefts" by attempting to steal points from their "opponents." There are nondeceptive alternatives to this paradigm. Most simply, the researchers could hire assistants to sit at a second computer that is connected to the participants' computer. This person could type in the responses that the computer program now enters, thus producing a nondeceptive study. Should IRBs require investigators to adopt this methodology instead? Is this study feasible and effective? Presumably, the person entering the data will make more mistakes than the computer and may not end up entering truly random responses. It follows that this alternative study design will require more resources. It will require hiring assistants and setting up a second computer in a different room. In addition, given the uncertainty regarding the data entry of the "responding" research assistant, the alternative study design will likely yield somewhat less powerful results.

Whether an IRB should mandate this alternative design depends on the balance of the potential harms of deception against the anticipated value of the study and the costs of requiring an alternative design. Some might argue that the risks of the study amount to the potential harm that might result from the participants' having their points stolen and how they respond to these thefts. The use of deception does not increase the risks of the study, hence there is no reason to require the investigators to pursue a more costly nondeceptive approach. In response, one could just as easily argue that this design offers a clear example of a deceptive study with a feasible, and effective, nondeceptive alternative. Granted, the alternative design introduces an extra variable. But the alternative study is relatively straightforward and the mistakes that the computer operator makes could be isolated and controlled for. Thus, on this view, one might conclude that the investigators should be required to pursue the nondeceptive alternative. To resolve this debate, we need to determine to what extent deception harms research participants.

Empirical Data on the Harms of Deception

A number of studies have found that deception does not upset most participants.[15–18] In a study of participants who had been deceived in psychology experiments, Epley and Huff found "little negative impact." Indeed, Smith and Richardson report that those who had been deceived in psychology experiments rated their overall experience as more positive than those who had not been deceived. Although these findings seem to suggest that deception itself poses no risk to participants, thus seeming to confirm Milgram's findings that the deception he used did not harm his participants, there are reasons to question the data and their relevance to clinical research. First, the data focus on healthy college undergraduates participating in psychology experiments. Yet healthy college students may have a different attitude toward being deceived than patients participating in clinical trials.[19] Second, it is estimated that approximately one-third to one-half of psychology experiments use deceptive techniques.[20,21] Given the prevalence of deception, combined with widespread debriefing, college students may *expect* psychology experiments to be deceptive.[22–25] Hence, the existing data may reflect the attitudes of participants who expect to be deceived, not the attitudes of those who assume they are participating in nondeceptive research.

Third, the relationship between investigators and participants in psychology studies may minimize the impact of deception. Deception is morally problematic in part because it involves a violation of trust in a relationship. The trusted deceiver manipulates the beliefs of the deceived and thereby undermines their ability to make autonomous decisions. On this analysis of the harm of deception, one would expect that the degree to which individuals are bothered by deception will depend in part on the extent to which they are dependent on the deceiver.[26–28] We expect those we trust and depend on to look out for our interests and support our making decisions for ourselves. As a result, we are more vulnerable to deception by them.

Young, healthy college students are unlikely to rely a great deal on psychology experimenters, whereas patients often invest a great deal of trust and hope in clinical investigators. Thus, deceiving patients in the research setting has the potential for greater harm, especially if it undermines patients' trust in physicians in general. For instance, in a study by Fleming and colleagues concerning alcohol use (discussed below), a majority of the individuals who were upset by being deceived stated that the use of deception would "lower their trust in the medical profession." In this way, investigators deceiving participants seems to conflict with physicians' obligations to earn and maintain the trust of their patients.[29]

Fourth, the majority of these studies assess the impact of deception by deceiving participants, debriefing them, and then asking whether they found the deception troubling. Because people do not like to view themselves as victims, under the control of others, they may downplay the effects of deception, particularly when asked by the individual who deceived them in the first place.[30,31] Finally, some of these studies assessed the impact of the deception after some time had elapsed. This is most clear in the case of Milgram's follow-up studies, which occurred years after the original experiment. It seems plausible to assume that any harms caused by deceiving participants would diminish over time.

These differences suggest that the psychology data provide little insight into the impact of deception on participants in clinical research. Moreover, despite the long history of deceiving participants in clinical research, few clinical investigators have attempted to gather data on its effects. To assess the generalizability of these data, IRBs that approve deceptive clinical studies should consider obtaining data on the impact of the deception, perhaps as part of the debriefing process. Indeed, it seems reasonable to argue that IRBs that approve deceptive studies should require the investigators to collect such data. These studies are being approved on the basis of assumptions about the harms caused by the deception. It seems reasonable for investigators and IRBs to systematically collect data to assess whether the IRBs' assumptions in this regard are accurate. Until such data are collected, assessment of the extent to which deceptive clinical research harms research participants must be based on more theoretical considerations.

It is worth noting a potential conflict between reducing the harms of deception versus reducing its wrongs. One might argue that debriefing remedies the wrong of deception to some extent by informing research participants that they were deceived. Debriefing may also limit the social harms of deceptive research by establishing a clear policy by which deceptive actions are disclosed, thereby notifying research participants in general that deception is not widespread and unreported. Debriefing, however, is likely to increase the extent to which deception harms research participants. Presumably, research participants who never realize and are never told that they were deceived will not experience psychological harm. Hence, some might argue that investigators should err on the side of no debriefing as a way to protect research participants from experiencing harm.

Theoretical Harms of Deceptive Clinical Research

Studies that fail to inform participants prospectively of the use of deception conceal the possibility that participants may experience distress once they are deceived. Those who learn that they were deceived may also lose trust in investigators, reducing the pool of potential research participants. Research participants may be harmed even when they are not upset by the use of deception. Being in control of one's life is central to human dignity and self-respect; hence, the fact that investigators fail to respect the autonomy of research participants by deceiving them may be harmful. The knowledge that medical researchers are sometimes deceptive may undermine the public's trust in the research enterprise. Finally, deceiving participants may have an adverse effect on clinicians, who are trained to promote the best interests of their patients.[32,33] These burdens may be exacerbated when participants inadvertently inquire about the misdescribed aspects of the study. To avoid such situations, researchers may minimize the opportunity for participants in deceptive studies to ask questions, further vitiating the informed consent process.

These concerns, although genuine, are largely theoretical. Hence, they leave IRBs in the position to choose, in the absence of sufficient data, whether to allow deceptive clinical research or not. Stopping all deceptive clinical research until sufficient data are collected would halt important research. Moreover, the effects of deception may be impossible to assess in the absence of deceptive studies that deceive participants and then assess the effects. Continuing to conduct deceptive clinical research also seems problematic, especially given social norms against deception and the possibility that use of deception may cause serious distress to some participants.

Regulations and Guidelines Governing Deception in Research

National and international guidelines regarding research with humans uniformly require participants' informed consent in most cases. Guidelines that mandate informed consent without exception may inadvertently prohibit deceptive research. For example, guidelines that require participants to be informed of the purpose of the research may effectively prohibit research whose validity depends on participants not being prospectively informed of the study's purpose.

Many guidelines do not address deception explicitly, but allow investigators to alter some or all of the elements of informed consent in some circumstances, typically when the risks are minimal. For example, U.S. research regulations allow IRBs to approve research that "does not include, or which alters, some or all of the elements of informed consent" provided that several conditions are satisfied, including the requirements that the risks are minimal and the research could not "practicably" be carried out without the alteration.[34] Hence, IRBs may approve deceptive studies provided they find that the studies pose no greater than minimal risk to participants.

Other guidelines address the issue of deception explicitly, typically leaving the decision of whether to approve the deception up to the reviewing IRB or research ethics committee. The research guidelines from Nepal state, "A special problem of consent arises when informing participants of some pertinent aspect of research that is likely to impair validity of the research. Such circumstances should be discussed with the [ethical review boards] who will then decide on the matter."[35] Similarly, the Brazilian regulations state that "when the merit of the research depends on some restriction of information to the subjects, such facts should be properly explained and justified by the research and submitted to the Committee of Ethics in Research."[36] And according to the Tanzanian guidelines, participants must be informed that treatments will be allocated at random, although "[e]xceptional cases are where there is an argument for not telling the patient the truth, and must be subject of the IRECs [institutional research ethics committee]."

Some guidelines draw a distinction between deception by lying to participants versus deception as the result of withholding pertinent information. The Indian guidelines state that "[d]eception of the subject is not permissible. However, sometimes information can be withheld till the completion of the study, if such information would jeopardize the validity of the research."[38] Guideline 6 of the guidelines produced by the Council for International Organizations of Medical Sciences (CIOMS; see Chapter 16) has one of the most extensive discussions of deception in research, arguing, "[a]ctive deception of subjects is considered more controversial than simply withholding certain information."[39] The CIOMS guidelines further state, "[d]eception is not permissible, however, in cases in which the deception itself would disguise the possibility of the subject being exposed to more than minimal risk" and stipulate that the "ethical review committee should determine the consequences for the subject of being deceived." The same approach is suggested by the Belmont Report (see Chapter 14), which allows investigators to "indicate to subjects that they are being invited to participate in research of which some features will not be revealed until the research is concluded." Importantly, the Belmont Report allows withholding information only when necessary and does not allow it in "cases in which disclosure would simply inconvenience the investigator."[40]

One of the most detailed guidelines regarding deception in research is the *Ethical Principles of Psychologists and Code of Conduct* produced by the American Psychological Association.[41] The *Principles* allow investigators to deceive subjects when the following four conditions are satisfied:

1. The use of deception is justified by the study's significant value.
2. Any equally effective, nondeceptive approaches are not feasible.

3. Deception is not reasonably expected to cause physical pain or severe emotional distress.
4. Any deception is explained to participants, preferably at the conclusion of their participation, but no later than the conclusion of the research, and participants are allowed to withdraw their data.

The second condition's requirement of *equal* effectiveness seems to conflict with the assumption that deception is prima facie unacceptable. If this assumption is correct, it follows that we might prefer a nondeceptive study even if it is somewhat *less* effective, because the harm incurred by the decrease in effectiveness might be outweighed by the good that is achieved in avoiding the deception.

The third condition attempts to address the concern that deception conflicts with respect for participants' autonomy by requiring that participants are not deceived in the context of studies that are reasonably expected to cause physical pain or severe emotional distress.

Briefly, we can think of harms as states of affairs that conflict with the interests of the individual harmed. For instance, physical integrity is in most individuals' interests. Therefore, states of affairs that involve destruction of physical integrity harm the person in question. States of affairs that conflict with individuals' moral interests, in contrast, are standardly understood not as harms, but as "wrongs." The third condition attempts to ensure that, as long as the use of deception does not conceal the potential for physical pain or severe emotional distress, it will not alter the enrollment decisions of prospective participants. In other words, as long as this condition is met, one might assume that participants who consent to a deceptive study would have consented even if that study had not been deceptive. This then leaves IRBs with the task of determining whether the social value of the research justifies the use of deception. One might assume that as long as the deception does not conceal risks of physical pain or severe emotional distress, then studies with essentially any social value can justify the deception, because the use of deception will not increase the risks to participants. This line of reasoning, however, ignores the possibility that the deception itself might pose a risk to participants.

Assessing Participants' Desire for Control

There are some data relevant to assessing the extent to which deception itself harms individuals. One example comes from alcohol research. Gathering accurate data on alcohol abuse is complicated by the fact that alcoholics often provide misleading information when asked direct questions about their alcohol use. To address this problem, some investigators have studied the acceptability of concealing the intent of alcohol abuse questionnaires by including questions about smoking, weight, exercise, and drug use. Under this design, participants are provided with "general health" questionnaires without being informed that the investigator's research interests are limited to the alcohol use questions.

At the end of one study, the investigators debriefed the participants and assessed the impact on them of the deception itself.[29] The data reveal that one-third of the participants were upset by the deception, but of these, two-thirds supported the study and said that they would be willing to participate again. The authors regard the relatively high number of participants who were willing to participate again, combined with the importance of accurate information on alcohol abuse, as showing that these kinds of deceptive studies are ethically acceptable.

But as previously noted, there are reasons to question whether individuals, once deceived, will accurately report how much the deception bothered them. Leaving that concern to the side for the moment, these same results tell us that one-ninth of the participants were upset by the deception to the point of refusing future participation. Importantly, these individuals had been told in advance the truth about the nature of the study, including its risks, the lack of expected benefit, the procedures involved, and the possible alternatives. The deception involved the minor point that the researchers were interested in a specific aspect of the participant's health, rather than the participant's health in general. And yet, a significant percentage of the participants were bothered enough to be unwilling to participate in such research again.

Presumably, many of these participants were upset not by the fact that the researchers were interested in alcohol use, but by the use of deception itself. This conclusion supports a piece of common sense: At least some people are upset by the mere fact of being deceived, independent of the nature of that deception, especially when the deception is for the benefit of others. It follows that no matter how carefully we minimize the *extent* of deception, for example along the lines of the American Psychological Association's *Principles*, deception still poses risks to some participants without their consent. Of course, most guidelines allow the use of deception only when the risks are minimal. However, this assessment is typically made by considering whether the deception conceals any significant risks from the participants, thus ignoring the possibility that the use of deception itself may pose risks to some participants.

Individuals who are upset by the use of deception per se are, presumably, those who place a high value on being in control of their lives. Therefore, taking control of these individuals' lives by deceiving them without their consent involves a contradiction of one of the values that is most important to them as persons. The fact that at least some are upset by deception per se establishes that even if the deception involved in a particular study does not conceal any risks that are present independently of that deception, the deception itself introduces a new risk into the study. And allowing studies that fail to inform participants of this risk contradicts the requirement that participants may not be put at risk without their consent. The most obvious way of avoiding this harm would be to treat the risk presented by the use of deception in exactly the same way that we treat all the other risks involved in research participation: Inform participants of the presence of that risk. The possibility suggests the need for "authorized" deception.

The Principle of Authorized Deception

It is widely assumed that deceptive clinical studies force investigators and IRBs to choose between respecting personal autonomy and collecting valid data. This assumption neglects the possibility that prospective participants can be informed of the deception and asked to consent to its use, without being informed of the nature of the deception. For instance, investigators who conduct deceptive research could include the following statement in the informed consent document:

You should be aware that the investigators have intentionally misdescribed certain aspects of this study. This use of deception is necessary to conduct the study. However, an independent ethics panel has determined that this consent form accurately describes the major risks and benefits of the study. The investigator will explain the misdescribed aspects of the study to you at the end of your participation.

For studies designed to deceive participants by *withholding* information, as opposed to providing false information, the first sentence might read: "You should be aware that the investigators have intentionally left out information about certain aspects of this study."

We have seen that deception per se presents a risk to participants; at least some are harmed when they are deceived, and others may have relevant idiosyncratic concerns that never get revealed because of the deception. Authorized deception warns participants of these risks. Therefore, potential participants who are bothered by deception per se will be able to avoid deceptive studies, those with idiosyncratic concerns will have the opportunity to reveal them, and others will have the opportunity to consent to being deceived. Authorized deception also removes any harm to the research team that is incurred when members of the team are required to deceive participants without their consent.

By alerting participants to the use of deception, authorized deception goes as far as possible in respecting the autonomy of research participants while permitting deception needed to generate scientifically valid data. Authorized deception also blocks the undermining of participants' and the public's trust in science and medicine by flagging those studies that are deceptive, and it justifies exposing participants to deception not in terms of the potential benefit to others but in terms of the participants' consent to that deception.

Objections to Authorized Deception

There are a number of possible objections to the use of authorized deception in clinical research. We raise and respond to three broad areas of concern below.

Concerns About Informed Consent

Some might argue that valid consent requires that participants know the exact nature of all the procedures they will undergo. On this view, people cannot provide valid consent, even when informed of the use of deception, because they do not know the true nature of the misdescribed procedures. In order to provide fully informed consent, they would have to know the nature of the deception as well. They would have to know what they are being deceived about.

We can grant that participants cannot provide fully informed consent as long as they are unaware of the nature of the deception and as long as we understand "fully" in a literal sense. However, as is widely acknowledged, participants never know everything there is to know about any study. There is simply too much to know. Therefore, in order to argue that authorized deception precludes informed consent, one would have to show that the information participants fail to obtain as the result of deception casts doubt on their consent in a way that the other information they never re-

ceive does not.[42] For instance, prospective participants need to be informed of the risks and potential benefits of study medications because most people care about this information and it might affect reasonable persons' willingness to participate; however, they typically need not be informed of the precise doses of the medication because this is a technical detail that is unlikely to affect their willingness to participate. This widely accepted analysis suggests that investigators can conduct deceptive clinical studies and still obtain valid consent as long as they do not deceive participants about any aspects of the study that would affect their willingness to participate or aspects of the study that individuals are likely to want to know prospectively.

To implement this approach, IRBs must decide which aspects of a given study might affect participants' willingness to participate. Because enrollment decisions depend upon the risks and benefits of the research, IRBs should approve deceptive studies only when the deception does not conceal significant risks or misleadingly promise significant benefits. The burden of proof should be on investigators to show why any deception regarding risks or benefits is necessary. In some cases, it may be acceptable to deceive participants about minimal risks.

When reviewing deceptive clinical research, IRBs should also consider whether the potential participants have idiosyncratic concerns that might affect their willingness to enroll. For instance, deceiving participants about the ingredients in a study drug typically would not affect their willingness to enroll. Yet such deception might be problematic if it conceals ingredients to which the participant population would strongly object, such as bovine-derived products for a Hindu population.

Authorized deception requires IRBs to use their judgment to assess what aspects of a given study might affect participants' willingness to participate. Of course, IRBs might get these judgments wrong in certain cases, and allow investigators to deceive subjects about aspects of the study that would have affected their willingness to participate. Given this possibility, IRBs should err on the side of caution, requiring investigators to accurately inform participants of all aspects that, in the judgment of the IRB, might affect their willingness to enroll.

Granting the potential for mistakes, it is important to note that this potential is not unique to deceptive studies. Informing participants of every aspect of a given study, including all the ingredients of every drug and every remote theoretical risk, would only confuse participants and undermine their informed consent. For this reason, investigators and IRBs must decide which aspects of the study might affect participants' willingness to participate every time they decide what information should be included in a consent form.

Similarly, most regulations allow IRBs to waive the requirement for informed consent when the research poses no greater than minimal risk and there are good reasons not to obtain informed consent. Assuming it can be ethical to conduct clinical research that the IRB deems to pose only minimal risks without consent at all, it seems acceptable to conduct otherwise ethically appropriate, deceptive research when the IRB judges that the use of deception poses no greater than minimal risks to participants.

Some might respond that this analysis ignores the fact that deceiving participants is different from withholding information from them. In cases of deception, participants fail to have certain information not because there is too much information to convey, but because they are being deceived. As a result, participants end up with false beliefs about the studies in which they are participating. Clearly, there is a difference between the two cases. However, it is not clear that this difference makes an ethical difference. Authorized deception informs participants of the use of deception, and provides them with the opportunity to consent to its use. Therefore, the deception per se will not make an ethical difference between the two cases. The participant, not the researcher, is in control of deciding whether the person participates in a deceptive study. In addition, the fact that the participant ends up with false beliefs, rather than no belief at all, does not seem to make an ethical difference either. It all depends on whether the issue in question is relevant to providing informed consent. And, as we have seen, relevance to informed consent gets decided using the same method in both cases: Is the information relevant to the participant's decision to enroll? If the answer is "no," then in both cases withholding that information does not cast doubt on the person's informed consent.

In some cases, however, there may be an important difference between a study that uses authorized deception and one that that simply does not inform participants of particular aspects of a study, on the assumption that the aspect is irrelevant to the decision of whether to enroll. In the latter case, investigators can solicit from prospective participants any individual concerns that might be relevant to the research. Of course, it may not occur to participants that a particular concern of theirs is relevant to the research. Hence, this approach is not guaranteed to uncover concerns. Yet some participants would likely reveal concerns. For instance, some Jehovah's Witnesses might present their views regarding receipt of various blood products.

In the case of research using deception, however, individuals might not reveal idiosyncratic concerns that happen to coincide with the aspects of the study relevant to the deception. If the study's informed consent form explicitly and inaccurately stated that participants would not receive any blood products or bovine-derived products, it seems unlikely that participants would reveal these concerns. The use of authorized deception might partly address this concern. When told that they are being deceived about some aspects of the study, potential participants might think to reveal these concerns. When it is felt that some participants might be especially bothered by some aspects of the study over which they are being deceived, the IRB could consider requiring a focus group of relevant participants to assess their views. For instance, a recent study of the impact of direct-to-consumer advertising on physician prescribing behavior failed to state in specific terms the purpose of the study.[43] It is unclear whether this is something that would bother these participants, a question that could be addressed by conducting a preliminary focus group of similar physicians.

Concerns About Study Data

Others might object that authorized deception could confound a study's data if informed participants tried to discover which aspects of the study have been misdescribed. Granting this possibility, the fact that many participants currently recognize the existence of deceptive studies suggests that this possibility may already be present.[44] Just as participants in placebo-controlled trials may try to guess whether they received the study drug or placebo, so informing participants about the use of decep-

tion might stimulate them to try to guess the nature of that deception.

There are several ways in which this effect can be reduced. First, researchers should make a clear offer of debriefing at the study's end. Knowing ahead of time that they can eventually learn the nature of the deception should reduce participants' desire to discover it for themselves. In addition, by disclosing the use of deception and explaining that it is necessary to generate valid data, researchers might enlist participant cooperation in maintaining the deception. For instance, participants can be asked ahead of time to focus on the procedures specifically asked of them, and researchers can explicitly limit any probing questions.

Some experimental evidence indicates that authorized deception would not necessarily bias the responses of research participants. For example, two groups of psychology students were exposed to a deceptive experiment in which they were falsely informed that they would receive two to eight "painful electric shocks" at random times after a red signal light appeared.[45] No shocks were actually administered. Measures of self-reported anxiety and physiological arousal (pulse and respiration rates) were obtained. Prior to the deceptive shock intervention, one experimental group was informed that deception is occasionally used in psychology experiments to assure unbiased responses. The other group exposed to the deceptive shock intervention did not receive any information about the possibility of deception. No outcome differences were observed for participants informed of the possibility of deception versus those not informed.

The information about deception in this experiment, however, falls short of the authorized deception approach that we recommend. It disclosed to prospective participants that deception is a possibility in "a few experiments" rather than informing them that deception would actually be employed for all or some participants in the particular experiment in which they were invited to enroll. In contrast, Wiener and Erker directly tested the authorized deception approach, described as "prebriefing," in an experiment evaluating attributions of responsibility for rape based on transcripts from an actual rape trial.[46] Participants (68 undergraduate psychology students) were either correctly informed or misinformed about the jury verdict regarding the defendant's guilt. Half of participants received an informed consent document stating "You may be purposefully misinformed." The other participants were not alerted to the possibility of deception. No differences on attribution of responsibility were observed depending on whether or not the participants were prebriefed about the use of deception.

The results of studies that use authorized deception, however, may not be comparable with the results of previous studies that did not use this approach. This is a genuine methodological concern, which must be weighed against the countervailing ethical concern. When preservation of data comparability is an issue, IRBs should decide whether it is of sufficiently compelling value to warrant waiving the requirement for authorized deception.

The use of authorized deception also may reduce accrual if people refuse to participate in studies they know to be deceptive. This possibility could undermine the generalizability of the data, especially if particular groups are more likely to avoid deceptive studies. Conversely, the use of authorized deception may increase the available pool of research participants in the long run, by reducing the number of those who refuse to participate in future research after being deceived. Currently, there are no data to make this assessment either way. On the other hand, there is clear evidence that deception upsets at least some people, violates respect for personal autonomy, and may cause problems for the research team. In addition, even if it turns out that authorized deception adversely affects accrual, it does not necessarily follow that authorized deception should be rejected. A finding that authorized deception substantially decreased accrual would suggest that people are especially bothered by the use of deception. Hence, we would have even more reason to argue that the use of deception *should* be revealed during the consent process.

Concerns About Harms

The argument for authorized deception assumes that people accurately gauge the extent to which being deceived will bother them. If this is not so—if, for instance, awareness of the use of deception concerns participants far more than actually being deceived would bother them—then authorized deception would make research less effective without making it significantly less harmful. In general, participants are more likely to be upset by the prospect of deception if they think that the deception might be concealing some risks involved in the study. The solution (to the extent that this is actually a problem) would be to explicitly state that the deception involved in the study does not conceal any risks. In the end, which alternative we should adopt depends upon how participants react to the use of authorized deception. Thus, a final decision will have to await the appropriate studies called for previously.

Conclusion

Deception in clinical research and valid informed consent are not necessarily incompatible, as is widely assumed. However, IRBs should consider allowing deceptive research only when the following conditions obtain: (1) the use of deception is necessary to achieve the goals of the study; (2) the use of deception is justified by the study's social value; (3) people are not deceived about aspects of the study that would affect their willingness to participate, including risks and potential benefits; (4) people are informed of the use of deception and consent to its use; and (5) people are informed of the nature of the deception at the end of their participation. To be sure, deception about the purpose of a study that is authorized in advance by participants is not *strictly* compatible with informed consent, because accurate disclosure about a study's purpose is a basic element of informed consent. However, if there is no reason to think that prospective participants would decline to participate if they knew the true purpose of the research, then authorized deception is compatible with respect for autonomy and thus with the spirit, if not the letter, of informed consent.

The use of authorized deception—an approach that generally has been neglected by researchers and IRBs—respects personal autonomy by putting participants in control of whether they are deceived; it minimizes the harms of deception to the participants; it removes the possibility that the use of deception will undermine one's willingness to participate in clinical research; it minimizes the possibility that the use of deception will undermine public trust in research; and it minimizes the burdens of conducting deceptive research on the research team.

Disclaimer

The opinions expressed are the authors' own and do not represent any position or policy of the National Institutes of Health, Public Health Service, or Department of Health and Human Services.

References

1. Wendler D, Miller F. Deception in the pursuit of science. *Archives of Internal Medicine* 2004;164:597–600.
2. Bok S. Informed consent in tests of patient reliability. *JAMA* 1992;267:1118–9.
3. Bok S. Shading the truth in seeking informed consent for research purposes. *Kennedy Institute of Ethics Journal* 1995;5:1–17.
4. Fost N. A surrogate system for informed consent. *JAMA* 1975;233:800–3.
5. Freedman B. The validity of ignorant consent to medical research. *IRB: A Review of Human Subjects Research* 1982;4(2):1–5.
6. Barnes M, et al. A randomized controlled trial of continuous positive airway pressure in mild obstructive sleep apnea. *American Journal of Respiratory and Critical Care Medicine* 2002;165:773–80.
7. Simmons MS, Nides MA, Rand CS, Wie RA, Tashkin DP. Unpredictability of deception in compliance with physician-prescribed bronchodilator inhaler use in a clinical trial. *Chest* 2000;118:290–5.
8. Miller FG, Kaptchuk TJ. Sham procedures and the ethics of clinical trials. *Journal of the Royal Society of Medicine* 2004;97:576–8.
9. Milgram S. Behavioral study of obedience. *Journal of Abnormal and Social Psychology* 1963;67:371–8.
10. Milgram S. Issues in the study of obedience: A reply to Baumrind. *American Psychologist* 1964;19:848–52.
11. Milgram S. Subject reaction: The neglected factor in the ethics of experimentation. *Hastings Center Report* 1977;7(5):19–23.
12. Vedantum S. Human responses to technology scrutinized: emotional interactions draw interest of psychologists and marketers. *The Washington Post* June 7, 2004:A14.
13. Wendler D. Deception in medical and behavioral research: Is it ever acceptable? *Milbank Quarterly* 1996;74:87–114.
14. Aristotle. *The Nicomachean Ethics*. Translated by J.A.K. Thomson. London, England: Penguin Books, 1955.
15. Fisher CB, Fyrberg D. College students weigh the costs and benefits of deceptive research. *American Psychologist* 1994;49:1–11.
16. Soliday E, Stanton AL. Deceived versus nondeceived participants' perceptions of scientific and applied psychology. *Ethics and Behavior* 1995;5:87–104.
17. Smith SS, Richardson D. Amelioration of deception and harm in psychological research: The important role of debriefing. *Journal of Personality and Social Psychology* 1983;44:1075–82.
18. Sieber JE, Iannuzzo R, Rodriquez B. Deception methods in psychology: Have they changed in 25 years? *Ethics and Behavior* 1995;5:67–85.
19. Korn JH. Judgments of acceptability of deception in psychological research. *Journal of General Psychology* 1987;114:205–16.
20. Adair JG, Dushenko TW, Lindsa RCL. Ethical regulations and their impact on research practice. *American Psychologist* 1985;40:59–72.
21. Korn JH. *Illusions of Reality: A History of Deception in Social Psychology*. Albany, N.Y.: State University of New York Press; 1997.
22. Fillenbaum S. Prior deception and subsequent experimental performance: The "faithful" subject. *Journal of Personality and Social Psychology* 1966;4:532–7.
23. Masling J. Role-related behavior of the subject and psychologist and its effects upon psychological data. *Nebraska Symposium on Motivation* 1966;14:67–103.
24. Kelman H. Human use of human subjects: The problem of deception in social psychology. *Psychology Bulletin* 1967;67:1–11.

25. MacCoun C, Kerr, NL. Suspicion in the psychological laboratory: Kelman's prophecy revisited. *American Psychologist* 1987;42:199.

26. Baumrind D. Research using intentional deception: Ethical issues revisited. *American Psychologist* 1985;40:165–74.

27. Holder AR. Do researchers and subjects have a fiduciary relationship? *IRB: A Review of Human Subjects Research* 1982;4(1):6–7.

28. Cupples B, Gochnauer M. The investigator's duty not to deceive. *IRB: A Review of Human Subjects Research* 1985;7(5):1–6.

29. Fleming MF, Bruno M, Barry K, Fost N. Informed consent, deception, and the use of disguised alcohol questionnaires. *American Journal of Drug and Alcohol Abuse* 1989;15:309–19.

30. Rubin Z. Deceiving ourselves about deception: Comment on Smith and Richardson's "Amelioration of deception and harm in psychological research." *Journal of Personality and Social Psychology* 1985;48:252–3.

31. Smith CP. How (un)acceptable is research involving deception? *IRB: A Review of Human Subjects Research* 1981;3(8):1–4.

32. Oliansky A. A confederate's perspective on deception. *Ethics and Behavior* 1991;1:14–31.

33. Murray TH. Learning to deceive: The education of a social psychologist. *Hastings Center Report* 1980;10(2):11–4.

34. Department of Health and Human Services, National Institutes of Health, and Office for Human Research Protections. The Common Rule, Title 45 (Public Welfare), Code of Federal Regulations, Part 46 (Protection of Human Subjects). [Online] June 23, 2005. Available: http://www.hhs.gov/ohrp/humansubjects/guidance/45cfr46.htm.

35. Nepal Health Research Council. *National Ethical Guidelines for Health Research in Nepal.* Kathmandu, Nepal: NHRC; 2001.

36. Ministry of Health of Brazil. National Board of Health. Resolution No. 196. October 1996.

37. Tanzania National Health Research Forum. *Guidelines on Ethics for Health Research in Tanzania.* Dar es Salaam, Tanzania: TNHRF; 2001.

38. Indian Council of Medical Research. *Ethical Guidelines for Biomedical Research on Human Subjects.* New Delhi, India: ICMR; 2000.

39. Council for International Organizations of Medical Sciences in collaboration with the World Health Organization. *International Ethical Guidelines for Biomedical Research Involving Human Subjects.* Geneva, Switzerland: CIOMS and WHO; 2002. [Online] November 2002. Available: http://www.cioms.ch/frame_guidelines_nov_2002.htm.

40. The National Commission for the Protection of Human Subjects of Biomedical and Behavioral Research. *The Belmont Report: Ethical Principles and Guidelines for the Protection of Human Subjects of Research.* Washington, D.C.: Department of Health, Education and Welfare; DHEW Publication OS 78-0012 1978. [Online] April 18, 1979. Available: http://www.hhs.gov/ohrp/humansubjects/guidance/belmont.htm.

41. American Psychological Association. *Ethical Principles of Psychologists and Code of Conduct,* Section 8.07. [Online] June 1, 2003. Available: http://www.apa.org/ethics/code2002.pdf.

42. Beauchamp TL, Childress JF. *Principles in Biomedical Ethics,* 5th ed. New York, N.Y.: Oxford University Press; 2001.

43. Kravitz RL, Epstein RM, Feldman MD, et al. Influence of patients' requests for direct-to-consumer advertised antidepressants: A randomized controlled trial. *JAMA* 2005;293:1995–2002.

44. Toris C, DePaulo BM. Effects of actual deception and suspiciousness of deception on interpersonal perceptions. *Journal of Personality and Social Psychology* 1984;47:1063–73.

45. Holmes DS, Bennett DH. Experiments to answer questions raised by the use of deception in psychological research: I. Role playing as an alternative to deception; II. Effectiveness of debriefing after a deception; III. Effect of informed consent on deception. *Journal of Personality and Social Psychology* 1974;29:358–67.

46. Wiener RL, Erker PV. The effects of prebriefing misinformed research participants on their attributions of responsibility. *Journal of Psychology* 1986;120:397–410.

Douglas L. Weed   Robert E. McKeown

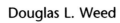

Epidemiology

Observational Studies on Human Populations

"Everyone wants to be an epidemiologist," declared the former chair of epidemiology at Harvard University. This rather bold claim, part of a plenary speech at a recent international meeting of epidemiologists, may come as a surprise to those who, quite happy with their current vocation, had never considered epidemiology a career option. The underlying premise of this distinguished cancer epidemiologist's message was that epidemiologic studies are increasingly at the center of nearly every public discussion of health and medicine. AIDS, SARS, avian flu, Agent Orange, Gulf War syndrome, the safety of silicone breast implants, and the value of hormone replacement therapy (HRT) are only a few examples of recent issues with epidemiologic studies at the center of the controversy. Add to this list the usual culprits responsible for most of the death and suffering of any community—heart disease, cancer, diabetes, injuries, accidents (now called unintentional injuries, as opposed to intentional injuries), conditions related to aging, and infectious diseases—and epidemiology's special relevance to public health becomes clearer.

Epidemiology, focusing its scientific method on the etiology and prevention of human disease, matters to the health of individuals and populations in a unique and powerful way. Those concerned about their health and the health of their communities need to appreciate the role that epidemiology plays in the science and practice of preventive medicine and public health. Epidemiologic methods, how results are interpreted, and what interventions arise from them have become increasingly important components of the education and training of health professionals. Physicians, nurses, public health practitioners, public policy makers, and those who will call themselves professional epidemiologists spend years learning the concepts, methods, and interpretative processes of epidemiology.

The legal profession is also interested in what epidemiologists do and what epidemiologic research means for their clients. Epidemiology rates its own chapter (alongside others on statistics, toxicology, and DNA evidence), in the Federal Judicial Center's *Reference Manual on Scientific Evidence.*[1] The epidemiologist's expertise in designing and interpreting studies of disease etiology and prevention has become a central (and often contentious) problem in deciding who should be compensated in toxic tort liability cases. Relating the population-based findings of epidemiologic research—general causation—to the cause of disease or death in an individual—specific causation—is at the heart of this difficult legal matter, with significant financial incentives for defendants, plaintiffs, and for their legal teams. The multibillion-dollar tobacco settlement is an excellent case in point.[2]

Epidemiology is also of great interest to the media. In the final weeks of writing this chapter, television, print, and web-related news companies reported the findings of a large epidemiologic study showing an association between taking antibiotics and subsequent increased risk of breast cancer. Reporters asked the investigators whether women should reconsider taking these medications if they are concerned about their risk of breast cancer. The long-winded answer (too long for the television sound bite) is that this finding could be a false alarm or it could be an early fair warning to women; deciding which explanation is more likely will require a careful examination of the results of other (earlier) studies, future analyses of similar data from different populations of women, and considerations of the so-called biological plausibility of the systematically collected and summarized findings, the time course of the relationship between onset of antibiotic usage and onset of cancer, and a host of other considerations to be discussed later in this chapter. Simply put, there is a sense—some might call it a misconception—in the media and in the public at large (two groups with relatively little understanding of the complexities and difficulties of interpreting observational epidemiological research) that a single "scientific" finding—in this case, an epidemiological finding—is true enough to warrant immediate public action. Rarely is that the case. More often, a single study provides the professional public health community with a starting point for further research, considerable discussion and debate, and (hopefully) the correct judgment regarding what should be done about it.

It is fair to say that misconceptions abound about the importance and nature of epidemiology among scientists and laypersons alike. Physical and biological scientists often have the impression that epidemiology is a severely limited, "soft" science, too weak to provide reliable, objective knowledge.[3] The public, on the other hand, is jokingly perceived among the ranks of epidemiologists as being so ignorant that it confuses the study of epidemics, disease causation, and disease prevention with dermatology (the medical specialty treating skin diseases). The media, whose role in society is to inform the public of interesting stories, does not have the responsibility for teaching the fine points of epidemiologic study design, analysis, and especially interpretation. Part of the problem is that epidemiology has traditionally been taught primarily at the graduate level as a specialty topic for healthcare professionals and for those who will use its population-based findings in public health or preventive medicine practice, as well as for future research epidemiologists. Small wonder the public is confused about the relevance and significance of epidemiologic findings.

Against this backdrop of wide relevance, keen interest, and unfortunate misunderstanding, we discuss the ethics of epidemiology. Understanding the ethics of epidemiologic research is important because, as we will describe in detail, public and private values and norms are intimately linked to the science and practice of epidemiology in public health and preventive medicine. For those who recognize epidemiology as their profession and for those who use epidemiologic methods, it is important to perform, interpret, disclose, and apply the results of these studies in the best ethical tradition. We believe therefore that there is a need to develop a deep understanding of the ethics of carrying out epidemiologic research and the ethics of applying that knowledge for the prevention and control of disease and for the promotion of health.

In this chapter, the ethical issues are discussed from the perspective of those who carry out the studies and those who practice epidemiology as a professional vocation. Not everyone who employs the methods of epidemiologic research—generally, observational methodologies—is a member of the profession. This situation leads to some interesting and provocative problems involving the societal roles and responsibilities of epidemiologists to be discussed later in this chapter.

What Is Epidemiology?

It is important to understand the definition of *epidemiology*. Epidemiology is the study of the distributions and (causal) determinants of health states in human populations and the application of the knowledge gained to health promotion as well as disease prevention and control.[4] Epidemiology is sometimes more narrowly defined in terms of its characteristic methods, but we will resist that temptation, emphasizing that for us epidemiology is a professional practice with its own evolving terminology, cardinal concepts, a characteristic methodological framework, and significant social responsibilities. We will not, however, describe its concepts and methods in detail, other than to distinguish observational studies (the sorts of studies referred to as *epidemiological*) from randomized controlled trials, whose ethical issues are discussed elsewhere in this text. The terminology of epidemiology and glossaries of ethical terms relevant to it can be found in recent publications,[4–6] and several textbooks provide excellent descriptions of epidemiological methodology.[7–13]

Epidemiologic studies are typically observational; the investigator does not intervene on an individual participant under study beyond physical measurements (such as drawing blood for analysis, taking blood pressure, or measuring height and weight) or questions about demographics (age, gender, ethnicity), social factors (income, education, marital status), lifestyle factors (diet, exercise, smoking) and medical history (previous heart attacks). For communities, epidemiologic studies assess environmental and contextual factors such as air quality, social cohesion, housing, availability of public health programs, and public policies. Epidemiologic study methodologies can be used to examine the impacts of interventions imposed upon (e.g., mandatory immunizations) or chosen by individuals (e.g., smoking cessation), communities (e.g., water treatment), and populations (e.g., dietary changes).

Epidemiologic studies are typically categorized as surveillance studies, cross-sectional surveys, case-control, and cohort studies with subtypes of each. They can be either retrospective (looking back in time) or prospective (looking forward). They can include measurements of molecular phenomena (e.g., the expression of DNA repair genes), personal habits (e.g., smoking behavior), environmental phenomena (e.g., air pollution), or social phenomena (e.g., income differentials between ethnic groups). Indeed, the genius of the epidemiologic approach is that it can integrate a broad range of potential health determinants and outcomes; in the past few years subspecialty areas within the discipline have emerged such as molecular epidemiology,[14] clinical epidemiology,[15–17] and social epidemiology,[18,19] adding to the traditional disease-oriented subdisciplines of chronic disease epidemiology,[20] psychiatric epidemiology,[21] and infectious disease epidemiology,[22,23] to name a few. Most epidemiologists pride themselves on their methodological expertise; a few have undertaken the task of describing the theoretical and philosophical foundations of the field; not many more have examined the ethical foundations of their practice. Indeed, a concerted effort to discuss ethics in epidemiology arose primarily within the professional ranks only as recently as the late 1980s.

Ethics is but one of several philosophical disciplines relevant to epidemiology. Epistemological problems and other issues related to the acquisition of knowledge and interpretation of evidence have received attention in the epidemiological literature.[24,25] Ontological and conceptual issues, such as the nature of causation, health, and disease, have also been examined. It is sometimes difficult to divorce epistemological and ontological issues fully from ethics, especially when discussing how epidemiologic studies should be designed and how epidemiologic results should be applied to populations. Underdetermination and its cousin, uncertainty, have important influences on any scientific discipline whose findings are applied and have such a profound impact on the well-being of human populations.[26] We will nevertheless focus primarily on ethics.

Major Categories of Ethical Concerns and a Brief History of Ethics in Epidemiology

For ease of presentation, we will discuss two major categories of ethical concerns: ethical issues in the conduct of observational studies, and ethical issues arising from the application of the scientific understanding—the knowledge—that emerges from epidemiologic research. It will be helpful to begin with a brief history of ethical inquiry applied to epidemiology.

One of the fundamental principles of bioethics is respect for persons, grounded in the Kantian imperative that people should always be treated as ends in themselves and never *merely* as means to an end. It is the major foundation for the obligation for informed consent in research and treatment, but it also informs decisions concerning study design and implementation.[5] (The emphasis is added to indicate that research participants are, in fact, means to an end, but they should not be treated *solely* as instruments for our ends.) In most bioethics discussions of this principle, the emphasis is on respecting autonomy, typically in the form of self-determination and freedom from coercion, and protecting persons with diminished autonomy. That is, people should be free to decide for themselves for or against a treatment or participation in research, and the decision must be voluntary, without coercion or fear.

Beyond this aspect of respect for persons, however, there is respect for the dignity of the individual, which means that research is culturally sensitive and refrains from demeaning or disrespectful actions or situations as well as from intentional physical harm, reflecting yet another bioethical principle: nonmaleficence. Nowhere in the history of epidemiology are these concerns for dignity, respect, and avoiding intentional harm more relevant than in what is widely considered to be the most infamous observational epidemiologic study ever undertaken: the Tuskegee Syphilis Study that came to public attention in 1972 (see Chapter 8). It is a classic example of an ethically reprehensible study and remains a sober reminder of the need for the appropriate ethical conduct of any scientific investigation of human subjects. There are many important ethical issues that arise from the Tuskegee experience: the choice of hypothesis, consent and coercion, the absence of benefit to participants, frank harm, a miscarriage of justice, and the responsibilities of professional "scientific" investigators toward the study participants. To this day, African Americans are reluctant to participate in some research studies due to the lingering effect of the Tuskegee disaster.

Yet despite the ethical importance of the Tuskegee Study as an exemplar, and despite the intense interest in it that was generated in the early 1970s, knowledge of its ethical significance remains outside the learning curves of many public health students; only 19% of graduate students surveyed at a major public health school in 1996 were aware of the ethical significance of the Tuskegee Study.[27] Part of the problem is that ethics in epidemiology has not yet been well incorporated into the curriculum of graduate epi-

demiology programs. In addition, ethics in epidemiology was not widely discussed in the literature before 1990 when a conference was held on the topic and a set of ethical guidelines was proposed by academic and industry leaders in the field, assisted by Tom Beauchamp and other leading scholars.[28–30] Several sets of ethics guidelines have appeared since that seminal conference,[31–35] and more recently the broader public health community in academia and government has produced codes and guidelines, books, and scholarly articles on related topics.[36–44] Other parallel developments such as the growth of the institutional review board (IRB) system, mechanisms for ensuring research integrity, and new federal privacy regulations on health-related information also impact the ethical practice of epidemiology.

The Nature and Ethics of Epidemiologic Studies

Contrasting observational epidemiological study designs to experimental (clinical trial) designs is a frequent point of departure for understanding the nature of epidemiologic studies and the ethics of conducting them. Observational epidemiologic research differs from clinical trials and community intervention trials primarily in the relationship of the investigator to the individuals or communities being studied. In trials, the protocol rather than the investigator determines the exposures given to research participants. In observational studies, as the name implies, the investigator only observes the effect of exposures or characteristics and does not manipulate or determine whether, how, when, where, and to what extent participants are exposed. The primary ethical implication of this difference has to do with the limitations on the exposures to which persons can be subjected in intervention trials research.

However, to assume that observational studies are thereby of less interest or have fewer ethical obligations is to overlook a number of rather profound issues. First, most intervention trials are undertaken with the possibility, if not the expectation, that at least some participants will derive benefit from the intervention. There are not similar added benefits from observational studies. That is not to say, however, that there are no benefits from observational studies. Sometimes observational study designs are used, for example, to study the impact of a voluntarily selected exposure with preventive potential, such as use of sunscreen as a skin cancer preventive. Typically, the direct benefits of observational research are small.[45] These studies are often justified in terms of the benefits to other persons similarly situated or to society more generally because of increased scientific understanding. However, the altruistic contribution of participating in a study for which one gains no direct therapeutic benefit can itself be a benefit to those who value making such contributions to society. Further, if the findings from the study are shared with the research participants, there is potential benefit both in increased understanding and, perhaps, even in risk reduction.

Another, less frequently emphasized difference between intervention trials and observational studies is that intervention trials assume a model of causality and test whether intervening in that causal web reduces adverse outcomes or enhances positive outcomes. Observational studies, in contrast, are typically directed toward elucidating the etiologic associations that make up the theoretical causal web, with much less attention paid to the form of the causal hypothesis in question. Counterfactual and other causal definitions are matters of interest for more theoretically inclined epidemiologists, but these have not had a major impact on the design or interpretation of epidemiologic studies to date.[46]

It is important to note that observational studies may involve sufficient contact with research participants that an intervention effect occurs. This goes beyond the classic Hawthorne effect (or the Heisenberg uncertainty principle as applied metaphorically to human research). There has been an assumption in some clinical circles, especially in cancer research, that patients enrolled in clinical trials have better outcomes, regardless of the arm to which they are randomly assigned, than those who are not trial participants.[47] However, the evidence for this "trial effect" is weak and, when it does occur, it seems to result from implementation of clear clinical protocols rather than participation in a clinical trial itself.[48,49] The latter explanation supports the possibility of this effect occurring also in observational studies. This is especially evident in cohort studies or studies requiring several phases of data collection or monitoring. For example, the enrollment and tracking of a cohort of participants over several years requires frequent contact and reinforcement to maintain the participants' continuing commitment to the study. That contact and the affirmation inherent in it constitute in themselves a kind of intervention. Newsletters may be used to maintain contact and as a way of providing feedback or useful information to participants.

Further, as the Tuskegee study so well illustrates, it is unethical for investigators managing an observational study to fail to respond if they detect adverse health problems in the study population. This means, for instance, that participants who suffer a serious problem during the course of a study should be referred for treatment. Even though such activities, along with the methods for tracking and retention, are not part of an intervention trial, they constitute a kind of intervention that might not otherwise have occurred for these participants. This means that investigators cannot assume that the natural history and etiologic associations observed in the study would directly duplicate the experience of a similar cohort who had not been part of such a study. However, the results would be applicable to participants if similar methods of screening, detection, diagnosis, referral, and continuing contact were to become general policy in communities, just as the use of standard clinical protocols in randomized trials may produce a "trial effect" that goes beyond the placebo effect. Such effects should also pertain to patients outside trials who receive the same protocol-driven treatment.

At the heart of the practice of epidemiology are methods and methodological decisions that often involve selection, trade-offs, evaluation, judgments, or other issues that evoke values or obligations and deserve ethical attention. The selection of a target population for an epidemiologic study requires considerations not only of suitability to the questions of interest and the availability or willingness of participants to be participants, but also the history of the populations. Is this a population that has been overburdened by research, without commensurate benefit or input into objectives, methods, implementation, or dissemination or application of results? Or is this a group that has been excluded or underrepresented in previous research, and therefore about which little is known?

Interest in understanding and addressing disparities in health status across population subgroups has grown in recent years. When previously overlooked groups are included in epidemiologic studies, such disparities become evident, as do avenues for research into causes of the disparity. In the United States, there are numerous examples of African Americans being excluded from research, especially clinical trials, or exploited in research.[50,51] This history of exclusion or exploitation has not only deprived the African American population and public health community of the benefits that could have resulted from ethically and methodologically sound studies, but has also contributed to the mistrust and reluctance to participate that make such research now more difficult.[52]

The principle of justice, as a basis for bioethical analysis, has two major domains, both related to distributive justice. The first has to do with the allocation of resources and the second with the burdens and benefits of research. It is this second aspect of the principle that concerns us here, though the first is relevant. For biomedical and epidemiologic research, this form of the principle of justice states that the burdens or risks and benefits of research should be fairly distributed within and across populations. No person or group should be asked to assume a greater share of the burden of research participation or the risks attendant to it without some ethical justification for that increased burden and without greater potential benefit commensurate with the increased burden or risk. All this assumes that the burden and risk is undertaken without coercion or deception and with full understanding, not only of what is being asked and of the attendant risks, but also that this person or group has been targeted for this research, and the justification for that focus.

Epidemiologists conducting observational studies should be sensitive to the history of populations studied and the risks and burdens they are asked to assume by participation, including risks of stigma related to findings. Further, researchers have an obligation to provide whatever benefit can be derived from the study to those who participate in the research. The nature of that benefit varies according to the nature of the study and the population, the resources available, and the findings. Indeed, a major argument of this chapter is that what we do with results of observational studies is an ethical issue deserving of greater attention.

In general, study design should take into account the particular needs and concerns of the population under study.[53] The elderly constitute another example of a population often either excluded or unnecessarily burdened by research because of a failure to account for their special needs or concerns. Special efforts may be required to respect their dignity, avoid embarrassment in data collection, or protect them from harms that might be of little concern to younger participants. Researchers should attend especially to issues related to consent, vulnerability, justice, and respect. Concerns of competence and comprehension may be obvious, but even considerations such as font size used in printed materials, allowing more time for building trust and for data collection, and providing a comfortable, reassuring setting may be critical.

The elderly may be particularly susceptible to even subtle coercion—a factor that should be taken into account during the consent process and in the wording and presentation of the research proposal. In addition to vulnerability related to consent, some elderly candidates may be at increased risk for harm from data collection that would otherwise be considered minimal risk, such as tests of balance, sensitive questions, and activities that could cause bruising. The special needs of the elderly may lead some researchers to exclude them, but that also raises questions concerning the implications of excluding a population subgroup who may have very different outcomes, exposures, or associations. On the other hand, the burdens of research may be viewed rather differently by elderly participants, some finding the data collection onerous or embarrassing, and others finding it stimulating, exciting, or providing them with a sense of contributing to science. As with all populations, the question must be raised, to whom do benefits accrue?

Finally, as with all persons, elderly research participants should be treated with respect and care. This means protecting their dignity as well as protecting them from physical and psychological harm. Engaging the elderly participant as a partner in research not only may enhance the quality of the data obtained, but also may contribute to greater participation rates and provide a benefit to the participant.

Data in observational research is often collected by interview or questionnaire. Epidemiologists focus on how to obtain valid and reliable data, especially on sensitive topics, but the ethical issues often receive less attention. If we recognize that research participants are the source of the data on which our work depends, and that their provision of very personal information is a significant contribution to that effort, then their role as participants gains value. The relationship of researcher and research participant then becomes one of mutual trust and confidence, which entails certain obligations on the part of the researcher. This perspective is grounded in a view of the researcher-respondent relationship as one of voluntary mutual trust and commitments. This concept of mutual trust and obligations may require some elaboration because, although it is implicit in the informed consent process, it is not typically made explicit.

When a person agrees to participate in a research project—whether a clinical trial or an observational study—that person places trust in (and sometimes entrusts his or her life to) the researcher. The typical requirements for disclosure, comprehension, competence, absence of coercion (voluntariness), and consent are expressions of respect for the autonomy and dignity of the person, but they are also the grounds on which the potential research participant bases a decision to place trust in this researcher. (Beauchamp has seven elements at three levels, adding a recommendation for a plan and dividing consent into the decision and the authorization, but the implication is the same.[54]) By consenting, the participant indicates a level of trust that the researcher has provided the information that is needed and will conform to the protocol outlined.

That we require justification for any deviation, such as deception, indicates that there is an implicit assumption that the participant can trust the researcher. Further, if participation in research carries risk or causes harm, then the researcher has an obligation to minimize the risk and rectify the harm, and that includes being sensitive to the impact the research may have on participants. If questions or procedures may evoke stress or anxiety, then the researcher is obligated by the relationship of trust to provide assistance. Studies that raise questions about or ascertain either mental problems (such as suicidality) or physical problems (such as abuse or disease state) should have in place procedures to respond, including additional measures for further assessment and referral.

Because the researcher typically is exposed to much less risk and stands to gain much more benefit in the way of information vital to his/her task than the participant in observational research,

then the greater obligation falls to the researcher. However, we contend that there are also certain obligations for the participant. Though there are always provisions for the volunteer to withdraw the consent, the agreement implies that, while participating, he/she will take part in all aspects of the protocol that are appropriate and not objectionable. There is, then, a level of commitment on the part of the research participant, though the commitment is less binding because the voluntariness of the commitment allows for the option of withdrawal.

The researcher enrolls a subject trusting that this person will, indeed, participate and will provide honest and accurate information to the extent possible. The researcher trusts that a participant will not intentionally subvert or sabotage the research and will not provide false or fabricated data. The researcher also trusts that the participant, when requested, will not disclose aspects of the research that may be proprietary, confidential, or could compromise the collection of data or recruitment of new participants. One example is in the conduct of qualitative research in which focus groups are employed. Participants are typically asked to maintain confidentiality of comments made in the group. This is an obligation to protect confidentiality on the part of research participants parallel to the obligation of the researchers themselves. Both the researchers and the other group members trust each participant to keep that information confidential.

We are suggesting that mutuality in the relation of investigator and research participant is important in the conduct of epidemiologic research and that both our ethical sensitivity and our epidemiologic methods can be enhanced by moving beyond the paternalism of the expert and embracing greater reciprocity in our relations with those we would study.

Beyond the principle of respect for persons, the values of human dignity and autonomy, and the obligations implied in a mutual agreement, there are also issues of character and the role of the virtues in ethical judgment and action. Good—ethically correct—research requires integrity, honesty, compassion, and trustworthiness among investigators.[5,6,55] Researchers should ask, "Are we presenting the process honestly?" "Are we considering the impact on the respondent?" "Are we acting so as to engender trust in us and in other researchers who may come after us?" To act ethically requires not only that we know how to determine the right thing to do, but also that we are disposed to act in conformity to that judgment. It is moral character that provides the impetus to do what is right. The formation of character is beyond the scope of this chapter, but it cannot be ignored as a critical component of ethics.

If epidemiologists embrace and strive to achieve the goal of improved health and well-being for the population, then steps toward that goal require continuing accumulation of knowledge about the determinants of health and disease in individuals and populations. Observational research comes into play because we cannot subject persons to randomization from the start, nor can we impose risk factors on persons, and the broad underlying structures and contexts that we increasingly understand to be critical for differences in incidence across populations do not lend themselves to randomized intervention research.

One of the chief advantages of randomized trials compared to observational studies is that randomization among the treatment groups is assumed to reduce confounding and some other types of bias. (Bias is a systematic error that may be due to study design or implementation, such as selection bias or information bias.)

Confounding can occur when there is a factor associated with both the outcome of the study and a specific factor of interest, such as exposure (like asbestos or pesticides), or personal characteristics (like income or education), or behavior (like diet or exercise). These associations, if not controlled for in either the design or analysis, can produce a biased estimate of the effect. Randomization is especially effective in preventing uncontrolled confounding. Randomization also reduces information (or misclassification bias) and is intended to protect from selection bias, although the rigid inclusion and exclusion criteria may mean the results will not apply to other population groups or the broader patient group that eventually receives a treatment. In general, it can be said that randomized controlled trials enhance the internal validity of a study, often at the expense of external validity. That is, the estimates are less likely to be biased with regard to the population actually studied, but may not apply to populations less rigorously selected.[56]

Random variability is quite distinct from bias, and applies to both randomized controlled trials and observational studies. Bias is a form of nonrandom variation. Random variations in measurements and estimates of effect do not constitute bias because they are not the result of systematic error, but they do contribute to our uncertainty about the accuracy of those measures. Researchers rely on statistical methods, with certain assumptions, to quantify uncertainty due to random variability. For randomized trials, that usually takes the form of hypothesis testing: Is treatment A better than treatment B (or better than no treatment)? The study typically proposes a null hypothesis that the two (or more) treatments are equally effective, or that a new treatment is no more effective than placebo. The researchers may believe the new treatment is superior; indeed, it is unlikely they would be conducting the trial if they did not have some evidence for a potential treatment advantage. If there is a difference observed between the two (or more) arms, then the researcher must decide if the difference is likely to be the result of random variability alone or reflects a real difference in effect.

Even if two randomized groups are given exactly the same treatment, we are likely to observe some difference in the point estimates of the outcome measures merely because of random variations in the measures. This is where statistical tests come into play. If the probability of obtaining a difference as large as or larger than the one actually observed (the P-value) is smaller than a previously established level of certainty (the alpha level) then the null hypothesis is rejected and we judge that the difference is unlikely to be due to chance. Note that the alpha level is determined ahead of time; that is, the researcher chooses the alpha level. (It is often set at 0.05, but the researcher must explicitly affirm that or another level.) If one rejects the null hypothesis, judging that there is a difference in treatments when, in fact, there is no difference, it is called a Type I error. If, on the other hand, one fails to reject the null hypothesis when it is false, meaning that the statistical test does not support a difference in treatment even though there really is one, it is called a Type II error. One can set the alpha level very low, reducing the likelihood of a Type I error, judging there to be a difference when there is none, but this increases the likelihood of a Type II error, judging there to be no difference when in fact one treatment is superior. The Type II counterpart to the alpha level is called beta, and 1-beta is the power, the probability of rejecting the null hypothesis when it is false.

In randomized trials and in observational studies, there is a trade-off between Type I and Type II errors. The trade-off is not simply a statistical one of balancing the seesaw of probabilities for one error or the other, but it is also potentially an ethical one. What is the cost of judging that a treatment is more effective when it actually is not, versus the cost of judging that a treatment is not more effective when in fact it is? What resources may be expended for a new treatment that provides no advantage, and what needs go unaddressed because of the diversion of those resources? Conversely, what suffering goes unmitigated because a treatment's advantage is not recognized?

The discussion thus far has used clinical trials to illustrate the potential ethical issues involved in what is typically thought to be purely statistical trade-offs in hypothesis testing, but similar concerns arise in observational studies, especially when they are used as the basis for decisions concerning policy and practice. Observational studies increasingly emphasize estimation with confidence intervals rather than hypothesis testing as a means of indicating the precision of the estimates; that is, how much confidence we have that an estimate of effect falls within some range of random variability. This approach may seem to reduce the concern over tradeoffs of Type I versus Type II error. However, when clinical decisions or public health policy decisions are made on the basis of observational studies, the concern about Type I versus Type II error becomes more pressing.

At some point a decision may be forced, and at that point we consider the trade-offs of one versus the other in light of the precision of our estimates and relative weighting of the cost of one type of error versus the other. It is easy to adopt alpha of 0.05 and beta of 0.2 (the predetermined critical probability of a Type II error) and some arbitrary difference in means or proportions or strength in the measure of association assumed to be clinically meaningful. More difficult is probing what difference it might make in policy or clinical decision making if the null hypothesis were erroneously rejected or, conversely, the null were not rejected when in fact there were true and meaningful differences or associations.

When one implements a decision to change some characteristic, program, or policy based on evidence that it will make a difference in the health of individuals or the population, when in fact it will make no difference, then resources are wasted that might otherwise have been used more effectively and, perhaps, lives are changed in unnecessary ways. On the other hand, if one fails to implement such changes because the evidence for an association does not meet some predefined, but arbitrary alpha level, when the changes would indeed result in enhanced individual or population health, then those people and the population are deprived of the benefits of healthier life and resources are expended that might otherwise be conserved to address the poorer health status. Deciding between these scenarios requires reflection on the resources and the values of those affected by the decision, as well as the obligations of those making the decision.

Power calculations are often used to estimate the probability of detecting a real difference of a certain size, if there is one, given a certain population size, or to estimate the sample size needed to observe an effect that is clinically meaningful at predetermined alpha and beta levels. There are a number of statistical assumptions required for power calculations, but our argument is that statistical analysis, even power calculations, as well as discussions of findings, require reflection on the implications for policy analysis or clinical decision making that rely on the data. Such reflections inevitably invoke values, principles, and obligations that are inherently ethical in nature. This raises the question of whether community input is needed even in observational research, not only concerning risks and benefits but where to err in judgments of effect. Consider research to determine the effectiveness of alternative programs that may subsequently be implemented as a matter of policy: Should the community be able to factor into their risk/benefit deliberations the probability of assuming that an ineffective intervention is effective, or conversely, assuming that an effective intervention is not?

Similar concerns can be raised in screening programs. For many screening tests, decisions must be made about appropriate critical values that define a positive test. The sensitivity measures how well the test detects the condition and is the probability the test will be positive given the person has the condition being screened (or the proportion of those with the condition who will have positive tests). The specificity measures how well the test screens out those without the condition and is the probability the test will be negative given the person does not have the condition being screened (or the proportion of those without the condition who will have negative tests).

For some tests, the critical value that defines a positive test can be chosen, typically to increase sensitivity at the expense of specificity or vice versa. These decisions must find a balance of sensitivity and specificity that is optimal for the outcome and population being studied. Although sensitivity (and 1 − sensitivity, the false negative proportion among those with the condition) and specificity (and 1 − specificity, the false positive proportion among those without the condition) are theoretically independent of the population, the predictive value of a screening test (the probability a person has the condition given a positive test, or the proportion of those with a positive test who actually have the condition) is a function of the pretest probability (the assumed probability that person has the condition before the test is given, or the prevalence of undiagnosed disease in the screened population). Decisions must be made on the relative importance and cost (in human terms as well as resources) of false negative versus false positive results.

It is commonly acknowledged among public health professionals that screening programs as a form of prevention should not be undertaken in the absence of demonstrated treatment options for those identified or other clear benefit as a result of screening. However, there is less agreement about the appropriateness or obligations of researchers conducting observational studies that function as de facto screening programs because of their identification of persons with (or likely to have) a disorder. We have previously argued that we believe researchers conducting observational studies that identify problems in participants have an obligation to have in place procedures for referral of those so identified.

Interpreting and Applying Observational Evidence: Ethics of Decisions and Interventions

We assume that the overarching purpose behind performing observational research (in the form of epidemiological studies) is to generate scientific understanding of disease etiology. There are, of course, other important purposes for epidemiologic studies:

For example, surveillance of disease incidence and mortality—measuring the demographics of disease of populations—is also an observational research activity. Similarly, monitoring the outcomes of medical (typically, therapeutic) interventions—often referred to as health outcomes research or health services research—relies heavily upon epidemiological methodologies and concepts. Our focus here will be on the use of epidemiological evidence for primary prevention—that is, the interpretation and application of epidemiological evidence to assess whether public health measures should be implemented for the identification and removal of disease-causing factors (exposures).

Although epidemiological research is at the center of the process of scientific interpretation, rarely are questions of causality answered solely with observational evidence on human populations. Evidence from other scientific disciplines, using quite different methodologies, notably biological (laboratory) studies, is often examined alongside epidemiologic evidence. One of the increasingly important considerations in causal interpretations of scientific evidence is *biological plausibility,* as discussed below.

It is also important to point out that certain categories of preventive interventions—for example, early disease detection technologies such as sigmoidoscopy for colon cancer, mammography for breast cancer, and many vaccinations for infectious diseases—are typically tested in randomized controlled clinical trials, a topic examined in detail elsewhere in this book. Active chemopreventive medications such as tamoxifen or raloxifene for the prevention of breast cancer, finasteride for the prevention of prostate cancer, and aspirin for the prevention of coronary heart disease are also tested in randomized trials, although these trials typically are undertaken after a variety of other types of studies have been performed, including laboratory, epidemiological, animal model, and preclinical studies for toxicity and acceptability.

Our focus here is on the interpretation and application of epidemiological evidence (often supplemented with evidence from biology) for primary prevention, the identification and removal of disease-causing factors and/or the promotion of so-called lifestyle factors and the social forces that affect them, such as physical activity (exercise), dietary interventions (e.g., eating fruits and vegetables), and safety devices such as seat belts or bicycle helmets.

Responsibility for Interpreting and Applying Epidemiologic Evidence for Primary Prevention

It may seem obvious that there are public health professionals willing to take on the responsibility of deciding whether the scientific evidence demonstrates a need for interventions or whether more evidence is needed before acting. By *need for interventions,* we mean that sufficient evidence exists to consider a factor a hazard and thus available for considerations of interventions, given that any intervention must also take into account the impact of the intervention on the community and on individual freedoms or rights, the benefit/risk horizon of the intervention, as well as a consideration of the populations who may warrant preferential consideration for intervention because they are vulnerable, underrepresented, or otherwise special.

However, the issue of responsibility for prevention has been hotly debated within the ranks of epidemiology, and it is one with prominent ethical roots.[57] Being responsible in this context means being accountable for decisions to intervene and being committed to improving the public's health, including but not limited to the health of individuals and the health of the communities in which they live.[58,59] Although it is widely accepted, for example, that physicians and other health-care professionals are responsible for decisions to intervene therapeutically—decisions ideally made with the full consent and cooperation of patients—it is less clear whose responsibility it is to prevent disease by offering preventive interventions to individuals not already ill or to populations with varying incidence rates or prevalence of disease, injury, birth defects, or other health-related conditions. In contemporary society, primary prevention is undertaken (even advocated for) by a host of different players: individual health professionals, some of whom are clinically trained and others who are not, institutions such as the American Cancer Society or the American Heart Association, government health agencies at the local, state, and national levels, regulatory bodies such as the Environmental Protection Agency, grass roots advocacy groups concerned about air or water pollution, and private, for-profit companies that, for example, impose no-smoking policies in the workplace.

As practicing professional epidemiologists, we have argued that we are responsible for directly connecting our research results with our communities through the complex and value-rich process of interpreting and applying epidemiologic evidence in preventive public health practice.[59]

Not everyone agrees. Some professional epidemiologists have countered that their responsibility ends with the causal interpretation of scientific evidence, providing information regarding the certainty with which one might accept or reject a given causal hypothesis, but providing no recommendation for public health (preventive) action.[57,60,61] A range of reasons for keeping epidemiologists free of the role of public health practitioner—some practical, others ethical—have been carefully examined elsewhere.[62] Among these are concerns that epidemiologists lack expertise in public health policy making, that advocating for public health policies negatively affects one's scientific objectivity, and finally, that the observational nature of epidemiologic science militates against applying that science to the real world. But these are not compelling reasons for limiting the role of epidemiologists to a scientific practice devoid of application.

Epidemiologists regularly participate in research and education policy making and therefore cannot be ignorant of the basics of policy making that is needed for public health practice. In addition, it has been argued that participation in public health policy making (and other forms of advocacy) may actually enhance epidemiologists' scientific objectivity by encouraging them to improve their methods of research synthesis, that is, their the methods of causal inference. And finally, it has been noted that public health applications regularly emerge from observational research, often coupled with evidence from the laboratory or clinical sciences. Decisions about interventions are unlikely to be solely dependent upon epidemiologic findings, but that fact does not mean that epidemiologists should not participate in (much less have a responsibility for) applications because the science is observational. Nevertheless, it is interesting and important to point out that some have recently argued for a rather strict separation of the role of researcher from that of clinical practitioner.[63] As Brody and Miller write, "There is an irreducible ethical tension between the roles of treating physician and investigator. In most

settings, this tension is best dealt with by *requiring* that the same physician not serve in both roles [emphasis added]."[63]

Such tension exists as much in prevention as it does in treatment scenarios, although the prime conflict appears to be the conflict between the duty to do one's best for a patient and the disruption in that duty that randomization creates in a clinical trial. Put another way, observational (epidemiological) research on treatment, or on factors that may cause or prevent disease, does not conflict with a practitioner's obligation to do his or her best for a patient or a community. Observational research does not disrupt the choice of intervention or the opportunity to avoid exposure that would be part of the joint responsibility of the health professional-researcher.

Causal Claims and Preventive Recommendations: Conceptual Rationale

The level (or strength) of evidence required to recommend a preventive intervention is not, in theory or practice, fixed. Clearly, if there is very strong evidence that some factor is causal and manipulable, then one must do all that is necessary to intervene to prevent further disease through further exposure. On the other hand, it would be in error to argue that "very" strong evidence of causation is necessary before any action to remove a purported causal factor can be recommended. In practice, those who are responsible for such recommendations need to know enough— just enough—to provide a warrant for the recommendation, taking into account, as described briefly above, the concomitant issues of the expected reduction in risk, the potential harm of the intervention, the acceptability and intrusiveness of the intervention, and the population or community the intervention will affect. In addition, we must consider the implications of being wrong in our recommendation, as noted in the discussion of Type I versus Type II errors. For all these reasons, we cannot act in a vacuum of information. We need to know something about the purported cause and its effects including the level of certainty we assign to our understanding.

We recognize that for different purported causal factors, the level of evidence required is likely to be different. We recognize that for some situations we may require an extensive understanding of the disease mechanisms, including how a purported causal factor such as exposure acts within those mechanisms. We recognize that for other situations we may require much less evidence. In terms of responsible action for prevention, we are, in essence, in a constant state of asking ourselves with each new piece of the evidentiary puzzle: Is it time to act, time to recommend a preventive intervention? Another way of putting this is to presume that we are looking for the least amount of evidence for causation, wherein that threshold (in any given situation) may be quite high indeed.

Causal Claims and Preventive Recommendations: Methodological Rationale for Interpreting Epidemiologic Evidence

Before describing the methodologies used in interpreting epidemiological evidence, it is important to point out that the practice of making causal claims and from them, preventive recommendations, is not only characterized by uncertainty, in a probabilistic sense, and by the epistemological condition of underdetermination, but also heavily influenced by values, both scientific and extrascientific. Although ideally one would expect an interpretative assessment of carefully collected scientific evidence to be objective and free—as much as possible—from the subjective influences of any individual reviewer, this may not be the case in the interpretation of epidemiologic evidence. Indeed, examples of nonscientific norms, such as antiabortion sentiments, affecting the process of causal interpretations of epidemiologic evidence, have been documented. The reason that such values can have such an effect is an important problem. The origin of this problem lies in the structure of the methods used to make causal claims, a mix of quantitative and qualitative strategies and components, as described below.

Causal claims are most often made in what are referred to as reviews of the scientific literature in which the available scientific evidence is summarized after a systematic collection from published sources. Some authors of reviews may choose to include previously unpublished (or nonpeer-reviewed) studies. Guidelines for systematic reviews emphasize the importance of clearly defining which studies were included (i.e., inclusion criteria), the methods used in summarizing the results of multiple studies (e.g., through pooled analyses or meta-analysis), and the overarching purpose of the review (e.g., to make research recommendations, causal claims, and/or preventive recommendations).

The most important types of observational study designs relevant to causal interpretations are the so-called analytic case-control and cohort studies. In a systematic review, these are tabulated separately with special attention paid to the characteristics of the study population, exposure measurements, results (often in terms of the relative risk of disease or death, estimated in case-control studies by the odds ratio), and a measure of statistical uncertainty, typically provided by a P value, or confidence interval, or both. The number of studies included in these tables depends upon factors such as when the reviewer happens to have undertaken his or her review in the historical context of studying the relationship between the exposure factor of interest and the disease or condition it is purported to cause; well-studied "associations" can generate tables with dozens of entries.

The interpretation of this body of evidence includes an assessment of statistical uncertainty and an assessment of the extent to which the findings (across all studies represented in the review) can be explained either by systematic biases or by unmeasured confounding factors. Although observational studies cannot, by their very nature, provide strong assurances that all potential confounders have been accounted for, or all other biases prevented or eliminated, a prominent part of the process of making causal claims from observational evidence is judging the extent to which the results could be "higher" or "lower" due to controlled confounding or presence of other biases. Though the possibility of bias affecting results is typically acknowledged in published epidemiologic studies, it is usually given less weight in evaluating the reliability of the results than the uncertainty due to random variability.

It is not uncommon for absolute decisions about associations to be based on whether p values exceed arbitrary alpha levels even when the degree of uncertainty can be quantified. The presence of bias, on the other hand, is often discussed in rather general terms and the impact of the bias on results is rarely assumed to negate the findings. Though methods of sensitivity analysis to quantify the impact of bias are available, they are only occasionally incorporated into the reporting of epidemiologic findings, whereas one can hardly conceive of an epidemiologic study being published without either p values or confidence intervals, sometimes both.

Assuming that a body of evidence successfully makes it through this initial assessment of statistical uncertainty, potential bias, and confounding, the reviewer then examines it from the perspective of what are referred to as causal "criteria," although the discipline recognizes that only one (of several used) can be considered a true criterion in the sense that it must be satisfied if causation is to be claimed. That criterion is temporality; the condition that a factor must precede its effect in time to be considered causal. Depending on the user's preference (and to an extent, the published source of these criteria), there are as many as eight and as few as no additional criteria used in causal assessments in practice. In theory—in other words, in the texts describing this methodology—there are typically nine criteria in all, including experimentation, by which it was meant a randomized controlled trial. This list includes the following: consistency, strength, dose-response, biological plausibility, specificity, coherence, temporality, experimentation, and analogy. A detailed description of each of these is not important for the purposes here. What is important is that each of these so-called criteria has an implicit rule of inference associated with it that can be easily manipulated by the individual (or group) writing the review. Put another way, causal claims from epidemiological evidence (and from the biological evidence used to assess the single criterion of biological plausibility) are dependent upon the rules assigned to these criteria as well as the number of criteria used and the priority assigned to them. Differing (often opposite) causal claims from the same epidemiological and biological evidence originate primarily from different interpretations of—that is, different rules of inference assigned to—these so-called causal criteria.[26]

Ethical Considerations in Translating Causal Claims Into Preventive Recommendations

Areas of ethical tension emerge when discussing the ethics of translating epidemiologic research into preventive action.[64] The first involves the balancing act between that which we need to know and that which needs to be done. Public health action aspires to be based on a strong foundation of scientific knowledge; evidence-based decision making has increasingly become the approach taken for all types of preventive (and most therapeutic) interventions. But science is a complex interdisciplinary phenomenon, neither fixed in stone nor free of subjectivity. Uncertainty flows through our understanding of human biology and pathophysiology at the individual and population levels encompassing biological, lifestyle, and social determinants of health and disease. The scientist's claim to objectivity is primarily supported by the validity and reliability of methodologies. Yet, as discussed above, the interpretation of evidence generated by observational methods of epidemiology requires not only judgment but often (if not always) consideration of evidence from biological (or social) sciences. The interpretative methods themselves are more qualitative than quantitative, allowing for subjectivity and a range of values to potentially influence those judgments.

Our search for what counts as truth (however tentative) and our duty to act to promote health and prevent disease in persons and populations are an important source of ethical tension. At its core lies a concern that we not err in our recommendations for preventive interventions. We should act neither too rashly nor too late. Unfortunately, there is no well worn path to assess our success or lack of it. It is one thing to say that we recommend an intervention because we are convinced of the causal attribution of the factor we plan to "remove" from a community so that a reduction in incidence or mortality can follow. It is quite another to demonstrate such a success, documenting the reduction.

Another source of tension involves the intervention itself— how the risks are balanced by the benefits and, perhaps most importantly for public health interventions, the extent to which individual freedoms have been sacrificed in the name of the common good. A contrast between individuals and populations is a prominent feature of most discussions of public health ethics, within which we place the ethics of epidemiologic practice. Observational research is characteristically performed on groups, sometimes defined by geography (e.g., women living in New York City), by occupation (e.g., nurses), or by social class (e.g., migrant farm workers). Although it is true that these groups are composed of individuals and that measurements are often (though not always) taken on each individual, the research results are characteristically presented in terms of the possible causal (or preventive) effects of the exposure on the population studied, rather than on any individual within that group. In a classic epidemiological paper contrasting research practices and preventive interventions for sick individuals and sick populations respectively, Rose made a strong point about the need for studying different populations that may be exposed, by choice or not, to quite different environmental factors and that could, as a result, manifest quite different disease distributions, impossible to discern within each population.[45]

Similarly, interventions are undertaken at the individual or population level for prevention, with smoking cessation (or tobacco control) a well worn but excellent example. Individuals can be encouraged to stop smoking in one-on-one sessions with therapists or physicians or friends, just as populations can be encouraged to stop smoking by regulations disallowing smoking in public places or worksites. It is this latter situation in which the ethical tension exists when the freedoms accorded to individuals in most contemporary societies are curtailed in the name of promoting the health of the community as a whole.[65] Starker examples involve preventive interventions that few individuals can avoid, such as fluoridation and chlorination of public water supplies, childhood immunizations, and seat-belt laws. Because the relationship with individual participants and populations is less direct and the benefits more distant or abstract for many observational studies, the ethical issues may not be as obvious.

Summary

The ethical issues facing epidemiology range from obligations to individual participants to epistemological challenges, reflections on causality, and policy formation. Epidemiologists, by the very nature of their research, cannot work in isolation from the populations they study, nor can they assume that the fruits of their labors are merely possible answers to interesting scientific puzzles.

Epidemiology is at the very heart of public health, providing a major cornerstone in its scientific foundation and taking responsibility for preventive action. The obligations this entails—to individuals, to populations, to the community of science, and to public health professionals and the entities where they work—are wide-ranging and profound.

References

1. Federal Judicial Center. *Reference Manual on Scientific Evidence,* 2nd ed. Washington, D.C.: Federal Judicial Center; 2000.
2. Gross CP, et al. State expenditures for tobacco-control programs and the tobacco settlement. *New England Journal of Medicine* 2002;347: 1080–6.
3. Taubes G. Epidemiology faces its limits. *Science* 1995;269:164–9.
4. Last JM, ed. *A Dictionary of Epidemiology,* 4th ed. New York, N.Y.: Oxford University Press; 2001.
5. Weed DL, McKeown RE. Glossary of ethics in epidemiology and public health: I. Technical terms. *Journal of Epidemiology and Community Health* 2001;55:855–7.
6. McKeown RE, Weed DL. Glossary of ethics in epidemiology and public health: II. Applied terms. *Journal of Epidemiology and Community Health* 2002;56:739–41.
7. Beaglehole R, Bonita R. *Public Health at the Crossroads.* New York, N.Y.: Cambridge University Press; 1997.
8. Friedman G. *Primer of Epidemiology.* New York, N.Y.: McGraw-Hill; 1994.
9. Rothman KJ, Greenland S. *Modern Epidemiology,* 2nd ed. Philadelphia, Penn.: Lippincott-Raven; 1998.
10. Gordis L. *Epidemiology,* 2nd ed. Philadelphia, Penn.: W.B. Saunders; 2000.
11. Szklo M, Nieto FJ. *Epidemiology: Beyond the Basics.* Gaithersburg, Md.: Aspen Publishers, Inc.; 2000.
12. Rothman KJ. *Epidemiology: An Introduction.* New York, N.Y.: Oxford University Press, 2002.
13. Koepsell T, Weiss N. *Epidemiologic Methods: Studying the Occurrence of Illness.* New York, N.Y.: Oxford University Press; 2003.
14. Schulte PA, Perera FP. *Molecular Epidemiology: Principles and Practices.* New York, N.Y.: Oxford University Press; 1993.
15. Fletcher RH, Fletcher SW. *Clinical Epidemiology: The Essentials,* 4th ed. Baltimore, Md.: Lippincott, Williams & Wilkins; 2005.
16. Sackett DL, Haynes RB, Guyatt GH, Tugwell P. *Clinical Epidemiology: A Basic Science for Clinical Medicine,* 2nd ed. Boston, Mass.: Little Brown; 1991.
17. Greenberg R, et al. *Medical Epidemiology.* Norwalk, Conn.: Appleton & Lange; 1996.
18. Berkman L, Kawachi I. *Social Epidemiology.* New York, N.Y.: Oxford University Press; 2000.
19. Kawachi I, Berkman LF, eds. *Neighborhoods and Health.* New York, N.Y.: Oxford University Press; 2003.
20. Brownson RC, Remington PL, Davis JR. *Chronic Disease Epidemiology and Control.* 2nd ed. Washington, D.C.: American Public Health Association; 1998.
21. Tsuang MT, Tohen M, eds. *Textbook in Psychiatric Epidemiology,* 2nd ed. New York, N.Y.: Wiley-Liss, Inc.; 2002.
22. Nelson KE, Williams CM, Graham NMH. *Infectious Disease Epidemiology: Theory and Practice.* Gaithersburg, Md.: Aspen Publishers, Inc.; 2000.
23. Giesecke J. *Modern Infectious Disease Epidemiology,* 2nd ed. New York, N.Y.: Oxford University Press; 2002.
24. Rothman KJ. *Causal Inference.* Philadelphia, Penn.: Little Brown; 1988.
25. Weed DL. Towards a philosophy of public health. *Journal of Epidemiology and Community Health* 1999;53:99–104.

26. Weed DL. Underdetermination and incommensurability in contemporary epidemiology. *Kennedy Institute of Ethics Journal* 1997;7: 107–27.

27. Coughlin SS, Etheredge GD, Metayer C, Martin SA Jr. Remember Tuskegee: Public health student knowledge of the ethical significance of the Tuskegee Syphilis Study. *American Journal of Preventive Medicine* 1996;12:242–6.

28. Susser M, et al. Ethics in epidemiology. *Annals of the American Academy of Political and Social Science* 1978;437:128–41.

29. Soskolne CL. Epidemiology: Questions of science, ethics, morality, and law. *American Journal of Epidemiology* 1989;129:1–18.

30. Beauchamp TL, et al. Ethical guidelines for epidemiologists. *Journal of Clinical Epidemiology* 1991;44(Suppl. 1):151S–169S.

31. Soskolne CL, Light A. Towards ethics guidelines for environmental epidemiologists. *The Science of the Total Environment* 1996;184:137–47.

32. Weed DL, Coughlin SS. New ethics guidelines for epidemiology: Background and rationale. *Annals of Epidemiology* 1999;9:277–80.

33. Bankowski Z, Bryant JH, Last JM, eds. *Ethics and Epidemiology: International Guidelines.* Proceedings of the 25th CIOMS Conference, 7–9 November 1990. Geneva, Switzerland: CIOMS; 1991.

34. American College of Epidemiology. Ethics Guidelines. *Annals of Epidemiology* 2000;10:487–97.

35. McKeown RE. American College of Epidemiology Ethics Guidelines: Filling a critical gap in the profession. *Annals of Epidemiology* 2000;10:485–6.

36. Pellegrino ED. Autonomy and coercion in disease prevention and health promotion. *Theoretical Medicine* 1984;5:83–91.

37. Gillon R. Ethics in health promotion and prevention of disease. *Journal of Medical Ethics* 1990;16:171–2.

38. Charlton B. Public health medicine—A different kind of ethics? *Journal of the Royal Society of Medicine* 1993;86:194–5.

39. Beauchamp D. Philosophy of public health. In: Reich W, ed. *Encyclopedia of Bioethics,* 2nd ed. New York, N.Y.: Simon & Schuster/ Macmillan; 1995:2161–6.

40. Coughlin SS, Beauchamp TL. *Ethics and Epidemiology.* New York, N.Y.: Oxford University Press; 1996.

41. Kass N. An ethics framework for public health. *American Journal of Public Health* 2001;91:1776–82.

42. Childress JF, et al. Public health ethics: Mapping the terrain. *Journal of Law, Medicine and Ethics* 2002;30:170–8.

43. Roberts M, Reich M. Ethical analysis in public health. *Lancet* 2002; 359:1055–9.

44. Thomas J, et al. A code of ethics for public health. *American Journal of Public Health* 2002;92:1057–9.

45. Rose G. Sick individuals and sick populations. *International Journal Epidemiology* 1985;14:32–8.

46. Parascandola M, Weed DL. Causation in epidemiology. *Journal of Epidemiology and Community Health* 2001;55:905–12.

47. Peppercorn JM, Weeks JC, Cook EF, Joffe S. Comparison of outcomes in cancer patients treated within and outside clinical trials: Conceptual framework and structured review. *Lancet* 2004;363:263–70.

48. Braunholtz DA, Edwards SJL, Lilford RJ. Are randomized trials good for us (in the short term)? Evidence for a "trial effect." *Journal of Clinical Epidemiology* 2001;54:217–24.

49. West J, Wright J, Tuffnell D, Jankowicz D, West R. Do clinical trials improve quality of care? A comparison of clinical processes and outcomes in patients in a clinical trial and similar patients outside a trial where both groups are managed according to a strict protocol. *Quality and Safety in Health Care* 2005;14:175–8.

50. Shavers-Hornaday VL, Lynch CF, Burmeister LF, Torner JC. Why are African Americans under-represented in medical research studies? Impediments to participation. *Ethnicity and Health* 1997; 2:31–45.

51. Shavers VL, Lynch CF, Burmeister LF. Racial differences in factors that influence the willingness to participate in medical research studies. *Annals of Epidemiology* 2002;12:248–56.

52. Thomas SB, Quinn SC. The Tuskegee Syphilis Study, 1932 to 1972: Implications for HIV education and AIDS risk education programs in the Black community. *American Journal of Public Health* 1991;81: 1498–1504.

53. Coughlin SS, Beauchamp TL. Ethics, scientific validity, and the design of epidemiologic studies. *Epidemiology* 1992;3:343–7.

54. Beauchamp TL. Informed consent. In: Veatch RM, ed. *Medical Ethics,* 2nd ed. Sudbury, Mass.: Jones and Bartlett, 1997, p.185–208.

55. Weed DL, McKeown RE. Epidemiology and virtue ethics. *International Journal of Epidemiology* 1998;27:343–8.

56. Walsh CR, Lloyd-Jones DM, Camargo CA Jr, Giugliano RP, O'Donnell CJ. Clinical trials of unfractionated heparin and low-molecular-weight heparin in addition to aspirin for the treatment of unstable angina pectoris: Do the results apply to all patients? *American Journal of Cardiology* 2000;86:908–12.

57. Anonymous. Discussion on the future of epidemiology. *International Journal of Epidemiology* 1999;28:1023.

58. Ogletree T. Responsibility. In: Reich WT, ed. *Encyclopedia of Bioethics,* 2nd ed. New York, N.Y.: Simon & Schuster/Macmillan; 1995: 2300–5.

59. Weed DL, McKeown RE. Science and social responsibility in public health. *Environmental Health Perspectives* 2003;111:1804–8.

60. Rothman KJ, Poole C. Science and policy making. *American Journal of Public Health* 1985;75:340–1.

61. Savitz D, et al. Reassessing the role of epidemiology in public health. *American Journal of Public Health* 1999;89:1158–61.

62. Weed DL, Mink P. Roles and responsibilities of epidemiologists. *Annals of Epidemiology* 2002;12:67–72.

63. Brody H, Miller FG. The clinician-investigator: Unavoidable but manageable tension. *Kennedy Institute of Ethics Journal* 2003;13: 329–46.

64. Weed DL, McKeown RE. Science, ethics and professional public health practice. *Journal of Epidemiology and Community Health* 2003;57:4–5.

65. Rose G. High-risk and population strategies of prevention: Ethical considerations. *Annals of Medicine* 1989;21:409–13.

Felice J. Levine   Paula R. Skedsvold

Behavioral and Social Science Research

Ethical issues in the conduct of behavioral and social science research with human participants involve considerations that are as diverse as the range of disciplines and fields that constitute these sciences. The methods, study populations, and issues being examined in studying behavioral and social processes all come into play in designing and implementing ethically sound research. This chapter provides an overview of the history of ethical considerations in the conduct of behavioral and social science research; addresses underlying ethical considerations that animate these fields of inquiry; unpacks the complexity of making ethical determinations, especially in the context of challenging circumstances, study populations, or methods; and raises issues—some unresolved—that merit consideration in planning for and reviewing research.

For all fields of human research, ethical determinations about the rights and interests of human research participants are an integral part of the research enterprise. Behavioral and social scientists undertaking research are informed by professional codes of ethics,[1-4] formal guidance enunciated in the Belmont Report,[5] and the Department of Health and Human Service's (DHHS) Policy for Protection of Human Research Subjects (45 CFR 46).[6] In the context of such guidance, scientists planning and implementing studies must make judgments about research participants, and thus need to apply ethical principles and rules responsibly to real-life circumstances in advance of and during the ongoing research process. This chapter examines how assessments about risk, harm, and benefit; confidentiality and privacy; disclosure and the processes of informed consent unfold in behavioral and social science research in relation to the substance of the study, the target population, and the specifics of the research method and design.

The social and behavioral sciences refer to a broad rubric of disciplinary and interdisciplinary fields dedicated to the scientific study of behavioral and social phenomena. Permeable at its boundaries, the term embraces fields ranging from anthropology, economics, political science, psychology, and sociology to linguistics, geography, demography, sociolegal studies, and education research, among others. Some disciplines like psychology have produced disciplinary subfields such as cognitive psychology or developmental psychology that also are quite interdisciplinary. Other fields, such as neuroscience, have interacted to create new arenas of scientific discovery and explanation. The richness and complexity of the behavioral and social sciences, the interdisciplinary synergism across these fields, and their growing interaction with the biological sciences can be seen in the conceptual framework used in volumes as early as the 1988 National Research Council report, *The Behavioral and Social Sciences,*[7] and more recently in the 2001 *International Encyclopedia of the Social & Behavioral Sciences.*[8]

In terms of health-related research, the Office of Behavioral and Social Sciences Research (OBSSR) at the National Institutes of Health (NIH) similarly conceives of behavioral and social science research to be a "large, multifaceted field" that is "not restricted to a set of disciplines or methodological approaches."[9] The OBSSR statement emphasizes the breadth of methodological approaches in these sciences, including surveys and questionnaires, interviews, randomized clinical trials, direct observation, physiological manipulations and recordings, descriptive methods, laboratory and field experiments, standardized tests, economic analyses, statistical modeling, ethnography, and evaluation. All of these methods come into play in behavioral and social science research on health—whether it is in the context of fundamental studies designed to further understanding of behavioral or social functioning or in the context of clinical research designed to predict or influence health outcomes, risks, or protective factors. Indeed, it is the methodology, rather than the specific field or purpose of the study, that tends to signal ethical issues worthy of attention.

The literature on ethical considerations in behavioral and social science research involving human participants focuses on the shared methods and complementary interests that cut across these fields. In work that was published during the same period that the Belmont Report and the federal regulations were issued, the emphasis was on methods, ethical concepts, and the newly emerging federal role in human research regulation. For example, chapters in the 1979 volume *Federal Regulations: Ethical Issues and Social Research*,[10] edited by Wax and Cassell for the American Association for the Advancement of Science Selected Symposium Series, addressed the complex ethical issues involved in qualitative as well as quantitative research. Similarly, contributions in the 1982 volume *Ethical Issues in Social Research*,[11] edited by Beauchamp, Faden, Wallace, and Walters, or in the two 1982 volumes edited by Sieber under the overarching title *The Ethics of Social Research*[12,13] focused on how ethical issues present themselves in the context of different research methods and examined key concepts such as benefit and harm, deception and consent, and privacy and confidentiality. More than 20 years later, in 2003, the National Research Council report *Protecting Participants and Facilitating Social and Behavioral Sciences Research*[14] also emphasized the link between research methods and key ethical concepts.

Emergence of Ethical Considerations

Ethical considerations in behavioral and social science research became an explicit topic of attention during the 1960s and 1970s. During this period, four types of activities emerged that over time intersected in terms of both substantive issues and networks of behavioral and social scientists working in these domains. Each contributed to heightened interest in research ethics. First, there was the emergence of a subfield of research (largely located within social psychology) giving systematic attention to the study of behavioral and social science research as a social process worthy of investigation. Second, researchers and scientific societies in behavioral and social science fields began focusing on the ethical practices and the ethical responsibility of researchers to human research participants. Some high-profile studies brought attention to these issues. Third, the federal government, largely in the context of biomedical research, but also including behavioral and social science research, turned to addressing the regulation of research with humans. Fourth, and not unrelated, interest in the regulation and ethics of research as well as the establishment of formal mechanisms stimulated some social science research addressed to these issues.

Social Psychology of Research

The social psychology of research involves examining the dynamics of research as a social process and the factors that could affect or bias results.[15] Research that commenced in the 1960s focused on the unintentional effects on research participants' responses of the investigators' knowledge of the hypotheses and experimental conditions (i.e., expectancy effects),[16] the impact of the nature of the information (e.g., the form or the wording of language) on outcomes,[17] the influence on results of simulated behaviors (e.g., role-playing behaviors of shorter or longer duration), and even whether volunteering or assumptions about the likelihood of deception (irrespective of ethical considerations) may reduce research participants' level of engagement with the research questions or tasks.[18] The desire of research participants to help, the social influence exerted in the situation, perceptions of the research participants and the researcher regarding socially appropriate responses,[19] participants' concerns about negative evaluations (i.e., not being a sufficiently "good" participant),[20] and the demand characteristics of the research situation are some of the factors that interested behavioral and social scientists because of their possible consequences for the validity of research.[21,22] Although most of this research focused on laboratory experiments (the context of much social psychological research), the questions being asked were germane to both fieldwork and social surveys. In addition, although this arena of research was directed to understanding the research enterprise and what contributes to, or erodes, its validity, the social processes being studied were quite central to ethical considerations (e.g., the amount of information disclosed to human participants and the social influence of research situations on participants' autonomous behavior).

Heightened Attention to Ethical Considerations

At about this same time, another strand of research in the behavioral and social sciences was directly addressing topics related to human values (e.g., conformity, obedience, stereotypes).[23,24] This work sought to better understand the impact of social situations, influences, and norms on human behavior using compelling research designs and tools. The visibility of such studies and the broader attention in this post–World War II era to the treatment of participants in research also led scientific associations, including professional societies in the social and behavioral sciences, to address ethical considerations in the conduct of research.

High-Profile Research

Much of the debate that unfolded about human research ethics in the behavioral and social sciences had its roots in notable work done in this period. A number of substantive studies raised questions about the appropriateness of the research procedures from the vantage point of the research participants. Although raising ethical questions about a study is distinct from judging a study to be ethically questionable, these two responses were frequently confounded. In many respects, the several studies that were particularly high profile were exemplars of a genre of behavioral and social science research of that time. Three studies—cutting across laboratory and field contexts—are most highly cited for leading those in the behavioral and social sciences to explore what constitutes viable ethical practices in their research and the conditions and criteria that should be applied in making such determinations.[25,26]

In the 1960s, experimental studies of obedience undertaken by Milgram involved research participants "believing" that they were administering painful shocks to others in the context of memory research. In reality, no shocks were being administered at all, despite participants being told that they were causing painful consequences to others.[27,28] The actual purpose of Milgram's research was to understand compliance with authority figures under varying conditions and to identify the factors that engendered resistance. The artificially constructed experimental situation encouraged participants to comply with authoritative instructions and continue to administer what they believed were painful shocks.

The scientific and social significance of Milgram's findings—that is, the propensity in certain situations for persons to obey authorities and override their sense of right and wrong—is generally acknowledged. Nevertheless, both the stress effects on participants of such compliance (resulting from "inflicted insights"[29]) and the deceptive scenario that placed them in this position, spawned significant discussion and debate in the research community, including by Milgram himself.[30–33] In many respects, Milgram was ahead of his time in explicitly addressing investigator's responsibilities to research participants. In his 1961 grant proposal to the National Science Foundation, for example, Milgram emphasized debriefing to put subjects at ease and to assure them of the adequacy of their performance. Conducting follow-up studies, he is credited with the first use of postexperimental procedures.[23] Although these studies showed that the vast majority of participants valued being in the study and only a few wished they had opted out, controversy continued to surround this research.

The 1971 prison simulation study by Zimbardo and associates[34,35] also framed ethical questions that engaged the attention of the research community.[26,36] Although there was no deception in this research, the long-term simulation of the role of prisoners or guards produced physical and psychological aggressive behaviors in "guards" and submissive behaviors in "prisoners." Participants became emotionally involved in their roles, leading to the experiment being terminated by the principal investigator because of concerns about psychological consequences.[35] Zimbardo's attention to research participant stress and the fact that he ended the study after six days are evidence of the care taken in the execution of this research. Though follow-up work identified no lasting adverse effects and yielded self-reports of benefits to participants, the study highlighted the larger ethical question of simulating behaviors that *could* induce sustained identity stress and potential psychological harm. How to weigh the potential risk of more than transitory stress in relation to the benefits of this form of research was, however, less a point of conversation than the behaviors that this simulation evoked.

The third inquiry conducted by Humphreys from 1965 to 1968 used participant observation and interview methods to study men who engaged in impersonal acts of fellatio in public restrooms (the "tearoom trade").[37] The research also included tracing car licenses to the homes of men Humphreys did not interview in the field in order to interview them subsequently without disclosing his true identity. He took this step to offset any social class bias, based on his observation that better educated men are more willing to talk about their lives and these sexual experiences in the field. Although the study contributed to understanding a highly stigmatized behavior and to reducing stereotypes about homosexuality, it simultaneously created considerable controversy about covert observation, deception, and potential harm, from emotional and interpersonal to legal.[38–40] Like the Milgram and Zimbardo studies, this field research generated debate in the behavioral and

social science community about the research procedures that Humphreys used. Although Humphreys sought to explicate the benefits of the research and reported that none of the participants subsequently expressed concerns about the deception or reported any harms, criticism about informed consent and deception eclipsed other issues.

Behavioral and Social Science Societies

During the 1960s, professional associations in the behavioral and social sciences also turned to a consideration of the ethical dimensions of research. The promulgation of ethics codes is perhaps the most tangible indicator of a commitment to articulate normative standards to guide and inform researchers in these fields. In taking up this task, scientific societies realized that periodic review of ethics codes would be necessary as knowledge evolved, methods developed, and contexts and issues emerged for study.

The American Psychological Association (APA) was the first professional association to take up this work and to use empirical methods to develop a code. The APA's critical incident method requested firsthand reports from some 7,500 members of decisions having ethical implications.[41,42] Instead of relying on a committee to identify issues, APA asked members to describe situations with ethical implications that they knew firsthand and to specify the ethical issues requiring decisions. Published in 1953, this code focused largely on psychologist-client relationships, in which the preponderance of incidents were reported.[43] In 1966, the APA established a Committee on Ethical Standards in Research that, also using the critical incident method, produced *Ethical Principles in the Conduct of Research With Human Participants,* which was adopted by APA Council.[44] The *Principles* became a new component of the APA Ethics Code published in 1972[45] and in all subsequent code revisions during that period.[46] The *Principles* was revised and reissued in 1982.[47] In 1992, the APA adopted a further revision of the code,[48] which was buttressed by publications related to human research participants.[49,50] The most recent revision of the Ethics Code appeared in 2002.[1]

By the late 1960s, other behavioral and social science societies took up this task as well. In 1967, the American Sociological Association (ASA) reactivated a process that had commenced in 1960, and by 1969, a Code of Ethics was approved by 88% of eligible members voting.[51] The ASA also saw its code as a dynamic document, with revisions being approved in 1982 and 1989, and enforcement procedures put in place by the ASA Council in 1983.[52] A major revision was approved in 1997.[2] The American Anthropological Association (AAA) initially addressed ethical issues in its 1967 Statement on Problems of Anthropological Research and Ethics.[53] By 1971, the AAA had adopted an ethics code, *Principles of Professional Responsibility,*[54] which was followed by amendments and a revision in 1990[55,56] and a further revision in 1998.[3]

The American Political Science Association (APSA) also addressed ethics in human research in the late 1960s. The APSA Committee on Professional Standards and Responsibilities issued a report in 1968 entitled "Ethical Problems of Academic Political Scientists," with a Standing Committee on Professional Ethics being established as a consequence.[57] Not until 1989, after a period of evolution, were these standards formalized;[4,58] they were further revised in 1998.[4] With funding from the Russell Sage Foundation in 1975–76, the APSA led 12 other social science associations[59] in undertaking a survey about confidentiality in social science research that yielded a statement, entitled "The Scholar's Ethical Obligation to Protect Confidential Sources and Data," and recommendations were approved by the APSA Council in 1976.[60]

Overall there was progress commencing in the late 1960s and 1970s in social and behavioral science societies' initiating activities and formalizing codes.[11] Nonetheless, some of the same ambivalence and tensions articulated by individual researchers about the balance between strengthening human research ethics and overregulation were also evident. Thus, the deliberations taking place in professional associations revealed an impulse to lead, but also to crystallize an evolving consensus in the formulation of ethical standards. Over time, for example, codes of ethics became much more explicit about informed consent[61] and about the use of students in research.[41] The evolution of federal regulations in this area similarly reflected an evolving consensus about ethical practices and how they should guide operational research.

Inclusion of Behavioral and Social Sciences Research in Federal Policy Making

Even in the earliest language and consideration of federal policy related to human research protection, discussions made reference to behavioral and social science research. Gray[62,63] traced the first inclusion of social and behavioral research back to a July 1966 revision of the February 1966 U.S. Public Health Service (PHS) policy that required institutional review of human research in all PHS awards.[64] Quoting from Gray,[62] the July 1966 revision stated that

> there is a large range of social and behavioral research in which no personal risk to the subject is involved. In these circumstances, regardless of whether the investigation is classified as behavioral, social, medical, or other, the issues of concern are the fully voluntary nature of the participation of the subject, the maintenance of confidentiality of information obtained from the subject, and the protection of the subject from misuse of the findings. . . . [social and behavioral sciences sometimes use procedures that] may in many instances not require the fully informed consent of the subject or even his knowledgeable participation.

Any ambiguity as to the intent of this language was further clarified in December 1966, when the U.S. Surgeon General, in response to a question, stated that the policy "refers to all investigations that involve human subjects, including investigations in the behavioral and social sciences." Furthermore, PHS policies issued in 1968 ("Public Health Service Policy for the Protection of the Individual as a Subject of Investigation") and 1969 ("Protection of the Individual as a Research Subject: Grants, Awards, Contracts") explicitly included behavioral and social science research, focusing in particular on risks that might be incurred due to breaches of confidentiality and misuse of findings. By 1971, in response to requests for better understanding of policy and the need for more uniformity in institutional review, the Department of Health, Education, and Welfare (DHEW), which preceded the DHHS, issued "The Institutional Guide to DHEW Policy on Protection of Human Subjects." This Guide dealt with concerns about physical, psychological, sociological or other harms and explicitly addressed harms, beyond physical harms, that could arise in behavioral and social science research.

The National Research Act of 1974 established the National Commission for the Protection of Human Subjects of Biomedical and Behavioral Research (National Commission) and required the establishment of a board to review biomedical and behavioral research involving human subjects at institutions that apply for funding from the PHS. The Act also affirmed the new DHEW regulations for the protection of human subjects (codified at 45 CFR 46) that required research to be reviewed and approved by committees as a prerequisite to funding. The behavioral and social science community expressed concerns about the potential suppression of research on controversial issues under the guise of ethical considerations; about the emphasis on a written document as part of informed consent, especially given ambiguous statements about waivers and documentation of consent; and about whether the regulations would be meaningfully extrapolated from biomedical and clinical settings to some of the challenging contexts and issues that animate social and behavioral science research (e.g., studying socially harmful behaviors or unsavory topics or persons). Concerns were also expressed about the very limited involvement of behavioral and social scientists on the National Commission or staff, although a number of papers were ultimately requested from these scientists by the National Commission.[62]

Over the four years that the National Commission worked (1974–78), behavioral and social scientists' level of engagement in research ethics increased. By 1979, when proposed revised regulations were published for comment in the *Federal Register,* the behavioral and social science community was better situated to respond. Comments ranged from encouraging ethical guidance that was better aligned with the designs and methods of the behavioral and social sciences to completely resisting any regulatory policy for social and behavioral science research. The federal regulations adopted in 1981 reflected the strengths of the National Commission's work and the urgings of the behavioral and social science community to specify a more nuanced understanding of risk, types of harm, and categories of review. Areas of research that could be exempt, areas that could be handled through expedited review, the capacity to waive documentation of consent, the definition of human subjects research to include *living* persons and identifiable *private* (not public) information were improved features of the 1981 revision. The National Commission's articulation of the core principles that formed the basis of the Belmont Report (i.e., respect for persons, beneficence, justice) as well as its openness to comments were important to the fuller integration of behavioral and social science research in federal policy.

Literature at that time[62,63,65] and later[14,66,67] provides an overview of the evolution of the 1981 federal regulations and the role of the National Commission in the development of these regulations. During the 1980s and the period that led to the adoption of the Common Rule (subpart A of the regulation) by federal agencies in 1991, behavioral and social science research operated within federal policy without much profile. By the late 1990s, with heightened public and policy attention to human research protection and the role and functioning of institutional review boards (IRBs), some of the same concerns expressed in the 1970s about one-size-fits-all solutions, the dominance of the biomedical model, and hyperregulation resurfaced in the behavioral and social sciences.[68,69]

Emerging Empirical Research on the Ethics of Research

Since the late 1990s, in addition to formal institutional responses in the form of new federal advisory committees, new National Academy of Sciences' committees, and initiatives of scientific societies, there have also been calls for better empirical knowledge about ethical aspects of human research in light of the methods and practices in these fields.[14,68,70] Assumptions abound about such issues as what research participants consider to be personal or private information, what they consider to be of risk or benefit, and what they believe they need to know before agreeing to participate in certain forms of research. To date, the literature on human research ethics largely remains more analytic or assumptive than empirical.

Work in the arena of survey research, addressed primarily to consent and confidentiality, is a major exception. Singer's work in particular stands out in this regard. Since the late 1970s, Singer has undertaken extensive research on such issues as the effect of the amount of information on consent and the impact of the request for and timing of written consent and confidentiality assurances (with sensitive and nonsensitive information) on response rates and response quality.[71–74] Singer reported that 8% of her sample refused to sign consent forms, but were willing to be interviewed—a finding consistent with a study by Ellikson and Hawes.[75] She also reported that when sensitive information is involved, confidentiality assurances matter in terms of willingness to respond and response quality, but confidentiality assurances have no significant effect when the content is not sensitive, complementing the findings of Turner[76] and of Boruch and Cecil.[77]

Much of the research in the 1970s was stimulated by the Privacy Act of 1974 and the 1974 federal regulations for the protection of research participants. In reflecting on this research in two review studies published in the 1990s,[78,79] Singer called for far more empirical inquiry on ethical issues in research. Over a wide range of issues and areas, the number of studies continues to be small in relation to the ethical questions about human research that could be informed by a critical mass of work. Singer's 2004 research, for example, has turned to the important issue of examining willingness to participate in surveys given perceptions of risk of disclosure, perceived harm, and perceived benefit.[80] Focusing on children and youth, Fisher has undertaken research on such issues as adolescents' assessment of investigators' use of varying options (such as maintaining confidentiality, reporting to parent/adult, encouraging self referral) under hypothetical conditions of investigators observing adolescents at various levels of jeopardy.[81] She has also been studying the capacity of children and youth to understand their rights, with younger children comprehending information but having less comprehension of their rights as research participants.[82] Others, like Hull and colleagues, are studying strategies for recruitment of family members in research in addition to the indexed participant.[83]

There has also been a resurgence of interest in studying IRBs, a topic that—despite its inherent interest and value—has received scant research attention[84] since the University of Michigan surveys undertaken by Gray and associates[63,85,86] as part of the work of the National Commission. Since the late 1990s, there have been additional commissions[87] and government reports[88] about IRBs that utilize or make reference to studies or data, but, over almost a 30-year period, only a modest number of studies has surfaced across a spectrum of issues. For example, in 1985, Ceci, Peters, and Plotkin reported on an experimental study of IRBs' responses to hypothetical proposals that differed in sociopolitical sensitivity and ethical concerns (e.g., presence or absence of deception, debriefing).[89] They found that when the purpose of the research was presented to IRBs as nonsensitive, the protocol was twice as likely to be approved. In 1995, Hayes et al. reported on a survey of IRB members at research universities, finding that over half received minimal or no training.[90] In 2003, Wagner, Bhandari, Chadwick, and Nelson reported on the costs of operating IRBs and economies of larger IRBs.[91] And in 2006, two studies were published that focused on investigator experiences, understandings, and perceptions of IRBs.[92,93]

Renewed attention and calls for empirical research on research ethics have been matched by some federal funding initiatives. In particular, the DHHS Office of Research Integrity commenced an extramural program of support in 2001. Also, the inauguration in 2006 of the *Journal of Empirical Research on Human Research Ethics* (JERHRE), dedicated to publishing empirical research and reviews of empirical literature on human research ethics, can be expected to further catalyze attention to inquiry on these issues.[94]

Ethical Issues in Research Contexts

The dearth of scientific knowledge about human research ethics adds to the challenge of undertaking research in all of the human sciences, including in the behavioral and social sciences. Nevertheless, absent deeper empirical knowledge, ethical considerations need to be weighed sensitive to the contexts of study and the fundamental principles of beneficence, respect, and justice specified in the Belmont Report and in codes of ethics. Key to making ethical decisions is to assess choices as part of the process of specifying the research design and methodology.

Complexity of Ethical Considerations

Behavioral and social science research draws on a range of research designs and methods in examining the complexities of human behavior—individually, in groups, in organizations and institutions, and in communities. Although different social science methods may be more frequently used or relied on by different behavioral and social science disciplines, almost every method is used to some degree in each behavioral and social science field. In addition, scientists increasingly draw on multiple methods in designing their research, even if there is primary reliance on a particular method.[95] The range of methods and multiple methods used in behavioral and social science research, the diverse populations under study, and the spectrum of issues (from mundane and everyday to highly sensitive and personal) make ethical considerations challenging and not amenable to easy characterization, generalization, or solution.

An emphasis on design and methods helps to identify ethical considerations across the behavioral and social sciences and between these sciences and the biomedical sciences—whether weighing autonomy, privacy, trust, benefit, or harm. Levine effectively dissected such issues in his 1976 paper "Similarities and

Differences Between Biomedical and Behavioral Research,"[96] prepared for the National Commission, and in his now classic volume *Ethics and Regulation of Clinical Research*.[97] Macklin also made an early and helpful contribution in her examination of disclosure in social science research.[98] Most comparisons between behavioral and social science research and biomedical research implicitly contrast the former to biomedical experimentation. It is from that vantage that behavioral and social science research is typically characterized as more likely to involve minimal risk for human participants because interventions in biomedical research have far greater potential for physical injury, harm, or adverse reaction.[14,99,100]

Leaving aside the additional complexity of research on special populations (e.g., children, prisoners), much of behavioral and social science research involves little interaction or intervention that could elevate risk beyond the minimal level, taking as the standard that the "probability and magnitude of harm or discomfort anticipated in the research are not greater in and of themselves than those ordinarily encountered in daily life or during the performance of routine physical or psychological examinations or tests."[6] Nevertheless, assessment of risks and benefits still comes into play in planning and implementing behavioral and social science research. Although the potential for physical harm or discomfort are rare, the risks are considered when appropriate— as is the potential for psychological, social, economic, or legal harm.[101,102] In some instances, the research activity itself could produce psychological discomfort or harm from feelings of being inconvenienced, embarrassed, or tired or from transitory stress or anxiety to more traumatic emotions or experiences. In most instances, risk of social, economic, or legal harms follows from insufficient protection of private information during the actual research or from breaches of confidentiality (including a person's anonymity) thereafter.

As suggested by the above, the substantive topics of inquiry may themselves cause psychological stress—from minor and transitory to more serious. For example, a research study on obesity that asks participants about their eating habits may cause minor and transitory stress. Research examining social support after the death of a loved one could cause a greater level of stress for participants because it evokes deep memories of sadness. Similarly, a retrospective study of adults who suffered child abuse could stimulate recollections that produce stress that is more than transitory or exceeds what persons would experience in everyday life. Research topics may also create the possibility of reputational, economic, legal, or physical harm that would exceed standards of low or minimal risk were there to be a breach of confidentiality. For example, a study of physicians charged with medical malpractice could produce reputational, economic, or legal harm were the identity of the physicians or the information they provided to researchers become known outside of the research setting. In each instance, precautions need to be taken to ameliorate or reduce the level of risk.

The biggest risk in behavioral and social science research most often relates to disclosure of a person's identity and information about him or her. Even in nonsensitive matters, a promise of confidentiality is typically part of the process of obtaining consent from research participants. How such consent will be obtained, whether the information will be preserved and for what purposes, who may have access to such data, and the consequences to research participants of any breach, even with seemingly quite everyday issues (e.g., a study of exercise practices at a gym that might reveal to an employer that the research participant was not home sick that day) need to be weighed in order to honor the explicit or implied agreement between research participant and researcher.

The next sections of this chapter address the operational processes involved in weighing ethical issues in research involving human participants. The emphasis is on considering the potential for risk and strategies for risk reduction in the context of planning and implementing research because, even in areas of minimal risk, it is incumbent upon researchers to design their research in ways that maximize benefits and reduce risk as well as protect against circumstances that could inadvertently raise risk levels. At least in principle, the responsibilities of investigators in this regard are generally quite well understood.

The attention to risk in these sections is not to eclipse consideration of the very real benefits that can flow from behavioral and social science research and that need to be weighed in a risk/benefit assessment. Indeed, behavioral and social science research can provide a wide range of benefits, including insights into human behavior or the practices of a particular culture, determinations regarding best therapeutic methods or educational practices, or strategies for addressing developmental challenges for children and the elderly. The results of this research may have a direct benefit for participants (e.g., decisions regarding work hours in an organizational setting) or may benefit society more generally by influencing broader public policy decisions (e.g., limited hours for workers in high-risk occupations). The benefits that derive from research are an important part of the equation in reviewing research and assessing risk and risk tolerance under varying circumstances.

A Heuristic Model for Guiding Ethical Considerations

A number of scholars have recognized the complexity of weighing ethical considerations and have sought to map the relationship between types of research and ethical issues. Kelman, for example, schematized the relationship between types of research, the concrete interests of participants, and potential effects of the research on participants and on larger social values.[26] Cassell also depicted the relationship between investigator, research participants, and research in the context of studies ranging from biomedical and psychological experimentation to fieldwork, nonreactive observation, and secondary analyses of data.[103] She characterized the contexts in which investigators have more (or less) power as perceived by participants or have more (or less) control over the context or setting of research. Using a more complex framework, Sieber, too, graphed how the assessment of risk (from mere inconvenience and social risk to legal, psychological, or physical risk) can best be assessed in the context of a scenario that takes into consideration aspects of the research activity (e.g., the research processes, use of research findings), the risk-related factors (e.g., privacy and confidentiality, deception and debriefing), and the vulnerability of the persons and institutions involved (e.g., those visible or public, those engaged in illegal activities).[104]

This chapter benefits from the ideas presented in these frameworks, but presents a three-dimensional model to inform ethical decision making that is more centrally focused on the core elements of the research: the methods, characteristics of the study population, and the type of inquiry. As noted in the introduction to this chapter, the ethical issues raised by the use of various methods are closely tied to the population under study and the type of inquiry. Figure 32.1 depicts the interaction between the degree of substantive sensitivity of the study, the level of methodological intervention, and the degree of vulnerability of the human participants. This three-dimensional model views the potential degree of risk to follow from a combination of the method used, person characteristics, and the nature of the research.

In Figure 32.1, the y axis characterizes the level of methodological intervention in relation to research participants. It varies from no interaction (e.g., the use of extant public data or records), to indirect or direct contact (e.g., survey or interview) to intervention (experiments). This continuum generally reflects the centrality of the intervention or interaction to the definition of human subjects research, as specified in 45 CFR 46.102(f).[6] Methods vary in the level of intervention with human participants (or their environments), and the level of research intervention can introduce risk. However, risk associated with methods is not a function only of the degree of intervention. Methods also vary in the amount of control an investigator has over the potential for risk (e.g., laboratory settings provide for a higher degree of investigator control than field studies) and in the degree of actual invasiveness

(e.g., video recordings in public places can be more invasive than a laboratory intervention on a relatively mundane issue). In selecting methods, investigators should weigh the scientific appropriateness of certain approaches cognizant of the value of minimizing or ameliorating the level of risk.

The x axis is the research population gradient and represents the level of human participant vulnerability. Any number of factors (biological, social, psychological, cultural) may influence where a research participant falls on the continuum. Federal law recognizes the vulnerability of certain populations of study (pregnant women, fetuses, and neonates; prisoners; and children), creating additional regulations for research involving these groups. The representation of participant vulnerability on a continuum allows viewing these and other potentially vulnerable groups (e.g., students, those in low-income brackets) on the same scale. It also permits depicting participants' vulnerability to heightened risks as a function of the characteristics of the population under study as distinct from any normative judgment about the desirability of protecting that population (e.g., studies of doctors engaged in insurance fraud or pharmacists engaged in illegal drug sales) or whether that population should otherwise receive any direct benefit at all. The responsibility of the investigator is to ensure that the vulnerability of human participants is not increased by virtue of being a part of the

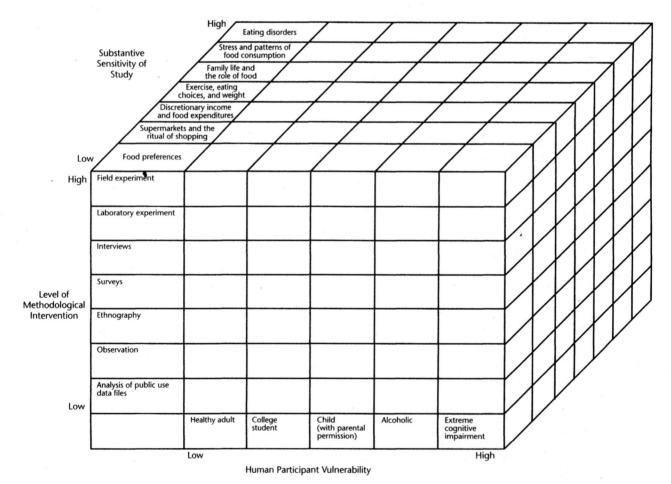

Figure 32.1. Risk in Research as a Function of Substantive Sensitivity of Study, Level of Methodological Intervention, and Human Participant Vulnerability.

research and being willing to contribute to the advancement of important knowledge.

The third dimension (z axis) displays the sensitivity of the study topic using, for heuristic purposes, illustrative studies about human interaction regarding food and consumption behavior. The sensitivity or the invasiveness of the research topic affects the level of risk in behavioral and social science research—from discomfort or embarrassment through anxiety, legal liability, and so forth. Figure 32.1 shows that risk level in matters of substance also interacts with the populations under study and the methods being employed. Although the invasiveness of the inquiry is often viewed alone in an analysis of risk, in reality it operates in concert with other factors that together shape risk.

The three dimensions highlighted above—level of methodological intervention, human participant vulnerability, and sensitivity of the study topic—interact to determine the level of risk. The next sections focus on factors that influence the risk of harm and consider the implications for the informed consent process and issues of confidentiality from the vantage point of different methodological approaches: experimental, observational, survey, interview, ethnographic, and analysis of public data files. The reader should note that although methodologies may overlap in any single study (e.g., the use of observation in experimental research), for purposes of clarity, each method is discussed separately.

Ethical Challenges

Experimental Methods

The experimental method provides a direct way of testing the cause and effect relationship between variables. Behavioral and social science experiments can occur in laboratories or in external field settings, including the school, community center, hospital, workplace, or neighborhood, to name but a few. This method, widely used by both biomedical and social scientists, is defined by the manipulation of a variable of interest, random assignment of participants, comparison of treatment or intervention and control conditions, and control of extraneous factors.

Take, for example, an experiment designed to test cognitive functioning under stress in older adults. The investigator gives experimental participants a task that is designed to tax their working memory and compares the results to those of a control group. First, the introduction of a manipulation of the environment alone raises ethical issues because such an intervention would not otherwise be experienced by the research participants. Because the researcher is changing the situation to which people would ordinarily be exposed, he or she has an obligation both to minimize any risks involved and to make those risks known to potential participants during the informed consent process.

The researcher who introduces and manipulates a variable must take care to examine the nature of the variable—its intensity and duration. In experimental research, investigators search for the level of intensity and duration that will produce an effect akin to what would occur in the lives of participants (referred to as experimental or mundane realism). An intervention may be positive, neutral, or negative and should not be assumed to be adverse. For example, the effect of relaxation exercises on workplace productivity for those in high stress jobs could be a very pleasant and satisfying intervention. The effect of group size and composition on problem solving may be a neutral manipulation. With inter-

ventions that may stimulate adverse states—such as tedium, anger, or performance anxiety—examination of the nature of the variable (both its intensity and duration) provides insights into the amount of invasiveness and its contribution to overall risk. If risk of an adverse state is beyond what might be expected in everyday life, the researcher may reduce the intensity of a planned intervention with the more limited goal of identifying triggers and mechanisms without risking substantial adverse behavior.

In planning and implementing experiments, the investigator needs to consider possible psychological and emotional consequences when germane. How is the manipulation of the situation viewed by the participant? Is the impact of the intervention (whatever its intensity or duration) transient? What will research participants be told about the research in advance of the study? Will debriefing return participants to their preexperimental state? In other words, does the manipulation increase risk for the research participant, and, if so, does the debriefing reduce it?

The design of the experiment can also have an impact on ethical considerations. A long-term sustained intervention may, in some instances, increase risk for research participants. For example, in an experiment designed to test the impact of images of aggression (e.g., shouting, pushing, hitting) on teenage behavior, those images that more closely approximate what teenagers experience in their daily life may pose less risk than those that exceed what they typically experience. Furthermore, the intensity and duration of the exposure may have an impact irrespective of the typicality of the depictions. Repeated exposure to a series of aggressive images may increase the level of fearfulness or of engaging in aggressive behavior. How participants may be affected by repeated exposures will be determined not only by characteristics of the methods, but also by individual factors. In this example, the risk to teenagers who have been abused or live in violent neighborhoods may be different in unknown directions than the risk to teenagers who have not had these experiences (e.g., at-risk teenagers may be desensitized or alternatively reaffirmed by the images).

Field experiments include randomized control trials and quasi-experimental designs that aim to test how modification of conditions can change behaviors or beliefs of individuals or groups. Experiments in the field alter the external environment (e.g., types of drug counseling, alternative strategies for teaching reading) that can affect the lives of those exposed to a treatment or control. The same ethical guidelines that apply to clinical medical trials apply here (e.g., one treatment should not offer more of a known benefit than another). Although experiments in the laboratory allow researchers to achieve a high degree of internal validity through careful controls, field experiments are introduced into real-world settings and thus have the potential for far greater external validity. Field experiments with randomized control designs are much more complex to plan and implement (from access to sites and agreements about the form of a manipulation to continuing follow-up to ensure consistent implementation of the treatment). Quasi-experimental designs are often introduced in the field when the context may require some alteration of a strict experimental design to be feasible. The classic texts by Campbell and Stanley[105] and by Cook and Campbell[106] provide more detailed descriptions of experimental and quasi-experimental design.

A field experiment might compare, for example, a novel intervention aimed at reducing risky sexual behaviors among teens with a control group that receives a standard educational intervention. The introduction of a variable into a natural as opposed to laboratory setting raises some unique ethical challenges: How is the variable introduced into the setting (e.g., individual education sessions or community wide)? Is the intervention visible to others, thus posing additional risks for human participants (e.g., being seen by neighbors or friends entering a clinic for treatment)? Does the intervention have a broader or spillover effect? If so, is the effect transient? Is the effect of the intervention desirable or undesirable? If the experiment is occurring in a natural setting, is there sufficient attention to privacy protection? If people are unaware that the research is occurring, is there sufficient respect for the autonomy of research participants to determine whether they wish to be part of the research? If research participants are members of a vulnerable group (e.g., prisoners, teens, at-risk teens), how, if at all, does this increase risk?

Naturalistic experiments also arise in the conduct of social and behavioral science research. A change in legal regulations about drug use, for example, may provide an apt opportunity for a before-after design or a case-control comparison to sites that have not had such change. Interventions may be person-made (as in the case of a change in regulations, policy, or practice) or may be naturally occurring. A naturally occurring event like a hurricane or other disaster affords an opportunity to study certain aspects of human behavior with a before-after design or through comparison (e.g., a study of the reactions of people at varying distances from the site of a disaster). In such an instance, risk in the form of emotional trauma may vary in terms of research participants' locations. It may be more intrusive to ask people to participate in a study than to observe their interactions with neighbors, police, or clergy. The researcher needs to examine carefully the methods, nature of the inquiry, and participant vulnerability in order to make an assessment regarding ethics in these different situations.[107] Obtaining the input of an independent group of scientists and community members as part of the IRB review process can serve as an important check on the process.[108]

Observational Methods

As with experiments, observational methods can be used in a range of research contexts from the carefully controlled setting of the laboratory to the field. In evaluating level of intrusion or possible risk, most researchers tend to focus on whether the behavior occurs in a public setting. However, the expectations of people in a particular setting also need to be considered. In using observational methods, researchers must consider (1) whether the setting is public or private and (2) whether the behavior is public or private. Although these variables can be placed on a continuum, in Table 32.1 we depict them in a 2 × 2 matrix for illustrative purposes.

Table 32.1 shows the interaction of public-private setting and public-private behavior through an example for each cell. Observations of spectators' consumption of alcohol at a baseball game would be considered public behavior in a public setting. Spectators enter this setting assuming that behavior will be observed by others and possibly even recorded (e.g., in photos or videos by other spectators). Observations of public behavior in a public setting are not considered invasive, and risk is generally considered minimal. However, how the behavior is recorded (e.g., field notes or video recording that serves as a permanent record) could potentially increase the invasiveness of the inquiry and the overall risk, and could make data that are otherwise unidentifiable potentially identifiable, thus transforming the observations into human subjects research as defined in the federal regulations at 45 CFR 46.102(f)(2).[6]

Even behavior in a public setting can easily be considered private when people's expectations change. The public setting–private behavior cell is probably the area that causes most concern for investigators. Behavior in a public setting can be considered public by a researcher, but the expectations of the participants in this setting need to be considered in making decisions about responsibilities to human participants in this research. For example, Internet chat rooms may be considered public settings in that any member of the public can access them and become involved in a conversation. However, a number of these chat room discussions involve highly personal and sensitive matters. Although one might argue that participants should consider their behavior public, their expectations may be otherwise. Humphrey's tearoom trade study,[37] mentioned earlier, provides another example of the public setting–private behavior overlap. Although the setting was a public restroom, most men probably considered their behavior private.

In an Internet chat room, the use of observational methods may involve no interaction or intervention (i.e., when the researcher's identity is concealed and participation is minimal to nonexistent), but the nature of the inquiry may still be considered invasive from the viewpoint of chat room users' expectations of what might reasonably be expected to occur in this situation. Those who are less aware that the setting is public (e.g., an elderly person with less knowledge of the Internet) are more vulnerable than those who realize its public nature. In addition, risk is increased if the sensitivity of the information can potentially harm research participants. If an investigator is monitoring and recording discussions of alcoholism in an Internet chat room, the information could have economic, social, and legal risks for the participant. Researchers can decrease the vulnerability of participants by recording observations in such a way that identities cannot be traced. In addition, although this setting can allow researchers to remain anonymous and this feature of the design can be important in understanding human behavior in real-life situations, the fact that a researcher's presence is unknown increases the level of invasiveness and risk for those involved because their ability to monitor and control self-presentation to fit the context is reduced.

In the private setting–private behavior cell, both setting and expectations combine to increase the potential risk to participants. First, the home itself is generally considered to be a private place. Second, most private behavior occurs in the home. Participants in

Table 32.1

Illustration of Interaction of Public and Private Dimensions in the Observational Method

		Setting	
		Public	*Private*
Behavior	*Public*	Observe alcohol use at baseball game	Observe alcohol use at open-house holiday party
	Private	Observe discussions of alcohol use in Internet chat room	Observe alcohol use in in-home family study

an in-home family study may consider the recording of observations about alcohol use to be intrusive despite their agreement to be involved. Special precautions should be taken to ensure fully informed consent and to plan confidentiality protections in advance. Here, privacy concerns are elevated, but proper informed consent can reduce ethical concerns about overstepping participants' expectations. In addition, taking steps to protect the confidentiality of the data can reduce the risk to participants.

Finally, observations of public behavior in a private setting should also be guided by participants' expectations. Although a home is typically considered private, behavior in the home may be considered "public" if, for example, a homeowner invites residents in the neighborhood into the home. One might reasonably expect that observations of alcohol use by other partygoers at an open-house holiday party could be discussed outside this setting. Still, a researcher's observation and recording of alcohol use at a party may be considered more intrusive than observations by party guests, and how such data are gathered can have different implications for the perceived intrusiveness of the inquiry. Making known a researcher's presence will decrease the perceptions of invasiveness and is more respectful of the autonomy of potential research participants who can decide whether to leave or stay. Acknowledged observation or participant observation in this context gives individuals more control over the situation than if the researcher fully conceals her or his identity. What form the research design should take and what the consent process should be (i.e., how much information should be revealed by the researcher in order to act ethically in obtaining valid data) need careful assessment by the researcher and independent assessment by an IRB, especially if the researcher seeks to waive some or all of the elements of informed consent.

Survey Methods

Survey research methods are widely known in the general public and are used in a range of studies from specific institutional or organizational contexts and small area population studies to major national or international surveys on general adult populations or on specialized populations of adults, children, or youths. Of behavioral and social science methods, survey research may be best known to the public because it is the social science method that has had the widest application outside of the social and behavioral sciences by, for example, commercial, political, and media organizations. The federal government also oversees many large-scale survey research projects. For example, in order to monitor the health and well-being of the population, the government regularly undertakes the National Health Interview Survey.

The level of risk in any survey is affected by several factors that may interact and affect overall risk. Specifically, the factors influencing the risk dimension include questionnaire content (sensitivity), mode of administration, recruitment strategies, mechanisms to increase participation, and the actual survey design (e.g., cross-sectional or longitudinal). Other factors influencing total risk are the population studied, anonymity of the responses, person or entity collecting the data, and data usage and storage. Together, these factors determine the level of risk in a survey. Each is described below.

The factor receiving most attention in survey research is the questionnaire content. Survey methods are used in a variety of substantive areas covering topics ranging from those with little or no sensitivity to those that may be considered highly sensitive. For example, questions about personal health information are generally considered more private or invasive than those that ask about product preference. Similarly, the mode of administration (e.g., telephone, mail, Internet, in person) affects whether participants think the procedure is more or less invasive. Mail surveys, especially anonymous ones addressed to "resident," are less intrusive than a face-to-face interview in the home. Telephone surveys and Internet surveys fall between these two points. Participants may perceive a certain degree of anonymity when responding to Internet surveys, thereby decreasing the perceived level of invasiveness (even if responses could ultimately be traced). From the human participants' perspective, the type of questions asked and how they are administered affect their view of the level of intrusion and the perceived risk associated with the survey.

Although surveys cover full populations under study, typically they are aimed at a sample of a population selected from a specified frame, however it is identified (often that means use of a list of potential participants who have attributes in common). If researchers access a publicly available list (e.g., a phone book) or obtain or construct a list from public information (e.g., a map of housing units in census track areas), participants are less likely to consider this an invasion of privacy because they know that the records are publicly available than if the researcher obtains a private list (e.g., a club membership list) that is not generally available. How potential respondents are identified (that is, the sampling frame from which they are drawn) and how they are approached are important in determining participants' perceptions of invasiveness and potential risk. Being asked to participate in a local or national household survey is less invasive and potentially less anxiety-arousing than being approached to participate in a survey as a cancer survivor or because a person is living in a community in which the water has a high lead content.

The quality of survey research is inextricably tied to the representativeness of the sample. Survey researchers employ a number of techniques in order to improve response rate such as callbacks, persuasive introductory or interviewing scripts, or incentives in the form of payments for research participants' time. Properly employed, these techniques can strengthen response rates without being overly intrusive, coercive, or infringing upon an individual's right to privacy. Interestingly, modern technologies such as unlisted cell phone numbers raise problems in sampling designs that can reduce the quality of the survey and thus, the benefits of conducting the research.

The design of the survey can also affect the potential level of risk. In longitudinal versus cross-section designs, there are many more scientific payoffs and potential benefits in terms of causal modeling and identifying patterns of behavior, but longitudinal research can require more from research participants in the amount of cooperation, and repeated follow-up can raise potential risk. Longitudinal designs that seek participation for long spans of time increase the opportunities for participants to be identified in contrast to cross-sectional designs (i.e., one-time-only collections of data), but sensitivity to how subsequent contacts are made and how data linkages are protected can avert increasing disclosure risk.

The level of potential risk is also affected by whether identifying information is obtained or retained. For example, if random-digit dialing is used in a telephone survey, individuals can remain anonymous. In household surveys, individuals are not anonymous; however, one's responses can be protected by data security and data access plans consonant with the level of sensitivity of the substance of the study. Despite these efforts to protect participants' identity and personal information, other inadvertent disclosures could occur. For example, during a phone or in-home survey, family members may overhear all or part of the conversation and convey that to others. Similarly, research assistants may inadvertently risk identification of participants by sharing examples of interesting cases with others outside the research team. In both instances, the risk level for participants is increased, but the rarity of such events and the nature of the harm or discomfort itself may not generally exceed the everyday standard of minimal risk.

Under federal regulations, surveys of healthy adult populations are exempt from review by IRBs if participation is anonymous and the topic of inquiry presents no more than minimal risk for respondents. Surveys that include identifier information may qualify for expedited review by IRBs if they are on healthy adult populations and if the topic of inquiry and the possibility of information disclosure involve no more than minimal risk. On the other hand, federal rules recognize the inherent vulnerability of children and, as such, require IRB review of surveys involving children. Even with adult populations, however, vulnerability and level of risk may vary. For example, paying low-income persons to participate in a study suggests a different level of potential coercion due to personal characteristics than providing the same payment to a middle-income person, and differential payments can raise questions about just and equitable treatment of human participants. Thus, the vulnerability of the population requires consideration in implementing the survey design and research.

Interview Methods

The level of risk in interviews is affected by many of the same factors as in surveys, such as the content of the questions, the population studied, and how the data are used and stored. There are, however, ethical factors that are more particularistic to the interview method. Surveys that are administered in person raise some of the same concerns. Four issues, in particular, need to be considered: degree of structure in the interview; unanticipated but sensitive responses; disclosure following group interviews; and recruitment through the use of interviews.

In behavioral and social science research, interviews can range from highly structured to unstructured formats. In some research, a list of questions is systematically designed, although not to the level of a survey instrument; in other studies, the interviews may be guided by only a general map. Alternatively, the researcher may prepare a general framework with specific questions that will vary depending on what issues are raised by the respondent in answering earlier questions. Follow-up questions may or may not be specified at the onset, depending upon the research training and tradition in which the investigator is grounded.

As one example, a researcher using a semistructured interview may create an "interview guide" that, for example, lists a range of questions by topic area: introduction (questions about the nature of the study and consent to participate), background (family, friends), and drug use (friends' drug use, personal drug use, multiple drug use), sexual experiences following drug use (who initiated, safe-sex practices). Here, subsequent stages of the interview would be guided by answers earlier in the interview. Questions about multiple drug use would be skipped if respondents indicate that they use only one drug. Similarly, questions about sexual experiences after drug use would be skipped altogether if respondents indicate that they do not use drugs.

In a structured or even a semistructured interview, the questions can be reviewed to determine the level of invasiveness (e.g., the sensitivity of the questions) as well as participant vulnerability (e.g., the appropriateness of the questions given the study population). In an unstructured interview, consideration must be given to the fact that a more open-ended procedure implies less control about what the interviewer might ask or what might be revealed by the participant, even if the level of invasiveness and the participant vulnerability remain unchanged. Unstructured interviews can also provide an opportunity for the interviewer to build rapport and a trusting relationship with research participants, enhancing the experience of participants and the quality of their responses.

Investigators conducting structured or unstructured interviews may be aware of the questions or type of questions they will ask, but respondents may provide unanticipated answers in an interview session. In surveys, the number of open-ended questions is constrained, and responses are typically selected from among those provided. In interviews, on the other hand, response options may not be given, and the length and type of responses may vary considerably. Generally, the response does not raise ethical issues, but it could if the response (1) indicates activity that a researcher is legally required to report (e.g., child abuse) or (2) reveals other sensitive information that should be protected. Given that the respondent freely communicates the information, the response does not per se affect the invasiveness of the inquiry, nor does the intrinsic vulnerability of the participant change. Nevertheless, the method used (here, open-ended interviews) increases the risk for participants. Investigators can decrease risk by indicating in the informed consent process what information can be protected, how it will be protected, and, depending on the topic, whether the researchers are legally required to disclose to authorities any information revealed by the participants.

An additional consideration when evaluating risk in interviews is whether the information will be collected in a group setting. For example, a group interview of early career faculty about professional transitions, coping strategies, multiple time demands, and mixed messages about performance expectations could enhance the quality of the insights and understandings that come from peer interaction; but a group interview could also make these professionals vulnerable were their views or feelings inadvertently to become known. Highly sensitive questions that could be considered invasive typically are not asked by researchers when interviews are conducted in groups, but respondents may provide answers that increase their risk if they assume the session is confidential. Researchers can protect the information provided, but they cannot ensure that other participants will refrain from intentionally or inadvertently disclosing a respondent's answers. Again, the level of risk is affected by the group interview format.

Researchers can decrease risk by describing the extent of the confidentiality protections during the informed consent process and by training interviewers to "head off" responses that increase risk. Similarly, in a group setting, participants' judgments can be influenced by others, and doing so could increase pressure on them to respond, respond in a particular way, or remain in the interview session when they would not do so were they alone. Researchers should consider the impact of subtle group influence on risk and implement steps to decrease it.

Finally, interviews can be used to screen participants for other research studies or follow-up phases of the current study. How, where, and by whom participants are approached can contribute to the invasiveness of the research and the degree of risk. For example, it is less intrusive to approach people by phone than in a waiting room of a health-related facility. However, if research is conducted on low-income residents, a phone may not be available in the home and approaching potential participants at a clinic may be the best way to obtain a representative sample that does not exclude certain populations from the study.

Under this scenario, who should approach these clinic patients? If a health professional conducts the screening, it will probably be considered less intrusive, but these professionals may not have the time if the research protocol is not a part of their job. Also, depending on how the approach is framed, contact by health professionals either could offer more autonomy for potential research participants to consent or refuse to consent, or could lead to undue influence to consent. Alternatively, assuming approval by the clinic, can the researcher approach potential participants in the clinic waiting room? Although the intrusiveness of the inquiry might be slightly higher, overall risk might be decreased by better protecting the identities of research participants. Discussions with a skilled interviewer may actually be a positive experience for participants, especially for those persons who are lonely or need to be heard on an issue. Of course, the positive aspect of an interview experience may also lead participants to reveal more private information, placing more obligations upon the researcher to ensure that all information is appropriately protected and that participants do not increase the risk of any subsequent harm or discomfort by revealing more than they wish others to know.

Participant vulnerability should also be considered in deciding on the best approach: Are people participating because they are ill and think the information learned in the interview will help them, or are they healthy persons who came to the clinic for an annual checkup? It should not, however, be assumed that vulnerable persons are unwilling or unable to discuss or provide information about certain topics. Investigators or IRBs determining that certain issues are off-limits for certain groups can be disrespectful of individuals, limit their autonomy to be part of studies, and reduce the benefit of having certain forms of knowledge on the most vulnerable populations. Taking care to ensure that research procedures do not add to risk does not mean that research topics should be avoided.

Ethnographic Methods

Ethnography is the in-depth study of individuals and groups in their own environments. The method itself involves the use of multiple methods including unstructured interviews, semistructured interviews, unobtrusive observations, participant observation, and document or audiovisual analysis. Although this method is employed by researchers in many disciplines, anthropologists have typically used it most to provide accounts of particular cultures, societies, or communities. Ethnographers may focus on a particular topic in conducting their research (e.g., child-rearing practices), or they may be interested in more holistic study of the context or setting.

Ethnographic methods typically involve more than one research strategy and more than one type of research participant (e.g., drug users, community leaders, health-care workers). In a study of domestic violence in a rural African village, for example, an investigator may begin preliminary work by speaking to people in the community over a period of months to learn about the cultural norms and practices that may contribute to the problem. The investigator may follow the informal discussions with a semistructured interview of couples in the region. Simultaneously, the investigator may observe husband-wife interaction in public places to identify normative practices and the limits of acceptable behavior. Information obtained from ethnographic phases of a study may also suggest culturally sensitive interventions that could be tested in a field experiment.

The ethical issues associated with the use of this method can also be placed within the contours of our model. The invasiveness of the inquiry depends on the subject matter of the research and the vulnerability of the human participants who are the focus of the study. The method itself (or the bundling of methods) may also raise ethical challenges and dilemmas. For example, use of participant observation—especially if the research is conducted over long durations of time—can lead to attachments between the researcher and participants. A researcher studying domestic violence who has created emotional bonds within the community may have access to more and better information from participants. Also, the attachment may increase benefits for participants if they feel more at liberty to share information that previously they have found hard to discuss or disclose (e.g., information regarding abusive experiences, long-held family secrets).

A fundamental feature of the ethnographic method is to build trust between the researcher and the research participants in the study. If rapport is not effectively established, the investigator's presence may lead to perceptions of intrusiveness. Usually, however, the fact that the researcher lives in the community and often does so for a period of time before beginning research—typically in an attempt to identify the research directions, possible participants, and cultural norms—enables the researcher to build trust with community members and may decrease the view that an inquiry, however broad, is invasive.

The degree of risk may also be affected by the level of control inherent in the method itself. For example, the actual beginning and end of the research may not be clear because the researcher may have conversations with community members about their practices and beliefs before deciding where to focus the research. The researcher studying domestic violence may observe and speak to community members regarding views of male and female roles, use of alcohol, and the role of extended family or religion in influencing behavior. At times, conversations may be casual and unrelated to research, may lead to research, or may be a part of the research (in which case the consent of participants should be obtained). In addition, the researcher may come and go from a community over a period of time, at times interviewing people and collecting data and at other times casually observing community members for purposes of deciding the next step in research. Although the nature of the research may signal a need for flexibility with the approach, researchers can decrease risk by ensuring that community members are aware of the research and their roles.

Given the nature of ethnographic research, the pool of human participants is not always identified at the onset. A researcher may begin discussions with community and religious leaders in trying to understand the high incidence of domestic violence in a community, but later move to discussions with employers to determine the role that job-related stress may play. As the researcher becomes immersed in a community and has a better understanding of it, he or she may choose to focus on certain members of the community. As the research progresses, other participants may also be identified. At these points, the researcher needs to engage potential participants in a conversation about the study and ascertain their interest in participating. If the discussions occur over a period of time, the researcher should continue to check the community members' willingness to participate. Thus, more than with other more targeted and time-bound methodologies, the consent process in ethnographic research is dynamic and ongoing—meeting the changing needs and circumstances of the research itself.

The risk associated with the method can be decreased by the use of a continuous consent process, as well as the flexibility to waive written consent when it would be culturally inappropriate, when participants are illiterate, or when use of consent forms could raise undue anxiety or place participants at risk. Indeed, in some cultures, being asked to sign a consent form may be considered an insult as a verbal agreement is valued. In some instances, it may also be appropriate to seek the consent of community leaders or elders, and community norms will suggest when this approach is congruent with human research protection or when it could elevate risk for research participants. Accounting for community norms, attending to the status of particular individuals in the community, and determining how consent should be obtained and whether it should be documented are elements of ethical decision making that can decrease overall risk.

Finally, as with other methods, the procedures used to collect, preserve, or store the information gathered can place participants at risk. Careful consideration of the protections available as well as individual and cultural expectations for the use and storage of the information can reduce the risk for research participants.

Analysis of Public Use Data Files

A great deal of information collected about individuals can be used in secondary analyses to examine important research questions, test rival hypotheses, verify findings, and so forth. For example, a wealth of information collected in periodic government surveys such as the Census, the National Education Longitudinal Survey, or the National Survey of Family Growth and in major national surveys such as the General Social Survey (GSS), the Panel Study of Income Dynamics (PSID), and the National Election Study (NES) can be accessed and used by other researchers. Some surveys like the GSS, the PSID, and the NES are undertaken to create data resources for multiuser analysis; other studies yield public use files that permit secondary study by other investigators (e.g., the National Longitudinal Study of Adolescent Health, the National Longitudinal Survey of Freshmen). The practice of creating public data files allows for greater use of a vast amount of data that would otherwise go unanalyzed and makes better use of limited resources to examine a range of behavioral and social science issues of scientific significance and societal importance.

By definition, public use data files refer to data that have already been collected and stripped of personal identifiers or altered to eliminate identifiable private information. Once these data files have been created and appropriately reviewed by an IRB or, in the case of a government agency, by a disclosure review board, they are no longer considered human subjects research as defined by 45 CFR 46(f),[6,109] although institutional IRBs individually act

on their status.[110] Because public use data provide essentially anonymous information to the secondary analyst, concerns about invasiveness of this work or risk of harm are not at issue, though the research offers general benefits to those whose information contributed to these data sets.

The most challenging ethical issue associated with public data files is their creation; that is, de-identification of the data. Federal agencies, research organizations, and public archives (e.g., the Inter-University Consortium for Political and Social Research) take extreme precautions to de-identify the data before making them publicly available via the Internet or other media. Federal agencies and research archives that are responsible for holding data and making them accessible have the responsibility to ensure that data are de-identified if they are to be in public data files. The agencies and research archives are responsible for removing direct or indirect identifiers which could individually or jointly identify a person, such as detailed geographic information, birth dates, Social Security numbers, and exact income. A number of techniques are used by these data providers to remove both direct and indirect identifiers including eliminating variables entirely, aggregating categories instead of using exact values (e.g., using income brackets) or adding random noise to variables. De-identifying data files can be a complex process, and obtaining the advice or assistance of experts in this area is wise if the data preparation work is not being done by a professional archive or other data provider.

The process of de-identification to permit researchers' access is applicable to other forms of protecting confidential information beyond what is obtained in surveys and other systematic studies. In accordance with provisions in the Health Insurance Portability and Accountability Act of 1996 (HIPAA), researchers may be provided with individual health information without the individual's authorization if the data have been de-identified, an IRB or a privacy review board waives authorization, and the research is of minimal risk.[111,112] Two approaches are available under HIPAA: the first identifies 18 categories of data elements that must be stripped (limiting the usefulness of the data), and the second requires a separate determination by a statistical expert attesting to the fact that the risk of identification from the data being sought is very small.

Although the use of de-identified public data poses little risk, researchers may at times want to combine a public data file with a nonpublic data file. An enhanced file can increase the risk of identifying people, so further analysis of disclosure risk and de-identification are in order if these data are to become public use files. In circumstances in which individuals can be identified through the secondary use of extant data, or through linking of public use data sets that are otherwise de-identified, further data protection procedures are required to reduce disclosure risk. Archives like the Inter-University Consortium for Political and Social Research work with investigators on data preservation, data sharing, and the forms of data release in order to maximize research access when threats of disclosure warrant stronger protections. Restricted use contractual data, site licenses, and secure data enclaves are vehicles for allowing access to identifiable data under strong guarantees of confidentiality.

Cross-Cutting Ethical Issues

The above discussion of ethical considerations, through the lens of the methods used in behavioral and social science research, emphasized issues of consent, privacy and confidentiality, and risk and harm. There are two other cross-cutting issues—deception and incentives—that merit additional consideration because they speak to the autonomy of human participants to determine whether to be part of research. Deception is best understood in the broader context of the amount of information available to research participants and at what point information is revealed consonant with ethical considerations. Incentives, too, have ethical implications because undue incentives may alter or influence the actual autonomy that research participants experience.

Deception

The provision of information about the nature and purposes of the research is intended to be respectful of the autonomy of persons to decide if they wish to be involved in a study and to allow them to make a meaningful decision. There has been a great deal of discussion and debate about the appropriateness of deception— providing misinformation—and the relationship between deception and partial or delayed information about the research. Willingness to participate in research and consent to do so require that research participants understand what they are being asked to do, even if they do not know at the outset the full purpose of the research. As summarized by Sieber,[104] typically researchers using deception seek to do the following: enhance stimulus control or random assignment; study responses to low-frequency events; obtain valid data without serious risk to subjects; or produce data that would otherwise be unobtainable. When deception is used, it is accompanied by debriefing at later stages of the study to inform participants about the fuller purposes of the research.

In *Planning Ethically Responsible Research,* Sieber allowed for the potential use of deception but considered alternatives including simulation studies and role playing.[104] She also set forth options in which information is concealed, but deception does not need to occur. These included informed consent to participate in one of various conditions, consent to be deceived, and consent to waive the right to be informed. The emphasis of these options is to gain agreement to participate, while making research participants aware that information about the study may be incomplete or inaccurate as an essential part of the work.

Federal regulations do allow the use of deception in research. Section 46.116(a)(1) of the federal regulations requires that participants be provided with a statement regarding the purpose of the research and the procedures involved. Yet Section 46.116(d) permits an IRB to waive elements of informed consent (even informed consent altogether) provided the IRB finds and documents that:

1. The research involves no more than minimal risk to the subjects;
2. The waiver or alteration will not adversely affect the rights and welfare of the subjects;
3. The research could not be practically carried out without the waiver or alteration; and
4. Whenever appropriate, the subjects will be provided with additional pertinent information after participation.[6]

Importantly, the regulations attempt to balance the risks to participants (e.g., allowing deception waivers only in minimal risk research that does not affect the welfare of the participants) with the need to understand how human beings behave. For example, an investigator may be interested in examining the effects of mood on memory. Informing participants of the purpose of the study would defeat its purpose. Such a full disclosure, for example, might tell participants something like this:

> In this study, you will first watch a videotape of either a happy or sad film in order to put you in a good or bad mood. Then you will see a list of words that you will rate on a pleasantness scale. We don't really care about the ratings but we want you to think about the words. Then you will do some math computations that we really don't care about either, but we need some time to pass for you to forget some of the words. Then we will test your memory for the words. We are trying to discover the relationship between mood and memory for items that have the same or opposite feeling as the mood you are in.[113]

Instead of such a frank and self-defeating disclosure of the study's aims, a researcher could inform the participant about the procedures involved and any risk associated with those procedures, and something about the overall goals of the study (i.e., to better understand memory), leaving the explanation of the full purpose until later in the study.

It is important to note that deception in research can be used only if the research procedures pose no more than minimal risk and if the information cannot practicably be obtained in another way. In addition, the investigator must make a case to the IRB and obtain its approval before deception (or delayed disclosure) may be used in research. The federal regulations, the principles articulated in the Belmont Report, and professional codes of ethics provide a framework for the investigator and IRB members when evaluating the risk and benefit to participants. Irrespective of the methodology, evaluating the sensitivity of the study topic and participant vulnerability can assist investigators and the IRB in determining whether a waiver of informed consent is appropriate.

Allowing the use of deception within ethical boundaries can yield important insights into human behavior. Indeed, in both biomedical and social science research involving experimentation, participants typically are not informed whether they will participate in the treatment or the control/placebo condition. Deception used for the purpose of gaining an individual's participation in research or obtaining information that participants do not wish to divulge is, however, outside of the boundaries of ethical research.

Incentives

Incentives should compensate participants for their time and serve as a means to thank them for participating, but must be structured such that they do not coerce participation. Researchers should consider when to pay participants, how often payments are to be made, how much of an incentive to provide, and what the meaning of the incentive is. Incentives can be financial or nonfinancial (gift certificates, provision of a service), and the type of incentive may have different meaning for different groups of people. For example, a $10 payment in cash may not be excessive in the United States, but may be so in a developing country. A lottery ticket may be an appropriate, inadequate, or excessive incentive depending on a participant's knowledge regarding the odds of winning. Similarly, deferring all payments until the end of the study may encourage participants to continue to expend the time, but it could also induce participants to complete a study when they would otherwise prefer to terminate their participation. Smaller incentives throughout the study might provide the right balance and decrease participant vulnerability.

In some instances, group-based incentives may be more appropriate. For example, when studying student behavior in a classroom, it may be more ethical to provide incentives to the entire class, rather than individual students. In this way, all students benefit, even those who do not wish to participate. In addition, when studying groups of any size, researchers must be aware that the decisions of a few (especially a vocal or popular few) may have a significant impact on others' decisions to participate (probably of most concern when studying adolescents). Although some degree of peer influence is probably acceptable, the researcher must consider whether the pressure to participate is a factor in the group process.

It is important to consider that incentives may be needed in order to ensure that the study population is sufficiently representative of the larger population from which participants are drawn. Just as vulnerable populations may be overincluded in studies because they are readily accessible or easier to manipulate, some populations may be underincluded because they do not have the wherewithal to travel to a research site, donate their time, or find the help they need with child care or elder care in order to participate. Incentives can serve to adjust for such imbalances. Because researchers are ethically obligated to ensure that the sample size is adequate for the research, incentives may ensure that the research as a whole is not undermined. Finding the right balance for encouraging, but not coercing, participation may not be easy, but it is ethically necessary.

Evolving Challenges

At any point in time, new scientific issues and methodological and technological advancements can raise ethical considerations in the conduct of human research that are uncharted, ambiguous, or controversial. As in the biomedical sciences, behavioral and social sciences face new ethical challenges, or understand old challenges differently, in the course of advancing knowledge in these fields. In our prior discussion of the use of observational methods in behavioral and social sciences research, for example, we raised issues regarding how investigators' use of video recording devices in public places, even when there is otherwise no interaction or intervention, changes the research from exempt to classified as human subjects research, as defined by 45 CFR 46, because recorded data are more readily identifiable. When new challenges first surface, ethical issues can seem formidable; typically, however, they become more tractable as scientists and those with expertise in the ethics of research unpack issues of risk of harm, privacy and confidentiality, and requirements of consent or the appropriateness of its waiver. A few illustrations make this point.

Internet Research

The Internet has expanded opportunities both to conduct research (e.g., surveys, experiments) and to study online behavior and human interaction. Earlier, we noted some of the complexities involved in using observational methods in the context of Internet chat rooms and considered the potential intrusiveness of such observation as well as the conditions under which Internet be-

haviors might be considered public or private. The Internet permits research on a global scale using extant data sources, using the Internet as a tool to collect data, and using the Internet context to study behavior in real-time and from web-based archives (e.g., transaction logs). Although the rapid transmission of information across time and space increases the salience of ethical considerations, the ethical issues that need to be weighed are not in general unique to Internet research.

Some Internet-based research presents few human research protection issues at all. If the data already exist as public records, there may be issues of appropriate reporting, but research on such records would typically fall outside of the regulatory definition of research with humans. In other instances, using the Internet to conduct research involves human research protection issues, including consent, confidentiality, and a weighing of benefits and risks. For example, when research is being conducted online, is awareness and continued participation a sufficient indicator of consent? Are there times when the sensitivity of the inquiry requires affirmative agreement to participate (for example, activating a radio button)? How can consent be documented especially given preferences for online anonymity and the frequent online use of pseudonyms? Are there areas in which Internet technology could increase risk (e.g., sharing of e-mail accounts, saving of documents by service providers)? And, do confidentiality protections need to be strengthened given the sensitivity of the data and the possibilities of compromising data security during data transmission or storage?

Internet technology also opens up new opportunities to study human behavior or interaction online. The nature of the Internet environment being studied; whether it might be presumed to be public or private (e.g., the rules governing the listserv, chat room, or discussion board); whether consent can or will be obtained; whether the confidentiality of the information can be protected (e.g., password protection for computers, encryption of data); and even how much the researcher reveals about her or his identity or presence all come into play in the ethical design and implementation of such research. The boundary between public and private is a particularly complex determination to be made in studying Internet communities, but rules of thumb are already being articulated to permit ethically responsible research in this environment (e.g., whether registration is required to be part of the forum; how many participants are in the forum; what are participants' perceptions of privacy).[114]

Most helpful in this rapidly emerging area of research on the Internet are the issues raised for investigators and for IRBs in reports by the American Association for the Advancement of Science (AAAS)[115] and the American Psychological Association (APA).[116] The AAAS and the APA reports point out the opportunities of using and collecting data and studying human interaction on the Internet. The AAAS report also addresses the basic principles of conducting human subjects research (e.g., informed consent, benefits and risk, privacy and confidentiality) in the context of this technology and also offers recommendations for undertaking research on the Internet and for undertaking studies and education that can further advance knowledge about human research ethics. The APA report, too, examines the benefits and challenges of conducting research on the Internet and provides advice on a wide-ranging set of issues from identifying potential harms and debriefing procedures to taking precautions when dealing with research involving minors.

Geospatial Measurements and Other Tracking Methods

In recent years, technological advancements in remote sensing and global positioning systems have permitted fine-grained geospatial measurements of latitude and longitude coordinates that allow for new and important studies of individuals over time and space.[117] Geospatial data on individuals' residences, workplaces, schools, or other locations are being linked with social surveys and other forms of social, environmental, and health data to study a range of issues from the distribution or transmission of disease[118] to how use of time is affected by travel and mobility patterns between locations.[119] Such data have enormous scientific potential, but also have embedded in them considerable potential for personal identification. In addition, unlike identifiers like name or Social Security number that can be more readily stripped from data sets, geospatial coordinates are themselves important data that can help to explain important behaviors and interactions and thus need to be preserved at some fine-grained level (even after statistical manipulation and masking) in order to remain of use.

As geospatial research has progressed, behavioral and social scientists are giving considerable attention to the ethical issues involved in working with such data aligned with other social data and how to maximize the scientific benefits of using this information while protecting the privacy of research participants or the confidentiality of the information obtained.[120] Primary data producers and researchers are addressing issues of consent and confidentiality at the data acquisition stage, and they and secondary users are examining the specification of strong data disclosure plans and strategies that can allow for meaningful data use while protecting data confidentiality. Because highly sensitive data can be involved, licensing agreements, enclaves that provide restricted access, and other mechanisms that maximize use yet minimize risk are being assessed by the behavioral and social science research community, including, in 2006–2007, the National Academies' Panel on Confidentiality Issues Arising from the Integration of Remotely Sensed and Self-Identifying Data.[121]

Although advanced technologies allow for the collection and preservation of very large amounts of geospatial measurements over large spans of geography, the ethical issues of confidentiality and risk reduction are akin to those that the behavioral and social sciences have been considering about microlevel data linkages for over a decade.[122] Even in this context, much research using such measurements is of minimal risk (depending upon the nature of the inquiry and the strength of the data protection plan). Yet behavioral and social scientists working in this milieu are giving considerable attention to how best to protect confidentiality and promote data use.

Beyond geospatial measurements, there are other new technologies for tracking behavior that have scientific potential for studying human interaction and social exchange. Some investigators have research participants use wearable computers to study how social relationships build and networks are formed. Sensor devices in computers permit recording sound, movement, and geographic locations with essentially continuous, fine time resolution for long periods of time over potentially large samples.[122,123] Researchers working in this domain are addressing both privacy and confidentiality concerns (for example, they intend to reduce privacy concerns by focusing on the patterns of talk and not the content of the talk). Some of the mechanisms being considered and honed for addressing privacy and confidentiality issues with geospatial data would have obvious relevance here.

Third Parties

The very nature of behavioral and social science research aims to understand how people act in their social contexts. For example, in order to fully comprehend the initiation and maintenance of drug use by young adults, a researcher may ask research participants about relationships with friends and family; contacts with social institutions such as a social or academic club, sports organization, or church; the strength of these associations; and the quality of social networks and relationships. The goal of such questions is to understand humans and their life circumstances, even though, in so doing, information about others is gathered from research participants in order to gain a more complete picture of these person's lives.

In 2001, a controversial case raised questions about the status of this information. The case, involving an adult daughter who provided a personal health history that included information about her father, raised questions about the appropriateness of providing this information without the father's consent. The term *third party* was used in this context to refer to the father, someone who was referenced by a research participant. Irrespective of particular aspects of this incident, the issue that became high profile was whether those who are referenced become research participants because someone in the study provided personal, identifiable information concerning them. The crux of the debate was about whether such persons met the regulatory definition of human subjects, and thus were entitled to the protections afforded by informed consent (unless a case is made for its waiver).

There is good reason to protect personal information provided by research participants—whether it is only about themselves or in relation to others in their social sphere. There is also good reason in terms of the integrity of research process and trust in science, as well as commitments to human participants, to be circumspect about alerting the identified human subjects in research. First, human subjects may be at increased risk if the fact of their participation in a study is known (e.g., study of victims in abusive marriage)—a necessity if third parties were required to give consent. Second, revealing participation of human subjects to others intrudes upon research participants' privacy and the confidential nature of information provided during the course of research. Thus, care must be taken to ensure that the rights of and responsibilities to human subjects are not compromised or eclipsed in considering whether consent from third parties should be sought.

The National Human Research Protections Advisory Commission (NHRPAC)[125]—the first advisory committee established in 2000 by then DHHS Secretary Donna Shalala to advise the Office for Human Research Protections—provided in our view sound recommendations about third parties, although the issue still remains unresolved. The NHRPAC clarification states that "neither reference to a third party in a research design, nor the recording of information about a third party in research records suggests that a third party must be regarded as a research subject." NHRPAC allowed for the possibility that third parties might be human subjects, but saw this determination to be a dynamic one to be made by IRBs based on the substance of the research and not on the fact that personal information provided by research participants may also be considered personal information relevant to others.

In locating the determination with IRBs, the NHRPAC statement makes clear that third parties who are referenced in research are not necessarily considered human subjects but that third parties may become human subjects if the IRB, through careful analysis of a number of factors, determines that the focus of the research is really also on the third party and not on (or not only on) the designated human subject. NHRPAC's statement also makes clear that the requirement of consent, or waiver of consent, pertains only to human subjects of research as defined by 45 CFR 46, and not to third parties unless IRBs determine that these third parties are human subjects as well.

Although this issue remains unresolved from a federal regulatory point of view, the thrust of the NHRPAC recommendation is compatible with the general emphasis on individuals as human research participants in 45 CFR 46, delegating to IRBs the final determination in contested or highly ambiguous circumstances as to when multiple parties are the subjects of research. In behavioral and social science research, multiple parties or groups (e.g., studies of gangs, work teams, governance boards) may be the subjects of research. Couples and family research, for example, can raise complex issues regarding privacy, confidentiality, and consent accorded to each individual while still being respectful of the family unit under study.[126] Thus, behavioral and social scientists have experience in protecting multiple human subjects under circumstances where more than one party is the subject of the research.

Conclusion

There is no doubt that new research questions, contexts of study, or technologies will raise new questions and challenge the best of investigators' ethical judgments. To develop researcher savvy on ethical issues, it remains important to include training in ethics and human research protection as an integral part of research training. It is also important to foster the empirical study of ethical issues so that decisions about consent, risk perception, potential for harm, strategies for risk reduction, and so forth can be assessed based on meaningful data. Ethical decision making is an ongoing, dynamic process that can require of researchers and research fields extrapolation and translation of ethical principles to addressing new research questions, examining new or rapidly changing circumstances or contexts for research, or using new research capacities. To the extent that behavioral and social scientists embed ethical considerations in the ongoing design and implementation of methods, they can achieve the dual goals of advancing science and protecting human participants in their work.

Acknowledgments

This chapter benefited from the ideas and discussions of the Social and Behavioral Sciences Working Group on Human Research Protections supported by a contractual services agreement from the Office of Behavioral and Social Sciences Research, National Institutes of Health, to the first author and chair of the Working Group.

References

1. American Psychological Association. *Ethical Principles of Psychologists and Code of Conduct. American Psychologist* 2002;57:1060–73. [Online] 2002. Available: http://www.apa.org/ethics/code2002.pdf.
2. American Sociological Association. *Code of Ethics.* Washington, D.C.: American Sociological Association; 1997. [Online] 1999. Available: http://www.asanet.org/galleries/default-file/Code%20of%20Ethics.pdf.
3. American Anthropological Association. *Code of Ethics of the American Anthropological Association.* Arlington, Va.: American Anthropological Association; 1998. [Online] 1998. Available: http://www.aaanet.org/committees/ethics/ethicscode.pdf.
4. American Political Science Association. *A Guide to Professional Ethics in Political Science.* Washington, D.C.: American Political Science Association; 1998. [Online] Available: http://www.apsanet.org/imgtest/ethicsguideweb.pdf.
5. The National Commission for the Protection of Human Subjects of Biomedical and Behavioral Research. *The Belmont Report: Ethical Principles and Guidelines for the Protection of Human Subjects of Research.* Washington, D.C.: Department of Health, Education and Welfare; DHEW Publication OS 78-0012 1978. [Online] April 18, 1979. Available: http://www.hhs.gov/ohrp/humansubjects/guidance/belmont.htm.
6. Department of Health and Human Services, Office for Human Research Protections. The Common Rule, Title 45 (Public Welfare), Code of Federal Regulations, Part 46 (Protection of Human Subjects). [Online] June 23, 2005. Available: http://www.hhs.gov/ohrp/humansubjects/guidance/45cfr46.htm.
7. Gerstein DR, Luce RD, Smelser NJ, Sperlich S, eds. *The Behavioral and Social Sciences: Achievements and Opportunities.* Washington, D.C.: National Academy Press; 1988.
8. Smelser NJ, Bates PB, eds. *The International Encyclopedia of the Social and Behavioral Sciences.* London, UK: The Elsevier Science Limited; 2001.
9. Office of Behavioral and Social Sciences Research, National Institutes of Health. *A Definition of Behavioral and Social Sciences Research for the National Institutes of Health.* Bethesda, Md.: NIH; 2001. [Online] Available: http://obssr.od.nih.gov/Content/About_OBSSR/BSSR_Definition/.
10. Wax ML, Cassell J, eds. *Federal Regulations: Ethical Issues and Social Research.* Boulder, Colo.: Westview Press; 1979.
11. Beauchamp TL, Faden RR, Wallace RJ Jr, Walters L, eds. *Ethical Issues in Social Science Research.* Baltimore, Md.: Johns Hopkins University Press; 1982.
12. Sieber JE, ed. *The Ethics of Social Research: Surveys and Experiments.* New York, N.Y.: Springer-Verlag; 1982.
13. Sieber JE, ed. *The Ethics of Social Research: Fieldwork, Regulation, and Publication.* New York, N.Y.: Springer-Verlag, 1982.
14. Citro CF, Ilgen DR, Marrett CB, eds. *Protecting Participants and Facilitating Social and Behavioral Sciences Research.* Washington, D.C.: The National Academies Press; 2003.
15. Rosenthal R, Rosnow RL, eds. *Artifact in Behavioral Research.* New York, N.Y.: Academic Press; 1969.
16. Rosenthal R. *Experimenter Effects in Behavioral Research.* New York, N.Y.: Appleton-Century-Crofts; 1966.
17. Duncan S Jr, Rosenberg MJ, Finkelstein J. The paralanguage of experimental bias. *Sociometry* 1969;32:207–19.
18. Rosenthal R, Rosnow RL. *The Volunteer Subject.* New York, N.Y.: John Wiley & Sons; 1975.
19. Alexander CN Jr, Sagatun I. An attributional analysis of experimental norms. *Sociometry* 1973;36:127–42.
20. Rosenberg MJ. The conditions and consequences of evaluation apprehension. In: Rosenthal R, Rosnow RL, eds. *Artifact in Behavioral Research.* New York, N.Y.: Academic Press; 1969:279–349.

21. Orne MT. On the social psychology of the psychological experiment: With particular reference to demand characteristics and their implications. *American Psychologist* 1962;17:776–83.

22. Orne MT. Demand characteristics and the concept of quasi-controls. In: Rosenthal R, Rosnow RL, eds. *Artifact in Behavioral Research*. New York, N.Y.: Academic Press; 1969:132–79.

23. Blass T. *The Man Who Shocked the World: The Life and Legacy of Stanley Milgram*. New York, N.Y.: Basic Books; 2004.

24. Kelman HC. *A Time to Speak: On Human Values and Social Research*. San Francisco, CA.: Jossey Bass Inc.; 1968.

25. Nelkin D. Forbidden research: Limits to inquiry in the social sciences. In: Beauchamp TL, Faden RR, Wallace RJ Jr, Walters L, eds. *Ethical Issues in Social Science Research*. Baltimore, Md.: Johns Hopkins University Press; 1982:163–73.

26. Kelman HC. Ethical issues in different social science methods. In: Beauchamp TL, Faden RR, Wallace RJ Jr, Walters L, eds. *Ethical Issues in Social Science Research*. Baltimore, Md.: Johns Hopkins University Press; 1982:40–98.

27. Milgram S. Behavioral study of obedience. *Journal of Abnormal and Social Psychology* 1963;67:371–8.

28. Milgram S. *Obedience to Authority*. New York, N.Y.: Harper & Row; 1974.

29. Baumrind D. Nature and definition of informed consent in research involving deception. In: National Commission for the Protection of Human Subjects of Biomedical and Behavioral Research. *The Belmont Report: Ethical Principles and Guidelines for the Protection of Human Subjects of Research*. Washington, D.C.: U.S. Government Printing Office (DHEW OS 78–0012); 1978:Appendix II, 23.1–23.71.

30. Baumrind D. Some thoughts on ethics of research: After reading Milgram's "Behavioral Study of Obedience." *American Psychologist* 1964;19:421–3.

31. Milgram S. Issues in the study of obedience: A reply to Baumrind. *American Psychologist* 1964;19:848–52.

32. Baumrind D. Research using intentional deception: Ethical issues revisited. *American Psychologist* 1985;40:165–74.

33. Elms EC. Keeping research honest: Justifying conditions for social scientific research strategies. In: Beauchamp TL, Faden RR, Wallace RJ Jr, Walters L, eds. *Ethical Issues in Social Science Research*. Baltimore, Md.: Johns Hopkins University Press; 1982:232–45.

34. Zimbardo PG, Haney C, Banks WC, Jaffe D. The psychology of imprisonment: Privation, power, and pathology. In: Rubin Z, ed. *Doing Unto Others*. Englewood Cliffs, N.J.: Prentice Hall; 1974:61–73.

35. Zimbardo PG. On the ethics of intervention in human psychological research: With special reference to the Stanford Prison Experiment. *Cognition* 1973;2:243–56.

36. Reynolds PD. *Ethical Dilemmas and Social Science Research*. San Francisco, Calif.: Jossey-Bass; 1979:133–9.

37. Humphreys L. *Tearoom Trade: Impersonal Sex in Public Places*. Chicago, Ill.: Aldine; 1970.

38. Sieber JE. Ethical dilemmas in social research. In: Sieber JE, ed. *The Ethics of Social Research: Surveys and Experiments*. New York, N.Y.: Springer-Verlag; 1982:1–29, p.1–3.

39. Warwick DP. Types of harm in social research. In: Beauchamp TL, Faden RR, Wallace RJ Jr, Walters L, eds. *Ethical Issues in Social Science Research*. Baltimore, Md.: Johns Hopkins University Press; 1982: 101–24, pp. 107–9.

40. Humphreys L. Social science: Ethics of research [letter]. *Science* 1980;207:712–3.

41. Canter MB, Bennett BE, Jones SE, Nagy TF. *Ethics for Psychologists: A Commentary on the APA Ethics Code*. Washington, D.C.: American Psychological Association; 1994.

42. Pope KS, Vetter VA. Ethical dilemmas encountered by members of the American Psychological Association: A national survey. *American Psychologist* 1992;47:397–411.

43. American Psychological Association. *Ethical Standards of Psychologists*. Washington, D.C.: American Psychological Association; 1953.

44. American Psychological Association, Ad Hoc Committee on Ethical Standards in Psychological Research. *Ethical Principles in the Conduct of Research With Human Subjects*. Washington, D.C.: American Psychological Association; 1973.

45. American Psychological Association. *Ethical Standards of Psychologists*. Washington, D.C.: American Psychological Association; 1972.

46. American Psychological Association. Ethical principles of psychologists. *American Psychologist* 1981;36:633–8.

47. American Psychological Association. *Ethical Principles in the Conduct of Research With Human Participants*. Washington, D.C.: American Psychological Association; 1982.

48. American Psychological Association. Ethical principles of psychologists and code of conduct. *American Psychologist* 1992;47: 1597–1611.

49. Sales BD, Folkman F, eds. *Ethics in Research With Human Participants*. Washington, D.C.: American Psychological Association; 2000.

50. Blank PD, Bellack AS, Rosnow RL, Rotheram-Borus MJ, Schooler NR. Scientific rewards and conflicts of ethical choices in human subjects research. *American Psychologist* 1992;47:959–65.

51. Rhoades LJ. *A History of the American Sociological Association: 1905–1980*. Washington, D.C.: American Sociological Association; 1981:45, 55.

52. Rosich KJ. *A History of the American Sociological Association: 1981–2004*. Washington, D.C.: American Sociological Association; 2005:10.

53. American Anthropological Association. Statement on Problems of Anthropological Research and Ethics. Washington, D.C.: American Anthropological Association; 1967. [Online] Available: http://www.aaanet.org/stmts/ethstmnt.htm.

54. American Anthropological Association. Principles of Professional Responsibility. Washington, D.C.: American Anthropological Association; 1971. [Online] Available: http://www.aaanet.org/stmts/ethstmnt.htm.

55. Hill JN. The committee on ethics: Past, present, and future. In: Cassell J, Jacobs S, eds. *Handbook on Ethical Issues in Anthropology* (Special Publication of the American Anthropological Association, No. 23). Washington, D.C.: American Anthropological Association; 1987. [Online] Available: http://www.aaanet.org/committees/ethics/ch2.htm.

56. Fluehr-Lobban C, ed. *Ethics and the Profession of Anthropology: Dialogue for a New Era*. Philadelphia, Pa.: University of Pennsylvania Press; 1991.

57. American Political Science Association Committee on Professional Standards and Responsibilities. Ethical problems of academic political scientists. *PS* 1968;1:3–29.

58. Reynolds PD, Frankel MS. Codes of ethics in the social sciences: Two recent surveys. *Newsletter on Science, Technology, and Human Values* 1977;18:15–9.

59. Carroll JD, Knerr, CR. A report of the APSA confidentiality in social science research data project. *PS* 1975;8: 258–61.

60. Carroll JD, Knerr CR. The APSA confidentiality in social science research project: A final report. *PS* 1976;9:416–9.

61. Fluehr-Lobban C. Informed consent in anthropological research: We are not exempt. *Human Organization* 1994;53:1–9.

62. Gray BH. Human subjects review committees and social research. In: Wax ML, Cassell J, eds. *Federal Regulations: Ethical Issues and Social Research*. Boulder, Colo.: Westview Press; 1979:43–59.

63. Gray BH. The regulatory context of social and behavioral research. In: Beauchamp TL, Faden RR, Wallace RJ Jr, Walters L, eds. *Ethical Issues in Social Science Research*. Baltimore, Md.: Johns Hopkins University Press; 1982:329–55.

64. U.S. Public Health Service. PPP #129, February 8, 1966.

65. Patullo EL. Modesty is the best policy: The federal role in social research. In: Beauchamp TL, Faden RR, Wallace RJ Jr, Walters L, eds.

Ethical Issues in Social Science Research. Baltimore, Md.: Johns Hopkins University Press; 1982:373–415.

66. McCarthy CR. The institutional review board: Its origins, purpose, function, and future. In: Weisstub DN, ed. *Research on Human Subjects: Ethics, Law and Public Policy.* Oxford: Pergamon Press; 1998:301–17.

67. Oakes JM. Risks and wrongs in social science research. *Evaluation Review* 2002;26:443–79.

68. Singer E, Levine FJ. Protection of human research: Recent developments and future prospects for the social sciences. *Public Opinion Quarterly* 2003;67:148–64.

69. Sieber JE, Plattner S, Rubin P. How (not) to regulate social and behavioral research. *Professional Ethics Report* 2002;15(2):1–4.

70. National Research Council. *Expanding Access to Research Data: Reconciling Risks and Opportunities.* Washington, D.C.: The National Academies Press; 2005.

71. Singer E. Informed consent procedures in surveys: Some reasons for minimal effects on response. In: Wax ML, Cassell J, eds. *Federal Regulations: Ethical Issues and Social Research.* Boulder, Colo.: Westview Press; 1979:185–216.

72. Singer E. Informed consent: Consequences for response rate and response quality in social surveys. *American Sociological Review* 1978;43:144–62.

73. Singer E. The effect of informed consent procedures on respondents' reactions to surveys. *The Journal of Consumer Research* 1978;5:49–57.

74. Singer E. Public reaction to some ethical issues of social research: Attitudes and behaviors. *The Journal of Consumer Research* 1984;11: 501–9.

75. Ellikson PL, Hawes JA. Active vs. passive methods for obtaining parental consent. *Evaluation Review* 1989;13:45–55.

76. Turner AG. What subjects of survey research believe about confidentiality. In: Sieber JE, ed. *The Ethics of Social Research: Surveys and Experiments.* New York, N.Y.: Springer-Verlag; 1982:151–65.

77. Boruch RF, Cecil JS. On solutions to some privacy problems engendered by federal regulation and social custom. In: Wax ML, Cassell J, eds. *Federal Regulations: Ethical Issues and Social Research.* Boulder, Colo.: Westview Press; 1979:173–84.

78. Singer E. Informed consent and survey response: A summary of the empirical literature. *Journal of Official Statistics* 1993;9:361–75.

79. Singer E, Von Thurn DR, Miller ER. Confidential assurances and response: A quantitative review of the experimental literature. *Public Opinion Quarterly* 1995;59:66–77.

80. Singer E. Principles and practices related to scientific integrity. In: Groves RM, Fowler FJ Jr., Couper MP, Lepkowski JM, Singer E, Tourangeau R. *Survey Methodology.* Hoboken, N.J.: John Wiley & Sons; 2004:345–76.

81. Fisher CB, Higgins-D'Alessandro A, Rau JB, Belanger S. Referring and reporting research participants at risk: Views from urban adolescents. *Child Development* 1996;67:2086–2100.

82. Bruzzese JM, Fisher CB. Assessing and enhancing the research consent capacity of children and youth. *Applied Developmental Science* 2003;7:13–26.

83. Hull SC, Glanz K, Steffen A, Wifond BS. Recruitment approaches for family studies. *IRB: Ethics and Human Research* 2004;26(4):12–8.

84. Bell J, Whiton J, Connelly S. Final Report: Evaluation of NIH Implementation of Section 491 of the Public Health Service Act, Mandating a Program of Protection for Research Subjects. Arlington, Va.: James Bell Associates; 1998.

85. Gray BH, Cooke RA, Tannenbaum AS. Research involving human subjects. *Science* 1978;201:1094–1101.

86. Gray BH. Institutional review boards as an instrument of assessment: Research involving human subjects in the U.S. *Science, Technology, and Human Values* 1978;4:34–46.

87. National Bioethics Advisory Commission. *Ethical and Policy Issues in Research Involving Human Participants: Vols. I, II.* Bethesda, Md.: NBAC; 2001.

88. Office of Inspector General, Department of Health and Human Services. *Institutional Review Boards: A Time for Reform.* OEI-01-97-00193. Washington, D.C.: DHHS; 1998. [Online] June 1998. Available: http://oig.hhs.gov/oei/reports/oei-01-97-00193.pdf.

89. Ceci SJ, Peters D, Plotkin J. Human subjects review, personal values, and the regulation of social science research. *American Psychologist* 1985;40:994–1002.

90. Hayes GJ, Hayes SC, Dykstra T. A survey of university institutional review boards: Characteristics, policies, procedures. *IRB: A Review of Human Subjects Research* 1995;17(3):1–6.

91. Wagner TH, Bhandari A, Chadwick GL, Nelson DK. The cost of operating institutional review boards (IRBs). *Academic Medicine* 2003;6:638–44.

92. Keith-Spiegel P, Koocher GP, Tabachnick B. What scientists want from their research ethics committee. *Journal of Empirical Research on Human Research Ethics* 2006;1(1):67–92.

93. Burris S, Moss K. U.S. health researchers review their ethics review boards: A qualitative study. *Journal of Empirical Research on Human Research Ethics* 2006;1(2):39–58.

94. Journal of Empirical Research on Human Research Ethics (JERHRE). [Online] Available: http://www.csueastbay.edu/JERHRE/.

95. Tashakkori A, Teddle C, eds. *Handbook of Mixed Methods in Social and Behavioral Research.* Thousand Oaks, Calif.: Sage; 2003.

96. Levine RJ. Similarities and differences between biomedical and behavioral research. Paper prepared for and published in agenda books for the National Commission for the Protection of Human Subjects of Biomedical and Behavioral Research, July 16, 1976.

97. Levine RJ. *Ethics and Regulation of Clinical Research,* 2nd ed. New Haven, Conn.: Yale University Press; 1986.

98. Macklin R. The problem of adequate disclosure in social science research. In: Beauchamp TL, Faden RR, Wallace RJ Jr, Walters L, eds. *Ethical Issues in Social Science Research.* Baltimore, Md.: Johns Hopkins University Press; 1982:193–214.

99. Diener E, Crandal R. *Ethics in Social and Behavioral Research.* Chicago, Ill.: University of Chicago Press; 1978.

100. Sieber JE. Planning research: Basic ethical decision-making. In: Sales BD, Folkman F, eds. *Ethics in Research With Human Participants.* Washington, D.C.: American Psychological Association; 2000: 13–26, p. 14.

101. Social and Behavioral Sciences Working Group on Human Research Protections. Risk and Harm, 2004. [Online] Available: http://www.aera.net/humansubjects/risk-harm.pdf.

102. Labott SM, Johnson TP. Psychological and social risks of behavioral research. *IRB: Ethics and Human Research* 2004;26(3):11–5.

103. Cassell J. Does risk-benefit analysis apply to moral evaluation of social research? In: Beauchamp TL, Faden RR, Wallace RJ Jr, Walters L, eds. *Ethical Issues in Social Science Research.* Baltimore, Md.: Johns Hopkins University Press; 1982:144–62.

104. Sieber JE. *Planning Ethically Responsible Research: A Guide for Students and Internal Review Boards.* Newbury Park, Calif.: Sage Publications; 1992:80–95.

105. Campbell DT, Stanley JC. *Experimental and Quasi-Experimental Designs for Research.* Chicago, Ill.: Rand McNally College Publishing; 1966.

106. Cook TD, Campbell DT. *Quasi-Experimentation: Design and Analysis Issues.* Chicago, Ill.: Houghton Mifflin Company; 1979.

107. Collogan LK, Tuma FK, Fleischman AR. Research with victims of disaster: Institutional review board considerations. *IRB: Ethics and Human Research* 2004;26(4):9–11.

108. Marshall PA, Rotimi C. Ethical challenges in community-based research. American *Journal of the Medical Sciences* 2001;322: 241–5.

109. National Human Research Protection Advisory Committee. Recommendations on Public Use Data Files, 2002. [Online] Available: http://www.hhs.gov/ohrp/nhrpac/documents/dataltr.pdf.

110. University of Wisconsin's Human Research Protections Program. Working With an Existing Data Set. [Online] Available: http://www.grad.wisc.edu/hrpp/view.php?id=10132&f=htm.

111. National Institutes of Health. *Institutional Review Boards and the HIPAA Privacy Rule.* NIH Publication No. 03–5428. Bethesda, MD: National Institutes of Health; 2003.

112. de Wolf VA, Sieber JE, Steel PM, Zarate AO. Part II: HIPAA and disclosure risk issues. *IRB: Ethics and Human Research* 2006;28(1):6–11.

113. Spellman BA. What and when of disclosure. Presentation on challenging issues in psychological sciences prepared for Course on Human Research Protections in Psychology and the Behavioral Sciences at the 15th Annual Convention of the American Psychological Society, May 29, 2003. [Online] Available: http://www.aera.net/humansubjects/courses/APS/Disclosure.ppt.

114. Eysenbach G, Till JE, Ethical issues in qualitative research on internet communities. *British Medical Journal* 2001;323:1103–5.

115. Frankel MS, Siang S. Ethical and legal aspects of human subjects research on the internet. A report of a workshop held on June 10–11, 1999 by the Scientific Freedom, Responsibility and Law Program of the American Association for the Advancement of Science, November. [Online] Available: http://www.aaas.org/spp/sfrl/projects/intres/report.pdf.

116. Kraut R, Olson J, Banaji M, Bruckman A, Cohen J, Couper M. Psychological research online: Report of board of scientific affairs' advisory group on the conduct of research on the internet. *American Psychologist* 2004;59:105–17.

117. VanWey LK, Rindfuss RR, Gutmann MP, Entwisle B, Balk DL. Confidentiality and spatially explicit data: Concerns and challenges. *PNAS* 2005;102:15337–42.

118. Rushton G, Armstrong MP, Gittler J, et al. Geocoding in cancer research: A review. *American Journal of Preventive Medicine* 2006; 30(Suppl.2):S16–S24.

119. Kwan MR, Lee J. Geovisualization of human activity patterns using 3D GIS. In: Goodchild MF, Janelle DJ, eds. *Spatially Integrated Social Science.* New York, N.Y.: Oxford University Press; 2004:18–66.

120. Levine FJ, Sieber JE. Ethical issues related to linked data. Paper prepared for the Panel on Confidentiality Issues Arising From the Integration of Remotely Sensed and Self-Identifying Date, Committee on the Human Dimensions of Global Change, The National Academies, December 6, 2005.

121. National Research Council. *Putting People on the Map: Protecting Confidentiality With Linked Social-Spatial Data. Panel on Confidentiality Issues Arising From the Integration of Remotely Sensed and Self-Identifying Data,* MP Gutmann, PC Stern, eds. Committee on the Human Dimensions of Global Change. Division of Behavioral and Social Sciences and Education. Washington, D.C.: The National Academies Press; 2007.

122. Duncan TG, ed. Special issue on confidentiality and data access. *Journal of Official Statistics* 1993;93:267–607.

123. Choudhury T, Kautz H, Kitts J, Fox D. Project Abstract: Creating dynamic social network models from sensor data. Prepared for 2005 Principal Investigators Meeting of the Human and Social Dynamics Emphasis Area, National Science Foundation, September 15–16, 2005. [Online] Available: http://www.nsf.gov/sbe/hsd/hsd_pi_mtg/abstracts/kautz.pdf.

124. Pentland A, Choudhury T, Eagle N, Singh P. Human dynamics: Computation for organizations. *Pattern Recognition Letters* 2004;26: 503–11.

125. National Human Research Protection Advisory Committee. Clarification of the status of third parties when referenced by human subjects in research, January 28–29, 2002. [Online] Available: http://www.hhs.gov/ohrp/nhrpac/documents/third.pdf.

126. Margolin G, Chien D, Duman SE, et al. Ethical issues in couple and family research. *Journal of Family Psychology* 2005;19:157–67.

Manish Agrawal   Ezekiel J. Emanuel

33

Phase I Oncology Research

Despite substantial improvements in treatments for individual cancers, 50% of people diagnosed with cancer—more than 550,000 per year in the United States—still die from it.[1] As the average age of developed country populations rises, both the absolute number and proportion of deaths from cancer will also rise in those countries. Therefore, research into finding novel therapies for most cancers remains an important priority. The process of translating basic research into clinical applications that could potentially lead to larger clinical trials and eventually to effective cancer therapies begins with Phase I oncology studies (see Table 33.1). Classic Phase I oncology studies are cohort studies in which patients are treated with increasing doses of investigational agents to learn about toxicities, maximum tolerated dose, and the pharmacokinetics of the agents, thereby permitting planning for Phase II studies of efficacy.[2,3]

In other areas of medicine, Phase I trials often enroll healthy volunteers to test the pharmacokinetics and safety of drugs. Because of the potentially serious toxicities of cancer drugs, Phase I oncology trials enroll only patients with cancer, usually with cancers that are refractory to other chemotherapeutic interventions and, therefore, are terminal but with good performance status—that is, relatively normal energy and activity levels.

Since the process of testing new cancer drugs was formalized after World War II, there have been fundamental concerns about the ethics of Phase I cancer trials. These ethical challenges usually can be categorized into two main issues: the risk/benefit ratio and informed consent.[4-9] One ethical challenge is that because Phase I oncology studies offer little therapeutic benefit but can have substantial, even life-threatening risks for patients, Phase I oncology studies seem to violate the ethical requirement for a favorable risk-benefit ratio. Enrolling patients in research with high risks and few benefits seems to entail exploitation. Furthermore, knowing about the risk and low chance of benefit, it seems irrational for patients to participate in Phase I oncology studies. That patients do consent to participate suggests there must be a problem with the consent process. Disclosure of information must be deficient, or the patients must fail to understand the information disclosed, or they are pressured and coerced into enrolling.

Are these claims valid? Are Phase I studies unethical because they are highly risky with little benefit? Are patients who enroll in Phase I oncology studies uninformed, misinformed, and/or coerced? What are the ethics of Phase I oncology research?[10-14]

Objections Based on the Risk-Benefit Ratio

A common concern regarding Phase I oncology studies is that they violate the ethical requirement for a favorable risk-benefit ratio. The purpose of Phase I studies is to evaluate safety and toxicity, not efficacy. Nonetheless, tumor response is often measured in Phase I studies, and tumor response is often seen as a benefit. Past meta-analyses of Phase I trials of anticancer drugs, mainly from research studies conducted between 1970 and 1987, showed an overall response rate of less than 5%[15-19] (see Table 33.2). The majority of these were partial responses, with less than 1% of patients experiencing a complete response—that is, when the tumor completely disappears based on radiological and other diagnostic evaluations.

Several more recent analyses of Phase I oncology research studies from the 1990s and early 2000s demonstrated similar

Table 33.1

Phases of Studies

Phase	Intent of Trial	Typical Size of Trial
I	Safety and defining short-term toxicities and side effects. Determining maximal tolerated dose for Phase II efficacy studies and clinical pharmacology of dosing, including pharmacokinetics and pharmacodynamics. Collecting anecdotal clinical antitumor activity.	20 to 80 patients
II	Efficacy. Seeing if experimental agent(s) or combinations of experimental and proven agents have antitumor activity. Additional assessments of toxicities and side effects.	100 to 300 patients
III	Effectiveness. Comparing, usually in a randomized controlled trial, experimental agent(s) or combinations of experimental and proven agents with existing standard treatment(s) or, if no treatment(s), placebo to assess antitumor activity and side effects.	More than 400 patients

response data. Among 213 trials of single agent, investigational cancer drugs published as abstracts and full papers between 1991 and 2002, the overall response rate was 3.8%[20] (see Table 33.2). An analysis of all Phase I studies sponsored by the National Cancer Institute (NCI) between 1991 and 2002 showed that among those evaluating a single investigational chemotherapy agent, the overall response rate was 4.4%, with 1.5% being complete responses (CR) and 2.9% being partial responses (PR)[21] (see Table 33.3).

What are the risks? Death from toxicity in Phase I studies is rare but definitely occurs. A study analyzing Phase I oncology studies between 1970 and 1987 showed an overall toxicity death rate of approximately 0.5%.[16] Subsequent studies confirmed this finding, documenting overall toxicity death rates between 0.54% and 0.57%[20,21] (see Table 33.2). Despite the perception that nausea, vomiting, and other debilitating side effects are common, their overall frequency, severity, and impact on quality of life have been poorly documented. One of the recent studies reported a rate of 10.3% for serious, that is grade 3 or 4, nonfatal, toxic events, although several toxicities could have occurred to a single patient[20] (see Table 33.2). Of these toxic events, 85% were reported as partially or completely reversible. The NCI data showed that for single investigational chemotherapy agents, 15.0% of patients had a grade 4—life-threatening—toxic event with an average of 1.6 grade 4 events per patient who experienced an event.[21] In addition to these serious risks, there are frequent blood draws, radiological evaluations, physician visits, biopsies, all of which require a substantial, but hitherto unquantified, commitment of time and resources from patients and their families.[5,6,22,23]

With a relatively low tumor response, a small but definite risk of death, severe life-threatening side effects, and substantial time commitment from patients, Phase I oncology studies have a very unfavorable risk/benefit ratio, according to critics. An unfavorable risk/benefit ratio violates the ethical requirements of clinical research, making Phase I oncology research inherently unethical. George J. Annas has claimed that under the guidelines of the Nuremberg Code and the Helsinki Declaration, "[Phase I] cancer drug research, for example, may not be performed on terminally ill subjects . . . because there is no reasonable probability that it will benefit the subjects."[22]

Response to Objections Based on the Risk-Benefit Ratio

Reassessing the Benefits of Phase I Oncology Research

Do the risk/benefit data as presented tell the whole story? What criteria ought to be used to evaluate whether a particular risk-benefit ratio is favorable or unfavorable?

In evaluating benefits, several additional considerations besides complete and partial tumor responses are relevant. An analysis of NCI Phase I studies between 1991 and 2002 found that the vast majority were not trials of single, novel, investigational chemotherapy agents (see Table 33.3). Many Phase I oncology research studies involved vaccines, immune modulators, antiangiogenesis

Table 33.2

Response and Toxic Death Rates and Other Side Effects of New Single Investigational Agents in Phase I Oncology Trials

Authors	Year Published	Number of Single Investigational Chemotherapy Agents	Total Number of Patients	Overall Response Rate	Complete Responses	Partial Responses	Toxic Death Rate	Rate of Serious Side Effects
Esty et al.[15]	1986	66	6,447	4.2%	0.7%	3.5%	N/A	N/A
DeCoster et al.[16]	1990	87	6,639	4.5%	0.3%	4.2%	0.5%	N/A
Von Hoff and Turner[18]	1991	N/A	7,960	6.3%	0.9%	5.4%	N/A	N/A
Itoh et al.[17]	1994	38	2,200	3.3%	1.1%	2.2%	N/A	N/A
Smith et al.[19]	1996	18	610	3.1%	N/A	N/A	N/A	N/A
Roberts et al.[20]	2004	213	6,474	3.8%	N/A	N/A	0.54%	10.3%#
Horstmann et al.[21]	2005	92	2,341	4.4%	1.5%	2.9%	0.57%	15%*

#These are grade 3 or 4 toxicities; *these are the grade 4—dose limiting—toxicities based on just 20 of the trials.

Table 33.3

Response Rates in NCI Sponsored Phase 1 Oncology Trials, 1991–2002[21]

	Number of Trials	Number of Assessable for Response	Overall Response Rate (CR + PR)	Complete Response Rate (CR)	Partial Response Rate (PR)	Stable Disease and Less than Partial Response Rate (SD + < PR)	Toxic Death Rate
Total	460	10,402	10.6%	3.1%	7.5%	34.1%*	0.49%
Chemotherapy Cytotoxic							
One investigational agent	92	2,341	4.4%	1.5%	2.9%	40.8%	0.57%
Multiple investigational agents	12	273	11.7%	1.5%	10.3%	27.5%	0.66%
Combinations with investigational and FDA approved agents	88	2,251	16.4%	5.6%	10.8%	31.3%**	0.77%
Trials including only FDA approved agents	29	792	27.4%	8.0%	19.4%	27.2%**	0.65%
Immunomodulator							
One investigational agent	13	203	11.3%	3.0%	8.4%	35.5%	0
Multiple investigational agents	28	651	6.9%	2.2%	4.8%	22.3%**	0.14%
Combinations with investigational and FDA approved agents	19	392	26.0%	5.6%	20.4%	26.7%**	0
Receptor/Signal Transduction							
One investigational agent	51	1,347	3.2%	0.7%	2.5%	39.3%	0.19%
Multiple investigational agents	7	81	7.4%	1.2%	6.2%	27.2%	2.02%
Combinations with investigational and FDA approved agents	61	935	11.7%	2.1%	9.5%	37.4%	0.74%
Antiangiogenesis							
One investigational agent	15	335	3.9%	0.6%	3.3%	31.0%	0
Combinations with investigational and FDA approved agents	9	135	14.8%	5.2%	9.6%	37.0%	0.58%
Gene Transfer							
One investigational agent	7	89	3.4%	0%	3.4%	30.3%	0
Combinations with investigational and FDA approved agents	1	3	0%	0%	0%	0%	0
Vaccine							
One investigational agent	15	265	3.4%	3.0%	0.4%	24.9%	0
Multiple investigational agents	7	198	1.0%	1.0%	0%	35.4%	0
Combinations with investigational and FDA approved gents	6	111	5.4%	2.7%	2.7%	19.8%	0

*For 630 of 10,402 participants, data on stable disease and less than partial response is not reported. The percentage is calculated using 9,772 as the denominator; **these percentages are calculated using a denominator adjusted to exclude participants for whom data on stable disease and less than partial response was unavailable.

factors, and signal transduction agents. These agents are widely perceived to be less toxic than chemotherapeutic agents, so the risk/benefit ratio may be different. In addition, their benefits may not be appropriately measured by evaluating tumor response; these agents usually control cancer growth rather than kill cancer cells, so different types of responses need to be assessed. Moreover, many of the 1991–2002 NCI Phase I studies combined investigational agents with proven chemotherapy drugs.[21]

When all these trials are aggregated, the overall response rate—including both complete and partial responses—was 10.6%. In addition to the complete and partial tumor responses, 34.1% of patients had stable disease or some minimal shrinkage of tumor, although less than the 50% tumor shrinkage that is required to be recorded as partial response (see Table 33.3). Although the significance of stable disease as a response to an investigational in-

tervention is controversial, it may well be a benefit to those patients whose tumors would otherwise be expected to grow.

Some critics object that response rate is not an important clinical outcome. At best, response rate is an "intermediate" or surrogate endpoint; what people care about is not whether their tumor shrunk but whether or not they will live longer. Since the 1980s, however, some data have emerged suggesting that at least for some cancers, such as lung cancer, response rate is related to prolonged survival. For instance, a 2004 study concluded that in non-small cell lung cancer, a 3.3% increase in response rate correlates with a one-week increase in median survival, and a 2% increase in response rate correlates with a 1% increase in one-year survival.[24] Consequently, response rate may be a reasonably good intermediate marker of benefit, or at least may be more meaningful than critics have hitherto acknowledged.

In a few notable cases, the benefits of Phase I research for patients have been more substantial. For example, when initially tested in Phase I studies in the 1970s, cisplatin for testicular cancer had a response rate of over 50%, and in a quarter of cases the tumor completely disappeared and was probably cured.[25] More recently, in Phase I testing, imatinib mesylate (Gleevec) for chronic myeloid leukemia demonstrated complete hematological response rates of 98%, of which 96% lasted beyond one year.[26,27]

Overall, saying that only 5% of patients respond in Phase I oncology studies fails to acknowledge that in some Phase I trials response rates are higher, that stable disease may be a valuable and meaningful outcome for patients, and that in some cases substantial clinical benefits, and even cures, have been achieved in Phase I oncology trials.

In addition, among some terminally ill oncology patients there can be other important physical, psychological, and social benefits from participation in cancer research trials. Well-being, especially in very sick and terminally ill patients, is "not merely the absence of disease or infirmity" but includes psychological, social, and other dimensions.[28] Empirical study of these aspects of well-being among participants in Phase I studies has been limited. In considering other physical benefits, some data show that chemotherapy provides symptom relief among terminally ill patients even better than does supportive care. In one study, patients with metastatic colorectal cancer who had already failed one chemotherapy regimen were given another chemotherapy regimen that was associated with longer survival, fewer symptoms, and higher quality of life.[29,30] Participating in Phase I oncology studies in some cases may stabilize patients' quality of life compared to patients who receive supportive care and who typically experience declines in functioning as their cancer progresses.[31-39] Most importantly, participating in Phase I studies does not exclude symptom management or palliative care. Participating in Phase I studies and focusing on quality of life are not necessarily—and should not be—inherently incompatible goals; indeed, enhancing quality of life should be one of the goals of Phase I studies.[40]

Data also suggest that some cancer patients in Phase I studies experience psychological benefit. Daugherty et al. reported that 65% of research participants said they believed they would receive psychological benefit from being in the Phase I study.[23] One study showed that for terminally ill cancer patients, chemotherapy improves emotional function on measures of quality of life.[41] For some participants, routine and regular physician contacts reduce psychological distress during a time of great uncertainty.[13,42] In another study, 78% of patients enrolled in Phase I studies reported at least a moderate amount of comfort from having study-related diagnostic tests and physician visits.[43] An additional 56% reported that participating in research studies with new drugs gave them hope. For other patients, participation allows them to exercise some control over a situation they did not choose. Some patients also receive comfort from knowing they are helping future patients with cancer:[11,13,43]

[There is] a complex relationship between knowing the reality of their situation (that they had incurable disease) and hoping that there still might be a treatment that would have a positive effect, even cure. . . . Patients do not seem to be harmed by their experience of participating in a Phase I trial and may experience benefits, albeit not in terms of tumor control.[13]

Finally, because of concern about potential risks, the dose escalation design of many of these trials is intended to minimize toxicity—which, ironically, ensures that the majority of participants are treated at doses that cannot produce responses in human tumors. Indeed, over 60% of participants in Phase I oncology studies appear to receive biologically inactive doses.[15] Consequently, participants face little risk, but also have little chance of benefits. Some investigators have proposed novel design strategies to allow more patients to be treated at biologically active doses, increasing the chances for a therapeutic response.[2,3,44-46] The aggregate response rates reported in the literature underestimate potential response rates that could be achieved with these design strategies. Ironically, less than 15% of Phase I studies use these innovative methods, largely because of a concern about minimizing toxicities.[2,20,47]

What Standard Determines a Favorable Risk-Benefit Ratio?

To determine when a risk-benefit ratio is favorable or unfavorable requires a standard of evaluation that is appropriate for patients with advanced cancer who are likely to decline clinically and die within months because of disease progression. What criteria should be used to define a favorable risk-benefit ratio for Phase I oncology studies?

No standard for what is an acceptable risk-benefit ratio for adult research subjects has been explicitly articulated.[7,48-50] One approach is to elucidate a standard based on socially accepted determinations of risk-benefit already used for cancer treatments, such as in FDA approval of cancer agents. For example, high-dose interleukin-2 (IL-2) is an FDA-approved treatment for metastatic renal cell carcinoma. This IL-2 regimen has a response rate of 14% (5% complete responses, 9% partial responses) with a median response duration of 20 months.[51] The possible toxicities of IL-2 are substantial, including a sepsis-like syndrome, requiring judicious use of fluids and vasopressor support to maintain blood pressure while avoiding pulmonary edema from capillary leak. Other chemotherapy treatments with relatively low response rates, such as topotecan with a 10% response rate for ovarian cancer, have also been approved by the FDA.[52] Irinotecan and Erbitux are two treatments approved for metastatic colon cancer on the basis of less than a two-month prolongation of overall survival.[53] Furthermore, gemcitabine is the FDA-approved treatment of choice for metastatic pancreatic cancer because of demonstrated quality-of-life benefits, despite a response rate of only 5.4%.[54] In all these cases, society, through the FDA, has deemed the relatively low increases in survival, and the risk-benefit ratio, acceptable for routine clinical care. This suggests that an even lower level of benefit might be acceptable in research.

For nonterminally ill cancer patients, the use of chemotherapy with limited benefits is also widely accepted even if debated. For instance, among patients with newly diagnosed Stage I breast cancer, for whom five-year overall survival is greater than 90%, a two- or three-drug chemotherapy regimen lasting four to six months, with its side effects, offers an absolute survival benefit of just 1–2%.[55,56] Yet the vast majority of women receive such chemotherapy.

The risk-benefit ratio found in many Phase I oncology studies is not clearly worse for individual participants—even excluding the benefit of social knowledge—than risk-benefit ratios used by the FDA as a basis for approval of many chemotherapeutic agents or by many nonterminally ill patients in their decision making. Among patients for whom all standard therapeutic interventions have failed, even a small chance of therapeutic benefit may be reasonable. The risk-benefit assessment requires consideration of the available alternatives.

Furthermore, when social knowledge is added to these evaluations of the risk-benefit ratio, it seems that participation in a Phase I trial is even more beneficial. A Phase I trial adds to social knowledge, which is a good. More important, the available data suggest that contributing to social knowledge is a benefit for people. Research participants value being altruistic and therefore gain benefit from contribution to others.[10,43] The focus on physical benefit by critics of Phase I research discounts this type of psychological benefit.

Who Decides What Constitutes a Favorable Risk-Benefit Ratio?

The lack of explicit criteria means that institutional review board (IRB) members and critics frequently rely on their intuitions to determine what constitutes an acceptable risk-benefit ratio for Phase I oncology studies.[57] But IRB members and critics tend to be healthy individuals. Substantial data demonstrate that patients facing serious illnesses make very different assessments of their own condition and the risks they are willing to confront than do healthy individuals. For instance, families consistently overestimate symptoms and underestimate satisfaction and quality of life of sick patients.[58–61] Furthermore, Slevin et al. found that patients with cancer were willing to undergo intensive chemotherapy with substantial side effects for a 1% chance of cure compared to oncology nurses who said they would need a 50% chance, doctors who would need a 10% chance, and the general public who would need a 50% chance of cure.[62] Healthy IRB members and critics are likely to view studies with few benefits and greater risks unfavorably, yet patients might view the same studies as having a risk-benefit ratio that they are willing to accept or even welcome.

It has been argued that in considering protocols involving vulnerable populations, such as children or patients with mental illness, IRBs should include such patients or their advocates as members to ensure their perspectives are included in deliberations.[63] Extending this logic suggests that the views of terminally ill cancer patients should inform IRB determinations of the acceptability of risk-benefit ratios for Phase I oncology studies. Just as having minorities or women on IRBs may expand the factors considered in evaluating a research protocol, having patients who are terminally ill and eligible for Phase I studies may expand the considerations of these IRBs. Such patients may not be narrowly focused on physical safety and might consider the psychological benefits to the patients, thereby viewing risk-benefit ratios more favorably.

Objections Based on Informed Consent

That patients consent to participate in Phase I oncology studies with such an unfavorable risk-benefit ratio is widely viewed as indicative of deficiencies in disclosure, understanding, or voluntariness in the informed consent process.[5,23,64–66] First, com-

mentators have claimed that physicians exaggerate the benefits while minimizing the risks of research participation. One bioethicist is quoted as having said, "Informed consent documents make Phase I studies sound like the cure for your cancer."[67]

To date, no studies directly document deficiencies in disclosure, exaggeration of benefits, or minimization of risks. Nonetheless, critics note that despite response rates of just 5%, most participants in Phase I oncology studies are motivated to participate by hopes for stabilization, improvement, or even cure of their cancer[12–14,42] (see Table 33.4). Such hope suggests that either patients are not given accurate information or they fail to understand the information they are provided. Perhaps researchers do not provide adequate disclosure because they themselves overestimate the potential benefits from Phase I oncology studies by three-fold.[8,66] "These exaggerated estimates may represent ignorance, itself a worrisome finding given that the physicians in this study were the ones to invite patients to participate."[68]

In addition, many consent documents do not make prospective research participants aware of their alternatives, especially for palliative care and hospice. For instance, a study of consent forms for Phase I oncology research revealed that less than 1% included mention of hospice care as an alternative.[69]

In addition to possible disclosure deficiencies, critics argue that most patients in Phase I studies have deficient understanding of the objectives, benefits, and risks of Phase I research. For instance, in one study 93% of the participants reported understanding most or all of the information given to them about the Phase I study in which they had agreed to participate, yet only 31% of them were able to state accurately the purpose of Phase I studies as dose-finding.[10] Another study found that although 90% of cancer patients who participated in research reported being satisfied with the informed consent process, few understood the potential for incremental risk or discomfort from participating in research, or the uncertainty of benefits to themselves.[11]

Finally, commentators also argue that even if patients are given accurate information and understand it, they are vulnerable, their judgment is clouded, and they are not to be trusted with their own decision making. Indeed, according to this argument, their decision to participate in such high-risk/low-benefit research is itself indicative of how vulnerable they are, their confused judgment, or coercion. As one critic put it, terminally ill patients who consent to Phase I oncology studies have "unrealistic expectations and false hopes."[66] Another claimed,

> Being ill brings with it a multitude of pressures, and a patient suffering from a life-threatening disease may feel as though she has little choice regarding treatment. Physicians should be aware of how vulnerable patients may be to the *coercive influence of unrealistic hope,* especially those suffering from chronic, life-threatening disorders [emphasis added].[70]

Cumulatively, concerns about disclosure, understanding, and voluntariness make some commentators argue that informed consent is simply not possible with terminally ill patients eligible for Phase I oncology research.

> Therefore, instead of being suspicious of experimentation, patients may demand access to experimental interventions as their right. . . . Respecting patient autonomy does not require that we accept demands for mistreatment, torture, or whatever the dying may want.[22]

Table 33.4

Studies Evaluating the Quality of Informed Consent in Phase I Oncology Trials

Authors	Year Published	Sample Size	Methods of Evaluation	Reasons for Participating	Awareness of Study Purpose and Design	Satisfied With Informed Consent Process	Would Participate Again
Rodenhuis et al.[14]	1983	10	Interview 1 week after treatment began	50% hope for improvement of their diseases; 30% pressure of family	60–80% recalled, "experimental," "so far only animal studies," "effect uncertain"	—	—
Itoh et al.[17]	1996	32	Questionnaire after enrollment but before drug administration	19% treatment benefit; 63% no benefit but participate anyway	43% knew goal is to determine recommended dose	81% said understood almost all information given to them	—
Yoder et al.[72]	1997	37	Quantitative and qualitative interviews at entry and exit of study	70% to get best medical care; 85% decreased tumor size	—	—	100%
Hutchison et al.[42]	1998	28	Interviews 2–4 weeks after consenting to participate	Majority hope for benefit		89%	—
Daugherty et al.[10]	2000*	144	Interviews within 1 week of receiving drug	73% seeking anticancer response	31% knew purpose	96%	—
Tomamichel et al.[71]	2000	31	Quantitative and qualitative analysis of taped interviews	59% possibility of medical benefit	—	96%	—
Moore et al.[13]	2000	15	Pre- and posttreatment questionnaire and structured interviews	3 themes: (1) need to try everything, (2) maintain hope; (3) help others	—	—	—
Schutta et al.[77]	2000	8	Quantitative and qualitative analysis of taped focus group	Hope for therapeutic benefit	—	—	—
Cheng et al.[66]	2000	30	Questionnaire after enrollment	60% expect to benefit			—
Joffe et al.[11]	2001	50**	Mail survey 1–2 weeks after consent		75% knew trials done to improve treatment of future patients; 71% knew may be no medical benefit to themselves	90%	77%
Meropol et al.[12]	2003	328; 260 enrolled in Phase I	In-person or phone survey within 3 days of signing consent or refusing participation in Phase I	77% estimated their chance of benefit was at least 50%; 39% thought maximal benefit was cure of cancer		78% reported discussing side effects of treatment; 79% reported discussing benefits of treatment; 29% reported discussing changes in length of life from treatment	
Agrawal et al.[43]	2006	163	In-person interview immediately after signing consent form		For 63% of patients, key information for deciding whether to participate in Phase I was whether drug killed cancer cells		90% even if 10% of dying from Phase I agent

*The initial publication by Daugherty et al.[23] of 27 patients is included in the 144 patients; **survey of patients participating in Phase I, II, and III studies. Total number of patients was 207 of which 50 were enrolled in Phase I studies. Unfortunately, the analysis of the responses failed to stratify according to phase.

Response to Objections Based on Informed Consent

Methodological Concern

Even though informed consent in Phase I oncology studies may be the most extensively empirically studied area of informed consent, the data are still limited (see Table 33.4). First, fewer than 1,000 total patients have been interviewed in 12 separate studies. Second, the studies are of limited size: All but three studies evaluated 50 or fewer patients in Phase I research trials, and all but two of the studies were from a single institution. Third, some studies combine responses from patients enrolled in Phase I, II, and III oncology studies making impossible interpretation relevant solely to Phase I studies.

More important, assessing understanding of patients is methodologically extremely complex. Most courts evaluating informed consent cases avoid trying to evaluate whether patients had adequate understanding because they do not know how to make this evaluation. One problem is timing. When the surveys are administered days or weeks after the patient signs the consent, these studies actually evaluate recall of information as opposed to the ethically relevant understanding at the time of decision making.

In addition to timing, people generally retain only the information salient to them, which may not be the same information ethicists and investigators think is important. In buying a house, for example, the information buyers care about is narrow and focused, and usually substantially less than the information the attorney describes about how the deed will be recorded or if the bank will sell the mortgage to another bank. Similarly, participants in Phase I oncology trials might not care about study design and might focus instead on factors they consider salient such as whether the drug kills cancer cells.

Finally, in the studies published to date, there are serious challenges involving question design and especially framing effects. Because there is no gold standard by which to judge the reliability or validity of questions about comprehension, they can be judged only on face validity. This places an even greater burden on the investigator to demonstrate that the questions asked are being interpreted and answered by the research participant in the intended manner. Many of the questions used to assess understanding by participants in Phase I research are posed primarily from an investigator's perspective rather than the patient's. The wording of the questions and interpretation of the responses fail to differentiate between two aspects of understanding: *comprehension,* that is, understanding of the factual components of the information, and *appreciation,* what the information means to a particular person. For example, one study asked, "Why did you decide to enter this research trial? (What was your main reason?)"[23] and reported that over 70% joined hoping for benefit. The fact that patients participate primarily for the chance of benefit is often seen as indicative of a deficiency in comprehension. Yet, this interpretation fails to recognize that patients could very well comprehend their limited chance for personal benefit and still hope that they may actually benefit.

The Quality of Disclosure

There are limited empirical data on the adequacy of disclosure of information to participants of Phase I oncology studies (see Table 33.4). One study evaluated the substantive content of 272 Phase I oncology consent forms and found that 99% explicitly stated the study was research and that in 86% this statement was prominent.[69] Furthermore, 92% indicated safety testing was the research goal. Overall, the mean length of the risks section was 35 lines in contrast with four lines as the average length of the benefit section; and, 67% of forms mentioned death as a potential consequence of participation in the study, whereas only 5% mentioned cure as a possible benefit. Only one consent form indicated that any benefits were expected. Although this study found that less than 1% of informed consent documents mentioned hospice as an alternative, 56% mentioned palliative or supportive care.

Defenders of Phase I oncology studies note that no empirical study has shown that physicians fail to accurately disclose the risk, benefits, and experimental nature of Phase I oncology trials. Although physicians may overestimate the response rates in Phase I studies, they overestimate the risk of death even more, by 20-fold.[23,66] Importantly, as Tomamichel et al.[71] report from recordings of physician-patient interactions, physicians told patients about the lack of known treatments and the investigational nature of the Phase I oncology study in over 90% of consultations, and about the lack of sufficient knowledge of toxicity of the drug in more than 80%. Two other studies report similar findings.[14,65] Furthermore, surveys of physicians and patients considering Phase I research trials indicate that many recall having discussed risks, benefits, and other aspects of the trial. For instance, 92% of physicians and 78% of patients recall having discussed possible side effects from the Phase I treatment. Similarly, 90% of physicians and 79% of patients recall discussing possible benefits.[12]

Although substantially more data are needed to evaluate the disclosure of information in Phase I oncology studies, available data do not support the notion that disclosure either in consent forms or by oncologists is systematically deficient or distorted.

More important, surveys of people who enrolled in Phase I research demonstrate that the formal disclosure in the informed consent process, whether by the documents or by discussion with researchers, is not the only way prospective research participants obtain information. For instance, in one study, 84% of participants were aware of palliative care and 81% were aware of hospice care as alternatives to participation.[43] This indicates that patients obtain information about Phase I research studies and alternatives outside of the formal disclosure processes of the informed consent document and discussion.

Do Terminally Ill Cancer Patients Misunderstand?

Recent data show that many patients are aware that the chance of benefit is low, but believe that they are likely to be among the beneficiaries. Indeed, it may be this very belief that they will be among the lucky ones that keeps them going. For instance, Daugherty et al.[23] found that 85% of patients were motivated to participate in Phase I studies for possible therapeutic benefit, but 78% were either unwilling or unable to state whether they believed they personally would receive benefit from participating in a Phase I trial. Similarly, Itoh et al.[65] found that 63% of participants did not expect any benefit but wished to participate anyway. Likewise, although Joffe et al.[11] concluded that misconceptions about cancer trials are frequent among trial participants, their data show that 71% of research participants recognized there may not be medical benefit to themselves from participation in the clinical trial, and 75% of them reported that the main reason cancer clinical trials are done is to improve the treatment of future cancer patients. Knowing the chances are low but believing that they could be among the few who do benefit is common. As other researchers put it, "Although subjects were told that fewer than 10% of patients in Phase I trials experience a tumor response, many of them believed that someone comprised the percentage of patients who experienced a response and that they might 'be in the lucky group.' "[72] Defenders of Phase I studies argue that such data suggest Phase I research participants do not misunderstand but have a form of adaptive denial that all people engage in to some degree.[9,43,72]

Similarly, studies show that although over 90% of patients felt they understood the information about the Phase I trial, only about a third were able to state accurately "what are the doctors trying to find out in the Phase I cancer research trial in which [they've] enrolled."[23] Defenders of Phase I studies argue that interpreting this as reflecting a lack of understanding by participants of Phase I oncology studies confuses the intent of a Phase I study and the probability of benefit from a Phase I study. Phase I studies are not designed or intended to produce benefit. Yet, what matters to patients is not the intent of a Phase I study but the probability of receiving benefit from participation. It is perfectly reasonable that investigators design and intend Phase I studies primarily to determine toxicity, whereas patients enroll because of a chance of benefit, without there being any misunderstanding.

Investigators and patients each may have their own purposes but they are not necessarily in conflict with one another and may in fact be complementary. If the patient's tumor shrinks it does not adversely affect the purpose of the Phase I study, and if the trial determines the toxicity it does not thwart the patient's goal of tumor response, although the goal may not be achieved. Thus patients' failure to state the purpose of the Phase I study as a dose-finding study probably demonstrates that patients care more about the probability of receiving benefit, the risks, and the requirements of the study than the scientific methodology or the researcher's intent in conducting the study. This interpretation is supported by data showing that although 84% of respondents reported that they read the consent form carefully, and 73% considered it an important source of information, only 37% considered the consent form important to their decision to participate in the Phase I study.[11]

Questions in prior studies evaluating understanding offer limited answer choices that force only one primary reason for participating in a Phase I study. But, as in most decisions, there are usually several reasons to participate even if one reason is more important than the others. For example, in their instrument Daugherty and colleagues list nine reasons that might have been motivations for patients to participate in Phase I studies. For each reason, a patient can circle "major," "minor," or "not" depending on the role that reason played in their decision making. Only 33% said helping future people with cancer was a major reason for participating, leading the investigators to conclude that "altruistic feelings appear to have a limited and inconsequential role in motivating participants to participate in these trials."[23] This interpretation fails to capture the multiplicity of motivations that drives the decision making of research participants. Other reasons—such as the need to do something, the comfort gained from the regularity of clinic visits, family circumstances, and re-

gaining a sense of control—which may contribute but may not be the main reason to enroll in the study, would not have been detected in prior studies because they were not asked.

Are Patients With Cancer Able to Choose Freely?

There is a widespread perception that even if patients with cancer are given full disclosure and understand the information, the fact that some still opt to receive experimental drugs is indicative that they are vulnerable, their judgment is clouded by their illness, or they are pressured into enrolling or unable to make truly voluntary decisions.[6,22,70]

According to advocates for Phase I oncology trials, the view that terminally ill cancer patients are vulnerable seems not to accurately reflect the actual data. It is certainly the case that people with life-threatening cancers face bleak choices. But this is different from being vulnerable in the sense of not being able to make free choices. Vulnerability in research is often understood as meaning that people are unable to make free choices because of their social position, thus vulnerable groups include oppressed minorities, the poor, or those who are poorly educated.[73] Whether or not such a presumption is accurate—that is, whether minorities or the poor should be presumptively considered unable to exercise free choice—this hardly fits the characteristics of participants in Phase I oncology research. Phase I oncology study participants are typically white, well-educated, well-off, and well-insured. For instance, in one multicenter study of Phase I participants, the average age was nearly 58, 88% of individuals considering research were white, 51% were college graduates or had postgraduate training, 62% had incomes over $50,000, and 96% had health insurance.[43] Other studies report similar demographic data.[12] This, it is argued, is not the picture of a vulnerable population.

Even if terminally ill patients who are considering Phase I oncology research are vulnerable in certain ways, it does not imply an inherent lack of capacity to give informed consent. When terminally ill patients draw up wills or request not to be resuscitated, these are treated as genuine, autonomous choices; the consent of patients that their organs be donated for life-saving organ transplants is not considered prima facie invalid because they are made by terminally ill patients who cannot think clearly. Advocates of Phase I studies claim that most people with advanced cancer are able to and do make rational, reasonable, and informed decisions. There will be some individuals who are unable to give adequate informed consent, just as is true for people without advanced cancer. But to conclude that patients with advanced cancer are, as a group, inherently vulnerable and therefore unable to give informed consent is demeaning.

To categorize the choice of patients with advanced cancer to participate in Phase I studies as inherently coerced is a serious confusion.[70] By definition, coercion is a credible threat exerted by one person that limits or adversely affects the options another person has available.[74-76] Presumably, no person associated with Phase I research is issuing irresistible threats to terminally ill patients. Patients may feel pushed by nature, fate, and their circumstances to enroll. However, being in a situation with limited and difficult choices does not itself constitute coercion.[75] Unless the adverse choice situation was created by another person, the choice made by the patient should not be labeled as coerced. Indeed having poor options can be consistent with making an autonomous or even laudable choice.[72,74]

Limited available data support this analysis. When asked, only 9% of patients enrolled in Phase I research studies reported moderate or a lot of pressure from family, and only 7% reported such pressure from the Phase I clinical researcher.[43] Conversely 75% reported "pressure" to enroll from the fact that their cancer was growing.[43] Whatever the pressure from a growing cancer is, it is not coercive because only people can coerce; nature cannot. Furthermore, many dying people want chemotherapy, even if there is very low chance of benefit and a reasonable chance of toxicity, because it offers them hope or fits with their life narrative to fight against the odds, to overcome challenges—because they feel that to die without trying everything would constitute being false to themselves and their values.[77] One participant in several Phase I oncology studies put it this way:

> Letting a patient choose the poisons (under professional guidance) adds something to the will to struggle. We who are struggling to escape cancer do not, obviously, want to die of it. The enemy is not pain or even death, which will come for us in any eventuality. The enemy is cancer, and we want it defeated and destroyed. This is how I wanted to die—not a suicide and not a passively accepting, but eagerly in the struggle.[78]

Advocates argue that these people are not coerced but have a different set of values from the critics.[9]

Conclusion

Phase I oncology trials are critical to improving the treatment of cancer. Critics have raised ethical concerns about the risk-benefit ratio and the adequacy of informed consent. A critical analysis of the risk-benefit ratio does not show it to be unfavorable. Empirical data on informed consent in Phase I oncology trials does not support the notion that consent is uninformed.

Disclaimer

The opinions expressed here are those of the authors alone and do not represent views of the National Institutes of Health, the Public Health Service, or the Department of Health and Human Services.

References

1. American Cancer Society. *Cancer Facts and Figures 2002*. Atlanta, Ga.: American Cancer Society; 2002. [Online] Available: http://www.cancer.org/downloads/STT/CancerFacts&Figures2002TM.pdf.
2. Arbuck SG. Workshop on Phase I study design. Ninth NCI/EORTC New Drug Development Symposium, Amsterdam, March 12, 1996. *Annals of Oncology* 1996;7(6):567–73.
3. Ratain MJ, Mick R, Schilsky RL, Siegler M. Statistical and ethical issues in the design and conduct of Phase I and II clinical trials of new anticancer agents. *Journal of the National Cancer Institute* 1993;85:1637–43.
4. Emanuel EJ. A Phase I trial on the ethics of Phase I trials. *Journal of Clinical Oncology* 1995;13:1049–51.
5. Lipsett MB. On the nature and ethics of Phase I clinical trials of cancer chemotherapies. *JAMA* 1982;248:941–2.
6. Miller M. Phase I cancer trials. A collusion of misunderstanding. *Hastings Center Report* 2000;30(4):34–43.
7. King NM. Defining and describing benefit appropriately in clinical trials. *Journal of Law, Medicine and Ethics* 2000;28:332–43.
8. Penman DT, Holland JC, Bahna GF, et al. Informed cons7ent for investigational chemotherapy: Patients' and physicians' perceptions. *Journal of Clinical Oncology* 1984;2(7):849–55.
9. Agrawal M, Emanuel EJ. Ethics of Phase 1 oncology studies: Reexamining the arguments and data. *JAMA* 2003;290:1075–82.
10. Daugherty CK, Banik DM, Janish L, Ratain MJ. Quantitative analysis of ethical issues in Phase I trials: A survey interview of 144 advanced cancer patients. *IRB: A Review of Human Subjects Research* 2000;22(3):6–14.
11. Joffe S, Cook EF, Cleary PD, Clark JW, Weeks JC. Quality of informed consent in cancer clinical trials: A cross-sectional survey. *Lancet* 2001;358:1772–7.
12. Meropol NJ, Weinfurt KP, Burnett CB, et al. Perceptions of patients and physicians regarding Phase I cancer clinical trials: Implications for physician-patient communication. *Journal of Clinical Oncology* 2003;21:2589–96.
13. Moore S. A need to try everything: Patient participation in Phase I trials. *Journal of Advanced Nursing* 2001;33:738–47.
14. Rodenhuis S, van den Heuvel WJ, Annyas AA, Koops HS, Sleijfer DT, Mulder NH. Patient motivation and informed consent in a Phase I study of an anticancer agent. *European Journal of Cancer and Clinical Oncology* 1984;20:457–62.
15. Estey E, Hoth D, Simon R, Marsoni S, Leyland-Jones B, Wittes R. Therapeutic response in Phase I trials of antineoplastic agents. *Cancer Treatment Reports* 1986;70:1105–15.
16. Decoster G, Stein G, Holdener EE. Responses and toxic deaths in Phase I clinical trials. *Annals of Oncology* 1990;1:175–81.
17. Itoh K, Sasaki Y, Miyata Y, et al. Therapeutic response and potential pitfalls in Phase I clinical trials of anticancer agents conducted in Japan. *Cancer Chemotherapy and Pharmacology* 1994;34:451–4.
18. Von Hoff DD, Turner J. Response rates, duration of response, and dose response effects in Phase I studies of antineoplastics. *Investigational New Drugs* 1991;9:115–22.
19. Smith TL, Lee JJ, Kantarjian HM, Legha SS, Raber MN. Design and results of Phase I cancer clinical trials: Three-year experience at M.D. Anderson Cancer Center. *Journal of Clinical Oncology* 1996;14:287–95.
20. Roberts TG, Jr., Goulart BH, Squitieri L, et al. Trends in the risks and benefits to patients with cancer participating in Phase 1 clinical trials. *JAMA* 2004; 292:2130–40.
21. Horstmann E, McCabe MS, Grochow L, et al. Risks and benefits of Phase 1 oncology trials, 1991 through 2002. *New England Journal of Medicine* 2005;352:895–904.
22. Annas GJ. The changing landscape of human experimentation: Nuremberg, Helsinki, and beyond. *Health Matrix* 1992;2:119–40.
23. Daugherty C, Ratain MJ, Grochowski E, et al. Perceptions of cancer patients and their physicians involved in Phase I trials. *Journal of Clinical Oncology* 1995;13:1062–72.
24. Shanafelt TD, Loprinzi C, Marks R, Novotny P, Sloan J. Are chemotherapy response rates related to treatment-induced survival prolongations in patients with advanced cancer? *Journal of Clinical Oncology* 2004;22:1966–74.
25. Higby DJ, Wallace HJ, Jr., Albert DJ, Holland JF. Diaminodichloroplatinum: A Phase I study showing responses in testicular and other tumors. *Cancer* 1974;33:1219–25.
26. Druker BJ, Talpaz M, Resta DJ, et al. Efficacy and safety of a specific inhibitor of the BCR-ABL tyrosine kinase in chronic myeloid leukemia. *New England Journal of Medicine* 2001;344:1031–7.
27. Druker BJ. Inhibition of the Bcr-Abl tyrosine kinase as a therapeutic strategy for CML. *Oncogene* 2002;21:8541–6.
28. Preamble to the Constitution of the World Health Organization as adopted by the International Health Conference, New York, 19–22

June, 1946; signed on 22 July 1946 by the representatives of 61 States (Official Records of the World Health Organization, no. 2, p. 100) and entered into force on April 7, 1948.

29. Cunningham D, Pyrhonen S, James RD, et al. Randomized trial of irinotecan plus supportive care versus supportive care alone after fluorouracil failure for patients with metastatic colorectal cancer. *Lancet* 1998;352:1413–8.

30. Simmonds PC. Palliative chemotherapy for advanced colorectal cancer: Systematic review and meta-analysis. Colorectal Cancer Collaborative Group. *British Medical Journal* 2000;321:531–5.

31. Melink TJ, Clark GM, Von Hoff DD. The impact of Phase I clinical trials on the quality of life of patients with cancer. *Anticancer Drugs* 1992;3:571–6.

32. Berdel WE, Knopf H, Fromm M, et al. Influence of Phase I early clinical trials on the quality of life of cancer patients. A pilot study. *Anticancer Research* 1988;8:313–21.

33. Quantin X, Riviere A, Daures JP, et al. Phase I–II study of high dose epirubicin plus cisplatin in unresectable non-small-cell lung cancer: Searching for the maximal tolerated dose. *American Journal of Clinical Oncology* 2000;23:192–6.

34. Cohen L, de Moor C, Parker PA, Amato RJ. Quality of life in patients with metastatic renal cell carcinoma participating in a Phase I trial of an autologous tumor-derived vaccine. *Urologic Oncology* 2002;7: 119–24.

35. Francis RJ, Sharma SK, Springer C, et al. A Phase I trial of antibody directed enzyme prodrug therapy (ADEPT) in patients with advanced colorectal carcinoma or other CEA producing tumors. *British Journal of Cancer* 2002;87:600–7.

36. Cox K. Enhancing cancer clinical trial management: Recommendations from a qualitative study of trial participants' experiences. *Psycho-Oncology* 2000;9:314–22.

37. Campbell S, Whyte F. The quality of life of cancer patients participating in Phase I clinical trials using SEIQoL-DW. *Journal of Advanced Nursing* 1999;30:335–43.

38. Sherliker L, Steptoe A. Coping with new treatments for cancer: A feasibility study of daily diary measures. *Patient Education and Counseling* 2000;40:11–9.

39. Hope-Stone LD, Napier MP, Begent RH, Cushen N, O'Malley D. The importance of measuring quality of life in Phase I/II trials of cancer therapy—The effects of antibody targeted therapy: Part I. *European Journal of Cancer Care* 1997;6:267–72.

40. Agrawal M, Danis M. End-of-life care for terminally ill participants in clinical research. *Journal of Palliative Medicine* 2002;5:729–37.

41. Doyle C, Crump M, Pintilie M, Oza AM. Does palliative chemotherapy palliate? Evaluation of expectations, outcomes, and costs in women receiving chemotherapy for advanced ovarian cancer. *Journal of Clinical Oncology* 2001;19:1266–74.

42. Hutchison C. Phase I trials in cancer patients: Participants' perceptions. *European Journal of Cancer Care* 1998;7:15–22.

43. Agrawal M, Fairclough D, Grady C, Meropol NJ, Maynard K, Emanuel EJ. Decision-making process of participants of Phase I oncology trials. *Journal of Clinical Oncology* 2006; forthcoming.

44. Simon R, Freidlin B, Rubinstein L, Arbuck SG, Collins J, Christian MC. Accelerated titration designs for Phase I clinical trials in oncology. *Journal of the National Cancer Institute* 1997;89:1138–47.

45. Frei E III. Clinical trials of antitumor agents: Experimental design and timeline considerations. *Cancer Journal from Scientific American* 1997;3(3):127–36.

46. Chen EX, Tannock IF. Risks and benefits of Phase 1 clinical trials evaluating new anticancer agents: A case for more innovation. *JAMA* 2004;292:2150–1.

47. Dent SF, Eisenhauer EA. Phase I trial design: Are new methodologies being put into practice? *Annals of Oncology* 1996;7:561–6.

48. Emanuel EJ, Wendler D, Grady C. What makes clinical research ethical? *JAMA* 2000;283:2701–11.

49. Weijer C. The ethical analysis of risk. *Journal of Law, Medicine and Ethics* 2000;28:344–61.

50. Meslin EM. Protecting human subjects from harm through improved risk judgments. *IRB: A Review of Human Subjects Research* 1990; 12(1):7–10.

51. Fyfe G, Fisher RI, Rosenberg SA, Sznol M, Parkinson DR, Louie AC. Results of treatment of 255 patients with metastatic renal cell carcinoma who received high-dose recombinant interleukin-2 therapy. *Journal of Clinical Oncology* 1995;13:688–96.

52. Creemers GJ, Bolis G, Gore M, et al. Topotecan, an active drug in the second-line treatment of epithelial ovarian cancer: Results of a large European Phase II study. *Journal of Clinical Oncology* 1996;14: 3056–61.

53. Saltz LB, Cox JV, Blanke C, et al. Irinotecan plus fluorouracil and leucovorin for metastatic colorectal cancer. Irinotecan Study Group. *New England Journal of Medicine* 2000;343:905–14.

54. Burris HA, 3rd, Moore MJ, Andersen J, et al. Improvements in survival and clinical benefit with gemcitabine as first-line therapy for patients with advanced pancreas cancer: A randomized trial. *Journal of Clinical Oncology* 1997;15:2403–13.

55. Fisher B, Dignam J, Tan-Chiu E, et al. Prognosis and treatment of patients with breast tumors of one centimeter or less and negative axillary lymph nodes. *Journal of the National Cancer Institute* 2001;93:112–20.

56. Lippman ME, Hayes DF. Adjuvant therapy for all patients with breast cancer? *Journal of the National Cancer Institute* 2001;93:80–2.

57. van Luijn HE, Musschenga AW, Keus RB, Robinson WM, Aaronson NK. Assessment of the risk/benefit ratio of Phase II cancer clinical trials by Institutional Review Board (IRB) members. *Annals of Oncology* 2002;13:1307–13.

58. Epstein AM, Hall JA, Tognetti J, Son LH, Conant L, Jr. Using proxies to evaluate quality of life. Can they provide valid information about patients' health status and satisfaction with medical care? *Medical Care* 1989;27(3 Suppl.):S91–S98.

59. McCusker J, Stoddard AM. Use of a surrogate for the Sickness Impact Profile. *Medical Care* 1984;22:789–95.

60. Magaziner J, Simonsick EM, Kashner TM, Hebel JR. Patient-proxy response comparability on measures of patient health and functional status. *Journal of Clinical Epidemiology* 1988;41:1065–74.

61. Rubenstein LZ, Schairer C, Wieland GD, Kane R. Systematic biases in functional status assessment of elderly adults: Effects of different data sources. *Journal of Gerontology* 1984;39:686–91.

62. Slevin ML, Stubbs L, Plant HJ, et al. Attitudes to chemotherapy: Comparing views of patients with cancer with those of doctors, nurses, and general public. *British Medical Journal* 1990;300: 1458–60.

63. National Bioethics Advisory Commission. *Research Involving Persons with Mental Disorders That May Affect Decisionmaking Capacity, Volume I.* Rockville, Md.: NBAC; 1998. [Online] December 1998. Available: http://www.georgetown.edu/research/nrcbl/nbac/capacity/TOC.htm.

64. Kodish E, Stocking C, Ratain MJ, Kohrman A, Siegler M. Ethical issues in Phase I oncology research: A comparison of investigators and institutional review board chairpersons. *Journal of Clinical Oncology* 1992;10:1810–6.

65. Itoh K, Sasaki Y, Fujii H, et al. Patients in Phase I trials of anti-cancer agents in Japan: Motivation, comprehension and expectations. *British Journal of Cancer* 1997;76:107–13.

66. Cheng JD, Hitt J, Koczwara B, et al. Impact of quality of life on patient expectations regarding Phase I clinical trials. *Journal of Clinical Oncology* 2000;18:421–8.

67. Stolberg SG. Teenager's death is shaking up field of human gene therapy experiments. *The New York Times* January 27, 2000.

68. Miller M. Phase I cancer trials: A crucible of competing priorities. International *Anesthesiology Clinics* 2001;39(3):13–33.

69. Horng S, Emanuel EJ, Wilfond B, Rackoff J, Martz K, Grady C. Descriptions of benefits and risks in consent forms for Phase 1 oncology trials. *New England Journal of Medicine* 2002;347:2134–40.

70. Berg JW, Appelbaum PS, Lidz C, Parker PA. *Informed Consent: Legal Theory and Clinical Practice,* 2nd edition. New York, N.Y.: Oxford University Press; 2001.

71. Tomamichel M, Sessa C, Herzig S, et al. Informed consent for Phase I studies: Evaluation of quantity and quality of information provided to patients. *Annals of Oncology* 1995;6:363–9.

72. Yoder LH, O'Rourke TJ, Etnyre A, Spears DT, Brown TD. Expectations and experiences of patients with cancer participating in Phase I clinical trials. *Oncology Nursing Forum* 1997;24:891–6.

73. Levine C, Faden RR, Grady C, Hammerschmidt D, Eckenwiler L, Sugarman J, on behalf of the Consortium to Examine Clinical Research Ethics. The limitations of "vulnerability" as a protection for human research participants. *American Journal of Bioethics* 2004;4(3):44–9.

74. Hawkins J, Emanuel EJ. Clarifying confusions about coercion. *Hastings Center Report* 2005;35(5):8–10.

75. Wertheimer A. *Coercion.* Princeton, N.J.: Princeton University Press; 1987.

76. Faden RR, Beauchamp TL, with King NMP. *A History and Theory of Informed Consent.* New York, N.Y.: Oxford University Press; 1986.

77. Schutta KM, Burnett CB. Factors that influence a patient's decision to participate in a Phase I cancer clinical trial. *Oncology Nursing Forum* 2000;27:1435–8.

78. Daugherty CK, Siegler M, Ratain MJ, Zimmer G. Learning from our patients: One participant's impact on clinical trial research and informed consent. *Annals of Internal Medicine* 1997;126:892–7.

Grant R. Gillett

Surgical Innovation and Research

Surgery, like all crafts, evolves to build on its successes and make use of changing materials and techniques. It is a craft in which physical or invasive methods are used to try to relieve a patient's suffering, and therefore the surgeon needs a certain confidence and assurance in his or her ability to do what needs to be done without the cure causing worse havoc than the disease. There are four quite different situations in which innovative surgery is used on real patients, who thereby become de facto subjects of medical experimentation even though no formal clinical trial might be in progress. These situations are as follows:

1. The one-off desperate case
2. The use of an established operation for a novel indication
3. The promising development that modifies a standard or widely practiced operation
4. The genuinely new operation

Before we discuss these possibilities, we need to introduce some basic features of clinical surgery that distinguish it in many ways from general medicine. In many areas of clinical treatment, we aim to correct an abnormality that is producing an illness. Sometimes finding the abnormality and figuring out how to correct it are easy, and this is the area of medicine in which we find surgeons (among others). So much is this the case that some physicians say that if surgery wasn't simple surgeons couldn't understand it.

When causes of disease are structural and easily visualized, surgeons devise means of correcting the structural abnormality in the hope that this will cure the problem. Most of these means are fairly simple-minded. Lumps are removed, blockages are cleared, stenoses are corrected, pressure that compromises function or causes pain is relieved, and infections are eradicated. Sometimes the corrective intervention is so obvious that there is no uncertainty, for example, removing a subdural hematoma causing pressure on the brain, cutting out a tumor obstructing the bowel, or clearing a blocked artery. These are transparently effective interventions: The clinician can see, at the time of surgery, that what was needed has been done well or badly. The standard of assessment can usefully be called *the appeal to the educated eye.*

Some diseases, however, are more complex than is apparent to the educated eye. Functional diseases, such as oversecretion of gastric acid or biochemical abnormalities, are detectable only by inference from tests indicating that something is going wrong in the body. In other cases the intervention's immediate or intended effect has gained it accepted status as good treatment, but its effect on the natural history of the disease requires clear and careful assessment. Procedures in this category include removal of prolactin-secreting adenomas of the pituitary, carotid endarterectomy for bruits, cholecystectomy, spinal decompression in malignant disease, endoscopic removal of bowel polyps, and so on. These accepted but unproven procedures are apparently effective, but we need more than the appeal to the educated eye because therapeutic efficacy must be gauged by some reliable method of tracking their impact on morbidity and mortality.

Some surgical techniques are supported by controversial theories, for example, gastric ulcer surgery, breast cancer surgery, hysterectomy for carcinoma in situ of the cervix, and so on. In such cases it is unclear whether a procedure is truly or only apparently effective. Once a question about the theoretical justification of a procedure is raised—usually because of evidence that seems to conflict with the theory—trials of that procedure must be done. But clinical trials of surgical procedures raise difficult ethical questions. Physicians' *duty of care*—the commitment to provide treatment that is at least as good as that the patient would otherwise have received—seems to require that such trials preserve the option of the best current treatment for those who need it. That would (prima facie) rule out the "gold standard" for evidence-based medicine—double-blind randomized controlled trials using placebos. Therefore, the ethical justification for trials of surgical techniques needs to be carefully examined in terms of the risks and benefits involved.

The Desperate Case

Surgical patients present unique challenges, some of which resemble but are not the same as those presented by other patients. The first time that it occurred to somebody that a heart could be transplanted to replace one that was failing the situation was indeed desperate, but the operations were doomed to failure.[1] If we project ourselves back into the life stories of patients with intractable heart failure due to severe valvular disease or high grade stenoses of the coronary arteries, we find ourselves contemplating dire prospects. Such a patient has not a lot to lose and a great deal to gain, but there are either no statistics to support the surgeon or very bleak reports of surgical deaths due to one or another of the many causes of failure for major heart surgery. In such a case, one can hardly deny the patient the faint hope offered by a procedure radical in nature and adventurous in the extreme but overwhelmingly likely, apart from the glimmer of hope, to result only in pain and death. Provided such patients understand the dire realities, then their decision to allow this throw of the dice on their behalf seems ethically unproblematic even though it clearly serves the interests of future potential patients and the surgeon in a more certain and evident way than it does the patient who is trying to defy the odds.

Here altruism, to which I shall come, clearly has a role, as does the fact that the journey to a new technique must begin somewhere even when the risks are stark and unattractive. Successive patients may face prospects not significantly different, but such is the nature of surgery that these "blood sacrifices" will almost certainly help to provide life-saving opportunities for those who follow. The relevant benefits differ considerably from a narrow assessment of statistical harms and benefits versus current therapeutic options presented to an individual patient. But the problem is capable of rational resolution as long as there is openness of information sharing and a genuine commitment to partnership in the surgeon-patient relationship.[2]

A New Indication

The development and extension of surgical techniques is consistent with Hippocratic injunctions about medical knowledge. The Hippocratics stressed the need for careful investigation of phenomena noted in the course of clinical practice along with a refusal to be biased by preformed theories. "Physicians," the writings say, "compare the present symptoms with similar cases they have seen in the past, so that they can say how cures were affected then."[3] The ability to transform chance observations into well-validated clinical therapies aimed at difficult problems is a valued aspect of surgery. The first treatments for Parkinsonism by lesions in the

basal ganglia followed this path, and the transition from observation to technique in an ethical way is centrally important for reflective surgical practice.

Indications can only be defined by carefully structured clinical trials of treatment versus nontreatment for various conditions. But for reasons already outlined, these trials are hard to do in surgery. Often when the chance observation occurs, some hypothesis about the functional interconnectedness of the system concerned suggests a tentative place for that observation in our corpus of medical knowledge and current understandings of pathophysiology. This may provide a rationale for what is done and a decision about new indications for the procedure, but often the place of the surgery remains unclear. This is an unhappy situation.

The Hippocratic writings describe the accumulation of careful clinical observations over time until conclusions can be drawn as to which methods are effective and which not. In surgery this is a somewhat varied business, so the gap between animal experiments and use of surgical techniques on humans tends to be filled by "informal research."[4] Evidence of safety and efficacy is often based on historical series despite the statistical hazards of such evidence.[5-7] A reported case of headache and neck stiffness from cervical spondylotic stenosis (CSS) followed this Hippocratic path, and its deficiencies against a placebo-controlled trial are evident.[8]

The surgeon began doing a posterior decompressive operation on the cervical spine for standard reasons, but out of a sense of partnership with his patients, he heard a lot about the operation and its effects. He noticed that many patients spontaneously reported resolution of tension-type headaches after their operations; for some, this was the most significant result of surgery. He began to regard severe and persistent cervicogenic or tension-type headaches as a relative indication for surgery. Eventually the results seemed so compelling that he operated on some patients who wanted the operation mainly in the hope of getting rid of their headache, with due warnings about the uncertainties and their entitlement to an alternative opinion quite possibly differing from his own. Patients were increasingly referred as "domino" cases: They or their doctor knew somebody with a similar syndrome who had been dramatically relieved.

What, from an ethical point of view, should the surgeon do at this point? Obviously, there are a number of people who seem to have gained a significant change in morbidity and functional status by opting for a relatively novel operation for controversial reasons. He cannot, in service of his Hippocratic duty of care, just ignore these observations. But it seems that he should do something to elucidate the safety and efficacy of the procedure in comparison with existing alternative treatments to ensure that he does not violate his duty to do no harm. In fact, it seems that the claim that symptom relief is truly related to surgery ought to be submitted to rigorous statistical testing in view of the subjective nature of the effect of surgery and the prevalence of placebo effects in the treatment of such symptoms.

Developing an Existing Technique

At this point we should note that some surgical techniques are no more than technical improvements on accepted treatments, which may themselves be well grounded in evidence or just accepted as normal practice. In such cases, it is reasonable to put considerable weight on the opinions of surgeons actually using the new technique as to whether it serves their surgical need better than the procedure it has replaced. However, in addition to the impressions of surgeons, a review of the outcomes of operations using both the new and traditional techniques—not necessarily a placebo-controlled, randomized trial—ought to be conducted to ensure that any modifications or technical improvements do not cause unforeseen complications and problems, perhaps at some time removed from the surgery.

The relevant studies would assess the new technique with respect to the achievement of the technical goals of the surgery and its safety, and in light of medical and surgical knowledge at the time. Thus the same doubts as to clinical indications and efficacy in altering the natural history (in terms of morbidity and mortality) would apply to the modification and to the basic technique.

Throughout the practice of surgery there is a strong presupposition in favor of a consensus of practicing surgeons (a standard of validation that has a very low ranking on the Cochrane scale of evidence). In fact this is not totally irrational when one considers that the techniques of surgery develop in a progressive manner and that initial attempts to correct an abnormality are likely to be refined by cumulative experience until surgeons can do the job safely and well. It is therefore a question of degree as to whether a modification of an existing technique requires only the educated eye test or a total reevaluation.

These facts make it understandable that a surgeon might do a certain kind of operation in a certain way and believe that it is superior in technical terms to his or her previous practice, without having good evidence either that the standard practice is beneficial or that the modification is a genuine improvement in anything more than intraoperative technique. We ought, therefore, to ask, why are modifications introduced?

A surgeon may notice that the existing techniques lack safeguards against common complications or deficiencies, or that they are time consuming and difficult, or that the morbidity of the operation can be obviated by a change of technique. In many such cases a technical comparison is appropriate, and the surgeons doing the operation should be consulted as to whether a new technique is better. But in other cases the new operation should be used only with suitable monitoring of the points of modification (and therefore of potential risk).

The Genuinely New Operation

An entirely new procedure may occur in two quite different situations:

1. The aim of surgery in terms of correction of abnormal structure has itself proven to be effective in treating the disease—as, say, in removal of a life threatening tumor of the brain.
2. The aim of the surgery has never itself been well proven but is a matter of accepted practice.

In both cases, the new technique should be compared in a clinical trial against the best available current treatment so that its advantages—or at least its equivalence—can be examined. But how should such a clinical trial be structured?

In order to compare the way we test surgical innovations with the more common clinical trials with which we are familiar, we should compare surgical trials with the phases of drug treatment trials. We cannot do early experimental operations on healthy volunteers, so Phase I studies of drugs have no counterpart in surgery—apart from animal trials and ancillary investigations, such as mechanical or laboratory testing.

Phase II studies investigate prima facie efficacy, and this is as far as formal trials of surgical innovations usually get. Surgical procedures are often introduced because they appeal to "the educated eye," which is attuned to a visible abnormality and a visible (or palpable) correction of that abnormality. There is no equivalent of the educated eye in nonsurgical medicine; biochemical and physiological functions are not surveyable in any obvious and simple way, and placebo-controlled trials are needed to prove the efficacy of an intervention aimed at a complex abnormality of function.

In surgery, Phase II success often leads directly to wide clinical adoption and, in effect, Phase IV testing. We seldom step back and ask whether correcting the obvious anomaly in accordance with the educated eye actually helps the patient. An audit of large numbers of procedures done as part of a Phase II demonstration of safety in patients might be the closest we usually get to a Phase III trial. Such an audit shows us something about risks and benefits of clinical use, but it lacks the evidential force of a proper clinical trial because of biases that a formal trial is designed to overcome.

Even though surgical techniques are commonly studied in something that looks like a Phase IV study, as Evans and Evans note: "We must try to pick out serious follow up work from mere marketing ploys."[9] Marketing ploys arise because innovation often involves new devices or marketable commodities, resulting in profits and royalties for their creators, and a common way to encourage widespread usage is to enlist surgeons in "research trials."

Placebo-Controlled Trials in Surgery

It is now time to turn to the reasons that placebo-controlled trials are needed for some surgical innovations. For most surgical procedures, a wide range of results have been reported and for a number of reasons, the interpretation of the relevant data is not at all straightforward. First, the indications for surgery often differ between surgical series, and they are not always clearly defined in published studies. Second, outcome measures vary from study to study and are often not reported in any detail. Third, assessment of the patient before and after surgery is often carried out by the surgical team doing the procedure, and therefore there is a well-recognized possibility of bias in the results. Fourth, we often are not told of inclusion and exclusion criteria for such a surgical series, nor whether there has, in fact, been a declared or undeclared selection of patients.

However, a controlled trial requires surgical equipoise, a contentious concept[10,11] (see Chapter 24). One might expect equipoise to exist when the clinician has no valid reason to believe that one of the treatments will confer any advantage. But this simple and rational definition is clouded by debates contrasting theoretical equipoise, somewhat vacuously defined as a condition in which the existing evidence is equally balanced between the two procedures, and clinical equipoise, a concept based on the existence of significant clinical disagreement.[12] Equipoise seems best defined as a position in which *there has been no clear-cut and sustained demonstration of the superiority of one treatment over another.* The standard then becomes objective and historically sensitive to the accretion of statistically valid evidence. In fact, we are often in this position, and surgeons tailor their advice to their own capabilities and to the opportunities open to a patient in their patient's position (because of geography, urgency, cost, antecedent clinical fitness for surgery, and so on). Prolonged debates about definitions of equipoise are therefore a waste of time, and the best we can do is note that in surgery, some disturbances of equipoise are based not on remote clinical outcomes but on factors proximate to the surgery, such as pain, time of operation, and worries based on the educated eye. And so we come to the nub of the problem.

Should We Perform a Randomized Controlled Trial of a New Surgical Procedure?

The question is difficult to answer for a number of reasons.

1. The surgeon has usually introduced the innovation for what he or she considers to be good reasons, so the surgeon is not in an equipoise condition unless that is narrowly interpreted overlooking, for instance, the educated eye and technical adequacy.

2. The fact that any given surgeon will have his or her own favored technique for a procedure means that the best comparisons that can be achieved are usually either prospective contemporaneous trials of patients allocated to different treatments nonrandomly or comparisons between historically distinct retrospective series. Both of these study designs present problems because they fail to control for the differing skills of different surgeons. Such trials also may fail to achieve comparability on other measures such as the clinical status and management of patients.

3. The idea of blinding and placebo control is hotly contested in surgery because placebo operations are ethically problematic.[13,14] I will consider this at length below.

Some of these problems can be ameliorated by such measures as careful attention to the clinical status of patients in each series, adjustment of morbidity and mortality statistics in retrospective series by using a marker procedure of similar difficulty to that contemplated (such as anterior discectomy rather than discectomy with implantation of an artificial disc), standardized questionnaires and instruments for measuring indications and outcomes, and careful assessment of diagnostic and other parameters used in the series. They are also addressed in part by what is known as the uncertainty principle.[15] This requires doctors to be genuinely reflective about the standard of evidence they have for their beliefs and—when they acknowledge that they are uncertain, or the evidence is inconclusive, about the best treatment—to seek to be part of a well-designed trial to address that uncertainty. This orientation is clearly needed in many areas of surgery, provided only that uncertainty is not defined in a way that neglects the collective wisdom of current practice.[11]

Placebo-Controlled Surgical Trials: The Problem of Sham Surgery

The idea of placebo arms of double-blind clinical trials in surgery makes most surgeons wonder what the world is coming to. However, when we consider the increasing move toward quality of life surgery and the importance of the placebo effect in that area, along with diminishing surgical morbidity, the idea of placebo-controlled trials looks more attractive. Adequate information and consent, the possibility of altruistic decision making, and the rational examination of surgical choices in the face of uncertainty may blunt some of the ethical worries that spring to mind. We should also recall, however, that prospective randomized double-blind placebo-controlled clinical trials may not be necessary for all surgical innovations because a considerable proportion of surgical innovation involves learning to operate in a less risky, more efficient, or more elegant way.

A 1999 issue of the *New England Journal of Medicine* addressed the ethics of placebo-controlled trials of surgery by examining the implantation of fetal brain cells in patients with Parkinson's disease.[16,17] All patients, both in the placebo and treatment groups, had a stereotactic frame fitted under general anesthetic, burr holes drilled in the skull, low dose cyclosporin for immune suppression, and repeated neurological assessment. But is submitting patients to the sham operation (and cyclosporin) as a placebo ethically justifiable? Ruth Macklin is quite clear that "it is unethical" to do operations that involve cutting into people and sewing them up again. She argues that sham surgery violates our duty to minimize the risk of harm to participants in research.[17]

The Tension Between Ethics and Science

Macklin contends that there is "a tension between the highest standard of research design and the highest standard of ethics."[17] This is an odd claim given that ethics concerns the making of good decisions and should attend to both the scientific merit of what we are doing and the best interests of the patient. Therefore the correct contrast can be only between good research design and the desire to minimize harm to the individual. But the risk of individual harm is not confined to the study. All surgical treatment is invasive and, if unproven, may cause harm without correlative benefit. So purely on the basis of harm, it is unethical to apply any unproven treatment to any patient. What is more, the wound associated with a sham operation is of a different order from the potential harm attendant on a full operation. Arguably, then, it is misleading to lump all surgical harm into one grab bag. It is not such an open-and-shut case as it initially appears, and some careful thinking is required about the ethics involved.

Why Placebo-Controlled Studies?

There is undoubtedly a need for rigorous testing of new procedures in surgery just as there is for new drug treatments. The baseline data against which new surgical techniques are assessed are problematic. We often rely on historical controls involving a range of different techniques and noncomparable clinical settings in terms of diagnostic facilities, surgical expertise, and the dynamic relationship between biomedical knowledge and the understanding of the indications and rationale for surgery. These problems are compounded by the lack of independent assessment of outcomes and inadequate reporting of the results of surgical series.

Moreover, two new developments are of particular relevance to placebo-controlled clinical trials of surgery. The first is the growth of surgery for quality of life indications—whose "success" requires subjective judgments that are particularly vulnerable to placebo effects—rather than for immediately life-threatening conditions whose outcomes are readily evident. Macklin discusses an operation aimed at controlling Parkinson's disease. It is similar to quality of life surgery in a number of other areas such as spinal surgery and orthopedic surgery in general, although the aim was to produce a cure. And as distinct from acute rescue or life-saving surgery, we might expect placebo responses to be particularly important. Therefore controlling for the placebo effect is a real issue in assessing many surgical innovations.

In addition, surgery is becoming safer. Operations have become cleaner, quicker, more closely monitored, and they threaten less morbidity and mortality than those in the past, a fact that justifies, at least for many patients, exploratory surgery with an uncertain promise of significantly improving quality of life. This fact also defuses, in part, the argument that placebo surgery is "too risky" to be ethically permissible. There are, however, other arguments that cannot be dealt with quite so definitively.

Vulnerable and Desperate Patients

People with diseases for which we have only relatively ineffective interventions are vulnerable and may be coerced by the hope of treatment, even when that hope is based on nothing but speculation or very poor evidence. We see this every day in clinical practice, when patients with cancer or AIDS turn to alternative and unproven treatments—or even barefaced quackery—searching for answers.

Despite the fact that the standards of evidence and efficacy for allopathic or orthodox medicine may not be fully applicable to the problems that present themselves to holistic practitioners, and despite misgivings about venerating the placebo-controlled trial, we do need clinical rigor. Significant worries about patient bias, placebo effects, observer bias, and subjective end points seem to require the use of placebos in some contexts. The articulation of ethical constraints on their use is therefore required.

General ethical considerations suggest that the first requirement is absolute honesty about the treatment proposed and the structure of the trial. Only disclosure of this kind allows the patient to give informed consent to participation. In a placebo-controlled study, such honesty demands an explanation of the actual chances of the surgery being "real" or "sham" and the importance of the use of placebos in the trial. It seems, however, that we cannot always rely on this being carried out well.

Macklin observes that "some researchers performed sham surgery without obtaining informed consent from patients" and notes that in a trial of coronary artery surgery, "the patients were told only that they were participating in an evaluation of this operation; they were not informed of the double blind nature of the study."[17] Notice that it is the use of placebos that is of most concern, and the probabilities must be clearly explained. Macklin recounts cases in which "the misconception that research is designed to benefit the patients who are the subjects is difficult to dispel," and she concludes that "the protection of human subjects cannot rest solely on the ethical foundation of informed consent."[17]

Before approving surgical research protocols, institutional review boards or other ethics committees should reassure themselves not only that patients will be appropriately informed, in an unbiased manner, but also that the surgeons involved are competent and held in good regard by other specialists in the relevant specialty. This would presumably include evidence that the technique had been presented at professional meetings and is subject to ongoing audit.

However, such an assessment could mean that some major medical advances might never have been made (for instance, in kidney transplantation and open heart surgery).[1] Therefore the needs of desperate patients and their willingness to contribute to future benefits for others must be balanced against the sometimes bleak prospects of the surgery that they are offered in its present state of development.

The Reasonableness of Ordinary Folk

Macklin identifies a tension that rests, in part, on the thought that people should never make self-harming choices. However, a moment's reflection reveals that this is not so. Consider, first, that surgeons often propose operations for which rigorous scientific evidence—in the form of a randomized placebo-controlled trial—is not available. The acceptability of most surgical procedures is based on favorable outcomes in historical series, not on evidence from placebo-controlled trials. Therefore, many patients opt for potentially harmful interventions that have never been strictly validated in terms of their efficacy or benefit. Refusing to allow volunteers to choose the minimal harm associated with placebo surgery would require many patients outside the clinical trial to go on submitting themselves to unproven (strictly speaking) and potentially harmful surgery, with no rigorously scientific way of determining the merits of that surgery. But it is clearly unethical to submit 1,000 people to an unproven and potentially harmful procedure when its merits or otherwise might be revealed by exposing 100 people (or, more probably, 50) to a much lesser risk than that involved in undergoing the real operation.

This is likely to be an ethically defensible approach when our general understanding of human function makes us sure that we are doing good, as, for instance, when we take out a blood clot that is killing a patient from raised intracranial pressure. In such a case the Hippocratics were content to allow the judicious use of reason to help good clinical decision making when we lacked the evidence to be more exact in our assessments of optimal management.[3] But recall that there is sometimes a gap between what seems intuitively to be the right thing to do and what can be proven beneficial by evidence, for example, lowering intracranial pressure after acute diffuse brain injury is intuitively correct but unproven in the management of acute head injury. Not only does the obtaining of good evidence make sense in terms of the greatest good for the greatest number, but it makes sense in terms of doing real good (not harm) in future individual cases.

Some thinkers are not swayed by the idea of collective harms and benefits even when the ultimate goal is to refine our ability to benefit identifiable individuals. They protest against utilitarian approaches on principle because they regard acting for the good of the individual as an absolute duty. At this point, we need to examine more closely the ethical basis of their claim.

It is clear that a narrow focus on the best interests of the individual gives certain weight to self-interest, autonomy, and paternalism. But the balance commonly struck is fraught with internal inconsistencies. Autonomy or self-rule generally means that we ought to respect the reasonable wants and intentions of an individual, in which a "reasonable" want or intention means that it is endorsable by a rational person and it is not unjust (in the sense that it does not infringe the rights of others). Among a person's reasonable interests are those which put a value on serving others, usually referred to as *altruistic intentions* and generally reckoned not only to be reasonable but morally commendable.

Given that concession, voluntary or even enthusiastic participation in a placebo-controlled surgical trial seems reasonable on at least two counts:

1. A 50% chance of a treatment that might help is arguably as good as a treatment whose effect is (strictly speaking) unknown.
2. The thought that our ignorance about the efficacy of a potentially helpful treatment would continue to dog future sufferers of a condition one suffers is itself unreasonable.

The chance of availing myself of the statistical opportunity of possible benefit (50%), combined with the possibility of uncovering important information for the treatment of others like me, arguably outweighs the harm of a relatively innocuous surgical intervention if I am in the 50% who get a placebo operation.

This might provide some people, and patients in particular, with a significant motivation for altruistic behavior. We have applauded altruism in the past, particularly in medical pioneers experimenting on themselves. But to deny patients the chance of participating in placebo-controlled surgical research would be to say, in effect, that altruism is no longer endorsable as a rational motive. The view of human motivation as narrow self-interest, which is reflected in (and possibly encouraged by) this ethical stance, is lamentable. It seems ironic that ethicists, of all people, should condemn altruism, which some would regard as a fundamental pillar of ethical behavior.

Safeguards for Patients

Despite the weaknesses in the argument against placebo-controlled surgery, there are safeguards that need to be in place for us to allow such a trial design to be ethically approved. The most important safeguard concerns patient information and consent. Patients should know that there is a 50% chance of undergoing sham surgery, but they should also be told that we do not actually know if the "real surgery" is of any benefit (which is why the study is being done in the first place) and that continuing in ignorance involves even more substantial risks not only to them but also to others. If the patient decides to go ahead and participate in the study, then it seems to me that a realistic "cooling off" period should be scheduled and/or that they should be provided with access to a medical opinion distanced from the surgical enthusiasts committed to doing the trial. If such conditions are met, then no reason remains to ethically disapprove of the altruistic participation of some patients in trials to advance the search for a well-grounded, scientifically proven response to their condition (given that they also have a chance of obtaining benefit from the experimental treatment).

Advances in Surgery and the Dogma of the Placebo-Controlled Trial

Placebo surgery addresses the question posed by the fundamentalism that venerates placebo-controlled trials above everything else in clinical medicine. This is not necessarily the core of evidence-based medicine, which is "the conscientious, explicit and judicious use of current best evidence in making decisions about the care of individual patients."[18] The fundamentalism involved is a product of clinical epidemiology conceived as a science wedded to the concept of provable causal efficacy from an equipoise situation.

However, medicine, and particularly its surgical arm, is a science-based art with elements of creativity and imagination involved, so flatfooted application of a generic and uniform intervention like a drug or a standardized procedure is not always appropriate. Many surgical procedures are, effectively, unique solutions tailored by the surgeon to suit the needs of the individual patient, although based on a generic technique. Of course we need evidence for the efficacy of these procedures, and we need to remove or negate potential biases in gathering that evidence. But surgery has a history of incremental innovation and cumulative refinement of its techniques and is therefore allied in some ways with the crafts practiced by skilled craftspeople. We must therefore ask when and what version of a technique or its refinements ought to be tested in a placebo-controlled trial. To some extent, surgeons are the best judges of this threshold, in the light of considerations such as those above about the possibility of new harms and benefits.

At one end of the continuum there are going to be new operations, even involving new, patented devices, which are better ways of doing the job that has to be done—as, for instance, might be the case with the current generation of aneurysm clips compared with their more remote ancestor devices. We then need to consider some developments, such as intra-arterial or interventional radiological occlusion of cerebral aneurysms, as alternatives to surgery when the procedures are so different that a comparative clinical trial could hardly proceed with equipoise except in relation to serious outcomes. In such a situation, some other kind of comparison is going to be required to establish exactly which patients will be more suitable for which procedures. But there are also interventions based on belief and theory, such as the use of prophylactic antibiotics, when the results are not always accessible to the intuitive technical judgment of a skilled practitioner and the solution is generic and uniform so that a standard clinical trial methodology is appropriate.

In between the innovations clearly in one camp and those clearly in the other, there are some that fall in the middle, like the resection of the gyrus rectus in clipping an aneurysm of the anterior communicating artery—a detail that is seemingly innocuous but which should be evaluated more thoroughly than just by making bedside assessments on a ward round. Similar points could be made in relation to developments in spinal fusion techniques, an area in which practice has shifted to suggest that active fusions are required in more and more cases without there ever having been a thorough validation of their necessity or effects.

Therefore the differences between the craft of surgery and the science of medicine in general suggest that we need to develop a more Hippocratic method of evolving and assessing techniques in surgery. Some techniques seem to confer technical advantages, but often the baseline of standard practice against which they are assessed is not well documented. In such a case we need to do what the Hippocratic practitioners did: document our baseline, do audits on our techniques, and document shifts in practice so that, despite the historical, nonblinded, nonplacebo-controlled methodology being used, we monitor what we are doing by careful case records and by audit (perhaps by independent assessors) of our results. There are some areas of surgery in which this approach, despite its nonconformity to the dogma of placebo-controlled trials, may be the correct way to proceed. In other cases, a placebo-controlled trial is the right way to go, and some groups are now using mixed designs that allow surgeons to exercise clinical judgment and yet study their techniques for efficacy.[15] In any event it seems after careful scrutiny that we cannot dismiss out of hand either way of proceeding in the evolution of surgery.

We now come to some general questions that should concern all surgeons involved in actual clinical innovation and research.

Do the Patients Concerned Understand That They Are Receiving Innovative Treatment?

This is the most important ethical consideration. However, the possible weakness of a focus solely on informed consent is the vulnerability of patients and the unequal power relationships in the clinical encounter, therefore further questions must be asked, in particular about the standard of information required.

Given that evidence about efficacy of existing treatments might be very poor by epidemiological standards, all that we can ask of surgeons is that they should be open with their patients about what they are going to do, they should reasonably believe that what they are doing is comparable to existing techniques, and they should submit their procedure to peer review. Such peer review depends on a careful audit of results and an attempt to do some kind of valid clinical comparison that will yield the best possible evidence as to the relative scientific merits of the technique used.

The patients should be told of their options and should appreciate how to position the surgeon's advice in relation to a representative body of medical opinion. Many clinicians, and surgeons in particular, are bad at this. They will decide their preferred mode of therapy but will not inform the patient about uncertainties or other options for treatment. But patients must be empowered to make their own decisions, especially when clinical facts do not unequivocally point to one approach—adjuvant chemotherapy for gliomas, for example. The patient should understand any sources of bias that would not be obvious and should be aware that surgery is a journey that may take many paths to the same destination.

If this is done, then patients become participants in designing (and owning) their own treatment regimes and monitoring their own outcomes. Such a partnership allows medical innovation to proceed in a very fruitful way because the patients feel permitted to contribute their own observations no matter how odd or unusual these seem to be. The ongoing audit of practice allows such observations to be a rich source of truly Hippocratic data, a branch of the tree of knowledge on which advances in medicine have hung for over 2,000 years.

It may be that a relatively new technique, unlike most surgical procedures, does not have a clear-cut scientific rationale. The lack of a theory explaining why the innovative technique works can be understandable and is not, in itself, an absolute barrier to doing the procedure; theory often lags behind data. However, some systematic investigation should be pursued—perhaps through anatomy, animal physiology, and so on, or perhaps with a placebo-controlled trial—to fill the gap in our knowledge, par-

ticularly in an area in which the results of surgery are partly assessed on the basis of quality-of-life criteria that are highly susceptible to the biases that a placebo-controlled trial is designed to eliminate. Once the observation or anecdotal finding is then established as a genuine finding, theory usually comes to grips with it and sets about elucidating it.

Conclusion

We need innovation in surgery to make techniques safer. We need good research to check on what we are doing and to refine our indications for using surgery in various clinical situations. Surgeons and their patients need to go into these trials and undertake their respective roles in these developments with an open mind and a careful attention to the need for the rigor that is to be had in a primarily healing art. They must do so in a spirit of open and informed partnership in which the maximum is done to address the imbalances that exist in the clinical setting and the patient is regarded as a coinvestigator. When significant innovation is being studied, an independent ethical review committee ought to oversee the trials that are conducted to develop and test that innovation.

Having said all this, we ought not to delay nor unnecessarily obstruct surgical innovation by always insisting on orthodox and rigid adherence to the tenets of the placebo-controlled trial, especially when an educated eye might inform us that a procedural variation is more technically adequate than an existing method. There are undoubtedly other ways of moving ahead, such as trials done under the principle of uncertainty or systematic case-matched reviews, which can achieve much the same result as a placebo-controlled trial.[5,6] But we should not altogether rule out the placebo-controlled trial on ethical grounds.

References

1. Jennett B. *High Technology Medicine.* Oxford, England: Oxford University Press; 1986.
2. Editorial. *British Medical Journal* 1999;319:717.
3. Lloyd GER, ed. *Hippocratic Writings.* London, England: Penguin; 1978:142.
4. Margo CE. When is surgery research? Towards an operational definition of human research. *Journal of Medical Ethics* 2001;27:40–3.
5. Benson K, Hartz AJ. A comparison of observational studies and randomized, controlled trials. *New England Journal of Medicine* 2000; 342:1878–86.
6. Concato J, Shah N, Horwitz RI. Randomized, controlled trials, observational studies and the hierarchy of research designs. *New England Journal of Medicine* 2000;342:1887–92.
7. Pocock SJ, Elbourne DR. Randomized trials or observational tribulations. *New England Journal of Medicine* 2000;342:1907–9.
8. Gillett G. Innovative treatments: Ethical requirements for evaluation. *Journal of Clinical Neuroscience* 1998;5:378–81.
9. Evans D, Evans M. *A Decent Proposal: Ethical Review of Clinical Research.* Chichester, England: John Wiley & Sons; 1996.
10. Freedman B. Equipoise and the ethics of clinical research. *New England Journal of Medicine* 1987;317:141–5.
11. Weijer C, Shapiro SH, Glass KC. Clinical equipoise and not the uncertainty principle is the moral underpinning of the randomised controlled clinical trial: For. *British Medical Journal* 2000;321:756–8.
12. Miller PB, Weijer C. Rehabilitating equipoise. *Kennedy Institute of Ethics Journal* 2003;13:93–118.

13. Gillett G. Unnecessary holes in the head. *IRB: Ethics and Human Research* 2001;23(6):1–6.

14. Edwards SJL, Lilford RJ, Hewison J. The ethics of randomized controlled trials from the perspectives of patients, the public and healthcare professionals. *British Medical Journal* 1998;317:1209–12.

15. Lindley RI, Warlow CP. Why and how should trials be conducted? In: Zeman A, Emanuel LL, eds. *Ethical Dilemmas in Neurology.* Edinburgh, Scotland: W.B. Saunders; 2000:87–100.

16. Freeman TB, Vawter DE, Leaverton PE, et al. Use of placebo surgery in controlled trials of a cellular-based therapy for Parkinson's disease. *New England Journal of Medicine* 1999;341:988–92.

17. Macklin R. The ethical problems with sham surgery in clinical research. *New England Journal of Medicine* 1999;341:992–6.

18. Sackett DL, Rosenberg WM, Gray JA, Haynes RB, Richardson WS. Evidence based medicine: What it is and what it isn't. *British Medical Journal* 1996;312:71–2.

Participant Selection

Section A. Fair Participant Selection

Leslie A. Meltzer   James F. Childress

What Is Fair Participant Selection?

Introduction: "Born in Scandal, Reared in Protectionism"

The U.S. regulations for the protection of humans in biomedical and behavioral research were, as Carol Levine notes, "born in scandal and reared in protectionism."[1] Other chapters in this volume identify and discuss research projects that were condemned because they imposed undue risks on research subjects or because they failed to obtain voluntary, informed consent. In addition, some were criticized as violations of standards of fairness, justice, and equity in the selection of subjects, now increasingly called "participants."

In Henry Beecher's 1966 exposé in the *New England Journal of Medicine* of 22 clinical trials in which researchers had engaged in "unethical or questionably ethical procedures,"[2] the vast majority of cases involved research on soldiers, hospital patients, institutionalized mentally retarded children, newborns, the elderly, and the terminally ill. These studies were not anomalies, Beecher demonstrated, but examples of mainstream science: All were published in prestigious medical journals and most were conducted at university or government facilities with federal funding.

Although Beecher's article accelerated the movement toward federal regulation of human experimentation in the United States, it was the media's discovery of the Tuskegee Syphilis Study in 1972 that ultimately led to many of the guidelines in place today. In an attempt to study the natural progression of untreated syphilis, the U.S. Public Health Service (PHS) had sponsored a 40-year trial in which close to 400 poor, African American men with syphilis were systematically deprived of established treatments and led to believe that the lumbar punctures they received were therapeutic,

not diagnostic[3] (see Chapter 8). Although this study was ethically flawed in several ways, one major ethical criticism focused on its unfair selection of subjects, a selection based in part on racist views that syphilis was a different disease in whites and in African Americans.[4]

In 1974, Congress responded to these and other scandals by passing the National Research Act,[5] which created the National Commission for the Protection of Human Subjects of Biomedical and Behavioral Research (hereafter, the Commission). The Commission was charged, first, with identifying the basic ethical principles that should underlie the conduct of research with human subjects, and, second, with developing guidelines to ensure that these principles were followed in the future. In carrying out these tasks, the Commission was directed to consider, for the first time, "appropriate guidelines for the selection of human subjects for participation in such research."[6]

Protection From the Burdens and Risks of Research

The Commission deliberated during a time in which clinical research involving humans had proven not only a risky enterprise but one that largely burdened vulnerable populations. An article published by Hans Jonas in 1969, which has since become one of the most anthologized essays in research ethics, is characteristic of this climate. One of the first authors to address the issue of subject selection directly, Jonas contended that in ruthlessly pursuing scientific progress, society had placed an excessively heavy burden on its most vulnerable members simply because they were readily available and easily expendable. He argued that in a rightly ordered society, physician-researchers, who have the motivation and understanding necessary to freely enter research, would be the primary source of research participants. Other members of society could participate in research in "descending order of permissibility," with society's most vulnerable members included in research only as a last resort.[7]

When the Commission released its Belmont Report in 1978, it echoed Jonas' protectionist attitude toward the selection of research participants (see Chapter 14). Recalling Tuskegee and other research scandals, the Commission wrote that

> [c]ertain groups, such as racial minorities, the economically disadvantaged, the very sick, and the institutionalized may continually be sought as research subjects, owing to their ready availability in settings where research is conducted. Given their dependent status and their frequently compromised capacity for free consent, they should be protected against the danger of being involved in research solely for administrative convenience, or because they are easy to manipulate as a result of their illness or socioeconomic condition.[6]

The Commission grounded its view in the principle of individual and social justice. Individual justice, the Commission wrote, requires "that researchers exhibit fairness" in the selection of participants. Accordingly, "researchers should not offer potentially beneficial research only to some . . . or select only 'undesirable persons' for risky research."[6]

The requirements of social justice added another layer to the conception of fairness. Social justice, the Commission stated, entails drawing a distinction between classes of people who should and should not participate in research "based on the ability of members of that class to bear burdens and on the appropriateness of placing further burdens on already burdened persons."[6] It also demands that research "not unduly involve persons from groups unlikely to be among the beneficiaries of subsequent applications of the research."[6] As a matter of social justice, then, researchers should prefer nonvulnerable populations to vulnerable ones and should not involve groups whose members do not stand to benefit from the results of the research.

In 1981, the Department of Health and Human Services (DHHS) and the Food and Drug Administration (FDA) issued separate federal regulations that reflected an attitude similar to the Commission's toward protecting vulnerable persons in research.[8–10] The DHHS regulations, Subpart A of which became the basis of the so-called Common Rule, required institutional review boards (IRBs) to ensure that the "selection of subjects is equitable." In studies "where some or all of the subjects are likely to be vulnerable to coercion or undue influence," the IRB reviewing the protocol is to ensure that "appropriate additional safeguards have been included in the study to protect the rights and welfare of these subjects." At its inception, Subpart A included children, prisoners, pregnant women, mentally disabled persons, and economically or educationally disadvantaged persons among the class of vulnerable persons. Specific guidance for research involving pregnant women, human fetuses, and neonates (subpart B); prisoners (subpart C); and children (subpart D) was also integrated into the DHHS regulations.[8] Most of the 18 federal departments and agencies that subsequently adopted the Common Rule, however, did not adopt subparts B, C, and D.

In the decade following Tuskegee, research participation was considered a heavy burden requiring stringent regulation. The paradigm was so-called nontherapeutic research; that is, research that does not offer the participant the prospect of direct benefit. The protectionist stances of the Belmont Report and the Common Rule, and their view of fairness in terms of the distribution of research burdens, reflect the era in which they were developed as well as the problems they faced. Looking back on this period, the Advisory Committee on Human Radiation Experiments indicated in 1996 that it "was troubled by the selection of subjects in many of the experiments we reviewed. The subjects were often drawn from relatively powerless, easily exploited groups, and many of them were hospitalized patients."[11]

Access to the Benefits of Research

By the mid-1980s, attitudes toward research participation had begun to change. Trials once regarded as burdensome and potentially dangerous came to be viewed as highly desirable opportunities for patients to access the latest benefits of medical science. Among the factors contributing to this transformed vision of clinical research were several studies demonstrating not only that research participation is relatively safe,[12,13] but also that research subjects often enjoy better health outcomes than their peers receiving the same therapy outside of the research setting.[14] At the time these data became public, the cost of health care in the United States was rising exponentially. Enrolling in a clinical trial was thus seen as a way to receive state-of-the-art medical care, improved disease monitoring, and access to the health-care system.[15]

Nowhere were the perceived benefits of participating in clinical research more pronounced than in the context of the HIV/AIDS crisis. First recognized in 1981, AIDS became one of the most feared diseases in modern times. Physicians had no standard treatment for the disease or the virus that caused it; and although antiretroviral therapy currently offers the best hope, the first antiretroviral drug was not available until 1986 and then only in clinical trials.

Individuals infected with HIV and those with AIDS clamored for access to clinical trials that offered even a slim chance at improvement. In the context of limited access to zidovudine (AZT), many HIV/AIDS activists argued that research was synonymous with health care, an argument that suggests there was a therapeutic misconception about the nature of these trials, many of which were placebo-controlled. Unlike critics of the previous decade who were preoccupied with protecting research participants from the burdens of research, the activist group AIDS Coalition to Unleash Power (ACT-UP) argued that people should have the right to decide for themselves what burdens to bear. From the perspective of AIDS activists, fairness demanded nothing less than unimpeded access to the potential benefits of research participation.[16]

Against this background, a different conception of justice in the selection of research participants began to emerge. The focus shifted from the fair distribution of research burdens and risks to the fair distribution of research benefits. Instead of asking how to protect certain vulnerable groups from the burdens of clinical research, the ethical question turned to how to ensure access to potentially beneficial research for vulnerable or underrepresented populations.[1] This ethical discourse occurred largely in the context of HIV/AIDS research.

Because AIDS was initially thought to be a disease primarily affecting gay men, those in the first several AZT trials were mostly white, homosexual men. The categorical exclusion of intravenous drug users from these trials, coupled with low inclusion rates for women and minorities, led to charges of discrimination and injustice.[17] Ethical analyses began to recognize that the protectionist regulations of the 1970s were limiting enrollment among many of the populations (e.g., women of childbearing age, prisoners, infants, prostitutes) that stood to benefit from participating in HIV/AIDS research.[18]

Subsequently, the U.S. Office for Protection from Research Risks issued guidance for IRBs concerning the fair distribution of benefits among potential research participants. Although not codified in the federal regulations, the guidance recommended that IRBs ask the following three questions when reviewing clinical protocols:

> To the extent that benefits to the subject are anticipated, are they fairly distributed? Do other groups of potential subjects have a greater need to receive any of the anticipated benefit? Has the selection process overprotected potential subjects who are considered vulnerable (e.g., children, cognitively impaired, economically or educationally disadvantaged persons, patients of researchers, seriously ill persons) so that they are denied opportunities to participate in research?[19]

This guidance illustrates the degree to which the ethics of clinical research had changed in just one decade. Instead of having to justify the *inclusion* of vulnerable populations in clinical trials, researchers were now asked to justify their *exclusion*. Fair selection in this ethical environment meant providing all prospective participants with equal opportunity for access to the potential benefits of participating in clinical research.

Proportional Representation in Research

In the early 1990s, an additional layer of ethical complexity was added to the discussion of fairness in the selection of participants. Several people argued that justice requires not only equal opportunity for access to benefits for individuals (through participation in research), but also equal opportunity for access to benefits for groups in the population at large (after the completion of research). To ensure fair or equitable distribution of the results of research among all groups, it was argued, people from those groups must be represented in the research. As numerous studies revealed, however, most research participants were middle-aged, white males who reported high or middle annual incomes[20]— hardly representative of the diverse groups who hoped to benefit from the results of research.

The early HIV/AIDS trials again provided the backdrop for these discussions. Because the participants in those trials were mostly white men, some argued that clinicians lacked important information about the efficacy of AZT in the wider population of HIV/AIDS patients.[17,18] Specifically, concern emerged that there could be relevant biological differences between white men and other groups with HIV/AIDS, such as women, racial minorities, and children.[21,22] The failure to include these latter groups in clinical trials left unanswered questions about the progression of the disease and the effective treatment dose in those populations.

When an experimental drug ultimately reached the market, it was argued, understudied groups might receive ineffective or even harmful treatment.[23]

In 1992, Rebecca Dresser's groundbreaking article demonstrated that the failure to include women and racial minorities in research was not limited to HIV/AIDS trials but, instead, was "ubiquitous."[24] During the 1970s and 1980s, for example, the National Institutes of Health (NIH) had funded several large-scale, male-only heart trials, including the now well known Coronary Drug Project,[25] Multiple Risk Factor Intervention Trial,[26] Coronary Primary Prevention Trial,[27] and Physicians' Health Study.[28] These studies systematically excluded women from participation; but even in studies that were not gender-restricted, female enrollment was low.[15,29] One reason given for women's underrepresentation in research was that "their hormonal fluctuations 'confound' or 'confuse' research results,"[30] but other articles suggested that low enrollment simply resulted from unreasoned sex biases in participant selection.[31,32] Just as these data were surfacing, so too were studies demonstrating that men and women respond differently to certain drug treatments.[33]

Racial minorities were also underrepresented in the vast majority of clinical trials at this time, and almost no clinical trials existed to study diseases that primarily afflicted minority populations.[34,35] There was also growing evidence that racial minorities respond differently from whites to certain drugs, such as antihypertensives,[36] and that they experience disease progression differently from whites, especially in the context of cancer.[37] As a result, there was legitimate concern that researchers were regularly extrapolating data from whites to racial minorities without any scientific justification for doing so.[38]

The use of children in research was similarly rare. In the mid-1990s, for example, only 20% of drugs approved in the United States had been labeled for use in infants and children, and only 37% of new drugs with the potential for pediatric use had pediatric labeling at the time of approval.[39] Off-label use of medications was thus the norm in pediatrics, but with it came the risk of exposing children to unexpected adverse reactions or suboptimal treatment.

The government responded to the exclusion and underrepresentation of women, racial minorities, and children in clinical trials in a series of personnel and policy changes that took effect throughout the 1990s. During the Senate confirmation hearings for Bernadine Healy, director of the NIH from 1991 to 1993, gender representation in biomedical research was the focus of discussion. Healy stated that her intent was to make women's health a central aspect of her administration, and as NIH director, she upgraded the status of the NIH Office of Research on Women's Health (ORWH). The office had been established in 1990, the same year in which the NIH required the inclusion of women and minorities in study populations unless researchers showed "a clear and compelling rationale" for their omission,[40] a standard that has since been tightened.

In 1993, the FDA and the NIH both took crucial steps toward ensuring the widespread applicability of research results. The FDA withdrew its previous prohibition against including women of childbearing age in early clinical trials and issued new guidelines stating that research participants "should, in general, reflect the population that will receive the drug when it is marketed."[41] This change in FDA policy dramatically affected drug companies, which were suddenly required to consider whether they had enrolled adequate numbers of women to detect gender-related differences in drug response.[42,43]

Echoing the FDA's message to researchers, Congress passed the NIH Revitalization Act of 1993, which mandated the inclusion of women and minorities in clinical research.[44] Under the Act, researchers conducting Phase III clinical trials were further obligated to enroll a sufficient number of women and minorities "such that valid analyses of differences in intervention effect can be accomplished."[45] The NIH justified this provision by pointing out that "[s]ince a primary aim of research is to provide scientific evidence leading to a change in health policy or a standard of care, it is imperative to determine whether the intervention or therapy being studied affects women or men or members of minority groups and their subpopulations differently."[45]

Federal efforts to encourage the inclusion of children in clinical trials developed more slowly. In 1995, Congress expressed concern that the NIH was devoting inadequate attention and resources to pediatric research it conducted and supported.[46,47] When a workshop convened by the National Institute of Child Health and Human Development and the American Academy of Pediatrics revealed that as many as 20% of clinical trials inappropriately excluded children,[48] Congress's fears were confirmed. In response to congressional demand, the NIH issued a policy in 1998 that required grant applicants seeking NIH support to include children in research, except in certain stated situations. The policy aimed "to increase the participation of children in research so that adequate data will be developed to support the treatment modalities for disorders and conditions that . . . affect children."[48] Following the same reasoning, the FDA implemented mirror regulations in 1998 that required all new drugs and biologics, absent a waiver, to be studied in pediatric research subjects.[49]

By the turn of the millennium, the concept of fairness in the selection of research participants had evolved substantially from its roots in protectionism. Policy experts, investigators, and ethicists alike acknowledged that a combination of overprotection and discrimination had created homogeneous study populations that did not reflect the full range of patients likely to receive a marketed therapy. Without information about how different groups responded clinically to research protocols, it was thought that physicians would not be able to provide equal care to all of their patients. In this context, fair selection meant ensuring that research cohorts resembled target clinical populations. Exclusion or underrepresentation of women, racial minorities, or children unjustly affected those groups by denying them access to the benefits of participating in research (the concern of the 1980s) and by failing to provide them with the benefits of applicable knowledge from research, such as information about how treatment regimens might affect them differently than the study population (the worry of the 1990s). Determining what exactly counts as proportional or fair representation in research remained an unanswered question.

Present Challenges

Researchers, ethicists, and others continue to grapple with the delicate balance between protecting vulnerable populations from the burdens of research and providing all individuals and groups with an equal opportunity to benefit from research, both in particular studies and after their completion. During the past 10 years, however, new challenges have suggested that achieving fairness in research may require fresh approaches. The continued underrepresentation of minorities in research, the exploitation of economically disadvantaged people, and the dearth of elderly research participants suggest that we need to look more thoughtfully at the factors that impede equitable participant selection. At the same time, the expansion of research in the international arena illustrates that although attention to participant selection is necessary for fairness in research, it is not always sufficient.

Ongoing Underrepresentation of Minorities

Despite U.S. federal regulations mandating the inclusion of racial minorities in clinical trials, recent studies demonstrate that African Americans, Hispanic Americans, and other minorities remain underrepresented.[50,51] One explanation offered for the low representation of minorities in research is that investigators do not know what the congressional legislation requires of them with regard to minority enrollment.[52,53] Although the 1993 NIH Revitalization Act was revised in 2000 and 2001, the provision that researchers must ensure the "appropriate inclusion" of minorities remains vague.

In highlighting this problem, one article suggested that "appropriate inclusion" could be interpreted in three different ways.[54] First, it could require researchers to use the burden of disease in a population to guide minority inclusion. If a group has a higher likelihood of disease, it should have greater representation in research, which translates into a greater likelihood of sharing in the benefits and burdens of the research. A second method for determining appropriate inclusion might be to use census data to guide the proportion of minorities included in research. On this view, a group's representation in a trial would be proportional to its representation in the population at large. A third option might be to use the demographic statistics of a region, rather than the country, to guide participant selection. This method would, for example, be more precise when the therapy being tested is intended to benefit people in a limited region of the country. Although these proposals demonstrate the need for clarity in the federal guidelines, the present ambiguity does not alone explain the continued underrepresentation of racial minorities in clinical trials.

An arguably larger impediment to minority enrollment in clinical trials is what has been called "the legacy of distrust"[55] or "Tuskegee fallout."[24] Both terms speak to the powerful deterrent effect that knowledge of past research scandals has on potential minority participation in research.[56,57] In one survey, African Americans stated that they avoid clinical research because doctors "always use our race as guinea pigs" so that others in society can benefit.[58] Other studies have similarly documented the pervasive distrust many African Americans have toward the medical establishment.[59] In part, because self-referral is a primary mechanism for enrollment in present-day clinical trials, skepticism and suspicion among potential participants have hindered minority representation.[60,61]

To be clear, the suspicion with which racial minorities view clinical research is not merely the result of research scandals from the 1960s and 1970s. Recent allegations of impropriety have likely increased the apprehension with which minorities view clinical research. In the mid-1990s, for example, it was revealed that the Centers for Disease Control and Prevention, in concert with Kaiser

Permanente of Southern California, had enrolled nearly 1,500 infants in a measles vaccine trial. The research subjects were largely members of minority groups: 44% were African American, 44% were Hispanic American, and 12% were from other unspecified groups.[62] Investigators did not inform any of the infants' parents that the vaccine was experimental or that it was not licensed for use in the United States. This trial further exacerbated the distrust that many minority populations already felt toward clinical research.

Although some minorities may choose not to participate in research, there is compelling evidence that many are never even offered the option of enrolling in a clinical trial.[15,60] Advertising for clinical trials on the Internet has increased self-referral among some populations, but many minorities do not have access to this information.[15] They enter clinical trials largely because they are recruited by investigators or referred by primary care providers.

Because many minority patients seek care at their neighborhood institutions, rather than at research centers, it is the rare few who come into contact with investigators recruiting for new trials.[60] Moreover, limited data suggest that health-care providers, like the rest of society, harbor prejudicial attitudes toward minority groups that influence their decisions about referrals.[50,63] Physicians may refer only "good study candidates" to trials: those who are likely to keep appointments, comply with drug dosing, and be otherwise reliable.[22] Patients who do not speak English,[64] or those with chaotic lifestyles—like single mothers, people with multiple jobs, or those with substance abuse problems or who lack transportation or housing—may not be referred to clinical trials because their primary care providers believe they will have trouble keeping appointments and following the experimental regimen. All too often, minorities are deemed bad study candidates, thereby further limiting their representation in clinical research.[22]

The reluctance among many minorities to participate in research, coupled with these impediments to minority recruitment, point to a need for greater education of both prospective research participants and researchers. Overcoming the pervasive distrust of the medical establishment among minorities will require substantial time and effort. Community-based education programs aimed at discussing concerns minorities have about research, providing information about federal safeguards intended to protect research participants, and sharing the results of relevant research with minorities are essential first steps. Including members of minority communities on research advisory boards, although rarer, has also proven an effective way to improve trust and communication between prospective participants and the research community.[65] At the same time, researchers must recognize that access to research participation is affected not only by eligibility criteria, but also by recruitment strategies and research biases.[66] Researchers must also be aware of and address prejudicial attitudes that prevent primary care providers from referring minorities to research trials.

Research With Economically Disadvantaged Persons

Although ethical analyses have devoted considerable attention to the underrepresentation of minorities in clinical research, far less has been written about the fair selection of those from economically disadvantaged populations. In 1978, the Belmont Report acknowledged that economically disadvantaged populations may be overrepresented in research, "owing to their ready availability in settings where research is conducted," and the ease with which they can be manipulated "as a result of their . . . socioeconomic condition."[6] The Common Rule, at 46.111, likewise includes economically disadvantaged persons as a subset of those "vulnerable to coercion or undue influence."[8] As such, it calls upon IRBs reviewing research involving economically disadvantaged participants to ensure (a) that the "selection of subjects is equitable" and (b) that "additional safeguards have been included in the study to protect the rights and welfare of these subjects" (46.111(a–b)).[8] A recent trial conducted on children in low-income housing suggests, however, that researchers, IRBs, and ethicists need to focus greater attention on the socioeconomic status of research participants and the meaning of the federal regulations designed to protect them.

In 1993 the Kennedy Krieger Institute (KKI), a Baltimore-based children's hospital affiliated with Johns Hopkins University, sought to measure the short- and long-term effectiveness of several different lead paint abatement procedures in low-income housing. KKI researchers estimated that as many as 95% of low-income housing units in Baltimore were contaminated with lead-based paint,[67] creating a risk for developing dangerous levels of lead in the blood of children who lived in those units. At low levels, lead poisoning can adversely affect cognitive development, growth, and behavior; extremely high lead levels can result in seizures, coma, and even death.[68]

Because the cost of safely removing lead-based paint from these low-income housing units often exceeded the cost of the units themselves, landlords frequently closed the properties rather than repairing them, thereby producing a shortage of low-income housing. Researchers at the KKI hypothesized that more economical lead abatement procedures could effectively reduce lead contamination in affected units, thus preserving the availability of low-income housing. In order to determine the effectiveness of various levels of lead abatement, KKI researchers wanted to measure the lead levels in the blood of children living in units that had undergone different degrees of lead abatement.

The two-year KKI study was approved by a Johns Hopkins University IRB and funded by the U.S. Environmental Protection Agency. The study classified 125 low-income Baltimore rental properties into five groups. Housing in the first three groups received varying degrees of partial lead abatement. Housing in the two control groups had either previously undergone full lead abatement or had been constructed without lead-based paint. KKI encouraged landlords to rent these properties, if they were vacant, to families with young children who intended to remain in the housing until the completion of the study.[67] In the event that young children already resided in a study property, their parents were encouraged to remain on the premises.[67]

KKI evaluated the success of each lead abatement method by measuring, at periodic intervals during the two-year period, lead levels in the blood of the children living in each housing group, and the extent to which lead dust remained in, or returned to, the housing. The consent forms signed by the children's parents indicated that lead poisoning in children was a significant problem in Baltimore, and stated that the purpose of the study was to measure the effectiveness of repairs that aimed to reduce, but not completely eliminate, the lead in their home.[67] In return for their participation, parents received periodic payments of $5 to $15 and were told that KKI would provide them with the results of their children's blood tests.

In 2001, the Maryland Court of Appeals permitted two families with minor children that had participated in the study to bring a negligence action against KKI. The parents alleged that they had not been completely and clearly informed of the risks of the research; that KKI had delayed informing them of tests that revealed their children had dangerously high levels of lead in their blood; and that their children had contracted lead-related health injuries during the study. In its defense, KKI claimed that it had no legal duty to protect the research participants from injury, and therefore could not be found negligent. The court disagreed with KKI and held that by virtue of the informed consent agreement entered into between the parents and the researchers, as well as the special relationship created between researchers and research participants, KKI had legal obligations to protect the participants in the study.[67] The court further held that in Maryland, parents cannot consent to their children's participation in "non-therapeutic research or studies in which there is any risk of injury or damage to the health of the subject."[67]

Most striking, though, was the court's comparison of the KKI study to the Tuskegee syphilis trial in its exploitation of economically vulnerable persons.[67] The court admonished the KKI researchers for recruiting families with limited access to low-income housing as research subjects, and it leveled strong words against the IRB that approved the research.[67] Although the court's comparison of the KKI study to the Tuskegee syphilis study has its limitations,[69] it serves as an important reminder that reliance on economically disadvantaged populations as a source of research participants is not merely a part of the past, but something we must actively safeguard against in the present and future. The disclosure in 2005 that NIH-funded researchers enrolled hundreds of mostly poor or minority foster children in HIV-related antiretroviral drug studies during the past two decades, often without advocates to act in the children's best interests, demonstrates the continued prevalence of economically disadvantaged children in research and underscores the need for safeguards to protect them.[70]

The Common Rule offers only limited guidance in this area; it specifies neither what counts as the equitable selection of vulnerable research participants nor what qualifies as an acceptable level of "additional safeguards" to protect them. To hold IRBs, research institutions, and investigators ultimately responsible for the research they approve and engage in, as the Maryland court did, the research community as a whole must take steps toward discussing and further specifying what constitutes fair research with economically disadvantaged persons.

Exclusion and Underrepresentation of Elderly Persons

In the next 25 years, the number of people in the United States who are over the age of 65 will double, and the number of those over 85 will quadruple. Recent literature suggests, however, that the elderly are often excluded and underrepresented in research, even in clinical trials targeting diseases that mostly affect older patients. For instance, in the United States, more than 80% of patients hospitalized with heart failure are aged 65 or older and more than 20% are 85 or older. Yet in a series of 59 clinical trials

conducted with more than 45,000 participants, nearly one-third of trials excluded elderly persons from enrollment.[71] Similarly, in a recent review of 1,522 people enrolled in cancer clinical trials, the enrollment rate for those aged 65 or older was unexpectedly low. Although 49% of breast cancers in the United States occur in people aged 65 or older, only 9% of women enrolled in breast cancer studies were aged 65 or older.[72]

Several factors contribute to the exclusion and underrepresentation of the elderly as research participants. Many clinical trials have enrollment criteria that strictly exclude elderly persons—not always with clear justification. Some trials exclude elderly participants because their comorbidities make them more likely than other participants to experience substantial side effects from experimental interventions. For similar reasons, trials may exclude elderly participants until preliminary dosing and safety data are available from research with the general population. Even when the formal study design does not require aged-based exclusion, criteria that exclude people with conditions that are disproportionately found in the elderly, or that exclude people using medications often taken by the elderly, often function to eliminate older people from the pool of research participants. Elderly patients are also less likely to know or to ask about trials, and because Medicare does not fully pay for experimental trials, many elderly patients may assume (sometimes correctly) that they must pay to participate. Among elderly patients who do want to enroll in research, decreased mobility may make participation more difficult.

Although federal guidelines address the inclusion of women, racial minorities, and children in research, they presently neglect the equally important challenge of enrolling elderly persons in research. Because age affects drug metabolism and disease progression, the lack of older persons in clinical trials limits the benefits of applying research knowledge to the elderly population. Conversely, elderly patients are at greater risk to experience toxic or suboptimal effects of medications that have not been tested for use in their age cohort. Medical advances that prolong life, coupled with the aging of the baby boom population, have rendered the unique health-care needs of the elderly a prime concern in the present era. Fairness in the selection of research participants demands that society consider mechanisms for proportionally representing them in research.

International Clinical Research

In the last decade, ethical controversy erupted about U.S.-sponsored, funded, and conducted clinical trials in the developing world. Such research is not new, however. In the 1950s, U.S. researchers enrolled poor Puerto Rican women in a study to test the effectiveness of the oral contraceptive pill without informing them that they were in research or that there was a risk they would become pregnant.[73,74] In the 1970s and 1980s, U.S. researchers conducted trials of Depo-Provera, a long-acting injectable contraceptive, on women in developing countries even though (and perhaps because) the FDA refused for safety reasons to license the drug in the United States.[75] But it was the work of U.S. researchers in the 1990s studying ways to reduce the perinatal transmission of HIV in the developing world that ultimately sparked the present controversy over the ethics of international clinical research. The debate quickly focused on whether the researchers had acted unethically when they used placebo controls instead of known, effective treatment for preventing perinatal HIV transmission, as would have been required had the research been conducted in the United States.[76,77]

Although that question remains critical to any discussion about the ethics of international research, and is indeed discussed at length in other chapters in this volume, it is equally important to address related concerns about fairness in participant selection. One commonly raised objection to international research is that it can exploit a vulnerable population, namely citizens of developing countries, when they are selected for research participation not for reasons related to the scientific question under study but rather because of their easy availability, their compromised position, and their ability to be manipulated by researchers.[78] To the extent that people living in developed countries are less likely to be exploited, international research often creates "an inequitable selection of research subjects across international boundaries."[75] This inequity is further exacerbated when disadvantaged populations from developing countries bear the burdens of research without the opportunity to enjoy the benefits that may result from its completion.

These concerns suggest the need for stringent guidelines to protect populations in developing countries. As the history of participant selection in the United States illustrates, however, adopting an overly protectionist attitude can prevent vulnerable populations from enrolling in clinical trials from which they may benefit. Fifty percent of people in developing countries do not have access to even the most basic drugs, arguably making participation in clinical trials an attractive way to gain access to physicians and medications otherwise unavailable.[79] Fair selection in this context therefore requires a delicate balance between protection from research harms and access to research benefits, both during the trial and after its completion.

Future Directions

Conceptions of fairness in research participant selection have evolved dramatically during the last 40 years. Ultimately, though, fair selection is just one component in ensuring fairness in the distribution of the burdens and benefits of research across the whole population. Each step in designing, conducting, and concluding a research study marks a moment in which fairness should be considered.[66] Setting research priorities, developing research questions, and distributing research funding all affect fairness in research by determining what counts as medically or socially beneficial research and who should be the participants in and beneficiaries of such research. A decision to address a disease that affects a large segment of the population, such as heart disease, may compete with studies that address a disease primarily affecting a minority population, such as sickle-cell anemia.

Study design and recruitment also shape the fairness of any research trial. Avoiding scientifically unnecessary exclusion criteria raises the probability that diverse populations will participate in research. Similarly, employing a variety of recruitment mechanisms increases the likelihood that people of different backgrounds will enroll in research. Certain recruitment methods, such as those requiring a computer, may limit access to trials, whereas flyers, classified ads, television commercials, and radio announcements may reach broader segments of the population.

At each stage in a clinical trial, researchers and IRBs should carefully consider the fairness of the study. Admittedly, the federal regulations offer far less guidance in this area than they do with regard to informed consent. And, to be sure, further conceptual, normative, and empirical work is needed to clarify and address exploitation as unfairly taking advantage of the circumstances, including the vulnerabilities, of particular populations.[80] Still, despite incomplete guidance and lingering ambiguities, investigators, IRBs, and research institutions must make practical efforts to ensure that research populations are selected equitably and represented proportionally. Any given research study should include people from diverse populations, where *not* scientifically inappropriate, without unduly burdening any particular population. Fairness in research demands nothing less than an ethically justified balance between protection and access.[81]

References

1. Levine C. Has AIDS changed the ethics of human subjects research? *Law, Medicine, and Health Care* 1988;16:167–73.
2. Beecher HE. Ethics and clinical research. *New England Journal of Medicine* 1966;274:1354–60.
3. Jones JH. *Bad Blood: The Tuskegee Syphilis Experiment*, 2nd ed. New York, N.Y.: Free Press; 1993 [1981].
4. Brandt AM. Racism and research: The case of the Tuskegee Syphilis Study. *Hastings Center Report* 1978;8(6):21–9.
5. U.S. Congress. National Research Act of 1974. Pub. L. No. 93–348, 93rd Congress, 2nd Session, July 12, 1974.
6. The National Commission for the Protection of Human Subjects of Biomedical and Behavioral Research. *The Belmont Report: Ethical Principles and Guidelines for the Protection of Human Subjects of Research.* Washington, D.C.: Department of Health, Education and Welfare; DHEW Publication OS 78-0012 1978. [Online] April 18, 1979. Available: http://www.hhs.gov/ohrp/humansubjects/guidance/belmont.htm.
7. Jonas H. Philosophical reflections on experimenting with human subjects. *Daedalus* 1969;98:219–47.
8. Department of Health and Human Services, National Institutes of Health, and Office for Human Research Protections. The Common Rule, Title 45 (Public Welfare), Code of Federal Regulations, Part 46 (Protection of Human Subjects). [Online] June 23, 2005. Available: http://www.hhs.gov/ohrp/humansubjects/guidance/45cfr46.htm.
9. Food and Drug Administration, Department of Health and Human Services. Title 21 (Food and Drugs), Code of Federal Regulations, Part 50 (Protection of Human Subjects). [Online] April 1, 2006. Available: http://www.gpo.gov/nara/cfr/waisidx_06/21cfr50_06.html.
10. Food and Drug Administration, Department of Health and Human Services. Title 21 (Food and Drugs), Code of Federal Regulations, Part 56 (Institutional Review Boards). [Online] April 1, 2006. Available: http://www.gpo.gov/nara/cfr/waisidx_06/21cfr56_06.html.
11. Advisory Committee on Human Radiation Experiments. *Final Report of the Advisory Committee on Human Radiation Experiments.* New York, N.Y.: Oxford University Press; 1996:502.
12. Arnold JD. Incidence of injury during clinical pharmacology research and indemnification of injured research subjects at Quincy Research Center. In: President's Commission for the Study of Ethical Problems in Medicine and Biomedical and Behavioral Research. *Compensating for Research Injuries: The Ethical and Legal Implications of Programs to Redress Injuries Caused by Biomedical and Behavioral Research.* Washington, D.C.: U.S. Government Printing Office; 1982.
13. McCann DJ, Pettit JR. A report on adverse effects insurance for human subjects. In: President's Commission for the Study of Ethical Problems in Medicine and Biomedical and Behavioral Research. *Compensating for Research Injuries: The Ethical and Legal Implications of Programs to*

Redress Injuries Caused by Biomedical and Behavioral Research. Washington, D.C.: U.S. Government Printing Office; 1982.

14. Lantos JD. The "inclusion benefit" in clinical trials. *Journal of Pediatrics* 1999;134:130–1.

15. Noah BA. The participation of underrepresented minorities in clinical research. *American Journal of Law and Medicine* 2003;29:221–45.

16. Levine RJ. The impact of HIV infection on society's perception of clinical trials. *Kennedy Institute of Ethics Journal* 1994;4:93–8.

17. Macklin R, Friedland G. AIDS research: The ethics of clinical trials. *Law, Medicine, and Health Care* 1986;14:273–80.

18. Levine C, Dubler NN, Levine RJ. Building a new consensus: Ethical principles and policies for clinical research on HIV/AIDS. *IRB: A Review of Human Subjects Research* 1991;13(1–2):1–17.

19. Department of Health and Human Services, Office for Health Research Protections. *Protecting Human Research Subjects: Institutional Review Board Guidebook.* Rockville, Md.: OHRP; 1993. [Online] Available: http://www.hhs.gov/ohrp/irb/irb_guidebook.htm.

20. Weijer C. Evolving ethical issues in selection of subjects for clinical research. *Cambridge Quarterly of Healthcare Ethics* 1996;5:334–45.

21. Levine C. Women and HIV/AIDS research: The barriers to equity. *IRB: A Review of Human Subjects Research* 1991;13(1–2):18–22.

22. Lynn LA. AIDS clinical trials: Is there access for all? *Journal of General Internal Medicine* 1997;12:198–9.

23. Committee on the Ethical and Legal Issues Relating to the Inclusion of Women in Clinical Studies. Justice in clinical studies: Guiding principles. In: Mastroianni AC, Faden R, Federman D, eds. *Women and Health Research: Ethical and Legal Issues of Including Women in Clinical Studies, Vol. I.* Washington, D.C.: National Academy Press; 1994: 75–83.

24. Dresser R. Wanted: Single, white male for medical research. *Hastings Center Report* 1992;22(1):24–9.

25. Coronary Drug Project Research Group. The coronary drug project: Design, method, and baseline results. *Circulation* 1973;47:I1–I50.

26. Multiple Risk Factor Intervention Trial Research Group. Statistical design considerations in the NHLI multiple risk factor intervention trial (MRFIT). *Journal of Chronic Diseases* 1977;30:261–75.

27. Lipid Research Clinics Program. Recruitment for clinical trials: the Lipid Research Clinics coronary primary prevention trial experience: Its implications for future trials. *Circulation* 1982;66:IV1–IV78.

28. Manson JE, et al. Baseline characteristics of participants in the Physicians' Health Study: A randomized trial of aspirin and beta-carotene in U.S. physicians. *American Journal of Preventative Medicine* 1991;7:150–4.

29. McCarthy CR. Historical background of clinical trials involving women and minorities. *Academic Medicine* 1994;69:695–8.

30. DeBruin DA. Justice and the inclusion of women in clinical studies: A conceptual framework. In: Mastroianni AC, Faden R, Federman D, eds. *Women and Health Research: Ethical and Legal Issues of Including Women in Clinical Studies, Vol. II.* Washington, D.C.: National Academy Press; 1994:127–50.

31. Resnik DR. Sex biases in subject selection: A survey of articles published in American medical journals. *Theoretical Medicine and Bioethics* 1999;20:245–60.

32. Weijer C, Crouch RA. Why should we include women and minorities in randomized clinical trials? *Journal of Clinical Ethics* 1999;10:100–6.

33. Gotay CC, Phillips PH, Cheson BD. Male-female differences in the impact of cancer therapy. *Oncology* 1993;7:67–74.

34. Allen M. The dilemma for women of color in clinical trials. *Journal of the American Medical Women's Association* 1994;49:105–9.

35. Mohiuddin SM, Hilleman DE. Gender and racial bias in clinical pharmacology trials. *Annals of Pharmacotherapy* 1993;27:972–3.

36. Svensson CK. Representation of American blacks in clinical trials of new drugs. *JAMA* 1989;261:263–5.

37. Dignam JJ, et al. Prognosis among African-American women and white women with lymph node negative breast carcinoma: Findings from two randomized clinical trials of the National Surgical Adjuvant Breast and Bowel Project. *Cancer* 1997;80:80–90.

38. Cotton P. Is there still too much extrapolation from data on middle aged white men? *JAMA* 1990;263:1049–50.

39. Nelson RM. Children as research subjects. In: Kahn JP, Mastroianni AC, Sugarman J, eds. *Beyond Consent: Seeking Justice in Research.* New York, N.Y.: Oxford University Press; 1998:47–66.

40. National Institutes of Health. Special instructions to applicants using form PHS 398 regarding implementation of the NIH/ADAMHA Policy Concerning Inclusion of Women and Minorities in Clinical Research Study Populations. *NIH Guide for Grants and Contracts* 1990;19:18–9.

41. Food and Drug Administration, Department of Health and Human Services. Guideline for the Study and Evaluation of Gender Differences in the Clinical Evaluation of Drugs; Notice. *Federal Register* 1993;58(139):39406–16.

42. Merkatz RB, et al. Women in clinical trials of new drugs: A change in Food and Drug Administration policy. *New England Journal of Medicine* 1993;329:292–6.

43. Cotton P. FDA lifts ban on women in early drug tests, will require companies to look for gender differences. *JAMA* 1993;269:2067.

44. NIH Revitalization Act of 1993, Pub. L. No. 103–43, 103rd Congress (June 10, 1993).

45. National Institutes of Health, Department of Health and Human Services. NIH Guidelines on the Inclusion of Woman and Minorities as Subjects in Clinical Research; Notice. *Federal Register* 1994;59(59):14508–13.

46. House of Representatives Report No. 209, 104th Congress, 1st session. 1995:80–1.

47. Senate Report No. 145, 104th Congress, 1st session. 1995:112.

48. National Institutes of Health. Policy and guidelines on the inclusion of children as participants in research involving human subjects. *NIH Guide for Grants and Contracts* March 6, 1998:26.

49. Food and Drug Administration, Department of Health and Human Services. 21 CFR Parts 201, 312, 314 and 601: Regulations Requiring Manufacturers to Assess the Safety and Effectiveness of New Drugs and Biological Products in Pediatric Patients; Final Rule. *Federal Register* 1998;63(231):66631–72.

50. King TE. Racial disparities in clinical trials. *New England Journal of Medicine* 2002;346:1400–2.

51. Gifford AL. Participation in research and access to experimental treatments by HIV-infected patients. *New England Journal of Medicine* 2002;346:1373–82.

52. Buist AS, Greenlick MR. Response to "Inclusion of women and minorities in clinical trials and the NIH Revitalization Act of 1993—The perspective of NIH trialists." *Controlled Clinical Trials* 1995;16:296–8.

53. Woolson R. Response to "Inclusion of women and minorities in clinical trials and the NIH Revitalization Act of 1993—The perspective of NIH trialists." *Controlled Clinical Trials* 1995;16:301–3.

54. Corbie-Smith G, Miller WC, Ransohoff DF. Interpretations of "appropriate" minority inclusion in clinical research. *American Journal of Medicine* 2004;116:249–52.

55. Gamble VN. A legacy of distrust: African-Americans and medical research. *American Journal of Preventive Medicine* 1993;9:35–8.

56. Shavers VL, Lynch CF, Burmeister LF. Factors that influence African-Americans' willingness to participate in medical research studies. *Cancer Supplement* 2001;91:233–6.

57. Gamble VN. Under the shadow of Tuskegee: African Americans and health care. *American Journal of Public Health* 1997;87:1773–8.

58. Corbie-Smith G, et al. Attitudes and beliefs of African-Americans toward participation in medical research. *Journal of General Internal Medicine* 1999;14:537–46.

59. Kass N, Sugarman J, Faden R, Schoch-Spana M. Trust: The fragile foundation of contemporary biomedical research. *Hastings Center Report* 1996;26(5):25–9.

60. El-Sadr W, Capps L. The challenge of minority recruitment in clinical trials for AIDS. *JAMA* 1992;267:954–7.

61. Burchard E, Ziv E, Coyle N, et al. The importance of race and ethnic background in biomedical research and clinical practice. *New England Journal of Medicine* 2003;348:1170–5.

62. Marwick C. Questions raised about measles vaccine trial. *JAMA* 1996;276:1288–9.

63. Stone VE, Mauch MY, Steger KA. Provider attitudes regarding participation of women and persons of color in AIDS clinical trials. *Journal of Acquired Immune Deficiency Syndromes and Human Retrovirology* 1998;19:245–53.

64. Hazuda HP. Non-English-speaking patients: A challenge to researchers. *Journal of General Internal Medicine* 1996;11:56–7.

65. Corbie-Smith G, Thomas SB, St. George DM. Distrust, race, and research. *Archives of Internal Medicine* 2002;162:2458–63.

66. Kahn JP, Mastroianni AC, Sugarman J. Implementing justice in a changing research environment. In: Kahn JP, Mastroianni AC, Sugarman J, eds. *Beyond Consent: Seeking Justice in Research.* New York, N.Y.: Oxford University Press; 1998:166–73.

67. *Grimes v. Kennedy Krieger Institute, Inc.,* 782 A.2d 807 (Md. Ct. App. 2001).

68. Centers for Disease Control and Prevention. Recommendations for Blood Lead Screening of Young Children Enrolled in Medicaid: Targeting a Group at High Risk. Advisory Committee on Childhood Lead Poisoning Prevention (ACCLPP). *Morbidity and Mortality Weekly Report* 2000;49(RR14):1–13. [Online] Available: http://www.cdc.gov/mmwr/PDF/rr/rr4914.pdf.

69. Mastroianni AC, Kahn JP. Risk and responsibility: Ethics, *Grimes v. Kennedy Krieger,* and public health research involving children. *American Journal of Public Health* 2002;92:1073–6.

70. Solomon J. AIDS drugs tested on foster kids. *CBS NewsOnline.* [Online] May 4, 2005. Available: http://www.cbsnews.com/stories/2005/05/04/health/main692980.shtml.

71. Heiat A, Gross C, Krumholz H. Representation of the elderly, women, and minorities in heart failure clinical trials. *Archives of Internal Medicine* 2002;162:1682–8.

72. Hutchins LF, et al. Underrepresentation of patients 65 years of age or older in cancer-treatment trials. *New England Journal of Medicine* 1999;341:2061–7.

73. Vaughan P. *The Pill on Trial.* New York, N.Y.: Coward-McCann; 1970.

74. Warwick D. Contraceptives in the third world. *Hastings Center Report* 1975;5(4):9–12.

75. Macklin R. Justice in international research. In: Kahn JP, Mastroianni AC, Sugarman J, eds. *Beyond Consent: Seeking Justice in Research.* New York, N.Y.: Oxford University Press; 1998:131–46.

76. Lurie P, Wolfe S. Unethical trials of interventions to reduce perinatal transmission of the human immunodeficiency virus in developing countries. *New England Journal of Medicine* 1997;337:853–6.

77. Angell M. The ethics of clinical research in the third world. *New England Journal of Medicine* 1997;337:847–9.

78. Barry M. Ethical considerations of human investigation in developing countries: The AIDS dilemma. *New England Journal of Medicine* 1998;319:1083–6.

79. Benatar SR. Distributive justice and clinical trials in the third world. *Theoretical Medicine and Bioethics* 2001;22:169–76.

80. Resnik D. Exploitation in biomedical research. *Theoretical Medicine and Bioethics* 2003;24:233–59.

81. Mastroianni A, Kahn J. Swinging on the pendulum: Shifting views of justice in human subjects research. *Hastings Center Report* 2001;31(3):21–8.

Neal Dickert   Christine Grady

Incentives for Research Participants

History

The practice of paying research participants dates back at least to the early 19th century, when William Beaumont provided Alexis St. Martin with room, board, and $150 per year for the use of his stomach in physiologic studies. St. Martin had been shot in the stomach and was left with a permanent gastric fistula, providing Beaumont with "access to the stomach and the opportunity to study the action of gastric juices."[1] Later, Walter Reed offered $100 in gold to participants in studies involving deliberate exposure to yellow fever. If successfully infected, participants received a $100 bonus (payable to their family if they died).[1] Although a long-standing practice, payment in research seems to be increasingly common with the growing volume of research conducted today.

Paying research participants, however, remains contentious. Ethical concerns have appeared in the literature since the 1970s and are far from resolved;[2–11] and the unfortunate deaths of Bernadette Gilchrist, Nicole Wan, and Ellen Roche have called attention to the practice of paying healthy participants.[12,13] Stories appearing in the mid-1990s about homeless participants in Phase I drug trials conducted by Eli Lilly and Co. raised concerns about offering money and other incentives to the homeless in exchange for research participation.[14] Analogous concerns have been raised with regard to the provision of otherwise unavailable health-care services when conducting research in the developing world.[15] In the United States, advertisements on television and radio, in newspapers, and on the Internet offer money, medications, free medical care, and other incentives in exchange for participation in all types of research. Ads recruit the young and the old, the sick and the healthy. There have even emerged a number of professional re-search participants, or "professional guinea pigs," who make a living participating in research. Online 'zines such as *Guinea Pig Zero* rate research facilities on criteria ranging from the amount of payment to the quality of food, and give potential research participants the "inside scoop" on how to be a successful participant.[16]

Core Conceptualization

Exchanging money and other goods for research participation can represent reimbursement or remuneration, compensation for time and effort, a gift or token of appreciation, or a recruitment incentive. These different ways of conceptualizing exchanges have distinct meanings and ethical implications. Here, we use the generic term *payment* to encompass all potential conceptualizations, and we discuss the different ethical implications of various conceptualizations.

Payment serves different purposes and occurs in numerous forms, many of which are nonmonetary. Payment has come in the form of sentence reduction for prisoners, academic credit for students, and toys or movie passes for children. Some studies offer free treatment for the condition under study or for unrelated medical conditions. Most literature has focused on cash payments, for two primary reasons. First, monetary exchanges are identifiable and fungible. Exchanges of health care or access to other studies may be less demarcated and even inseparable from the research. Second, there is a particular concern about offering money in a traditionally volunteer relationship, especially when patients who are ill are involved.[7,17–19] For any research project, whether health care or other benefits are offered, participants must make the same type of decision as when money is offered. They must decide whether to accept the risks, benefits, and inconvenience of research participation in exchange for valuable goods. The following discussion thus pertains to payment in multiple "currencies."

It is important to consider why payment is offered in the first place. First, payment may encourage or allow individuals to perform a needed service. It may aid recruitment by lessening the burden of participation or presenting an opportunity for "profit." The extent to which payment actually facilitates recruitment, however, is not well documented. Payment is known to facilitate response to surveys, but the relevance of such data to clinical research is uncertain.[20] The second reason payment may be offered is to recognize and compensate for the time, inconvenience, cost, or even risk of participation. Rather than paying to achieve recruitment goals, investigators may seek to recognize participants' contributions and to thank them for it.

Elsewhere we have described three core models for paying research participants: a market model, a wage payment model, and a reimbursement model.[3] We will review the ethical advantages and disadvantages of these models, as well as those of an additional posttrial appreciation model.[21] Table 36.1 presents some core features of each of the models.

Market Model

If the primary purpose of payment is recruitment, the intuitively appropriate model is the market model. This model relies on the principle of supply and demand to decide the amount and type of incentive needed to recruit a sufficient number of qualified research participants in the desired time frame.[3,22] If research is risky or unpleasant, incentives increase. If research is desirable, as in studies of new medications for diseases for which no treatment existed previously, payment may be low or nonexistent. Likewise, payment may increase or decrease relative to other local studies recruiting similar participants, or it may vary based on the time frame within which studies must be completed. Pay might be contingent on completion of the study or might increase over the course of the study as an escalating incentive. Although money is the paradigm, any "currency" can fit this model. Free physical examinations, medications, or academic credit can all be scaled to meet demand.

Wage Payment Model

The wage payment model regards research participation as akin to unskilled labor for which participants are paid an amount close to the standard hourly wage for other unskilled jobs in the geographic area in which the research is conducted.[2,3,23] Completion bonuses or increases for inconvenience or discomfort may be employed, but payment is essentially based on the amount participants "work." Wages can clearly act as incentives; however, the unskilled labor market sets wages, rather than individual preferences or pure market demand, and pay across studies is relatively standardized.

Reimbursement Model

The reimbursement model allows only for reimbursement of expenses actually incurred, based on the idea that research should be "revenue neutral." This model could be applied in radically different ways. Out-of-pocket expenses such as parking and transportation could be reimbursed. Or research participants could be paid what they are normally paid for their work as reimbursement for wages lost while participating in research. If the latter standard were applied, a homemaker might receive nothing, whereas an executive would receive quite a lot of money for the same contribution to research. However, no participant would profit, supply and demand do not influence payment, and nonmonetary expenses, such as inconvenience or discomfort, are not reimbursed.[3]

Posttrial Appreciation Model

A fourth model is a posttrial appreciation model in which participants receive a gift or reward upon completion of a study. This model can apply to research with adults, but it is most popular in pediatric research in which the appreciation gift might be a toy or game.[24–26] Although gifts are not always a surprise, in this model participants are not typically informed of the gift during the consent process or the study. To the extent that investigators keep potential research participants from knowing about the gift during decision making, the gift will not be an incentive to participate; it is a reward for participation. However, as rewards become known to potential participants, either through prior participation or word of mouth, they could also operate as incentives.

Table 36.1
The Four Models of Payment

	Market Model	Wage Payment Model	Reimbursement Model	Posttrial Appreciation Model
Justification for payment	Recruitment of research participants is vital to research; monetary incentives help to recruit the needed research participant pool	Participation in research requires little skill but takes time, effort, and endurance of uncomfortable procedures	Participation in research should not require financial sacrifice by research participants	Participation in research is a valuable service that merits recognition and appreciation
Function of payment	Pure incentive	Working wage	Reimbursement for expenses	Recognition of service
Strategy employed	Payment based on supply and demand; employment of completion bonuses and other end-loaded incentives	Payment based on standard wage for unskilled labor; augmented for particularly uncomfortable procedures	Payment determined by research participant's expenses; can be payment for lost wages or for other expenses incurred	Goods of any kind offered to research participants after participation is finished; research participants not informed at time of consent

Ethical Concerns

These four models represent the essential conceptualizations surrounding the payment of research participants. Some may propose further divisions, and actual practice may employ variations or combinations;[21] however, considering each model individually allows isolation of ethical concerns associated with each strategy. Table 36.2 presents the principal advantages and disadvantages of the four models.

Coercion and Undue Inducement

The principal concerns cited in the literature on payment relate to the possibility of coercion or undue inducement.[6,7,10,11,22,27] Unfortunately, these terms are often confused or used inappropriately. Coercion is defined by the presence of a threat of harm or force that could make the coerced person worse off in some way.[28] Undue inducement, on the other hand, is not associated with threats but with offers.[11,30] What makes certain offers undue is a subject of significant debate. We suggest that offers are unduly influential if they are so attractive that they lead individuals to participate in research studies to which they would normally have important objections.

True and morally problematic coercion in research is a rare phenomenon. Few investigators overtly threaten to make anyone worse off for refusing to participate in a study. Coercion may be an important concern in research with prisoners or other captive populations, in which refusal to participate in research could be met with punishment or retaliation. Though technically possible whenever a power differential exists between investigator and participant, most institutional review boards (IRBs) scrupulously prohibit threats of harm for refusal. People may sometimes fear that they will be treated worse for not participating in research, even when no threat exists. Such perceived coercion is a crucial consideration, but neither perceived nor real coercion has any direct or consistent connection to payment because payment is never (or should never be) a threat itself. In some cases, refusal to participate in a paid study could indirectly result in harm. For example, if the spouse of someone refusing to participate in a paid study threatens the refusing spouse, payment might facilitate third-party coercion, but the investigators themselves could not be charged with coercion. In a doctor-patient relationship, payment may actually reduce perceived coercion by transforming the exchange into one that is less personal, and unrelated to medical care.

Some writers have discussed omissive coercion, based on the concern that society "threatens" to remove or does not provide the

Table 36.2
Potential Advantages and Disadvantages of the Four Models

Model	Advantages	Disadvantages
Market	• Ensures sufficient research participant pool in desired time • Increases likelihood of research participants completing the study • Research participants profit from performing a social good • Lessens financial sacrifice of participation	• High offers may be unduly influential • May provide an incentive to remain uninformed • May provide an incentive to conceal information • May particularly influence poor populations • May lead to recruitment of research participants with no concern for the ends of research • Leads to interstudy competition based on research participant payment • Commodifies research participation
Wage payment	• Offers profit commensurate with other unskilled jobs • Standardizes payment across studies • Lessens financial sacrifice of participation • Ensures minimum wage for paid research participants • Research participants may profit performing a social good	• May not recruit sufficient research participant pool in desired time • Presents profit only to poorer populations • Requires financial sacrifice for wealthier populations • Commodifies research participation
Reimbursement	• Precludes undue influence from money • Provides no incentive to conceal information • Provides no incentive to remain uninformed • Does not preferentially induce poorer populations • Lessens financial sacrifice of participation	• May not recruit a sufficient research participant pool in desired time • Requires financial sacrifice for uncompensated time *If time is reimbursed:* • May lead to targeting poorer populations • May increase the cost of conducting research • Pays differentially for the same function
Posttrial appreciation	*If hidden:* • Allows for profit with no potential for undue inducement • Rewards a valuable service • Expresses appreciation without undermining volunteerism *If not hidden:* • Rewards a valuable service • Expresses appreciation without undermining volunteerism • May allow for sufficient recruitment within time goals (if treated as a recruitment device)	*If hidden:* • May not recruit sufficient research participant pool in desired time • May still require financial sacrifice • No basis for determining the magnitude of "reward" *If not hidden:* • No constraints on reward may lead to undue inducement • May lead IRBs to ignore potential power of the offer • Does not ensure volunteerism, which is its primary goal • No basis for determining the magnitude of "reward"

means to obtain certain basic goods unless those individuals participate in research.[31] Although this is a legitimate concern, investigators' responsibility for background social conditions seems minimal, and calling this situation coercive seems a misnomer. Individual vulnerabilities resulting from societal failures are crucial considerations, but we believe these are really concerns about possible exploitation, not coercion. We discuss this further below.

Undue inducement is the predominant ethical concern in the literature and the focus of the sparse guidance in the U.S. Common Rule, as well as guidance issued by the Food and Drug Administration (FDA), the Office for Human Research Protections (OHRP) in the Department of Health and Human Services, and the Council for International Organizations of Medical Sciences (CIOMS).[32–35] Yet there is significant ambiguity and disagreement about what constitutes undue inducement and how to avoid it.[22,30,36,37] The classic scenarios involving undue inducement are studies that pose significant risk of harm and offer considerable incentives to research participants who often have limited means and opportunities. For example, a trial that administers general anesthesia to healthy research participants may pay quite a bit of money and involve significant risk. A challenge study investigating psychiatric disease may provide psychiatric treatment in exchange for the risk of a research challenge and enroll individuals with little or no access to health care. Although all concerns about undue inducement refer to attractive offers, different reasons have been put forth regarding when and why such offers are problematic. Some accounts have to do with the quality of judgment or voluntariness of decisions, whereas others focus on risks to research participants or to scientific integrity.

Several writers have expressed concern about the effect of payment on the quality of judgment or decision making.[6,33,37,38] There are two ways that a participant's decision might potentially be compromised in the setting of significant inducement.[11] First, a research participant may ignore the risks of a study. A homeless man may be so eager to make $500 that he neglects to read the consent form or ignores a research coordinator's description of study risks. Strictly speaking, his decision might be voluntary, but it would be uninformed and based on incomplete understanding. However, even though data show that informed consent is less than adequate in many ways, there are no data that show that payment exacerbates these inadequacies. In fact, some data suggest that it does not.[38] Furthermore, if the worry is about understanding, the more immediate remedy would be to take extra steps to ensure that participants are well informed rather than to ban payment for research participation.[30,39]

Other concerns about the quality of judgment have more to do with the voluntariness of decisions.[11] The disagreement over this concern can hardly be understated. Some writers worry that large incentives may control individuals' decisions in a way that is morally objectionable,[6] though exactly what constitutes "control" over decisions is unclear. Others have argued that it is absurd to talk about reducing voluntariness by giving someone what they want.[22,27] After all, we rarely say that people offered a high salary for a job are being unduly induced. The fact that people "cannot refuse" an attractive offer speaks to the appeal of the offer and not to nonvoluntariness. Although we do not dismiss all concerns about undue inducement, we agree with the view of those who argue that voluntariness is not the right way to frame this concern.

Most worries about attractive offers likely stem from the view that money and other incentives ought not to be the only reasons that an individual participates in research. At the heart of research ethics is a moral tension about "using" a person's body for research, rooted in the Kantian prohibition against treating other people merely as means. Many believe that research participants ought, in some way, to accept the ends of the research as their own.[40] However, there are deep questions about this view.[30]

First, why are monetary or other goals advanced by payment illegitimate compared with the goals of the research? Second, Kantian theory particularly prioritizes respect for individuals' ability to determine their own values and to make autonomous, rational decisions. Although concerns about payment compromising voluntariness seem misdirected, using forms of payment to overcome important values that people hold is potentially problematic. A rich conception of respect for persons as autonomous agents, we believe, does include sensitivity to individuals' fundamental values and strong preferences. It thus entails a certain responsibility to allow people to live lives in accordance with their values and preferences, a responsibility that may be incompatible with making certain offers that knowingly challenge those values.

Consider, for example, a safety study of an investigational blood substitute that is derived from human blood but does not have to be matched. Investigators are conducting this study in an area in which a very high proportion of the population are Jehovah's Witnesses. Despite the fact that the new blood substitute is not whole blood, the use of this agent would constitute a major violation of this population's religious beliefs. Because investigators know that few people in the area will want to take part in this study, they decide to offer $20,000 to participants, knowing that this amount of money will likely lead enough Jehovah's Witnesses to participate in the study because of the promise of significant financial reward.

We do not assert that Jehovah's Witnesses who would make this choice would be acting in an irrational, uninformed, or involuntary manner; nor would we necessarily criticize them for making the choice to enroll. We do, however, have deep concerns that the practice of offering such a reward with the aim of encouraging people to overcome important and deeply held values fails to respect those persons and their values in an important way. For the same reasons that many would suggest conducting the study in an area in which fewer people would find it objectionable, we submit that raising the offer to an amount that might induce people to set aside deeply held values in order to recruit an adequate sample is not compatible with respecting participants.

Other writers reduce the concern for undue inducement to a concern about risk to participants.[7,30] Emanuel, for example, argues that undue inducement cannot occur in an appropriately approved study, because risks should not be unreasonable relative to the benefits for participants or society.[30] It does seem that essentially risk-free studies do not raise concerns about undue inducement; however, even in appropriately approved studies, risk-based concerns remain relevant for three reasons. First, IRBs must make determinations based on what reasonable people consider to be acceptable risks. Potential participants, however, lie on a spectrum from extreme risk aversion to extreme risk tolerance. Any given level of risk will surely carry different meanings for different participants. Second, actual risks vary among individual participants, and some risks are idiosyncratic. Third, risk tolerance may be an important aspect of individuals' values and preferences. Large amounts of payment at the end of the spectrum of approvable risk might induce individuals who are actually quite averse to risks, or more susceptible to risks, to participate in studies that are otherwise problematic for them. For these reasons, concerns about undue inducement cannot simply be dismissed based on an IRB's finding that the level of risk is reasonable.

Another concern about undue inducement is that individuals, enticed by large offers, may conceal information about themselves that might otherwise disqualify them from studies (e.g., past medical history or medications). Similarly, they may be reluctant to report adverse events out of fear that they may be removed from the study and not receive their payment. The concern is that such misrepresentation may expose participants to increased risk or that it may compromise the data.[3,6,27,32,36,39] One study suggests that people are unlikely to hide information in studies they perceive as risky but may be more likely to misrepresent themselves in lower-risk studies.[41] The degree to which these concerns are real is largely unknown, and they warrant further empirical investigation and attention.

In sum, we argue that undue inducement may occur when offers are so attractive that they lead individuals to participate in research studies to which they would normally have strong objections, based on risk or other important values or preferences. This account has some similarities to that of Grant and Sugarman.[36] Importantly, a decision to participate does not have to be irrational or less than fully voluntary in order to be unduly induced. Rather, the key determinant is that the activity is one that participants find objectionable in a significant way. The proper focus of scrutiny is thus more on the research, and the likely participants, than on payment itself. Although the incidence of undue inducement is an empirical question, relatively few people are likely to have true, strong objections to most research projects, making real undue inducement a rare occurrence. IRBs should nevertheless consider its possibility—especially at the end of the spectrum of approvable risks and when people are likely to have strong values or preferences that conflict with the research. At the same time, IRBs also cannot avoid all potential cases of undue inducement, because strong objections to research may be very individual and idiosyncratic and therefore hard to predict.

On any account of undue inducement, the degree to which it is a concern varies by payment model. Because the market model contains no constraints on incentives, those most concerned about undue inducement will likely find the market model problematic. The reimbursement model, in which only actual expenses are reimbursed, and the posttrial appreciation model, in which the reward is not offered at the time of consent, do not raise the possibility of undue inducement. The wage payment model limits concern about undue inducement by capping, though not eliminating, the degree of incentive provided to participants and offering an inducement commensurate with other unskilled jobs available elsewhere. Although wage-like amounts of money may possibly be more attractive to low-income participants, the amount is unlikely to cause many people to compromise deeply held values or preferences.

Justice

Two considerations of justice are relevant when offering payment for research participation. First, justice requires that benefits and burdens of research be distributed equitably; therefore no population should bear a disproportionate burden. Second, justice requires that similar people be treated similarly.[27,29]

Because incentives may be more attractive to poorer individuals, there could be overrepresentation of poor individuals in research.[2,3,39] If so, an already disadvantaged segment of the population could bear a disproportionate share of the research burden. On the market model, it is easy to meet the "price" of poor people. On the wage payment model, unskilled wages are likely to be preferentially attractive to the poor. Even the reimbursement model might preferentially attract poorer research participants, as reimbursement is likely to provide more meaningful reductions in opportunity costs for poorer research participants.[3] Similarly, the attractiveness of gifts, if known at the time of consent, may differ for members of different socioeconomic classes.[24]

How much should we worry about differential effects of payment according to socioeconomic status, and how much is this concern borne out in practice? Wilkinson and Moore clarify the distinction between the question of group-level justice, which they term "pattern equity," and concerns about exploitation, which involves inappropriately taking advantage of the predicaments of others. The pattern equity concern refers to the distribution of burdens and benefits across the population of potential research participants.[27] Most importantly, they argue, many paid research participants view participation and payment as beneficial, so it is strange to speak of a maldistribution of burden. In addition, poverty and the consequent attractiveness of research participation are problems with the way society distributes goods, not necessarily problems with the conduct of research.[27] Payment may even be a way to advance justice by increasing enrollment of underrepresented groups in research.[36,37] Real ethical worries about enrolling poor participants are likely concerns about exploitation rather than pattern equity.

The second demand of justice, that similar cases be treated similarly, conflicts with concerns about pattern equity because one solution to pattern equity concerns is differential payment to different groups.[2,3,36] Treating similar people similarly is arguably more important than pattern equity.

The concerns and demands of justice have different implications for various payment models. A market model could allow vastly different amounts of payment per participant or per study, depending upon supply and demand, and could allow for preferential recruitment of any type of person. The wage payment model is largely premised on the notion that similar work should be paid similarly, but low, standardized payments could preferentially attract poor people.[2,3,36,39] A posttrial appreciation model might offer the same gift to each participant within a study but might not standardize across studies and could preferentially induce people with greater need or desire for the gift. Contrary to the assertions of Dunn and Gordon,[39] it seems that the only way to be sure to avoid preferential recruitment of poor people (and its consequent impact on justice and scientific integrity) would be to employ a strict reimbursement model involving different payments to every person in the study.

Exploitation

An important concern, often confused with and sometimes overlapping with concerns about undue inducement, is the potential for payment to be exploitative. Concerns about exploitation are often raised when investigators conduct research in developing countries or enroll poor individuals or sick patients who do not have access to care. Though commonly discussed, the word *exploitation* is often loosely used, and there remains debate about exactly what constitutes exploitation. Alan Wertheimer argues that exploitation occurs in circumstances in which "A takes unfair advantage of B." Simply put, unfair-advantage exploitation involves an unfair distribution of harm and benefit between the two parties, a possibility even in cases when both parties benefit.[42] Wilkinson and Moore argue that payment for research participation is not exploitative in this sense, because it is not clear that research participants ought to be paid more. They also note that imbalances in benefits exist in almost every type of transaction.[22] Furthermore, they claim, as Emanuel does, that the obvious fix to unfair exchange would be to pay participants more, not less.[22,30] This solution illustrates an important tension between unfair-advantage exploitation and undue inducement, a tension clearly recognized in the *IRB Guidebook* in its discussion of payment to prisoners. Prisoners represent a population with few options for making money; thus they have the potential to be exploited by being significantly underpaid for their work. On the other hand, any offer to a prisoner is likely to be exceedingly attractive and eagerly accepted, resulting in concerns about undue inducement.[32]

Although paying more may be appropriate in some situations, it may not always eliminate exploitation. Raising payment when recruiting and paying research participants with restricted options may make the transaction fairer in strict economic terms, but it ignores the potential incommensurability of payment with certain values that people hold. In this sense, the concern for exploitation closely parallels and may magnify concern for undue inducement. Wilkinson and Moore counter that investigators are simply not responsible for the background conditions that, often unjustly, leave people in such a state of need. Further, denying paid research opportunities will only exacerbate already existing needs[22] (see Chapter 20).

Not surprisingly, different payment models address concerns about exploitation differently. The market model dismisses it as a concern because individuals are free to negotiate their price and investigators the amount they are willing to pay. Yet in the market model, poor research participants could still be exploited by being paid very little because of their weak bargaining position. A wage payment model sets a floor and a ceiling on the amount research participants are paid, limiting how much the situation of particular research participants can be exploited. Yet setting the limit too low may be taking advantage of people with few opportunities. Importantly, prohibiting payment to such research participants in the interest of "protecting" them is also exploitative, if one believes that participants provide a valuable service that can warrant some form of payment.[3,22,30]

Commodification

In an often cited but now dated piece, Max Wartofsky likens the payment of research participants to prostitution. Just as sex ought not to be traded, Wartofsky argues that one's body is not an appropriate "commodity" for use in research.[43] Similar arguments have been used against paid organ donation and surrogacy—assertions that these practices fail to respect or value human bodies in the appropriate way.[44] Providing incentives for any service involves, to some extent, "commodifying" people. Paying

for research participation and the accompanying risks does not seem inherently different from many other paid transactions accepted as normal parts of life. Modeling, sports, police work, and firefighting, for example, all involve the use of human bodies, and some entail significant risk. Furthermore, research participation is not as intensely personal as sexual intimacy or pregnancy. As with undue inducement, however, commodification may be a concern when individuals have important objections to research participation.

A related view conceptualizes research participation as an instance of gift giving.[9,18,19] In his discussion of blood donation, Richard Titmuss argues that preserving gift giving is an important part of our social structure, and that commercialization can erode the social fabric of mutual dependency and altruism that is important for societal flourishing.[19] We find these arguments unpersuasive with regard to payment for research participation. First, anyone can refuse to accept payment; volunteering for research without pay is still an option. The personal value of volunteering may even increase for some if payment is offered and refused. Second, payment does not necessarily obviate altruism. It may facilitate gift giving by making sacrifices less demanding. Finally, any potential harm to the social fabric should be weighed against the benefit of quality research with adequate numbers of participants. Empirical research could play an important role in assessing the effect of payment on total rates of participation, as well as on important elements of the social fabric.

If preserving volunteerism is the major concern, the market model might be particularly offensive. The wage payment model may enable gift giving for some, but treating research participation as a job may be viewed as insulting. The reimbursement model is unlikely to be objectionable, and posttrial gifts may be superfluous but not offensive.

Incentives for Risk

A common theme throughout the literature on payment, and echoed within national and institutional guidance, is that payment should not compensate for risk.[7,45] In particular, researchers conducting risky studies should not offer more money than those conducting less risky studies involving similar effort or inconvenience. Some justify this view by arguing that risk simply ought not to be incentivized.[7] Others have argued that allowing risk-based payment could reduce investigators' incentive to minimize risks.[3] On the other hand, proponents of payment for risk argue that prohibiting such payments constitutes simple, unjustified paternalism. More compensation is often offered for risky jobs, and prohibiting payment for risk in research fails to respect people's ability to make decisions about acceptable levels of risk.[22]

Although disagreement exists about whether risk ought to figure into payment amounts, there is widespread agreement that IRBs ought to consider whether the balance of risks to potential benefits of a given project is reasonable independent of payment.[30] Payment will thus not *make* any study approvable. Whether incentives can or should be offered to make otherwise approvable, but riskier, studies more attractive to potential participants is a matter of significant disagreement.

Opponents of risk-based incentives will find the market model most offensive, as payment could be increased until it overcomes any aversion to risk. The wage payment model does not base payment on risk, focusing instead on the nature of the "work" research participants do. Some may argue, however, that risk is an important determinant of the value of "work."

Special Populations

Certain populations present particular concerns regarding payment for research participation. Prisoners and other captive populations may be susceptible to coercion. Worries about justice and exploitation focus on the poor and homeless, as well as on participants in developing countries. Two populations, however, raise unique concerns: patients and children.

Patients

It is sometimes assumed that only healthy research participants are paid for participation in research and not patients with the condition being studied. This belief is simply incorrect. A review of protocols at major academic institutions and independent IRBs showed that over half of paid studies involved patients.[46] Some writers, nevertheless, argue that patient-participants differ from healthy research participants because they are particularly vulnerable and may benefit medically from participation.[17,47] Patients' vulnerability stems either from an inability to distinguish between clinical care and research[48] or from a power differential between patients and investigators. Payment does not exacerbate either source of vulnerability in principle.[3] Paying patients may in fact call attention to activities not designed to advance their medical interests by signifying that investigators are not functioning only as physicians providing medical care. Payment could also depersonalize the exchange, making it easier for patients to refuse and putting them on more equal bargaining terms with investigators. Though noncash "payment" by means of free or reduced-cost medical treatment may be thought to be more appropriate than other currencies, health-related offers have the potential to exacerbate any therapeutic misconception.

That patient-participants may already receive benefits from participating in some research should not warrant a prohibition of payment to patients. Many studies involving patients offer no potential for direct benefit. It seems odd to assert that patients ought not to receive payment in these cases while allowing payment for healthy participants. And although studies offering potential benefits may not need to pay to recruit patients, it is unclear why payment would be unethical.

Children

Payment certainly magnifies ethical challenges involved in conducting research with children. Several key factors make payment challenging in this setting. First, parents are the primary decision makers, but they are expected to make research decisions based primarily on children's interests. The greatest worry is that parents will use children as a source of revenue.[49] Consequently, payments to parents are often discouraged or limited. Incentive payments, in particular, have been flatly banned in Europe, a position echoed in a U.S. Institute of Medicine (IOM) report in 2004.[49,50] The extent to which this concern is well-founded, however, is unclear. In addition, parents are more likely than the child to incur opportunity costs, and having a child participate in a study can be quite inconvenient. Wendler et al. argue that carefully calculated compensatory payments to parents for inconvenience and time, if calibrated to the resources of the least well-off families

among potential participants, are acceptable and unlikely to result in significant distortions in parental decisions, even if they result in some profit. Concerns about profit-minded parents, they argue, are also reduced by the strict limits on allowable risk in pediatric research regulations.[24] The IOM report, on the other hand, insists that compensation cover only actual expenses.[49] Other groups, such as the Therapeutics Development Network of the Cystic Fibrosis Foundation, support a standardized payment schedule resembling the wage payment model that likely entails small profit for some participants.[49,51]

Paying children directly is another approach, and these are not mutually exclusive. Knowing how to pay children is difficult, particularly because children of different ages view payment differently, and children's roles in research decisions are often unclear. The American Academy of Pediatrics (AAP) recommends a posttrial appreciation model, suggesting that gifts not be disclosed at the time of consent.[26] This model allows giving children gifts that only they would appreciate, such as a toy or a stuffed animal. By not disclosing the gift at the time of consent, investigators make sure that children do not give their assent because of the gift. Wendler et al. have questioned the legitimacy of this method, asserting that parents and children are quite likely to be aware of posttrial gifts. They also point out that this method may lead IRBs to ignore the potential power of the gifts that are offered.[24] The 2004 IOM report also supports up-front disclosure of any payment, and it is known that many institutions ignore the AAP's approach.[25,49]

When and how to pay children and their parents for research participation merits further empirical and conceptual study. Wendler and colleagues suggest that the acceptability of the payment should not depend on ignorance of payment at the time of consent, and that it may be appropriate to pay children and adults differently when both populations are enrolled in the same study. They also suggest using forms of payment that are unlikely to entice adults, avoiding large lump-sum payments and putting the money in an account to be accessed by the child at an older age.[24] The IOM report concurs on many levels. It also recommends that institutions develop policies on this issue and explicitly allows for "reasonable, age-appropriate compensation based on the time involved in research that does not offer the prospect of direct benefit."[49] The primary discrepancy between these sets of suggestions seems to be tolerance for parental profit. Although there is no principled reason why parental profit should be prohibited, empirical work could help to determine whether the concerns with parental profit are borne out in practice.

Other Concerns

Additional concerns are practical in nature but carry significant ethical implications. As mentioned, the effect of payment on the quality of scientific knowledge is an important question warranting further investigation. Other practical concerns also have ethical implications. The market model, for example, could lead to competition among investigators for research participants, driving up research costs and potentially compromising the ability to recruit adequately for projects with smaller budgets. These outcomes are speculative and subject to dispute.[3,27] Several writers have asserted that the wage payment model would require regulations more in keeping with other types of employment. For example, unionization, overtime, and health benefits may be needed if research participants are treated as workers.[52] Although the extension of the employment analogy is helpful in certain respects, such as the need for safe working conditions, most individuals do not participate in studies on a long-term basis or frequently enough to justify being considered employees warranting health insurance coverage or overtime.

Empirical Data

Though deep conceptual disagreements exist, the controversy over payment is perpetuated by the paucity of empirical data about the extent to which ethical concerns are borne out in practice.

Perhaps the most basic question is simply how payment affects recruitment. Are monetary incentives more effective than medications or health services? To what extent do completion bonuses retain participants? What amount of payment will maximize recruitment? These questions are largely unanswered. Conversations with representatives from contract research organizations (CROs) and private Phase I drug development units suggest that they have conducted local studies in developing their own policies, but these data are proprietary. Response rates to surveys are affected by both the amount and timing of payment.[53] However, few studies have looked explicitly at the effect of incentives in clinical research. Korn and Hogan showed some effect of increasing academic and small monetary rewards for participation in hypothetical experiments of varying types, but the effects were relatively small. The aversiveness of the intervention being tested had a much more important effect on willingness to enroll than the incentive offered.[54] In sum, we know very little about how payment affects recruitment for different types of clinical research.

Several studies have attempted to measure paid research participants' motivations for participating in research. Bigorra and Banos found that healthy participants from the general population were likely to report solely monetary reasons (90%) as the motivation to participate in research, in contrast to healthy medical students, who were more likely to report other motivations as primary (only 5% reported money as a primary reason).[55] Other studies have found that healthy research participants join research primarily for money (78.4 % to 93%).[56,57] Van Gelderen et al. found that younger research participants seemed more interested in monetary payment, and older research participants in free medical examinations.[57] Older studies with healthy subjects reveal similar variation in the importance of money.[58–60] Aby et al. asked individuals participating in Phase III studies of allergy and asthma interventions to rate different potential motivations on a five-point scale of importance to their decision. Participants rated all "altruistic" reasons highly, and payment ranked fifth among nonaltruistic reasons. Health-related reasons were consistently more important.[61]

Conclusions from these studies are limited. First, only Aby et al. interviewed anyone other than healthy research participants. Second, the studies have important methodological differences and flaws. In many cases, people were asked only for their primary motivation to participate; there are surely multiple reasons why people decide to join a study. Only the Novak and Aby studies asked about a range of motivations. And in none of these studies is it really apparent how payment factored into participants' actual decisions. Most importantly, none assessed what types of trade-offs research participants are willing to make for varying amounts or types of pay. This information, however, is crucial to assessing undue inducement.

Halpern et al. attempted to assess the effect of payment on willingness to participate.[38] They asked individuals eligible for participation in hypertension research to rate their willingness to participate in studies involving varying amounts of payment, likelihood of adverse effects, and chance of placebo assignment. They found that payment did increase willingness to participate at every level of risk, but the effect of payment remained relatively constant over different levels of risk. Thus, they argued that payment did not disproportionately affect willingness to participate in higher-risk studies. It is unclear, however, exactly what influence one would expect payment to have and what level of willingness to participate should be expected at any given level of risk.

Another study attempted to ascertain what level of payment adolescent asthma patients and their parents found to be appropriate in different types of hypothetical asthma studies.[62] Researchers found, not surprisingly, that adolescents considered as "fair compensation" lower levels of payment than their parents did, as did participants with lower versus higher income. Participants' estimates of fair compensation were more likely to be greater than actual compensation in low-risk studies. The study shows that expectations regarding reasonable levels of payment differ based on the nature of the study, the socioeconomic situation, and age (parent vs. adolescent) of the potential participant.

Other empirical questions in need of further study are the effect of payment on informed consent and the extent to which payment leads to lying or concealing information in order to prevent exclusion or discontinuation from studies. Bentley and Thacker attempted to address both questions in a study involving U.S. pharmacy students.[41] They found that payment did not impact participants' understanding of risks entailed by hypothetical studies. Payment appeared, however, to increase participants' willingness to conceal relevant facts about themselves in low-risk studies, but not their willingness to report adverse effects. The generalizability of this study, however, is limited in that pharmacy students are likely to have a more sophisticated understanding of research than the general public and may not be the best population in which to test the effect of payment on informed consent.

Other work has focused on institutional policies and practices regarding payment. In our study of U.S. research institutions, most endorsed the notion of payment for time, travel, and inconvenience; there was less agreement about payment for risk (31%) or as an incentive (58%). Few institutions (25%) had any prescribed, standardized method of determining when and how much to pay research participants; most IRBs and investigators make decisions with little substantive guidance. Moreover, few institutions track studies that offer payment. Institutions generally require that payment be explicitly described in consent forms, typically in a separate section, and that payments be prorated if individuals withdraw. And institutions usually pay healthy participants and patient-participants similarly.[45] A 2002 review of policies for payment of children revealed a significant division among institutions with respect to the AAP's recommendation that payment not be mentioned at the time of enrollment in the study.[25]

A review of protocols at major academic institutions and independent IRBs demonstrates several important practice trends with regard to payment.[46] First, there is variability, within and across institutions, in the amount offered for particular procedures, with little rationale given in protocols or consent documents for how payment is determined. Patients are paid for participation in many types of studies, including both potentially therapeutic Phase II and III studies and clearly nonbeneficial biologic or physiologic studies. Finally, although the range is wide, the amount of payment offered was usually relatively modest (median = $155; range $5 to $2,000).

Policy Implications

Though contentious, payment to research participants is common and takes many forms. On the simplest level, payment enables and rewards individuals for making a valuable contribution to medical science. Prohibiting payment seems unnecessary and inappropriately paternalistic.

Because paying research participants has important ethical implications, there is a need for policy guidance. Existing data show that research participants are paid on a haphazard and inconsistent basis. In the United States, a national policy or set of guidelines with more substance than those currently in place, and which promotes standardization while allowing appropriate variation according to local conditions, would be helpful to investigators and IRBs. In the absence of a national policy, individual institutions might develop local policies to promote internal consistency and guide investigators and IRB members. Explicit attention to research regarding children and patient-participants should be included.

We believe that the wage payment model most effectively balances the needs to recruit and protect research participants. This model recognizes that payment may be one appropriate consideration in a decision to participate in research and compensates research participants at a level similar to other jobs requiring similar levels of skill, effort, and inconvenience. It also reduces concern about undue inducement and provides standardization within and across studies, reducing competition between investigators and avoiding further escalation in research costs.[3]

Unanswered Questions

Policy formulations are difficult to make because of currently unanswered conceptual and empirical questions. Deeper conceptual analysis of exploitation is warranted, particularly the tensions between exploitation and undue inducement. Another important conceptual question is the legitimacy of treating research participation as a job. Many are uneasy about the wage payment model precisely because it treats research participation as a form of unskilled labor. Yet why research participation is or should be different is unclear. More analysis of the ethical acceptability of providing incentives to children and their parents is also needed, as there is divergence within the field and a small body of literature on the topic.

Perhaps the most immediate need is for careful empirical work on issues related to payment at both institutional and individual participant levels. There is a surprising lack of institutional data tracking studies and participants, resulting in very little information about the demographics of the research participant pool. We do not know who participates in studies or how paid research participants differ, if at all, from unpaid participants. The percentage of studies that pay participants, how much of the research budget is used, and the range of incentives employed in different regions are important data in assessing the large-scale impact of payment practices.

We also know little about how payment affects decisions to participate or to refuse participation in research studies, and what types of trade-offs research participants make for various types or amounts of payment. There are no data on whether paid research participants understand less about the studies in which they actually enroll than unpaid participants, and it is unknown how often research participants misrepresent their health status to meet eligibility criteria or to remain in paid studies if they experience adverse events. Finally, though we have argued that there is no inherent reason to treat patients and healthy participants differently, it would be valuable to study whether payment exacerbates or reduces any vulnerability that patient-participants might have.

Disclaimer

The views expressed here are the authors' own and do not represent any positions or policies of the National Institutes of Health, the Public Health Service, or the Department of Health and Human Services.

References

1. Rothman DJ. Research, Human: Historical Aspects. In: Reich WT, ed. *Encyclopedia of Bioethics*. 2nd ed. New York, N.Y.: Macmillan; 1995: 2248–58.
2. Ackerman TF. An ethical framework for the practice of paying research subjects. *IRB: A Review of Human Subjects Research* 1989;11(4): 1–4.
3. Dickert N, Grady C. What's the price of a research subject? Approaches to payment for research participation. *New England Journal of Medicine* 1999;341:198–203.
4. Fagot-Largeault A. Discussion paper on the compensation of human volunteers. In: Champey Y, Levine RJ, Lietman PS, eds. *Development of New Medicines—Ethical Questions*. Proceedings of a conference sponsored by Fondation Rhône-Poulenc Santé; 2 December 1988. London, United Kingdom: Royal Society of Medicine Services; 1988:63–9.
5. Levine R. What should consent forms say about cash payment? *IRB: A Review of Human Subjects Research* 1979;1(6):7–8.
6. Macklin R. Due and undue inducements: On paying money to research subjects. *IRB: A Review of Human Subjects Research* 1981; 3(5):1–6.
7. McNeill P. Paying people to participate in research: Why not? A response to Wilkinson and Moore. *Bioethics* 1997;11:390–6.
8. Morris RC. Guidelines for accepting volunteers: Consent, ethical implications, and the function of a peer review. *Clinical Pharmacology and Therapeutics* 1976;13:782–6.
9. Murray T, Robbins FC. Human subjects of research give us a gift. *The Plain Dealer* (Cleveland, Ohio). Jan. 2, 1997;B9.
10. Newton L. Inducement, due and otherwise. *IRB: A Review of Human Subjects Research* 1982;4(3):4–6.
11. Grady C. Money for research participation: Does it jeopardize informed consent? *American Journal of Bioethics* 2001;1(2):40–4.
12. Kolata GB. The death of a research subject. *Hastings Center Report* 1980;10(4):5–6.

13. Darragh A, Kenny M, Lambe R, Brick I. Sudden death of a volunteer. *Lancet* 1985;325:93–4.

14. Cohen LP. To screen new drugs for safety, Lilly pays homeless alcoholics. *The Wall Street Journal* Nov. 14, 1996;Sect.A1:c01.6.

15. National Bioethics Advisory Commission. *Ethical and Policy Issues in International Research: Clinical Trials in Developing Countries, Vol. I: Report and Recommendations*. Bethesda, Md.: NBAC; 2001. [Online] April 2001. Available: http://www.georgetown.edu/research/nrcbl/nbac/clinical/V011.pdf.

16. Guinea Pig Zero: A Journal for Human Research Subjects. [Online] Available: http://www.guineapigzero.com/.

17. Lemmens T, Elliott C. Guinea pigs on the payroll: The ethics of paying research subjects. *Accountability in Research* 1999;7:3–20.

18. Chambers T. Participation as commodity, participation as gift. *American Journal of Bioethics* 2001;1(2):48.

19. Titmuss RM. *The Gift Relationship: From Human Blood to Social Policy*, expanded and updated edition; Oakley A, Ashton J, eds. New York, N.Y.: The New Press; 1997 [1971].

20. Berry SH, Kanouse DE. Physician response to a mailed survey: An experiment in timing of payment. *Public Opinion Quarterly* 1987;51: 102–14.

21. Sears JM. The payment of research subjects: Ethical concerns. *Oncology Nursing Forum* 2001;28:657–63.

22. Wilkinson M, Moore A. Inducement in research. *Bioethics* 1997;11: 373–89.

23. McGee G. Subject to payment? *JAMA* 1997;278:199–200.

24. Wendler D, Rackoff JE, Emanuel EJ, Grady C. The ethics of paying for children's participation in research. *Journal of Pediatrics* 2002;141: 166–71.

25. Weise KL, Smith ML, Maschke KJ, Copeland HL. National practices regarding payment to research subjects for participating in pediatric research. *Pediatrics* 2002;110:577–82.

26. Committee on Drugs, American Academy of Pediatrics. Guidelines for the ethical conduct of studies to evaluate drugs in pediatric populations. *Pediatrics* 1995;95:286–94.

27. Wilkinson M, Moore A. Inducements revisited. *Bioethics* 1999;13: 114–30.

28. Wertheimer A. *Coercion*. Princeton, N.J.: Princeton University Press; 1987.

29. The National Commission for the Protection of Human Subjects of Biomedical and Behavioral Research. *The Belmont Report: Ethical Principles and Guidelines for the Protection of Human Subjects of Research*. Washington, D.C.: Department of Health, Education and Welfare; DHEW Publication OS 78-0012 1978. [Online] April 18, 1979. Available: http://www.hhs.gov/ohrp/humansubjects/guidance/belmont.htm.

30. Emanuel EJ. Ending concerns about undue inducement. *Journal of Law, Medicine, and Ethics* 2004;32:100–5.

31. Wilkinson S. The exploitation argument against commercial surrogacy. *Bioethics* 2003;17:169–87.

32. Department of Health and Human Services, Office for Health Research Protections. *Protecting Human Research Subjects: Institutional Review Board Guidebook*. Rockville, Md.: OHRP, 1993. [Online] Available: http://www.hhs.gov/ohrp/irb/irb_guidebook.htm.

33. Council for International Organizations of Medical Sciences in collaboration with the World Health Organization. *International Ethical Guidelines for Biomedical Research Involving Human Subjects*. Geneva, Switzerland: CIOMS and WHO; 2002. [Online] November 2002. Available: http://www.cioms.ch/frame_guidelines_nov_2002.htm.

34. U.S. Food and Drug Administration. Information Sheets: Guidance for Institutional Review Boards and Clinical Investigators: Payment to Research Subjects. [Online] 1998. Available: http://www.fda.gov/oc/ohrt/irbs/toc4.html#payment.

35. Department of Health and Human Services, National Institutes of Health, and Office for Human Research Protections. The Common Rule, Title 45 (Public Welfare), Code of Federal Regulations, Part 46 (Protection of Human Subjects). [Online] June 23, 2005. Available: http://www.hhs.gov/ohrp/humansubjects/guidance/45cfr46.htm.

36. Grant RW, Sugarman J. Ethics in human subjects research: Do incentives matter? *Journal of Medicine and Philosophy* 2004;29:717–38.

37. Faden RR, Beauchamp TL, with King NMP. *A History and Theory of Informed Consent*. New York, N.Y.: Oxford University Press; 1986.

38. Halpern SD, Karlawish JHT, Casarett D, Berlin JA, Asch DA. Empirical assessment of whether moderate payments are undue or unjust inducements for participation in clinical trials. *Archives of Internal Medicine* 2004;164:801–3.

39. Dunn LB, Gordon NE. Improving informed consent and enhancing recruitment for research by understanding economic behavior. *JAMA* 2005;293:609–612.

40. Jonas H. Philosophical reflections on experimenting with human subjects. *Daedalus* 1969;98:219–47.

41. Bentley JP, Thacker PG. The influence of risk and monetary payment on the research participation decision making process. *Journal of Medical Ethics* 2004;30:293–8.

42. Wertheimer A. *Exploitation*. Princeton, N.J.: Princeton University Press; 1996.

43. Wartofsky M. On doing it for money. In: National Commission for the Protection of Human Subjects of Biomedical and Behavioral Research. *Research Involving Prisoners: Appendix to Report and Recommendations*. DHEW Publication No. (OS) 76–132. Washington, DC; 1976:3:1–3:24.

44. Anderson ES. Is women's labor a commodity? *Philosophy and Public Affairs* 1990;19:71–92.

45. Dickert N, Emanuel E, Grady C. Paying research subjects: An analysis of current policies. *Annals of Internal Medicine* 2002;136:368–73.

46. Grady C, Dickert N, Jawetz T, Gensler G, Emanuel E. An analysis of U.S. practices of paying research participants. *Contemporary Clinical Trials* 2005;26:365–75.

47. Yaes RJ. What's the price of a research subject? [letter] *New England Journal of Medicine* 1999;341:1551; author reply:1552.

48. Appelbaum PS, Roth LH, Lidz CW, Benson P, Winslade W. False hopes and best data: Consent to research and the therapeutic misconception. *Hastings Center Report* 1987;17(2):20–4.

49. Institute of Medicine. *Ethical Conduct of Clinical Research Involving Children*. Washington, D.C.: National Academies Press; 2004.

50. Directive 2001/10/ec of the European Parliament and of the Council of 4 April, 2004, on the approximation of the laws regulations, and administrative provisions of the member states relating to the implementation of good clinical practice in the conduct of clinical trials, in Article 4(d).

51. Therapeutics Development Network, Cystic Fibrosis Foundation. Guidelines for reimbursement to study subjects. In: *Cystic Fibrosis Foundation, Manual of Operations*. Bethesda, Md.: Cystic Fibrosis Foundation; 2003:P, F–2.

52. Anderson JA, Weijer C. The research subject as entrepreneur. *American Journal of Bioethics* 2001;1(2):67–9.

53. Martinson BC, Lazovich D, Lando HA, Perry CL, McGovern PG, Boyle RG. Effectiveness of monetary incentives for recruiting adolescents to an intervention trial to reduce smoking. *Preventive Medicine* 2000; 31:706–13.

54. Korn JH, Hogan K. Effect of incentives and aversiveness of treatment on willingness to participate in research. *Teaching of Psychology* 1992;19:21–4.

55. Bigorra J, Banos JE. Weight of financial reward in the decision by medical students and experienced healthy volunteers to participate in clinical trials. *European Journal of Clinical Pharmacology* 1990;38: 443–6.

56. Vrhovac R, Francetic I, Rotim K. Drug trials on healthy volunteers in Yugoslavia. *International Journal of Clinical Pharmacology, Therapy, and Toxicology* 1990;28:375–9.

57. van Gelderen CE, Savelkoul TJ, van Dokkum W, Meulenbelt J. Motives and perception of healthy volunteers who participate in experiments. *European Journal of Clinical Pharmacology* 1993;45:15–21.

58. Novak E, Seckman CE, Stewart RD. Motivations for volunteering as research subjects. *Journal of Clinical Pharmacology and New Drugs* 1977;17:365–71.

59. Martin DC, Arnold JD, Zimmerman TF, Richart RH. Human subjects in clinical research—A report of three studies. *New England Journal of Medicine* 1968;279:1426–31.

60. Hassar M, Weintraub M. "Uninformed" consent and the wealthy volunteer: An analysis of patient volunteers in a clinical trial of a new anti-inflammatory drug. *Clinical Pharmacology and Therapeutics* 1976; 20:379–86.

61. Aby JS, Pheley AM, Steinberg P. Motivation for participation in clinical trials of drugs for the treatment of asthma, seasonal allergic rhinitis, and perennial nonallergic rhinitis. *Annals of Allergy, Asthma and Immunology* 1996;76:348–54.

62. Scherer DG, Brody JL, Annett RD, Hetter J, Roberts LW, Cofrin KM. Financial compensation to adolescents for participation in biomedical research: Adolescent and parent perspectives in seven studies. *Journal of Pediatrics* 2005;146:552–8.

Franklin G. Miller

Recruiting Research Participants

Clinical research promotes social value by means of producing scientific knowledge that can lead to improvements in public health and medical care. The social value that justifies clinical research also justifies using techniques of recruitment to enroll eligible participants in research protocols. However, recruitment strategies pose ethical issues insofar as they threaten to distort the physician-patient relationship, exploit potential research participants, interfere with informed consent, or violate confidentiality or privacy. As compared with study design and informed consent, participant recruitment has received relatively little attention in the bioethics and medical literatures. It is an important topic because recruitment techniques represent the initial communication or contact between potential participants and investigators or other members of the research team, which may influence participants' understanding of research and the voluntariness of their participation.

This chapter will address three ethical issues in the recruitment of research participants: (1) the role of physicians in recruiting their own patients for clinical research; (2) respecting confidentiality and privacy in the recruitment process; and (3) the use of advertisements to recruit potential participants. I will focus here mainly on the recruitment of "patients"—that is, individuals with a disorder under investigation. Recruitment of patients is ethically complex because research participation involves a status change from being a patient with a given medical condition, often seeking treatment in the context of clinical trials, to being a research participant in a study aimed at developing generalizable knowledge. Recruitment messages and interactions can either clarify or confuse the ethically important differences between medical care and clinical research.

Recruitment by Treating Physicians

Patients are recruited for clinical research by a variety of mechanisms. They may be referred by their treating physician to researchers conducting a study relevant to the patient's medical condition; they may respond to advertisements for clinical research in newspapers, on television or radio, in advocacy group publications, or posted in public areas; or they may learn about available research by examining Internet web sites. In addition, physician-investigators employed by academic medical centers traditionally have recruited their own patients for enrollment in clinical research. In recent years patients have increasingly been recruited by community physicians to participate in industry-sponsored clinical trials.[1,2] Although this latter practice of treating physicians recruiting their own patients for research in which the physicians are involved is widely accepted and probably necessary to maintain adequate enrollment in valuable clinical research, it raises ethical questions that deserve careful consideration.

Historically, clinical research has been conducted in the context of the physician-patient relationship.[3] The ethos of scientific medicine has made the activities of medical care and clinical research seem inextricably and properly connected.[4] Prior to the late 1960s, physician investigators typically saw no ethical problems in enrolling their patients in clinical investigations without obtaining informed consent.[5] Recognition of the ethically significant distinction between therapy and research has led to the understanding that there is a potential conflict of roles and role obligations between acting as a treating physician and acting as an investigator.[6] The treating physician is devoted to promoting the medical best interests of his or her patients; the investigator is devoted to producing generalizable knowledge about well-defined groups of patients. In some cases, research participation can be seen as promoting the medical best interests of a particular patient, for example, when the patient has failed to respond to available standard therapies and has a reasonable prospect of receiving medical benefit from an investigational treatment available only in the context of a clinical trial. In many cases, however, research participation will not serve the medical best interests of patients.

It does not follow that recruiting patients for research that is not likely to be medically beneficial (for some or all participants) is unethical. The question remains whether it can be ethical for a treating physician to request his or her patient to consider enrolling in a study when research participation does not offer the patient a prospect of net medical benefit that is as good as or better than standard medical care. It would seem that under these circumstances, loyalty to the best medical interests of one's patients would preclude a treating physician from inviting his or her patient to enroll in research. Recruitment is only one dimension of this issue of role conflict; the responsibility to monitor the condition of enrolled participants poses tensions between the duty to care for patients and the commitment to complete valuable research.

One response to this problem is to invoke the principle of clinical equipoise as a guide to when it is ethical for treating physicians to enroll their own patients in clinical research.[7] As long as there exists uncertainty or an honest disagreement within the expert medical community between the experimental and control treatments being evaluated in a randomized clinical trial, then physicians can maintain their therapeutic obligations to their patients when inviting enrollment in the trial. The duty of competent medical care and enrollment in a clinical trial are alleged to coincide when clinical equipoise obtains.[8]

Apart from theoretical and practical difficulties with clinical equipoise (see Chapter 24), this solution to the problem fails for two reasons. First, it applies only to randomized clinical trials. Clinical equipoise has no bearing on clinical research that is not aimed at evaluating treatments. One might argue, accordingly, that treating physicians should not be permitted to recruit their patients for "nontherapeutic" research. This, however, would make it difficult, if not impossible, to conduct valuable studies aimed at improving the understanding of rare diseases in which the only available and competent investigators and eligible patients are those who stand in a therapeutic physician-patient relationship.

Second, clinical trials that satisfy the principle of clinical equipoise will often include research procedures such as blood draws, lumbar punctures, and biopsies that are aimed at determining participant eligibility, characterizing the study population, or measuring outcomes. These procedures carry some degree of risk without any compensating medical benefits to the enrolled participants. It is difficult to see how recruiting patients for research containing such nonbeneficial components is compatible with the obligation of the treating physician to always promote the medical best interests of the patient.

This ethical problem is also recalcitrant to a procedural solution by means of review and approval by an institutional review board (IRB). Competent independent review will endeavor to minimize risk to participants and determine that any risks not compensated by medical benefits are justified by the anticipated value of the knowledge to be gained from the research. Nevertheless, this will not guarantee that research participation is in the best medical interests of patients who are recruited by their treating physicians, leaving the problem of divided loyalties intact.

We seem to be faced with a dilemma. On the one hand, precluding treating physicians from recruiting their patients would greatly hamper the conduct of valuable clinical research. On the other hand, permitting treating physicians to recruit their patients into clinical research often appears to violate the fundamental norm of medical ethics—prescribing unswerving loyalty of treating physicians to the best medical interests of their patients. There is no escaping the problem of divided loyalty when treating physicians recruit their patients for clinical research (and monitor them during research participation). Nonetheless, I suggest that the problem is ethically manageable if physicians who are subject to this divided loyalty face squarely the fact that their situation poses inherent ethical tensions, if they strive to help patients understand how research participation differs from patient care, if they are committed to protecting patients from harm, and if they respect the patients' right to withdraw from research without penalty.[9,10] As Henry Beecher noted long ago, an important ethical safeguard relevant to this problem is "the presence of an intelligent, informed, conscientious, compassionate, responsible investigator."[11]

Managing the tensions of divided loyalty with integrity requires that physician-investigators are honest with themselves and with patient-participants about how clinical research differs ethically from patient care. Across the range of ethically justifiable clinical research studies it is not possible to have it both ways—that is, to maintain fidelity both to promoting the medical best interests of patients and to conducting valuable research. It is tempting to see the relationship between physician-investigators and patient-participants as a fiduciary relationship, comparable to the doctor-patient relationship in medical care.[12] But this flies in the face of the fact that nearly all clinical research includes procedures that pose risks to participants without compensating medical benefits to them. Thus, physician-investigators cannot, and should not, promise explicitly or implicitly that during the course of research they will be functioning as a treating physician dedicated to promoting the medical best interests of their patients. What investigators can promise is that they will endeavor to protect the research participant from serious harm as a result of research participation and will always respect the right of the patient to withdraw from research.

A related problem associated with physicians recruiting their patients for clinical research is the potential for the prior physician-patient relationship to place undue pressure on patients to agree to research participation, thus compromising informed consent. If physicians are permitted to enroll their patients in clinical research, this potential for undue influence cannot be eliminated. Any recommendation by a physician to a patient to consider research participation may be perceived as pressure, because it comes from an authority figure whom patients are interested in pleasing or to whom they feel a debt of gratitude. This situation is most worrisome when the physician is directly involved in conducting the research in question. Nevertheless, informed consent does not require the absence of influence; rather, it is incompatible with controlling influence.[13]

Established guidance on this issue has been promulgated by the World Medical Association, in its Declaration of Helsinki, and by the Council on Ethical and Judicial Affairs of the American Medical Association (AMA). Principle number 23 of the Declaration of Helsinki states "When obtaining informed consent for the research project the physician should be particularly cautious if the subject is in a dependent relationship with the physician or may consent under duress. In that case the informed consent should be obtained by a well-informed physician who is not engaged in the investigation and who is completely independent of this relationship."[14] The AMA's ethical position is that "the physician who has treated a patient on an ongoing basis should not be responsible for obtaining that patient's informed consent to participate in a trial to be conducted by the physician. . . . Instead, after the physician has identified that a patient meets a protocol's eligibility and recommends that a patient consider enrolling in the trial, someone other than the treating physician should obtain the participant's consent."[15]

These two statements differ in details. The Declaration of Helsinki provision is less restrictive in one respect and more restrictive in another. On the one hand, the qualification that the patient is in a "dependent relationship" suggests that the separation between recruitment and obtaining informed consent is not required in all cases for treating physicians who desire to enroll their patients in research. The AMA's position lacks any such qualification. On the other hand, when separation of recruitment and informed consent is indicated, Helsinki requires that consent be obtained by a physician not associated with the research. The AMA position permits another member of the research team to obtain informed consent, provided that he or she does not have a treating relationship with the patient. As the main concern is separating the informed consent process from the influence of a prior therapeutic relationship, the AMA position appears to offer more sound ethical guidance.

It is not clear, however, whether this separation between recruitment and informed consent constitutes a genuine protection for participants. The AMA statement notes in defense of its position that "patients may feel indebted to their physician or may hesitate to challenge or reject their physician's advice to participate in research." But these forms of pressure may be present regardless of whether it is the treating physician who obtains informed consent. An interview survey of 1,882 patients in medical oncology, radiation oncology, and cardiology clinics found "little evidence that patients felt coerced or manipulated by health care providers or scientific investigators to participate in research."[5] No data were reported comparing those with and without a prior physician-patient relationship with investigators. Empirical research is needed to clarify whether patients with a prior physician-patient relationship with the investigator feel greater pressure to consent than those lacking such a relationship and whether separation between recruitment and obtaining informed consent makes any difference in perceived pressure.

Undue influence is not the only ethical concern associated with physicians recruiting their own patients. The tendency of patient-participants to confuse research participation with medical care, known as "the therapeutic misconception," is a widely discussed issue in the ethics of clinical research.[16,17] It seems plausible to assume that this confusion, with the potential to interfere with informed consent, is likely to be more prevalent when physicians recruit their own patients into research as compared with recruitment that does not involve any prior therapeutic relationship. Whether this is true is a factual issue that could be addressed by empirical research. In any case, clarifying, or at least not obscuring, the differences between research participation and routine

medical care is an important component of the processes of recruitment and informed consent. The issue of the therapeutic misconception is discussed further below in the context of addressing advertising for clinical research.

Habiba and Evans have recently argued that treating physicians breach confidentiality when they use private information obtained from patients seeking their care for the purpose of recruiting these patients to participate in research.[18] They assert that "to approach patients for recruitment into research based on information about them held by their treating physician infringes on their privacy because the information is used *outside the confined circumstances* for which it was given. . . . In other words, the principle of confidentiality should apply not only to prevent a patient's records from being disclosed to others, including researchers, but also to constrain a doctor from making use of it himself if acting in a different capacity, such as that of a representative of a commercial health insurer *or* that of a clinical researcher."

This is a novel and dubious construal of the concept of confidentiality. Breaches of confidentiality in professional contexts essentially involve an interpersonal communication by a professional who has a right to know private information about a client or patient and a duty not to disclose this to others who have no right to know this information without the consent of the client or patient. When the investigator who seeks to recruit his patient for research is the same person as the treating physician who is entitled to know the patient's diagnosis, there is no disclosure of private information to another outside the therapeutic relationship. Hence, no breach of confidentiality is at stake in this invitation to participate in research. The shift from the therapeutic to the research role may be ethically problematic; however, it is not confidentiality that explains the ethical problem.

Instead of being seen as breach of confidentiality, this role shift might be viewed as an instance of exploitation. Alan Wertheimer analyzes exploitation as the situation of person A taking unfair advantage of person B.[19] Treating physicians who endeavor to recruit their patients for research certainly take advantage of their therapeutic relationship in making the invitation to participate in research. In this situation, it is by virtue of the therapeutic relationship that the physician has access to an eligible patient who may consent to research participation. The ethical question is whether the use of one professional role to pursue a different professional role is unfair. When there is no ongoing therapeutic relationship, there is nothing wrongful or unfair in physician-investigators recruiting persons with a medical diagnosis for valuable clinical research. Indeed, clinical research is a socially valuable activity that requires the expertise of physicians and the participation of patients. It is unclear why a prior physician-patient relationship should make recruitment unfair provided that valid informed consent is obtained, which requires respecting the right of the patient to refuse without any penalty to the therapeutic relationship.

I conclude that that the issues of divided loyalty and potential pressure on patients to consent make research recruitment by treating physicians ethically problematic but not necessarily unethical. Other things being equal, it is better for recruitment and enrollment in research to be separated from a prior therapeutic physician-patient relationship. A strict separation should not be mandated, however, because it would unduly constrain the conduct of valuable clinical research. A vital safeguard against abuse in this situation is the professional integrity of the physician-nvestigator.[9] Concern with avoiding undue influence to participate by other members of the research team, such as nurses, may also contribute to participant protection.

Preserving Confidentiality and Privacy in Recruitment

Although U.S. federal regulations governing research with humans provide no explicit guidance about recruitment, they do address confidentiality and privacy. Among the "criteria for IRB approval of research" is the following stipulation: "When appropriate, there are adequate provisions to protect the privacy of subjects and to maintain the confidentiality of data" (§46.111(a)(7)).[20] Strictly speaking, this language does not clearly apply to the recruitment process, which involves contact with potential participants prior to enrollment in research. Yet the spirit of this requirement makes it applicable to IRB review of the recruitment process, in which genuine breaches of confidentiality may occur.

The following example illustrates the importance of IRB review of mechanisms of participant recruitment with an eye to protecting confidentiality. A protocol submitted to an IRB proposed to recruit patients hospitalized following motor vehicle accidents for the purpose of studying acute stress disorder, a psychiatric condition that often progresses to the chronic condition of posttraumatic stress disorder. Upon questioning by members of the IRB, it became clear that the investigators planned to station a member of the research team at a nearby community hospital who would receive from hospital staff the names of potentially eligible patients in order to approach them concerning their interest in participating in the research. Although this represented a convenient means of gaining access to patients for recruitment, the communication of the names of patients being treated for injuries after motor vehicle accidents was viewed by IRB members as violating the confidentiality of these patients. The recruitment plan of communication between hospital staff and the research team would have violated patient confidentiality because a researcher not connected with the care of these patients had no right to information about their presence in the hospital or their reason for being there.

Fortunately, in this situation a somewhat less convenient alternative recruitment plan was available. Clinicians involved in the care of potentially eligible patients could give them a flyer describing the research with a check-off box indicating willingness to be approached by a member of the research team. Under this approach, approved by the IRB, researchers would endeavor to recruit only those patients who previously consented to contact with the research team, thus preserving privacy and confidentiality. Because the details of recruitment plans may not be spelled out in protocols submitted to IRBs, it is incumbent on IRB members to raise questions about recruitment techniques so as to assure the protection of research participants.

Ethical concerns may arise about invading privacy in the recruitment process when no breach of confidentiality is involved. The issue of recruiting family members of participants enrolled in genetics research has recently received systematic attention by the Cancer Genetics Network Bioethics Committee.[21] The authors note that a "central challenge in any approach is to provide appropriate protections while promoting sufficient recruitment to achieve scientific goals." A variety of recruitment approaches are considered ethical. As a general rule, this group recommends that initial contact with family members come from enrolled participants who are provided with written material concerning the research with a mechanism for the family members to either opt in or opt out of being contacted.

Advertising for Clinical Research

Advertising is an established method to recruit people for research. This practice, however, has received little ethical attention. The regulations of the U.S. Department of Health and Human Services concerning the protection of humans in research do not mention advertisements for clinical research as within the purview of IRBs; however, guidance issued by the U.S. Office for Human Research Protections directs IRBs to review recruitment materials as part of initial review of research protocols.[22] For research under its jurisdiction, the U.S. Food and Drug Administration (FDA) requires that IRBs review and approve advertisements to recruit human participants.[23] The FDA "considers direct advertising for study subjects to be the start of the informed consent and subject selection process."[23] Because advertisements may set the stage for interactions between patient volunteers and investigators and influence the quality of informed consent, they should be subject to IRB scrutiny and approval for all research with humans.

For many research participants, initial interest may be stimulated by advertisements. This first, anonymous communication between researchers and patient volunteers may tap motivations, foster beliefs, and create expectations that influence research participation in ethically significant ways. Commentators on the ethics of clinical research have noted the need to balance the traditional normative framework of protecting the rights and welfare of research participants with the more recent goal of promoting access to clinical trials.[24] Advertising to recruit research participants serves the latter goal; however, the accuracy of advertisements about clinical research and the nature of the inducements they offer raise ethical issues pertaining to participant protection.

Miller and Shorr examined weekly issues of the *Washington Post* "Health" section from December 1, 1998 through February 16, 1999.[25] They identified a total of 111 advertisements addressed to persons suffering from particular diseases or specific symptoms. Sponsors of the advertisements included institutes of the National Institutes of Health, academic medical centers, for-profit research firms, physician practice groups, and individual investigators. Nearly all the observed advertisements mentioned that volunteers were being recruited for a study or for research. More significant than the bare fact of disclosing that volunteers were being recruited for research was the overall tenor of the message of the advertisements and the motivations to which they were directed. In most cases, advertisements for patient volunteers began with bold type referring to a disease and/or symptoms. In the case of psychiatric research, these advertisements sometimes included pictures of people showing signs of psychic distress. The advertisements typically noted that study medications and medical examinations or evaluations would be provided free of charge. It appears that the predominant intent was to gain the attention of persons who were suffering (or their families) and to offer personal benefit. The appeal to suffering patients risks creating unrealistic expectations

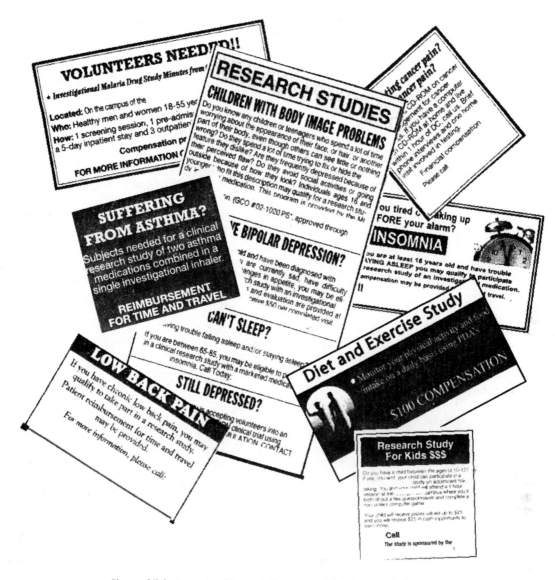

Figure 37.1. Examples of Research Recruitment Advertisements in Newspapers

for medical benefit, because there is no guarantee that patients will benefit from research participation. On the other hand, none of the observed advertisements appealed to altruistic motivations—to contribute to scientific knowledge that might benefit future patients.

Even though advertisements almost always disclose that persons are being recruited for research, they typically appeal to prospective research participants as patients seeking needed treatment rather than as volunteers invited to join investigators as partners in research. A major difficulty in this appeal to personal suffering and benefit is that it fosters the expectation that clinical research has the same individualized, patient-centered orientation as clinical care, whereas clinical research is designed primarily to produce generalizable knowledge about a class of patients. Accordingly, the prevailing focus of advertisements may contribute to the therapeutic misconception, confusing clinical research and standard clinical care.[16] Some commentators see the therapeutic

misconception as a pervasive characteristic of clinical research that compromises informed consent.[17]

In a large-scale survey of patients participating in clinical research, it was found that altruistic motivations were reported no less often than self-interested motivations. Of those patients in treatment studies, 76% indicated a "way to help others" and 69% "advance medical science" as major reasons for research participation; 69% indicated "gave hope" and 67% "chance to get better treatment."[26] These data suggest that advertising appealing to altruistic motivations, such as to contribute to scientific research and to help future patients, might prove as effective as the prevailing appeal to individual benefit.

Advertisements for clinical research also should be evaluated with respect to what they fail to communicate. None of the observed advertisements mentioned any risks of study participation.[25] Detailed disclosure of risks is a matter for conversations between investigators and potential research participants and for written consent documents. However, it is arguable that advertisements should at least mention that risks of study participation will be disclosed and discussed before enrollment begins. Indeed, the fact that advertisements mention potential benefits suggests that they should not omit any mention of risks. Such omission may skew the perception of what is involved in research participation.

Another significant omission in observed advertisements is reference to the use of placebos. There is no way of knowing the nature of the study design from most observed advertisements. It would be surprising, however, if none of them involved placebo controls, given the frequency of their use in randomized trials. Investigators may fear that the mention of placebos might dissuade some from inquiring about research participation. On the other hand, advertisements that create the expectation of benefit and offer free treatment might incline patients to decide in favor of research participation without careful thought about the meaning of enrolling in a placebo-controlled trial. Unrealistic initial expectations may be fostered that are not dispelled by the subsequent informed consent process, even when the use of placebos and how this makes a clinical trial different from standard clinical care are adequately disclosed.

Clinical trials sometimes require that patient volunteers stop prior treatment for a period of time before they receive medications under investigation. A few of the observed advertisements mentioned that patients must be free of medications as a condition of enrollment.[25] It is not clear, however, whether this requirement was disclosed for all studies involving a drug washout.

IRB oversight should aim at ensuring that advertisements strike a reasonable balance between the legitimate goal of recruitment and the adequacy of disclosure about the nature of clinical research. Accordingly, IRBs should review proposed advertisements in the light of the following questions:

- Does the advertisement make clear that participants are being recruited for research?
- Does the message of the advertisement have the potential to contribute to confusion between research participation and standard clinical care?
- Are the suggested benefits of research participation consistent with the scientific protocol and consent forms?
- Does the advertisement disclose important features of the study design that may influence enrollment: for example, the use of placebos or the requirement for prior medication withdrawal?
- Does the advertisement mention that risks will be disclosed prior to study enrollment?

Conclusion

Beginnings matter. Recruitment is the first stage of research participation, which can set the moral tone for the relationship between investigators and research participants. When physician-investigators enroll their own patients into clinical research the problem of divided loyalty between patient care and scientific investigation cannot be eliminated; however, it can be managed ethically by conscientious investigators. The process of recruitment deserves greater ethical attention in both conceptual and empirical research.

Disclaimer

The opinions expressed are the author's own. They do not represent any position or policy of the National Institutes of Health, Public Health Service, or Department of Health and Human Services.

References

1. Bodenheimer T. Uneasy alliance: Clinical investigators and the pharmaceutical industry. *New England Journal of Medicine* 2000;342: 1539–44.
2. Rettig R. The industrialization of clinical research. *Health Affairs* 2000;19:129–46.
3. Reiser SJ. Human experimentation and the convergence of medical research and patient care. *Annals of the American Academy of Political and Social Science* 1978;437:8–18.
4. Miller FG, Rosenstein DL. The therapeutic orientation to clinical trials. *New England Journal of Medicine* 2003;348:1383–6.
5. Advisory Committee on Human Radiation Experiments. *Final Report of the Advisory Committee on Human Radiation Experiments.* New York, N.Y.: Oxford University Press; 1996.
6. Levine RJ. Clinical trials and physicians as double agents. *Yale Journal of Biology and Medicine* 1992;65:65–74.
7. Weijer C. The ethical analysis of risk. *Journal Law, Medicine, and Ethics* 2000;28:344–61.
8. Freedman B. Equipoise and the ethics of clinical research. *New England Journal of Medicine* 1987;317:141–5.
9. Miller FG, Rosenstein DL, DeRenzo EG. Professional integrity in clinical research. *JAMA* 1998;280:1449–54.
10. Brody H, Miller FG. The clinician-investigator: Unavoidable but manageable tension. *Kennedy Institute of Ethics Journal* 2003;13: 329–46.
11. Beecher HK. Ethics and clinical research. *New England Journal of Medicine* 1966;274:1354–60.
12. Miller PB, Weijer C. Rehabilitating equipoise. *Kennedy Institute of Ethics Journal* 2003;13:93–118.
13. Faden RR, Beauchamp TL, with King NMP. *A History and Theory of Informed Consent.* New York, N.Y.: Oxford University Press; 1986:256–62.
14. World Medical Association. *Declaration of Helsinki: Ethical Principles for Medical Research Involving Human Subjects.* Tokyo, Japan: WMA; October 2004. [Online] 2004. Available: http://www.wma.net/e/policy/b3.htm.
15. Morin K, Rakatansky H, Riddick FA, et al. Managing conflicts of interest in the conduct of clinical trials. *JAMA* 2002;287:78–84.
16. Appelbaum PS, Roth LH, Lidz CW, Benson P, Winslade W. False hopes and best data: Consent to research and the therapeutic misconception. *Hastings Center Report* 1987;17(2):20–4.
17. Lidz CW, Appelbaum PS. The therapeutic misconception: Problems and solutions. *Medical Care* 2002;40(Suppl.):V55–V63.
18. Habiba M, Evans M. The inter-role confidentiality conflict in recruitment for clinical research. *Journal of Medicine and Philosophy* 2002;27:565–87.
19. Wertheimer A. *Exploitation.* Princeton, N.J.: Princeton University Press; 1996.
20. Department of Health and Human Services, National Institutes of Health, and Office for Human Research Protections. The Common Rule, Title 45 (Public Welfare), Code of Federal Regulations, Part 46 (Protection of Human Subjects). [Online] June 23, 2005. Available: http://www.hhs.gov/ohrp/humansubjects/guidance/45cfr46.htm.
21. Beskow LM, Botkin JR, Daly M, et al. Ethical issues in identifying and recruiting participants for familial genetic research. *American Journal of Medical Genetics* 2004;130A:424–31.

22. Department of Health and Human Services, Office for Human Research Protections. Guidance on Written IRB Procedures. [Online] July 11, 2002. Available: http://www.hhs.gov/ohrp/humansubjects/guidance/irbgd702.htm.

23. U.S. Food and Drug Administration. FDA Information Sheets: Guidance for Institutional Review Boards and Clinical Investigators; Recruiting Study Subjects. [Online] 1998. Available: http://www.fda.gov/oc/ohrt/irbs/toc4.html.

24. Brody BA. Research on the vulnerable sick. In: Kahn JP, Mastroianni AC, Sugarman J, editors. *Beyond Consent*. New York, N.Y.: Oxford University Press; 1998:32–46.

25. Miller FG, Schorr AF. Advertising for clinical research. *IRB: A Review of Human Subjects Research* 1999;21(5):1–4.

26. Sugarman J, Kass NE, Goodman SN, Perentesis P, Fernandes P, Faden RR. What patients say about medical research. *IRB: A Review of Human Subjects Research* 1998;20(4):1–7.

Participant Selection

Section B. Special Populations

Colleen Denny   Christine Grady

38

Research Involving Women

As of July 2005, the U.S. Census Bureau estimated that there were approximately 150,410,658 women living in the United States, a little less than 51% of the total population.[1] This percentage is not a new phenomenon; due to a greater death rate in men of a number of age groups, women have long been the majority sex in the United States.[2] Yet despite this majority, women have long found themselves excluded or at least underrepresented in many areas of society, including academia, the business sector, and the political arena.

What has recently come to be recognized, however, is that women have long been underserved in the context of modern medicine as well. Since the United States began seriously engaging in clinical research in the mid-20th century, views on women as participants and as a source of valuable research questions have changed enormously, fluctuating from a sort of indifference, to active exclusion, to today's state of deliberate inclusion. This oscillation is in large part attributable to the unique ethical dilemmas that surround the participation of female subjects in clinical research: Not only might women in general be subject to particular pressures and risks due to their status as a historically oppressed population, but their biological capacity to become pregnant and gestate may also put both them and future human beings at risk of dignitary and/or physical harm. Balancing these unspecified risks with the desire to enable research participation in hopes of more fairly distributing research's benefits has been a difficult and ongoing struggle.

Recent conceptual and empirical work has the potential to aid researchers and institutions grappling with these complex dilemmas. Data are still lacking on many important questions, yet existing information can enable clinical researchers to better analyze the conflicting obligations and grasp the practical nature of the problem at hand. Data and discussions also serve to illuminate the

creation of overarching policies and strategies for study design, bringing them more in line with contemporary thinking. To understand the maelstrom of ethics, empirical data, and policy questions that surround the issue of women's participation in clinical research, we start from the historical vantage point.

History

The history of women's involvement in modern medical research reflects a shift in society's priorities concerning sex differences. Whereas early researchers and research institutions sought to protect women and their potential unborn offspring from the hazards of research participation, more contemporary women's rights activists and research ethicists stress the importance of women's participation in order to fairly distribute both the direct and indirect benefits of medical research. The establishment and subsequent dismantling of the protectionist approach to women's research participation during the last quarter of the 20th century was marked by scandals, changing policies, reports, legislation, and a growing awareness in the health-care community of the important role research participation plays in overall health-care equity.

Protectionist Era of Women in Clinical Research

Scandals in Women's Health

Advocacy for women-specific health care, prominent in the modern debate over women's research participation, dates back to the popular health movement of the 1800s. Early activists organized lectures and "conversationals" designed to educate women about diverse topics such as hygiene, proper diet and exercise, and family planning.[3] Indeed, women activists protesting the sale of addictive "tonics" for female health problems were the main impetus for the creation of the Food and Drug Administration's (FDA) predecessor in 1906.[4] However, little attention was specifically paid to the role of women in clinical research until the blossoming of research in the mid-20th century. As the number of new drugs and medical treatments available in the health-care market began to explode, a series of scandals related to women's health, particularly maternal and fetal health, led to the institutionalization of a default exclusion of female research subjects in many types of clinical trials.

Perhaps the most infamous drug tragedy in the modern research age revolved around the discovery of the teratogenic effects of thalidomide, an antinausea drug being prescribed mainly for pregnant women with morning sickness. Though the drug was widely available in Europe throughout the late 1950s, the application for U.S. marketing approval was still pending at the FDA in 1961, when scientists publicly confirmed reports of thalidomide-induced birth defects such as stunted fetal limb development and damage to other organ systems.[5] The visual impact of thousands of European thalidomide babies focused American attention on enhancing the FDA's ability to protect consumers through more stringent requirements in the approval of new pharmaceuticals. This popular support for increased regulation of the pharmaceutical industry, in turn, proved to be the final boost Congress needed to pass the Kefauver-Harris Drug Control Act in 1962. Among other things, this legislation empowered the FDA to require drug manufacturers to prove the effectiveness of their products as well as their safety, to report adverse events to the FDA, and to ensure that advertisements to physicians disclosed the risks as well as the benefits of their products. Informed consent was also now required from participants in clinical studies. The FDA was given jurisdiction over prescription drug advertising and marketing techniques, the types of trials done on experimental drugs, and more.[4,6] Although the new amendments did not specifically address the issue of women's role as clinical research subjects, the tragedy of thalidomide boosted the FDA's power significantly, paving the way for increased scrutiny of clinical research practices.

Though the thalidomide disaster occurred outside the realm of research and affected only pregnant women, another scandal in New Zealand illustrated how women generally could suffer unethical treatment in the context of clinical research. In 1966, the National Women's Hospital of New Zealand began a study of cervical carcinoma in situ (CIS) in hopes of proving that a positive result on the newly developed Pap smear test should not be taken as a sign of imminent cervical cancer.[7] Though common medical wisdom at the time held that positive Pap smears necessitated swift preventive measures (including hysterectomy) to ensure long-term health, the physician in charge of the National Women's Hospital study allowed hundreds of women with positive test results to go untreated. The primary investigator, Herb Green, strongly agreed with the traditional view that hysterectomies for CIS needlessly compromised women's core identities by depriving them of their reproductive capacity; he claimed that a sterilized woman had "thrown away a unique possession" and betrayed her "heritage" by having her uterus removed.[7] Thus, Green and his researchers did not inform untreated women that they were being included in a research trial or that ignoring a positive Pap smear

was not the current standard of practice. Dozens of female patients died before the study was finally stopped in 1984. Although many details of the scandal emerged too late to significantly affect legislative changes in the United States, exposure of the trial in the popular media gave strength to the belief that female patients were at heightened risk of harm or exploitation in clinical research and required special protection.

Despite increased FDA supervision in the United States, several additional health-care scandals in the early 1970s resulted in significant harm for female patients and/or their offspring, further driving the campaign for greater protection of women research subjects. First, in 1971 the FDA announced that diethylstilbestrol (DES), a synthetic hormone often prescribed to pregnant women, had been found to be strongly associated with the risk of an extremely rare and aggressive reproductive cancer, clear cell adenocarcinoma (CCA), in female offspring.[8] Despite a 1951 study that failed to demonstrate DES's efficacy in preventing miscarriages, physicians had continued to administer the drug to women for another two decades, exposing an estimated 5 million to 10 million women and their unborn fetuses to DES and resulting in a spate of CCA diagnoses.

The uproar surrounding the Dalkon Shield, an intrauterine device first marketed nationwide in the United States in January 1971, was another medical product with unexpected dire consequences for female patients. Approximately 2.8 million Dalkon Shields were sold in the United States before 1974, when the manufacturer pulled the devices from the shelves after reports of increased infection and pregnancy complications. Subsequent reports revealed that users of the Dalkon Shield had a five-fold increased risk of pelvic inflammatory disease and a greater chance of medically complicated pregnancies.[9] These two health-care tragedies contributed to the growing consensus among clinical and research institutions that women's exposure to experimental or even relatively new approved procedures should be limited, both to avoid unforeseen health consequences for them and their potential offspring and to limit liability for drug manufacturers. By and large, women in the late 1960s and early 1970s reacted to these scandals by protesting the unethical inclusion of women in research.[10]

Beyond the specific realm of medicine, other social forces at work in the early 1970s contributed to the creation of a default exclusion of women from many types of research trials. The vocal pro-life community, galvanized in the wake of the U.S. Supreme Court's 1973 Roe v. Wade decision, expressed concern for unborn fetuses by pushing for stringent limits on women's research participation.[10] Additionally, the revelation of the Tuskegee Syphilis Trial in the early 1970s and the subsequent convening of the National Commission for the Protection of Human Subjects in Biomedical and Behavioral Research attracted further attention to the potential of medical research to exploit populations of lower social status (see Chapters 8 and 14). Charged with identifying the core ethical principles that should govern the conduct of research with human subjects, the National Commission also proposed additional extra protections for populations it deemed to be historically vulnerable in light of past tragedies, including pregnant women and fetuses.[10]

Establishment of Protectionist Legislation

The series of particularly visible women's health disasters, in conjunction with greater social and political focus on protecting historically oppressed populations from unfair treatment, culminated in the adoption of several new guidelines designed to more strictly regulate women's participation in clinical research. First, in 1977 the FDA passed Guideline 77–3040, significantly proscribing research participation for "women of childbearing potential." According to these regulations, fertile women were not to participate at all in early clinical studies such as Phase I or Phase II trials, and should only be included in later clinical trials if animal studies had already been performed to investigate the reproductive effects of the investigational drug or device.[4] The passage of this regulation effectively excluded a large majority of women from serving as research subjects in many types of clinical studies.

A second set of regulations, adopted by the U.S. Department of Health and Human Services (DHHS) in 1978 (revised in 2001), made official policy of many of the National Commission's proposals regarding research with populations previously designated as vulnerable.[11] In 45 CFR 46 Subpart B, the DHHS specifically delineated the types of research that were permissible with pregnant women and fetuses. Unless the proposed research had the potential to directly benefit a pregnant woman, she was not permitted to enroll in research that would pose greater than minimal risk to her fetus. Additionally, if research participation was thought to have the potential to directly benefit the fetus alone, informed consent was required from the biological father as well as the mother (unless "he is unable to consent because of unavailability, incompetence, or temporary incapacity or the pregnancy resulted from rape or incest").[11] Although these regulations applied only to research sponsored by the DHHS, they significantly curtailed the ability of pregnant women to enroll in clinical research.

The adoption of these two sets of regulations by government agencies marked the strongest moment of the protectionist approach to women's participation in clinical research. Faced with a series of public tragedies involving women as medical subjects, many officials felt that anything less than a stringent attitude toward women's participation in clinical research would only invite further disaster. Barred from almost all research if they were pregnant or of "childbearing potential," women found themselves generally excluded from research "for their own good" and the good of their potential offspring. Yet although women were now thought to be protected from future potentially harmful experimental products in the vein of thalidomide, DES, and the Dalkon Shield, a growing opposition movement began to point out and protest the dearth of information about women's health that resulted from their research exclusion.

Dismantling the Protectionist Approach

Changes in Public Opinion

One of the earliest signs of the sea change in public opinion regarding women's participation in potentially riskier endeavors was the 1978 passage of the Pregnancy Discrimination Act, an amendment to the Civil Rights Act of 1964. Passed just one year after the FDA instituted its policies excluding women from most forms of clinical research, the new legislation defined discrimination on the basis of pregnancy, childbirth, or related medical conditions as a form of unlawful sex discrimination prohibited under Title VII of the Civil Rights Act. Both married and unmarried women affected by pregnancy or related conditions were to be treated in the same

manner as other employees or applicants with similar abilities or limitations.[12] Pregnancy in itself could no longer be a legal reason for excluding women from the workplace.

Echoing the general reversal of public attitudes and policies toward fertile women's exclusion from the workplace, several political action groups in the early 1980s weighed in on the debate regarding the inclusion of women in clinical research. Regulations once thought to be protective were now increasingly deemed "paternalistic" and "discriminatory."[10] As women of the baby boomer generation began to reach adulthood (and, in some cases, graduate from medical school), they became increasingly concerned with the significant lack of research with women and its impact on women's health.[10] In response to data indicating that both pregnant and nonpregnant women were frequent users of pharmaceuticals that had never been tested in female research subjects, activists and ethicists pointed out that excluding women from research participation seemed actually to exacerbate the likelihood of harm; women would be taking the drugs either way, but were currently doing so without any evidence base or professional supervision.[13–15] Furthermore, commentators observed that women's health, as a subspecialty, had long been conflated with women's reproductive health; little research attention had been paid to the ways in which the sexes varied outside the realm of obstetrics and gynecology.[10]

The widespread absence of women in studies of heart disease, for example, was one of the most glaring omissions in research on nonreproductive health issues: Large-scale studies such as the Coronary Drug Project (CDP), the Coronary Primary Prevention Trial (CPPT), the Multiple Risk Factor Intervention Trial (MRFIT), and the Physicians' Health Study (PHS) all recruited solely male subjects.[16] Inspired by AIDS activists, who through the 1980s lobbied successfully for greater access to experimental drugs by stressing the fair distribution of the benefits of research participation, activists for women's rights began applying the same logic to encourage the greater inclusion of female clinical research subjects.[10] Gathering pressure eventually led to the creation of a two-year public health task force, charged with investigating the effects of exclusionary policies on women's health.

New Mandates for Inclusion

The report of the Public Health Service Task Force on Women's Health Issues, published in 1985, was a watershed event in the debate regarding women's participation as clinical research subjects, marking the beginning of a 15-year flurry of government reports, policies, and legislative acts (see timeline, Figure 38.1). The task force report declared that "the historical lack of research focus on women's health concerns has compromised the quality of health information available to women as well as the health care they receive,"[17] a perspective providing official credence to activists' claims. The National Institutes of Health (NIH), faced with pressure from both popular and government sources, enacted the first of its policies designed to dismantle the protectionist approach: the 1986 Policy Concerning the Inclusion of Women in Study Populations. This policy encouraged, but did not mandate, the inclusion of women in clinical trials.[10] NIH administrators hoped that the lenient new guidelines would appease women's rights activists without creating animosity among those researchers who claimed that the addition of female subjects would beget greater costs and difficulties with study design.[10]

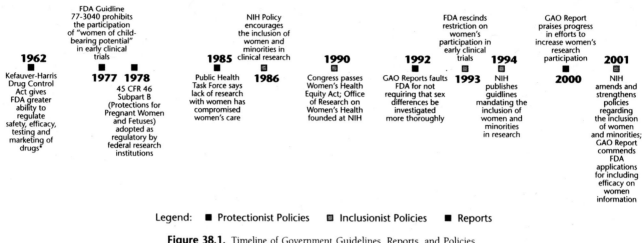

Legend: ■ Protectionist Policies   ▨ Inclusionist Policies   ■ Reports

Figure 38.1. Timeline of Government Guidelines, Reports, and Policies

Despite this new policy, a General Accounting Office (GAO, now the Government Accountability Office) report issued four years later had the NIH scrambling to revise its policies toward female subjects yet again. After a thorough review of NIH policies and practices, the GAO concluded that, despite the 1986 policy change, NIH clinical studies were failing to include women at an appropriate rate.[18] The report received a great deal more public attention than the earlier Public Health Service Task Force on Women's Health Issues, provoking a louder outcry from the general population and spurring reconsideration of many older policies regarding women's research participation.

Public reaction was so great as to prompt Congress to take action. Shortly after the official publication of the 1990 GAO report, the Congressional Caucus on Women's Issues, with Sen. Barbara Mikulski (D-Md.) as the primary sponsor, introduced the Women's Health Equity Act, calling for "greater equity in the delivery of health care services to women through expanded research on women's health issues, improved access to health care services, and the development of disease prevention activities responsive to the needs of women."[19] The bill also mandated the creation of five contraceptive and fertility research centers as well as an Office of Research on Women's Health to serve as a "focal point for women's health research at the NIH."[20]

The Supreme Court's 1991 decision in *United Autoworkers* v. *Johnson Controls* reflected the widespread growing resistance to the previous protectionist ideology even outside the research arena. In a unanimous decision, the justices wrote that the Johnson Controls manufacturing company's blanket prohibition banning fertile and/or pregnant women from working in positions potentially harmful to their reproductive capacities was in violation of Title VII of the Civil Rights Act.[21] The decision held that the company's policy discriminated against women, as it did not prohibit fertile men from the same positions, despite the fact that lead exposure had also been proved hazardous to male reproductive systems; further, the potential for fetal harm due to lead exposure did not prevent women from doing any of the essential tasks required to perform their jobs. This ruling established that even well-intentioned employment policies meant to protect women and fetuses were forbidden if they resulted in the discriminatory exclusion of women.[21]

The NIH Revitalization Act of 1993 (P.L. 103–43) further encouraged the inclusion of women in research by including a provision requiring NIH to ensure that (1) women and minorities were to be included in all clinical research, (2) women and minorities were to be included in Phase III trials in numbers adequate to allow for analysis of gender and group differences, (3) cost was not an acceptable reason for excluding these groups, and (4) programs would be initiated to recruit and retain women and minorities for clinical research.[22] In 1994, the NIH revised its policy to meet the legislative mandate, publishing "Guidelines on the Inclusion of Women and Minorities as Subjects in Clinical Research," and charged the NIH Office of Research on Women's Health with monitoring adherence to this policy.[23] A 1993 Institute of Medicine report offered numerous arguments regarding the need for women's inclusion, simultaneously tackling concerns about the resulting rising costs of studies by laying out strategies for designing efficient and scientifically appropriate research subject groups.[24]

Having successfully spurred the NIH into action, the GAO turned its attention to the exclusionary policies of the FDA. In 1992, the GAO issued a second report, entitled "Women's Health: FDA Needs to Ensure More Study of Gender Differences in Prescription Drug Testing," strongly recommending that the agency revise its policy of excluding women from early trials in the pharmaceutical approval process so as to better serve the needs of women's health.[25] After a year's deliberation in July 1993, the FDA adopted many of these suggestions in its "Guideline for the Study and Evaluation of Gender Differences in the Clinical Evaluation of Drugs." This policy overrode the previous protectionist policy of 1977 and described the agency's new high expectations for pharmaceutical sponsors regarding the inclusion of both genders in clinical drug trials.[26] An FDA Office of Women's Health was established by congressional mandate in 1994.

With these dramatic changes at two major federal agencies, the protectionist approach to female research subjects quickly fell from favor. New GAO reports released at the end of the 1990s commended the NIH and FDA efforts to increase women's inclusion in clinical research, though the GAO warned that some newly approved pharmaceuticals still lacked sufficient safety data from women.[27] Some scientific journals even began publicly calling on researchers to analyze their data for sex and ethnicity differences, though this trend has yet to become the norm at all biomedical publications.[28,29]

By the beginning of 21st century, official and institutional policies toward women's research participation had undergone drastic changes in the space of a few decades, reversing and dismantling the protectionist approach popular in the 1970s. Although regulation 45 CFR 46 (Subpart B) still strictly limits the participation of pregnant women in federally funded clinical research, most barriers to the participation of nonpregnant women as research subjects have been removed. However, notwithstanding federal regulations, both researchers engaged in the daily work of clinical trials and ethicists attempting to parse the implications of women's participation still face a number of challenges. Despite a new official attitude regarding women's research participation, important ethical questions raised by the inclusion of women, particularly pregnant women, have not yet been laid to rest.

Ethical Issues

The fundamental ethical dilemma regarding women's participation in research centers on the question of balancing inclusion and protection. As women's rights activists point out, there are numerous reasons to include women in as much and the same types of research as men: The availability of research participation's benefits should not depend on sex alone, and women have many sex-specific health concerns that have received short shrift in past decades. On the other hand, as legislators faced with tragedies in the 1960s and 1970s realized, there are also reasonable arguments for excluding women from research. Most significantly, as illustrated by the fallout from thalidomide and DES, risks undertaken by women may be propagated to future or currently gestating fetuses. Additionally, women have long been a relatively powerless group in most societies, possibly making them more vulnerable than men to exploitation and other forms of unethical treatment. Greater inclusion of women has also been attacked from a resource allocation standpoint: Mandating inclusion may increase the costs of studies, jeopardizing other worthwhile research ventures. These conflicting concerns weigh on all those attempting to make participation policies as equitable as possible without unduly exposing women (and potential fetuses) to risk.

Ethical Issues With Women in General

Though the rhetoric about the ethical hazards of including women as research subjects often focuses primarily on the potential harm to gestating fetuses, there are also ways in which including women, regardless of their reproductive capabilities, brings up ethically difficult questions. Should women be considered vulnerable subjects who incur particular risks in the research setting? How should the possibility of increased costs because of inclusion be viewed? Should some research projects be discouraged for their potential social harm to an already oppressed group? And do women have claims to greater research participation?

"Vulnerability" and Resulting Risks

A discussion of the ethics of women's inclusion in clinical research necessarily requires consideration of the ethics of including or excluding any population or group from research. Fundamental ethical principles of justice require that both the risks and benefits of research participation should be fairly distributed throughout the general population, an imperative that makes the exclusion of certain populations from research unethical without scientific or harm-based reasons.[15,30] Faced with the prospect of exposing a possibly vulnerable population to unnecessary risk or harm in the context of clinical studies, many researchers and research institutions might be tempted to err on the side of caution by excluding members of that population from participation as a default option. However, such exclusion may be unfair when one takes into account the significant benefits that research participants may receive. These benefits can be both on a personal level, such as when participants receive early access to promising new drugs months before they are available on the general market, and on the population level, such as when new findings about subpopulations are reflected in better-tailored medical care and treatments. This general reasoning clearly applies to the exclusion of women from clinical research: If the reasons for their exclusion are not adequately justified by scientific validity concerns or particular risk of harm, barring their participation in research is not defensible.

The concession that women may be excluded from research for scientific validity reasons seems relatively straightforward; women might justifiably be excluded from studies of prostate cancer, for example. The principle that populations may be excluded if they are susceptible to a "particular risk of harm" not present in the wider population, however, leads to debate about what sort of harms women may be uniquely at risk for and/or vulnerable to. Are there good reasons to think that women should be considered a "vulnerable" population? Although many authors in the bioethics literature have tackled the question of how to deal with vulnerable populations in clinical research, the meaning and scope of *vulnerability* remains somewhat unclear.[31] As the Council for International Organizations of Medical Sciences (CIOMS) argues in its commentary on Guideline 13, vulnerability is perhaps best conceived as the relative or absolute inability to protect one's own interests.[32] This definition offers a starting point for discussion of whether women should be considered vulnerable in the context of clinical research, and, if so, in what particular situations.

What sort of factors, if any, might make women relatively or absolutely unable to protect their own interests in the research setting? Women as a group have historically been an oppressed and underprivileged population; as such, it has been argued, women's ability to protect their own best interests as research subjects may be compromised, creating vulnerability. This lack of power may be reflected in women's inferior social status, their socialization to defer to more powerful groups in society, and/or their lack of political and socioeconomic resources, all of which could make them vulnerable to particular risks and harms in the research setting. The nature of these risks may be manifested differently according to the nature of the research scenario.

For example, as a population that both holds less sociopolitical power and has been long socialized to defer to socially powerful groups such as physicians, women may be at greater risk for exploitation in the research setting. They also may be inclined to accept offers of unfair benefits in exchange for research participation.[33,34]

Additionally, because of their lack of economic resources and power within relationships, women might be at risk of being "unduly induced." If women are offered particular goods or services that they lack and need in exchange for enrollment, the worry is that they might disregard the risks of study participation or give the risks insufficient weight in their decision-making process. Concern about undue inducement often emerges in research with economically disadvantaged populations; authors have examined whether offers of access to medical treatment, money, free health care, and so forth, can beget irrational decision making in poorer communities.[35] Similarly, certain benefits offered in exchange for research participation might serve as undue inducements for female research subjects. The offer of free health care for female research subjects' children, for example, may be so attractive for new mothers who lack health insurance as to hinder their ability to objectively weigh the risks and benefits of research participation. In another example, women who otherwise lack the social power to demand monogamy or safe sexual practices from their partners may be unduly attracted to an experimental vaccine for a sexually transmitted disease.[36]

Although these scenarios predicting heightened risk for women are theoretically possible, it is not clear that all or even most women actually feel powerless to protect their own interests in the research setting, even given their historical oppression and particular needs. Some research, for example, has noted the particular resilience and resourcefulness that populations lacking socioeconomic power often demonstrate in response to stressful situations.[37] Women as a population face many of the same hypothetical risks of exploitation and undue inducement in daily life that they might encounter in the research setting; research participation does not necessarily present more of a threat to them than their everyday experiences. Given the CIOMS definition of vulnerability as the relative or absolute inability to protect one's own interests against risks and harms,[32] the application of the term *vulnerable* to women as a whole population remains contentious.

Further, not all members of a "vulnerable" or "historically oppressed" group are equally vulnerable or oppressed. For example, there are women who may be doubly or triply disadvantaged by virtue of age, race, ethnicity, education, and so forth. On the other hand, a white English-speaking woman of high socioeconomic status might be less vulnerable in research than a poorer Hispanic woman for whom English is difficult to understand. However, although it is overly simplistic to assume that all women have the same sets of needs and vulnerabilities in the research setting, it is also extremely difficult for researchers and policy makers to create written regulations that account for each individual's specific needs.

Increased Costs of Research

Mandatory inclusion of women as research subjects, some NIH spokespersons pointed out in the early 1990s, could significantly increase the overall costs of some studies. Requiring statistical power to detect differences based on sex would require a significantly greater number of research subjects, leading to greater budget requirements.[10] The increased costs of including women could in turn become an ethical difficulty if money would therefore be unavailable to fund other valuable research studies. Given this tension, how should limited funding be spent? Is the inclusion of women as research subjects always more ethically important than enabling other avenues of research? Although opponents protest that full inclusion of all subpopulations (gender as well as age, race, ethnicity, etc.) would produce astronomical research costs,[38] those in favor of women's inclusion argue that research recruitment ought to reflect the diversity of the wider population (whose tax dollars fund public research) and particularly the distribution in the general populace of the condition under study.[24,39] For research involving specific diseases, advocates argue that the makeup of the research participant population logically ought to reflect the makeup of the disease population.[24] Empirical evidence on the costs of including women is lacking, a point that will be discussed further in the next section.

"Validating" Female Stereotypes

Some concerns about including women echo those raised with other minority or historically oppressed populations. For example, because minority groups are often saddled with negative public stereotypes, there may be special risk from research results that give leverage to harmful generalizations that minorities have long worked to overcome. In the particular case of women, researchers might reveal data that reinforce long-held beliefs that women are more emotional due to hormonal cycles, or that women have fewer neurons in sections of the brain thought to moderate math and science learning.[15] These sorts of findings are far from hypothetical; recent data support a number of female stereotypes, such as that women are disinclined to adopt "warrior" mindsets[40] and that men are better able to understand and manipulate rule-based systems.[41] If data such as these might contribute to the oppression of an already disempowered group, how should researchers proceed? Should such studies not be permitted for fear of giving leverage to historical oppression? Though complete suppression of research on sex differences and any resulting discoveries is inappropriate, the potential for such data to negatively affect oppressed groups inevitably influences decisions about dissemination of research findings.

Legal Rights and Entitlement Issues

Might women or any other population of research subjects have a constitutional right as U.S. citizens not to be unfairly denied research participation? Some authors have argued that because barring women from research participation has the effect of denying the known benefits of government-sponsored research to them as a class, this exclusion is unconstitutional without sufficient justification for such disparate treatment.[42,43] The traditional justification for exclusion—that fertile women may potentially become pregnant during the course of research—is viewed as decidedly insufficient by proponents of this view. Although the exclusion of women on the basis of sex alone might not be unconstitutional in privately funded research, rational arguments exist for believing that sex-based exclusion from federally funded research violates constitutional entitlements, given that research participation can be thought of as a government-provided potential benefit.[42]

Additionally, does the past exclusion of women from research entitle them to greater consideration than men in the current federal research agenda? In compensation for this history of unnecessary exclusion, several feminist authors have argued that women and other oppressed groups in society "should have a privileged place in studies that are likely to be of specific benefit to members of the group investigated" and have called for greater support for research on women's health concerns.[33] The U.S.

government has in some sense acquiesced to this demand, funding such projects as the Women's Health Initiative,[44] but there is some resistance to this policy. Critics claim that excessive attention and funding given to women's health issues works to the disadvantage of other groups in society, both privileged and underprivileged. Although women's rights proponents stress the importance of "catching women up" in terms of gender-specific research data, others emphasize the need to consider the lot of other groups in a research agenda with limited resources.

The range of ethical issues associated with the research participation of women in general is extensive, including ethical issues associated with all minority or historically oppressed groups as well as those specific to women. However, women's capacity to become pregnant and give birth adds a further set of ethical difficulties.

Ethical Issues Specifically With Pregnant Women

What aspects of pregnancy and bearing children might add greater ethical complexity to women's participation in research? First, the pregnant woman herself might have special needs and susceptibilities to risk by virtue of her pregnancy that are not shared by other minority or historically oppressed groups, including nonpregnant women. Second, fetuses and biological fathers have their own interests regarding pregnant women's research participation that may conflict with those of the woman herself. We now consider some of the main dilemmas researchers working with pregnant subjects may encounter; this is not meant to be an exhaustive list, but rather a collection of the concerns about pregnant research subjects that loom largest.

Pregnant Women as Vulnerable Subjects?

Although many oppose the classification of women in general as a "vulnerable population," regulations frequently label *pregnant* women as vulnerable and in need of special protections, including DHHS regulations governing federally funded research with human subjects.[11] This label, however, seems to confuse what entity is vulnerable and at risk. There does seem to be a widely held intuition among both researchers and the general public that pregnant women require greater protection than do nonpregnant human beings, but support for that intuition is often unclear, particularly in the research setting. Most regulations and guidelines offer no explanation for these special protective measures, and those that do usually refer to the risk of fetal rather than maternal harm during research participation.[45] Although teratogenicity constitutes an important ethical concern, many women's rights activists and ethicists have pointed out that the potential of a medical treatment to harm a gestating fetus should not be conflated with the potential for pregnant women themselves to become incapable of protecting their own interests.[10] As one researcher writes, "Sometimes the obvious needs to be repeated: Being pregnant does not by itself result in diminished decision-making capacity."[46]

Conflicts of Maternal and Fetal Interests

Yet whereas concern over pregnant women's particular vulnerability to coercion, exploitation, or undue influence in the research setting may be misguided, the ethical difficulties of potentially conflicting interests of a woman and her fetus are less easily put aside. Although some authors have questioned whether the image of maternal-fetal conflict is the most useful way to portray this dilemma,[47] there is clear potential for contradictory needs on the part of the two entities.

Some regulations have attempted to tackle this potential conflict by establishing a hierarchy of dominant interests. DHHS regulations, for example, state that research on pregnant women may be permitted when

> [t]he risk to the fetus is caused solely by interventions or procedures that hold out the prospect of direct benefit for the woman or the fetus; or, if there is no such prospect of benefit, the risk to the fetus is not greater than minimal and the purpose of the research is the development of important biomedical knowledge which cannot be obtained by any other means.[11]

Although the guidelines establish a hierarchy of interests, difficulties remain in their implementation. First, even a guideline like this one, which attempts to cover all possible conflicts, cannot clear up all ambiguity, because it leaves to the researcher and the institutional review board (IRB) the determination of what constitutes a "direct benefit" or "minimal risk." Second, uncertainty about what these regulations require and fear of contravening them may result in fewer studies that include pregnant women. Exclusion of pregnant women in turn leaves important questions unanswered about how to treat a variety of illnesses and conditions in pregnant women and may unjustly skew the distribution of research's benefits.[30]

Regulations and guidelines regarding the inclusion of pregnant women are often understandably influenced by the religious and political debate over the moral status of the fetus. Without overtly stating their justifications, regulations like the one quoted above often give weight to both fetal and maternal interests while granting ultimate precedence to the concerns of the mother; this is consistent with the widely held sentiment in public and legal opinion that an unborn fetus has inferior moral status to its living mother. Several authors in the bioethics literature have attempted to form a coherent rationale and conceptual framework to support giving more weight to maternal interests than to those of the fetus, with varying degrees of success. One intriguing framework suggests the unborn fetus has "dependent moral status"—that is, the fetus is only granted status as a person with legitimate interests by the personal preference of its mother, not out of her obligation to do so.[46] This granting of dependent moral status is closely correlated with the expectation that a given fetus will later achieve the moral status of a child with rights.

Research With Fetuses to Be Aborted

However, this raises another ethical dilemma: Should research involving pregnant women who are planning to abort be governed by different guidelines? The National Commission for the Protection of Human Subjects of Biomedical and Behavioral Research concluded in the 1970s that the future of the fetus—that is, whether the pregnant woman planned to give birth or abort—was immaterial to the regulation of fetal research; it argued that if there were no potential of direct benefit for mother or fetus, only minimal-risk research should be permitted.[48] However, some authors have questioned the logic behind this statement. If the regulations for research with pregnant women are justified to protect the interests of a future child who could suffer or be impaired as a result of teratogenic procedures, the regulations seem nonsensical when there will be no future child to protect.[14]

Fathers' Input

The role, influence, or veto power that a potential father should have in such research participation is another ethical concern specific to the situation of pregnant women. The National Commission occasionally referred to the need for consent from fathers without overtly detailing the nature and limits of their power, stating, for example, that "nontherapeutic research on the pregnant woman or on the fetus *in utero* may be conducted or supported, provided . . . the father has not objected."[48] DHHS regulations (45 CFR 46, subpart B) state that the consent of the father, in addition to the mother, is necessary for any research with the possibility of direct benefit solely for the fetus, unless the father cannot give consent for reasons of "unavailability, incompetence, or temporary incapacity or the pregnancy resulted from rape or incest."[11] The father's consent is not necessary, however, for research that holds out the prospect of direct benefit for the pregnant woman or for both the pregnant woman and the fetus, or when research involves only minimal risk but aims to develop important biomedical knowledge that cannot be otherwise obtained; the consent of the pregnant woman is still required in these situations (45 CFR 46.204). These variations partially reflect the public debate about men's say in abortion decisions, as demonstrated in the controversy over spousal notification laws.[49]

Although relatively little has been written about men's role in the research participation decisions of their pregnant partners, some authors, particularly those more oriented toward feminist ideology, are reluctant to give fathers much say in the decision.[14] They argue that although fathers might have a legitimate interest in preventing a pregnant woman who is not planning to abort from participating in a study potentially risky to the fetus, pregnant women would not be enrolled in these types of studies according to current regulations anyway.[14] Alternatively, if the pregnant woman plans to terminate her pregnancy, these authors echo the general women's rights sentiment that denies men's veto power.[14]

Liability Concerns

One common concern in research with pregnant women is a particularly legal one: Sponsors worry about incurring liability for the possible injury of a fetus in the course of a research trial. Although data regarding the frequency and likelihood of legal action seem to indicate that suits on behalf of fetuses are unlikely (a point that will be discussed in the next section), the fear of liability remains significant among researchers and is probably one of the primary contributors to women's exclusion from clinical studies.[15,45,46,50] However, even if fear of liability is justified by legal theories and practices, a number of scholars have pointed out that company sponsors and research institutions might also incur liability for *excluding* women from trials, given that drugs in the postmarketing phase will expose more women to the possibility of unexpected and adverse reactions to the treatment.[43,51] Fear of liability among researchers must be scrutinized for its validity and directly addressed with clearly established regulations and policies so as to avoid unnecessary exclusion of pregnant and potentially pregnant female subjects.

Women as "Potentially Pregnant" Persons

Women with established pregnancies clearly present a host of difficult ethical problems unique to their biological condition, but an ethically grayer area involves the nature of fertile women as *potentially* pregnant entities. Although the FDA's 1977 regulations prohibiting all "potentially pregnant" women from early clinical research seemed to unjustly bar women from the personal and population-based benefits of research participation, the knowledge that fertile women may become pregnant in the course of research participation brings up difficult questions regarding how to anticipate and plan for this possibility. Specifically, should women's attitudes toward contraceptive use be factored into the decision about whether to enroll them in a given research trial?

To give an example, researchers studying a serious chronic disease want to evaluate the antiinflammatory effects of the known teratogen thalidomide. Should the use of birth control during the course of the study be mandatory? If there is a nonnegligible chance that women could become pregnant with severely deformed fetuses as a result of study participation, researchers might reasonably consider excluding women who would refuse to use contraception; on the other hand, this criterion would necessarily exclude particular subgroups of women who, for religious or other reasons, do not believe in artificial contraception.

At its core, the question over whether to make contraceptive use an inclusion criterion can be construed as balancing a woman's autonomy against beneficence-based and justice-based obligations to a hypothetical future child.[52] Although researchers may sometimes be able to work with a woman to reduce the chances of pregnancy without violating her religious or moral beliefs, this will not always be a viable option. Rather, it has been suggested that requiring contraception use or abstinence as an inclusion criterion ought to be evaluated in light of the potential benefits of participation in a particular study. Although researchers may exclude a woman not using birth control from a trial that has little potential for her medical benefit and uses teratogenic substances, they might relax inclusion criteria if the woman could potentially greatly benefit from trial participation that involved experimental treatment unavailable outside of the research setting. Likewise, the greater the potential for teratogenicity in a trial, the more stringent the requirement for contraceptive use should be.

In the actual event of an unexpected pregnancy, women's rights advocates in the bioethics literature stress women's autonomy, contending that although fertile women should be explicitly informed during the consent process that an experimental drug/device has teratogenic potential, the choice to enroll and a possible subsequent choice regarding pregnancy termination should be left to the woman herself.[46,53] Though some authors have also noted the ethical tensions that antiabortion researchers themselves might feel if faced with a pregnant participant in a study of teratogenic pharmaceuticals, they assert that researchers of both pro-choice and pro-life views should feel ethically comfortable with neutrally referring pregnant subjects to a obstetrician/gynecologist.[46]

Although the gray area involving potentially pregnant women in possibly teratogenic studies has its own set of ethical difficulties, these dilemmas seem best managed on an individual study basis. Rigorous attention during the informed consent process to possible harms to the fetus from experimental agents or interventions, as well as counseling to help participants deal with unexpected pregnancies, may assist conscientious research planning.

Researchers ought to continue opening doors to female research participants, including those who are pregnant, but these ethical debates suggest that they should proceed with a certain amount of caution. Women's status both as a historically oppressed group and as the biological gestators of new human beings contributes to the ethical complexity inherent in involving them in an enterprise generally and necessarily fraught with risks for harm. The significant potential benefits from such involvement, however, strongly compel the research enterprise to seek ways of justly including female research subjects.

Empirical Data

Given the many ethical issues raised by the participation of pregnant and nonpregnant women in clinical studies, it is of the utmost importance to gather empirical evidence regarding the nature and effects of women's inclusion as research subjects. Data from many academic fields, including sociological, epidemiological, biological, and medical disciplines inform deliberations about the appropriate inclusion of female research subjects. Bioethics debates often benefit from population-based data that clarify the nature of disparities, opinions, and day-to-day realities that characterize the research environment.[54] In the particular case of women's research participation, existing empirical data can both buttress arguments for greater inclusion of women and help determine solutions to some of the problems created by their participation.

Evidence of Physiological Sex Differences

Empirical evidence establishes the need for female research subjects by illustrating the widespread and significant ways that male and female biology differ. In recent years, scientists have accrued a staggering list of conditions and general physiological characteristics that vary by sex (see Table 38.1). Though sex differences in physical and biological characteristics directly related to reproduction have long been acknowledged, researchers in recent decades have also begun to uncover sex differences that occur in other bodily systems or in the course of various illnesses.[55] Some conditions vary in prevalence by sex: Urinary incontinence, for example, is significantly more likely in women, as are type 2 diabetes, irritable bowel syndrome, chronic fatigue syndrome, musculoskeletal diseases such as osteoarthritis, and major depression; alternatively, autism, learning disabilities, and attention deficit hyperactivity disorder (ADHD) are significantly more common in men.

Sex differences are also seen in the presentation and natural history of some diseases. Women have a significantly lower initial HIV viral load than do men, for example, and they generally demonstrate lower pain tolerance. Men and women may also differ in their reactions to specific treatments and medications: Women react more positively to certain opioid analgesics for pain management than their male counterparts, for example, and pharmacologic agents used to treat cardiovascular disease induce different responses depending on sex. (See chart for citations.) This litany of physiological differences is not meant to be comprehensive, but rather to indicate the many and varied subfields of medicine in which sex differences exist, illustrating the vast extent of physiological variation between men and women for which there is empirical evidence.

Table 38.1

Selected Studies Demonstrating Medical Differences Between the Sexes

Condition	Details	Findings Published
Urinary incontinence	2:1 more common in women than men[56]	2001
AIDS and HIV	Initial viral load in women is significantly lower than in men, though both sexes develop AIDS at the same rate[57]	2001
Pain management	Women appear to have lower pain thresholds and tolerances than men;[58] certain opioids are much more effective analgesics in women[59]	2001, 1996
Type-2 diabetes	More prevalent in women than men, especially after age 65[60]	2000
Irritable bowel syndrome	3:1 more common in women than in men[61]	2001
Chronic fatigue syndrome	Nearly 2:1 more common in women than in men[62]	2001
Musculoskeletal diseases (osteoporosis, osteoarthritis, sports injuries)	More common in women than in men[63]	2000
Autoimmune diseases	More common (and deadly) in women than in men[64]	2000
Cardiovascular diseases	Differences in severity, incidence, importance of age, presentation, efficacy of treatment[44]	1999–2006
Depression	Twice as common in women as in men[65]	2000
Autism, learning disabilities, ADHD	More common in men[66]	2001

Extent and Effects of Research Exclusion

Given that women often differ from men in their presentation of disease and reaction to treatments, it is important to analyze how these sex differences interact with women's past exclusion from clinical research to affect them as a group. Data provided by numerous population-based studies strongly support the claim that less research has been done, and to a lesser degree continues to be done, with female populations than with male, particularly in studies of specific diseases.[67–69] Though some authors question the actual size of the disparities in the current research agenda,[16] several gaps appear to exist in the amount of research done with women in a number of medical fields.[24] Disparities exist not only in research on diseases unique to women, but also in areas unrelated to the reproductive system, such as chronic conditions like

Alzheimer's disease and obesity, genomic studies, musculoskeletal disorders, cancer, addictions, and more.[70]

This lack of research data from female subjects, in turn, has been demonstrated to have a sizeable negative impact on women's health "downstream" because it impairs the quality of women's primary care. When new medications and procedures are tested only in one subgroup of the population, there is a heightened danger that other subgroups will experience unexpected and potentially adverse reactions to the same treatment.[24,71] This is especially true given the documented physiological differences between women and men, who made up the bulk of study participants, particularly in older research studies. Historical examples abound: Male-only studies of heart disease and cholesterol led to widespread recommendations of a diet that could actually exacerbate the risk of heart disease for women;[15] efficacy of certain approved psychological medications was later demonstrated to oscillate significantly over the course of the menstrual cycle;[72] women with schizophrenia and bipolar disorder were found to exhibit different responses to treatment that had been found effective in studies using only men;[66] and so forth.

The impact of exclusion from research is also apparent with pregnant women. For a widespread example, little to no psychopharmaceutical research has been done with pregnant subjects.[73,74] Consequently, physicians treating pregnant women suffering from psychosis and other mental disorders have little information about the teratogenicity of various psychopharmaceuticals. Prescribing such drugs anyway, without evidence of safety and teratogenicity, puts women and fetuses at unknown risk.[75] Fear of teratogenicity and unexpected side effects may make some physicians reluctant to prescribe untested drugs at all, potentially leading to the undertreatment of serious psychiatric disease during pregnancy. Empirical data thus lend objective credence to the claims that exclusion from research may impair the quality of women's clinical care for a number of medical conditions.

Prevalence of the "Male Norm/Bias"

If evidence indicates that sex differences do exist, even in many supposedly "gender neutral" diseases, and that women and men experience different symptoms and have different optimal treatment regimens, what sort of obstacles might prevent the embrace of more gender-tailored medicine and greater numbers of female research subjects? One such barrier might be physicians' conscious or unconscious adoption of a "male norm" of health and disease. One physician provided this comparison: "If a 50-year-old man goes to the doctor complaining of chest pains, the next day he will be on a treadmill taking a stress test. If a 50-year-old woman goes to the doctor and complains of chest pains, she will be told to go home and rest."[76] Although this statement could be written off as anecdotal or as one isolated physician's opinion, evidence indicates that many health care professionals operate with "a *male bias* (observer error caused by adopting a male perspective and habit of thought) and/or the *male norm* (the tendency to use males as the standard and to see females as deviant or problematic, even in studying diseases that affect both sexes)."[77] Proving that such norms and biases exist and are in practice is difficult; after all, many physicians and researchers may not realize they are employing them. It may sometimes be inferred, however, that biases or inappropriate norms are at work in health care pro-

fessionals' opinions. For example, in reaction to the 1985 Public Health Service Task Force's report, some researchers publicly opposed new guidelines mandating the inclusion of female research subjects, claiming that women's menstrual cycles add an "extra variable" and thus extra work in their analyses. This argument, however, assumes that a nonmenstruating (male) body is the "normal" human body, exemplifying the thinking behind the "male norm." Determining what counts as "extra" depends on how the baseline is viewed.[10,15,38] Though more empirical research on this topic is clearly needed, researchers' and physicians' beliefs about the sexes may influence their research designs and their treatment of patients.

Female Subject Recruitment

Empirical data may also prove useful in untangling ethical dilemmas related to women's inclusion in research. For example, how might recruitment and retention of female research subjects differ from that of male research subjects? Should recruiters utilize certain tactics to attract female subjects, or be particularly concerned about certain influences on a female subject's decision to continue or withdraw? Several studies suggest that the roles and responsibilities women commonly assume in U.S. society may influence their decision to enroll and continue to participate in research studies.

Often charged with the care of children, women may be less likely to enroll in research if there is no option for child care or if the study has an extremely inflexible research appointment schedule.[78] Similarly, elderly women in particular may be less likely to drive or to have sufficient income to absorb the cost of taxi fares.[78] Recruiters ought to be sensitive to any potential stigma that may be attached to certain studies for female participants. For women in rural Africa, for example, participating in an HIV vaccine trial could offer personal benefits; however, the social stigma associated with being mistakenly viewed as HIV-positive and/or engaging in extramarital relationships is sufficient to keep many women from enrolling.[36] In a less serious but similar situation, one research study discovered that using the word *menopause* on recruitment flyers had a deterrent effect on recruitment in a major metropolitan U.S. center, because menopause and aging have salient negative connotations in Western society.[78] In light of evidence demonstrating that women are faced with a different set of daily obligations, difficulties, and taboos than men, female subjects may warrant somewhat different recruitment strategies.

Recruiting and retaining women of color in clinical research might be even more challenging. African American, Hispanic, and other minority women contemplating research participation face not only the obstacles shared by ethnic minority men but also additional difficulties by virtue of their specific status as minority *women*. Much has been written about researchers' difficulties in recruiting participants of either gender from ethnic minority groups, including the widespread suspicion and distrust of research institutions among minorities, stronger spirituality that may make minorities unlikely to seek treatment for conditions that are "God's will," and the difficulty of committing to time-consuming studies for individuals of low socioeconomic status.[38,79,80] Minority women may also have greater difficulties than white women due to child care responsibilities: Women of color are more likely both to be single parents and to adhere to traditional child caring roles in the home.[79] Armed with empirical information about the barriers faced by women—and particularly minority women—researchers may be better able to increase recruitment and retention of female subjects, further patching the holes in knowledge about women's health.

Liability Concerns

As previously noted, a major concern in research with female participants is the fear of liability for any injuries that may occur during the course of trial participation. Though there is always a potential for the woman herself to be injured and sue in clinical research, this situation is no different from the potential liability researchers assume with male subjects. Rather, researchers and sponsors worry about assuming additional legal responsibility for a *fetus* harmed during the course of the trial. Although available information cannot completely assuage this fear, it can dampen the concern. Suits by patients injured in the course of research are rare,[43,45] and suits on behalf of children injured in the course of their mother's research participation are even less common.[45] Although a few state courts have ruled in favor of prenatally injured children in lawsuits unrelated to research participation,[43] the extensive research consent process coupled with disagreement about the fetus's status as a rights-bearing human being lead some legal experts to doubt the success and even likelihood of any such lawsuit.[15,50,52]

Effects of Increased Attention to Research on Women's Health

Despite difficulties with past exclusion as well as practical and psychological barriers to women's research participation, empirical data demonstrate the clear beneficial impact that greater inclusion of women in clinical research can have on the quality of clinical care. NIH's Women's Health Initiative (WHI), for example, a long-term, multimillion dollar research project, supported a large-scale study of hormone replacement therapy for post-menopausal women. Though previously believed to be harmless or even beneficial, WHI research demonstrated that estrogen-progesterone therapy was correlated with an increase in the risk of stroke, heart attack, and breast cancer, a discovery which led the U.S. Preventive Services Task Force of the U.S. Agency for Healthcare Research and Quality (AHRQ) to issue a recommendation against chronic estrogen and progestin therapy in post-menopausal women.[44,70] Genomic studies of breast cancer, and the discovery of the *BRAC1* and *BRAC2* genes, have led to a number of new clinical preventive approaches for women found to be at genetic risk.[81,82] Empirical data have revealed important sex differences in the symptoms and optimal treatment for cardiovascular disease, including the particular ways women present with myocardial infarction[83] and a sex-specific reduction in stroke for women taking aspirin regularly.[84] Despite the relative youth of the movement for greater inclusion of women in clinical research, large gains have already been achieved that may be translated into primary care.

Avenues for Future Empirical Research

Additional empirical data in yet uninvestigated areas could help administrators and researchers to create sensible policies regard-

ing female research subjects. For example, in response to the claim that the compulsory inclusion of women in research trials leads to extremely elevated costs,[10,38] it would be helpful to know both the actual costs of adhering to the NIH inclusion guidelines and the estimated future costs of unnecessary or ineffective treatment of women—and lost productivity—because of the underrepresentation of women in clinical trials. Similarly, data on the primary care effects of women's research exclusion would be informative, such as the percentage of drugs taken by pregnant women that have been actively investigated for teratogenicity, or the extent to which female patients are still receiving the typical "male" treatment for diseases despite demonstrated sex differences in reaction to treatments. Information about the progress of recruiters in enrolling and retaining female subjects, particularly from racial minority groups or the elderly, would also benefit policy makers attempting to allocate resources appropriately. Finally, additional data revealing sex differences in responses to treatment or in disease manifestation are critical. Each upstream discovery in a specific field has the downstream potential to provide women with a higher quality of care and life. Further empirical evidence on these and a host of other questions will continue to enrich debates about the ethics of women's research participation.

Policy Implications

The historical record of women's exclusion and gradual inclusion in research studies, the ethical issues raised by their participation, and empirical evidence that supports or weakens the ethical debates all aim to influence public policy. Without a method of translating conceptual and empirical work into policy, however, academic studies will not affect the way women relate to and experience medical research. The success of this translation rests on how researchers and administrators use empirical findings and ethical clarification to shape both "big picture" policy decisions, such as issues of resource allocation and official research agendas, and more mundane policy questions such as how researchers design their studies and interpret existing ethical principles.

Major Policy Decisions

Establishing Priorities on the Research Agenda

One of the primary "big picture" policy concerns is how women's health needs should affect the ordering of research priorities, particularly for federally funded research. Several arguments support giving women's health problems at least some priority when competing for scarce funding resources. First, for conditions that affect both men and women, less research has focused on women—what treatments work for them, what symptoms they exhibit at the onset of the disease or condition, the usual clinical progression of the condition, and so forth.[67] Thus, compared to men, women with certain conditions are at a disadvantage in the doctor's office; they are more likely to receive inadequate treatment than their male counterparts for problems such as cardiovascular disease, for example.[70] Consequently, some argue, priority should be given to narrowing gender-based gaps in clinical care for diseases found in both sexes by investing greater resources in research on women's experiences with these conditions, with the aim of raising the quality of women's health care to equal status with that of men.[15]

However, other conditions that affect women—such as breast cancer, endometriosis, pregnancy, and so forth—simply do not occur in men, or occur predominantly in women. Thus, the call for greater research on these issues cannot be based on the imperative to equalize quality of care for men and women suffering the same illnesses. Rather, increased research on women-specific health issues might be justified as a means of improving the quality of women's health care overall, not just for specific conditions.[46]

Some argue that resource allocation for research on specifically female issues is desirable in order to "make up" for past exclusionary practices.[15] Critics liken such a policy to affirmative action in other sectors of society; research programs would be funded not for their merit alone, but in an attempt to make up for historical injustices. Though the affirmative action comparison does not exactly hold—men's health would not directly regress because of more research with women, in the way that men may actively lose jobs to women under employment-oriented affirmative action programs—these complaints stress the need for careful consideration of policies that put women's health issues at a premium, recognizing that other potentially worthy research projects may be unfunded as a consequence.

A tangential debate over research priorities springs from the widespread dearth of information on the teratogenicity of many widely prescribed treatments. Though some treatments are known to cause birth defects, many have never been studied for possible harmful affects on gametes and developing fetuses, leading women's research advocates to push for more funding for the investigation of drugs' and procedures' mutagenic potential.[53,85] However, experimental pharmaceuticals and treatments may have mutagenic effects on the gametes of both sexes. If our research agenda stresses a closer examination of the teratogenic effects of new treatments, it seems logical to examine the effects on the reproductive systems of both women and men.[14,15]

Eliminating Bias in Institutional Policy

Another important issue for policy change revolves around the idea of eliminating the male norm or male bias in official research regulations and guidelines.[77] Although it is hard to know precisely how often this bias is operative, advocates concerned with the persistence of views defining men as the "default" and women as "variations" urge policy makers to closely examine seemingly gender-neutral policies for the presence of these biases. Regulations that exclude women from research because of biological conditions found in most women—menstrual cycles, for example—are said to be operating under the assumption that women's differences from men are "extra" or "variations from the norm."[10] Though these policies may be based on a desire to keep costs and necessary analyses down, they represent a perspective on sex differences that many claim is unjust. Policy makers ought to carefully consider the reasoning behind regulations that seek to exclude women on the basis of a given biological difference.

Regulations Governing Research With Pregnant Women and Fetuses

Policy makers also ought to recognize the intentions and implications behind important barriers that exist in research with pregnant women and fetuses. For example, as previously noted, many current regulations and guidelines do not permit anything more than minimal risk for fetuses in clinical research if there is no potential for benefit for mother and/or fetus, regardless of whether the woman plans to carry the pregnancy to term.[11,48] Such limits on permissible risks in fetal research seem to be justified for protecting the interests of a future child, but is it logically consistent to extend these same limits to research on fetuses that will be aborted?[14,86] At the very least, some clarification seems to be necessary regarding the reasoning behind the similar or differential treatment of fetuses based on whether the pregnancy is expected to be brought to term.

Similarly, policy makers might examine policies regarding prehuman animal studies that must occur in order to gauge the teratogenicity of new treatments. Although the federal regulations prohibit research with pregnant women and fetuses unless "appropriate" preclinical studies have been done with animals to assess risks, the text of the regulations offers little guidance on what studies are appropriate.[11] Different types of experimental treatments might necessitate different types of animal studies to best evaluate possible teratogenicity. In addition, inherent differences in biology and anatomy can make it difficult to predict how animal reactions to treatments will be reflected in human beings. Chemicals such as the rubella vaccine have been found to cross the placental membrane in humans but not in nonhuman primates.[14] Animal data alone is insufficient to determine how a new pharmaceutical or treatment will affect a human fetus. Acknowledging that different types of animal studies might be necessary to properly assess the risks and benefits of study participation in a given research project, and that animal studies are not a sure indicator of teratogenicity in humans, policy makers ought to specify the types of information they actually hope to gain from animal studies and clarify existing regulations accordingly.

Daily Research Practices

Attitudes Toward Liability Concerns

Data regarding liability for research-related injuries might inform policy and practice at the day-to-day level of study design. We have already discussed empirical statistics that suggest legal action resulting from prenatal injuries is decidedly rare.[45] Furthermore, from a pragmatic viewpoint, there are the two previously discussed arguments claiming that excluding women could incur more liability than including them. First, because women have a constitutional right to equal protection under the law, they could bring lawsuits claiming unfair exclusion from studies.[43] Second, the liability that a drug sponsor assumes during the course of a research trial involving women is several orders of magnitude less than the liability a manufacturer could face if an unexpectedly teratogenic pharmaceutical enters widespread and unmonitored use.[50] Acknowledging the relevant data and logical arguments, research institutions ought to feel relatively confident about their current methods of reducing liability by disclosing information in the consent process and providing care for research-related injuries. Accordingly, potential liability from unexpected fetal defects should not be a reason for categorically excluding pregnant and potentially pregnant women from research trials.

Interpreting Ambiguous Regulations

IRBs and researchers might benefit from academic work, specifically in the ethics field, in their attempts to interpret policy regulations that use ambiguous or undefined terms. According to

U.S. federal regulations, for example, the permissibility of research depends to some extent on whether study participation "holds out the prospect of direct benefit to the pregnant woman," but the phrase "direct benefit" is not defined.[11] Is there prospect of direct benefit even if the expected benefit is small or the chances of the woman actually responding to the treatment are slim?[86] Some ethicists have dealt with the question of what should be considered a "prospect of direct benefit" under the federal regulations by focusing instead on the sort of benefit that would be necessary to justify potential harm to a fetus; that is, although we might agree that a potentially teratogenic new acne medication technically has the prospect of providing a "direct benefit" to a woman, we still might conclude that this benefit is too minor to justify the significant risk to a developing fetus.[86] This approach calls for an individual calculation of the benefits and potential risks for the woman and the fetus with each research project.

A similar problem of definition exists with the federal regulations' minimal risk standard. Research permissibility may depend on there being only "minimal risk" to the fetus; but what risks should be considered minimal? Although the federal regulations attempt to clarify *minimal risk* as "the risks of daily life," this definition only raises the question of what "daily life" consists of.[11] IRBs have been found to vary enormously in their interpretation of the minimal risk standard, leading to further confusion among researchers.[87] Although the definition of minimal risk remains a live question, scientists trying to design and categorize their studies might gain some guidance from recent ethics work attempting to quantify the risks of *daily life* by using data on the risks of driving in a car or engaging in common sports.[88]

Study Design

Conceptual and academic work on women's participation in clinical research also has ramifications for research study design. These design strategies concern both the mechanisms by which women can be included fairly as participants in clinical research and the means of mitigating some of the more ethically difficult situations that can occur with female participants.

Creating Equitable Research Participant Populations

The first and most important consideration is how to ensure that women are not unnecessarily excluded from research participation at the level of study design. Women ought to be fairly included in clinical studies so as to fairly distribute the benefits of research—both the personal benefits of research participation and the general benefits that result from being able to tailor diagnoses and therapies to sex-specific differences.[15,30] In addition, research designs that recruit sufficient female subjects to enable sex and gender comparisons are crucial to equalizing the "downstream" quality of health care between men and women.[10,17,24,67]

Thought should be given to how to fairly include various subgroups of women as well, such as minority and elderly women, in acknowledgment of the possibility of relevant differences among different types of women. However, it is clear that at some point cost and complexity become limiting factors; if researchers were required to have equal numbers of every possible subgroup, research costs would become prohibitively expensive, and the an-

alyses might become so unwieldy as to be unworkable. To balance subgroup representation and finite resources, researchers should consider how the biological feature of interest expresses itself in the wider population, then aim for the research subject population to reflect this incidence appropriately.[24]

Recruiting and Retaining Female Subjects

Researchers should also consider implementing different styles and methods of subject recruitment that may be more likely to attract women. Evidence suggests that women are more likely to enroll and stay with trials that cater to women's particular needs, such as providing child-care options (particularly with ethnic minority women), maintaining a flexible appointment schedule, and providing transportation for subjects unable to arrange it themselves.[78] Additionally, recruiters ought to be alert to the potential stigma that can occur for women involved in certain cases of clinical research and should consider presenting the study in a different way to avoid negative reactions. For example, in the menopause studies mentioned earlier, recruitment materials were altered to focus on the positive need for more research on women's heart disease. Often, by making relatively small changes, study recruiters faced with policies mandating greater inclusion of women in clinical research trials can make participation more appealing for female subjects.

Planning for unexpected developments during the course of women's research participation should also be considered.[52] In anticipation of the chance that fertile women may become pregnant during the investigation of a possibly teratogenic treatment, researchers involved in the consent process should take special care to (1) clearly communicate the risks a given study's protocol would have for a potential fetus, (2) explain how women can successfully avoid pregnancy during the course of the trial, and (3) discuss what actions will be taken if the woman does unexpectedly become pregnant. Rather than excluding women opposed to birth control for fear of causing possible harm to a fetus, advocates for women's clinical research participation urge researchers to provide sufficient information during the consent process so that women are sufficiently empowered to make their own choices about participation.[52] This approach not only respects women's ability to make autonomous choices, but makes it less likely that researchers will be found legally liable in the event of a research injury to the woman or fetus.[50]

Conclusion

Women as a population hold a unique and thorny place in the arena of clinical research. Though women cannot technically be considered a minority, because they comprise more than half the total population, they have historically suffered discrimination and unfair treatment at the hands of many U.S. institutions, including the research enterprise. Despite the inclination to protect women, given their status as both a relatively disempowered population and the sex who share their bodies with future new human beings, society has come to realize the important role research participation has in improving the quality of health care and the general promotion of justice. The ethical difficulties that necessarily surround women's research participation should not be underestimated and cannot be easily resolved. But in recent years both conceptual and empirical work have driven significant improvements in both clarifying issues and delineating interests and concerns that should take priority in official policies and regulations.

The protective approach to women and pregnant women in clinical research has been difficult to debunk and is still reflected in many contemporary guidelines, but significant progress has been made in increasing women's opportunities to participate. These efforts have had an important impact on the creation of more equitable policies and study designs, which in turn has had and will continue to have a tangible influence on the quality of women's medical care. It is imperative to continue in this tradition to assure the fair distribution of research's benefits.

References

1. United States Census Bureau. Annual estimates of the population by sex and five-year age groups for the United States: April 1, 2000 to July 1, 2005.

2. Cromie WJ. Why women live longer than men. *Harvard University Gazette* Oct. 1, 1998. [Online] Available: http://www.hno.harvard.edu/gazette/1998/10.01/WhyWomenLiveLon.html.

3. FDA Office on Women's Health and PHS Coordinating Committee on Women's Health. The Women's Health Movement: The History and Future of Women's Health. [Online] Available: http://www.4woman.gov/owh/pub/history/2centurya.htm.

4. FDA Office of Women's Health. FDA Milestones in Women's Health. [Online] 2001. Available: http://www.fda.gov/womens/milesbro.html.

5. Center for Drug Evaluation and Research, Food and Drug Administration. Thalidomide: Important Patient Information. [Online] July 7, 2005. Available: http://www.fda.gov/cder/news/thalidomide.htm.

6. Center for Food Safety and Applied Nutrition, Food and Drug Administration. The Story of the Laws Behind the Labels: Part III: 1962 Drug Amendments. [Online] Available: http://www.cfsan.fda.gov/~lrd/histor1b.html.

7. Covey S. *The Unfortunate Experiment: The Full Story Behind the Inquiry Into Cervical Cancer Treatment.* Auckland, New Zealand: Penguin Books; 1988.

8. Centers for Disease Control and Prevention. DES History. [Online] Available: http://www.cdc.gov/des/consumers/about/history.html.

9. Centers for Disease Control and Prevention. Elevated risk of pelvic inflammatory disease among women using the Dalkon Shield. *Morbidity and Mortality Weekly Report* 1983;32(17):221–2.

10. Johnson T, Fee E. Women's participation in clinical research: From protectionism to access. In: Mastroianni AC, Faden R, Federman D, eds. *Women and Health Research: Ethical and Legal Issues of Including Women in Clinical Studies, Volume 2. Workshop and Commissioned Papers.* Washington, D.C.: National Academy Press; 1994:1–10.

11. Department of Health and Human Services, National Institutes of Health, and Office for Human Research Protections. The Common Rule, Title 45 (Public Welfare), Code of Federal Regulations, Part 46 (Protection of Human Subjects), Subpart B: Additional Protections for Pregnant Women, Human Fetuses and Neonates Involved in Research. [Online] June 23, 2005. Available: http://www.hhs.gov/ohrp/humansubjects/guidance/45cfr46.htm#subpartb.

12. The U.S. Equal Employment Opportunity Commission. Facts About Pregnancy Discrimination. [Online] http://www.eeoc.gov/facts/fs-preg.html.

13. Kinney EL, Trautmann J, Gold JA, Vesell ES, Zelis R. Underrepresentation of women in new drug trials: Ramifications and remedies. *Annals of Internal Medicine* 1981;95:495–9.

14. Steinbock B. Ethical issues related to the inclusion of pregnant women in clinical trials (II). In: Mastroianni AC, Faden R, Federman D, eds. *Women and Health Research: Ethical and Legal Issues of Including Women in Clinical Studies, Volume 2. Workshop and Commissioned Papers.* Washington D.C.: National Academy Press; 1994:23–8.

15. Dresser R. Wanted: Single, white male for medical research. *Hastings Center Report* 1992;22(1):24–9.

16. Meinert CL, Gilpin AK, Ünalp A, Dawson C. Gender representation in trials. *Controlled Clinical Trials* 2000;21:462–75.

17. U.S. Public Health Service. Report of the Public Health Service Task Force on Women's Health Issues. *Public Health Reports* 1985;100(1):73–106.

18. Statement of Mark V. Nadel, Associate Director, National and Public Health Issues, Human Resources Division. Subcommittee on Health and the Environment, Committee on Energy and Commerce. Washington, D.C., 1990.

19. U.S. Congress. Women's Health Equity Act of 1990. H.R. 5397, S.2961, 101st Congress, 2nd Session, 1990.

20. National Institutes of Health. Office of Research on Women's Health. [Online] Available: http://orwh.od.nih.gov/index.html.

21. *United Automobile Workers* v. *Johnson Controls, Inc.,* 499 U.S. 187 (1991).

22. U.S. Congress. NIH Revitalization Act of 1993. Pub. L. 103–43, June 10, 1993.

23. National Institutes of Health, Department of Health and Human Services. NIH Guidelines on the Inclusion of Women and Minorities as Subjects in Clinical Research; Notice. *Federal Register* 1994;59(59):14508–13.

24. Institute of Medicine, Board on Health Sciences Policy. *Inclusion of Women in Clinical Trials: Policies for Population Subgroups.* Washington, D.C.: National Academies Press; 1993.

25. General Accounting Office. Women's health: FDA needs to ensure more study of gender differences in prescription drug testing. GAO/HRD-93-17. Washington, D.C.: GAO; 1992.

26. Food and Drug Administration, Department of Health and Human Services. Guideline for the Study and Evaluation of Gender Differences in the Clinical Evaluation of Drugs; Notice. *Federal Register* 1993;58(139):39406–16.

27. Gesensway D. Reasons for sex-specific and gender-specific study of health topics. *Annals of Internal Medicine* 2001;135:935–8.

28. Arnold K. Journal to encourage analysis by sex/ethnicity. *Journal of the National Cancer Institute* 2000;92:1561.

29. Vidaver RM, Lafleur B, Tong C, Bradshaw R, Marts SA. Women subjects in NIH-funded clinical research literature: Lack of progress in both representation and analysis by sex. *Journal of Women's Health and Gender-Based Medicine* 2000;9:495–504.

30. Emanuel E, Wendler D, Grady C. What makes clinical research ethical? *JAMA* 2000;283:2701–11.

31. Levine C, Faden RR, Grady C, et al. The limitations of "vulnerability" as a protection for human research participants. *American Journal of Bioethics* 2004;4(3):44–9.

32. Council for International Organizations of Medical Sciences, in collaboration with the World Health Organization. *International Ethical Guidelines for Biomedical Research Involving Human Subjects.* Geneva, Switzerland: CIOMS and WHO; 2002. [Online] November 2002. Available: http://www.cioms.ch/frame_guidelines_nov_2002.htm.

33. Sherwin S. Women in clinical studies: A feminist view. In: Mastroianni AC, Faden R, Federman D, eds. *Women and Health Research: Ethical and Legal Issues of Including Women in Clinical Studies, Volume 2. Workshop and Commissioned Papers.* Washington, D.C.: National Academy Press; 1994:11–7.

34. Wertheimer A. *Exploitation.* Princeton, N.J.: Princeton University Press; 1996.

35. Emanuel E, Currie XE, Herman A. Undue inducement in clinical research in developing countries: Is it a worry? *Lancet* 2005;366:336–40.

36. Mills E, Nixon S, Singh S, Dolma S, Nayyar A, Kapoor S. Enrolling women into HIV preventive vaccine trials: An ethical imperative but a logistical challenge. *PLoS Medicine* 2006;3(3):e94.

37. Leffers JM, Martins DC, Brown DG, Mercer J, Sullivan MC, Viau P. Development of a theoretical construct for risk and vulnerability from six empirical studies. *Research and Theory for Nursing Practice* 2004;18:15–34.

38. Roan S. Sex, ethnic bias in medical research raises questions. *Los Angeles Times* August 3, 1990.

39. Society for the Advancement of Women's Health Research. Annual Report: Women's Health Research: Prescription for Change. Washington, D.C.: Society for the Advancement of Women's Health Research; 1991.

40. Reuters. Researchers identify "male warrior effect." Sept. 8, 2006.

41. Baron-Cohen S. The extreme male brain theory of autism. *Trends in Cognitive Sciences* 2002;6(6):248–54.

42. Charo RA. Brief overview of constitutional issues raised by the exclusion of women from research trials. In: Mastroianni AC, Faden R, Federman D, eds. *Women and Health Research: Ethical and Legal Issues of Including Women in Clinical Studies, Volume 2. Workshop and Commissioned Papers*. Washington, D.C.: National Academy Press; 1994:84–90.

43. Legal Considerations. In: Mastroianni AC, Faden R, Federman D, eds. *Women and Health Research: Ethical and Legal Issues of Including Women in Clinical Studies, Volume 1*. Washington, D.C.: National Academies Press; 1994:128–74.

44. National Heart Lung and Blood Institute. Women's Health Initiative. [Online] Available: http://www.nhlbi.nih.gov/whi/.

45. Kass NE, Taylor HA, King PA. Harms of excluding pregnant women from clinical research: The case of HIV-infected pregnant women. *Journal of Law, Medicine, and Ethics* 1996;24:36–46.

46. McCullough LB, Coverdale JH, Chervenak FA. A comprehensive ethical framework for responsibly designing and conducting pharmacologic research that involves pregnant women. *American Journal of Obstetrics and Gynecology* 2005;193(3 Suppl.1):901–7.

47. Merton V. Impact of current federal regulations on the inclusion of female subjects in clinical studies. In: Mastroianni AC, Faden R, Federman D, eds. *Women and Health Research: Ethical and Legal Issues of Including Women in Clinical Studies, Volume 2. Workshop and Commissioned Papers*. Washington, D.C.: National Academy Press; 1994:65–83.

48. The National Commission for the Protection of Human Subjects of Biomedical and Behavioral Research. *Research on the Fetus*. Bethesda, Md.: DHEW; 1975.

49. The Pew Research Center for the People and the Press. Public opinion supports Alito on spousal notification even as it favors *Roe v. Wade*. [Online] November 2, 2005. Available: http://people-press.org/commentary/display.php3?AnalysisID=122.

50. Clayton EW. Liability exposure when offspring are injured because of their parents' participation in clinical trials. In: Mastroianni AC, Faden R, Federman D, eds. *Women and Health Research: Ethical and Legal Issues of Including Women in Clinical Studies, Volume 2. Workshop and Commissioned Papers*. Washington, D.C.: National Academy Press; 1994:103–12.

51. Flannery E, Greenberg SN. Liability exposure for exclusion and inclusion of women as subjects in clinical studies. In: Mastroianni AC, Faden R, Federman D, eds. *Women and Health Research: Ethical and Legal Issues of Including Women in Clinical Studies, Volume 2. Workshop and Commissioned Papers*. Washington, D.C.: National Academy Press; 1994:91–102.

52. McCullough LB, Coverdale JH, Chervenak FA. Preventive ethics for including women of childbearing potential in clinical trials. *American Journal of Obstetrics and Gynecology* 2006;194:1221–7.

53. Beran RG. The ethics of excluding women who become pregnant while participating in clinical trials of anti-epileptic medications. *Seizure* 2006;15:563–70.

54. Halpern SD. Towards evidence based bioethics. *British Medical Journal* 2005;331:901–3.

55. Executive Summary. In: Institute of Medicine (Wizemann TM, Pardue M-L, eds.). *Exploring the Biological Contributions to Human Health: Does Sex Matter?* Washington, DC: National Academy Press; 2001.

56. Romanzi LJ. Urinary incontinence in women and men. *Journal of Gender Specific Medicine* 2001;4(3):14–20.

57. Sterling TR, Vlahov D, Astemborski J, Hoover DR, Margolick JB, Quinn TC. Initial plasma HIV-1 RNA levels and progression to AIDS in women and men. *New England Journal of Medicine* 2001;344:720–5.

58. Hoffman DE, Tarzian AJ. The girl who cried pain: A bias against women in the treatment of pain. *Journal of Law, Medicine, and Ethics* 2001;29:13–27.

59. Gear RW, Miaskowski C, Gordon NC, Paul SM, Heller PH, Levine JD. Kappa-opioids produce significantly greater analgesia in women than in men. *Nature Medicine* 1996;2:1248–50.

60. Campaigne BN, Wishner KL. Gender-specific health care in diabetes mellitus. *Journal of Gender Specific Medicine* 2000;3(1):51–8.

61. Horwitz BJ, Fisher RS. The irritable bowel syndrome. *New England Journal of Medicine* 2001;344:1846–50.

62. Natelson BH. Chronic fatigue syndrome. *JAMA* 2001;285:2557–9.

63. Gwinn DE, Wilckens JH, McDevitt ER, Ross G, Kao T-C. The relative incidence of anterior cruciate ligament injury in men and women at the United States Naval Academy. *American Journal of Sports Medicine* 2000;28:98–102.

64. Walsh SJ, Rau LM. Autoimmune diseases: A leading cause of death among young and middle-aged women in the United States. *American Journal of Public Health* 2000;90:1463–6.

65. Desai HD, Jann MW. Major depression in women: A review of the literature. *Journal of the American Pharmacists Association* 2000;40(4):525–37.

66. Blehar MC. The NIMH women's mental health program: Establishing the public health context for women's mental health. *Trends in Evidence-Based Neuropsychiatry* 2001;3:42–3.

67. Pinn VW. Sex and gender factors in medical studies: Implications for health and clinical practice. *JAMA* 2003;289:397–400.

68. NIH Advisory Committee on Women's Health Issues. Women's Health Issues Research Report: FY 1985–1987. Bethesda, Md.: NIH; 1989.

69. Vidaver RM, Lafleur B, Tong C, Bradshaw R, Marts SA. Women subjects in NIH-funded clinical research literature: Lack of progress in both representation and analysis by sex. *Journal of Women's Health and Gender-Based Medicine* 2000;9:495–504.

70. Pinn VW. Research on women's health: Progress and opportunities. *JAMA* 2005;294:1407–10.

71. Rademaker M. Do women have more adverse drug reactions? *American Journal of Clinical Dermatology* 2001;2:349–51.

72. Jensvold MF, Reed K, Jarrett DB, Hamilton JA. Menstrual cycle-related depressive symptoms treated with variable antidepressant dosage. *Journal of Women's Health* 1992;1:109–15.

73. Frank E, Novick DM, Kupfer DJ. Beyond the question of placebo controls: Ethical issues in psychopharmacological drug studies. *Psychopharmacology* 2003;171:19–26.

74. Howard L, Webb RT, Abel KM. Safety of antipsychotic drugs for pregnant and breastfeeding women with non-affective psychosis. *British Medical Journal* 2004;329:933–4.

75. Mattison D, Zajicek A. Gaps in knowledge in treating pregnant women. *Gender Medicine* 2006;3(3):169–82.

76. Manson JE, Stampfer MJ, Colditz GA, et al. A prospective study of aspirin use and primary prevention of cardiovascular disease in women. *JAMA* 1991;266:521–7.

77. Executive Summary. In: Mastroianni AC, Faden R, Federman D, eds. *Women and Health Research: Ethical and Legal Issues of Including Women in Clinical Studies, Volume 1.* Washington, D.C.: National Academy Press; 1994:1–25.

78. Stoy DB. Recruitment and retention of women in clinical studies: Theoretical perspectives and methodological considerations. In: Mastroianni AC, Faden R, Federman D, eds. *Women and Health Research: Ethical and Legal Issues of Including Women in Clinical Studies, Volume 2. Workshop and Commissioned Papers.* Washington, D.C.: National Academy Press; 1994:45–51.

79. Mitchell JL. Recruitment and retention of women of color in clinical studies. In: Mastroianni AC, Faden R, Federman D, eds. *Women and Health Research: Ethical and Legal Issues of Including Women in Clinical Studies, Volume 2. Workshop and Commissioned Papers.* Washington, D.C.: National Academy Press; 1994:52–6.

80. List JM. Histories of mistrust and protectionism: Disadvantaged minority groups and human-subject research policies. *American Journal of Bioethics* 2005;5(1):53–6.

81. Ford D, Easton DF, Stratton M, et al. Genetic heterogeneity and penetrance analysis of the BRCA1 and BRCA2 genes in breast cancer families. The Breast Cancer Linkage Consortium. *American Journal of Human Genetics* 1998;62:676–9.

82. Narod SA. Modifiers of risk of hereditary breast cancer. *Oncogene* 2006;25:5832–6.

83. Merz NB, Johnson BD, Kelsey PSF, et al. Diagnostic, prognostic, and cost assessment of coronary artery disease in women. *American Journal of Managed Care* 2001;7:959–65.

84. Ridker PM, Cook NR, Lee I-M, et al. A randomized trial of low-dose aspirin in the primary prevention of cardiovascular disease in women. *New England Journal of Medicine* 2005;352:1293–1304.

85. Webb RT, Howard L, Abel KM. Antipsychotic drugs for non-affective psychosis during pregnancy and postpartum (Cochrane Review). *Cochrane Database of Systematic Reviews* 2004;2:CD004411.

86. Robertson J. Ethical issues related to the inclusion of pregnant women in clinical trials (I). In: Mastroianni AC, Fader R, Federman D, eds. *Women and Health Research: Ethical and Legal Issues of Including Women in Clinical Studies, Volume 2. Workshop and Commissioned Papers.* Washington, D.C.: National Academy Press; 1994:18–22.

87. Shah S, Whittle A, Wilfond B, Gensler G, Wendler D. How do institutional review boards apply the federal risk and benefit standards for pediatric research? *JAMA* 2004;291:476–82.

88. Wendler D. Protecting subjects who cannot give consent: Toward a better standard for "minimal" risks. *Hastings Center Report* 2005;35(5):37–43.

Bernard Lo   Nesrin Garan

39

Research With Ethnic and Minority Populations

Historical Background

Egregious misconduct in clinical research has often centered on ethnic and minority populations. The Nazi "experiments" involved disregard for the lives of Jewish, Gypsy, and other subjects whom the Nazis considered racially inferior. The Tuskegee study was flagrantly unethical because of its lack of informed consent, its deception, and its exploitation of poor, often illiterate African Americans. The legacy of Tuskegee persists today among many African Americans, who are largely mistrustful of medical research and often unwilling to participate in clinical trials.[1] Specifically, a number of studies show that African Americans are more likely than people from other ethnic backgrounds to believe that researchers would lie to them about research and would expose them to unnecessary risks.[1-3] In addition, African Americans tend to believe that to give informed consent for research is to sign away their rights.[2] Furthermore, African Americans view research in the context of broader concerns about racism and remain skeptical that research would provide any benefits to them as a group.[1,4]

Some ethnic and minority communities also fear that research will support political and social policies that will be detrimental to them. For example, many genetics researchers in the late 19th and early 20th centuries supported eugenic public policies including immigration restrictions and forced sterilization.[5] In retrospect, much of this research and the conclusions drawn from this research were flawed and biased. Because of this history, many ethnic and minority communities today remain concerned about the policy implications of research. This chapter will focus on racial groups such as African Americans, and religious groups such

as Ashkenazi Jews, but not minority populations of other kinds such as gay men or sex workers.

Current Interest in Research With Ethnic and Minority Populations

Certain diseases disproportionately affect minority groups. Worldwide, the vast majority of cases of HIV infection occur in sub-Saharan Africa and Asia, whereas in the United States, new cases of HIV, end-stage renal disease, lead poisoning, and other conditions are significantly more common in African Americans.[6] Health disparities are another driving force for research on ethnic and minority populations; in the United States, racial and ethnic minorities tend to have poorer health-care outcomes, lower quality of care, and worse access to care than nonminority populations.[6] These disparities are compounded because racial and ethnic minorities tend to have economic and social disadvantages that are also associated with worse health outcomes. However, studies find that health disparities persist even when minorities have similar access to care; thus, research is essential to clarify the reasons for these disparities. A recent Institute of Medicine report found evidence that bias and stereotyping by health-care providers and the health-care system contribute to unequal treatment.[6]

Researchers sometimes enroll members of ethnic and minority groups because it is necessary to include such individuals in order to adequately understand or ameliorate a serious condition that disproportionately affects them. For example, in the United States HIV infection in Caucasians most commonly results from men having sex with other men, whereas HIV infection in persons of color results primarily from injection drug use or heterosexual intercourse with injection drug users. Hence prevention and clinical trials of HIV infection that enroll primarily Caucasian participants may not provide reliable data on HIV infection in minority communities because of differences in risk behaviors and adherence to therapy.

Studies targeting persons in ethnic and minority groups are justified when they are designed to improve the circumstances that lead to serious risks or illness in their lives.[7] However, even when the disproportionate inclusion of persons from ethnic and minority groups is justified, such disproportionate enrollment can lead to concerns about or the perception of inequitable selection of subjects. For example, in the context of HIV research, the ethical concern is that minority persons in developing countries may be being used as research subjects to test vaccines or drugs that they may not have access to after research is completed.[8] Indeed, the concern may be that if research shows the intervention to be effective and safe, people in industrialized countries will be the primary beneficiaries, because they will be able to afford it.

Populations from different geographical origins may differ in their physiological response to medications.[9,10] Some groups have less favorable responses to standard medications for certain conditions. For example, some African Americans have a less favorable response to beta-blockers and ACE inhibitors in hypertension.[11] However, the effect is small, and the vast majority of African Americans have responses to these medications that are similar to those found in Caucasians. Similarly, African Americans may have less favorable responses to ACE inhibitors in congestive heart failure than Caucasians.[11] There are many potential explanations for this finding, including the selection of endpoints and the presence of comorbid conditions such as diabetes, as well as genetic differences between the groups. More research is needed to understand such differences.

Ethnic and racial minorities are underrepresented in research.[12] As a result, rigorous evidence is lacking regarding safety and efficacy of therapies in these populations. Hence clinical recommendations for such populations are based on weak scientific evidence. Such underrepresentation may be due to lack of access to clinical trials or unwillingness to talk to researchers about a clinical trial, rather than unwillingness to enroll in a trial once asked do so.[13]

In the genomics era, there is a strong scientific rationale for conducting research on ethnic and minority populations. Genes for conditions of interest are more likely to be identified in populations that have a high prevalence of genetic disorders and/or low genetic diversity. Researchers who study human population genetics also need samples from diverse populations. In both instances, ethnic and minority populations may provide scientifically important data.

Research With Ashkenazi Jewish Populations

Over several decades, researchers have studied Tay-Sachs disease, the role of BRCA1 and BRCA2 genes in breast cancer, and the role of the APC gene in colon cancer in Ashkenazi Jewish populations. Researchers studying these diseases have worked closely with community and religious leaders and carried out extensive programs of community outreach and education. In addition to informed consent from individuals, researchers have obtained the support of rabbis and community advisory committees for their studies.

Researchers have had to address concerns that individuals who are identified as carriers of a disease or at risk for an adult-onset disease would suffer stigmatization and discrimination. In the case of Tay-Sachs disease, individuals and community leaders feared that carriers would become unmarriageable.[14] In the case of susceptibility to cancer, there were concerns about discrimination against at-risk individuals by health insurance companies and employers, particularly if confidentiality were breached.[15] Researchers, in conjunction with community leaders, have addressed these concerns in innovative ways. With Tay-Sachs disease, researchers initiated extensive community education about the disease. After the ethical and social issues were widely discussed in the community, a nonprofit group called Dor Yeshorim was organized to carry out confidential and anonymous genetic testing for Orthodox Jewish couples considering marriage, and to inform them if either or both partners were carriers.[14] In cancer genetics research, researchers offered participants the option of participating in research studies without learning the results of their own genetic tests.

Some Ashkenazi Jewish community leaders raised concerns about stigmatization of the group even if confidentiality of individual research participants were maintained. These leaders worried that the Jewish community might be labeled "bad gene carriers" because of news reports that perpetuated the idea that Jews are particularly susceptible to cancer and other conditions. Researchers found, however, that the Jewish community was not homogeneous regarding such concerns about group stigmatization. Although there was considerable concern in some cities, in others there was relatively little.[16] Researchers therefore were able to successfully recruit participants in the communities that believed the potential benefits of the research outweighed the risks of group harm.

Research With Amish and Mennonite Communities

Amish and Mennonite communities have several characteristics that are advantageous in studying genetic diseases.[17,18] They experience high rates of particular genetic diseases because of a founder effect (many members of the community can trace their ancestry to a single individual) and inbreeding. In addition, they are relatively small populations that remain geographically localized, have large families, and keep excellent genealogical records.

Research has been successfully carried out in these communities in large measure because the main researchers live within the communities and have made a commitment to public service.[19] Physicians established the Clinic for Special Children in Pennsylvania to provide diagnostic services and therapy as well as to identify cases for research.[17] The Amish and Mennonites do not buy medical insurance, nor do they accept public funding for medical care; therefore, the clinic carries out fundraising to help pay patients' medical bills. The researchers thus have made a long-term commitment to provide crucial health-care services to the community, rather than simply to collect research samples and data. Physicians also hold meetings to educate the community about the diseases under study, their research findings, and potential new therapies.

In order to study and treat this population, researchers must take into account the community's pervasive cultural values about science and technology. These groups traditionally shun modern technology, including automobiles and electricity. Children with Crigler-Najjar syndrome, a congenital disorder that prevents the usual metabolism of bilirubin, which can then lead to kernicterus and brain damage, require extensive daily exposure to special blue lights. More advanced cases may require liver transplantation. In explaining the need for these therapies and for research on such high-tech interventions as gene transfer, researchers and physicians had to respect families' concerns about technology. Most families have accepted such research and therapies. They have accommodated these medical technologies, while continuing to reject most other technologies.[19] Often the blue phototherapy lamps are the only electrical appliances in the home.[20]

The Human Genome Diversity Project

The Human Genome Diversity Project (HGDP) proposes to study the variation within the human genome by collecting, storing, and analyzing samples from diverse populations.[21] This project would be useful in identifying alleles that cause or predispose to disease and in ascertaining how genetic variation affects the response to drugs. The HGDP would also provide crucial information for human population genetics and about human migration and evolution.

The project has remained on hold, however, because of lack of funding, disagreements over what information should be collected about individuals, and opposition from activist organizations on behalf of native and aboriginal communities.

Critics attacked the HGDP as biocolonialism and biopiracy, because genes from indigenous peoples could be patented and developed into commercial products, yielding profits to corporations in the developed world.[21] To address concerns about exploitation, HGDP investigators were urged to "seek ways in which participation in the HGDP can bring benefits to the sampled individual and their communities," for example through health screening, medical care, or education.[22] Proponents of the project also declared that it would "work to ensure that the sampled population benefit from the financial return" from any commercial products that may be developed.[22] Ironically, no medical or phenotypic information would be collected from donors, making the likelihood of developing commercial products actually very low.[22]

One of the most contentious matters has been the issue of consent from groups as well as from individual participants who might donate samples for the HGDP. The North American investigators concluded that collective consent from groups was required through their "culturally appropriate authorities." The rationale was that the group itself was subject of the study and thus bore the risks of research.[23] In North America, the researchers were dealing with Native American tribes that have formal political authorities with the power to give or withhold such group consent. However, critics argued that group consent was generally impractical, particularly when there was no legitimized group government. Moreover, in their view, group consent reinforced the mistaken idea that there were significant genetic differences among populations with different cultures.[24–26]

Use of Racial and Ethnic Categories in Clinical Research

In the United States, racial and ethnic minorities tend to have worse health-care outcomes, lower quality of care, and worse access to care than nonminority populations.[6] These disparities, as well as the history of racial discrimination against African Americans, form the background for U.S. controversies over the use of ethnic and racial categories in research. The Institute of Medicine report called for ongoing collection of racial and ethnic data in outcomes research and clinical care in order to monitor these disparities and to evaluate measures intended to reduce them.

Going beyond outcomes research, some clinical trials are targeted specifically to certain ethnic populations. Historically, racial and ethnic minorities have been underrepresented in clinical trials, despite efforts by the National Institutes of Health (NIH) to increase their participation. As a result, the evidence base for the care of minority populations remains weak. In response to data suggesting that African Americans may respond differently to cardiac drugs, a randomized clinical trial that enrolled only African Americans showed in 2004 that a combination of hydralazine and isosorbide dinitrate added to standard therapy for congestive heart failure decreased mortality.[9] This combination did not appear effective when added to standard therapy in a racially heterogeneous population. FDA approval was sought and given for use only in African Americans.[27,28]

This study and its approach of using the participant's own categorization of his or her ethnicity in studies of race-based therapies have been sharply criticized. The sponsor of this trial obtained a patent to use two generic drugs in combination in African Americans. Hence the cost to patients and insurers of this patented combination drug, BiDil, is far greater than if the component drugs were sold as in generic formulations.[27] A more profound issue is the use of race as a proxy for the specific genetic variations, which have not yet been discovered, responsible for different responses to the drug being studied.[10] More generally, testing for specific genetic polymorphisms would be a more reliable guide to therapeutic decisions for individual patients than is the use of race. These polymorphism markers are likely to be present in many but not all African Americans, and they will also be present in some persons who self-identify as Caucasian rather than as African American. Hence using racial categories to determine who should be prescribed a drug can lead to two errors: prescribing the drug to some patients who will not benefit, and not prescribing it to other patients who will benefit. However, the patent system offers the manufacturer of BiDil little incentive to carry out research to identify the specific genetic variations that cause patients to respond to the drug.

The BiDil example illustrates controversies over the use of racial and ethnic categories in clinical research. Some critics argue that ethnic and racial categories are outmoded in the genomics era and should no longer be used in research, because race and ethnicity are too imprecise to guide clinical decision making for individual patients.[29] Most genomic variation occurs within populations rather than across populations. A population may have a higher or lower probability of being at risk for a condition or of having a successful response to therapy; however, for an individual, the likelihood of being at risk or responding to therapy by virtue of being a member of the population is not sufficient to guide clinical decisions. Further testing or trials of therapies are generally needed to guide individual care. According to this line of reasoning, testing of individuals for specific alleles associated with disease susceptibility or response to therapy may be a better approach to genomics research and medical care than self-identified ethnic and racial categories. Such individualized testing will be increasingly possible as genomic variations and their effects on disease and treatment are better understood and as microarrays for DNA testing become feasible. Moreover, the continued use of race in scientific publications reinforces the mistaken idea that race is a valid scientific category. In reality, its meaning is contested and overlaid with social and cultural values. Critics warn that race-based genomics research will be used or misused to reinforce existing racial stereotypes.

Others argue that racial and ethnic categories are useful in genomics research and clinical care.[30] For certain conditions, genetic variability accounts for medically important differences in disease frequency and outcome among racial and ethnic groups. In addition, some clinically important alleles occur almost exclusively in certain ethnic populations. Pharmacogenomics may be a fruitful area in which genetic variation is particularly likely to have clinically meaningful implications. Hence these scholars advocate using race and ethnicity as starting points for further research.

Special Considerations in Research With Minority Populations

The analytical framework of the Belmont Report—its focus on the assessment of the risks and potential benefits of research, respect for persons, and justice—provides a useful way to think about how minority populations raise special issues regarding research ethics.

Risks and Potential Benefits of Research

The risks of research participation may be greater for minority populations than for the general population. For example, in those minority populations that live within a small and tightly knit community, the participation of individuals in studies may not remain confidential. Mere participation in a research project may be stigmatizing; for example, others might infer that the participant has the condition under study. Thus, in a study of familial breast or colon cancer in an Ashkenazi Jewish community, some may conclude that an individual who participates in the study has a family history of cancer or is particularly susceptible to cancer.

Furthermore, even if individual confidentiality is maintained, the group as a whole may suffer psychosocial harms. A group that is perceived as vulnerable to disease may be viewed by others as inferior, or may cause individuals to suffer loss of self-esteem and self-image.[16] From an ethical perspective, such harms would be particularly troubling if they occurred in groups that were already disadvantaged because of racial discrimination or because of co-existing low socioeconomic status.

Native American populations have raised specific concerns about group harms.[31–33] Some tribes are concerned that findings from genetic research may undermine their beliefs about creation and tribal origins, the cultural history of their people, or their definition of membership within a group. Thus, some Native Americans oppose research that may result in these kinds of harms to the community, even though confidentiality of individual participants is maintained. Research may also violate cultural norms of some tribes. For example, some tribes have taboos against the handling of body specimens by persons of the opposite gender or against disclosing a name and location of a particular community to

outsiders, even in a research publication. But these problems, once identified, can be addressed by changes in the research protocol; for example, only the general geographical location, rather than the name of the community, need be mentioned in publications.

Some writers have rejected such intangible group risks as speculative or unimportant.[25] However, from the point of view of the ethnic or minority group, these harms may be considered serious because they disrupt long-standing traditions and core beliefs of the group. Generally, the perspective of the person who would suffer the harm should guide the protocol; in research trials, it is the participant's evaluation of the degree of risk, not the researcher's, that is determinative. Moreover, all risks are matters of probability and thus in some sense speculative rather than certain. Even a small risk of a very serious harm deserves attention.

The risks of research participation may also be different in kind, not just in magnitude, for minority populations. If there is a history of perceived exploitation, groups may be skeptical that the prospective benefits of research will actually occur. They may fear that minority and ethnic groups will disproportionately bear the risks of research but not gain from the fruits of that research.[4] For example, members of an economically disadvantaged group may doubt that they will have access to new treatments developed from the research. In the case of genomics research with blood samples, they may believe that their participation in research will primarily benefit drug and biotech companies, which will reap profits from their biological materials and information. In addition, Native American and other groups may object to patenting natural materials, which may be perceived as tribal property or as beyond the control of human beings.[33]

Respect for Persons

Research with minority and ethnic populations that have a distinctive culture may also raise special concerns about respect for persons and about the informed consent process. When U.S. researchers carry out studies in other countries, it is not sufficient to simply translate consent forms into the language used in the community. In the culture of the community, the biomedical model of health and illness may not be accepted.[8] For example, some hold the view that disease is caused by spirits or by an individual's failure to observe prescribed rituals. In this case, it would be difficult to articulate the rationale for research to potential participants. It may also be a challenge to reconcile the concepts of genomics with the community's cultural views of ancestry and family. Furthermore, if the authority of healers typically is not questioned, it may be difficult for potential research participants to accept that healers do not know the best course of treatment, which is an ethical prerequisite for a randomized clinical trial. Moreover, in cultures in which the patients do not give consent for therapy, the idea of explaining what the research involves and asking for consent may seem bizarre. Furthermore, key concepts in clinical trials, such as blinding and randomization, are difficult to explain to highly educated persons, let alone to individuals with low health literacy. Investigators have found that community groups and representatives often can suggest how to explain these concepts to participants in the particular study in a clear and comprehensible manner.[4,34]

The concept of individual informed consent may also be alien to a community's culture.[8] Participants may feel obligated to consult with others, rather than making independent decisions about participating in research. In some cultures, individuals regard themselves primarily as members of a family, community, or culture, in contrast to the view that individuals mold their own autonomous identities. Thus, asking participants to give individual consent effectively asks them to disregard their primary affiliation and sense of self. In such cultures, it may be important to give participants the option of consulting with others about the decision to participate in research.

When participants consult with others about their participation, researchers need to distinguish two situations regarding consent. First, an individual may not want to participate in research, but someone else in a controlling social role—such as a husband, father, or group leader—may want them to participate. This situation is often gender-specific; women in some cultures traditionally defer to their husbands, fathers, or group elders. The individual herself may decide to consult with others and believe that she cannot contravene their wishes, but ultimately the individual must be permitted to refuse to participate in research. That is, others in the community may not give permission to enroll her in the study over her objections. Researchers must observe the ethical guideline of respect for individual autonomy.[8] It would be desirable for researchers to devise a consent process that would provide the refusing individual some protection against reprisal. For example, in a study of home-based HIV counseling and testing in sub-Saharan Africa, researchers were careful to have the home interview take the same amount of time, whether or not the prospective subjects agreed to testing.

Second, an individual may want to participate in research although group leaders object to the project. Group leaders or advocacy groups may not have legal veto power unless they have political authority. However, it may not be feasible for researchers to pursue the project in the face of widespread and determined opposition. HIV prevention trials of preexposure prophylaxis with the drug tenofovir were halted in Cambodia and in several sub-Saharan African countries because of strong opposition from advocacy groups.[35] Similarly, an individual may want to participate but her spouse may object. Researchers need to ascertain that the participant understands the psychosocial risks she may face in this situation. Researchers should also take steps in the protocol to minimize those risks, for example, by implementing additional measures to protect confidentiality. However, researchers should allow informed persons to enroll themselves in the study.

Justice

Justice is pertinent to research with minority and ethnic populations in several senses. First, the selection of research participants should be equitable. On the one hand, recruitment targeted to specific ethnic/minority groups requires justification. Mere convenience or access to subjects is not an adequate rationale for targeting minority and ethnic communities. An increased burden of disease or a heightened importance of the research topic for the group is a necessary condition, but not a sufficient one. Beyond the burden of disease, it must be plausible that the research will lead to benefits for the group itself, as opposed to benefits that accrue primarily to others or throughout the population as a whole. Minority and ethnic populations may also have concurrent conditions that make them vulnerable as research subjects, such as low literacy, poor education, poverty, low social status, and so

forth. On the other hand, including minority and ethnic groups in research is essential to obtain reliable evidence on which to base clinical care. When minority and ethnic communities are disproportionately likely to suffer from a disease, they need to be included in research so that scientists can learn how to provide them with better care. Researchers will need to devise outreach, recruitment, and educational procedures that overcome barriers to the participation of minority and ethnic communities and individuals in clinical research. Community and advocacy groups can be invaluable in planning such activities.[4]

Second, justice as reciprocity requires researchers and sponsors of research to give participating individuals and communities their due. Researchers need to address concerns that minority and ethnic communities may raise about the history of exploitative research projects. To be sure, researchers cannot predict what they will find, nor can they be responsible for how others use their findings. However, the process of conducting research in minority and ethnic communities can address these concerns. The project can try to hire members of the community as research staff and provide them opportunities for training and advancement. Moreover, in conjunction with the project, researchers can carry out community service, such as outreach, educational initiatives, and screening programs. Finally, ethnic or minority communities that are economically disadvantaged may not be able to afford drugs that are proven effective in clinical trials. Although the issue of access has been raised primarily in terms of access to HIV drugs that are studied in resource-poor countries, it is an issue in all countries, including the United States.[6,36] Researchers should take reasonable steps to help the groups that participate in clinical trials obtain access to the intervention after the trial.[8]

Recommendations for Research With Minority and Ethnic Populations

Community Involvement in Research

The primary goals of community involvement in research are to show respect for the community, to identify and minimize risks to participants and to the community, and to strengthen informed consent.[4] Community involvement can also benefit researchers, for example, by enhancing the enrollment in studies. Alternatively, strong opposition from respected community leaders may make a research study impractical to carry out.

A community may be involved in research in a variety of ways.[4,37] On the most basic level, researchers should provide information about the topic and purpose of research and the specific project to the communities targeted for participation. Furthermore, after the study is completed, researchers should communicate their findings to the community. These activities should be required of all research, and especially that which targets ethnic and minority populations.

On the next level, researchers can discuss the study design and protocol with community representatives, who can give feedback on the risks and burdens of research in the particular setting, ways to minimize those risks, and ways to enhance informed consent. This interaction is most appropriate when an ongoing series of research projects is envisaged. A similar process commonly occurs with disease-specific research where researchers have learned to work with advocacy groups, such as those who advocate for research on HIV, breast cancer, and rare genetic conditions. Such interactions provide benefits to researchers as well as project participants and the community. The discussions often strengthen the protocol scientifically by focusing on the research questions that will make a difference in clinical decision making, and by balancing the potential benefits and risks more favorably. Suggestions for changes in the protocol from community members often enhance recruitment and follow-up. Community support may also help researchers obtain funding and recruit subjects.[4]

Problems may arise from the range of views within a community. There may be a disconnect between the views of community leaders and those who are affected with the condition under study or who are providing services to them. In addition, there is the potential for co-option if researchers pick community representatives who are likely to agree with them. These problems are not specific to this situation but also occur with any process of selecting community members, as in the selection of lay and community members for institutional review boards (IRBs), as required under the Common Rule. Difficulties and potential pitfalls in implementing a policy in good faith should not be viewed as a justification for rejecting the policy completely.

Even greater involvement occurs in community-based participatory research using community-based organizations. Studies of cancer screening and prevention have been organized among African Americans through churches, which are important and respected institutions in those communities.[38] Researchers have involved church leaders and members in the design of research and writing of grant applications, as well as in recruitment. This kind of involvement often necessitates changes in protocol. One such study involved a nutritional intervention. Although a usual-care control group was originally planned, researchers decided to give the control group a delayed intervention in response to community objections. At a follow-up visit, researchers found that over 90% of individuals in the intervention group and over 85% of those in the control group expressed high levels of support for the research project.[38] The researchers ascribed the high levels of trust, satisfaction, and perceived personal benefit to active community participation in the design of the study.

The highest level of community involvement is formal approval from the community. Some ethnic or minority communities have authorized political leadership, are localized geographically, or have clear rules for group membership. Native American tribes, for example, are like sovereign nations. In this situation, formal approval from the tribal government may be required to carry out research. Community involvement is more controversial and more complex, however, if the community has no political authority, is geographically dispersed, and has cultural heterogeneity and ambiguous criteria for group membership.[37] In the latter situation, it is difficult to determine who has legitimacy to speak on the community's behalf. In the absence of such formal authority, critics object to a requirement for community consultation and to allowing a community to have veto power over individual members' decisions to participate in research.[24,39,40]

Several practical issues regarding community involvement need to be addressed. Researchers have considerable latitude in determining who speaks for a community. They should not choose community representatives based on the likelihood that the representatives will agree with researchers and approve the projects. Rather, researchers should appreciate the need to elicit different perspectives and moreover should be sensitive to patterns of social interaction that may make it difficult for individuals to speak up in a public forum. Communities may have customs about deferring to elders or to persons in certain social roles. Thus, individuals who have conflicting points of view may not speak up in a meeting when first asked to do so.[41]

Heightened Review by IRBs and Funding Agencies

Recruitment targeted to specific ethnic/minority groups should trigger special IRB review because of the possibility that the protocol represents research with a vulnerable population. The targeting may be intentional or may result from a recruitment strategy that appears, but is not, neutral regarding recruitment of ethnic and minority groups. Some questions that the IRB should ask are the following:

- Is the targeting of these groups as research participants justified?
- Are these groups at particular risk in this study?
- Are there special informed consent issues in these groups regarding the study?
- Are there additional issues that are salient in the ethnic or minority group? For example, a study to collect and store samples for DNA testing and use in future research studies in an African American population would need to address issues of trust in research and researchers.[4]

Federal regulations require IRBs to take into account local considerations in assessing risks and potential benefits and approving consent procedures. However, IRBs may not have sufficient expertise among their members regarding the perspectives of ethnic and minority groups. Thus IRBs may need to add ad hoc reviewers who are from the communities being studied.[4] For example, someone both fluent in the language and knowledgeable about the culture must review recruitment advertisements and consent forms in a foreign language. This additional review would be similar to ad hoc scientific reviewers with particular technical expertise, or reviewers from a disease advocacy group for a rare condition with which an IRB is not familiar.

Peer review by funding agencies should also include reviewers who are knowledgeable about conducting the particular type of research in the targeted populations.[41] Such review would help assure that the proposed project is feasible and is likely to have an ultimate impact on clinical care.

Responsibilities of Researchers

Researchers who carry out research with minority and ethnic communities have special obligations to vulnerable populations to assure that the balance of risks and potential benefits in the study is acceptable. One reason is that communities may fear that such research might be misinterpreted or misused in ways that adversely impact the groups. Moreover, such communities may believe that in the past, their participation in research has not led to improvements in their health or social conditions; that is, they have not derived any long-term benefits from participating in research.[4] Furthermore, because of the suspicion that some minority and ethnic communities have about research, researchers need to overcome mistrust in order to carry out the study. Researchers can fulfill these obligations in several ways as we discuss below.

Investigators should involve the affected minority and disadvantaged community in the planning of the research project.[4] Researchers should elicit community concerns about the project and respond to them. Scientists need not make all changes in the study requested by community stakeholders, but they need to listen to the concerns and explain why they do not agree with the requests.[4] This process shows respect for community members and groups and helps to build trust.

As previously discussed, researchers should provide community education about the project and the topic of research. In addition, researchers ought to make some effort to use their expertise for the well-being of the subjects and communities. This can involve providing scientific information to help communities pursue changes in public policy and helping community groups write grant applications to obtain funding for needed social services.[4]

Researchers need to use due care in presenting and publishing their findings, particularly in light of the history of misinterpretations and abuses of research with ethnic and minority communities. Researchers need to point out the limitations of their findings, making clear that their results apply only to the condition and population that they studied. They should distinguish their empirical findings from hypotheses for future research, implications for theories and models, and policy recommendations.

Researchers also should take some responsibility for helping to disseminate their study findings in the lay media. Scientists are sometimes reluctant to give media interviews about their work, believing that peer-reviewed publications speak for themselves. However, by helping to write press releases and by providing reporters with clear explanations of their work in lay terms, scientists can increase the likelihood of accurate coverage in the press. Scientists also have some responsibility to speak out when others misinterpret their data in ways are likely to harm the community or participants in the study. Although researchers cannot be responsible for the social and political uses to which findings are put, they are responsible for using their expertise and authority to try to correct misunderstandings and distortions of their work. This responsibility may involve giving interviews to the press and testifying before government committees. Although all researchers have such responsibilities, they are particularly important in the context of long-standing health disparities that in part result from widespread public misunderstanding, unfounded group stereotypes, and bias and stereotyping by health-care professionals.

Conclusion

In summary, ethnic and minority communities may mistrust researchers because of a history of unfavorable experiences with research projects. However, there may be cogent reasons to target such communities for research and research may also benefit these communities. Researchers must be sensitive to the particular ethical issues that arise in research with such communities and must take steps to ensure that their projects meet high ethical standards.

References

1. Freimuth VS, et al. African Americans' views on research and the Tuskegee Syphilis Study. *Social Science and Medicine* 2001;52:797–808.

2. Corbie-Smith G, et al. Attitudes and beliefs of African Americans toward participation in medical research. *Journal of General Internal Medicine* 1999;14:537–46.

3. Corbie-Smith G, Thomas SB, St. George DM. Distrust, race, and research. *Archives of Internal Medicine* 2002;162:2458–63.

4. Lo B, O'Connell ME, eds. *Ethical Considerations for Research on Housing-Related Health Hazards Involving Children*. Washington, D.C.: National Academy Press; 2005.

5. Kevles DJ. *In the Name of Eugenics: Genetics and the Uses of Human Heredity*. New York, N.Y.: Alfred A. Knopf, 1985.

6. Committee on Understanding and Eliminating Racial and Ethnic Disparities in Health Care. *Unequal Treatment: Confronting Racial and Ethnic Disparities in Health Care*. Washington, D.C.: National Academies Press; 2003.

7. Wendler D, Emanuel E. A framework for assessing the ethics of housing research with children. Paper commissioned by the Committee on Ethical Issues in Housing-Related Health Hazards Research in Children, Youth and Families, National Academy of Sciences, 2004.

8. National Bioethics Advisory Commission. *Ethical and Policy Issues in International Research: Clinical Trials in Developing Countries, Vol. I.* Bethesda, Md.: NBAC; 2001. [Online] 2001. Available: http://www.georgetown.edu/research/nrcbl/nbac/clinical/Vol1.pdf.

9. Taylor AL, et al. Combination of isosorbide dinitrate and hydralazine in blacks with heart failure. *New England Journal of Medicine* 2004; 351:2049–57.

10. Bloche MG. Race-based therapeutics. *New England Journal of Medicine* 2004;351:2035–7.

11. Barr DA. The practitioner's dilemma: Can we use a patient's race to predict genetics, ancestry, and the expected outcomes of treatment? *Annals of Internal Medicine* 2005;143:809–15.

12. Freedman LS, et al. Inclusion of women and minorities in clinical trials and the NIH Revitalization Act of 1993—the perspective of NIH clinical trialists. *Controlled Clinical Trials* 1995;16:277–85; discussion: 286–9, 293–309.

13. Wendler D, et al. Are racial and ethnic minorities less willing to participate in health research? *PLoS Medicine* 2005;3(2):e19.

14. Bach G, Tomczak J, Risch N, Ekstein J. Tay-Sachs screening in the Jewish Ashkenazi Population: DNA testing is the preferred procedure. *American Journal of Medical Genetics* 2001;99:70–5.

15. Lehmann LS, Weeks JC, Klar N, Garber JE. A population-based study of Ashkenazi Jewish women's attitudes toward genetic discrimination and BRCA1/2 testing. *Genetics in Medicine* 2002;4:346–52.

16. Nelson NJ. Ashkenazi community is not unwilling to participate in genetic research. *Journal of the National Cancer Institute* 1998;90:884–5.

17. Morton DH, et al. Pediatric medicine and the genetic disorders of the Amish and Mennonite people of Pennsylvania. *American Journal of Medical Genetics* 2003;121C:5–17.

18. Puffenberger EG. Genetic heritage of the Old Order Mennonites of southeastern Pennsylvania *American Journal of Medical Genetics* 2003;121C:18–31.

19. Belkin L. A doctor for the future. *New York Times Magazine* November 6, 2005.

20. Grady D. At gene therapy's frontier, the Amish build a clinic. *New York Times* June 29, 1999; Sec. F1.

21. Greely HT. Human genome diversity: What about the other human genome project? *Nature Reviews Genetics* 2001;2:222–7.

22. Human Genome Diversity Committee of HUGO. Summary Document (incorporating the HGD Project outline and development, proposed guidelines, and report of the International Planning Workshop held in Porto Conte, Sardinia, Italy. September 9–12, 1993. [Online] Available: http://www.stanford.edu/group/morrinst/hgdp/summary93.html.

23. North American Regional Committee of the Human Genome Diversity Project. Proposed model ethical protocol for collecting DNA samples. *Houston Law Review* 1997;33:1431–73.

24. Juengst ET. Groups as gatekeepers to genomic research: Conceptually confusing, morally hazardous, and practically useless. *Kennedy Institute of Ethics Journal* 1998;8:183–200.

25. Reilly PR. Rethinking risks to human subjects in genetic research. *American Journal of Human Genetics* 1998;63:682–5.

26. Committee on Human Genome Diversity, Commission on Life Sciences, National Research Council. *Evaluating Human Genetic Diversity.* Washington, D.C.: National Academy Press; 1997.

27. Sankar P, Kahn J. BiDil: Race medicine or race marketing? *Health Affairs* 2005;Oct.11:W5– 455–63 (web exclusive).

28. Carlson RJ. The case of BiDil: A policy commentary on race and genetics. *Health Affairs* 2005;Oct.11: W5– 464–8 (web exclusive).

29. Cooper R, Kaufman J, Ward R. Race and genomics. *New England Journal of Medicine* 2003;348:1166–70.

30. Burchard E, et al. The importance of race and ethnic background in biomedical research and clinical practice. *New England Journal of Medicine* 2003;348:1170–5.

31. Foster MW, Freeman WL. Naming names in human genetic variation research. *Genome Research* 1998;8:755–7.

32. Foster MW, et al. The role of community review in evaluating the risks of human genetic variation research. *American Journal of Human Genetics* 1999;64:1719–27.

33. Dalton R. When two tribes go to war. *Nature* 2004;430:500–2.

34. Woodsong C, Karim QA. A model designed to enhance informed consent: experiences from the HIV prevention trials network. *American Journal of Public Health* 2005;95:412–9.

35. The editors. The trials of tenofovir trials [editorial]. *Lancet* 2005;365:1111.

36. Curran J, Debas H, Arya M, Kelley P, Knobler S, Pray L, eds. *Scaling Up Treatment for the Global AIDS Pandemic.* Washington, D.C.: National Academies Press; 2005.

37. Weijer C, Emanuel EJ. Protecting communities in biomedical research. *Science* 2000;289:1142– 4.

38. Corbie-Smith G, et al. Trust, benefit, satisfaction, and burden: A randomized controlled trial to reduce cancer risk through African-American churches. *Journal of General Internal Medicine* 2003; 18:531– 41.

39. Juengst ET. What "community review" can and cannot do. *Journal of Law, Medicine and Ethics* 2000;28:52– 4, 3.

40. Reilly PR. Public concern about genetics. *Annual Review of Genomics and Human Genetics* 2000;1:485–506.

41. Lo B, Bayer R. Establishing ethical trials for treatment and prevention of AIDS in developing countries. *British Medical Journal* 2003;327:337–9.

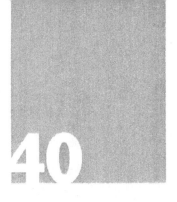

Carol Levine

Research Involving Economically Disadvantaged Participants

A hypothetical institutional review board (IRB) meets to discuss three hypothetical protocols. In the first, investigators propose to study the effectiveness of a new antianxiety drug that has been shown to be safe in Phase I trials. Participants will be eligible if they demonstrate high levels of stress on a validated screening instrument, are not currently taking another antianxiety drug, and have no significant medical problems. The procedures include several blood draws, physical exams, and hour-long interviews over the course of six months. The participants will be paid $500 on completion of the study. The IRB approves the study with only a few minor changes to the consent form.

The second protocol involves a comparison of a long-lasting formulation of an antihypertensive drug and the standard shorter-lasting version to see if the new version improves adherence. The participants are already taking the standard formulation and there are no additional risks. They will be paid $25 each visit for a blood pressure check and other basic tests. The IRB has many questions about the protocol and with some reluctance approves it.

In the third protocol investigators are studying a new and expensive drug for vascular complications of diabetes. No payment will be offered to participants. There are some known risks as well as unforeseeable ones. The IRB decides that the risk-benefit ratio is acceptable and that the consent form is clear and accurate. Yet it sends the protocol back to the investigator for further revisions.

What accounts for this hypothetical IRB's seemingly inconsistent decisions? Economic disadvantage played a different role in each protocol. In the first, the antianxiety drug for highly stressed people, the participants were medical students. Their low income and burgeoning debt were not seen as problems in obtaining consent, nor was $500 seen as an "undue inducement." In the second protocol, a study of an antihypertensive drug, most of the participants would be unemployed drug users recruited from a public hospital clinic. Some IRB members worried that the payment, modest though it was, would be spent on alcohol or drugs. Investigators in the third protocol, studying the expensive diabetes medication, planned to recruit participants from private physicians' offices. In this case the IRB felt that this plan did not provide for equitable selection of participants, especially because it would not reach many men and women with diabetes who come from poor, ethnic minority communities.

Poverty Matters, but How Much and In What Ways?

What does *economically disadvantaged* mean in the context of the ethics of clinical research? From the relatively sparse literature, one can conclude that there is a consensus that poverty matters. However, it is not as clear to what extent economic disadvantage is a significant factor to be weighed on its own or is rather an indicator of other factors such as low educational level or language barriers, which might impede full understanding and voluntariness. In the United States, where poor people often have limited access to health care because they lack insurance, there is a particular concern that uninsured people will be induced to enter research studies to obtain basic health care.[1] Internationally, the concern goes beyond the potential for exploitation of poor people as individuals or as members of minority groups to include entire populations in resource-poor countries and regions.[2-4]

On the other hand, some advocates who speak for economically disadvantaged groups in the United States are concerned that poor people are being deprived of the opportunities to benefit from clinical trial participation and that information gathered from other groups will not be applicable to them. For example, Stephen Sodeke, interim director of Tuskegee University's National Center for Bioethics in Research and Health Care, acknowledges that historical abuses have led to mistrust of the health-care system among African Americans and other economically disadvantaged populations. Yet, he believes, "We have a responsibility to assist the community to understand why research is done and how it can help individual members of the community. . . . The only way to get the best information is to involve more of the various populations of people that make up a community in the research process. This means we must involve them as research subjects in clinical trials as well as in community groups and as community representatives."[5]

Economic disadvantage has come to be seen as a marker of *vulnerability*, a signal that an IRB needs to take special care in the selection of research participants and in the approval of the protocol. It is helpful to review how this linkage came about, and how it has been interpreted.

Vulnerability and Economic Disadvantage in Clinical Research

A fundamental assumption underlies the modern history of research ethics: Certain categories of people are more likely than others to be misled, mistreated, or otherwise taken advantage of as participants in clinical research. These populations are deemed *vulnerable*, a status that imposes a duty on researchers, review committees, and regulators to provide special protections for them. Although other basic tenets of research ethics—informed consent and risk-benefit analysis, for example—have been the subject of extensive discussion and debate, until recently the concept of vulnerability has been relatively unexamined. The only significant questions raised have been whether or not to include a particular group in the vulnerability category, and to a lesser degree, what kinds of protections are needed.

Vulnerability is typically explained in terms of examples, rather than being explicitly defined. Although used freely in the *IRB Guidebook* produced by the U.S. Department of Health and Human Services' Office for Human Research Protections, vulnerability is not defined in the Guidebook's extensive glossary.[6] However, other "special classes of subjects" are highlighted for special consideration. These include cognitively impaired persons; traumatized and comatose patients; terminally ill patients; elderly/aged persons; minorities; students, employees, and normal volunteers; and participants in international research.

The U.S. federal regulations (45 CFR 46) provide special protections for what they call "particularly vulnerable populations": children; prisoners; pregnant women, fetuses, and neonates.[7] "Economically disadvantaged" persons as such are not included in these designated categories, although they are listed in the regulations as "vulnerable" (CFR 46.111(a)(3)).[7] They are "vulnerable" but not "particularly vulnerable," whatever that distinction may mean in practice. In what would be a broad expansion of the regulations, Howard Stone suggests that economically and educationally disadvantaged people—the "invisible vulnerable"—

should be given additional protections under a new subpart of the U.S. regulations. These protections, he says, should limit their participation to studies that present minimal risk to participants or to research that holds out the potential of directly benefiting the individual participants.[8]

In the international arena, the most recent revision of the World Medical Association's Declaration of Helsinki simply states, "Some research populations are vulnerable and need special protection" (see Chapter 13). The Declaration advises that the "particular needs of the economically and medically disadvantaged must be recognized. Special attention is also required for those who cannot give or refuse consent for themselves, for those who may be subject to giving consent under duress, for those who will not benefit personally from the research and for those for whom the research is combined with care."[9] Inclusion of this latter group suggests to me a similar concern as in the United States: Poor people will agree to participate in research in order to obtain basic care.

With an even more specific list, the 2002 guidelines of the Council for International Organizations of Medical Sciences (CIOMS) include as vulnerable "junior or subordinate members of a hierarchical group," such as "medical and nursing students, subordinate hospital and laboratory personnel, employees of pharmaceutical companies, and members of the armed forces or police"[10] (see Chapter 16). Furthermore, the guidelines describe elderly people as "likely to acquire attributes that define them as vulnerable." The commentary on Guideline 13 also includes other categories such as "residents of nursing homes, people receiving welfare benefits or social assistance and other poor people and the unemployed, people in emergency rooms, some ethnic and racial minority groups, homeless persons, nomads, refugees or displaced persons, prisoners, patients with incurable disease, individuals who are politically powerless, and members of communities unfamiliar with modern medical concepts."[10] Some of these groups are by definition poor; others are probably also in that category.

The concept of vulnerability that has become so firmly fixed in the ethics vocabulary was established in the 1979 Belmont Report, a product of the U.S. National Commission for the Protection of Human Subjects of Biomedical and Behavioral Research, which formed the basis for the U.S. regulations[11] (see Chapters 14 and 15). The Belmont Report addressed vulnerability in the context of the principle of justice as applied to the selection of research participants. Vulnerable groups, the report stated, should not bear unequal burdens in research. The report explained that its examples of vulnerable populations—"racial minorities, the economically disadvantaged, the very sick, and the institutionalized"—may continually be sought as research participants because of their "ready availability in settings where research is conducted." These groups require special protections because of their "dependent status and frequently compromised capacity for free consent."[11]

Concern about "economic disadvantage" creating vulnerability is thus directly tied to the venerable Belmont Report, although it was never codified in regulation. However, the Belmont Report, written at a time when most research was conducted in clinics or academic medical centers, focused on the "ready availability" of poor people in these settings and their "dependent status." It did not anticipate the situation today: A much broader sponsorship and dispersion of research, as well as a strong belief (primarily but not exclusively among the economically well-off) that research participation is not a burden but rather that it offers benefits such as early access to promising investigational drugs and additional monitoring. In the early years of the HIV/AIDS epidemic, early access to promising drugs was not just a slogan but a war cry. Those who led the charge were primarily gay, white, middle- and upper-class men and their advocates. They accelerated the pendulum swing in research ethics from protection to inclusion.[12]

From the available data it appears that economically disadvantaged people are not overrepresented in U.S. clinical trials today, although they undoubtedly were in the 1970s, when the National Commission wrote the Belmont Report. A few studies do show that people without health insurance enter trials when free medical care is an incentive.[13] However, this does not seem to be typical. Because many trials at best pay only for the care associated with the research itself, besides providing the study drug, the participant's health insurance, the institution, or the participant must directly pay for much of the additional care.[1] (Consent forms are supposed to point this out.) Studies that require high investments from participants arguably discriminate against those without resources. On the whole, those who are male, white, insured, middle-class, and well-educated are more likely to participate in research studies than are women and men from lower socioeconomic groups. Wendy Rogers points out that as a result of the general observation that people in trials fare better than those outside of them, "lack of participation in trials effectively removes this benefit from disadvantaged groups." More important, however, is the paucity of research evidence about which interventions are effective in these groups.[14]

The concept's prominence in the Belmont Report and its staying power in clinical research ethics undoubtedly derive from post–World War II history. Revulsion against the abuses of research on captive populations in World War II by the Nazis (and, as later revealed, by the Japanese as well) profoundly affected the development of international codes of research ethics.[15] However, the impetus for the creation of the National Commission for the Protection of Human Subjects of Biomedical and Behavioral Research in 1974 was a series of domestic scandals, first revealed by Henry Beecher in his 1966 *New England Journal of Medicine* article.[16] These scandals included the Jewish Chronic Disease Hospital study, in which elderly patients were injected with live cancer cells without their consent, and the Willowbrook hepatitis vaccine studies, in which some institutionalized children were accepted as patients only if their parents consented to the studies. The U.S. Public Health Service syphilis studies of poor black men in Tuskegee, Alabama, which had numerous ethical violations, played a major role in supporting a regulatory climate in which protection was paramount[17] (see Chapters 6–8). Research came to be seen as a risky enterprise, from which institutionalized or cognitively impaired individuals in particular needed protections that they were not able to provide for themselves.

Although the early guideline and regulation drafters were reacting to a series of specific historical events, the more recent history of vulnerability in biomedical research seems based more on general concerns about political, economic, and social inequality. Here economic disadvantage comes much more to the fore. In the international context, the 2002 CIOMS guidelines for biomedical research define, if not vulnerability, then at least vulnerable persons: "those who are relatively or (absolutely) incapable of protecting their own interests" because they may have "insufficient power, intelligence, education, resources, strength,

or other needed attributes."[10] Commenting on an earlier draft of the CIOMS guidelines from 2000, Deborah Zion and her colleagues define vulnerable people in political terms: "those who lack basic rights and liberties that make them particularly open to exploitation."[18]

Beyond individuals or groups, Ruth Macklin suggests that whole communities or countries may be vulnerable to exploitation, particularly if "investigators or sponsors are from a powerful industrialized country or a giant pharmaceutical company and the research is conducted in a developing country."[2] A Pakistani researcher points to widespread poverty in South Asia as one potential cause of tension between the aims of the researchers and the needs of the community; the others are illiteracy, male dominance, a hierarchical society, lack of health care, and corruption.[19]

In arguing against double standards in research in multinational studies—permitting research in destitute countries that would not be approved in wealthy ones—Michael Kottow distinguishes between vulnerability and susceptibility. Vulnerability, he says, applies to everyone; what really matters in research ethics is susceptibility, which means being poor, undernourished, and lacking in medical care and therefore predisposed to additional harm.[3]

These definitions and comments reflect concerns that poor people in developing countries will be used, as they have been in the past, to test drugs that are destined for developed country markets, without compensating benefit to the participants or their communities in terms of improved access to health care. International research protocols, on this view, should be evaluated not just with regard to the impact on the individuals who enroll but also on the health-care needs and power imbalances in the country. Research thus becomes not just a scientific effort, but a tool for social and economic reforms as well.

Social Science Research and Economic Disadvantage

It is instructive to look at social science research, which also addresses economic disadvantage in the selection of research participants, because economic disadvantage plays an even more significant role in many of these studies. Although there does not seem to be a single definition of vulnerability in social science research, there is some overlap with definitions in biomedical research. The characteristics of a vulnerable population in social science research are typically described in terms of a group's social status, powerlessness, and potential for exploitation. Social status and powerlessness are also described as sources of vulnerability by the CIOMS guidelines for biomedical research. Similarly, Jacquelyn Flaskerud and Betty Winslow define vulnerable populations in health services research as "social groups who experience limited resources and consequent high relative risk of morbidity and premature mortality."[20] Among the groups "recognized as vulnerable" are "the poor; persons subject to discrimination, intolerance, subordination and stigma; and those who are politically marginalized, disenfranchised, and denied human rights."[20]

Recognizing both the individual and social aspects of vulnerability, Robert Chambers notes that "vulnerability has two sides: an external side of risks, shocks and stress to which an individual or household is subject; and an individual side which is defenselessness, meaning a lack of means to cope without damaging loss."[21] Martin Watts and Hans-Georg Bolhe offer three coordinates of vulnerability: "The risk of being exposed to crisis situations (exposure), the risk of not having the necessary resources to cope with these situations (capacity), and the risk of being subjected to serious consequences as a result of the crises (potentiality)."[22]

In reviewing the ethical implications of vulnerability for participants in research conducted by the Substance Abuse and Mental Health Services Administration (SAMHSA), Thomas McGovern claims, "Vulnerability is a universal and ongoing human experience. The awareness of being wounded and the potential for same gnaws at our sense of security. We are capable of being hurt at many levels: physical, mental, emotional, and spiritual. . . . Our greatest vulnerability centers on assaults from within and without that threaten our integrity and dignity as persons."[23] In bioethics terminology, vulnerability in this sense involves not just the risk of being harmed physically, socially, or psychologically but also the risk of being wronged—of being treated in ways that assault one's dignity or one's personhood. Poor people may or may not be at heightened risk of harm in particular protocols; but given the unjust conditions in which they live and are treated in society, they are surely at heightened risk of being wronged.

The mental health literature often links vulnerability with its opposite or antidote—resiliency. In 1996, the Basic Behavioral Science Task Force of the U.S. National Advisory Mental Health Council posed the question, "Why do some people collapse under life stresses while others seem unscathed by traumatic circumstances, such as severe illness, the death of loved ones, and extreme poverty, or even by major catastrophes such as natural disasters and war?"[24] In seeking to answer this question, the Task Force developed, if not a definition, a good description of vulnerability: "Studies to date suggest that there is no single source of resilience or vulnerability. Rather, many interacting factors come into play. They include not only individual genetic predispositions, which express themselves in enduring aspects of temperament, personality, and intelligence, but also qualities such as social skills and self-esteem. These, in turn, are shaped by a variety of environmental influences."[24] Taking this holistic view, economic disadvantage can lead to vulnerability, but also to inner strength and resolve.

In brief, then, the concept of vulnerability as it is used in clinical research emphasizes limitations to an individual's or a group's decision-making capacity and the potential for coercion among populations that are literally or figuratively "captive."[25] In social science research, by contrast, *vulnerable* most often describes people who may have decision-making capacity but who lack the power and resources to make truly voluntary choices. Economic disadvantage is but one factor among many to consider.

Economic Disadvantage as a Group Characteristic

As a matter of justice, the concept of vulnerability stereotypes whole categories of individuals without distinguishing between individuals in the group who indeed might have special characteristics that need to be taken into account and those who do not. Particular concerns have been raised about considering all poor people, all pregnant women, all members of ethnic or racial mi-

norities, and all people with terminal illness as inherently unable to know their own best interests and to make appropriate choices for themselves.

Debra DeBruin makes this argument from a philosophical perspective. She claims that "vulnerability ought not to be conceived of as a characteristic of groups. Rather, certain traits may render certain persons vulnerable in certain situations."[26] On this view, putting poor people or poorly educated people in the class of vulnerable participants treats them as less capable of asserting their autonomy than those who are better off. The argument that people with life-threatening illnesses can still make their own health-care and research decisions has been made most forcefully by people with HIV/AIDS, but it is by no means limited to them.

Furthermore, some people may be vulnerable in certain ways or circumstances but not in others. After all, the mythic archetype of the vulnerable person is Achilles, immortal except for that one little spot on his heel that his goddess mother failed to dip in the sacred waters of the River Styx. Just as "decision-making capacity" for health-care decisions is now generally understood to depend on the question being asked and the consequences of the decision, an individual's need for special protections in the research context depends on the kind of study, the implications of participating or not participating, and the alternatives available. An economically disadvantaged person may have become extraordinarily adept at "gaming" the system to obtain medical care and other benefits, whereas a person with far greater resources may be naïve and overly sanguine about the goals of research and the demands of the protocol. Having had to look out for their own interests, poor people may well be more astute at judging whether to enter a particular research protocol than people who have come to believe that the system always works or can be made to work in their favor. Some skepticism about the research enterprise is often a rational response.

Weighing Economic Disadvantage

In their ethical analysis of enrolling uninsured people in clinical trials, Christine Pace and her colleagues weigh the competing issues of susceptibility to undue inducements and the right of the uninsured to "fair consideration for research participation." They conclude that enrolling uninsured research participants "is not inherently exploitative and that, in fact, excluding such participants without scientific reason is unfair." The risks that the participants will lack access to effective treatment after the trial and of undue inducement, they assert, do not justify a categorical exclusion of those without health insurance.[1]

Using an economic model, Laura Dunn and Nora Gordon point out that "rational potential research participants make decisions based on expected costs and benefits of participation."[27] These include the opportunity cost of forgoing another way of spending one's time, transaction costs such as transportation and child care, and potential discomfort of adverse responses. Although most concern about payment has focused on the idea that higher payment will disproportionately encourage poor people to participate, these authors argue that "relatively low compensation levels would do the same because wealthier research participants have higher opportunity costs and value their last dollar earned less than poorer participants."[27] They conclude that trust and perceived fairness, not economic status per se, are central to ethical recruitment.

In considering the weight that ought to be given to economic disadvantage in terms of the protections afforded research participants, several aspects should be considered. For example, what is the purpose of the protocol? If it is a study that is designed to test a drug for a disease that affects the potential participant, or that is prevalent in that person's community, the socioeconomic status of the participants might not be a particular cause for worry. If, on the other hand, it is a physiologic study in which the investigators are looking for normal healthy volunteers, and in which the participants are drawn from a pool of unemployed people who consistently volunteer for the money alone, some more thought about the relevance of socioeconomic status to the selection process is warranted.

As with all studies, the level of risk to which research participants will be subject is another important consideration. As noted earlier, Stone suggests limiting research recruitment among poor people to studies with minimal risk,[8] but this proposal draws the line too narrowly and may deprive individuals of potential benefit and the opportunity to contribute to research of benefit to future patients. Nevertheless, when moderate or significant risk is known or can be anticipated, it is essential that potential participants fully understand and accept the risks. For example, in some cases in which the risks may be unknown or unknowable, some form of "special scrutiny"—a specially-focused review—may be warranted.[28]

In many but not all instances, economic disadvantage is accompanied by lower educational status; in such cases, informed consent processes must be carefully developed and monitored. The setting of the research, including factors such as the availability of transportation and child care, are critical factors that must be considered. Any features of the research setting that might make participants feel that they have limited options to decline, such as in emergency rooms or drug abuse clinics, bear further consideration. Other factors might include whether the participant has a regular physician with whom he or she can discuss the protocol and to whom he or she can be referred for follow-up; whether there is adequate provision for care in case of adverse effects; and what possibilities exist after the research ends for obtaining the study drug if it proves beneficial.

In studies in which it is important for scientific or ethical reasons to increase the participation of economically disadvantaged people, some concrete actions can be taken. Research studies can be discussed in community settings, such as churches and social service agencies, in which community leaders and potential participants can ask questions and raise concerns. Research opportunities can be widely disseminated, so that poor people are not being singled out for enrollment. Subsidies can be built into the funding so that participants do not incur additional financial burdens on account of their participation.

Logistical barriers to participating—lack of child care, transportation, and so on—can be reduced. Flexible plans can be instituted for contacting study participants who may not have telephones or be able to receive calls at work. Using experienced patient-education staff to provide health information as well as information about study requirements may build trust. In a cervical cancer prevention trial, for example, Joanne Bailey and her colleagues found that multiple strategies were needed to recruit and retain economically disadvantaged women. These included "expansion to five geographically distinct clinical sites, the use of nurse practitioners focused primarily on patient issues, extremely

flexible study hours and location, honorariums, support for transportation and child care, and creativity in maintaining contact with study participants."[29] Using these strategies, 90% of eligible patients consented to participate in the study.

In international studies, the rationale for the study and its design should be subjected to particular scrutiny because of the potential for exploitation that is noted in all statements of U.S. and international bodies and individual advocates (see Chapters 64–67). Only when a protocol has been deemed acceptable on these grounds should the methods of recruitment, consent, and other aspects come under consideration. Although in my view it is unrealistic and unfair to hold the research enterprise responsible for reforming the health-care system and repairing underlying inequities in a country, it is nevertheless important to create something of value for the communities from which the participants are drawn.

Conclusion

Economic disadvantage is a deceptively simple criterion on which to make an ethical judgment about the selection of research participants. Poor people can indeed be vulnerable to exploitation and undue inducements; yet to consider them, on the basis of poverty alone, incapable of making decisions about their own best interests, fails to recognize their autonomy and treats them with condescension. Researchers, sponsors, and IRBs have to weigh all the factors in a protocol judiciously, and when economic disadvantage plays an inordinate role, work to minimize its impact.

Acknowledgments

Some of the material in this chapter appeared in Levine C, Faden R, Grady C, Hammerschmidt D, Eckenwiler L, Sugarman J., The limitations of "vulnerability" as a protection for human research subjects, *American Journal of Bioethics* 2004;4(3):44–9, and was derived from discussions in the Consortium to Explore Clinical Research Ethics (CECRE), funded by the Doris Duke Charitable Foundation. The other CECRE members are not responsible for the views expressed here.

References

1. Pace C, Miller FG, Danis M. Enrolling the uninsured in clinical trials: An ethical perspective. *Critical Care Medicine* 2003;31(3 Suppl.): S121–S125.
2. Macklin R. Bioethics, vulnerability, and protection. *Bioethics* 2003;17: 472–86.
3. Kottow MH. The vulnerable and the susceptible. *Bioethics* 2003;17: 460–71.
4. Dickens BM, Cook RJ. Challenges of ethical research in resource-poor settings. *International Journal of Gynaecology and Obstetrics* 2003;80:79–86.
5. Interview with S. Sodeke, Protecting vulnerable populations, 2003. Available at U.S. Department of Energy Protecting Human Subjects website: www.science.doe.gov/ober/humsubj/fal103.pdf.
6. Department of Health and Human Services, Office for Human Research Protections. *Protecting Human Research Subjects: Institutional Review Board Guidebook*. Rockville, Md.: OHRP; 1993. [Online] Available: http://www.hhs.gov/ohrp/irb/irb_guidebook.htm.

7. Department of Health and Human Services, National Institutes of Health, and Office for Human Research Protections. The Common Rule, Title 45 (Public Welfare), Code of Federal Regulations, Part 46 (Protection of Human Subjects). [Online] June 23, 2005. Available: http://www.hhs.gov/ohrp/humansubjects/guidance/45cfr46.htm.

8. Stone TH. The invisible vulnerable: The economically and educationally disadvantaged subjects of clinical research. *Journal of Law, Medicine, and Ethics* 2003;31:149–53.

9. World Medical Association. *Declaration of Helsinki: Ethical Principles for Medical Research Involving Human Subjects*. Tokyo, Japan: WMA; October 2004. [Online] 2004. Available: http://www.wma.net/e/policy/b3.htm.

10. Council for International Organizations of Medical Sciences in collaboration with the World Health Organization. *International Ethical Guidelines for Biomedical Research Involving Human Subjects*. Geneva, Switzerland: CIOMS and WHO; 2002. [Online] November 2002. Available: http://www.cioms.ch/frame_guidelines_nov_2002.htm.

11. The National Commission for the Protection of Human Subjects of Biomedical and Behavioral Research. *The Belmont Report: Ethical Principles and Guidelines for the Protection of Human Subjects of Research*. Washington, D.C.: Department of Health, Education and Welfare; DHEW Publication OS 78-0012 1978. [Online] April 18, 1979. Available: http://www.hhs.gov/ohrp/humansubjects/guidance/belmont.htm.

12. Levine C. Changing views of justice after Belmont: AIDS and the inclusion of "vulnerable subjects." In: Vanderpool HY, ed. *The Ethics of Research Involving Human Subjects: Facing the Twenty-First Century*. Frederick, Md.: University Publishing Group; 1996:105–26.

13. Gorkin L, Schron EB, Handshaw K, et al. Clinical trial enrollers vs. nonenrollers: The Cardiac Arrhythmia Suppression Trial (CAST) Recruitment and Enrollment in Clinical Trials (REACT) Project. *Controlled Clinical Trials* 1996;17:46–59.

14. Rogers WA. Evidence-based medicine and justice: A framework for looking at the impact of EBM upon vulnerable or disadvantaged groups. *Journal of Medical Ethics* 2004;30:141–5.

15. Katz J, with Capron AM, Glass ES. *Experimentation With Human Beings*. New York, N.Y.: Russell Sage Foundation; 1972:633, 1007–10.

16. Beecher HK. Ethics and clinical research. *New England Journal of Medicine* 1966;274:1354–60.

17. Rothman DJ. *Strangers at the Bedside: A History of How Law and Bioethics Transformed Medical Decision Making*. New York, N.Y.: Basic Books; 1991.

18. Zion D, Gillam L, Loff B. The Declaration of Helsinki, CIOMS and the ethics of research on vulnerable populations. *Nature Medicine* 2000; 6:615–7.

19. Jafarey AM. Conflict of interest issues in informed consent for research on human subjects: A South Asian perspective. *Science and Engineering Ethics* 2002;8:353–61.

20. Flaskerud JH, Winslow BJ. Conceptualizing vulnerable populations health-related research. *Nursing Research* 1998;47(2):69–78.

21. Chambers R. *Rural Development: Putting the Last First*. London, England: Longman; 1983.

22. Watts MJ, Bolhe G. Hunger, famine, and the space of vulnerability. *Geojournal* 1993;30(32):117–25.

23. McGovern TF. Vulnerability: Reflection on its ethical implications for the protection of participants in SAMHSA programs. *Ethics and Behavior* 1998;8:293–304.

24. Basic Behavioral Science Task Force of the National Advisory Mental Health Council. Basic behavioral science and research for mental health: Vulnerability and resilience. *American Psychologist* 1996; 51:22–8.

25. Moreno J. Convenient and captive populations. In: Kahn J, Mastroianni AC, Sugarman J, eds. *Beyond Consent: Seeking Justice in Research*. New York, N.Y.: Oxford University Press; 1998: 111–30.

26. DeBruin D. Reflections on "vulnerability." *Bioethics Examiner* 2001;5(2):1,4,7. [Online] Available: http://www.bioethics.umn.edu/publications/BE-2001-summer.pdf.

27. Dunn, LB, Gordon, NE. Improving informed consent and enhancing recruitment for research by understanding economic behavior. *JAMA* 2005;293:609–12.

28. Levine C, et al., on behalf of the Consortium to Examine Clinical Research Ethics. "Special scrutiny:" A targeted form of research protocol review. *Annals of Internal Medicine* 2004;140:220–3.

29. Bailey JM, Bieniasz, MD, Kmak D, Brenner DE, Ruffin MT. Recruitment and retention of economically underserved women to a cervical cancer prevention trial. *Applied Nursing Research* 2004;17:55–60.

Donald L. Rosenstein   Franklin G. Miller

41

Research Involving Those at Risk for Impaired Decision-Making Capacity

Medical conditions that impair a person's ability to make decisions (e.g., dementia, stroke, schizophrenia) are devastating for affected individuals and their families. Too often, modern medicine provides only modest symptomatic improvement for patients with these disorders. Much-needed progress in the diagnosis, treatment, and prevention of these illnesses depends on clinical advances through research. However, the conduct of research exposes these individuals to the possibility of exploitation precisely because they may not be able to make informed decisions about participation.

This chapter employs a process-oriented and practical approach to the ethics of research with adults who may not be able to provide informed consent because of impaired decision-making capacity (DMC). Neither emergency research nor research with children will be addressed. The chapter is organized into the following sections: a brief history of ethical aspects of research with those who are decisionally impaired; our conceptualization of DMC as it relates to the ethics of clinical research; a review of empirical data on research subjects who have, or are at risk for, impaired DMC; policy and study design implications; and unresolved empirical issues regarding the ethics of DMC and clinical research. Throughout the chapter, we emphasize the integral relationship between research methodology (i.e., subject selection, the nature of the proposed research interventions, and specific protocol details) and the ethical analysis of a given research proposal.

History

Concerns about clinical research with decisionally impaired subjects received serious consideration following revelations of Nazi experimentation with mentally disabled individuals during World War II (see Chapter 2). Although they are more infamous for participating in the extermination of hundreds of thousands of mentally ill patients, Nazi physicians also conducted unauthorized experiments (e.g., infection with malaria, sterilization) on mentally disabled prisoners.[1–3] Indeed, the Nuremberg Code begins with the following two sentences:

> The voluntary consent of the human subject is absolutely essential. This means that the person involved should have legal capacity to give consent; should be so situated as to be able to exercise free power of choice, without the intervention of any element of force, fraud, deceit, duress, overreaching, or other ulterior form of constraint or coercion; and should have sufficient knowledge and comprehension of the subject matter involved so as to enable him to make an understanding and enlightened decision.[4]

A literal interpretation of the Nuremberg Code would preclude all research involving incompetent persons, including children and incapacitated adults. As noted by other commentators,[5–7] it is not clear whether this was the intent of the judges of the Nuremberg tribunal. Subsequent research codes and guidelines (e.g., more recent versions of the Declaration of Helsinki; the Council for International Organizations of Medical Sciences' *International Ethical Guidelines for Biomedical Research Involving Human Subjects;* and the U.S. Code of Federal Regulations)[8–10] explicitly allow the enrollment of those who are unable to provide informed consent provided that other conditions are met (e.g., permission by a legally authorized representative).

In the years following World War II, several cases of research abuse in the United States were revealed, including the exploitation of decisionally impaired subjects. Henry Beecher's classic 1966 article in the *New England Journal of Medicine* detailed 22 cases of research ethics violations, several of which involved subjects with, or at risk for, impaired DMC.[11] These examples of exploitation of the mentally disabled provided the backdrop for a 1978 report by the U.S. National Commission for the Protection of Human Subjects of Biomedical and Behavioral Research entitled "Research Involving Those Institutionalized as Mentally Infirm."[12] In this report, the Commissioners called for the adoption of specific federal regulations governing research with the "mentally disabled," as they later did for children in 1983. However, their proposed framework was never incorporated into the U.S. regulations governing federally funded research.

Current U.S. regulations make minimal specific references to the mentally disabled, including the following: "When some or all of the subjects are likely to be vulnerable to coercion or undue influence, such as children, prisoners, pregnant women, mentally disabled persons, or economically or educationally disadvantaged persons, additional safeguards have been included in the study to protect the rights and welfare of these subjects."[10]

The regulations do not provide a definition of what constitutes a mental disability. As a result, variable practice exists within the research community regarding who is considered decisionally impaired due to a mental disability. Furthermore, the only specific guidance regarding "additional protections" included in the regulations is the requirement that a legally authorized representative provide permission for research participation if the subject is unable to do so.

In the early 1990s, allegations were made against schizophrenia researchers at the University of California, Los Angeles following the death of a former research subject. The investigators were accused of conducting "high-risk" research with "vulnerable" subjects and without adequate informed consent. This case, and its subsequently well-publicized federal investigation, ushered in a period of intense ethical scrutiny and criticism of research involving mentally ill subjects. In 1995, the National Bioethics Advisory Commission (NBAC) was established and charged with providing recommendations on bioethics (including research with the mentally disabled), to the National Science and Technology Council. Following extensive public testimony and investigation, NBAC released its 1998 report, "Research Involving Individuals With Mental Disorders That May Affect Decisionmaking Capacity."[13] Although these recommendations have not been incorporated into U.S. research regulations or adopted by the research community in any coherent fashion, they have stimulated much debate and research relevant to those at risk for impaired DMC.

Core Conception and Methodological Rationale

The principal ethical concern raised by research involving subjects with impaired DMC is the potential exploitation of such individuals. An inherent tension exists between the danger of exploitation and the compelling need for improvements in the clinical care of patients who suffer from medical, neurological, and psychiatric illnesses that impair DMC. Because progress through research requires the participation of subjects at greatest risk of exploita-

tion, an ethical assessment of these studies depends critically on how they are conducted.

Clearly, some medical conditions are associated with predictable impairment of DMC (e.g., advanced dementia, massive head trauma, delirium). However, we contend that a diagnosis-based approach to the ethics of research with subjects at risk for impaired DMC is not supported by existing data and, further, that such an approach stigmatizes the millions of people who suffer from mental illness. Data summarized below demonstrate that many, if not most, of these individuals are quite capable of providing informed consent for research participation. Furthermore, impaired DMC represents just one of several ways in which research subjects can be "vulnerable." There exists no consensus about what constitutes adequate informed consent for any research, let alone research with those thought to be vulnerable. Consequently, we advocate a process-oriented and protocol-driven approach as described below.

Our approach to the ethical analysis of research with decisionally impaired subjects is based on four core concepts. First, DMC is a complex and modifiable clinical phenomenon. As such, the domains of competency, DMC, and the ability to provide informed consent must be understood as closely related yet distinct. Despite the complexity of DMC, the clinical research review and approval processes require the rendering of categorical determinations about inherently continuous phenomena. Although individuals vary in their decisional capacity and their actual understanding of a given research protocol, they must be judged to be capable or incapable of giving informed consent and as having or lacking sufficient understanding to qualify as providing valid consent. Ultimately, these decisions require some measure of "clinical judgment," but our approach mandates that DMC is viewed as a continuous variable. Second, those judged to be at substantial risk for impaired DMC are appropriately considered vulnerable in the research context and deserving of additional safeguards. Consequently, the default position of investigators and institutional review boards (IRBs) should be to conduct studies with volunteers who clearly are able to provide informed consent. If an IRB concludes that important research requires the enrollment of subjects who may not be able to make capacitated decisions, then additional safeguards must be incorporated into the design and conduct of the study to protect those subjects. Third, distinctions between the provision of standard medical care and clinical research participation have important implications for decisionally impaired subjects. Fourth, as a practical matter, the ethical analysis of research with decisionally impaired subjects should be anchored to the IRB oversight process and considered on a protocol-by-protocol basis.

Throughout most of the developed world, adults are presumed competent to make autonomous decisions. A judgment that someone is incompetent is made by formal judicial ruling and rendered in the context of the person's ability to make specific decisions (e.g., choices concerning medical care, management of finances, designation of a substitute decision maker, execution of a will). From a legal perspective, persons are either competent to make decisions for themselves or incompetent, in which case someone else makes decisions on their behalf. Furthermore, the threshold for incompetence varies depending upon the task an individual is called upon to perform. Unfortunately, limited empirical data are available to help determine appropriate thresholds. Therefore, competency determinations are made on a case-by-case basis.

The evidence upon which a judicial determination of competence relies includes the formal assessment of decision-making abilities by professionals with appropriate expertise. This clinical evaluation is generally referred to as the assessment of DMC. Few human activities are as complex and individually determined as how we make decisions. Core components of DMC include intellectual ability, emotional state, memory, attention, concentration, conceptual organization, and aspects of executive function such as the ability to plan, solve problems, and make probability determinations. Most of the literature on DMC in the clinical research setting focuses on cognitive functions and uses psychometric approaches to the study of individuals with neuropsychiatric illnesses such as dementia, psychosis, major depression, and bipolar disorder.[14] Psychologists, cognitive neuroscientists, and economists have contributed to an extensive parallel literature through studies of healthy volunteers in which various experimental manipulations are used to probe the dynamics of decision making (e.g., the effects of time pressure on risk-taking and information-processing strategies).[15,16] Despite this rapidly expanding body of evidence, the manner in which individuals assign relative importance to a particular cognitive strategy when making decisions remains poorly characterized.

The contributions of mood, motivation, and other mental processes on risk assessment and decision making have direct implications for the process and quality of informed consent for research. However, the extent to which these factors, and less discrete concepts like intuition, trust, duty, or altruism, influence someone's choice to enroll in a study is not known. Cutting across all of these determinants is the fact that decisions about participating in research typically take place within the context of relationships between research subjects and investigators. How characteristics of these relationships impact DMC and the informed consent process are also unknown. Although much work remains to better understand decision making and informed consent, it is clear that focusing exclusively on measures of cognitive impairment is insufficient.

In the medical setting, it is common for patients to manifest diminished DMC in some domains but retain the ability to make autonomous decisions in others. For example, a patient with schizophrenia may suffer from delusions or hallucinations yet still adequately attend to activities of daily living and manage her financial affairs. However, even in cases of patently impaired DMC, it is unusual for such patients to undergo formal competency evaluations and judicial proceedings. Informal judgments about competence based on these capacity assessments are generally accepted as reasonable proxies for judicial review. In this chapter, we use the terms *capacity* and *impaired capacity* to refer to findings from a clinical evaluation and *competence* and *incompetence* to refer to the status of individuals to make their own legally binding decisions. In the clinical research setting, a judgment that a person is capacitated means that he or she is able to provide informed consent for the specific research protocol under consideration.

In contrast to the dichotomous nature of competency determinations, DMC is more accurately conceptualized as a skill set that varies along a continuum from incapacitated to fully capacitated (see Figure 41.1). For example, individuals in the early stages of dementia may be unable to provide informed consent for a complicated clinical trial but retain the ability to appoint a trusted family member or friend to serve as the holder of a durable power of attorney (DPA) for medical and research decisions. Despite this spectrum of DMC, clinical researchers routinely make yes or no determinations as to whether a subject understands the risks and benefits of a study "well enough" to provide informed consent. Indeed, there are several examples relevant to clinical research in which categorical decisions are made with respect to continuous phenomena. Research regulations typically require that a sharp line of demarcation be drawn between childhood and adulthood despite the wide variability and uneven maturation among adolescents and young adults in their cognitive and emotional development. Similarly, IRBs make categorical risk determinations (i.e., minimal risk and more than minimal risk) for research-related harms and discomforts that actually reflect continuously distributed probabilities. IRBs face multiple challenges when reviewing protocols designed to enroll subjects with variable DMC into research that poses a range of risks and offers an uncertain prospect of direct medical benefit.

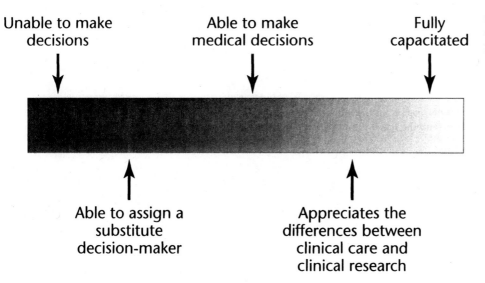

Figure 41.1. Decision-Making Capacity as a Continuous Phenomenon

One straightforward approach to protecting vulnerable research subjects is to require that incapacitated adults be enrolled in research only when their participation is necessary to answer the scientific question posed. This requirement has been termed the *necessity clause* and has been articulated best by Wendler and colleagues.[17] In our experience, this fundamental question of whether it is scientifically necessary to enroll subjects who are unable to provide informed consent is often inadequately addressed in the IRB review process. Investigators may argue that excluding subjects who are unable to provide informed consent will result in a selection bias (i.e., enrolling healthier subjects) that compromises the scientific validity of the study. Another objection to the necessity clause is that it will result in unacceptably long recruitment time and/or make the study impracticable. Our position is that the investigator is responsible for explicitly justifying the enrollment of subjects who are unable to provide informed consent. The IRB must then make an independent judgment regarding whether this justification is acceptable.

An IRB determination about the acceptability of a research project likely to enroll individuals at risk for impaired DMC raises several further questions. How will the subjects be recruited? What is the probability that subjects will be unable to provide informed consent? Who will evaluate DMC? What methods will be employed in this assessment? How will questionable cases of DMC be resolved? Will research authorization be permitted by surrogates if the subject is unable to provide informed consent? If so, is there a need to assess the capacity or appropriateness of the surrogate for this task? Because individual research subjects can manifest impaired DMC at any time during a study, whether or not this was anticipated by the IRB, is there a mechanism in place for the evaluation and protection of subjects with unanticipated incapacity?

The answers to these questions vary widely among individual investigators and research institutions. In contrast to the research setting, a clinical and legal framework for the assessment of DMC in the medical setting is well-established. Within this framework, several important points of consensus have emerged for determining decisional capacity in the treatment context and making medical decisions for incompetent adults.[18]

First, competence is understood as relative to the type and complexity of the treatment decision at stake. Some decisionally impaired patients are competent to make simple treatment decisions but incompetent to make complex ones that require weighing and balancing the risks and benefits of alternative treatments and factoring in uncertainty about outcomes. The assessment of capacity, which informs decisions about competence, includes assessing the abilities: (1) to make and express a choice; (2) to understand information relevant to the treatment decision; (3) to appreciate the significance of this information for the individual's own situation; and (4) to reason with the relevant information in weighing options.[19]

Second, thresholds for competence to make treatment decisions should adopt a "sliding scale."[20] The thresholds for competence should become more demanding as the risks of a treatment intervention, the uncertainty of its benefits, and/or the complexity of the research increase.

Third, assessing DMC is the responsibility of the treating physician. In cases in which capacity is called into question, a psychiatric or neurological consultation to more formally assess DMC may be indicated and helpful.

Fourth, when patients are judged incapable of making treatment decisions, surrogate decision makers must be engaged. Two legal and ethical standards govern surrogate decision making.[21] If the prior preferences of the patient are known, then the surrogate should make a "substituted judgment" that he or she believes the patient would have made if able; if not known, the surrogate together with the physician chooses the option believed to promote the patient's best interests. Exceptions include emergency interventions or when surrogate decision makers cannot be found, in which case physicians make treatment decisions for the patient. Surrogate decision makers may be designated by patients through a DPA. Additionally, written guidance about the patient's treatment preferences may be available in the form of an advance directive or living will. The vast majority of patients have not engaged in such formal advance planning, although many may have informally communicated their preferences to others. If no surrogate has been designated in advance, next of kin are generally considered appropriate surrogate decision makers and recognized as such by law. It is presumed that they know best the preferences and values of the patient that should determine or inform treatment decisions and that they will be concerned to promote the patient's best interest.

Differences between clinical care and clinical research affect the applicability of the framework developed for clinical care of incapacitated adults to the research setting. Four specific issues deserve attention: (1) DMC must include the ability to appreciate key differences between clinical care and clinical research—clinical research is designed to develop scientific knowledge concerning diseases and their treatment, not to promote optimal medical care for particular patients; (2) levels of risk that are justified in medical care may not be justifiable in clinical research; (3) a formal plan for capacity assessment may be necessary in some research protocols; and (4) surrogate decision making should take into account the differences between clinical care and clinical research.

Although the same types of abilities that constitute capacity to consent to treatment are relevant to capacity to consent to research,[22] capacity assessment in research is complicated because patient-volunteers may have a "therapeutic misconception" in which they see various research interventions as directed to individualized diagnostic or therapeutic benefit.[23–25] No agreement exists on how realistic it is to expect sick patients deciding to enroll in clinical research to be able to fully appreciate the differences between personal care and research participation. Nonetheless, the ability to appreciate these differences may be so impaired that some individuals, who may be capable of making treatment decisions, should be judged incapable of making research decisions.

Individuals who lack capacity to give informed consent may be capable of assent—a less demanding standard of research authorization.[26] Along with the requirement for parental permission, the U.S. federal regulations on research with children allow children to give assent for research in accordance with their capacities for understanding, appreciation, and reasoning.[10] Adults who are incapable of giving informed consent may similarly have sufficient ability to assent to research participation. Soliciting assent shows respect for the capacities that they retain as well as for their former autonomy.

Just as incapacitated individuals are often unable to provide valid consent to research, they are similarly unable to decide to withdraw from research. Dissent is widely accepted as sufficient grounds for withdrawing from research. However, it is also generally assumed that valid dissent is a result of a rational decision-making process. It is much harder to know how to respond to behavior suggesting dissent that is not the result of a rational decisional process, for example, dissent that might be voiced by an individual in an acute paranoid psychosis or postconcussive state. Behaviors suggesting objection in these types of cases may represent anxiety, confusion, or ambivalence rather than a rational decision to decline participation. Although there is no consensus on what to do when faced with these situations, withdrawing the individual from the research may not always be the most ethically appropriate course of action. Halting the particular procedure and considering reapproaching at a different time may be an appropriate alternative. A surrogate decision maker can sometimes be helpful in making these types of determinations. However, persistent objection should be respected by withdrawing the individual from research.[27]

Given the ethical and procedural complexity of research with decisionally impaired subjects, it is not surprising that efforts to craft definitive policy and legislation have been largely unsuccessful. Nonetheless, one tangible outcome from extensive public deliberations over the past decade has been a significant increase in the number and quality of studies of DMC in the research setting.

Empirical Data

Potential research subjects may be considered at risk for impaired DMC for several reasons. The most common cause for concern is the nature of the underlying medical, neurological, or psychiatric disorder under study.[13,14,23,28–37] Frequently cited conditions include dementia, delirium, psychotic disorders, depression, mania, and intoxication with alcohol or illicit substances. The nature of the research protocol, rather than the disorder being studied, might also render research subjects at risk for impaired DMC. For example, an oncology trial for malignant melanoma in which individuals receive high dose interleukin-2, a cytokine associated with central nervous system toxicity, places otherwise capacitated subjects at risk of losing DMC. In this case, the concern is less about adequate informed consent on the "front end" of the study than it is about subjects losing their ability to provide adequate ongoing informed consent after receiving interleukin-2.

Although investigators and IRBs are charged with making their best judgments about "high-risk" study populations and protocols, intuitions about DMC are not always confirmed by research findings. Several methodologically sound studies of DMC suggest the following three important findings:

1. DMC is variable within and between diagnoses. A wide range of patient groups (e.g., those with dementia, schizophrenia, depression, Parkinsonism, HIV/AIDS, delirium, and diabetes mellitus) have been studied with respect to their ability to provide informed consent for either an actual clinical trial or a hypothetical investigation. Several studies have confirmed that some patient groups are at higher risk for impaired DMC than samples of healthy controls or other medically ill comparison groups.[29,38–41] However, each of these studies reported substantial overlap in measures of DMC between comparison groups and suggested that diagnosis alone was inadequate for differentiating between subjects who were and were not able to give informed consent for the study. More importantly, despite predictable cognitive and deci-

sional deficits, only a minority of subjects from these "high-risk" samples (e.g., those with schizophrenia, dementia, or depression) were determined to be incapable of providing informed consent for clinical care or a research study.[29,32,38,40,42–49] Interestingly, certain aspects of neurocognitive deficits (e.g., working memory, "negative" symptoms of apathy, avolition, and inappropriate affect) are more predictive of impaired DMC than psychotic symptoms (e.g., hallucinations and delusions).[29,39,43,44]

2. DMC can be improved through educational interventions. An important finding replicated by several independent research groups is that educational interventions for at-risk patients designed to improve informed consent are effective. Typically, the most robust improvements in DMC, as they relate to the informed consent process, are observed in the domains of *understanding* and *reasoning.* Some investigators reported that following an educational intervention, subjects with impaired baseline DMC performed as well as healthy comparison subjects on tests of DMC. Several different educational approaches were used in these studies, and it remains uncertain whether specialized educational programs provide additional improvement in decisional capacity beyond standard subject education.[29,39,46,50–52]

3. Surrogate consent is acceptable for some research. Not surprisingly, proxy decision makers report ambiguity in their role and experience this activity as psychologically burdensome.[53] Still, the majority of "at-risk" subjects and caregivers are supportive of this mechanism of research authorization for low-risk research that offers a prospect of direct medical benefit to subjects.[54–56] Fewer data exist regarding the willingness of proxy decision makers to enroll decisionally impaired subjects in higher risk research. However, in a related study, Wendler et al. queried healthy individuals who had a close relative with Alzheimer's disease about their attitudes toward research advance directives.[54] They found that of the 39 healthy respondents who filled out a research advance directive, 20 were willing to participate in research with greater than minimal risk and no potential benefit.

Policy and Study Design Implications

Several policy and study design implications stem from the conceptual considerations and empirical data relevant to DMC. First, it is unlikely that one simple policy will address the scope and complexity of this aspect of research. Although some studies propose the enrollment of subjects known to be incapacitated, others will enroll only capacitated subjects onto a trial of a medication that will lead to loss of capacity in susceptible individuals. A single approach to such different studies is inappropriate. Policies on DMC in research will need to be flexible enough to allow for both a wide range of studies and individual cases of protocol-emergent loss of capacity. Second, current research guidelines provide insufficient detail as to appropriate additional safeguards and how they should be implemented.[57–60] Third, investigators should build specific educational interventions into their protocols. Fourth, the greater use of advance directives and a DPA for research participation should be encouraged by IRBs (or mandated for high-risk studies). Fifth, the protection of decisionally impaired subjects may be strengthened by more specific research regulations similar to those for children.

Although there are no regulations governing risk-benefit assessment for research with incompetent adults, the federal policy framework for research involving children offers valuable guidance (see Chapter 42). Under this framework, research that provides a prospect of benefit to the child-subject and/or poses minimal risk to subjects is allowed.[10] (The regulations define *minimal risk* as "the probability and magnitude of harm or discomfort anticipated in the research are not greater in and of themselves than those ordinarily encountered in daily life or during the performance of routine physical or psychological examinations or tests."[10])

Research that presents a minor increase over minimal risk and does not hold the prospect of benefit for the child-subject may also be justifiable if it fulfills the following conditions: (a) "the intervention or procedure presents experiences to subjects that are reasonably commensurate with those inherent in their actual or expected medical, dental, psychological, social, or educational situations"; (b) "the intervention or procedure is likely to yield generalizable knowledge about the subjects' disorder or condition which is of vital importance for the understanding or amelioration of the subjects' disorder or condition"; and (c) "adequate provisions are made for soliciting assent of the children and permission of their parents or guardians."[10] Proposed research that has greater than a minor increase over minimal risk and no prospect of benefit for the subjects must be approved by the Secretary of Health and Human Services. We believe that these risk-benefit categories are also reasonable to apply to research with incompetent adults, even though there debate continues about how best to interpret the definitions for the various risk levels.[61,62]

Because the presence of a diagnosis is neither necessary nor sufficient to identify an individual in need of protections above and beyond those in place for all research subjects, we suggest that additional safeguards should be considered for any subject or class of subjects who are either unable to provide informed consent or who are at risk of being unable to do so for a particular study. With this approach, investigators, IRBs and others charged with monitoring research can make determinations of vulnerability and the need for additional safeguards on a protocol-by-protocol basis or for individually identified subjects.

Protocol Review and Determination of Appropriate Safeguards

Despite a substantial literature on the subject of research with decisionally impaired subjects, there exists little practical guidance for IRBs with respect to the kinds of safeguards that can be employed to protect decisionally impaired subjects.[13,28–30,33,38,63–66] Protocols must include a description of how informed consent will be obtained and are expected to include additional procedural details when subjects are likely to have impaired DMC. The IRB, in turn, makes its own determination as to the adequacy of these plans.

Many commentators on this issue have called for the assessments of DMC to be performed by someone independent of the research team. This was a key recommendation in NBAC's report which stipulated that this assessment of capacity to consent should be made by an "independent, qualified professional" when studies pose more than minimal risks.[13] The commissioners did not specify how investigators and IRBs were to decide who that professional should be, their requisite degree of independence, what methods of evaluation should be used, and how this process would be administered within a research setting.

For protocols enrolling subjects who might have decisional impairment but who are not at particularly high risk in this regard, the IRB can require that the informed consent discussion between the subjects and the investigators be observed by someone who is not part of the research team (i.e., consent monitor). If the consent monitor has concerns about the subject's ability to provide informed consent, then a more formal capacity evaluation of that subject would be indicated.

Obtaining informed consent from a research participant is an early, ongoing and integral component of what should be a trusting relationship between investigator and subject. As such, it should not be interfered with without cause. The presence of a consent monitor is, no doubt, an intrusion and could influence the informed consent process in both positive and negative ways. However, if all parties (i.e., investigator, IRB, consent monitor, and subject) are clear about the purpose and function of consent monitoring, this intrusion can ultimately serve to improve this fundamental research contract with minimal disruption to what has been historically a private and highly variable conversation.

In contrast to consent monitoring, independent capacity assessment should occur after the initiation of discussions about a study but prior to signing the informed consent document. It is essential that the person or team that performs these evaluations has clear authority and administrative backing to prevent the enrollment of subjects who are unable to provide informed consent.

Safeguards other than consent monitoring and assessment of DMC can be employed by the IRB. For research institutions that provide a bioethics consultation service, review of a research protocol or a specific subject's participation by an individual or group independent of the research team can provide meaningful protection for subjects. The use of an independent clinician to manage clinical care separately from the research care of subjects has also been proposed as a safeguard for high-risk studies with vulnerable subjects. An infrequently employed safeguard is the enforcement of a specific hospital policy on research with decisionally impaired or potentially impaired research subjects. Despite the obvious guidance such policies can provide to investigators and IRBs, only a few exist.[67,68]

Which safeguards are chosen for which protocols should depend on the level of risk posed by the research and the nature of the anticipated decisional impairment of subjects. For example, although it is reasonable for the IRB to require independent assessment of DMC for potential subjects in a more than minimal risk schizophrenia clinical trial, this same requirement would make little sense for a minimal risk MRI study in advanced Alzheimer disease. A more appropriate safeguard in this latter case would be for the IRB to stipulate the assignment and active involvement of a legally authorized representative in providing surrogate permission.

Some researchers have instituted a procedure by which individuals likely to have declining capacity prepare an advance directive at the time of enrollment that includes assigning a surrogate decision maker to take an increasingly active role in decision making as the subject's own abilities decline.[69] Although this model will not work in all protocols, it may be a useful way to incorporate surrogate decision makers into a system of safeguards for at-risk subjects.

Areas in Need of Further Research

One of the more pressing needs for empirical data is to examine methods and tools with which to identify individuals who are decisionally impaired and who are thus unable to provide adequate informed consent. In our view, the MacArthur Competence Assessment Tool for Clinical Research (McCAT-CR) employs the most meaningful framework currently available for the assessment of DMC for research participation. The McCAT-CR is a modification of the DMC model described earlier and addresses the domains of understanding, appreciation, reasoning, and the ability to express a choice. To date, the McCAT-CR has been used predominantly as a research tool[29,31,32,34,38,43–45,47–50] and is limited by the need to customize it each time it is used for a new protocol. Some research programs have piloted the use of the McCAT-CR modified in such a fashion that a short version can be rapidly adapted for a new protocol. One facet of the McCAT-CR model, the concept of appreciation, has not been well explicated. In this context, appreciation is generally understood as the extent to which subjects understand the relevance of the research activity to their particular circumstances. For example, knowledge that a clinical trial includes both a placebo and an active medication arm demonstrates "understanding." In contrast, a full awareness that one may actually receive placebo and as a result forgo other available treatments is an example of "appreciation." What constitutes appreciation and how it should be assessed remain key unanswered questions.

A related issue in need of empirical research is a framework for assessing the adequacy of surrogate permission to enroll incapacitated individuals in research. Just as we need more systematic studies of the motivations and experiences of research participants, we need the companion data relevant to surrogate decision makers. Only then will we be in a position to know what constitutes adequate or appropriate understanding by a proxy decision maker. Current policy at the National Institutes of Health's Clinical Center requires an ethics consultant to assist in the selection of surrogates for incapacitated adult prospective research subjects.[66] Like patient-volunteers, surrogates may be subject to the therapeutic misconception that confuses clinical research with individualized medical care. Education for surrogates as well as consultation with a neutral professional or lay advocate may help prepare them for their responsibility to make informed choices on the behalf of incapacitated subjects.[70] Clearly, there is much to be learned about the factors involved in deciding for others in the research setting.

Several other important questions related to the protection of vulnerable subjects remain unanswered. With so much attention and effort being directed at decisional capacity determinations at the "front end" of research participation, there has been little discussion of optimal ways to protect those subjects who are able to provide informed consent at the start of the study but who then lose that capacity during the study. The use of a research advance directive or prospective authorization for research is a logical strategy in this regard but one that has yet to be widely implemented. As research programs move toward the systematic implementation of additional safeguards for vulnerable research subjects, there will be a growing need for data on how to construct the most efficient and effective programs to protect research subjects. Finally, research into novel and effective methods of training clinical investigators holds out the promise of improving the ethical conduct of virtually every aspect of human subjects research, including specific protections for decisionally impaired subjects.[71,72]

Conclusion

One of the major conclusions to emerge from a decade of debate on research involving individuals with compromised DMC is that it is both inaccurate and stigmatizing to conclude that all or most individuals with a psychiatric diagnosis are unable to make decisions for themselves. Nonetheless, for certain types of studies involving subjects judged to be at risk for impaired DMC, there are compelling reasons to consider them vulnerable and therefore in need of additional safeguards. As is true for any clinical study, when a member of the research team encounters any subject, at any time during the conduct of the study, who presents with questionable DMC, that subject should be carefully evaluated and either managed according to the dictates of the protocol or removed from the study.

The ethical framework applicable to enrolling incapacitated adults in clinical research deserves more systematic exploration and articulation. Although the framework for treatment decision making for incompetent adults and the framework for research with children are helpful, they fail in several ethically important ways as described above. More systematic empirical data are needed to better understand the extent to which adults in a variety of conditions have impaired ability to give informed consent to research participation. In addition, too little is known about surrogate decision making, for example, the motivations of surrogates for enrolling incapacitated persons in research, their understanding and appreciation of what research participation involves, their knowledge about the research-relevant preferences and values of the incapacitated individuals whose research participation they authorize, and the extent to which they are involved in monitoring research participation. Programmatic experimentation and evaluative research are needed in the areas of enhancing the capabilities of decisionally impaired individuals to give informed consent, formal methods of capacity assessment, independent capacity assessment, consent monitoring, advance directives for research participation, evaluation and education of surrogates, and the use of lay advocates. Funding sources for clinical research involving decisionally impaired individuals should support initiatives to improve the protection of these vulnerable research subjects and to conduct well-designed, ethics-related empirical research.

Acknowledgments

The research was supported by the Intramural Research Programs of the NIMH and the NIH.

Disclaimer

The views expressed here are those of the authors alone and do not represent any position or policy of the National Institutes of Health, Public Health Service, or Department of Health and Human Services.

References

1. Lifton RJ. *The Nazi Doctors: Medical Killing and the Psychology of Genocide.* New York, N.Y.: Basic Books; 1986.

2. Eckart WU, Vondra H. Malaria and World War II: German malaria experiments 1939– 45. *Parassitologia* 2000;42:53–8.

3. Annas GJ, Grodin MA, eds. *The Nazi Doctors and the Nuremberg Code.* New York, N.Y.: Oxford University Press; 1992.

4. The Nuremberg Code. In: *Trials of War Criminals Before the Nuremberg Military. Tribunals Under Control Council Law No. 10. Volume 2.* Washington, D.C.: U.S. Government Printing Office; 1949:181–2. [Online]. Available: http://www.hhs.gov/ohrp/references/nurcode.htm.

5. Berg JW, Appelbaum PS, Lidz CW, Parker LS. *Informed Consent: Legal Theory and Clinical Practice.* New York, NY: Oxford University Press; 2001:249–78.

6. McCormick RA. Proxy consent in the experimentation situation. *Perspectives in Biology and Medicine* 1974;18:2–20.

7. Perley S, Fluss SS, Bankowski Z, Simon F. The Nuremberg Code: An international overview. In: Annas GJ, Grodin MA, eds. *The Nazi Doctors and the Nuremberg Code.* New York, N.Y.: Oxford University Press; 1992:149–73.

8. World Medical Association. *Declaration of Helsinki: Ethical Principles for Medical Research Involving Human Subjects.* Tokyo, Japan: WMA; October 2004. [Online] 2004. Available: http://www.wma.net/e/policy/b3.htm.

9. Council for International Organizations of Medical Sciences, in collaboration with the World Health Organization. *International Ethical Guidelines for Biomedical Research Involving Human Subjects.* Geneva, Switzerland: CIOMS and WHO; 2002. [Online] November 2002. Available: http://www.cioms.ch/frame_guidelines_nov_2002.htm.

10. Department of Health and Human Services, National Institutes of Health, and Office for Human Research Protections. The Common Rule, Title 45 (Public Welfare), Code of Federal Regulations, Part 46 (Protection of Human Subjects). [Online] June 23, 2005. Available: http://www.hhs.gov/ohrp/humansubjects/guidance/45cfr46.htm.

11. Beecher HK. Ethics and clinical research. *New England Journal of Medicine* 1966;274:1355–60.

12. National Commission for the Protection of Human Subjects of Biomedical and Behavioral Research. *Research Involving Those Institutionalized As Mentally Infirm.* Washington, D.C.: U.S. Department of Health, Education, and Welfare; 1978.

13. National Bioethics Advisory Commission. *Research Involving Persons with Mental Disorders That May Affect Decisionmaking Capacity, Vol. I.* Rockville, Md.: NBAC; 1998. [Online] December 1998. Available: http://www.georgetown.edu/research/nrcbl/nbac/capacity/TOC.htm.

14. Chen DT, Miller FG, Rosenstein DL. Enrolling decisionally impaired adults in clinical research. *Medical Care* 2002;40:V20–V29.

15. Ernst M, Paulus MP. Neurobiology of decision making: A selective review from a neurocognitive and clinical perspective. *Biological Psychiatry* 2005;58:597–604.

16. Maule AJ, Hockey GRJ, Bdzola L. Effects of time-pressure on decision-making under uncertainty: Changes in affective state and information processing strategy. *Acta Psychologica* 2000;104:283–301.

17. Wendler D, Shah S, Whittle A, Wilfond BS. Nonbeneficial research with individuals who cannot consent: Is it ethically better to enroll healthy or affected individuals? *IRB: A Review of Human Subjects Research* 2003;25(4):1– 4.

18. Buchanan AE, Brock DW. *Deciding for Others.* New York, N.Y.: Cambridge University Press; 1989.

19. Grisso T, Appelbaum PS. *Assessing Competence to Consent to Treatment.* New York, N.Y.: Oxford University Press; 1998.

20. Drane JF. The many faces of competency. *Hastings Center Report* 1985;15(2):17–21.

21. Beauchamp TL, Childress JF. *Principles of Biomedical Ethics,* 5th ed. New York, N.Y.: Oxford University Press; 2001.

22. Appelbaum PS, Roth LH. Competency to consent to research: A psychiatric overview. *Archives of General Psychiatry* 1982;39:951–8.

23. Appelbaum PS, Roth LH, Lidz CW, Benson P, Winslade W. False hopes and best data: Consent to research and the therapeutic misconception. *Hastings Center Report* 1987;17(2):20– 4.

24. Joffe S, Cook EF, Cleary PD, Clark JW, Weeks JC. Quality of informed consent in cancer clinical trials: A cross-sectional survey. *Lancet* 2001;358:1772–7.

25. Horng S, Grady C. Misunderstanding in clinical research: Distinguishing therapeutic misconception, therapeutic misestimation, and therapeutic optimism. *IRB: A Review of Human Subjects Research* 2003;25(1):11–6.

26. Leikin S. Minors' assent, consent, or dissent to medical research. *IRB: A Review of Human Subjects Research* 1993;15(2):1–7.

27. Redmon RB. How children can be respected as 'ends' yet still be used as subjects in non-therapeutic research. *Journal of Medical Ethics* 1986;12:77–82.

28. Bonnie RJ. Research with cognitively impaired subjects: Unfinished business in the regulation of human research. *Archives of General Psychiatry* 1997;54:105–11.

29. Carpenter WT, Gold JM, Lahti AC, et al. Decisional capacity for informed consent in schizophrenia research. *Archives of General Psychiatry* 2000;57:533–8.

30. Cherniack EP. Informed consent for medical research by the elderly. *Experimental Aging Research* 2002;28:183–98.

31. Kim SYH, Caine ED, Currier GW, Leibovici A, Ryan JM. Assessing the competence of persons with Alzheimer's disease in providing informed consent for participation in research. *American Journal of Psychiatry* 2001;158:712–7.

32. Kim SYH, Karlawish JHT, Caine ED. Current state of research on decision-making competence of cognitively impaired elderly persons. *American Journal of Geriatric Psychiatry* 2002;10:151–65.

33. National Bioethics Advisory Commission. *Research Involving Persons with Mental Disorders That May Affect Decisionmaking Capacity, Vol. II.* Rockville, Md.: NBAC; 1998. [Online] December 1998. Available: http://www.georgetown.edu/research/nrcbl/nbac/capacity/volumeii.pdf.

34. Palmer BW, Nayak GV, Dunn LB, Appelbaum PS, Jeste DV. Treatment-related decision-making capacity in middle-aged and older patients with psychosis: A preliminary study using the MacCAT-T and HCAT. *American Journal of Geriatric Psychiatry* 2002;10:207–11.

35. Elliott C. Caring about risks: Are severely depressed patients competent to consent to research? *Archives of General Psychiatry* 1997;54:113–6.

36. Casarett DJ. Assessing decision-making capacity in the setting of palliative care research. *Journal of Pain and Symptom Management* 2003;255:S6–S13.

37. Misra S, Ganzini L. Capacity to consent to research among patients with bipolar disorder. *Journal of Affective Disorders* 2004;80:115–23.

38. Kim SYH, Cox C, Caine ED. Impaired decision-making ability in subjects with Alzheimer's disease and willingness to participate in research. *American Journal of Psychiatry* 2002;159:797–802.

39. Dunn LB, Lindamer LA, Palmer BW, Schneiderman LJ, Jeste DV. Enhancing comprehension of consent for research in older patients with psychosis: A randomized study of a novel consent procedure. *American Journal of Psychiatry* 2001;158:1911–3.

40. Griffith HR, Dymek MP, Atchison P, Harrell L, Marson DC. Medical decision-making in neurodegenerative disease: Mild AD and PD with cognitive impairment. *Neurology* 2005;65:483–5.

41. Jeste DV, Depp CA, Palmer BW. Magnitude of impairment in decisional capacity in people with schizophrenia compared to normal subjects: An overview. *Schizophrenia Bulletin* 2006;32:121–8.

42. Karlawish JHT, Casarett DJ, James BD, Xie SX, Kim SYH. The ability of persons with Alzheimer disease (AD) to make a decision about taking an AD treatment. *Neurology* 2005;64:1514–9.

43. Stroup S, Appelbaum PS, Swartz M, et al. Decision-making capacity for research participation among individuals in the CATIE schizophrenia trial. *Schizophrenia Research* 2005;80:1–8.

44. Moser DJ, Schultz SK, Arndt S, et al. Capacity to provide informed consent for participation in schizophrenia and HIV research. *American Journal of Psychiatry* 2002;159:1201–7.

45. Palmer BW, Dunn LB, Appelbaum PS, et al. Assessment of capacity to consent to research among older persons with schizophrenia, Alzheimer disease, or diabetes mellitus: Comparison of a 3-item questionnaire with a comprehensive standardized capacity instrument. *American Journal of Psychiatry* 2005;62:726–33.

46. Wirshing DA, Wirshing WC, Marder SR, Liberman RP, Mintz J. Informed consent: Assessment of comprehension. *American Journal of Psychiatry* 1998;155:1508–11.

47. Appelbaum PS, Grisso T, Frank E, O'Donnell S, Kupfer DJ. Competence of depressed patients for consent to research. *American Journal of Psychiatry* 1999;156:1380–4.

48. Lapid MI, Rummans TA, Poole KL, et al. Decisional capacity of severely depressed patients requiring electroconvulsive therapy. *Journal of ECT* 2003;19:67–72.

49. Moser DJ, Reese RL, Schultz SK, et al. Informed consent in medication-free schizophrenia research. *American Journal of Psychiatry* 2005;162:1209–11.

50. Lapid MI, Rummans TA, Pankratz VS, Appelbaum PS. Decisional capacity of depressed elderly to consent to electroconvulsive therapy. *Journal of Geriatric Psychiatry and Neurology* 2004;17:42–6.

51. Wirshing DA, Sergi MJ, Mintz J. A videotape intervention to enhance the informed consent process for medical and psychiatric treatment research. *American Journal of Psychiatry* 2005;162:186–8.

52. Stiles PG, Poythress NG, Hall A, Falkenbach D, Williams R. Improving understanding of research consent disclosures among persons with mental illness. *Psychiatric Services* 2001;52:780–5.

53. Sugarman J, Cain C, Wallace R, Welsh-Bohmer KA. How proxies make decisions about research for patients with Alzheimer's disease. *Journal of the American Geriatrics Society* 2001;49:1110–9.

54. Wendler D, Martinez RA, Fairclough D, Sunderland T, Emanuel E. Views of potential subjects toward proposed regulations for clinical research with adults unable to consent. *American Journal of Psychiatry* 2002;159:585–91.

55. Kim SY, Kim HM, McCallum C, Tariot PN. What do people at risk for Alzheimer disease think about surrogate consent for research? *Neurology* 2005;65:1395–1401.

56. Ferrand E, Bachoud-Levi AC, Rodrigues M, Maggiore S, Brun-Buisson C, Lemaire F. Decision-making capacity and surrogate designation in French ICU patients. *Intensive Care Medicine* 2001;27:1360–4.

57. Wendler D, Prasad K. Core safeguards for clinical research with adults who are unable to consent. *Annals of Internal Medicine* 2001;135:514–23.

58. Dresser R. Planning for future research participation: Ethical and practical considerations. *Accountability in Research* 1999;7:129–36.

59. DeRenzo E. Surrogate decision making for severely cognitively impaired research subjects: The continuing debate. *Cambridge Quarterly of Healthcare Ethics* 1994;3:539–48.

60. Silverman HJ, Druml C, Lemaire F, Nelson R. The European union directive and the protection of incapacitated subjects in research: An ethical analysis. *Intensive Care Medicine* 2004;30:1723–9.

61. Freedman B, Fuks A, Weijer C. In loco parentis: Minimal risk as an ethical threshold for research upon children. *Hastings Center Report* 1993;23(2):13–9.

62. Kopelman LM. Children as research subjects: A dilemma. *Journal of Medicine and Philosophy* 2000;25:745–64.

63. Dunn LB, Candilis PJ, Weiss Roberts L. Emerging empirical evidence on the ethics of schizophrenia research. *Schizophrenia Bulletin* 2006;32:47–68.

64. Sugarman J, McCrory DC, Hubal RC. Getting meaningful informed consent from older adults: A structured literature review of empirical research. *Journal of the American Geriatrics Society* 1998;46:517–24.

65. Rosenstein DL. IRB review of psychiatric medication discontinuation and symptom-provoking studies. *Biological Psychiatry* 1999;46:1039–43.

66. Fletcher JC, Dommel FW, Cowell DD. Consent to research with impaired human subjects: A trial policy for the intramural programs of the National Institutes of Health. *IRB: A Review of Human Subjects Research* 1985;7(6):1–6.

67. Candilis PJ, Wesley RW, Wichman A. A survey of researchers using a consent policy for cognitively impaired human research subjects. *IRB: A Review of Human Subjects Research* 1993;15(6):1–4.

68. Sunderland T, Dukoff R. Surrogate decision making and advance directives with cognitively impaired research subjects. In: Pincus HA, Lieberman JA, Ferris S, eds. *Ethics in Psychiatric Research*. Washington, D.C.: American Psychiatric Association; 1998:107–27.

69. Dukoff R, Sunderland T. Durable power of attorney and informed consent with Alzheimer's disease patients: A clinical study. *American Journal of Psychiatry* 1997;154:1070–5.

70. Fins JJ, Miller FG. Enrolling decisionally incapacitated subjects in neuropsychiatric research. *CNS Spectrums* 2000;5:32–42.

71. Rosenstein DL, Miller FG, Rubinow DR. A curriculum for teaching psychiatric research bioethics. *Biological Psychiatry* 2001;50:802–8.

72. Beresin EV, Baldessarini RJ, Alpert J, Rosenbaum J. Teaching ethics of psychopharmacology research in psychiatric residency training programs. *Psychopharmacology* 2003;171:105–11.

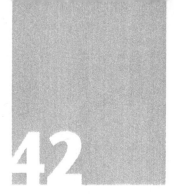

Alan R. Fleischman   Lauren K. Collogan

Research With Children

In the developed world, biomedical and public health research during the 20th century resulted in dramatic changes in maternal and infant mortality rates, the near eradication of infectious causes of death in childhood, and the conquering of many serious diseases affecting children. The development of vaccines to prevent diphtheria, polio, and measles; pharmacologic treatment regimens to change leukemia, other cancers, and human acquired immunodeficiency disease from uniformly fatal to chronic or even curable diseases; and the application of technology and molecular biology to the treatment of the consequences of profound prematurity are a few examples of the successes of scientific progress combined with clinical research involving children.

The great benefits of research involving children are tempered by concerns that children require added protection from the risks of research. Unlike adults, children cannot consent to place themselves at some level of risk with uncertain benefit in a research setting for the purpose of generating new knowledge that will likely help future children. Some commentators have questioned whether it is ever ethical to use children in research.[1,2] Most agree that we should be willing to place some children at risk for the sake of all children, but we must develop the necessary methods to protect those children who are enrolled in research so as not to place them at undue risk without compensating direct benefit. Research with animals, and research with adults and older children who can participate in the decision-making process should, when feasible, precede research with young children and infants. Yet the distinct aspects of childhood diseases, the need to consider the broad range of childhood growth and development, children's unique metabolism, and unexpected drug toxicities require that research be conducted with children in order to create the scientific and medical advances expected by society to enhance the health and well-being of children.

The history of research involving children reveals that the interests of child participants were not always protected and some children were exploited by researchers.[3,4] Since the 1970s, a system of regulation and supervision of research involving children has developed in the United States that allows advances in the understanding of the physical, psychological, and social growth and development of children and the pathophysiology and treatment of diseases and disorders that affect them, while protecting children from unnecessary and uncompensated risks and discomfort. The benefits to children of research advances and the need to study proposed and standard interventions and therapies in order to identify unanticipated harms make it imperative to have a system of research regulation that enables research involving children to go forward.

History of Research With Children

Medical research with children is not well documented prior to the 18th century and the development of pediatrics as a medical specialty. Although the history of medicine with children begins with references to specific childhood conditions in texts from ancient Egyptian, Greek, and Roman physicians, most of these references are observational in nature and do not explore the unique physiological status of children and adolescents.[3] Discussion of children and their medical conditions continued into medieval times, and some writing on the subject emerged, particularly after the introduction of printing in the 1400s. However, most of the pediatric writing until the late 1600s centered on observations, folklore, and suggestions based on informal trial and error. Infant mortality during these times was extremely high and considered unalterable.

The 17th century saw a rebirth of medicine, and physicians began to take a greater interest in children. Entire texts devoted to the treatment of childhood conditions began to appear, and European medical schools began to include instruction in pediatrics. The 17th century also saw the beginning of modern medical research, "the study of disease by the recording and correlating of clinical phenomena."[3] This type of formal clinical observation led to advances in medicine, including the introduction of inoculation for smallpox in the 18th century. Children, who were highly susceptible to smallpox, were among the first to be inoculated in England when members of the British royal family began having the procedure performed on their offspring. In 1796, Edward Jenner conducted his famous smallpox vaccination experiment using cowpox on an 8-year-old patient and other children in his village.[5] Jenner saw his work as highly beneficial, particularly to families, and although he discussed the risks with his subjects and attempted to minimize them, he did not seem troubled by the use of children in experimentation. Jenner's trials, as other early research with children, had its roots in a sincere desire to benefit society and help a group that had historically been ignored by medical practitioners.

Pediatric medicine became a recognized medical specialty in the 19th century, and medical societies in the United States and Europe began to form pediatric sections in the 1880s.[6] A growing interest in child health led to the creation of pediatric hospitals, which, along with orphanages, provided investigators with a ready population of children on whom to experiment.[7] These types of institutions often had rapid outbreaks of various communicable diseases, and their readily available populations made useful subjects for a growing number of investigations.[4] There was little concern about securing informed consent from children or their parents, and few objections within the medical community to research involving institutionalized children. Most saw the societal benefits of the research as outweighing the potential risks to subjects, particularly for institutionalized children whose risk of contracting a communicable disease was very high.

Research with children continued into the 20th century. As with earlier research, many of these U.S. studies focused on highly communicable diseases that spread rapidly in institutions, such as smallpox, molluscum contagiosum, tuberculosis, pertussis, measles, and polio.[8–13] Other studies examined new diagnostic techniques such as spinal taps or looked at child physiology such as stomach emptying in an attempt to understand differences between children and adults.[14,15] However, in contrast to Jenner, investigators during the early 1900s rarely discussed the risks or discomfort associated with the research, and rarely mentioned any ethical concerns about using children in research. Furthermore, the subjects in these studies were often poor or abandoned children who were provided to researchers by doctors working in orphanages and asylums, and these studies contain no mention of obtaining consent.

Although most medical professionals did not voice objection to the use of children in research, the antivivisectionist movement, which had long protested the use of animals in medical research, objected to the use of children in research beginning in the late 19th century. Antivivisectionists opposed the "research imperative" and "experiments on live animals" or on children.[16] These protests included journals devoted to citing research cruelties and pamphlets arguing against research involving children. The protests prompted some lawmakers to propose antivivisection bills that attempted to formally regulate or ban research with live animals and with children.

As the 20th century progressed, protests against research with children remained confined to antivivisectionists, and research continued mostly unobserved and unhindered. Some investigators were concerned with safety and attempted to obtain prior consent from subjects, but investigators were rarely criticized for experiments that put children at undue risk.[17] The advent of World War II and concern over injury and illness among soldiers overseas created an urgent need for medical research, and the number of research studies in the United States dramatically increased.

Moving Toward Research Regulation

Numerous medical experiments were conducted on humans by Nazi doctors in concentration camps during World War II (see Chapter 2). Many of these experiments had dubious, if any, scientific bases, and experimenters made no attempt to solicit consent or to explain the purpose of the studies. Many of these experiments resulted in tremendous suffering, disability, and death. Children were not exempt from experimentation; indeed, some Nazi physicians specifically sought children for studies. Josef Mengele, a Nazi doctor and scientist, tortured and murdered numerous children in the name of science.[18] For example, in "germ warfare" experiments, one child, a twin, would be injected with bacteria, become deathly ill and be allowed to die, and the healthy twin would be killed in order to examine differences between organs of the two children. These children, like all of the prisoners who were experimented upon, had no way of knowing that they were being used as guinea pigs, nor could they refuse participation.

Nuremberg Code

After the liberation of the concentration camps and the end of the war, 23 of the physicians and Nazi officials who had performed experiments were brought to trial at Nuremberg. The U.S. judges at the trial issued the Nuremberg Code, a list of 10 governing principles to guide medical experimentation with humans (see Chapter 12). The Code was intended to be a universal statement to ensure the ethical conduct of research and was adopted by the judges due to a lack of commonly accepted practices in this area. In addition to mandating sound scientific experimental methods and appropriate risk-to-benefit ratios, the Code required the voluntary consent of every person who participated in research. It insisted that the "voluntary consent of the human subject is absolutely essential" and that consent was valid only if the person giving it had the legal capacity to do so.[19] This requirement would have effectively prohibited any research with children, as well as with other incapacitated individuals, such as those with mental illness or physical ailments that affect capacity to consent, and it was largely ignored in the United States. Not only did Americans view Nazi doctors and the situation of the Holocaust as removed from the reality of medicine and experimentation in the United States, but to adhere to the Code would have meant ending all ongoing research with children.[20] Accordingly, research with children continued in the United States without any real attempts at regulation for the next 20 years.

Declaration of Helsinki

In the early 1960s, the World Medical Association (WMA) set about to create and promulgate a universal set of professional guidelines to aid investigators in conducting ethically sound research. Given the largely indifferent response to the Nuremberg Code and its prohibition of research with children, these guidelines were created by physicians for physicians and would help the progress of research as it sought to standardize its practices. The result of the WMA's work was the Declaration of Helsinki, which first appeared in 1964 and has since undergone many revisions, most recently in 2000 (see Chapter 13). Key in the Declaration was the distinction between therapeutic research (research combined with medical care) and nontherapeutic research (research performed on healthy individuals to gain generalizable knowledge).[21] Furthermore, the final, adopted version of the Declaration allowed for both types of research to be performed using minors, provided that consent was obtained from the minor's representative and assent was obtained from the minor him- or herself whenever appropriate. Thus, the Declaration was far more tolerant of research with children than the Nuremberg Code, and was widely supported, particularly by researchers in the United States. However, though the Declaration was an influential document, particularly in that it was internationally recognized, there were still no regulations to govern research with humans in the United States.

Evolution of U.S. Federal Regulations on Research With Children

Although research involving children continued without formal regulation in the United States even after the adoption of the Declaration of Helsinki, there was a growing awareness among professionals, government agencies, and members of the public that some form of research oversight was needed. After it was discovered that the use of the experimental drug thalidomide by pregnant women caused severe birth defects, the Food and Drug Administration (FDA) mandated in 1962 that experimental drugs be tested in standardized trials using formal consent procedures.[22] In 1963, the director of the National Institutes of Health (NIH) created a committee to examine research under the auspices of the NIH to study problems of consent and unethical practices in research protocols. This committee developed several proposals for consideration by the U.S. Public Health Service (PHS) that resulted, in 1966, in a memorandum from the U.S. Surgeon General, William H. Stewart, to all institutions receiving federal funds. The memorandum stated that no research involving humans would be funded by the PHS unless the grantee had indicated that the grantee institution had provided prior review by a committee of "institutional associates" to assure an independent determination of the rights and welfare of the research participants, the appropriateness of the methods used to secure informed consent, and the risks and potential benefits of the investigation.[23]

Willowbrook and Tuskegee

Two studies exposed in the early 1970s made the public aware of questionable research practices and instigated the creation of government research regulations. Studies on the transmission of hepatitis in institutionalized children were conducted over a number of years at the Willowbrook State School, a large hospital for mentally disabled children in Staten Island, New York. Hepatitis was endemic at Willowbrook, and investigators were working to find a way to prevent its spread, much as scientists had done for centuries in other institutions.[24] This research program was criticized when published studies indicated that children at the institution had been deliberately infected with hepatitis virus as a means of studying the potential to develop a vaccine for the disease.[25] The investigators defended their work and argued that exposing children to hepatitis while following a protocol and keeping them in a special hepatitis unit entailed "less risk than the type of institutional exposure where multiple infections could occur."[26] Although permission of the children's parents had been solicited, critics argued that deliberately infecting healthy children was mere exploitation of an institutionalized population[27] (see Chapter 7).

The Tuskegee Syphilis Study was funded in 1932 by the U.S. PHS as a natural history study of the progression of syphilis in 400 black men in Alabama. Although the Tuskegee study did not include children, its exposure focused attention on the potential for exploitation of vulnerable populations in the context of research. The study was not a secret in the medical community or to the government sponsors; over the years, several papers were published with updated results and observations.[28–30] However, in 1972, when a reporter for the Associated Press wrote an exposé documenting the study, there was a great deal of public criticism[31,32] (see Chapter 8).

These two studies and the resultant public outcry prompted an examination of the problem of research abuses and creation of standards for the protection of research participants. The Department of Health, Education and Welfare (DHEW)—now the Department of Health and Human Services, DHHS—implemented the *Institutional Guide to DHEW Policy,* which was more detailed than previous NIH/PHS policies and highlighted "at-risk" research populations, including children. The FDA applied the new DHEW policy to research protocols for new drugs, and in 1974, Congress strengthened the DHEW policy and required institutional review of any protocol under DHEW purview.[33]

Paul Ramsey and Richard McCormick

In addition to the general public's concern about research practices, there was a vigorous debate in the 1970s among health-care providers, researchers, and ethicists about the morality of involving children in research. Paul Ramsey, a Protestant theologian, wrote that research involving children was only justified if it furthered the medical interests of that child.[34] He argued that research without the potential for benefit should never be performed without the informed consent of the subject. Richard McCormick, a Catholic theologian, argued on the other hand that research with children was necessary to improve the health and well-being of children and that parental consent was sufficient to protect the interests of individual children exposed to research risks even without compensating benefits.[35]

McCormick argued further that individuals, even infants, ought to value human life and the health of others. If they were able to make informed decisions, he asserted, children would most likely choose to participate in experiments that held the potential of contributing to knowledge, provided that the risks to themselves were not too great. Thus, he maintained that parents and guardians, in the interest of serving what would be the choices of their children, should be able to consent to the participation of their children in research. McCormick and others, including William Bartholome—a leading figure in the development of pediatric research ethics, for whom the American Academy of Pediatrics has named an annual award—believed that parents not only should be allowed to consent to research involving their children because of the future benefits to children in general, but should contribute to their children's moral development by consenting to their participation in research without the prospect of benefit, as an altruistic gesture to society.[36]

Ramsey vehemently disagreed with McCormick's arguments and maintained that to enroll children in research because they "ought" to help others was to impose adult morality on a population that lacked the capacity to make such decisions.[37] He maintained that being involved in research could not contribute to the moral growth of children because their participation was unconscious and unwilled. He argued that any nontherapeutic research participation by those persons unable to provide consent, no matter how small the potential risk, was ethically untenable.

The U.S. National Commission

As a result of substantial public concern about the research enterprise, Congress passed legislation in 1974 to create the National Commission for the Protection of Subjects of Biomedical and Behavioral Research (hereafter, the National Commission) to make recommendations about how research should be regulated in the United States. Research involving children was among the most pressing concerns of the National Commission.

The Belmont Report—perhaps the most respected explication of the principles of research ethics ever published in the United States—was published by the National Commission in 1979 and laid out a broad justification of research involving children (see Chapter 14). The report states the following: "Effective ways of treating childhood diseases and fostering healthy development are benefits that serve to justify research involving children—even when individual research subjects are not beneficiaries."[38] The report goes on to mention another justification for research involving children: "Research also makes it possible to avoid the harm that may result from the application of previously accepted routine practices that on closer investigation turn out to be dangerous." However, the report is quite clear in describing children as potentially vulnerable and in need of protection from undue influence and coercion. Concerning this issue, in defining the principle of respect for persons, the report incorporates two ethical convictions: first, that individuals should be treated as autonomous agents, and second, that persons with diminished autonomy are entitled to protection. Children, unable to consent for their own participation in research, are entitled to protection. Invoking the authority of parents as surrogate decision makers is seen as only one aspect of that protection. Careful scrutiny of the level of risk to which child participants might be exposed in the research context, and minimizing risks in research whenever possible, were two additional protective approaches described in the report.

The National Commission released *Research Involving Children,* its report that examined the ethical aspects of research with children, in 1977. The commissioners noted that the most pressing concern about involving children in research is their "reduced

autonomy" and "incompetency to give informed consent," leaving them vulnerable and unable to protect themselves against unscrupulous research practices.[39] The National Commission's support of research involving children was based on the fact that in many instances, there is no suitable alternative population of research participants. Additionally, the prohibition of such research would impede innovative efforts to develop new treatments for diseases that affect children, decrease knowledge of the antecedents of adult disease, and result in the introduction of practices in the treatment of childhood diseases without the benefit of research or evaluation.

The report defines children as "persons who have not attained the legal age of consent to general medical care as determined under the applicable law of the jurisdiction in which the research will be conducted." Such a definition recognizes the local implementation of federal guidelines or regulations and implies that the recommendations made in the report would vary in their applicability, depending on local and state laws. The definition also focuses on ability to consent as a distinguishing factor between children and adults, one that is not dependent on chronologic age. The definition exempts individuals who might be younger than a designated "age of majority" from the recommended protective restrictions, depending on applicable local statutes regarding consent for medical treatment.

The National Commission directly addressed Ramsey's arguments against allowing research with children that has no therapeutic intent and rejected his views as overly restrictive and unnecessary to protect the rights and interests of children. The Commission did, however, recommend specific limitations on research with children, requiring that a local institutional review board (IRB) determine that:

A. The research is scientifically sound and significant.
B. Where appropriate, studies have been conducted first on animals and adult humans, then on older children, prior to involving infants.
C. Risks are minimized by using the safest procedures consistent with sound research design and by using procedures performed for diagnostic or treatment purposes whenever feasible.
D. Adequate provisions are made to protect the privacy of children and their parents, and to maintain confidentiality of the data
E. Subjects will be selected in an equitable manner, and
F. The conditions of all applicable subsequent recommendations are met.[39]

Subsequent recommendations include discussions of permissible levels of risk, the balancing of risks and potential benefits, the role of parental permission and child assent, and the involvement in research of children who are institutionalized or wards of the state.

U.S. Federal Regulations Regarding Research With Children

In 1981 Congress adopted the DHHS Policy for Protection of Human Research Subjects, regulations that were revised in 1991 and now referred to as the Common Rule and codified at 45 CFR 46.[40] The regulations require institutional review of all research with humans as well as voluntary informed consent from research participants or their guardians. This chapter will focus on the special protections afforded to children that were adopted in 1983 as subpart D of the regulations, titled Additional Protections for Children Involved as Subjects in Research (codified at 45 CFR 46.401–409),[40] and those adopted as subpart B, titled Additional Protections for Pregnant Women, Human Fetuses and Neonates Involved in Research, revised in 2001 (codified at 45 CFR 46.201–207).[40]

The regulations in subpart D have also been adopted (with one notable exception concerning waiver of parental permission) by the FDA for application to clinical drug trials.[41,42] The National Commission's report, *Research Involving Children,* had a significant impact on the creation of this part of the regulations. Much like the National Commission's Belmont Report, subpart D, at 45 CFR 46.402(a), defines children as "persons who have not attained the legal age for consent to treatments or procedures involved in the research, under the applicable law of the jurisdiction in which the research will be conducted."[40] This definition has significance particularly for adolescents, who in many jurisdictions may consent for clinical care and treatment for sexually transmitted diseases, pregnancy and its prevention, and mental health services. Although permitting adolescents to give such consent is somewhat controversial and not universally applied, when local statutes permit, IRBs may consider research on these issues involving adolescents to be reviewed as if the prospective participants were not children but rather autonomous adults who may consent for participation in research without parental involvement. Forgoing parental permission is not permitted in research regulated by the FDA. The general issue of consent in adolescents will be discussed later in the chapter.

Over the past several years, there has been increased recognition of the need for more pediatric research. Health-care decisions for children are often based on extrapolation from adult data because limited evidence exists regarding treatment of children.[43] Recent policy and regulatory changes have encouraged the involvement of children in research. The Food and Drug Administration Modernization Act of 1997 created pediatric exclusivity incentives, allowing the FDA and the NIH to encourage companies to perform more pediatric clinical trials of drugs that may provide health benefits to children.[44] In 1998, the NIH published guidelines requiring the inclusion of children in clinical research unless there were scientific or ethical reasons to exclude them.[45] In 2002, the U.S. Best Pharmaceuticals for Children Act reauthorized the pediatric studies provisions of the Food and Drug Modernization Act, and directed the National Cancer Institute to expand and intensify research on treatments for pediatric cancers.[46] The Pediatric Research Equity Act of 2003 requires research on pediatric uses of new drugs and biological products.[47] In 2006, the European Union Parliament and Council adopted a regulation on medicines for children that creates a pediatric committee, extends patent protection for pharmaceutical companies, and requires companies to present a "pediatric investigation plan," among other things.[48,49] All of these initiatives have resulted in an expanding number of pediatric studies and in studies that include children. None of these initiatives to increase research involving children include any provisions to decrease the strong protections that exist for children participating in research. Nevertheless, with the expansion of pediatric research comes a greater need to ensure that programs and activities that protect the rights and safety of children enrolled in research are performing well.

The federal regulations create four categories of permissible research involving children. First, research is permitted if the level of risk is no greater than minimal, regardless of whether there is the prospect of direct benefit to the child. Second, research that holds out the prospect of direct benefit to individual subjects is permitted as long as the risks are minimized and justified by the level of anticipated benefit. Third, research is permitted even if it involves greater than minimal risk and no prospect of direct benefit to individual children, provided that the level of risk is a minor increase over minimal, the intervention or procedure presents experiences to subjects that are commensurate with actual or expected medical, dental, psychological, social, or educational situations, and the research is likely to yield generalizable information of vital importance about the subjects' disorder or condition. Fourth, research that is not otherwise approvable under the first three categories but presents an opportunity to understand, prevent, or alleviate a serious problem affecting the health or welfare of children may be permitted by the secretary of the DHHS after expert consultation and opportunity for public review. This regulatory framework imposes a significant limit on the discretion of investigators and parents to permit the participation of children in research that entails more than minimal risk, but at the same time it allows much research of importance to the health and well-being of children. Each of these categories requires interpretation of various terms and requirements. Figure 42.1 depicts Robert Nelson's algorithm that is useful in applying the regulations and understanding the components of each category.[50]

Research Not Involving Greater Than Minimal Risk (45 CFR 46.404)

According to 45 CFR 46.102 of the regulations, a risk is considered *minimal* if "the probability and magnitude of harm or discomfort anticipated in the research are not greater in and of themselves than those ordinarily encountered in daily life or during the performance of routine physical or psychological examinations or tests."[40] This definition has been controversial and open to differing interpretations since its adoption over 20 years ago. A study of pediatric researchers and department chairs in 1981 revealed broad disagreement on the level of risk represented by common procedures performed in pediatric practice.[51] A more recent survey of IRB chairs confirmed the continued lack of agreement on this fundamental definition and revealed wide variation in perceived risk levels of such research procedures as confidential surveys and simple blood draws.[52]

Several commentators have criticized the definition for its use of comparisons to the risks encountered in daily life.[53,54] Clearly, there is a wide range of socially acceptable behaviors that normal, healthy children encounter in their daily lives that are quite risky. These include traveling in cars and buses, bicycle and horseback riding, and playing sports. Few researchers or IRBs have been confused by the intention of the regulations even if the words allow for misinterpretation. For a procedure to be considered minimal risk, it must have an exceedingly low likelihood of significant or sustained discomfort, irreversible harm, or substantial embarrassment.

Recent reports by two federal advisory committees to the secretary of the DHHS[55,56] and the Institute of Medicine (IOM)[57] have attempted to clarify the definition of minimal risk. These reports concur that minimal risk should be an objective standard,

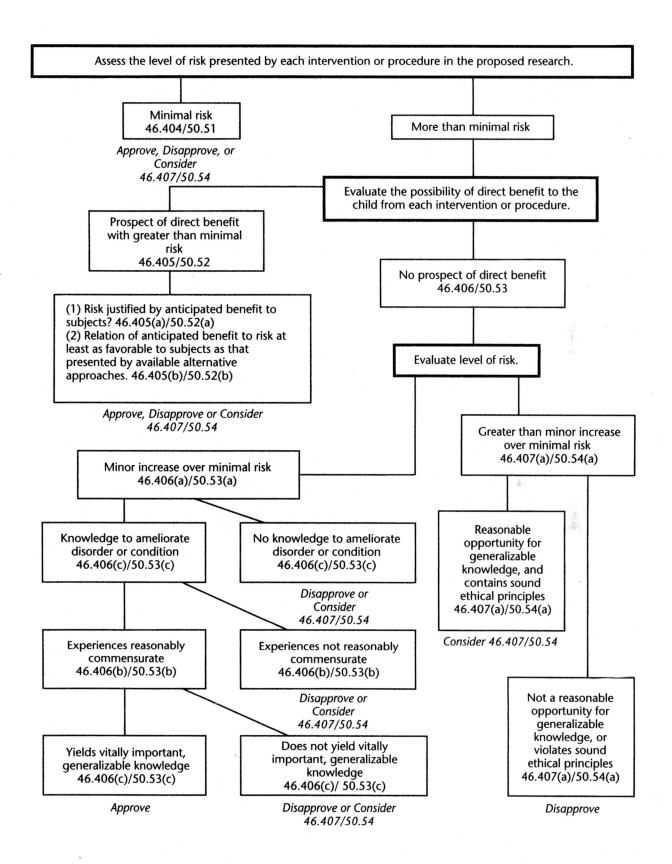

Figure 42.1. Algorithm for Making Assessments of Research Protocols as Required by 45 CFR 46.404–407 and 21 CFR 50.51–54.[50]

that is, related neither to the level of illness of the child not to the social circumstances in which the child finds him- or herself. Risks should include all harms, discomforts, indignities, embarrassments, and potential breaches of privacy and confidentiality associated with the research, and minimal risk should be that level of risk associated with the daily activities of a normal, healthy, average child. Indexing the definition of minimal risk to the lives of healthy, average children eliminates considering those higher risks that are routinely experienced by sick children or children exposed on a daily basis to greater risks because of social circumstances.

This definition does, however, allow the concept of minimal risk to take into account the changing risks normally experienced by children of different ages. The daily risks encountered in the life of an infant or toddler who is rarely, if ever, left unattended by an adult differ dramatically from the risks encountered by an adolescent who attends school, might drive, plays sports, and engages in many independent activities. Thus, research that might be considered to pose greater than minimal risk for a younger child might be consistent with the risks ordinarily encountered in the daily lives of an older child and thus might be considered minimal risk for that population.

The definition of minimal risk also includes those experiences encountered by normal, healthy, average children in routine physical and psychological examinations such as during routine visits to the doctor or dentist, or routine psychological testing and observations in school. This allows research procedures such as simple blood draws, noninvasive urine collections, questionnaires, and interviews with healthy children to be permissible as minimal risk under this section of the regulations. However, when procedures performed once are deemed to be consistent with the definition of minimal risk, the same procedure performed serially or repetitively over a short period may or may not still constitute minimal risk.

The definition of minimal risk need not be interpreted literally as only those risks encountered in the actual daily lives of children or during their visits to a doctor's office, but may include risks thought to be *equivalent* to those routinely encountered in the daily lives and experiences of normal, healthy, average children. What research procedures fit into this interpretation of the definition is left to individual IRBs.

Prospect of Direct Benefit to Individual Subjects (45 CFR 46.405)

IRBs may approve research that entails more than minimal risk to a child if the intervention or procedure holds out the prospect of direct benefit for the child or may contribute to that child's well-being. Any risks must be justified by the anticipated benefits, and the relation of the anticipated benefit to the risk must be at least as favorable to the child as that presented by alternative available approaches.[40] Most clinical trials fall under this category of research. Many such research studies are targeted to benefit participants afflicted with serious diseases while exposing the participants to a substantial level of risk. This is the crucial balancing required of IRBs. When determining whether a research proposal offers the prospect of direct benefit to individual participants, IRBs should ensure that the benefits accrued are from the research interventions themselves and not from the collateral benefits often associated with participation in research. Furthermore, the provision of standard clinical care not otherwise available to individ-

uals, or monetary compensation for research participation, should, in and of itself, not be considered benefits that warrant exposing participants to risks greater than minimal.

Each procedure in a study, if greater than minimal risk, must be evaluated independently to assure that there is a prospect of direct benefit to the participant from that procedure. If a specific risky procedure (e.g., bone marrow aspirate, spinal tap, imaging with sedation) has no potential to benefit the participant and is performed only to collect data that is not of clinical relevance, the IRB may not approve that portion of the research based on the regulatory standards of 45 CFR 46.405—the category of "prospect of direct benefit" research. Such a procedure might be considered and possibly approved under the standards of 45 CFR 46.406—the category of "minor increase over minimal risk" research.

When assessing the risks imposed by research participation, it is also important to distinguish between those risks associated with research interventions or procedures and risks inherent in standard diagnostic approaches and treatments of disease.[58] To assist in defining the incremental risks of the research itself and determining whether the risks to children of research participation are reasonable in relation to anticipated benefits, IRBs can do a component analysis. Through component analysis, the IRB examines each procedure and intervention to determine the prospect of benefit, level of risk and whether the risks have been sufficiently minimized. This approach can help define incremental risk and assist IRBs to fulfill their obligations to protect children who are the participants in research.[59]

Research Involving Greater Than Minimal Risk and No Prospect of Direct Benefit to Individual Subjects (45 CFR 46.406)

Research that involves greater than minimal risk to children with no prospect of direct benefit is permissible only under certain conditions. The research must involve risk that is only a minor increase over minimal risk; the intervention or procedure must present experiences to the children that are reasonably commensurate with those inherent in their actual or expected medical, dental, psychological, social, or educational situations; and the research must be likely to yield generalizable knowledge about the child's disorder or condition that is of vital importance for the understanding or amelioration of that disorder or condition.

The concept of a *minor increase over minimal risk* is contingent upon the interpretation of the definition of minimal risk. The level of risk contemplated by the regulations as a minor increase over minimal risk is a small increment over that level of risk experienced by normal, healthy, average children in their daily lives and experiences. It is not intended that a minor increase over minimal risk be defined as the level of risk generally experienced by children who are ill or in socially compromised circumstances. In addition, it is the role of the investigator to make the case and the role of the IRB to review the evidence that research proposed under this category meets the standard of providing generalizable information of vital importance and that the procedures are reasonably commensurate with the prior or expected experiences of the potential research participants.

The definition of *disorder or condition* also requires interpretation, and there is some disagreement. In our view, a condition affecting children should be understood more broadly than a specific disease or diagnostic category; it refers to a specific set of physical, psychological, neurodevelopmental, or social characteristics that have been shown to affect children's health and well-being or their risk of developing a health problem in the future. This definition of *condition* can include a genetic or familial predisposition to future illness or even a social circumstance that has been linked to a potential deficit in future health and well-being, as long as the investigator can substantiate that there is an established body of scientific evidence or clinical knowledge to support that association.

Research Not Otherwise Approvable That Presents an Opportunity to Understand, Prevent, or Alleviate a Serious Problem Affecting the Health and Welfare of Children (45 CFR 46.407)

The regulations are intended to limit research that involves significant risks without compensating benefit to individual children. However, the regulations create a process for review of credible research that may not be approved at the local level under the three categories outlined above but has the potential to significantly affect child health and welfare. An IRB may determine that a proposed study may not be approved under the minimal risk (45 CFR 46.404), prospect of direct benefit (45 CFR 46.405), or minor increase over minimal risk (45 CFR 46.406) categories, yet find that the research has a reasonable opportunity to further the understanding, prevention, or alleviation of a serious problem affecting the health or welfare of children. The IRB may then send the proposal to the DHHS Office for Human Research Protections (OHRP) and request review and approval by the secretary of the DHHS. The secretary must consult with a panel of experts and assure public review and comment before determining whether the research should be permitted to proceed. This procedure has been used sparingly in the past and more frequently in recent years; an efficient process has been developed to facilitate timely review.[60]

Minimizing Risk

According to 45 CFR 46.111(a)(1), it is the duty of the investigator and the IRB to ensure that risks are minimized in all research.[40] This is particularly relevant to research involving children. Even in research studies that involve minimal risk or a minor increase over minimal risk, every attempt should be made to minimize risk. Research procedures should be integrated with clinical care and diagnostic procedures whenever feasible in order not to duplicate uncomfortable procedures and interventions. Procedures should only be performed by professionals skilled with children. Protocols should include specific rules setting limits on the number of unsuccessful attempts at a procedure or the length of time for completion of a questionnaire. And appropriate methods should be used to accustom children to the research environment and to decrease potential anxiety and discomfort whenever possible.

In determining whether a proposed procedure has minimized risks, the IRB should take into consideration the context in which the research will be performed. The population under study, the experience of the investigator and the professionals performing the procedures, as well as the research environment, may influence the level of risk of each proposed procedure. Some groups of children may perceive certain interventions or procedures as involving more risk, anxiety, or discomfort as compared to other groups. For example, children who are mentally challenged, emotionally disturbed, or mentally ill may experience a simple procedure, such as a blood draw, as extraordinarily disconcerting. Because of their likely reaction, a blood test with such children might be considered more than minimal risk research, unless efforts could be made to ameliorate their distress.

Examples of Risk Levels Associated With Common Research Procedures

Table 42.1, reproduced from the final report of the National Human Research Protections Advisory Committee, aims to clarify specific portions of subpart D of the federal regulations and provide some examples of the level of risk of common research procedures.[55]

The National Human Research Protections Advisory Committee report also highlights the importance of several factors that go into interpreting the level of risk in common procedures. For example, the level of risk of the insertion of an intravenous catheter or an injection may be considered minimal, but the risk level may increase based on the length of time the needle will remain in place, the substance being injected or infused, the age and cognitive capacity of the child, and the experience of the investigator performing the procedure. Another common research procedure, an MRI imaging test, may be minimal risk if no sedation is required for the procedure, but the level of risk increases if procedural sedation or general anesthesia is required in order to perform the test.

Parental Permission and Child Assent (45 CFR 46.408)

Informed consent remains the cornerstone of protection for humans in research, even when the research participant is a child. However, because children are generally not capable of providing informed consent, the process of obtaining consent for children is best thought of as parental permission with child assent sought as appropriate.[61] Parental permission is required, except in specific circumstances, for all research involving children. An IRB may determine that permission of one parent is sufficient for research approvable under 46.404, involving minimal risk, or under 46.405, providing the prospect of direct benefit to the individual child. However, the permission of both parents is required when research is approved under 46.406, involving a minor increase over minimal risk and no prospect of direct benefit, or when the research requires the approval of the DHHS secretary under 46.407. Exceptions include when one parent is deceased, unknown, incompetent, or not readily available, or when only one parent has legal responsibility for the care and custody of the child.

Waiver of parental permission may be approved in circumstances similar to the waiver of informed consent for adult participants in research found at 45 CFR 46.116(c)-(d).[40] These circumstances include research conducted by local governments to evaluate public benefit or service programs, or research that involves no more than minimal risk and that could not practicably be carried out without the waiver. In this circumstance, the waiver must not adversely affect the rights and welfare of the children, and whenever appropriate, the children or their parents

Table 42.1
Common Research Procedures by Category of Risk[55]

| | Category of Risk | | |
Procedure	Minimal	Minor Increase Over Minimal	More Than a Minor Increase Over Minimal
Routine history taking	X		
Venipuncture/fingerstick/heelstick	X		
Urine collection via bag	X		
Urine collection via catheter		X	
Urine collection via suprapubic tap			X
Chest X-ray	X		
Bone density test	X		
Wrist X-ray for bone age	X		
Lumbar puncture		X	
Collection of saliva	X		
Collection of small sample of hair	X		
Vision test	X		
Hearing test	X		
Complete neurological exam	X		
Oral glucose tolerance test	X		
Skin punch biopsy with topical pain relief		X	
Bone marrow aspirate with topical pain relief		X	
Organ biopsy			X
Standard psychological tests	X		
Classroom observation	X		

Note: The category of risk is for a single procedure. Multiple or repetitive procedures are likely to affect the level of risk.

should be provided with additional pertinent information after participation.

There are additional circumstances that may permit waiver of parental permission. Although it is generally beneficial to include parents in decisions about the care of their children, there are situations in which involving parents in the medical care of their child may be detrimental to the child's best interest.[39] This has been recognized by laws in virtually every state that permit medical treatment for specific conditions in adolescents (such as sexually transmitted disease, mental illness, and pregnancy) with the consent of the young person and without informing parents.[62] Waiving parental involvement in consent can be appropriate in the research context as well. Federal regulations, at 45 CFR 46.408(c), permit IRBs to waive parental involvement in research when "parental or guardian permission is not a reasonable requirement to protect the subjects."[40] This could permit waiver of parental permission in research involving child abuse or neglect or when adolescents might be hurt by revealing certain behaviors or illnesses to their parents. In each case the IRB must ensure that the investigator will both assess the capacity of the adolescent to understand the research and his or her research rights and has created appropriate procedural safeguards (such as the availability of a counselor independent of the research) to protect the interests of the adolescent participants. At present, parental permission may not be waived in any research regulated by the FDA.

In addition to obtaining parental permission, researchers working with children must also solicit the child's assent when appropriate. Assent is defined at 45 CFR 46.402(b) as "a child's affirmative agreement to participate in research."[40] IRBs must take into account the age, maturity, and psychological state of the children involved in the research when determining whether assent will be required or can be waived. IRB practices vary widely in the interpretation of the regulations concerning assent.[63] If a child does not provide affirmative agreement or fails to respond, assent cannot be assumed. Not all children, especially those who are very young, are able to provide assent. IRBs may determine that all children in a particular protocol must assent to participate; that children above a certain age (such as 7) must assent; or that each child must be assessed individually for the capacity to provide assent. Such individualized decisions are left to the IRB. Assent is not required if the research intervention or procedure involved holds out the prospect of direct benefit that is important to the health or well-being of the participants and is available only in the context of the research. Assent from children may be waived by IRBs just as informed consent may be waived for adults.

The assent process must be age- and developmentally appropriate and should be an empowering and respectful experience. It does not directly parallel the informed consent process for adults, and there is no need to duplicate all the essential elements required in adult informed consent during the assent process.[57] Obtaining assent from children includes making them aware of their condition (when appropriate), informing them about what will happen and what to expect, assessing their ability to understand their situation, and asking them whether or not they are willing to take part in the research.[64] Assent need not include a written form or a signature. The assent process should describe what will happen from the perspective of the child and what discomforts might be involved in the research. Of course, as children become older, assent information should become more substantive and specific and should begin to resemble an adult informed consent.

In the case of research that provides the prospect of direct benefit available only in the context of the research, assent is not a requirement. In such cases, children should still be informed about the research but they should not be asked for their assent if lack of affirmative agreement to participate will not be respected. It is disrespectful of children to ignore their preferences after they have been solicited. This can result in lack of trust in the research enterprise and significant tension among the parents, children, and investigators.

Wards (45 CFR 46.409)

The final section of subpart D concerns research with children who are wards. There is no definition of wards in the regulations, but it is taken to mean children who do not have a parent or legal guardian from whom to obtain permission for enrollment in the research. Such children may be institutionalized or in foster care. The regulations permit wards to be enrolled in research that involves no greater than minimal risk or has the prospect of direct benefit without additional protections. However, according to 45 CFR 46.409(a), research that involves a minor increase over minimal risk with no prospect of direct benefit, or research approved by the secretary of DHHS, may be conducted with wards only if the research is related to the child's status as a ward or is to be "conducted in schools, camps, hospitals, institutions, or similar settings in which the majority of children involved as subjects are not wards."[40] Such research also requires the appointment of an advocate to act in the child's best interests during the child's participation in the research. The advocate may not be associated with the research, the investigators, or the institution legally responsible for the child.

Incentives, Compensation, and Payment

Compensation of pediatric research participants and their families has long been a controversial issue.[65] Federal regulations regarding the protection of humans in research do not explicitly mention compensation and payments related to participation in research studies. However, investigators often believe that financial inducements are essential to enhance recruitment and retention, particularly in studies that provide no benefit to participants. Some commentators believe that children should never be paid for research participation because this may be an undue inducement that affects the voluntariness of their participation.[66] Similarly, some commentators argue that parents ought not to be paid to enroll their children in research, for fear that children will be used as commodities and placed at undue risk for the sake of parental financial gain. A survey of factors that influenced parental views on enrollment of their children in clinical studies in one U.S. city found that financial factors had some influence on parental judgment about participation, even if it was not one of the most important factors in the decision.[67]

The basic concern is to balance the need to make participation in studies attractive to children and their parents, particularly when there is no prospect of individual benefit, with the desire to protect children from the potential risks of research and to ensure that parents remain free of inappropriate influences on their decisions about the interests of their children.[57] Compensation of participants and their parents may be considered in two general categories: reimbursement of incremental costs of participation in the research, and inducements to participate.

It seems unfair to ask parents and children to bear additional costs that result from participation in research. Reimbursement for expenses directly related to research participation such as travel, parking, meals, and child care seem warranted and can be calculated based on real out-of-pocket costs to the families or based on a reasonable estimate of average costs. Payment of lost wages for the older child and parent as a result of participation in the research is sometimes considered a reasonable reimbursement, because lost wages will undoubtedly be a substantial disincentive to participation. However, determining a fair level of reimbursement in this area can be difficult and should not exceed the actual lost income due to participation.

There are three types of inducements to participate: compensation for time spent in participation; enticements for recruitment and retention; and gifts of appreciation at the completion of the study. It is generally agreed that individuals who participate in research with the major motivation of benefiting others with no prospect of direct benefit to themselves may receive some additional incentive for participation. A small token gift to the child as a "thank you" for participation in research is common in such settings. Because larger gifts to the parent or child may unduly influence participation, it seems acceptable only to vary the value of the gift based on the length of time required by the research, not based on the level of risk. A modest incentive for each activity in a study is a common practice but may become an undue inducement if the cumulative amount is excessive and able to influence voluntary participation.

The OHRP's *IRB Guidebook* discusses IRB responsibilities in assuring that consent is truly voluntary, uncoerced, and not unduly influenced by external factors, including payment.[68] In some of its review and criticism of institutional compliance with federal regulations, OHRP has argued that enrollment procedures should minimize the possibility of undue influence and that IRBs must recognize the provision of free care as a potential undue influence on voluntary participation. However, there is little specific guidance about providing payment or free care in research involving children.

The FDA has specific guidelines for review of compensation in the case of clinical drug trials.[69] The FDA requires that IRBs review and approve all amounts, methods, and timing of payments to research participants to assure that there is no coercion or undue influence on participation. Additionally, any credit for payment should accrue as the study progresses and not be contingent upon the person completing the entire study. However, a reasonable bonus for the completion of the study is acceptable as long as the IRB determines that the amount is not so large as to unduly induce people to stay in the study when they would otherwise have withdrawn. The American Academy of Pediatrics suggests that if remuneration is to be given directly to the child in the research, it is best if it is not discussed until after the study so as not to affect voluntary participation.[64] The Academy also states that medical costs associated with treatment under a research protocol may be permitted in certain circumstances. Because health-care insurance is not available to all children, this practice may be coercive and an undue influence on participation for children living in poverty. But in some circumstances, when the research requires the provision of specific care, provision of medical costs may be warranted. The potential of this type of compensation to unduly influence poor and uninsured families to be part of research studies must be considered by the IRB in its deliberations.

Compensation for Injury

Section 45 CFR 46.116(a)(6) of the U.S. federal regulations require that for research involving more than minimal risk, informed consent include a statement concerning whether any compensation or medical treatment will be available if injury occurs as part of the research, and stating where further information about such compensation may be obtained.[40] No federal law or regulation requires or provides compensation for research-related injury. Most research involving children does not offer compensation for nonnegligent injury that might occur during a research study. Although this issue is not unique to child participants in research, it seems unfair that children who are enrolled in research without their autonomous consent might be subject to long-term disability due to the research without any compensation from the investigators or sponsors. A 2004 IOM report concerning research with children recommended that research organizations and sponsors pay the medical and rehabilitation costs for children injured as a direct result of research participation, without regard to fault.[57] This practice is unlikely to become commonplace unless there is federal regulation requiring it and a no-fault insurance pool is developed for such purposes.

Special Populations

Adolescents

Although the federal regulations regarding research with children apply to all individuals under the legal age of consent to medical treatment for the procedures involved in the research (18 years old for most medical treatment in the United States), there has been a growing concern about how these protections ought to pertain to adolescents. Adolescents are individuals between 10 and 21 years of age, and their constant state of physiological and psychological development sets them apart from younger children and adults.[70,71] This population has a number of unique health-related needs and behavioral risks that deserve the attention of the research community.[72] Many adolescents are also unwilling to take part in research if disclosing their illness, condition, or behaviors to their parents or guardians is required.[73,74] As a result, studies that involve substance abuse, mental health, sexual activity, and pregnancy often lack sufficient adolescent participation, and development of interventions in these areas to address adolescent concerns may be lacking.

Some adolescents do not require the involvement of parents in decision making about their medical care or research participation because they are legally emancipated. Emancipated minors are individuals below the age of majority who have the legal status of adults.[70,75] Historically, minors became emancipated when they married, enrolled in the military, or were financially independent and living apart from their parents. The emancipation process used to be conducted in the courts, but many states now have laws describing specific conditions warranting emancipation. Because of their legal status as adults, emancipated minors may consent to medical treatment and presumably participation in research, although not all states explicitly include this right in their emancipation statutes.

Another potential exception to parental permission in research comes through the mature minor doctrine. This doctrine has evolved in the courts in the context of medical treatment so that minors who possess the decisional capacity necessary to provide informed consent may do so in certain circumstances and receive treatment without parental permission; and doctors who treat them cannot be held liable for providing care without consent.[62] This generally includes minors who are not emancipated from their families. Some states have passed laws explicitly defining a mature minor and cite certain characteristics such as age, educational level, marriage status, living situation, financial independence, being a parent, and whether or not an individual is incarcerated or has previously been emancipated. However, beyond these explicit standards, the courts have also invoked the doctrine to allow treatment without parental permission in cases in which the minor patient seemed capable of providing informed consent.[62]

In addition to the mature minor doctrine, all states have statutes that allow minors to consent to treatment based on certain specific types of treatment they are seeking. The conditions for which minors are allowed to seek medical and mental health treatment without parental permission vary from state to state, but states often permit adolescents to consent to treatment for conditions about which they might be reluctant to inform their parents. These conditions generally include sexually transmitted diseases, mental illness, substance abuse, pregnancy, and birth control.[62] Because the definition of *children* in the federal regulations includes those not legally allowed to consent to treatment involved in the research, an IRB may waive the requirement for parental permission and accept the consent of a mature minor for enrollment in certain research studies that wish to enroll adolescents who may legally consent for the type of treatment being studied.

For most adolescents, parental permission is required ostensibly to protect those who do not have adequate capacity to provide informed consent; but there is evidence to suggest that many adolescents under the age of 18 (the nearly universal age of legal consent to treatment) have the decisional capacity necessary to consent to medical treatment and research participation.[76–78] Most minors under the age of 14 lack the developmental and emotional maturity required to provide informed consent.[76,79] Adolescents older than 14 may lack life experience and may be more easily influenced than adults (particularly regarding physical appearance and social concerns), but there is evidence that they can provide meaningful informed consent for treatment and research participation in the proper environment.[80] As a result, a number of health-care providers, researchers, educators, and other professionals, including the Society for Adolescent Medicine, have advocated allowing older adolescents to provide full informed consent for participation in research by increasing the use of waivers of parental permission.[57,72,81]

The IOM report on research involving children recommends that IRBs consider waivers of parental permission in informed consent for research when (1) the research is important to the health and well-being of adolescents and cannot be reasonably or practically carried out without the waiver, or (2) the research involves treatments or procedures that state laws permit adolescents to receive without parental permission. In addition, the investigator is required to present evidence that the adolescents are capable of understanding the research and their rights as research participants, and that the research protocol includes appropriate safeguards to protect the interests of the adolescent consistent with the risk presented by the research. This approach, consistent with the Common Rule,[40] has been controversial but has received widespread support.

Neonates

In November 2001, a revised section of subpart B of the federal regulations was published and codified at 45 CFR 46.201–207 concerning nonviable neonates or neonates of uncertain viability involved in research.[40] These additional regulations have the potential to be confusing because of some overlap with subpart D that specifically addresses regulations for all children (including neonates) involved in research. The primary purpose of subpart B is to regulate research involving pregnant women and fetuses and, in addition, regulate research pertinent to nonviable fetuses after delivery. However, definitions in this subpart create some new challenges for pediatric research.

A *nonviable neonate* is defined at 45 CFR 46.202(e) of the regulations as "a neonate after delivery that, although living, is not viable."[40] And at 45 CFR 46.202(h), *viable* is defined as "being able, after delivery, to survive (given the benefit of available medical therapy) to the point of independently maintaining heartbeat and respiration."[40] The difficulty for pediatric investigators and IRBs is that much neonatal research involves extremely premature neonates at gestational ages of 23 to 26 weeks whose long-term viability is considered very uncertain. The regulations in subpart D (Additional Protections for Children Involved as Subjects in Research) have adequately protected the interests of these babies who participate in research, but now provisions of subpart B (Additional Protections for Pregnant Women, Human Fetuses and Neonates Involved in Research) must also be applied to this population.

For research involving these neonates of uncertain viability, subpart B requires that the research hold out the prospect of enhancing the probability of survival of the neonate to the point of viability, or that the purpose of the research is the development of important biomedical knowledge that cannot be obtained by other means and there will be no added risk to the neonate resulting from the research. This provision of subpart B could be interpreted to be in direct conflict with the minimal risk and minor increase over minimal risk standards of subpart D. Thus, for research that does not offer the prospect of direct benefit to neonates at the threshold of viability, IRBs must utilize the "no added risk" standard of subpart B rather than the "minimal risk" standard of subpart D. This may result in an IRB being unwilling to approve important research involving premature neonates that could have been approved under the 46.406 provision in subpart D, which permits research that has a level of risk just a minor increase over minimal.

Economically or Educationally Disadvantaged Children

Federal regulations, at 45 CFR 46.111, admonish investigators and IRBs to provide additional safeguards when subjects are likely to be vulnerable to coercion or undue influence because of being economically or educationally disadvantaged.[40] Many of the most important illnesses and conditions affecting children are disproportionately represented in those who are economically or educationally disadvantaged, and much important research is focused on preventing and ameliorating these conditions. Children who are economically disadvantaged have multiple vulnerabilities, including living in poor neighborhoods in substandard housing, lacking access to health care, and being educated in lower quality schools. Their families are more likely to be immigrants or members of minority groups who may have suffered and continue to experience racism and discrimination. These factors make research with disadvantaged children fraught with potential ethical problems. The relative lack of social, economic, and political power of low-income families can affect the voluntariness of informed consent. The educational disadvantage of such families may affect understanding of the nature of the research and may increase the likelihood that participant families will suffer from a therapeutic misconception, conflating research studies with clinical care.[82]

One approach might be to exclude socioeconomically vulnerable children from research in order to protect them from the potential for exploitation and harm. This approach may protect some children but would result in depriving the children who need help the most from the knowledge gained and the potential benefits of research. Research can be viewed as a burdensome enterprise with substantial risk, but it also can be seen as an activity that provides potential benefits to individuals and affected populations. Vulnerable populations should be permitted to participate in research when appropriate, but additional scrutiny and procedural safeguards may be required to assure their protection from harm.[83] Fairness requires that all children who are affected by a condition, whether rich or poor, be offered the opportunity to be potential participants in research. The burdens of the research and the benefits of the findings should be distributed among all those who may benefit. It is important, however, to involve disadvantaged children in studies that have the potential to improve the circumstances in which they live and provide knowledge about the social determinants of their health.

IRBs responsible for review of research involving multiply vulnerable poor and minority children must give special scrutiny to these proposals to ensure that the balance of risks to benefits in the research are acceptable and that parents are well informed and assisted in making a truly voluntary choice about the participation of their children in the research.[82]

Conclusion

Over the past few years, several regulatory and legislative initiatives have increased funding for research involving children in the United States and have created incentives for the pharmaceutical industry to study drugs in children.[45–47,84,85] The pediatric research community and many advocates for children have applauded these changes as long overdue programs to enhance the health of children. Pediatricians note that clinical research is required because many medications used in children have never been studied in appropriate populations, and because translating knowledge gained from recent advances in developmental biology, genetics, and neuroscience into improved diagnostic tests and treatments for children is possible only through research.

Others have voiced concern about increasing research in children because they believe the present system for protecting human research participants is generally inadequate to protect the interests of all participants.[1] Children, particularly vulnerable because of their limited capacity for informed consent, require additional special protections. These concerns are reinforced by a Maryland court decision that questioned the authority of parents to consent for children to be enrolled in studies that include any level of risk without "therapeutic" benefit,[2] and by reports of healthy children exposed to "risky" medications solely for research purposes.[86]

Those who criticize the system for protection of children involved in research claim that increased federal funding and incentives to pharmaceutical companies result in healthy children being subjected to undue risks and sick children being enrolled in trials that provide more benefit to the pharmaceutical industry sponsor than to the child participants. They argue that IRBs are not properly evaluating the level of risk in protocols and are approving studies not in the interests of participants. However, none of the recent initiatives to increase research in children has weakened the federal regulations that have governed research involving children since 1983. Clearly there are aspects of the system to protect child participants in research that would benefit from modification, as has been suggested in recent reports from the National Bioethics Advisory Commission[83] and the IOM,[87] but the fundamental structure of the system to protect children as participants in research is sound and appears to work pretty well.[88,89]

The quality of IRB review of individual protocols varies greatly, and there is general agreement about a need for accreditation of IRBs and better education of IRB members to increase uniformity and accountability, as well as for development of performance measures to evaluate the system.[90] Few IRBs provide the kind of detailed guidance on their web sites that might help pediatric investigators to ensure ethically designed and implemented protocols.[91] Specifically, for children in research, there is a need for clarification of the present regulations and assurance of qualified pediatric expertise on IRBs. There is also a need for federally promulgated guidance about several controversial issues, such as waiver of parental permission in research involving adolescents and compensation for children who are research participants and their families.

Well-designed and well-executed research involving children is essential to improve children's health. Investigators, IRBs, research institutions, and government policy makers and regulators all play critical roles in facilitating excellence in research while assuring the protection of children who are participants.

References

1. Sherav VH. Children in clinical research: A conflict of moral values. *American Journal of Bioethics* 2003;3(1):W12–W59.
2. *Grimes v. Kennedy Krieger Institute, Inc.* 782 A.2d 807 (Md. Ct. of App., 2001).
3. Still GF. *The History of Paediatrics: The Progress of the Study of Diseases of Children Up to the End of the 18th Century.* London, England: Oxford University Press; 1931.
4. Lederer SE, Grodin MA. Historical overview: Pediatric experimentation. In: Grodin MA, Glantz LH, eds. *Children as Research Subjects: Science, Ethics, and Law.* New York, N.Y.: Oxford University Press; 1994:3–25.
5. Jenner E. *An Inquiry into the Causes and Effects of the Variolae Vaccinae.* London: Sampson Low; 1798.
6. Shulman ST. A history of pediatric specialties: The history of pediatric infectious diseases. *Pediatric Research* 2004;55:163–76.
7. Grodin MA, Alpert JJ. Children as participants in medical research. *Pediatric Clinics of North America* 1988;35:1389–1401.
8. Hess AF. The use of a series of vaccines in the prophylaxis and treatment of an epidemic of pertussis. *JAMA* 1914;63:1007–9.
9. Knowles FC. Molluscum contagiosum: Report of an institutional epidemic of 59 cases. *JAMA* 1909;53:671–3.
10. Kolmer JA, Klugh GF, Rule AM. A successful method for vaccination against acute anterior poliomyelitis. *JAMA* 1935;456–60.
11. Sternberg GM, Reed W. Report on immunity against vaccination conferred upon the monkey by the use of the serum of the vaccinated calf and monkey. *Transactions of the Associations of American Physicians* 1895;10:57–69.
12. Von Ruck C. A practical method of prophylactic immunization against tuberculosis. *JAMA* 1912;58:1504–7.
13. Shaffer MF, Rake G, Stokes J, O'Neill GC. Studies on measles: II Experimental disease in man and monkey. *Journal of Immunology* 1941;41:241–57.
14. Roberts MH. The spinal fluid in the new-born with especial reference to intracranial hemorrhage. *JAMA* 1925;85:500–3.
15. Pisek GR, LeWald LT. The further study of the anatomy and physiology of the infant stomach based on serial roentgenograms. *Archives of Pediatrics* 1913;30:150–65.
16. Illinois Anti-Vivisection Society. *Anti-Vivisection: Opposed to Experiments in Live Animals in Medical Colleges and Elsewhere, Vol. III.* Aurora, Ill.: Illinois Anti-Vivisection Society; 1896.
17. Lederer SE. Children as guinea pigs: Historical perspective. *Accountability in Research* 2003;10:1–16.
18. Annas GJ, Grodin MA, eds. *The Nazi Doctors and the Nuremberg Code.* New York, N.Y.: Oxford University Press; 1992.
19. The Nuremberg Code. In: *Trials of War Criminals Before the Nuremberg Military Tribunals Under Control Council Law No. 10. Volume 2.* Washington, D.C.: U.S. Government Printing Office; 1949:181–2. [Online]. Available: http://www.hhs.gov/ohrp/references/nurcode.htm.
20. Moreno JD, Reassessing the influence of the Nuremberg code on American medical ethics. *Journal of Contemporary Health Law and Policy* 1997;13:347–60.
21. World Medical Association. *Code of Ethics of the World Medical Association: Declaration of Helsinki.* Helsinki, Finland: WMA; June 1964. British Medical Journal 1964;2:177.
22. U.S. Congress. Kefauver-Harris Drug Amendments of 1962, Pub. L. No. 87–781, 76 Stat 780, 87th Congress (codified in scattered sections of 21 USC), October 10, 1962.
23. Memorandum of the Surgeon General William H. Stewart to the Heads of Institutions Conducting Research with Public Health Grants, February 8, 1966.
24. Krugman S. Experiments at the Willowbrook State School. *Lancet* 1971;297:966–7.
25. Krugman S, Giles JP, Hammond J. Infectious hepatitis: Evidence for two distinct clinical, epidemiological, and immunological types of infection. *JAMA* 1967;200:365–73.
26. Krugman S. The Willowbrook hepatitis studies revisited: Ethical aspects. *Reviews of Infectious Diseases* 1986;8:157–62.

27. Beecher HK. *Research and the Individual*. Boston, Mass.: Little Brown and Company; 1970.

28. Olansky S, Simpson L, Schuman SH. Untreated syphilis in the male negro: Environmental factors in the Tuskegee study. *Public Health Reports* 1954;69:691–4.

29. Schuman SH, Olansky, S, Rivers E, Smith CA, Rambo DS. Untreated syphilis in the male negro: Background and current status of patients in the Tuskegee study. *Journal of Chronic Diseases* 1955;2:543–58.

30. Rockwell DH, Yobs AR, Moore MB. The Tuskegee study of untreated syphilis: The 30th year of observation. *Archives of Internal Medicine* 1964;114:792–8.

31. Heller J. Syphilis victims in U.S. study went untreated for 40 years. *New York Times* July 26, 1972.

32. Curran WJ. The Tuskegee Syphilis Study. *New England Journal of Medicine* 1973;289:730–1.

33. Department of Health, Education, and Welfare. Protection of Human Subjects, 45 CFR 46: Final rule. *Federal Register* 1974;39(105):18914–20.

34. Ramsey P. *The Patient as Person*. New Haven, Conn.: Yale University Press; 1970.

35. McCormick RA. Proxy consent in the experimentation situation. *Perspectives in Biology and Medicine* 1974;18:2–20.

36. Bartholome WG. Parents, children, and the moral benefits of research. *Hastings Center Report* 1976;6(6):44–5.

37. Ramsey P. Children as research subjects: A reply. *Hastings Center Report* 1977;7(2):40–2.

38. The National Commission for the Protection of Human Subjects of Biomedical and Behavioral Research. *The Belmont Report: Ethical Principles and Guidelines for the Protection of Human Subjects of Research*. Washington, D.C.: Department of Health, Education and Welfare; DHEW Publication OS 78-0012 1978. [Online] April 18, 1979. Available: http://www.hhs.gov/ohrp/humansubjects/guidance/belmont.htm.

39. The National Commission for the Protection of Human Subjects of Biomedical and Behavioral Research. *Research Involving Children: Report and Recommendations*. Washington D.C.: U.S. Government Printing Office; 1977. [Online] Available: http://www.bioethics.gov/reports/past_commissions/Research_involving_children.pdf.

40. Department of Health and Human Services, National Institutes of Health, and Office for Human Research Protections. The Common Rule, Title 45 (Public Welfare), Code of Federal Regulations, Part 46 (Protection of Human Subjects). [Online] June 23, 2005. Available: http://www.hhs.gov/ohrp/humansubjects/guidance/45cfr46.htm.

41. Food and Drug Administration, Department of Health and Human Services. Title 21 (Food and Drugs), Code of Federal Regulations, Part 50 (Protection of Human Subjects). [Online] April 1, 2006. Available: http://www.gpo.gov/nara/cfr/waisidx_06/21cfr50_06.html.

42. Food and Drug Administration, Department of Health and Human Services. Title 21 (Food and Drugs), Code of Federal Regulations, Part 56 (Institutional Review Boards). [Online] April 1, 2006. Available: http://www.gpo.gov/nara/cfr/waisidx_06/21cfr56_06.html.

43. Caldwell PHY, Murphy SB, Butow PH, Craig JC. Clinical trials in children. *Lancet* 2004;364:803–11.

44. U.S. Congress. Food and Drug Administration Modernization Act of 1997, Pub. L. No. 105–115, 105th Congress, 1st Session (codified as amended in scattered sections of 21 U.S.C.). [Online] January 7, 1997. Available: http://www.fda.gov/cder/guidance/s830enr.txt.

45. National Institutes of Health. NIH Policy and Guidelines on the Inclusion of Children as Participants in Research Involving Human Subjects. [Online] March 6, 1998. Available: http://grants.nih.gov/grants/guide/notice-files/not98–024.html.

46. U.S. Congress. Best Pharmaceuticals for Children Act, Pub. L. No. 107–109, S. 1789, 107th Congress, 1st Session (codified as amended in scattered sections of 21 U.S.C. and 42 U.S.C.). [Online] Jan. 4, 2002. Available: http://www.fda.gov/opacom/laws/pharmkids/contents.html.

47. U.S. Congress. Pediatric Research Equity Act of 2003, Pub. L. No. 108–155, S. 650, 108th Congress, 1st Session. [Online] Jan. 7, 2003. Available: http://www.fda.gov/cder/pediatric/S-650-PREA.pdf.

48. European Public Health Alliance. The EU adopts a regulation on medicines for children. [Online] June 30, 3006. Available: http://www.epha.org/a/1451.

49. Editorial. Clinical trials in children, for children. *Lancet* 2006;367:1953.

50. Nelson RM. Algorithm for subpart D analysis. Pediatric Advisory Subcommittee Meeting, Food and Drug Administration, 2003. In: Institute of Medicine. *Ethical Conduct of Research Involving Children*. Washington D.C.: National Academies Press; 2004:119.

51. Janofsky J, Starfield B. Assessment of risk in research on children. *Journal of Pediatrics* 1981;98:842–6.

52. Shah S, Whittle A, Wilfond B, Gensler G, Wendler D. How do institutional review boards apply the federal risk and benefits standards for pediatric research? *JAMA* 2004;291:476–82.

53. Kopelman L. Children as research subjects: A dilemma. *Journal of Medicine and Philosophy* 2000;25:745–64.

54. Wendler D, Belsky L, Thompson KM, Emanuel EJ. Quantifying the federal minimal risk standard: Implications for pediatric research without the prospect of direct benefit. *JAMA* 2005;294:826–32.

55. National Human Research Protections Advisory Committee (NHRPAC), Children's Workgroup. Final Report: Clarifying specific portions of 45 CFR 46 subpart D that governs children's research. [Online] Available: http://www.hhs.gov/ohrp/nhrpac/documents/nhrpac16.pdf.

56. Department of Health and Human Services, Secretary's Advisory Committee on Human Research Protection. Minutes April 18–19, 2005. [Online] Available: http://hhs.gov/ohrp/sachrp/mtgings/mtg04–05/mtg04–05.htm.

57. Institute of Medicine. *Ethical Conduct of Research Involving Children*. Washington, D.C.: National Academies Press; 2004.

58. Freedman B, Fuks A, Weijer C. Demarcating research and treatment: A systematic approach for the analysis of the ethics of clinical research. *Clinical Research* 1992;40:653–60.

59. Weijer C, Miller PB. When are research risks reasonable in relation to anticipated benefits? *Nature Medicine* 2004;10:570–3.

60. Office for Human Research Protections. Children Involved as Subjects in Research: Guidance on the HHS 45 CFR 46.407 ("407") Review Process. [Online] May 26, 2005. Available: http://www.hhs.gov/ohrp/children/guidance_407process.html.

61. Kodish E. Informed consent for pediatric research: Is it really possible? *Journal of Pediatrics* 2003;142:89–90.

62. English A, Kenney KE. *State Minor Consent Laws: A Summary*, 2nd ed. Chapel Hill, N.C.: Center for Adolescent Health and the Law; 2003.

63. Whittle A, Shah S, Wilfond B, Gensler G, Wendler D. Institutional Review Board practices regarding assent in pediatric research. *Pediatrics* 2004;113:1747–52.

64. American Academy of Pediatrics Committee on Drugs, Guidelines for the ethical conduct of studies to evaluate drugs in pediatric populations. *Pediatrics* 1995;95:286–94.

65. Wendler D, Rackoff JE, Emanuel EJ, Grady C. The ethics of paying for children's participation in research. *Journal of Pediatrics* 2002;141:166–71.

66. Grodin MA, Glantz LH, eds. *Children as Research Subjects: Science, Ethics, and the Law*. New York, N.Y.: Oxford University Press; 1994.

67. Rothmeir JD, Lasley MV, Shapiro GC. Factors influencing parental consent in pediatric clinical research. *Pediatrics* 2003;111:1037–41.

68. Department of Health and Human Services, Office for Human Research Protections. *Protecting Human Research Subjects: Institutional Review Board Guidebook.* Rockville, Md.: OHRP; 1993. [Online] Available: http://www.hhs.gov/ohrp/irb/irb_guidebook.htm.

69. Food and Drug Administration. Guidance for institutional review boards and clinical investigators: Payment to Research Subjects. [Online] 1998. Available: http://www.fda.gov/oc/ohrt/irbs/toc4.html#payment.

70. English A. Treating adolescents: Legal and ethics considerations. *Medical Clinics of North America* 1990;74:1097–112.

71. Fleming, M, Towey K, Jarosik J. *Healthy Youth 2010: Supporting the 21 Critical Adolescent Objectives.* Chicago, Ill.: American Medical Association; 2001.

72. Santelli JS, Rogers AS, Rosenfeld WD, et al., for the Society for Adolescent Medicine. Guidelines for adolescent health research—A position paper of the Society for Adolescent Medicine. *Journal of Adolescent Health* 2003;33:396–409.

73. Ford CA, English A. Limiting confidentiality of adolescent health services: What are the risks? *JAMA* 2002;288:752–3.

74. Reddy DM, Fleming R, Swain C. Effect of mandatory parental notification on adolescent girls' use of sexual health care services. *JAMA* 2002;288:710–4.

75. Campbell AT. State regulation of medical research with children and adolescents: An overview and analysis. In: Institute of Medicine. *The Ethical Conduct of Clinical Research Involving Children.* Washington D.C.: National Academies Press; 2004:320–87.

76. Grisso T, Vierling L. Minors' consent to treatment: A developmental perspective. *Professional Psychology* 1978;9:412–27.

77. Weithorn L, Campbell S. The competency of children and adolescents to make informed treatment decisions. *Child Development* 1982;53:1589–98.

78. Piaget J. The stages of the intellectual development of the child. *Bulletin of the Menninger Clinic* 1962;26:120–8.

79. Weithorn L. Children's capacities to decide about participation in research. *IRB: A Review of Human Subjects Research* 1983;5(2):1–5.

80. Leiken SL. Minors' assent or dissent to medical treatment. *Journal of Pediatrics* 1983;102:169–76.

81. Collogan LK, Fleischman AR. Adolescent research and parental permission. In: Kodish E, editor. *Ethics and Research With Children.* New York, N.Y.: Oxford University Press; 2005:77–99.

82. National Research Council and Institute of Medicine. *Ethical Considerations for Research on Housing-Related Health Hazards Involving Children.* Washington D.C.: National Academies Press; 2005.

83. National Bioethics Advisory Commission. *Ethical and Policy Issues in Research Involving Human Participants.* Bethesda, Md.: NBAC; 2001. [Online] Available: http://www.bioethics.gov/reports/past_commissions/nbac_human_part.pdf.

84. Food and Drug Administration, Department of Health and Human Services. Regulations Requiring Manufacturers to Assess the Safety and Effectiveness of New Drugs and Biological Products in Pediatric Patients: Final rule. *Federal Register* 1998;63:66632–72.

85. U.S. Congress. Children's Health Act of 2000, Pub. L. No. 106–310, H.R. 4365, 106th congress, 2nd Session, October 17, 2000. [Online] Available: http://frwebgate.access.gpo.gov/cgi-bin/getdoc.cgi?dbname=106_cong_public_laws&docid=f:pub1310.106.pdf.

86. Montero D. Minority children were singled out in drug tests. *New York Post* June 11, 1998:2.

87. Committee on Assessing the System for Protecting Human Research Participants, Institute of Medicine (Federman DD, Hanna KE, Rodriguez LL, eds.). *Responsible Research: A Systems Approach to Protecting Research Participants.* Washington, D.C.: National Academies Press; 2002.

88. National Human Research Protections Advisory Committee (NHRPAC). Children's Workgroup Report, April 5, 2001. [Online] Available: http://www.hhs.gov/ohrp/nhrpac/mtg04–01/child-workgroup4–5–01.pdf.

89. Lantos JD. Pediatric research: What is broken and what needs to be fixed? *Journal of Pediatrics* 2004;144:147–9.

90. Emanuel EJ, Wood A, Fleischman AR, et al. Oversight of human participants research: Identifying problems and evaluating solutions. *Annals of Internal Medicine* 2004;141:282–91.

91. Wolf L, Zandecki J, Lo B. Institutional Review Board guidance on pediatric research: Missed opportunities. *Journal of Pediatrics* 2005;147:84–9.

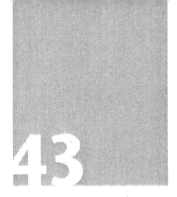

Valerie H. Bonham   Jonathan D. Moreno

Research With Captive Populations
Prisoners, Students, and Soldiers

Today, respect for persons is a bedrock principle governing research with humans. But although Americans have long held the belief, as Justice Cardozo declared in 1914, that "every human being of adult years and sound mind has a right to determine what shall be done with his own body,"[1] they have not always applied this notion equally or scrutinized its significance without prejudice. Following World War II, for example, Americans condemned the Nazi experiments on concentration camp prisoners but asked strikingly few questions about the status of participants in their own research activities. Into the 1960s, the popular understanding of captive populations in research often overlooked the influence of captivity, or inequality of physical, financial, educational, or social status, in making many captive populations seem more willing to participate in research than other groups in society.

This complacency ended in the late 1960s and 1970s. At that time, widespread challenges to the ethics of the medical profession dovetailed with public reports of abuses in U.S. prisons. Consequently, public policy toward captive human research participants, particularly those who were imprisoned, ricocheted from an unquestioning presumption that they were "volunteers" to the restrictive conclusion that, for most research participants, captivity itself precluded voluntarily consent. Society also became more sensitive to the ways in which other groups may in effect be "captive," and therefore in need of special protection to ensure that they have free choice to participate in research, if possible. For example, the exercise of free choice is often in direct conflict with the command structure of military duty. Despite numerous longstanding regulations and policies mandating soldiers' voluntary participation in research, national interests may sometimes supersede individual interests. Students too may be denied free

choice, if, for example, they are required to participate in research as a condition of completing their coursework, or if their choice to participate in research is unduly driven by their financial needs.

The tacit and uncritical assumptions that governed medical research with captive populations before the 1970s, and the challenges that continue to appear, reflect a tension between competing interests. The interests of the group—including the interests of future patients and the scientific community—compete with the interests of an individual in exercising autonomous choice over the use of his or her body. Without doubt, most researchers respect and seek to advance the rights and welfare of those who participate in their experiments, including the right to free choice. Less clear, however, is what level of scrutiny is given to appreciating the effects of captivity on a person's ability to function as a true volunteer. Even today, when informed and voluntary individual consent is a central tenet of the research enterprise, group interests may supplant (or override) individual interests.

I. Captivity and Research

The Meanings of Captivity

What does it mean to be a "captive" population? Perhaps the most essential common element is that captive populations in some critical sense lack the ability to exercise free choice. For one reason or another, their individual autonomy is limited. The most obvious of these limits, frequently, is physical. Captive populations are separated, often physically or through other means, from the general population. They often live, with little or no choice, in

461

institutions. Prisoners are kept in locked cells established by the state to prevent them from interacting with society at large. They sleep, eat, dress, and work together in groups with no freedom to leave. Soldiers are often housed in barracks or on bases where uniforms, room, and board are provided, and they are free to leave only after their commander consents. Students, although relatively free to move amidst the general population, often live together in dorms or other student housing. They are separated by their location, their dress, and often their resources from the rest of society. The physical isolation that each of these captive populations faces suggests that they may be more easily manipulated and coerced into research participation.

Less obvious than physical restraints, but often more influential, is that captive populations have limited choices and are to some degree under the control of others. Restrained behind locked prison gates, prisoners must do what their guards and wardens instruct. They cannot seek outside employment or otherwise exercise independence. Soldiers are subject to the military command structure and obligated, sometimes upon threat of grave physical consequences, to follow orders issued from above. Students are often limited in their ability to exercise free choice because of financial needs or academic and professional goals that keep them beholden to their teachers. Each of these groups is dependent upon and subject to the commands of others. They are unequal players.

In the medical research arena, the effect of this power differential is compounded by the traditional, and often closely guarded, authority that medical professionals routinely exert. Since the time of Hippocrates, physicians have vowed, as a condition of sharing in the knowledge of medical science, "to help, or at least to do no harm" and to "abstain from all intentional wrong-doing and harm."[2] This oath leads many patients to assume that their physicians, first and foremost, will protect them, an assumption that is a key reason for the trust that patients put in their doctors. Patient trust is grounded also in the mystery that surrounds the practice of medicine. Compared with the general population, medical professionals undergo extensive training and licensing that separates them from laypeople and requires the uninitiated to defer to them. For prisoners, soldiers, and students, this deference can be magnified by their limited opportunities to select among physicians (or teachers) and the other indicia of captivity that often make them especially attractive candidates for research.

The Advantages Captive Populations Offer in Research

Captive populations offer special advantages for medical research. Typically, health information about these groups is centrally maintained, and investigators may be able to access it more easily than information about the general population. Certainly recruitment can be more efficient. Advertisements seeking males and females aged 18 and over are commonplace on university campuses for just this reason. Moreover, research participants who are physically confined are less likely to be lost for follow-up examination. Soldiers and their medical records are readily located. Students can be expected to complete their role in a study, especially if they are enrolled in the investigator's course. For similar reasons, participants from captive groups may also be especially cooperative and compliant with protocol requirements. They are accustomed to being monitored or graded and they are used to completing duties or tasks that others assign.

In addition to being efficiently recruited and retained, captive populations may be more motivated to participate in research than the general population. For example, research may offer greater or more immediate access to income than other options. Students can fit participation in a trial into irregular school schedules and may be paid a higher hourly wage than is offered by more typical work-study opportunities. Prisoners, and to some extent soldiers, may find research to be one of only a few feasible ways to supplement their existing income. But financial rewards are not the only, nor necessarily the primary, reason for participation in research.

Captive populations also may be motivated to participate in research to respond to many other needs in their lives. Prisoners have reported joining a study as a way to repay some of their debt to society, or to obtain other nonmonetary benefits.[3] They may also receive better medical care and attention when they participate in research. Soldiers may see research as a necessary component of supporting their fellow troops and establishing and maintaining an effective and safe fighting force. Students may want a favorable grade, or if they are planning to enter the research field or training to practice medicine, they may believe that participating in research will enable them to better understand the research process, be more successful in their later careers, or impress those who may support their applications. As captive populations, each of these groups has reasons for participating in research that are separate from financial rewards or other factors that may ordinarily motivate the general public.

The Moral Hazards of Research With Captive Populations

For the very reasons that captive populations can offer special advantages for researchers, they also present particular moral hazards. Isolated and under the direction of others, captive groups are limited in their ability to exercise choice. Absent free choice, it cannot be said that a participant is a "volunteer" in any meaningful sense of that term, and thus, a researcher's use of that person is morally suspect. This idea is widely recognized, at least in theory. For example, writing in a 1916 edition of the *Journal of the American Medical Association* in language nearly identical to that of Justice Cardozo, pioneering experimental physiologist Walter Cannon stated that "there is no more primitive and fundamental right, which any individual possess than that of controlling the use to which his own body is put."[4]

In medical ethics discourse over the past 50 years, many thoughtful commentators have examined and expanded upon the basis for Cannon's conclusion. In its seminal report on the ethical principles for research with humans, commonly called the Belmont Report, the National Commission for the Protection of Human Subjects of Biomedical and Behavioral Research (National Commission) explained the idea as "respect for persons," which, in the research context, "demands that subjects enter into the research voluntarily and with adequate information"[5] (see Chapter 14). The challenge when captive populations become research participants is that they are unequal players and may thereby have a diminished ability to exercise free choice, which may lead them to be coerced or manipulated into participation. Soldiers or students required by superior officers or professors to participate in research, for example, cannot be said to be choosing freely. Prisoners facing few or nonexistent alternatives to participation face similar illusory choices.

An additional moral concern that may arise with captive populations is that expediency may diminish scrutiny of a participant's capacity to volunteer. In some cases, the needs of others and a social consensus that certain subgroups are unequal can seem to justify experimentation that otherwise might not occur. Unequal bargaining power, legal philosopher H.L.A. Hart observed, is morally problematic not only because it may limit an individual's free choice but also because it defies accepted social ideals of equality. Hart explained that "most modern societies" assume that all people are "entitled to be treated alike and that differences of treatment require more to justify them than just an appeal to the interests of others."[6] But, Hart noted, society often falls short of this paradigm. It is "plain," Hart wrote, "that neither the law nor the accepted morality of societies need extend their minimal protections, and benefits, to all within their scope, and often have not."[6]

The history of research with captive populations confirms that at times, and often unreflectively, society views and treats certain subgroups differently from others. For example, a 1962 study addressing prisoners' participation in research identified this disparity: "When the public hears that inmates are [participating in a seemingly very hazardous study], they rationalize 'Well, I wouldn't do it, but it's all right with prisoners.'"[7] More recently, researchers at the University of Rochester exposed a healthy student to four times the maximum anticipated dose of an anesthetic drug in order to obtain tissue samples in a cancer study. In the military, special pressures relating to protecting and arming troops can affect judgments about voluntariness. For example, during and after World War II, uncertainty about the effects of radiation, combined with the increasing demands for knowledge about its risks, led the military to sponsor experiments in which soldier-participants, among others, were not informed about or given the choice to decline participation.[7] Military exigencies—the need to protect fighting forces and civilians—continue to put strains on policies to protect individual autonomy, as we describe below.

Despite a general presumption that the interests of others should not justify treating subgroups differently, the interests of others have frequently provided a significant rationale for research with captive populations, if only implicitly or in part. Among these others are fellow soldiers, future patients, the public, investigators, and research institutions. Policy efforts to protect captive populations have aimed, in part, to mediate the risk that the capacity for voluntary consent may be compromised when captive populations participate in research.

Policy Efforts to Protect Captive Populations

To ensure that individuals truly choose to participate, and to combat the risks of coercion, manipulation, and exploitation that fueled many tragedies in clinical research over the last century, policy makers have crafted various rules requiring that research participants be "volunteers" who make informed choices to participate. Among the best known of these rules is the Nuremberg Code, promulgated in 1947 by the judges presiding over the trial of Nazi physicians charged with human rights abuses perpetrated on concentration camp inmates during World War II. The code's famous first sentence reads: "The voluntary consent of the human subject is absolutely essential."[8] To ensure that consent is volun-

tary, the code requires that subjects "should be so situated as to be able to exercise free power of choice."[8] Absent from this guidance, however, are specific standards for evaluating whether particular populations are so situated (see Chapter 12).

Later codes proposed more concrete guidance, sometimes specifically targeted to captive populations. For example, the 1961 draft Code of Ethics of the World Medical Association, which later became the Declaration of Helsinki, proposed that research intended solely to advance science, but offering no prospect of medical benefit for the participant, should not be conducted with those who are (a) "in a dependent relationship to the investigator, such as a medical student to a teacher . . . ," (b) "prisoners of war, military or civilian . . . ," or (c) "in prisons, penitentiaries, or reformatories."[9] These specifics were deleted from the final draft, although the document retained a general admonition that an investigator should be cautious "if the subject is in a dependent relationship to the investigator."[10]

Current U.S. regulations—codified at 45 CFR 46, and generally referred to as the Common Rule—expand upon the framework established in these earlier codes. Human testing is generally prohibited absent the person's informed consent or the consent of a legally authorized representative, which must be obtained in "circumstances that provide the prospective subject or the representative sufficient opportunity to consider whether or not to participate and that minimize the possibility of coercion or undue influence."[11] In setting forth the elements of a valid informed consent (at 45 CFR 46.116(a)(1)-(8)), the federal rules expressly require prospective participants to be informed that their participation is voluntary and that they cannot be denied any benefit to which they are legally entitled if they decline to participate.[11] They also limit research with certain captive populations, namely, prisoners because, as the regulations explain at 45 CFR 46.302, "prisoners may be under constraints because of their incarceration which could affect their ability to make a truly voluntary and uncoerced decision" to participate in research.[11] As discussed below, international standards are equally, and sometimes even more, stringent.

II. Prisoners

Prisoners, perhaps the paradigm of a captive population, have long been a desirable group for medical research. From ancient history through the 20th century, societies have used prisoners to experiment on human health. Often prisoners were used because their welfare and interests were unilaterally and routinely subordinated to those of society as a whole. However, even in societies in which prisoners were not viewed as mere means to advance the interests of others, they have been sought for research because of their captive status. Describing the benefits of working in prisons, researchers writing in the *Journal of the American Medical Association* in 1967 explained:

> One of the chief advantages of [working in prisons] is that it permits selection of men of any given age, height, and weight. By screening, the investigator can select persons who have a specific disorder. . . . He can select subjects with any characteristic that might commonly be found within a prison population. These subjects can then be hospitalized in the metabolic ward under combined prison and research discipline or in the clinical research center under

similar supervision for the time necessary to complete an experiment.[12]

Prisoners are an especially attractive population because their captive status means that, generally, they eat the same food, sleep in the same conditions, undertake the same amount of exercise, and are readily observable. In addition to the opportunity for close monitoring and a controlled environment, the authors of the 1967 article found that prisoners were willing research participants: "The level of compliance by prisoners with research rules and regulations has been surprisingly high. They have eaten strange diets, swallowed tubes, submitted to repeated venipunctures, and participated in a wide variety of physiological tests with a commendable degree of good humor and cheerfulness."[12]

In justifying their use of prisoners for research, these researchers, like many before them, relied on expediency. They explained that they needed participants "urgently" and that the "ideal circumstances" of the prison made their activities appropriate.[12] As was common when referring to prisoner participants, they added that participation in research "enables the participants to feel they are serving a useful function."[12] Thus, the history and still evolving public policy of prisoners in research provides useful insight into the ways captive populations are used in research.

Twentieth-Century Experience

Before World War II, prisoners were used in research in relatively small numbers and with little controversy.[13] In the early 1900s, Harvard professor Richard Strong tested experimental vaccines for cholera and plague in prisoners awaiting death in the Philippines. In one of these experiments, 13 of 26 participants died. The U.S. Public Health Office induced pellagra in 12 Mississippi prisoners in 1915 and used 500 prisoners in San Quentin in testicular transplant experiments from 1919 to 1922.

During and after World War II, however, revelations about horrific exploitation and torture of prisoners in Nazi concentration camps, ostensibly in the name of advancing science and fortifying the war effort, brought the use of prisoners into new light. Telford Taylor, the lead prosecutor during the Nuremberg Doctors' Trial, argued that the Nazi researchers were "not ignorant men," but that they were instead "callous to the suffering of people regarded as inferior."[14] At Dachau concentration camp, for example, they conscripted prisoners for high altitude or low pressure experiments that involved locking the victims in chambers, reducing air pressure to simulate high altitude and depriving them of oxygen until they died, a half hour later. Other prisoners received oxygen, but were pummeled by severe atmospheric changes designed to replicate falls from over 47,000 feet. Dachau prisoners were also used in freezing experiments, in which they were stripped and left standing in below-freezing temperatures for nine to 14 hours, or immersed in freezing water for up to three hours at a time. Many died[14] (see Chapters 2 and 12).

These examples are only a few of the numerous ways in which the Nazis used human beings as a means to advance their scientific, military, and medical goals. In other cases, prisoners were infected with malaria, typhus, yellow fever, smallpox, cholera, epidemic jaundice, and other contagious diseases. These, along with thousands of sterilization experiments, phosphorous burn studies, and others, shocked the Allies' consciousness when they came to light following the war. (Although not widely known at the time,

Japanese researchers also made ready use of prisoners. From 1938 to 1945, Japanese immunologist Ishii Shiro tested anthrax and cholera as a means for biological weapons on thousands of Chinese prisoners in Harbin and Ping Fan Prison in Manchuria, known as Unit 731.)[15]

Ironically, given the prominent role that Americans played in prosecuting the Nazi doctors and formulating the standards that would be used to convict them, Americans, too, used prisoners for research during and after World War II. However, the prisoners used in the U.S. experiments were in the regular domestic prison system, not in concentration camps or prisoner-of-war camps. Moreover, U.S. experimenters often paid little attention to whether the prisoners were—in the words of the Nuremberg Code—"so situated as to be able to exercise free power of choice." Much of the interest in prisoner research came from the military, which needed to identify and protect troops from health risks, especially infectious diseases to which they were exposed in fighting overseas. For example, malaria presented a serious threat to forces fighting in the Pacific, and the United States sponsored numerous treatment and prevention studies in prisons in the 1940s. Prisons in Illinois, Georgia, and New Jersey provided many hundreds of humans for this research, which continued into the 1950s. The prisoners participated without compensation or promise of pardon or sentence reduction, and they were celebrated for their patriotism.[7]

Recognizing the risks these prisoner-participants faced, and perhaps sensitive to public opinion, Illinois Governor Dwight H. Green in 1946 appointed a committee to consider whether to pardon or reduce these prisoners' sentences "as a reward for service in addition to that ordinarily allowed because of good conduct."[16] The committee was chaired by Andrew Ivy, a physician who served as Taylor's chief medical ethics expert in the Nazi doctors' trial and drafted the standards that formed the basis for the Nuremberg Code. Ivy's committee anticipated the Nuremberg Code's mandate for voluntariness and characterized it this way: "when a person is able to say 'yes' or 'no' without fear of being punished or of being deprived of privileges due him in the ordinary course of events."[16] Although the committee acknowledged that reduction of sentences might be an inducement for prisoners, it did not reject the idea altogether. Instead, because prisoners who participated in research showed "a social consciousness of high order," the committee objected only to any "excessive reduction in sentence which would exercise undue influence in obtaining the consent of prisoners."[16]

But even though the Nuremberg Code, the Illinois committee, and occasional published literature insisted that prospective research participants must be true volunteers, the prison experiments increased after World War II—with little attention to the circumstances motivating prisoners' participation. In 1956, Albert Sabin tested experimental polio vaccine on 133 prisoners in Ohio.[17] From the 1950s into the 1970s, hundreds of Pennsylvania prisoners participated in experiments for viral hepatitis, psychopharmacological testing, skin research, and various diseases[18] (see Figure 43.1). As with the wartime experiments, these experiments offered the prisoners no prospect of medical benefit and the popular press continued to support the "volunteer" prisoners and celebrate their generosity.[19]

In 1962, the demand for prison research rose sharply after federal legislation required manufacturers applying for drug approval to give the U.S. Food and Drug Administration (FDA) data

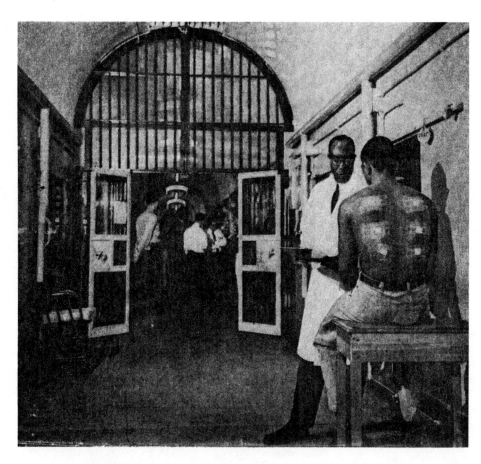

Figure 43.1. Solomon McBride, medical administrator of Holmesburg Prison's human research, questions an unidentified prisoner/research subject in H block in Feb. 1966. Source: Urban Archives, Temple University. Reproduced with permission.

from at least two "adequate and well controlled" clinical studies.[20,21] To meet this new demand, pharmaceutical companies began performing early (Phase I) safety testing of drugs almost exclusively on prisoners.[22] The research involved exposing prisoners to new compounds to determine the level at which they might harm human health. The testing offered no prospect of clinical benefit, though prisoners generally received small cash payments to participate. Prisons were in a unique position to supply the large number of humans needed for this testing, and throughout the country, many thousands of prisoners participated. By 1976, roughly 85% of Phase I testing was being conducted in prisons.[13]

The risk of coercion, abuse, and conflict of interest in these studies was high. For example, in one program involving three state prison systems, the company running the studies paid the prisoners, the prison systems, and the prison physicians for participation. One doctor received supplemental income that exceeded his annual salary by more than 250%—$20,000 versus $8,000—and others were shown later to own the company conducting the research. As a result of these activities, between 500 and 1,000 prisoners in these systems contracted hepatitis and 4 died.[23]

Government agencies also continued experimenting on prisoners, again with no promise of direct benefit to them. For example, from 1963 through 1973, Carl G. Heller and C. Alvin Paulsen conducted government-sponsored testicular irradiation experiments on prisoners in Oregon and Washington to better understand the health effects of exposure to radiation in space

flight, in weapon and nuclear plants, and during battle.[7] These experiments included multiple testicular biopsies and required a vasectomy at the close of the research (to prevent the prisoners from fathering children with possible chromosomal anomalies). Payments of $25 per biopsy and for the vasectomy meant that many prisoners received payments of $100 or more when their prison salary for, say, laundry work, was about 25 cents a day.[7] Reviewing these studies in 1995, the President's Advisory Committee on Human Radiation Experiments found "little doubt that the financial incentives offered for participation" in the studies were "the main reason most inmates volunteered."[7]

Americans' social acquiescence to prisoner research began crumbling in the late 1960s and early 1970s. As various reports of abuse and tragedy surfaced,[24,25] researchers began expressing a more specific appreciation for the effects of incarceration on prisoner "choices" than had earlier investigators. One writer in the *Journal of the American Medical Association* in 1974, explained: "Judgment about an acceptable degree of risk requires contact with the free world as opposed to the prison environment. What may be perceived as an acceptable risk for a person inside prison may be totally unacceptable for the same person outside."[26]

Politics and the courts also came into play. As publicity concerning abuses in the prison system emerged, many prisoners filed lawsuits alleging lack of informed consent and poor oversight.[7] In January 1973, the Oregon Corrections Division shut down all prison research programs in the state after the chief prison administrator found that prisoners could not freely consent.[7] In late 1973, Massachusetts Senator Edward M. Kennedy convened hearings to examine research with prisoners and other groups.[27] In 1976 the Federal Bureau of Prisons announced plans to suspend all prisoner research by the end of that year.[13] Today, the Federal Bureau of Prisons allows research to occur, under tight conditions.[28]

The National Commission for the Protection of Human Subjects of Biomedical and Behavioral Research also reviewed the ethics of prisoner research in 1976. The members failed to reach consensus about banning prison research, but they proposed that it should proceed rarely and only under strict conditions to ensure that the prisoners volunteered freely. The U.S. Department of Health, Education, and Welfare (now the Department of Health and Human Services, DHHS) was statutorily required to respond to the Commission's recommendations. Finding that "most testimony before the Commission opposed the use of prisoners in any form of medical research not intended to benefit the individual prisoner,"[29] the agency promulgated regulations in 1978 that significantly limited prisoner involvement in federally funded research.[29]

The 1978 regulations, which today remain largely unchanged (and are found at 45 CFR 46, Subpart C),[11] brought research with prisoners to a virtual standstill in the United States. But they were controversial and arguments for and against prisoner research persisted. For example, in 1980 the FDA prepared to issue regulations to prohibit using prisoners in clinical trials, including Phase I research, but some prisoners objected, based on a perceived "right" to participate. These objections led FDA to stay the final rule, which by early 2006 had yet to appear.[30]

Ethical Assessment and Current Policies

Respect for persons requires that individual autonomy be promoted and protected. One interpretation of respect for persons requires society to permit prisoners to participate in whatever kind of research they want. This is the view advanced by those who objected to the FDA's proposed regulations to ban clinical research with prisoners. It generally discounts suggestions of "undue" influence arising from prisoners' living conditions or financial resources, especially when prisoners are "free" to decline participation through some form of consent process. It objects to perceived paternalism in regulations aimed at reducing such influences. But, in so doing, this interpretation largely ignores the historical record of abuse in research with prisoners and ignores the reality of many prisoners' everyday lives.

The National Commission favored a different view. Because "prisoners are, as a consequence of being prisoners, more subject to coerced choice and more readily available for the imposition of burdens which others will not willingly bear,"[13] the National Commission concluded that "the appropriate expression of respect [for persons] consists in protection from exploitation."[13] In other words, in the National Commission's view, respect for persons recognizes that external conditions may motivate people "to engage in activities which, were they stronger or in better circumstances, they would avoid," and demands "that they be protected against those forces that appear to compel their choices."[13] This view, the basis for current federal law governing prisoner research, seeks to balance the risks of exploitation with the necessity for free choice.

Undoubtedly, the prospect of higher income and better living conditions for people who have few, if any, other choices can lead them to make choices and accept risks that they would not or-

dinarily accept. Various studies in the late 1960s and 1970s confirmed that prisoners' decisions to participate in research often arose squarely from the circumstance of their prison life. At the same time, however, prisoner-participants reported a sense of importance and higher self-esteem among their peers, and many participated out of a sense of patriotism or desire to make amends for their crimes.[31] These interests cannot be ignored.

In weighing the need to protect prisoners from exploitation versus the need to enable them freely to determine the uses to which their bodies will be put, U.S. federal rules, adopted in 1978 and applicable today, strongly favor reducing the risk of coercion and exploitation. These regulations, which apply to all entities receiving federal funding for research from DHHS, presume that prisoners "because of their incarceration" may be unable "to make a truly voluntary and uncoerced decision whether or not to participate" in research. Therefore, the regulations—at 45 CFR 46.306(a)(2)—generally limit research to the following four areas: (1) the possible causes, effects, or processes of incarceration and criminal behavior; (2) the prison as an institution or prisoners as incarcerated persons; (3) conditions particularly affecting prisoners as a class—for example, hepatitis vaccine trials or alcoholism research; and (4) practices that intend and have a reasonable probability to improve the health or well-being of the prisoner-participant.[11] Procedural limitations for findings of "minimal risk" or DHHS approval further protect prisoner interests. Following complaints from public health researchers that these categories unduly limited low-risk epidemiological research, the U.S. Office for Human Research Protections (OHRP), which administers and oversees the DHHS regulations, announced a waiver that essentially added a fifth category in 2003.[32] Through the waiver, DHHS funds can be used to conduct or support epidemiological research with prisoners so long as prisoners are one of many populations studied and not an exclusive target group.[32] The waiver permits research related to chronic diseases, injuries, and environmental health—for example, surveys involving all HIV-infected persons in a state—so long as the research involves no more than minimal risk and no more than inconvenience to the prisoner participants.[32]

These regulations reflect a heightened sensitivity to the ways in which individual circumstances can affect the choice to participate in research that was absent from public debate before the 1970s. Defending the policy, one commentator explained: "Correctional institutions, with their stated aims of confinement, are inherently coercive . . . and the introduction of research [adds] one more element to benefit the strong, punish the weak, encourage the extortionist, and further undermine fairness and even-handedness in administration."[33] Still, as the 2003 waiver shows, public policy in this area is evolving.

In 2006 the Institute of Medicine (IOM) of the National Academies of Science completed a report on the rules that currently apply to federally supported prison research, with recommendations for reform.[34] The report, "Ethical Considerations for Research Involving Prisoners," was developed at the request of OHRP. The current regulations had not been revised since their creation 25 years before and the OHRP found them difficult to interpret and apply to modern prison conditions. Among the IOM recommendations were that the current definition of prisoner be expanded to include all those whose liberty has been restricted, that the same rules should apply to all prisoners regardless of which jurisdiction they may fall under (federal, state or local), that assessments of research proposals be based on risks and benefits, that a concept of collaborative responsibility be added to the framework of research protections, and that systematic oversight of research involving prisoners be enhanced. These recommendations could result in a modification of the current federal regulations concerning prison research.[34]

In Europe the Nuremberg Code's requirement for "free choice" seems to have precluded most prison experiments and bright line standards continue.[13,35] The 1993 recommendations of the Council of Europe state with regard to prisoners that "persons deprived of their liberty may not undergo medical research unless it is expected to produce direct and significant benefit to them." Like U.S. regulations, this standard reflects the notion that prisoners are generally limited in their capacity to give informed consent. Other international bodies have adopted similar standards, but sometimes with different ethical underpinnings. For example, the Council for International Organizations of Medical Sciences, an organization formed by the World Health Organization and the United Nations Educational, Scientific and Cultural Organization, claims in its International Ethical Guidelines for Biomedical Research Involving Human Subjects that prisoners generally should not be used in research because historically they participated in experimentation disproportionately: "The central problem . . . is that such plans [to use prisoners and other "vulnerable" populations in research] may entail an inequitable distribution of the burdens and benefits of research participation."[36]

In the United States, individual state laws can be even more restrictive. For example, §3505 of the California Penal Code prohibits most biomedical research with prisoners and permits behavioral research only when it concerns the "causes, effects and processes of incarceration," "prisons as institutional structures," or "prisoners as incarcerated persons."[37] And other regulatory provisions in California permit biomedical research only when a physician determines that it is in the "best medical interest" of the prisoner, the prisoner gives informed consent according to specific standards, and the state Department of Corrections approves the research.[38,39]

III. Students

Although the use of prisoners in research is a fairly well documented and closely examined practice, with concern about coercion and exploitation rigorously debated during the past 30 years, the use of students is less studied. Little attention is paid to students as research participants because the vast majority of studies that recruit students are low-risk, survey research studies. In a historic practice that continues, many introductory courses in the behavioral sciences seem to require students to serve as research subjects in order to receive a grade. Students seem generally to be offered the option of writing a paper instead of participating in a study, but many students may find this option singularly unattractive. This required participation is in minimal risk research but when participation in research is a condition of completing a course and, therefore, successful completion of the student's major, one may argue that the participation is less than fully voluntary.

Students make a desirable research population for some of the same reasons that prisoners are attractive. Most students are within a defined age group. At universities there are often thousands of possible participants from whom to choose, and students usually have time to participate during the day. They are often highly

motivated. Some students are compelled to participate, but many studies recruit students outside of class, through flyers and advertisements in student papers. Considering that students' finances are often strained, they generally respond favorably to financial compensation offers, which helps ensure that students will return to complete the study.

Science students, in particular, are often highly educated, schooled in scientific methods, and interested in the professional advancement that may result from working with the researchers who experiment upon them. Describing medical students' traditional involvement in research, historian Susan Lederer explains that "students were readily available for experiments and they did not require elaborate explanations of the goals, needs, and risks of the research."[40] This ready supply of students for research, however, in rare cases has led to tragic consequences.

From Routine to Tragic

It is not surprising that many scientists are willing to expose themselves to potentially great heath risks to accomplish their goals. Whether they are, or only strive to be, a part of "the research team," many students share these risks and goals with their mentors. Other students participate in research for more mundane, though no less manipulable, reasons. They need money or a grade; participating in research solves these problems.

Historically, college health departments have been a locus of research involving students as subjects.[41] According to historian Heather Munro Prescott, Harold S. Dielh, then director of student health at the University of Minnesota, explained in 1927 that research by health center staff served to "stimulate scholarship" and "prevent the day's work from becoming routine and monotonous."[41] Frequently, this research examined diseases and conditions commonly found in student populations, including childhood infectious diseases and alcohol abuse.[41] Other studies used student populations to identify "standards of normality" for various health characteristics, including body type, blood pressure, metabolism, and psychology.[41] Many researchers saw students as a uniquely useful pool of potential research participants. As Prescott notes, Oberlin College's R.W. Bradshaw opined in 1929 that "[t]here is no other large group of people who can be so well molded into an experiment as the average college student body."[41]

Students also are a convenient population. Large numbers of students can be assembled quickly and efficiently. To be sure, research on students has nearly always occurred without harm and with little popular attention or concern.[41] But several well-publicized incidents illustrate how students may be selected as participants *because* they are young, perhaps impressionable, and more willing than their elders to undertake certain activities and risks.

In the early 1960s, Harvard professors Timothy Leary and Robert Alpert conducted research involving hallucinogenic psilocybin, a mushroom derivative, with numerous undergraduate and graduate students in Boston. In response to university concern about the health effects of the drug, the researchers at first agreed to suspend experiments with undergraduates, but, later, they were dismissed for continuing the experiments. Another example of research perhaps especially suited to a student population is the "prison life experiments" in which students role-played as inmates and guards in a "prison" in a Stanford University basement. The student-guards' actions were so severe and brutal, for example, in meting out punishment to the student-inmates, that the researchers stopped the study after only six days.[42] A third study that was little noticed at the time it was performed in 1962 gained notoriety in 2000 when it was revealed that Ted Kaczynski, popularly known as the "Unabomber," participated in it as an undergraduate. The study sought to test how the students would respond when their self-described personal beliefs were systematically attacked by an authority figure who aimed to undermine them. Recalling their experiences over 25 years later, some participants described shock, anger, and "unabating rage."[43]

Although some of the most shocking stories of student research involve studies that would not likely be approved by an institutional review board (IRB) today, tragic stories of students injured while participating in research can still be heard. In 1996, a 19-year-old undergraduate at the University of Rochester, Nicole Wan, died two days after participating as a "normal," or healthy, volunteer in a study examining bronchial cell defense mechanisms. The investigators recruited participants from local colleges and offered Wan $150 for her participation in the study, which involved bronchoscopy and brush biopsies to obtain cell samples. To prevent pain, the researchers administered lidocaine, a topical anesthesia. However, before finishing the protocol, which called for ten bronchial brushings, the researchers had undertaken 28 brushings and given Wan what was later found to be more than four times the maximum dosage for lidocaine. The medical examiner concluded that she died from lidocaine poisoning.[44]

After Wan died, critics charged, among other things, that the protocol failed to state whether participants would receive the promised compensation, an apparent incentive to participate, if they withdrew or failed to complete the study. Although the injuries resulted from failure to follow the study protocol, and may theoretically have occurred with any subject, Ms. Wan's death illuminated how students, more than some other groups in society, may face such risks. State officials later directed the university to develop guidelines to protect "vulnerable populations," which in the state's view included "college students [who] may be especially vulnerable to the inducement of a substantial honorarium for participating in a professor's research project."[44]

Ethical Assessment and Current Practices

As public doubts about the ethics of medical research in prison populations evolved during the last half of the 20th century, discourse about students in research also increased, though on a much smaller scale. This discussion regularly focused on the students' educational "opportunities" and generally downplayed the risk that financial or academic inducements could unduly influence students' choices. However, even as many denied these risks, the mere recognition of these confounding variables in students' motivations constituted an important shift in thinking that opened the door to the development of policies to limit students' risks. Nicole Wan's death vividly illustrates that students who "choose" to participate in research may face tragic consequences. Today, although there are no federal rules expressly prohibiting or limiting the use of students as research participants, many academic centers have policies aimed at reducing the risk that students, by virtue of their status as students, can be exploited or manipulated into participating in research.

The key ethical issues arising from the use of students as research participants concern financial inducements, academic inducements such as grades or extra credit, and academic pressures such as professors asking or otherwise communicating a desire to have students volunteer. The issue of financial inducements was the first and perhaps the easiest to be recognized. In 1956, Harvard Medical School adopted a policy for student participation that framed the issue as one of preserving students' ability to succeed academically. "Motivation should stem from an opportunity to learn and to contribute," Harvard stated, "rather than from a financial inducement per se."[45–47] Thus, "payment should not ordinarily be made to the student for participating as a subject in an experiment," but payment could proceed for students "collaborating" in a project, participating as a subject "during vacation periods," or "under special circumstances at other times during the research year" and to student research fellows.[46] Despite this laudable design, the reality, acknowledged by some researchers and the school even then, was that financial interests clearly influenced students' choices to participate.[48]

Defending the role of financial incentives, some have argued that students would not be willing to participate without compensation.[45] Proponents of paying students have argued that "[e]arning money from participation in research is at least as reputable a way as a variety of others available to students, such as selling their blood, tending bar, or babysitting for a faculty member's children."[49] Moreover, critics of special protections to limit or deny payments to students have argued that disparate treatment of students, as compared with the rest of the general population, is elitist.[49,50] According to Angoff they ask, "Why is it acceptable to ask the masses to accept risk in the name of science but not the very people [e.g., medical students] whose futures are linked to the successful perpetuation of biomedical research?"[49] They also contend that students, like the rest of the population, ought to be free to participate in research as an expression of their own autonomy.

Generally missing from these criticisms, however, is acknowledgment that students like Nicole Wan may be and frequently are situated differently from the "masses." As Shannon writes, because many students "need the stipends offered for their participation" they may be induced to do things they would not otherwise do.[51] They are not necessarily "free" choosers.

Academic interests and pressures also create circumstances that may undermine students' ability to exercise free choice. In the 1960s and 1970s, researchers began expressing conflicting views as to how students' academic requirements could undermine, if not preclude, voluntary consent. One researcher concluded that so long as participation in experiments "was not a requirement" of a course, the students "had volunteered" even if they did "receive two points credit towards their final grade for having taken part."[52] But, another researcher opined, "if a student in a classroom is asked to volunteer by his instructor, there is at least the implied threat of loss of affection (and decreased academic grade) if the student fails to volunteer."[53] A medical student writing about this phenomenon in 1979 explained that "[m]edical students are vulnerable to undue pressure from an investigator whose dual role as instructor makes it difficult for the student to refuse [a request to participate]."[50] When these requests are attached to course requirements or offers of extra credit, the pressure to accept may be overwhelming.

Today, some universities have promulgated policies to ameliorate some of these inequities. For example, one institution explains that the "relationship of teacher and student is inherently of unequal power" and, consequently, if the researcher is "a professor of the student or is in another position of authority" he or she is to proceed cautiously.[54] Another university, which expressly aims to "reduce the element of coercion or influence in any use of students as subjects" in research, requires professors to inform students before course enrollment if they may be asked to serve as research participants and give "alternative ways" to satisfy participation requirements.[55]

Other institutions apply more scrutiny to academic "alternatives," including extra papers, book reports, or quizzes, because these may not mitigate coercion when they require additional study and they involve greater uncertainty because the teachers will still grade them.[56] One university requires preapproval for all alternatives and will likely reject, for example, "the choice of either volunteering for a 30-minute experiment involving filling out a questionnaire or writing a 5-page paper." The university views this choice "as coercive, since writing a 5-page paper involves considerably more time, effort, and stress."[57]

Although modest compared with the procedures for prisoners and soldiers used in research, these university policies represent a significant step toward understanding a little-discussed problem. The ethical issues for this research are mainly of inequity and coercion, not death or serious injury. But historical examples like Leary's Harvard experiments and the Stanford "prison" experiments show that students can sometimes face unusually high health risks. Moreover, tragedies like Nicole Wan's death highlight the more dramatic risks that students, like other research participants, may face. Researchers may not always fully appreciate these risks, perhaps because they depend heavily on student populations, and also because they view participation as valuable for the student, at least for medical students or others in research training. But justifying a research intervention on the ground that it benefits the subject, the researcher, or other interests can obfuscate risks to individual autonomy. Key examples of this hazard are provided in the history of soldier-participant experiments.

IV. Soldiers

Problems of Research Consent in the Military

Today, the U.S. Department of Defense (DOD) requires that potential research participants give informed consent, except in certain "minimal-risk" research studies. Carefully drawn parameters, aimed to ensure voluntariness, govern when and how consent is obtained. But these policies have evolved from many years of contentious debate and even today, military planners face unusual and often unique challenges. These challenges stem largely from the circumstances of soldiers' lives and the role they play in society. The command and control framework of military operations means that soldier-participants can be ordered to participate in activities like research or find themselves the recipients of an experimental product administered without their knowledge when their supervisors determine that the action is necessary to protect the safety of the force or accomplish military goals.

As has been well documented elsewhere,[7] the military leadership wrestled with how and whether to obtain consent from soldiers throughout the middle part of the last century when it faced unknown health threats from new atomic, biological, and chemical weapons. Having convened the Nuremberg trial in 1946,

the military had every reason to know of the Nuremberg Code and its principles for research. In 1953 then-Defense Secretary Charles Wilson issued a memorandum that effectively adopted the Nuremberg Code and set written, voluntary consent as the Pentagon's policy for research in atomic, biological, and chemical warfare. The "voluntary consent of the human subject is absolutely essential," the document stated, and voluntary consent required "that the person involved should have the legal capacity to give consent; should be so situated as to be able to exercise free power of choice, without the intervention of any element of force . . . duress . . . or other ulterior form of constraint or coercion."[7] Wilson's directive would seem to eliminate any questions about the need to obtain voluntary consent before testing a new product or treatment modality, but the history is much more complicated.

Evidence shows that the DOD did not implement the Wilson policy or communicate it effectively down the chain of command. Part of the reason for the disparity between the military's written policy and its field activities arises from questions about what is a "medical experiment" versus, for example, necessary treatment in the face of uncertain risks or a required training exercise. Another reason is that imminent attack or health threats may change the calculus in balancing the needs of the group and the interests of any individual.

Landmark Cases

The military has a long tradition of experimenting with soldiers and other populations. Faced with soldiers dying from yellow fever in Cuba in 1900, the U.S. Army ordered Walter Reed to identify the vector of the virus. Reed's team asked American soldiers and local workers to agree to be exposed to mosquitoes that had just feasted on yellow fever blood.[58] Reed was apparently the first researcher to require participants to sign a contract memorializing their status as volunteers, though the agreement bears little resemblance to the detailed informed consent forms used in research today[58] (see Chapter 1).

Early military requirements for "voluntary" participation appeared to reflect the view that when an activity posed an especially high and often unknown or hard to calculate risk, soldiers should have freer choice whether to participate. In 1925 the Army established a policy requiring that "volunteers" be used in "experimental research" involving infectious diseases.[7] In 1932, the Navy established a policy permitting early diving experiments with "informed volunteers."[7] However, the fear of punishment for insubordination and the desire to serve may have undermined servicemen's ability to make truly free and uncoerced decisions.

The onset of World War II created new demands for human testing from many sources. Recognizing that many of these experiments would be dangerous, and that some might fall outside soldiers' ordinary duties, military planners articulated a requirement for voluntariness, though liability concerns also appeared. In one early letter, the head of the military's research coordinating group, the Committee on Medical Research, explained, "When any risks are involved, volunteers only should be utilized as subjects . . . and these only after the risks have been fully explained and after signed statements have been obtained which shall prove that the volunteer offered his services with full knowledge and that claims for damages will be waived."[7] Despite this clear statement, the military undertook substantial research without following these principles.[7]

For example, in 1942, the military began a series of gas experiments to test protective gear against chemical weapons, including, for example, mustard gas, one of the deadliest chemicals used during World War I. Mustard gas, also called sulfur mustard, causes severe skin blistering, vomiting, eye swelling, blindness, and internal and external bleeding, and in many cases during World War I, threatened slow and painful death. Then, as today, no known antidote existed. To combat mustard gas, the military developed masks and protective clothing and tested this equipment and troops' abilities when wearing it.

In its 1993 report on military gas experiments during World War II, the National Academy of Sciences concluded that "although the human subjects were called 'volunteers,' it is clear from the official reports that recruitment of the WW II human subjects, as well as many of those in later experiments, was accomplished through lies and half-truths."[59] Some of these experiments, which the soldiers swore to keep secret, occurred in gas chambers. Soldiers were outfitted with the protective clothing and locked in the gas chambers for one to four hours while gas was pumped in around them.[58] Afterward, they were required to wear the clothing and masks for up to 24 hours, and then the experiments were repeated until the soldiers developed skin reactions.[58] A contemporaneous Navy report of these tests explained how dissenters were managed: "Occasionally there have been reports of individuals or groups who did not cooperate fully. A short explanatory talk, and if necessary, a slight verbal 'dressing down,' has always proven successful. There has not been a single instance in which a man has refused to enter the gas chamber."[58]

Field tests also were conducted. To test protective gear in tropical battlefield conditions in 1944, 150 soldiers marched into a jungle area near Panama shortly after two U.S. bombers dropped 200 gas-filled bombs on the region. Describing the test, military reports later explained that the soldiers "had only to look about them to see the shining mustard on the foliage, to see the pools of mustard in bomb craters around their position."[58] Some of the soldiers reacted poorly, and "there were moments when panic or mass hysteria seemed close to the surface" among the troops.[58] But, as in the chamber tests, declining to participate was not an option.

After the war, the U.S. military continued using soldiers in an array of tests designed to better understand new atomic, biological, and chemical weapons. Experiments were often conducted without the person's knowledge or opportunity to make an informed decision about whether to participate. In part, this deception arose from a sense of expediency and a failure to distinguish among soldiers used as research participants and others exposed to similar conditions during mandatory service activities. For example, in 1946, the Navy and the Army Air Force jointly conducted the first underwater explosion of an atomic bomb during Operation Crossroads in the Marshall Islands.[60] As part of the test series, which aimed to test the survivability of ships and equipment, medical personnel also monitored the health risks to servicemen who were exposed to radiation during the tests and posttest surveillance of the area.

Servicemen did not "volunteer" for this duty. It was assigned in the normal course of business. Indeed, throughout the 1940s and 1950s, as the military developed its nuclear arsenal, medical researchers mined soldiers' training experiences to evaluate protective clothing designs and understand "how much radiation penetrated the human system" during, for example, mushroom cloud fly-throughs.[58] These activities were not considered "human experiments," and soldiers were not asked to consent or given a choice not to participate.

At the same time, however, other soldiers participating in human research—for example, flash blindness studies to test visual impairment after exposure to a nuclear blast—were asked for consent and informed of the experiment's risks.[58] One research participant later explained that "[w]hen the time came for ophthalmologists to describe what they thought could or could not happen, and we were asked to sign a consent form, just as you do in the hospital for surgery, I signed one."[58] Thus, it is clear that in some cases the military, even in the middle of the last century, undertook serious efforts to obtain informed consent before soldiers participated in research.

But tempting though it is to look for patterns in the military's consent practices during this time, they are hard to find. The line between military operations and medical research was often muddy and military planners, although generally affirming the principle of voluntary consent for experimentation, did not apply it consistently or across activities.

In the early 1960s, military regulations for human research became somewhat clearer, though the tension between operations and research continued. For example, the U.S. Army's 1962 regulation, AR 70–25: Use of Volunteers as Subjects of Research, required "voluntary consent" for research when "human beings are deliberately exposed to unusual or potentially hazardous conditions"—defined as conditions "which may be reasonably expected to involve the risk, beyond the normal call of duty, of privation, discomfort, distress, pain, damage to health, bodily harm, physical injury, or death."[61] Exempted from this policy were activities "encountered as part of training or other normal duties," experiments "wherein disclosure of experimental conditions to participating personnel would reveal the artificial nature of such conditions and defeat the purpose of the investigation," and "investigations involving the basic disease process or new treatment procedures conducted by the Army Medical Service for the benefit of patients." In some respects, these exceptions swallowed the rule and experiments sometimes occurred without regard to obtaining voluntary consent and often without telling the individual.[7]

Among the most famous, or infamous, government-sponsored research activities during this time were the Army and Central Intelligence Agency (CIA) experiments involving the hallucinogen lysergic acid diethylamide, or LSD. Code named "MKULTRA" in the CIA, the studies exposed military personnel and others to LSD without their knowledge or consent. Among other victims, CIA scientist Frank Olsen received the drug during a staff retreat in 1953. After his death was tied to the LSD experiments more than 20 years later, Olsen was said to have suffered a severe psychiatric reaction to the experiment and shortly thereafter fell to his death from the 10th floor of the Statler Hilton in New York City.[58] The precise circumstances of Olson's death are still a matter of disagreement.

Thousands of military personnel were used in the LSD experiments. Master Sergeant James Stanley volunteered in 1958 to participate in a study to combat chemical weapons but instead the Army gave him LSD. Stanley suffered years of unexplained personal turmoil thereafter. Only after congressional investigations in 1975 revealed the LSD testing, mustard gas studies, and other secret experiments involving soldiers did Stanley learn the truth about the drugs he ingested. Stanley sued the government to compensate him for his injuries.[58] Ultimately, the Supreme Court, in a 5–4 ruling, dismissed the case as barred by the long-standing doctrine that prohibits military personnel from suing for damages incurred incident to service.[62] But, in dissent, Justice O'Connor rejected the majority's conclusion in prose that echoes Justice Cardozo's clear affirmation 70 years earlier. Calling the research "so far beyond the bounds of human decency that as a matter of law it simply cannot be considered a part of the military mission," Justice O'Connor concluded that "[n]o judicially crafted rule should insulate from liability the involuntary and unknowing human experimentation alleged to have occurred in this case."[62] Although Stanley and other soldiers were unable to redress their grievances in the courts, the revelations of MKULTRA and other hidden experiments involving military personnel fueled debate about human experimentation that, as with prisoners and students, led to greater public sensitivity about what it means for a research participant to volunteer.

Gulf War Illness and Post–Desert Storm Controversy

Military policies, by the time of the *Stanley* decision in 1987 and today, support the notion that human participants should be informed volunteers.[7] But the sense of necessity and urgency that motivated many of the military's human experiments with unconsenting and uninformed soldiers has not disappeared. Instead, these tensions continue to arise as the United States faces new security threats.

In planning for Operation Desert Storm in 1990, for example, the military faced serious questions and concerns about the effects of Iraq's chemical and biological weapons on soldiers' safety and effectiveness. To combat these risks, new vaccines and drugs were tested. The military wanted to use them, but given concerns about the feasibility of obtaining informed consent from the hundreds of thousands of troops to be stationed in the Gulf, and about the possibility that some soldiers might decline to participate, the military asked the FDA for a waiver of the consent requirements for investigational products.[20] The military argued that it needed the waiver because of the imminent battlefield risks: "[M]ilitary combat is different. If a soldier's life will be endangered by nerve gas, for example, it is not acceptable from a military standpoint to defer to whatever might be the soldier's personal preference concerning a preventive or therapeutic treatment that might save his life, avoid endangerment of other personnel in his unit and accomplish the combat mission."[63]

After lengthy internal and interagency discussions, the FDA agreed and in December 1990 issued a new, interim regulation to permit the military to administer investigational drugs and biologics to military personnel without obtaining informed consent.[63,64] Under the regulation, the FDA could issue waivers, on a case-by-case basis, when a military physician, the investigational product's sponsor, and an IRB find a waiver to be "ethically justified" in a particular combat-related situation. Each must also find that informed consent is "not feasible" and that "withholding treatment would be contrary to the best interests of the military personnel."[63] This policy was premised on the conclusion that the exigencies of war could justify forced participation: "Military combat (actual or threatened) circumstances in which the health of the individual or the safety of other military personnel may require that a particular drug or biologic for prevention or treat-

ment be provided to a specified group of military personnel, without regard to any individual's personal preference for no treatment or for some alternative treatment."[63] Subsequently, the FDA approved the military's proposed use of two investigational products: (1) pyridostigmine bromide to be administered in tablet form every eight hours to protect against the effects of nerve gas, and (2) injected botulinum toxoid to vaccinate against botulism.[65]

The FDA's policy choice angered many critics. Many found the military's rationale for the waiver—battlefield exigencies—to be insufficient to justify jettisoning the fundamental respect for persons embodied in the requirement for informed consent.[66] Others felt that the military did not need the waiver to accomplish many of its goals. For example, one of the drugs, pyridostigmine bromide, was approved for other uses and therefore (technically) available for any treatment use, and the vaccine for botulism was ultimately administered on a voluntary basis, demonstrating that consent was obtainable.[66] Within several weeks after the FDA issued the interim rule, a soldier stationed in Saudi Arabia and his wife filed suit to enjoin the military from using unapproved products without obtaining consent.[65] The U.S. District Court for the District of Columbia dismissed the case, *Doe v. Sullivan*, in favor of the government in January 1991, 16 days after the Gulf War began. The court concluded that "judicial interference" in the military's "strategic decision would not be proper," once the military had explained that using the unapproved products would "improve the survival rate of troops that may encounter chemical and biological weapons," which, in turn, would "increase the safety of servicemen in the field and . . . decrease the medical burden of treating victims."[65]

Reflecting the long-standing tension of distinguishing *research* and *operations*, the court found that the planned action was not *research,* subject to separate DOD statutory prohibitions on using humans in experiments without prior informed consent, because the "primary purpose of administering the drugs is military, not scientific" and because "the DOD has responded to very real circumstances and chosen what it views as the best alternative given current knowledge."[65] Moreover, the court concluded that the military's interest in "successfully accomplishing the military goals of Operation Desert Storm" as well as its desire to protect the troops "constitute legitimate government interests that may counterbalance an individual's interest in being free from experimental treatment without giving consent."[65] The U.S. Court of Appeals for the District of Columbia affirmed the lower court's analysis.[67]

Ethical Assessment and Current Practices

As the *Doe v. Sullivan* case illustrates, in some respects, the concept of informed consent that today is an accepted prerequisite for voluntary participation in medical research is unsuited to the military context. Military regulations intentionally deny individual soldiers' autonomy in order to preserve and advance the fighting force. Thus, it is no surprise that U.S. history includes not only groundbreaking policies to ensure that soldiers participate in research only if they volunteer but also examples showing that the concept of voluntariness has not been well understood or executed.

The question of waiving informed consent for military use of experimental agents during wartime remains a live issue. In 1997, the FDA sought public comment on its Gulf War waiver provisions.[68] The following year, in 1998, Congress passed a law prohibiting the administration of experimental drugs and drugs unapproved for their intended use to service members without their informed consent.[69] The only exception to this policy was through presidential waiver based on a finding that consent is not feasible, is contrary to the soldier's best interests, or is contrary to national security.[69] President Bill Clinton issued an executive order in 1999 reiterating these standards.[70]

Shortly thereafter, the FDA repealed its Gulf War waiver provisions and issued a new interim rule to establish criteria for the president to apply when considering a waiver in accord with the law.[71] But, after the terrorist attacks of Sept. 11, 2001, and the onset of operations in Afghanistan and Iraq, Congress went further. In 2004 Congress authorized use of unapproved medical products, or products unapproved for particular uses, pursuant to an "emergency use authorization" (EUA) issued by the FDA after an emergency or potential for emergency involving heightened risk of attack with a specific biological, radiological, nuclear, or chemical agent is identified.[72] At the same time, however, Congress required that all individuals to whom products are to be administered under an EUA be given information about risks and benefits and have the option to refuse administration.[72]

The DOD's Anthrax Vaccination Immunization Program (AVIP), which provides anthrax vaccine to service members, became a test case for these provisions. In a suit brought by six active duty military personnel, the U.S. District Court for the District of Columbia in 2004 enjoined the military from requiring personnel to receive anthrax vaccines in the absence of "informed consent or a Presidential waiver."[73] But, in April 2005, following passage of the 2004 law and declaration of an EUA, the court allowed the military to resume anthrax vaccinations under certain conditions. The court specified, consistent with the law, that members of the armed forces receive education on the program and be given the option to refuse the vaccination without penalty.[74] The following year, after the FDA designated the vaccine as "safe and effective" to combat anthrax inhalation exposure, the need for the EUA and the court's injunction dissolved.[75]

As the challenges to the AVIP program illustrate, when the circumstances of military life require a soldier to participate in an experiment or accept an unproven therapy against his or her will, it cannot be said that the soldier is "volunteering." More than any other of the captive populations we have discussed, soldiers live in circumstances in which the command structure may force them to participate and the needs of the whole may override the interests of the few. As the military stated during the Gulf War, ingestion of an experimental vaccine may be necessary to ensure that the entire force will be protected. This paternalistic usurpation of an individual's expressed, and presumably informed, judgment can only be justified in rare circumstances, if at all. The history of involuntary research with uninformed soldiers, especially in dual-purpose activities in which research and training occur together, demonstrates how military expediency may be used, albeit subconsciously, to authorize research in soldiers that would not be permitted in the general population.

Excepting situations in which competing group interests may outweigh respect for individual choices to decline participation, the military setting does not per se preclude the possibility of free choice. For soldiers to truly "volunteer" they must feel that they can decline without suffering adverse consequences. When soldiers are informed about the risks of participation and are given genuine options to decline, the risk that a soldier will misunderstand the research or feel pressured to participate is reduced. In these circumstances, soldiers are like their nonmilitary counterparts who volunteer for research. So long as the soldiers do not face or perceive career limits for opting not to participate, voluntary consent is feasible. Today's military has many provisions in place to ensure that soldiers who volunteer truly are "volunteers."

Conclusion

Captive populations are different from the general society. Often they are physically separated, sometimes locked behind prison walls or concentrated on military bases. At other times they are separated by their dress, lifestyle, or financial opportunities. Together, they live in circumstances and share interests that may make them especially vulnerable to coercion and exploitation. Moreover, and perhaps most important, society generally has looked at captive populations through colored lenses that failed to scrutinize, or even recognize, how these differences could affect captive populations' ability to "volunteer" for research. Ironically, having condemned the Nazi crimes, the United States in the mid-20th century at least by its silence condoned extensive prisoner research at home without considering whether the terms of the Nuremberg Code—the concept of genuinely free choice—held any relevance to the lives of prisoners who were not in the extreme circumstances of concentration camp inmates.

During the last half of the 20th century, the United States examined the effects of captivity with more precision. For some captive groups, like prisoners, policy makers judged that the conditions of their captivity effectively precluded voluntary consent in most cases and found that often the risks of research far outweighed its potential benefits. In other cases, like the military's consent exception during the Gulf War, the benefits for the group may outweigh individual choices. What is essential in examining research with captive populations is to recognize how the conditions of captivity can influence whether a participant truly "volunteers" for research, and how the interests of others, including investigators, fellow soldiers, or the scientific enterprise, may influence what sorts of risks participants are allowed to accept.

References

1. *Schloendorff* v. *Society of New York Hospital* (105 N.E. 92, 93; N.Y., 1914).
2. Hippocrates. The Oath. In: *Hippocrates, Volume 1,* trans. Jones WHS. Cambridge, Mass.: Loeb Classical Library of Harvard University Press; 1923.
3. Tannebaum AS, Cooke RA. Research in prisons: A preliminary report. In: National Commission for the Protections of Human Subject of Biomedical and Behavioral Research. *Research Involving Prisoners: Appendix.* DHEW Pub. No. (OS) 76–132. Washington, D.C.: DHEW; 1976.
4. Cannon WB. The right and wrong of making experiments on human beings. *JAMA* 1916;67:1372–3.
5. The National Commission for the Protection of Human Subjects of Biomedical and Behavioral Research. *The Belmont Report: Ethical Principles and Guidelines for the Protection of Human Subjects of Research.* Washington, D.C.: Department of Health, Education and Welfare; DHEW Publication OS 78-0012 1978. [Online] April 18, 1979.

Available: http://www.hhs.gov/ohrp/humansubjects/guidance/belmont.htm.

6. Hart HLA. *Law and Morals.* Oxford, England: Clarendon Press, 1965, p.181–207. In: Reiser SJ, Dyck AJ, Curran WJ, eds. *Ethics in Medicine: Historical Perspectives and Contemporary Concerns.* Cambridge, Mass.: MIT Press; 1977:104–13.

7. Advisory Committee on Human Radiation Experiments. *Final Report of the Advisory Committee on Human Radiation Experiments.* New York, N.Y.: Oxford University Press; 1996. [Online] Available: http://www.eh.doe.gov/ohre/roadmap/achre/report.html.

8. The Nuremberg Code. In: *Trials of War Criminals Before the Nuremberg Military Tribunals Under Control Council Law No. 10. Volume 2.* Washington, D.C.: U.S. Government Printing Office; 1949:181–2. [Online]. Available: http://www.hhs.gov/ohrp/references/nurcode.htm.

9. Ethical Committee of the World Medical Association. *Draft Code of Ethics on Human Experimentation.* Helsinki, Finland: WMA; September 1961. *British Medical Journal* 1962;2:1119.

10. World Medical Association. *Code of Ethics of the World Medical Association: Declaration of Helsinki.* Helsinki, Finland: WMA; June 1964. *British Medical Journal* 1964;2:177.

11. Department of Health and Human Services, National Institutes of Health, and Office for Human Research Protections. The Common Rule, Title 45 (Public Welfare), Code of Federal Regulations, Part 46 (Protection of Human Subjects). [Online] June 23, 2005. Available: http://www.hhs.gov/ohrp/humansubjects/guidance/45cfr46.htm.

12. Hodges RE, Bean WB. The use of prisoners for medical research. *JAMA* 1967;202:513–5.

13. National Commission for the Protection of Human Subjects of Biomedical and Behavioral Research. *Research Involving Prisoners: Report and Recommendations.* DHEW Publication No. (OS) 76–131. Washington, D.C.: DHEW; 1976. [Online] Available: http://www.bioethics.gov/reports/past_commissions/Research_involving_prisoners.pdf.

14. Taylor T. Opening statement of the prosecution, December 9, 1946. In: Annas GJ, Grodin MA, eds. *The Nazi Doctors and the Nuremberg Code.* New York, N.Y.: Oxford University Press; 1992:67–93.

15. Williams P, Wallace D. *Unit 731: Japan's Secret Biological Warfare in World War II.* New York, N.Y.: The Free Press; 1989.

16. Ivy AC. Ethics governing the service of prisoners as subjects in medical experiments: Report of a committee appointed by Governor Dwight H. Green of Illinois. *JAMA* 1948;136:447–58.

17. Sabin AB. Behavior of chimpanzee-avirulent poliomyelitis viruses in experimentally infected human volunteers. *American Journal of the Medical Sciences* 1955;230:1–8.

18. Hornblum A. *Acres of Skin: Human Experiments at Holmesburg Prison.* New York, N.Y.: Routledge; 1998.

19. Shuster A. Why human "guinea pigs" volunteer. *New York Times Magazine* Apr. 13, 1958.

20. U.S. Congress. Federal Food, Drug, and Cosmetic Act (codified in scattered sections of 21 U.S.C.). [Online] Available: http://www.fda.gov/opacom/laws/fdcact/fdctoc.htm.

21. Food and Drug Administration, Department of Health and Human Services. Title 21 (Food and Drugs), Code of Federal Regulations, Part 314 (Applications for FDA Approval to Market a New Drug), Sections 314.125(b)(5) and 314.126. [Online] April 1, 2006. Available: http://www.access.gpo.gov/nara/cfr/waisidx_06/21cfr314_06.html.

22. Merrill RA. The architecture of government regulation of medical products. *Virginia Law Review* 1996;82:1753–1866.

23. Drug Investigation Committee of the Medical Association of the State of Alabama, (Harrison TR, Chairman). The use of prisoners for drug trials in Alabama. In: Katz J, with Capron AM, Glass ES. *Experimentation With Human Beings.* New York, N.Y.: Russell Sage Foundation; 1972:1041–5.

24. Mitford J. *Kind and Usual Punishment.* New York, N.Y.: Alfred A. Knopf; 1973.

25. Burt RA. Why we should keep prisoners from the doctors. *Hastings Center Report* 1975;5(1):25–34.

26. Bach-y-Rita G. The prisoner as an experimental subject. *JAMA* 1974;229:45–6.

27. U.S. Congress, Senate Committee on Labor and Public Welfare, Subcommittee on Health. Hearings on Quality of Health Care—Human Experimentation, 93rd Congress, 1st Session, March 7, 1973. Washington, D.C.: Government Printing Office; 1973.

28. U.S. Department of Justice, Federal Bureau of Prisons. Program Statement 1070.07; Research. Washington, D.C.: Federal Bureau of Prisons; 1999. [Online] May 12, 1999. Available: http://www.bop.gov/policy/progstat/1070_007.pdf.

29. Department of Health, Education, and Welfare. Additional Protections Pertaining to Biomedical and Behavioral Research Involving Prisoners as Subjects; Supplementary Information and Final Rule. Federal Register 1978;43(222):53652–6.

30. *Fante et al. v. Department of Health and Human Services* (U.S. District Court, Eastern District of Michigan, Southern Division, Civil Action No. 80–72778, 1978.)

31. Martin DC, Arnold JD, Zimmerman TF, Richart RH. Human subjects in clinical research. *New England Journal of Medicine* 1968;279: 1427–8. In: Katz J, with Capron AM, Glass ES. *Experimentation With Human Beings.* New York, N.Y.: Russell Sage Foundation; 1972: 1024–5.

32. Office of Human Research Protections, Department of Health and Human Services. Waiver of the Applicability of Certain Provisions of Department of Health and Human Services Regulations for Protection of Human Research Subjects for Department of Health and Human Services Conducted or Supported Epidemiologic Research Involving Prisoners as Subjects: Final Action on Waiver. *Federal Register* 2003; 68(119):36929–31.

33. Dubler N. The burdens of research in prisons. *IRB: A Review of Human Subjects Research* 1982;4(9):9–10.

34. Committee on Ethical Considerations for Revisions to DHHS Regulations for Protection of Prisoners Involved in Research, Institute of Medicine (Gostin LO, Vanchieri C, Pope A, eds.). *Ethical Considerations for Research Involving Prisoners.* Washington, D.C.: National Academies Press; 2006.

35. Jaffe M, Snoddy C. An international survey of research in volunteers. In: National Commission for the Protections of Human Subject of Biomedical and Behavioral Research. *Research Involving Prisoners: Appendix.* DHEW Pub. No. (OS) 76–132. Washington, D.C.: DHEW; 1976.

36. Council for International Organizations of Medical Sciences, in collaboration with the World Health Organization. *International Ethical Guidelines for Biomedical Research Involving Human Subjects.* Geneva, Switzerland: CIOMS and WHO; 2002. [Online] November 2002. Available: http://www.cioms.ch/frame_guidelines_nov_2002.htm.

37. State of California. California Penal Code, Title 2.1 (Biomedical and Behavioral Research), §3505.

38. State of California. California Penal Code, Title 2.1 (Biomedical and Behavioral Research), §3502.5(a).

39. State of California. California Code of Regulations, Title 15 (Crime Prevention and Corrections), Article 9.1 (Research of Inmates/Parolees), §3369.5 (Research), December 31, 2004.

40. Lederer S. *Subjected to Science: Human Experimentation in America Before the Second World War.* Baltimore, Md.: The Johns Hopkins University Press; 1995:19.

41. Prescott HM. Using the student body: College and university students as research subjects in the United States during the twentieth century. *Journal of the History of Medicine* 2002;57:3–38.

42. Zimbardo PG. The power and pathology of imprisonment. Congressional Record. (Serial No. 15, October 25, 1971). Hearings Before

Subcommittee No. 3, of the Committee on the Judiciary, House of Representatives, 92nd Congress, 1st Session on Corrections, Part II, Prisons, Prison Reform and Prisoner's Rights: California. Washington, DC: U.S. Government Printing Office; 1971.

43. Chase A. Harvard and the making of the Unabomber. *Atlantic* 2000; 285(6):41–65.
44. New York State Department of Health. Case report on death of University of Rochester student issued. Albany, N.Y.: New York State Department of Health; 1996. [Online] September 30, 1996. Available: http://www.health.state.ny.us/press/releases/1996/wan.htm.
45. Christakis N. Do medical student research subjects need special protection? *IRB: A Review of Human Subjects Research* 1985;7(3):1–4.
46. Berry GP. Memorandum: Harvard Medical School Rules Governing the Participation of Medical Students as Experimental Subjects, 1968. In: Katz J, with Capron AM, Glass ES. *Experimentation With Human Beings.* New York, N.Y.: Russell Sage Foundation; 1972:1036.
47. Office for Research Subject Protection, Harvard Medical School. *Rules Governing the Participation of Medical Students as Experimental Subjects in Research Studies* (approved by Faculty Council, May 20, 1986). Boston, Mass.: Harvard Medical School; 1986. [Online] Available: http://www.hms.harvard.edu/orsp/doc/rules_student_partic.DOC.
48. Lasagna L, von Felsinger JM. The volunteer subject in research. *Science* 1954;120:359–61.
49. Angoff NR. Against special protections for medical students. *IRB: A Review of Human Subjects Research* 1985;7(5):9–10.
50. Nolan KA. Protecting medical students from the risks of research. *IRB: A Review of Human Subjects Research* 1979:1(5):9–10.
51. Shannon TA. Should medical students be research subjects? *IRB: A Review of Human Subjects Research* 1979;1(2):4.
52. Ring K, Wallston K, Corey M. Mode of debriefing as a factor affecting subjective reaction to a Milgram-type obedience experiment—An ethical inquiry. In: Katz J, with Capron AM, Glass ES. *Experimentation With Human Beings.* New York, N.Y.: Russell Sage Foundation; 1972:395–400.
53. Lasagna L. Special subjects in human experimentation. *Daedalus* 1969;98:449–57.
54. Purdue University Committee on the Use of Human Research Subjects. Students as subjects. West Lafayette, Ind.: Purdue University Human Subjects Office. [Online] Available: http://www.irb.purdue.edu/studentsubjects.shtml.
55. Columbia University Human Research Protection Program. Use of Columbia University students as study subjects in research. New York, N.Y.: Columbia University Human Subjects Review Committee. [Online] June 26, 2003. Available: http://www.columbia.edu/cu/irb/policies/StudentSubjectsPolicy_062603.html.
56. Gamble HF. Students, grades, and informed consent. *IRB: A Review of Human Subjects Research* 1982:4(3):7–10.
57. Indiana University Office of the Vice Provost for Research, Bloomington Campus, Bloomington Human Subjects Committee. Students as subjects. [Online] Available: http://www.research.iu.edu/rschcomp/stusub.html.
58. Moreno JD. *Undue Risk: Secret State Experiments on Humans.* New York, N.Y.: W. H. Freeman and Company; 2000.
59. Committee to Survey the Health Effects of Mustard Gas and Lewisite, Division of Health Promotion and Disease Prevention, Institute of Medicine (Pechura CM, Rall DP, eds.). *Veterans at Risk: The Health Effects of Mustard Gas and Lewisite.* Washington, D.C.: National Academy Press; 1993.
60. Weisgall J. *Operation Crossroads: The Atomic Tests at Bikini Atoll.* Annapolis, Md.: Naval Institute Press; 1994.
61. Headquarters, Department of the Army. *Army Regulation 70–25: Use of Volunteers as Subjects of Research.* Washington, D.C.: Department of the Army; 1962. [Online] Available: http://ethics.iit.edu/codes/coe/us.gov.army.research.1962.html.
62. *United States* v. *Stanley,* 483 U.S. 669 (1987).
63. Food and Drug Administration, Department of Health and Human Services. Informed Consent for Human Drugs and Biologics: Determination That Informed Consent Is NOT Feasible; Interim Rule and Opportunity for Public Comment. *Federal Register* 1990; 55(246):52814–7.
64. U.S Senate (John D. Rockefeller IV, Chairman). Is Military Research Hazardous to Veterans' Health? Lessons Spanning Half a Century: A Staff Report Prepared for the Committee on Veterans' Affairs, S. Prt. 103–97, 103rd Congress, 2nd Session, Dec. 8, 1994.
65. *Doe* v. *Sullivan,* 756 F. Supp. 12 (D. D. C. 1991).
66. Annas GJ. *Some Choice: Law, Medicine, and the Market.* New York, N.Y.: Oxford University Press; 1998.
67. *Doe* v. *Sullivan,* 938 F. 2d 1370, 1381 (D.C. Cir. 1991).
68. Food and Drug Administration, Department of Health and Human Services. Accessibility to New Drugs for Use in Military and Civilian Exigencies When Traditional Human Efficacy Studies Are Not Feasible; Determination Under the Interim Rule That Informed Consent Is Not Feasible for Military Exigencies; Request for Comments. *Federal Register* 1997;62(147):40996–41001.
69. U.S. Congress. 10 U.S.C. 1107: Title 10 (Armed Forces), Subtitle A (General Military Law), Part II (Personnel), Chapter 55 (Medical and Dental Care), §1107: Notice of use of an investigational new drug or a drug unapproved for its applied use.
70. The President. Executive Order 13139—Improving Health Protection of Military Personnel Participating in Particular Military Operations. *Federal Register* 1999;64(192):54175–8.
71. Food and Drug Administration, Department of Health and Human Services. Human Drugs and Biologics; Determination That Informed Consent Is NOT Feasible or Is Contrary to the Best Interests of Recipients; Revocation of 1990 Interim Final Rule; Establishment of New Interim Final Rule; Opportunity for Public Comment. *Federal Register* 1999;64(192):54179–89.
72. U.S. Congress. Project BioShield Act of 2004, Pub. L. No. 108–276, 108th Congress, S. 15, H.R. 2122, July 21, 2004.
73. Doe v. Rumsfeld, 341 F. Supp. 2d. 1, 16 (D.D.C. 2004
74. Doe v. Rumsfeld, 2005 WL 1124589 (D.D.C. 2005).
75. Doe v. Rumsfeld, 172 Fed. Appx. 327 (D.C. Cir. 2006).

Morris W. Foster   Richard R. Sharp

Research With Identifiable and Targeted Communities

Most research studies that involve human participants target specific categories of people through inclusion/exclusion criteria. Some of those targeted categories are defined by scientific criteria, such as people with a diagnosis of a particular disease or people without the disease who can serve as "healthy" controls. Other targeted categories are defined by demographic criteria, used either as proxies for specific life experiences, exposures, or incidence rates or as measures of inclusiveness. As an example of the latter, even studies that recruit members of the "general public" often use social identities such as gender, race, or ethnicity to ensure that a sample resembles the makeup of that larger general population.

Some of the categories of people targeted for study recruitment may be more vulnerable than others to harms associated with taking part in research, requiring special considerations in the evaluation of and protection against potential research risks. Prisoners, for example, are more vulnerable to coercion because of their incarcerated status, whereas children and the mentally incapacitated may not be able to fully understand what they are giving consent to do. Other categories of people, such as pregnant women and the elderly, may have health risks greater than other participants. Ethical review committees and institutional review boards have historically provided higher levels of protection for such vulnerable persons, including greater scrutiny of studies that target them, additional protections from potential risks, and the inclusion of advocates for them on such committees and boards.

These examples of populations typically considered more vulnerable to research risks are designated as such because of functional attributes that may affect their ability to consent or that may pose special physical risks; that is, prisoners have less individual autonomy than others, children and the mentally impaired tend to

have less well developed abilities to make autonomous decisions, and pregnant women and the elderly tend to have greater health risks than other healthy adults.

Other groups, though, such as Native American tribes and other indigenous groups around the world, have also been proposed for special consideration as targeted populations.[1–3] Two primary arguments have been made for extending a special status to them: (1) that their members are readily identifiable as such, so that research findings associated with a named group or community can have consequences for all identifiable members of the group or community, and (2) that their shared identities indicate collective moral, cultural, and/or legal authorities that are recognized by most persons whom those identities label as having some license to regulate or sanction individual claims to group membership and appropriate behaviors in group contexts, and so should be consulted and respected when targeted by a research study.[4,5] Because of these collective implications and qualities, some ethicists and group members have proposed higher levels of scrutiny and special protections for populations targeted because of shared social identities.[6,7]

Studies that target such populations often present risks to individuals outside the researcher/research participant relationship, and so can introduce a number of distinctive ethical challenges.

First, studies in which targeted communities are identified in research reports may inadvertently reinforce existing stereotypes about the community and its members. For example, studies of existing health disparities—such as studies of a particular locale or workplace—may reinforce local perceptions of a community as unsafe or unhealthy. These negative images of a community or its members may be associated with forms of social devaluing such as decreased property values, individual discrimination such as decreased access to employment opportunities, and stigma, leading to decreased opportunities for social interaction with individuals outside the community. These considerations are particularly noteworthy in contexts in which there are histories of social disadvantage or pervasive social divisions that are the result of existing stereotypes regarding a targeted community.

Second, studies of targeted communities may cause a range of disruptions within a targeted community. For example, intracommunity discussions about taking part in a study of a condition that has the potential to be publicly prejudicial, such as alcoholism or HIV, or in a study that uses a methodology about which some segments of the public are suspicious, such as genetics, can become polarizing issues that divide community members. Despite a sincere intention to improve the health of community members, these disruptions to existing social relationships may be considered by those persons affected to be a significant harm resulting from the research.

Third, studies of targeted communities may suggest an inappropriate image of the community as static or one-dimensional. Most targeted communities are heterogeneous and diverse with regard to a range of variables that may be associated with increased health risks. When studies of targeted communities present data suggesting an association between one aspect of the community and a particular health risk, this may be understood by some as suggesting that *all members* of the community are at increased risk. Such studies may thus undermine efforts to increase sensitivity to important variability within communities with a common collective label such as "Italian American" or "elementary school teachers."

These and other risks to people indirectly affected by studies of targeted communities may be difficult to anticipate in advance. As a result, researchers may fail to disclose all salient risks to prospective participants or to community leaders during the informed consent process. When histories of profound mistrust of medical researchers exist, researchers may find that it is difficult to communicate the full range of potential benefits and risks associated with a study to community members whose past experiences condition them to anticipate the worst possible harms. In addition, researchers may inadvertently present research findings in a manner that is insensitive to potential harms to affected third parties or otherwise fail to establish adequate protections for individuals placed at risk. When the risks at issue are closely tied to the unique social histories of the community under investigation, and the investigators conducting the study are not intimately familiar with those histories, it may be especially difficult to identify the potential harms at stake without substantial community participation in the design and development of a research protocol.

Indeed, to a considerable extent, most discussions of the ethical significance of collective risks and interests have been linked with discussions about processes for involving communities and their members in evaluating these risks and interests. The involvement of communities recognizes that researchers and ethics committees cannot evaluate the risks and interests unilaterally because they often lack information about how members of other communities perceive those risks and interests.[8,9] Thus, taking account of the collective implications that a research study may have (that is, the implications for all those who share a targeted identity whether they take part in the study or not) is necessarily a combination of conceptual and empirical approaches. In particular, various forms of group or community consultation have been proposed as supplements to individual informed consent to manage the additional level of risks that may be associated with collective identities as well as to recognize the importance of engaging those collective entities in studies that specifically target their members. These include community consultations, in which some community members are engaged in discussions about a proposed study before it is undertaken, and in some cases community consent, in which some formal approval is obtained from a community in which formal decision-making processes exist, such as in Native American tribes.[10–12]

In some instances, requirements for community consultation and/or consent have been adopted by local ethics committees, government agencies, and international organizations.[13,14] However, there is a continuing debate about the kinds of existing social groups and communities that merit such special protections and the extent to which collective concerns should be weighed alongside individual concerns about taking part in research.[15–17] In this chapter, we review approaches and guidelines that have been proposed, outline the issues that have arisen in this developing area of research ethics, and anticipate future directions in which those might lead.

Current Standards and Guidelines

For some time, communitarian frameworks have been available within research ethics as alternatives to the dominant focus on individual autonomy. Innovations in the ethics of the collective implications of research, however, have grown out of more practical concerns about research that focuses on tribes and indigenous groups rather than from philosophical critiques of individualism. Many aboriginal groups have or assert unique legal statuses within larger nation-states in addition to having experienced long histories of discrimination and stigmatization that often include having been subjected to medical studies that would today be considered unethical.[18] That combination of assertions of collective authority and experiences of past abuses contributed to a series of guidelines for research from indigenous peoples in Canada,[19] Australia,[20] and the United States.[21] Some of these guidelines were motivated by heightened concerns about the implications of genetic research for group identity, particularly the use of genetic information to rewrite population history. Other concerns included the ownership of intellectual property arising from the development of gene-based diagnostics and therapeutics that might be commercialized.[22]

Many of the principles articulated in those guidelines are common to what has become community-based, participatory research (CBPR). CBPR brings targeted communities into the planning of a study, focusing on a community's research priorities rather than the researcher's, structuring a study to build capacity within the community, making provisions to share any benefits from the study with community members and presenting research findings back to the community.[23] Other provisions deal with the collective authority or jurisdiction of the group and include such issues as whether the group has the right to approve or veto proposed studies, whether manuscripts must be approved by the group before publication, and whether data generated by the study are owned by the group rather than by researchers, their institutions, or the agency that funded the study.[24,25]

These latter claims are best understood in the context of similar legal and political negotiations, in which many indigenous peoples also have been engaged, about land claims, treaty rights, ownership of natural resources, self-determination, control of cultural symbols and heritage, and sovereignty, as well as the health disparities and limited access to care that such groups continue to experience. Some indigenous groups have succeeded in establishing their own ethics committees that review proposed studies and also have begun to build their own research infrastructure, often in collaboration with outside institutions.[26] Some local ethics committees now require separate tribal approval for studies that target members of specific native communities. In addition, increasing numbers of researchers negotiate conditions of data ownership and publication with indigenous groups prior to beginning a study with their members.[27] Although some controversies continue to arise, often based on older studies,[28] research practices increasingly recognize that indigenous groups have some legitimate claim to collective authority when a study specifically targets group members for participation.

This growing recognition, however, has not been codified into a single set of consensus standards or best practices that can be applied generally, despite various efforts to do so. A primary reason for this failure is that the unique cultural and historical positions of different native groups are more conducive to situational negotiations than to a single policy. At the same time, notions of collective authority and collective implications have been extended beyond indigenous groups to include a broader range of social entities. These extensions include localities in which emergency medical studies are subjected to local community approval,[29] the common interests of groups of people defined by a shared disease status such as HIV/AIDS,[30] and local community consultation for genetic samples that are used as proxies for larger ethnic and continental populations.[31] Different levels of collective interests and authority are also routinely recognized in international research, ranging from national governments to ethnic, cultural, and religious subgroups to localities.[32]

These extensions raise a number of questions about the organizational capacity and moral authority of social groups and categories that, unlike most indigenous communities, lack a long-standing tradition and process of collective decision making. Both Weijer and Emanuel[11] and Sharp and Foster[10] have proposed systematic frameworks for evaluating whether different social entities have appropriate capacities and authorities for the consideration of collective ethical implications. Weijer and Emanuel emphasize the importance of social cohesion within a group for establishing the moral authority considered necessary for true communal consent or approval of a study. They consider this kind of social cohesion rare in examples outside aboriginal communities or localized geographical communities that have legitimate mechanisms for political representation and decision making. Community consultation—stopping short of formal consent—is treated as a lesser level of protection, but one that also requires some degree of cohesion, as might exist in the case of religious communities that share a common cultural framework and communication network but lack centralized decision-making processes.[11]

Sharp and Foster also note the importance of social cohesion to establishing moral authority, but they explore the ways in which social science methods can be used to sample the range of views that exist within more dispersed, less centralized communities or populations.[10] A strong case can be made for considering the collective implications of studies that target certain larger geographically dispersed populations such as African Americans, for example, because of their history of discrimination as well as specific examples of abuse in clinical research[33,34] (see Chapter 8). However, such populations are socially and culturally diverse, at least more so than localized, centrally organized entities, and have multiple levels of organization and leadership, none of which can speak definitively for the whole.

Empirical examples of community consultation are primarily situated at local levels and emphasize repeated face-to-face interactions between researchers and community members, arguably a necessary dynamic to encourage interaction and build trust.[35] For studies that involve implications that are generalized beyond the immediate communities from which participants are recruited, however, the localized dynamics of consultation may limit the extent to which the range of views of the immediate community can be considered to represent the larger population views, depending on how representative the local community is of the larger group.

Perhaps the highest-profile example of community consultation has been the engagement with three local communities—in Tokyo, Beijing, and Ibadan, Nigeria—leading up to DNA sample collection for the International HapMap Project.[31] In a series of individual interviews, focus groups, surveys, and public meetings, these communities were consulted about their preferences for how donors would be recruited, how their communities were to be named in labeling the samples and in subsequent publications that identified them, and how community advisory groups were to be set up to monitor future uses. A primary focus of these consultations was the collective implications of findings from the HapMap. Those implications included both the immediate communities in which samples were obtained and the larger ethnic and continental populations for which the samples served as proxies in seeking common patterns of human genetic variation. At best, though, consulting with members of local communities enabled researchers only to tailor their recruitment procedures, social labels, and framing of study findings to the ways in which some Japanese, Han Chinese, and Yoruba understood those collective implications, given the practical difficulties of sampling larger populations with millions of members each.

The HapMap experience suggests that collective implications and interests of populations targeted for research might be divided into two categories: (1) those of the larger population to which findings are generalized and (2) those of the local community or communities from which participants are recruited. Protections for the latter category will necessarily provide some benefit for the former as well, but may not fully address all concerns about implications for the larger population. Nonetheless, the advantage of focusing ethical protections for collective interests on local communities from which participants are to be recruited is that these are the settings within which collective and individual considerations will intersect in actual decisions to take part in research studies. That local intersection supports the goals of community consultation that Dickert and Sugarman have delineated: protection of participants' welfare and interests, enhancement of benefits for participants and their communities, ethical and political legitimacy for the study, and shared responsibility for the research through establishing a truly collaborative partnership between researchers and the communities they study.[36] Still, a number of conceptual and methodological issues remain in incorporating the evaluation and protection of collective interests of targeted populations and communities into clinical research ethics.

Issues to Be Resolved

How can we satisfy both individual autonomy and collective interests? This is perhaps the central conceptual challenge in incorporating the collective interests of targeted populations into research ethics. When community consent is appropriate, as in the case of politically organized tribes, a collective decision to disapprove a research project in effect denies individual tribal members the opportunity to take part in a study that some might consider valuable. Moreover, some group members may not subscribe to the authority of leaders to approve manuscripts that describe study findings or to have oversight over future uses of biological samples or other data. Even in cases in which consultation is undertaken without the possibility of community consent, some individual members may strongly disagree with the political or moral authority of those whose views were solicited to speak on their behalf.

This moral conflict becomes particularly acute in the case of members who live outside the territorial jurisdiction or homeland of the population or community in question. Should the authority of the parent population be respected, or should emigrants who may not recognize that authority be given the opportunity to make individual choices about studies that target those who share a particular identity? That problem arises not only with respect to members of indigenous groups who move to urban areas, but also to members of a variety of national, cultural, ethnic, and other populations who emigrate outside their ancestral homeland, often to other countries, and are approached by researchers as proxies for those ancestral populations. Despite their geographical and social separation, their shared social identity can subject both emigrant and ancestral populations to the same implications of research findings.

How can we weigh differing views of a population's collective interests? Different local communities can have very different views about the collective implications of a proposed study, particularly in the case of large, geographically dispersed populations.[10] Moreover, organizations that claim to represent the interests of larger populations across localities, and that may do so in some part, also can have different views either with one another or with some local communities. For example, several national and international Native American organizations have called for prohibitions on genetic research with tribal members, whereas some sovereign tribal governments have approved genetic studies and even themselves invested in genetic projects.[37] A similar situation, of course, can arise in the case of targeted populations or communities that lack the political organization of tribes. In either instance, researchers and ethics committees are left to weigh those differing views in deciding whether and how to protect the varying representations of collective interests at issue.

Does a consultative focus on local communities constitute forum shopping? Given the possibility that some local communities or organizations within a targeted population may have few concerns about a specific study whereas others may have considerable concerns, researchers might be accused of forum shopping in collaborating with the former rather than dealing with the stronger objections of the latter. So long as choosing to consult with a particular local community does not violate the political or moral authority of some other entity within which that locality is encapsulated, however, it is difficult ethically to fault researchers and communities for collaborating based on greater shared interests. The test of encapsulation is also useful in defining a community to approach for consultation. Preexisting communities should evidence some degree of shared, and therefore bounded, social and moral regulation among their members, even if that regulation is only informal and relatively weak and is focused primarily on claims to and symbols of a common identity.[38] Although *community* is a concept that can be defined at many different scales, any claim to consult members at a particular level should include some rationale for involving or sampling those who can be said to speak for whatever diversity of views exists within that social universe.

Are collective risks more a matter of perception than reality? Although many concerns have been raised about the collective risks of genetic research, for instance, there are in fact few documented examples of collective harms based on shared social identities.[15] Nonetheless, three responses can be made to this question. First, ethical evaluation and protection are premised on anticipating the reasonable potential for harm, not as responses after harm has been shown to occur. Second, history is replete with examples of people who have been harmed or killed due solely to their social identities. Third, perceptions of risk often are culturally constructed, so that what may be perceived as a minor matter to an outside researcher or ethics committee may be a much more significant risk to members of a particular cultural community. For this reason, involving members of populations or communities targeted for research in evaluating proposed studies often is a necessary empirical exercise in weighing the ethical significance of collective interests.[39–41]

What is the threshold for requiring community consultation beyond those communities that have centralized political processes capable of community consent? For the most part, consultations tend to be undertaken in populations or communities that have experienced histories of discrimination and health disparities—and/or that have cultural frameworks different from those of researchers—are more likely both to be vulnerable to collective harms and to have perceptions of collective implications or interests that may not be anticipated by outsiders.[4] Community consultation also may be appropriate for those groups that have strong collective interests in the risks and benefits of the study being conducted because they themselves may be affected by its conduct and/or outcome. Examples include people with HIV/AIDS, who have shared interests in studies focused on that disease, or those who reside in localities in which emergency medical studies may be conducted without individual consent and who could themselves end up as unconsenting participants.

Who is an appropriate representative for a community that does not have centralized political processes capable of community consent? Researchers most often try to identify leaders of local organizations such as churches or educational institutions when approaching a community for collaboration. Relying on local leaders alone, though, may not provide a sufficient perspective on community members' views, because leaders often have a self-interest in augmenting their positions by acting as intermediaries between members and outsiders. Sampling methods developed by social scientists offer more reliable means for consulting a cross section of local community members, but may require greater time and effort to complete than simply dealing with local leaders.

What kinds of community concerns are sufficient to force abandonment of a proposed study? As with risks to individuals, risks that may significantly harm collective interests, and for which protections cannot be devised, should be considered reasons to abandon targeting a particular population or community. However, before that question reaches an ethics committee, it is likely that consultation with community members will make evident the nature of the collective risks and the difficulty that those collective considerations will impose in recruiting participants, an early indication to researchers that a proposed design may be inappropriate for that community.[4] Similarly, consultations that provoke strong arguments among community members, leading to disruptions in their interactions with one another, provide evidence that carrying out the proposed study could cause further disruptions.[39] The consultation process should enable researchers and community members to collaboratively work out modifications in a study protocol that will reduce both collective and individual risks.

Does community consultation mistakenly define social identities as biological categories? An influential criticism of community consultation in genetics research has been that using social identities to evaluate studies that investigate biological categories contributes to the conflation of the social with the biological.[42] Indeed, using social identities for such purposes may tend to support the idea that racial, ethnic, and other categories are biologically defined. There are two difficulties with this critique. First, social categories can have biological relevance, as when socially labeled populations have differing frequencies of particular alleles. Second, most clinical studies recruit and label participants, and report findings, using social identities—and especially racial and ethnic identities—due both to a history of using those identities to document population-based health disparities and, in the United States, to legal mandates for inclusion of specific racial and ethnic minorities in federally funded studies.[43] So long as those practices continue, the collective interests of the social groups involved are appropriate subjects for ethical analysis.

Future Directions

The focus on collective interests of populations and communities targeted by clinical research has benefited from the convergence of several coincident trends: an emerging focus on population-specific patterns of genetic variation, coupled with special funding opportunities for research on ethics in genetics; the increasing involvement of disease-specific advocacy groups in scientific policy and planning; and heightened interest in and funding for community-based, participatory research. This convergence will continue to provide a growing number of opportunities for researchers, ethicists, funders, and community members to innovate standards and processes for community involvement in the planning and oversight of clinical research studies, with special attention to the collective interests of populations targeted for those studies. In addition, the ongoing debate over the relevance of racial and ethnic identities in clinical research and practice will ensure that collective interests continue to be at issue in interactions between researchers and study participants.[44,45]

It is unlikely, however, that a single standard or process will be established for all populations or all kinds of studies, due mainly to differences in forms of social organization and moral authority by which different populations construct communities to regulate their shared identities (with greater and lesser degrees of social cohesion). Differences in the cultural frameworks by which collective implications are perceived also make standardization difficult. What is likely, though, is that communities will increasingly expect researchers to demonstrate respect for the moral authority of community-specific social practices and cultural beliefs and to consult members about studies that target them as those protocols are planned and carried out. That expectation will require researchers and ethicists to develop a flexible set of best practices for involving communities in research as well as for evaluating and weighing information about collective interests produced through that involvement.

At the same time, technological advances and emerging health issues may contribute to new kinds of communities based on shared disease status, as happened in the emergence of a community focused on HIV/AIDS, or on shared genetic characteristics, as may happen in the case of those who have lower response rates to specific drugs because of polymorphic variation, and so have shared interests in the development and availability of alternative therapies to which they will respond. Populations defined in these ways have specific collective interests in research that targets their members, but few have social and cultural frameworks for constituting communities with sufficient social cohesion and moral authority to engage with researchers in pursuing those interests. Nonetheless, a variety of disease-based advocacy groups have had a growing influence on research policy and also have been involved in the planning of specific clinical studies and trials. That increasing level of involvement may support the development of greater social cohesion and authority among persons affected by a common disorder.

Future developments in the ethics of collective implications and interests of populations targeted for research will continue to require a combination of conceptual innovation and empirical investigation to better understand and involve the diverse, dynamic social and cultural entities that researchers engage in clinical research studies. It is difficult to imagine an approach to the ethics of research with communities that does not maintain that necessary link between empirical and conceptual activities.

References

1. Weijer C, Goldsand G, Emanuel EJ. Protecting communities in research: Current guidelines and limits of extrapolation. *Nature Genetics* 1999;23:275–80.

2. Sharp RR, Foster MW. Community involvement in the ethical review of genetic research: Lessons from American Indian and Alaska Native populations. *Environmental Health Perspectives* 2002;110:145–8.

3. Sharp RR, Foster MW. An analysis of research guidelines on the collection and use of human biological materials from American Indian and Alaskan Native communities. *Jurimetrics* 2002;42:165–86.

4. Foster MW, Sharp RR, Freeman WL, et al. The role of community review in evaluating the risks of human genetic variation research. *American Journal of Human Genetics* 1999;64:1719–27.

5. Kaufman CE, Ramarao S. Community confidentiality, consent, and the individual research process: Implications for demographic research. *Population Research and Policy Review* 2005;24:149–73.

6. Greely HT. The control of genetic research: Involving the "groups between." *Houston Law Review* 1997;33:1397–430.

7. Dukepoo FC. The trouble with the Human Genome Diversity Project. *Molecular Medicine Today* 1998;4:242–3.

8. Foster MW, Eisenbraun AJ, Carter TH. Communal discourse as a supplement to informed consent for genetic research. *Nature Genetics* 1997;17:277–9.

9. Weijer C. Protecting communities in research: Philosophical and pragmatic challenges. *Cambridge Quarterly of Healthcare Ethics* 1999;8:501–13.

10. Sharp RR, Foster MW. Involving study populations in the review of genetic research. *Journal of Law, Medicine, and Ethics* 2000;28:41–51.

11. Weijer C, Emanuel EJ. Protecting communities in biomedical research. *Science* 2000;289:1142–4.

12. Freeman WL, Romero FC. Community consultation to evaluate group risk. In: Amdur RJ, Bankert EA, eds. *Institutional Review Board: Management and Function.* Sudbury, Mass.: Jones and Bartlett Publishers; 2002:160–4.

13. Canadian Institutes of Health Research, the Natural Sciences and Engineering Research Council of Canada, and the Social Sciences and Humanities Research Council of Canada. *Tri-Council Policy Statement: Ethical Conduct for Research Involving Humans.* [Online] 1998 (with 2000, 2002 and 2005 amendments). Available: http://www.pre.ethics.gc.ca/english/policystatement/policystatement.cfm.

14. Council for International Organizations of Medical Sciences, in collaboration with the World Health Organization. *International Ethical Guidelines for Biomedical Research Involving Human Subjects.* Geneva, Switzerland: CIOMS and WHO; 2002. [Online] November 2002. Available: http://www.cioms.ch/frame_guidelines_nov_2002.htm.

15. Reilly PR. Rethinking risks to human subjects in genetic research. *American Journal of Human Genetics* 1998;63:682–5.

16. Juengst ET. What "community review" can and cannot do. *Journal of Law, Medicine, and Ethics* 2000;28:52–4,3.

17. Juengst ET. Community engagement in genetic research: The "slow code" of research ethics? In: Knoppers BM, ed. *Populations and Genetics: Legal and Socio-Ethical Perspectives.* Leiden, The Netherlands: Brill Academic Publishers; 2003:181–98.

18. Manson SM, Garroutte E, Goins RT, Henderson PN. Access, relevance, and control in the research process: Lessons from Indian country. *Journal of Aging and Health* 2004;16(5 Suppl.):S58–S77.

19. Royal Commission on Aboriginal Peoples. *Report of the Royal Commission on Aboriginal Peoples, Volume 5. Renewal: A Twenty-Year Commitment.* Appendix E: Ethical Guidelines for Research. Ottawa, Canada: RCAP; 1993.

20. Australia National Health and Medical Research Council. *Guidelines for Ethical Conduct in Aboriginal and Torres Strait Islander Health Research.* Canberra, Australia: NHMRC; 2003.

21. American Indian Law Center. Model Tribal Research Code. Albuquerque, N. Mex.: American Indian Law Center; 1994.

22. Davis DS. Groups, communities, and contested identities in genetic research. *Hastings Center Report* 2000;30(6):38–45.

23. Macaulay AC, Commanda L, Freeman WL, et al. Participatory research maximizes community and lay involvement. *British Medical Journal* 1999;319:774–8.

24. Schnarch B. Ownership, control, access, and possession (OCAP) or self-determination applied to research: A critical analysis of contemporary First Nations research and some options for First Nations communities. *Journal of Aboriginal Health* 2004;1(1):80–97.

25. Castellano MB. Ethics of aboriginal research. *Journal of Aboriginal Health* 2004;1(1):98–114.

26. McCabe M, Morgan F, Curley H, Begay R, Gohdes DM. The informed consent process in a cross-cultural setting: Is the process achieving the intended result? *Ethnicity and Disease* 2005;15:300–4.

27. Caldwell JY, Davis JD, Du Bois B, et al. Culturally competent research with American Indians and Alaska Natives: Findings and recommendations of the First Symposium of the Work Group on American Indian Research and Program Evaluation Methodology. *American Indian and Alaska Native Mental Health Research* 2005; 12(1):1–21.

28. Andrews L. Havasupai Tribe sues genetics researchers. *Law and Bioethics Report* 2004;4(2):10–1.

29. Morris MC, Nadkarni VM, Ward FR, Nelson RM. Exception from informed consent for pediatric resuscitation research: Community consultation for a trial of brain cooling after in-hospital cardiac arrest. *Pediatrics* 2004;114:776–81.

30. Morin SF, Maiorana A, Koester KA, Sheon NM, Richards TA. Community consultation in HIV prevention research: A study of community advisory boards at 6 research sites. *JAIDS: Journal of Acquired Immune Deficiency Syndromes* 2003;33:513–20.

31. International HapMap Consortium. Integrating ethics and science in the International HapMap Project. *Nature Reviews Genetics* 2004; 5:467–75.

32. Dawson L, Kass NE. Views of U.S. researchers about informed consent in international collaborative research. *Social Science and Medicine* 2005;61:1211–22.

33. Harris Y, Gorelick PB, Samuels P, Bempong I. Why African Americans may not be participating in clinical trials. *Journal of the National Medical Association* 1996;88:630–4.

34. Corbie-Smith G, Thomas SB, St. George DM. Distrust, race, and research. *Archives of Internal Medicine* 2002;162:2458–63.

35. Foster MW, Bernsten D, Carter TH. A model agreement for genetic research in socially identifiable populations. *American Journal of Human Genetics* 1998;63:696–702.

36. Dickert N, Sugarman J. Ethical goals of community consultation in research. *American Journal of Public Health* 2005;95:1123–7.

37. Reardon J. *Race to the Finish: Identity and Governance in an Age of Genomics.* Princeton, N.J.: Princeton University Press; 2005.

38. MacQueen KM, McLellan E, Metzger DS, et al. What is community? An evidence-based definition for participatory public health. *American Journal of Public Health* 2001;91:1929–38.

39. Foster MW, Sharp RR. Genetic research and culturally specific risks: One size does not fit all. *Trends in Genetics* 2000;16:93–5.

40. Parker DB, Barrett RJ. Collective danger and individual risk: Cultural perspectives on the hazards of medical research. *Internal Medicine Journal* 2003;33:463–4.

41. Jenkins GL, Sugarman J. The importance of cultural considerations in the promotion of ethical research with human biologic material. *Journal of Laboratory and Clinical Medicine* 2005;145:118–24.

42. Juengst ET. Groups as gatekeepers to genomic research: Conceptually confusing, morally hazardous, and practically useless. *Kennedy Institute of Ethics Journal* 1998;8:183–200.

43. Sankar P, Cho MK. Toward a new vocabulary of human genetic variation. *Science* 2002;298:1337–8.

44. Burchard EG, Ziv E, Coyle N, et al. The importance of race and ethnic background in biomedical research and clinical practice. *New England Journal of Medicine* 2003;348:1170–5.

45. Cooper RS, Kaufman JS, Ward R. Race and genomics. *New England Journal of Medicine* 2003;348:1166–70.

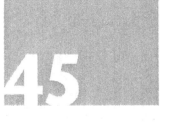

Albert R. Jonsen   Franklin G. Miller

Research With Healthy Volunteers

In the winter of 2005, at a time when fear of a global influenza pandemic galvanized public concern, healthy young people were volunteering to test the safety and efficacy of an experimental vaccine derived from an avian influenza virus.[1] Scientific research with the potential to have a great public health impact thus depends on the willingness of healthy individuals to volunteer the use of their bodies. In addition to testing experimental vaccines, healthy volunteers are needed for early-phase safety testing of pharmaceutical agents, to evaluate the efficacy of various agents to prevent common diseases that cause substantial mortality and morbidity, for a wide range of studies aimed at understanding normal human biology, and as a comparison group for research aimed at understanding the nature of diseases and better ways to treat them.

A healthy volunteer, sometimes historically referred to as a *normal volunteer,* may be a person who appears to be free of any disease or health-compromising condition, or one who may have some health-compromising condition but not the condition under study in the protocol. Healthy volunteer is not synonymous with *control* because in some research, controls are chosen who are not healthy; they may have a disease that is relevant to the study but is not its direct object, for example, a diabetic without heart disease who serves as a control in a study of the cardiac complications of diabetes.

The research ethics literature has little to say about *normal subjects* or *healthy volunteers.* Although the ethics literature and regulations pay attention to special classes of vulnerable subjects, the healthy subject merits little notice, often not even appearing in the indices of books on research ethics. The use of the word *healthy* may suggest that these subjects can take care of themselves and

need little attention or protection. This is an unfortunate misunderstanding. *Healthy* or *normal* may not mean healthy and normal in all respects. Indeed, one institution's research policy statement declares that "[t]here are no federal regulations that address the participation of normal volunteers in research protocols. However, this class of subjects could be considered vulnerable, and special precautions must be taken to ensure that their rights and welfare are adequately protected."[2] Although healthy subjects should not immediately be considered vulnerable and in need of special precautions, some healthy volunteers may be vulnerable for particular reasons.

The promise of research involving healthy volunteers must be assessed against the perils of such human experimentation, including abusive experiments of the past and the rare but disturbing fatal outcomes of some contemporary research. In a high-profile case that occurred in 2001 at Johns Hopkins University, a healthy volunteer died as the result of receiving a pharmacologic agent administered in a study of the pathophysiology of asthma.[3] From an ethical perspective, clinical research with healthy volunteers underscores the fundamental moral concern of human experimentation, namely, that some are exposed to risks and burdens for the sake of benefits to future patients and society. Although this concern applies to all clinical research, it is apt to be obscured in research involving subjects who are also patients, especially clinical trials that evaluate treatments and thus offer participants a prospect of direct medical benefit.[4] Subjects are prone to confuse clinical trials aimed at developing generalizable knowledge about the treatment of disease with personalized medical care—a phenomenon known as *the therapeutic misconception* (see Chapter 58).

Moreover, the ethics of clinical research may be confused, or conflated, with the ethics of medical care because of failure to recognize the ways in which clinical research necessarily departs from the physician-patient relationship. In medical practice, risks to patients can be justified only by anticipated medical benefits. In clinical research with healthy volunteers, however, research participants are exposed to risks and burdens solely for the benefit of others. Recognizing this fact helps to focus attention on the fundamental challenge posed by the ethics of human investigation. It also helps to reinforce the insight that the relationship between investigators and research participants throughout clinical research is not equivalent to or completely continuous with the doctor-patient relationship in medical care. Finally, despite such terms as *beneficence* and *risk-benefit ratios* that apply appropriately to both medical care and clinical research, research with healthy volunteers demonstrates that this central ethical terminology does not have exactly the same meaning in clinical research as in medical care. Healthy volunteers receive no direct medical benefits from their research participation, and there is comparatively little chance that their participation will have indirect or ancillary health benefits for them.

Historical Background

There is a long history of biomedical and behavioral research in healthy people, some of whom were vulnerable in other respects. In one of the earliest historical references to medical research, the Roman medical writer Celsus reported in the 2nd century that two prominent Egyptian physicians were allowed to perform vivisection on condemned criminals in order to study normal anatomy and observe physical processes in vivo.[5] In the early 19th century, the American military physician William Beaumont took advantage of a fistula in the stomach of his indentured servant, Alexis St. Martin, to perform experiments to test the acidity of gastric juices.[6]

A major milestone for research with healthy volunteers was the famous yellow fever research led by Walter Reed.[7,8] At the turn of the 20th century yellow fever was an untreatable, often fatal disease. In order to demonstrate the mode of transmission of yellow fever, healthy volunteers were exposed to mosquitoes in Cuba, where yellow fever was rampant. Most of the recruited volunteers got yellow fever but none died; however, one of Reed's coinvestigators who participated in the experiments died as a result. An ethically important innovation associated with this research was the use of written "contracts" to designate voluntary consent for a potentially life-threatening experiment. This research has been considered heroic, although it is doubtful that research of comparable risk to healthy volunteers would be considered ethically approvable according to current standards (see Chapter 1).

Certain forms of research by their nature require healthy subjects. Inoculation and vaccination must be tested on healthy subjects, for example, because vaccines are intended to prevent the onset of an infectious disease by stimulating a protective immune response. Thus, a vaccine's first use amounts to an experiment to determine whether it is safe and immunity can be achieved. In the early 18th century, Zabdiel Boylston in Boston inoculated his own son and some slaves against smallpox;[9] and in 1796, Edward Jenner vaccinated an eight-year-old healthy boy, James Phipps, and finally a group of orphan children in preparation for vaccination of the royal children.[10] Children dwelling in orphanages and asylums were common subjects of vaccine research in the 19th and early 20th centuries. The development of polio vaccines in the 1940s and 1950s required experimental use in thousands of healthy children, and a few children died in these experiments[8] (see Chapter 5). In this sort of research, the subjects are physiologically healthy but often vulnerable because they are children or institutional residents.

The Nazi medical experiments are important for the ethics of research with healthy participants for two major reasons (see Chapter 2). First, they represent the extreme of human experimentation for the sake of developing biomedical knowledge. Second, the Nuremberg Code was promulgated at the war crime trials of Nazi physician-researchers (see Chapter 12). The Nazi experiments were performed in concentration camps, of course, and did not involve volunteers. But many involved prisoners who were selected as biologically normal humans, rather than as subjects with a disease. These experiments illustrate the potential for the objectifying gaze of science to treat humans as laboratory material—guinea pigs—to be manipulated without concern for their suffering and deliberately killed for the sake of developing biomedical knowledge.

In one of the most brutal experiments, prisoners at Dachau were immersed in a tank of ice water for up to three hours to investigate the body's reactions to hypothermia, with the aim of learning how to save the lives of German pilots forced to parachute into the North Sea. The opening statement of the prosecution at the 1946 Nuremberg Trial quoted a 1942 report of Dr. Sigmund Rascher, who supervised hypothermia experiments:

> Electrical measurements gave low temperature readings of 26.4° in the stomach and 26.5° in the rectum. Fatalities occurred only when the brain stem and the back of the head were also chilled. Autopsies of such fatal cases always revealed large amounts of free blood, up to ½ liter, in the cranial cavity. The heart invariably showed extreme dilation of the right chamber. As soon as the temperature reached 28°, the experimental subjects died invariably, despite all attempts at resuscitation.[11]

Noteworthy is the detached, objective language describing torture and murder in the context of scientific investigation. Hubert Markl, president of the Max Planck Society for the Advancement of Science, aptly observed in a remarkable 2001 address concerning the Nazi experiments: "The guilt for utilizing human beings as laboratory animals can be specifically placed on biomedical science that was robbed of every moral boundary."[12]

The Clinical Center of the National Institutes of Health (NIH), which opened in 1953, admitted patients suffering from particular diseases to serve as subjects in NIH research projects, and also recruited "normal volunteers" to serve as control subjects and subjects of physiological and pharmacological research on their healthy bodies. In the beginning, these normal, healthy volunteers were often employees of the Clinical Center, and during the 1960s also convicts from local prisons. The major pool of healthy volunteers, however, were conscientious objectors from the traditional "peace churches," such as the Mennonites and the Church of the Brethren, who were allowed to fulfill their Selective Service obligations by participating in research. In 1957, an NIH report stated that 173 volunteers had provided 18,329 days of research service: 59% were under 21 years of age and 12% were female. The volunteers received living accommodations and a small stipend (about $10/month). Soon the need for volunteers outgrew this source and NIH sought recruits from among college students, particularly those in the health sciences.

The NIH program continues to recruit "residents of the local community who respond to advertisements in the media or visit the Clinical Research Volunteer Program office and review information about protocols that need healthy volunteers. A small cadre of healthy clinical research volunteers is available through selected colleges, which permit their students to participate in long-term inpatient studies."[13] During 2004, the NIH Clinical Center healthy volunteer program registered 9,926 participants who received a total compensation of $2 million. Compensation averages $40 per day for inpatient studies and about $7 per hour for outpatient studies; allowances for travel and inconvenience are also provided. Some participants are college science students who also were enrolled in preceptorships.[14]

The earliest NIH Clinical Center policies distinguished between patients admitted for the study and treatment of their diseases and healthy volunteers. Patients were considered protected by the physicians who cared for them, bound by the traditional duty to seek the benefit of their patients (the fact that these physicians were also investigators and thus susceptible to possible conflict with regard to that duty was not considered problematic). Healthy volunteers, on the other hand, were recognized as unprotected by this traditional medical duty. An explicit policy of requesting them to sign a written consent as research subjects was adopted in the 1950s. This distinction prevailed until the revisions of NIH policy in the mid-1960s made written consent universal.[15]

One of the largest groups of healthy subjects participating in U.S. clinical research was inmates in U.S. prisons who were, for many years, recruited into research projects. For example, in the 1950s, the testicles of prison inmates were irradiated to study the effect of X-rays on sperm production. These prisoners were "normal" in that they were healthy adults; they were also volunteers. However, they were also vulnerable subjects because they were susceptible to coercion due to their incarceration. The practice of using prisoners for research greatly expanded in the United States during World War II when prisoners were asked to participate in studies of infectious diseases affecting American troops. These incarcerated volunteers were given public praise but were not granted pardons or shortened sentences as enticement, as often believed. After the war, many pharmaceutical companies set up prison programs for Phase I drug testing. In 1975, a survey reported that 16 of 51 reporting drug companies used incarcerated persons: 3,600 prisoners participated in 100 protocols studying 71 substances.[16] Since the National Commission for the Protection of Human Subjects of Biomedical and Behavioral Research's investigation of research with prisoners in the mid-1970s, federal regulations have limited permissible research involving prisoners.

An example of healthy subjects who appear less vulnerable occurred in the venerable practice of scientists serving as experimental subjects in their own research, as did the yellow fever researchers.[17] From the earliest days of pharmacological research, investigators ingested or injected new drug formulations in their own bodies before inviting others to take them. Cardiac catheterization began in 1929 when Walter Forssmann, then a medical student in Germany, inserted a catheter into his own heart. This practice of "auto-experimentation" was considered ethically proper and recognized in the first major formulation of research ethics.

Provision 5 of the Nuremberg Code states that "No experiment should be conducted where there is an *a priori* reason to believe that death or disabling injury will occur; except, perhaps, in those experiments where the experimental physicians also serve as subjects."[18] Hans Jonas, in a pioneering essay on the ethics of research, took the position that researchers, who most fully identified with the goal of the research and understood its risks, should be the first to volunteer.[19]

In some historical cases, normal, healthy persons have been subjected to research without being volunteers. In the 1950s, offshore Navy ships sprayed *Serratia marcescens* bacteria over San Francisco and thousands of residents unknowingly inhaled it. The purpose was to study the efficacy of such a mode of delivery of biological weapons. Although the bacterium was then thought to be harmless, 11 persons became ill and 1 died. Similar experiments were performed in Florida, Minnesota, and in the New York subways.[20] Such research is unquestionably a violation of current standards of research ethics. Nonetheless, this experiment starkly poses a current ethical question: In an era when biological warfare and pandemic infection are real threats, how should large-scale studies be carried out? Ethical problems associated with research on communities of subjects have not been well delineated. Community consent has been proposed but methods of gaining such consent have yet to be perfected, and the validity of community consent may be questioned when risks fall upon individuals. The ethics of research, however, has focused almost exclusively on the autonomy and protection of the individual; the principle of justice, although confirmed as one of the basic principles of research ethics in the Belmont Report, has not been seriously explored as a basis for evaluating such forms of research.

Ethical Guidance

The Nuremberg Code remains a central source of ethical guidance for human investigation, especially for research with healthy participants.[18] The first principle declares that "The voluntary consent of the human subject is absolutely essential." Few, if any, commentators subscribe to this principle without qualification, as it would rule out all research with children or incapacitated adults, as well as valuable minimal-risk research for which informed consent is impossible to obtain. Yet informed, voluntary research participation in the case of competent adults is the moral norm, and the burden of proof rests on investigators who propose to deviate from this standard.

In addition, the Nuremberg Code requires that proposed research must have potential social value, that "the anticipated results will justify the performance of the experiment," that appropriate animal experimentation should precede human investigation, that scientifically unnecessary physical and mental suffering and injury should be avoided, that due care should be taken in experimental design and conduct so as "to protect the experimental subject against even remote possibilities of injury, disability, or death," that subjects should be free to withdraw from research, and that the responsible investigator must stop the experiment if there is reason to believe that a participant is likely to experience injury, disability, or death. Accordingly, the Nuremberg Code is the source of much of the basic ethical guidance for subsequent codes and regulations, such as the requirements to minimize risks, justify risks by the social value of the anticipated knowledge from research, obtain informed consent, and protect subjects from undue risks of harm during the course of research. The Nuremberg Code differs from some other prominent ethical guidance, such as the Declaration of Helsinki and the U.S. federal regulations, by placing an upper limit on allowable risks: "No experiment should be conducted where there is an *a priori* reason to believe that death or disabling injury will occur."[18] This principle will be examined below. An important omission in the Nuremberg Code, in view of subsequent developments, is the absence of any requirement for prior review and approval by an independent ethics committee.

Although the Declaration of Helsinki is primarily concerned with research conducted by physician-investigators with patient-subjects, it contains a few provisions specifically concerning research with healthy participants.[21] It stipulates that special attention is required "for those who will not benefit personally from the research," but explicitly states that medical research involving healthy volunteers should not be precluded. After declaring that "Medical research involving human subjects should only be conducted if the importance of the objective outweighs the inherent risks and burdens to the subjects," the Declaration of Helsinki observes that "This is especially important when the human subjects are healthy volunteers."[21] Presumably, this derives from the fact that healthy volunteers, unlike many patient-subjects enrolled in clinical trials, have no prospect of direct benefit to their health from participation in medical research. These various statements in the Declaration of Helsinki suggest that research with healthy volunteers is inherently a matter of ethical concern, though vital to the progress of biomedical knowledge. The Declaration relaxes the highly restrictive first principle of the Nuremberg Code by allowing research on children, including healthy children (and incompetent adults), provided that there is informed consent for these subjects from "the legally authorized representative." It also stipulates prior review and approval by an independent committee, which also should have the authority to monitor ongoing research to protect subjects.

The U.S. federal regulations refer throughout to human subjects, without stipulating any requirements for healthy volunteers as distinct from patient-subjects.[22] There are, however, special provisions for research involving prisoners and for children, among whom are included healthy participants. The regulations governing research with children allow institutional review boards (IRBs) to approve research involving healthy children only if it poses minimal risks. In contrast, children who are patient-subjects can be enrolled in greater than minimal risk research if it holds out a prospect of direct benefit to them (subject to additional constraints). Furthermore, children with a medical disorder or condition can be exposed to research interventions that pose "a minor increase over minimal risk." Whether this differential risk-benefit standard for healthy children and those who are patient-subjects is ethically defensible is open to question. As mentioned above, the federal regulations do not stipulate any limitations for allowable risk for adult subjects. Rather, they state that IRBs must determine that "Risks to subjects are reasonable in relation to anticipated benefits, if any, to subjects, and the importance of the knowledge that may reasonably be expected to result."[22] As there are no anticipated benefits for healthy participants, in principle, any level of risk might be justified so long as risks are minimized "consistent with sound research design"—that is, they are no greater than necessary to provide a scientifically valid answer to the research question—and they are judged by an IRB to be reasonable with respect to the knowledge to be gained from the research.

A risk threshold for research with healthy participants was adopted in a 1986 report of the Royal College of Physicians of London, which stated that "a risk greater than minimal is not acceptable in a healthy volunteer study."[23] The report defined *minimal risk* as including the following two types of situations: "The first is where there is a small chance of a recognized reaction which is itself trivial, e.g., a headache or feeling of lethargy. The second is where there is a very remote chance of a serious disability or death."[23] The first situation relating to discomfort produced by research procedures is unduly restrictive, as it would appear to prohibit a considerable range of valuable research with healthy volunteers such as Phase I toxicity studies and challenge experiments.

Ethical Issues in Research With Healthy Volunteers

Research with healthy volunteers is subject to the same ethical requirements as all clinical research. However, the nature of and history of research with healthy volunteers suggest that particular emphasis should be given to risk-benefit assessment, especially the evaluation of acceptable risks, and to fair selection of subjects.

Risk-Benefit Assessment

Satisfying the key ethical requirement for a favorable risk-benefit ratio in a study enrolling healthy participants involves the sequential steps of identifying the risks posed by research interventions, minimizing these risks, and judging that the potential benefits of the research to society justify the risks. The identification of risks involves three domains of assessment: probability, magnitude, and duration of harm. Accordingly, three questions must be addressed in assessing the level of risk posed by a study. First, what is the chance or probability that the research interventions will produce various harms to the health or well-being of participants? Second, how serious is the potential harm from study interventions? Third, how long is the potential harm expected to last if it occurs, and is it treatable or reversible? Risk assessment includes consideration of temporary discomfort or distress associated with research interventions as well as lasting physical harm.

Data on Adverse Events

Little systematic data are available concerning the extent of adverse events in research with healthy volunteers. A 1998 study of adverse events in Phase I drug studies of healthy volunteers in a single center in France over a 10-year period reported data on 1,015 healthy volunteers.[24] The incidence of adverse events, defined as the ratio between the number of adverse events and the number of days of follow-up, was 12.8% (1,558/12,143). Ninety-seven percent of these adverse events were rated as "of minor intensity," and 3% as "severe." Out of the 43 severe adverse events, nine were rated as "worrying," requiring hospitalization in two cases. A recent similar single-center study of Phase I drug testing in Germany, involving 1,559 healthy participants over 29,664 follow-up days, found an incidence of adverse events (defined in the same way as the previous study) of 8.8%.[25] Nearly all of these

(99.2%) were rated as of mild or moderate intensity, and only six were rated as severe.

Given that Phase I studies aim to determine the maximum tolerated dose of new pharmacologic agents, adverse events are expected. However, these data suggest that, on the whole, this common method of research with healthy volunteers is safe. Nevertheless, serious adverse events do occasionally occur, and the authors of the French report noted that a review of the extant literature revealed case reports of four deaths of healthy volunteers in Phase I research and five life-threatening events.[23]

Minimizing Risks

The requirement to minimize the risks of research involving healthy volunteers does not mean that these risks must be "minimal." Risks must be minimized within the context of designing and conducting valuable and rigorous clinical research. Accordingly, minimizing risks requires an inherently comparative assessment. A proposed research plan should be evaluated in the light of alternative ways to provide a rigorous answer to the scientific question that pose less risk to subjects. If the question can be answered by an alternative study design with lower risk to subjects or without including a procedure that carries significant risks to subjects, then this alternative should be adopted and/or the unnecessary procedure omitted.

Multiple dimensions of the design and conduct of clinical research are relevant to the requirement to minimize risk. Exclusion criteria for eligible participants should rule out those who can be predicted to be at increased risk from research interventions. Experimental procedures posing higher risks of physical harm or serious discomfort need to be carefully scrutinized to judge whether they are necessary to produce valuable data. Investigators must thoroughly review the literature to determine if drugs or procedures proposed for use in research have been associated with serious adverse events and take steps to obviate or minimize such risks. Failure of due diligence in reviewing the literature on the safety of research interventions was a major factor contributing to the death of a healthy volunteer in the Johns Hopkins asthma experiment.[3] Alternative, less risky ways to test study hypotheses should be explored. For example, imaging studies without the use of ionizing radiation, such as MRI, are preferable to those that use radiation, such as PET scans, provided that data of adequate quality can be obtained. When radiation use is scientifically necessary, the lowest dose needed to test research hypotheses should be administered. Finally, to minimize risks, careful procedures must be in place to monitor the condition of research participants and to intervene to counteract adverse events. Investigators should be prepared to end the study participation for particular subjects or terminate the study to protect subject safety.

Screening of Volunteers

Medical screening of prospective healthy participants is important both to assure the scientific validity of research and to protect subjects. Healthy volunteers are often recruited for studies as a comparison group to patients diagnosed with a given disease or condition. If prospective healthy subjects are not normal with respect to the medical conditions under investigation, then the data derived from studying these subjects may be invalid or biased. However, it is not necessary, or feasible, for healthy volunteers to be free of any medical condition. The point of screening for scientific validity is to assure that volunteers do not have conditions that would confound the research.

Screening is also essential to minimize the risks of harm to participants. Volunteers who present themselves as healthy may upon medical examination turn out to have evidence of a condition that would put them at excessive risk of harm from the research procedures used in a given study. Many studies recruiting healthy participants may enroll repeat volunteers, who participate in research as a source of income.[26] Whereas the risk of harm from participating in a single study may be minor, risks might be of greater concern for individuals who have repeatedly volunteered for research. For example, when studies include procedures involving radiation, the cumulative exposure of prospective subjects to radiation in previous research participation needs to be assessed.

Does the Importance of the Knowledge Justify the Risks?

After identifying the risks posed by a proposed study and taking care to minimize risks, the final step of risk-benefit assessment is to determine whether the potential benefits of the knowledge to be gained justify the risks to subjects. A difficult and unsettled issue of risk-benefit assessment is whether there exists an upper threshold on allowable risk for research involving healthy volunteers.[27] As the risks from proposed studies increase, the value of the potential knowledge needed to justify these risks certainly must also increase. Are some studies too risky to conduct no matter how much potential benefit in clinically relevant knowledge they offer? Neither the U.S. federal regulations nor the Declaration of Helsinki place any definite limits on the risks to which research participants can be exposed. In contrast, the Nuremberg Code stipulates, "No experiment should be conducted where there is an *a priori* reason to believe that death or disabling injury will occur; except, perhaps, in those experiments where the experimental physicians also serve as subjects."[18] The Nuremberg Code does not make clear what antecedent probability of death or disabling injury from a research intervention should rule out a study enrolling healthy volunteers. For some research procedures, such as an exercise stress test, there is a known but very remote risk of death.

In view of the risks that people routinely take in daily life, including activities aimed to help others, it seems unreasonable to exclude research procedures with an extremely low risk of death, especially when adequate precautions are taken to minimize risks. On the other hand, it is not clear that higher risk research that would not otherwise be justifiable might be approvable on the condition that investigators also participate as subjects. (This possible exception for research involving self-experimentation was included in the Nuremberg Code with an eye to Walter Reed's famous yellow fever research.[28])

The inherent uncertainty of research deserves attention in considering the issue of stipulating limits to research risks in the case of healthy participants. The social value of a research protocol depends crucially on the ability of the proposed investigation to provide a compelling answer to the research question, and also on the actual answer provided. Both "positive" findings confirming study hypotheses and "negative" findings that affirm the null hypothesis are scientifically and socially valuable. However, a positive finding that demonstrates a breakthrough in the understanding, treatment, or prevention of disease will obviously have greater social value than a negative finding that runs contrary to the study hypotheses. Because the answer is unknowable in advance of research, the value of the knowledge that will be generated by a study is uncertain. Moreover, on the whole, any given research study is likely to provide at best an incremental increase in biomedical knowledge. When research procedures pose risks of death, serious injury, or disability that are known to have more than a remote or very small chance of occurring, it is difficult to see how they can be justified by the uncertain prospects of benefit from the knowledge to be gained.

It might be objected that it is unjustifiably paternalistic to preclude informed, altruistic, healthy volunteers from knowingly risking their health or life for the sake of highly important medical research. The justifiability of paternalism is a complex issue in moral philosophy. Yet it is not clear that affirming an upper limit on allowable risk is necessarily taking a paternalistic stance. At stake ethically in this issue are both the professional integrity of conscientious scientific investigators, who must take responsibility for the anticipated consequences of their research, and the integrity of biomedical research. Public trust, necessary for the conduct of biomedical research, may erode if healthy volunteers are sacrificed, even with their informed consent, for the sake of science. All things considered, placing a heavy burden of proof on the conduct of high-risk research involving healthy volunteers seems reasonable.

How, then, in the final analysis, can it be determined whether the potential value of knowledge to be gained from a given study can justify the risk posed to research subjects? There are no formulas available. The assessment calls for carefully considered and deliberated judgments by research sponsors, investigators, and IRBs.

Fair Subject Selection

Healthy subjects selected for research participation may also be members of a vulnerable population or perceived as particularly vulnerable to undue influence or exploitation. These include the economically disadvantaged, prisoners, employees of research institutions, and students. Ethical concerns about recruiting members of such groups generally center on the voluntariness of their participation and fair distribution of the burdens and benefits of research. But there is controversy over the propriety of designating any particular population as vulnerable. For example, employees and students may be quite intelligent and competent, and they may have a wide range of choices. At the same time, they may be subject to certain sorts of discrimination, influences, and sanctions arising from a dependent relationship. The extent to which these considerations actually relocate a subject from normal to vulnerable is often a matter of discretion rather than generalization.

People volunteer as research subjects for many reasons. Some may be highly altruistic individuals who are motivated only to help unknown others. Some may be interested in particular diseases because they have a family member or friend who is afflicted. Some may be motivated by fascination with research or by offers of compensation. Although a few studies have examined volunteer motivations, relatively little is known about who healthy volunteers are, how many there are, or why they volunteer. Advertisements inviting health professional students to participate can be found on the bulletin boards of medical, dental, and nursing

schools, and many research projects post notices on web sites. Increasingly, attractive invitations appear in newspaper, magazine, radio, and television ads. IRBs customarily scan such advertisements but many may escape scrutiny. Large research institutions may have a pool of persons who show up regularly as volunteers, and in some places there are small cadres of "professional" research volunteers who make their living by participating in research studies.

Beauchamp and colleagues have presented a detailed ethical analysis of research involving one of the most vulnerable groups of healthy volunteers, namely, homeless individuals recruited for Phase I pharmaceutical research.[29] They argue that categorical exclusion of the homeless would be unjust discrimination and would unfairly deny them an opportunity to earn appropriate monetary compensation from participation. However, to avoid exploitation, according to these authors, the homeless should not be targeted for such research; nor should they be disproportionately represented among research participants. With respect to payment, Beauchamp and colleagues contend that "The key is to strike a balance between a rate of payment high enough that it does not exploit subjects by underpayment and low enough that it does not create an irresistible inducement."[29]

Whether scientists and others invested in the research should be allowed to take risks in auto-experimentation that affect only themselves is another relevant question. First, although it can be supposed that these subjects are, as Jonas says, the most informed and the most committed, they may also be the most indiscreet. Their enthusiasm for their project may entice them to take risks that are beyond what is reasonable. Rash decisions leading to disastrous results for the investigator might constitute harm to others because the event could cast research in a bad light or lead to compromise or even abandonment of a promising line of research. An IRB might, on these grounds, prohibit the researcher from taking highly risky steps. Walter Reed's scientific colleagues and Werner Forssmann might object that taking these risky steps in a free, informed manner is precisely what has advanced science and benefited health. A corollary of this problem is the possibility that auto-experimentation, particularly when highly risky, may entice the investigator to biased interpretation of the data and thus taint the experiment. Auto-experimentation, although noble in intent, deserves careful scrutiny by prudent consultants and review bodies.

Community volunteers do not have the same investment and understanding of the research as do investigators. Their generosity in offering themselves should be matched by particularly careful protection from risks as discussed above, and by informed consent.

Informed Consent

On the whole, there is less ethical concern about the quality of informed consent in the case of healthy volunteers than with patient-subjects, who may harbor therapeutic misconceptions that lead them to confuse research participation with standard medical care. Additionally, healthy volunteers do not suffer from potential impairments in cognition and judgment associated with being ill, which can complicate or make impossible informed consent. However, in higher-risk research, it may be desirable to institute formal measures to test the comprehension of healthy volunteers with respect to the risks and discomforts associated with research interventions.

One issue related to informed consent of healthy participants, which is widely considered to raise ethical concern, is payment for participation. When, if ever, does the level of payment for research participation constitute "undue inducement," particularly for those who are economically disadvantaged? The major concern is that participants may discount the risks and discomforts of study participation because of their need for money (see Chapter 36).

Conclusion

Research with healthy volunteers is a necessary component of biomedical research. It evokes ethical concern especially because healthy volunteers face risks of discomfort and physical harm but have no prospect of benefiting directly from research participation. Accordingly, as in all clinical research, careful attention to risk-benefit assessment is ethically required to conduct research with healthy volunteers. Members of the public owe a debt of gratitude to healthy volunteers, and to patient-subjects, for contributing to medical progress.

Disclaimer

The opinions expressed here are those of the authors alone and do not represent policies of the National Institutes of Health, the Public Health Service, or the Department of Health and Human Services.

References

1. Levine S. Taking a shot for science: Volunteers in vaccine study help doctors combat bird flu. *Washington Post* December 8, 2005:B1.
2. Wayne State University, Human Investigation Committee. HIC Policy: Vulnerable Participants: Normal Volunteers. Wayne State University, October 30, 1998. [Online] Available: http://www.hic.wayne.edu/hicpol/volun.htm.
3. Steinbrook R. Protecting research subjects—The crisis at Johns Hopkins. *New England Journal of Medicine* 2002;346:716–20.
4. Miller FG, Rosenstein DL. The therapeutic orientation to clinical trials. *New England Journal of Medicine* 2003;348:1383–6.
5. Scarborough J. Celsus and human vivisection in Ptolomaic Alexandria. *Clio Medica* 1976;11:25–38.
6. Numbers RL. William Beaumont and the ethics of human experimentation. *Journal of the History of Biology* 1979;12:113–35.
7. Bean WR. Walter Reed and the ordeal of human experiments. *Bulletin of the History of Medicine* 1977;51:75–92.
8. Lederer SE. *Subjected to Science: Human Experimentation in America Before the Second World War.* Baltimore, Md.: The Johns Hopkins University Press; 1995.
9. Howard-Jones N. Human experimentation in historical and ethical perspective. *Social Science and Medicine* 1982;16:1429–48.
10. Baxby D. *Jenner's Smallpox Vaccine: The Riddle of Vaccinia Virus and Its Origins.* London, UK: Heinemann; 1981.
11. Annas GJ, Grodin MA, eds. *The Nazi Doctors and the Nuremberg Code.* New York, N.Y.: Oxford University Press; 1992: p. 74.
12. Nicosia FR, Huener J, eds. *Medicine and Medical Ethics in Nazi Germany.* New York, N.Y.: Berghahn Books; 2002: p. 137.
13. National Institutes of Health Clinical Center. Guidelines for Protocol Preparation, n.d., n.p.
14. Personal communication, Dorothy Cirelli, Chief Patient Recruitment, NIH Clinical Center, Feb. 28, 2005.
15. Frankel M. The development of policy guidelines governing human experimentation in the United States: A case study of public policy making for science and technology. *Ethics in Science and Medicine* 1975;2:41–59.
16. Pharmaceutical Manufacturers Association. Survey: Use of prisoners in drug testing, 1975. In: National Commission for the Protection of Human Subjects of Biomedical and Behavioral Research. *Research Involving Prisoners: Appendix to Report and Recommendations.* DHEW Publication No (OS) 76–131. Bethesda, Md.: Department of Health, Education and Welfare; 1976.
17. Altman LK. *Who Goes First? The Story of Self-Experimentation in Medicine.* Berkeley, Calif.: University of California Press; 1998 [1987].
18. The Nuremberg Code. In: *Trials of War Criminals Before the Nuremberg Military Tribunals Under Control Council Law No. 10. Volume 2.* Washington, D.C.: U.S. Government Printing Office; 1949:181–2. [Online]. Available: http://www.hhs.gov/ohrp/references/nurcode.htm.
19. Jonas H. Philosophical reflections on human experimentation. *Daedalus* 1969;98:219–47.
20. Carlton J. Years ago, the military sprayed germs on U.S. cities. *Wall Street Journal* Oct. 22, 2001.
21. World Medical Association. *Declaration of Helsinki: Ethical Principles for Medical Research Involving Human Subjects.* Tokyo, Japan: WMA; October 2004. [Online] 2004. Available: http://www.wma.net/e/policy/b3.htm.
22. Department of Health and Human Services, National Institutes of Health, and Office for Human Research Protections. The Common Rule, Title 45 (Public Welfare), Code of Federal Regulations, Part 46 (Protection of Human Subjects). [Online] June 23, 2005. Available: http://www.hhs.gov/ohrp/humansubjects/guidance/45cfr46.htm.
23. Royal College of Physicians. Research on healthy volunteers. *Journal of the Royal College of Physicians of London* 1986;20:243–57.
24. Sibille M, Deigat N, Janin A, et al. Adverse events in phase-I studies: A report in 1015 healthy volunteers. *European Journal of Clinical Pharmacology* 1998;54:13–20.
25. Lutfullin A, Kuhlmann J, Wensing G. Adverse events in volunteers participating in phase I clinical trials: A single-center five-year survey in 1,559 subjects. *International Journal of Clinical Pharmacology and Therapeutics* 2005;43:217–26.
26. Tishler CL, Bartholomae S. Repeat participation among normal healthy research volunteers: Professional guinea pigs in clinical trials. *Perspectives in Biology and Medicine* 2003;46:508–20.
27. Miller FG. Clinical research with healthy volunteers: an ethical framework. *Journal of Investigative Medicine* 2003;51(Suppl.1):S2–S5.
28. Advisory Committee on Human Radiation Experiments. *Final Report.* U.S. Government Printing Office; 1995:134.
29. Beauchamp TL, Jennings B, Kinney ED, Levine RJ. Pharmaceutical research involving the homeless. *Journal of Medicine and Philosophy* 2002;27:547–64.

Ronald M. Green

Research With Fetuses, Embryos, and Stem Cells

Biomedical research involving the human embryo or fetus raises a host of ethical questions. Because the embryo or fetus cannot consent to be a research subject, who is morally entitled to authorize research involving it? The fetus has a unique relationship to the mother, and their interests can sometimes conflict. How should these different claims be balanced? Intensifying all these questions are sharp disagreements over the moral status of the embryo and the fetus, raising the question of whether either really has any claims on us. All these questions make embryo and fetal research one of the most controversial topics in biomedicine today.

Following a definitional preface, this chapter begins by examining the array of issues surrounding fetal research. For a variety of reasons, there is greater consensus about the norms governing this area of research than any other. Next, the chapter turns to human embryo research, which has been a topic of controversy for 25 years. More recently, controversy about embryo research has been intensified by the progress of human embryonic stem cell and therapeutic cloning research. This will be treated as a separate arena of moral and legal debate. As each issue is discussed, the leading moral debates will be placed against a background of existing laws and regulations both in the United States and elsewhere.

Definitions

For scientific purposes, *embryo* is usually defined as the product of conception until eight weeks gestation. From that point onward, the term *fetus* is used. However, these definitions are not pertinent to the major legal and ethical debates about research. For example,

the U.S. regulations governing fetal research define *fetus,* at 45 CFR 46.203(c), as "the product of conception from the time of implantation . . . until a determination is made, following expulsion or extraction of the fetus, that it is viable."[1] Because implantation occurs in vivo at about five to six days of gestational age, this identifies as a fetus what science describes as an embryo. In ethical terms, there is an important distinction between entities produced by in vitro fertilization (or flushed from a uterus following natural fertilization) and which exist in vitro, and those that have implanted in a womb, in which research necessarily implicates the gestational mother. For this reason, following Tauer and others,[2,3] this chapter will define the *embryo* as "the product of conception (whether produced in vitro or flushed from a uterus) as it exists in the laboratory and that has not undergone transfer to a woman" (see Figure 46.1). The *fetus,* accordingly, is "the product of conception existing in a womb" and comprises both in vivo embryos and fetuses. These definitions bypass the question of the organism's developmental stage. However, because it is not possible to culture an embryo in vitro for more than five or six days, a limit not likely to be exceeded soon, the term *embryo* as used here describes the early product of conception—that is, a mass of largely undifferentiated cells with no body form or organs—whereas the term *fetus* usually refers to a more developed entity undergoing organogenesis and possessing an incipient nervous system. In debates about embryo research, the terms *preembryo* or *preimplantation embryo* have been used for the ex utero embryo. This chapter will use the more general term *embryo* for this entity.

These definitions leave some issues unresolved. What are we to make of the phrase *product of conception* in an era when it is possible, by means of somatic cell nuclear transfer (cloning)

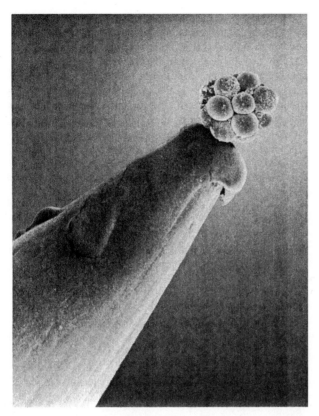

Figure 46.1. Human Embryo. Colored scanning electron micrograph (SEM) of a human embryo at the 10-cell stage on the tip of a pin. The ball of cells of the embryo is known as a *morula,* a cluster of almost identical, rounded cells each containing a central nucleus. This 10-cell embryo is about three days old. It is at the early stage of transformation from a single cell to a human composed of millions of cells. The cells multiply by repeated cleavage divisions (mitosis) and will form a hollow ball of cells (the blastocyst). Development of the blastocyst occurs before the embryo implants into the wall of the uterus (womb). Magnification: x130 at 6 x 7cm size. Magnification: x450 at 8 x 10 inch size. Credit: Dr. Yorgos Nikas/Photo Researchers, Inc.

technology, to produce organisms that are capable of developing to birth and adulthood without fertilization having occurred? Although no human being has yet been produced in this way, the possibility cannot be ruled out. Are the human cell clusters that result from cloning *embryos?*[4] Should they be accorded the same moral protections given to sexually produced embryos? Another question is how we should regard parthenotes, human eggs that have been induced by electrical or chemical means to cleave and develop in vitro. Because human parthenotes lack the paternal imprinting needed for the proper development of placental tissues, it is unlikely that they could ever develop to birth even if transferred to a womb. Nevertheless, both primate and human parthenotes have been cultured in vitro up to the blastocyst stage.[5,6] Should we regard parthenotes as merely sex cells, like sperm or eggs that do not merit protection as research subjects, or should they be accorded the same ethical consideration as embryos or fetuses? The Dickey-Wicker amendment to the Balanced Budget Downpayment Act of 1996, an annual appropriation measure repassed each year since 1996 by the U.S. Congress, forbids

federal funding for any research that destroys an embryo. It further defines *embryo* as "any organism . . . that is derived by fertilization, parthenogenesis, cloning, or any other means from one or more human gametes."[7] Adopting this expansive definition for moral and legal analysis would have the effect of blocking many research and clinical directions.

At what point should an embryo be regarded as coming into being? Although many people speak of the *moment of conception,* it is now well known that conception/fertilization is not a discrete event but a process that takes places over many hours or days.[8] Beginning with the transmission and reception of chemical signals between egg and sperm while they are still apart, it progresses to sperm penetration of the outer layers of the egg; the migration of male and female pronuclei to the egg's center; syngamy (the lining up of the pronuclei in their complementary configuration at about 22 hours after sperm penetration); cleavage (which does not occur until at least 24 hours after sperm penetration); and, finally, the appearance at the two-cell stage of the first cells with a normal envelope around their nuclear material. Further complicating matters is the fact that continued development is entirely governed by oocyte genes until the six- to eight-cell stage, approximately two days after penetration of the egg by sperm. Only then does the paternal genetic component begin to influence development.

Thus, there are at least several candidate *events* that might be used to mark conception/fertilization. The choice among them determines whether the organism is an embryo or a sex cell and can significantly alter our moral and legal conclusions with regard to specific research protocols. For example, regulations in the State of Victoria in Australia define fertilization as occurring at syngamy,[9] whereas British regulations hold that fertilization is complete at the appearance of "a two cell zygote."[3] Although slightly different, both of these definitions open the door to significant studies on the development of the early embryo as well as the efficacy of some contraceptive measures. A definition of *fertilization* that stressed "sperm penetration of the egg" would be even more limiting.

This chapter will not try to resolve these issues, other than to say that, for definitional purposes, we should probably be guided by reasonable intuitions. Thus, entities having approximately the same viability and developmental potential as sexually produced embryos should be regarded as embryos for ethical and legal purposes. This would bring cloned human organisms under the rubric of human embryo research, whereas it would exclude both parthenotes and pluripotent stem cells from the definition of *embryo.* As far as the commencement of the embryo is concerned, jurisdictions that have looked closely at the issue tend to regard syngamy as the earliest point at which a novel organism can be said to exist.

Research on the Human Fetus

Although our abortion debates reveal that there are sharp disagreements in our society about the moral status of the fetus, several considerations have muted these disagreements when fetal research is concerned and have tended to produce more consensus about ethical and regulatory matters than is true for embryo research. One is the more advanced developmental stage of the fetus, including the presence of bodily form, a heartbeat, and early neural development (with the possibility of sentience). Another is the possibility that the fetus might go on to term. This brings it under similar protections afforded to children who are born. Finally, the presence of the fetus in the mother's body accentuates the willingness to extend protections to it because research-related harms can implicate the mother's life, health, and decisional freedom.

Three distinct research areas come under the heading of fetal research: (1) direct research on the fetus itself; (2) research directed toward pregnant women or the condition of pregnancy, for which the fetus is an indirect subject of research; and (3) fetal tissue transplantation research. For each of these research areas, existing U.S. regulations identify the major moral issues involved and, with one or two exceptions, also reflect the international moral consensus on these issues.[10]

Direct Research on the Fetus

When research on the fetus itself is concerned, current U.S. federal regulations, at 45 CFR 46.208, governing federally funded or conducted research and FDA-regulated drug research distinguish between research directed at the health needs of a particular fetus and research not directed to the health needs of the fetus.[1] In the former case, institutional review boards (IRBs) may approve a protocol if the fetus will be placed at risk only to the minimum extent necessary to meet such needs. An example is research on a new technique for fetal transfusion for Rh incompatibility. When the health needs of the fetus are not at issue, however, research is permitted if the risk to the fetus imposed by the research is minimal and the purpose of the activity is the development of important biomedical knowledge that cannot be obtained by other means.[1] As in pediatric and other research with humans, the U.S. federal regulations define *minimal risk* at 45 CFR 46.102 to mean that "the probability and magnitude of harm or discomfort anticipated in the research are not greater in and of themselves than those ordinarily encountered in daily life or during the performance of routine physical or psychological examinations or tests."[1] Examples of minimal risk research might include studies of minor changes in maternal diet (daily life) or the use of ultrasonography (routine tests).

The U.S. standard for research on the fetus in utero is somewhat stricter than that which applies to research on children. Regulations permit research on children that represents no prospect of direct benefit to individuals and a minor increase over minimal risk if, according to 45 CFR 46.406(c), the intervention or procedure is likely to yield "generalizable knowledge about the subjects' disorder or condition which is of vital importance for the understanding or amelioration of the subjects' disorder or condition."[1] However, when research on the fetus is concerned, there is no such permission for a minor increase over minimal risk unless the mother's health is at issue. Not all nations hold to this strict standard, which partially reflects heated U.S. debates over abortion and the moral status of the fetus. Finland, for example, broadly permits research on the fetus not directly to its benefit if the research "is likely to benefit the health of people related to the woman or the foetus" (Finnish legislation does not clarify the meaning of the word *related* here).[3] Because the Dickey-Wicker amendment extends the same protections to embryos, as defined by that legislation, as it does to fetuses, this very high level of protection also applies to federally funded in vitro research on embryos, parthenotes, and cloned organisms.

United States regulations, and those of most other nations, do not to distinguish between a fetus destined for abortion and one intended to be carried to term. At first sight, it might seem reasonable to permit some degree of increased risk when the termination of the pregnancy is in prospect and when useful research can be done. An example is an experiment to see whether a teratogenic agent passes through the placenta. However, endangering the fetus in such cases will either limit a woman's freedom to change her mind about abortion or result in harm to the child if she should choose to continue the pregnancy to term. The unacceptability of either of these alternatives commends a standard of similar treatment of all fetuses. It is important to note, however, that once this standard has been met, nothing prevents preferential use of fetuses intended for abortion when minimal risk research is concerned.

Direct research can also take place on the fetus ex utero following a spontaneous or induced abortion. A viable fetus is treated by existing U.S. regulations as a premature infant and comes under the protections of regulations governing research on children. The fetus is judged to be viable, according to 45 CFR 46.203(d), if it is able to survive (given the benefit of available medical therapy) to the point of independently maintaining heartbeat and respiration.[1] In general, a fetus that has not attained a gestational age of 20 weeks and does not exceed 500g in weight is judged to be nonviable.[11] Independent medical assessment of nonviability is required when these limits are exceeded. A nonviable fetus may be involved in research only when (1) its vital functions are not artificially maintained; (2) experimental activities that of themselves would terminate its heartbeat or respiration are not employed; and (3) the purpose of the activity is the development of important biomedical knowledge that cannot be obtained by other means. According to 45 CFR 46.209, until it is ascertained whether or not a fetus ex utero is viable, it may not be involved in research unless (1) there will be no added risk to the fetus resulting from the activity, and the purpose of the activity is the development of important biomedical knowledge that cannot be obtained by other means; or (2) the purpose of the activity is to enhance the possibility of survival of the particular fetus to the point of viability.[1]

Because fetuses normally have male and female progenitors, the question arises as to whose consent is required for such research. The need for the mother's consent is evident and is recognized in all jurisdictions. Perhaps reflecting our debates on maternal-paternal consent for abortion, in the United States the father, as coprogenitor, is also required to consent. However, U.S. federal regulations at 45 CFR 46.208(b) and 209(d) permit exceptions to this rule if the father's identity or whereabouts cannot reasonably be ascertained, if he is not reasonably available, or if the pregnancy resulted from rape.[1]

The Fetus as an Indirect Subject of Research

Research directed at women who are pregnant necessarily implicates the fetus. At 45 CFR 46.207, the U.S. federal regulations specify that no pregnant woman may be involved in research unless either (1) the purpose of the activity is to meet the health needs of the mother, and the fetus will be placed at risk only to the minimum extent necessary to meet such needs, or (2) the risk to the fetus is minimal.[1] In such cases, research may proceed only if the mother and father are legally competent and have given their informed consent. The father's consent is not required, however, if the purpose of the research is to meet the health needs of the mother or if the three exceptions to paternal consent mentioned in connection with research directed at the fetus apply.

Regulatory protections also apply to nonpregnant women of childbearing age. The regulations codified at 45 CFR 116(b)(1) require that, when appropriate as part of the informed consent process, women be provided "a statement that the particular treatment or procedure may involve risks to the subject (or to the embryo or fetus, if the subject is or may become pregnant) which are currently unforeseeable."[1]

These regulations raise several ethical questions. Research whose primary purpose is to meet "the health needs of the mother" requires a determination of whether a procedure, drug, or dosage level imposes risk on the fetus "only to the minimum extent necessary." Because some procedures, drugs, or dosage levels may enhance maternal outcomes while increasing fetal risk, this can create a dilemma for investigators and IRBs, putting them in a situation of having to weigh the mother's welfare against that of the fetus. The very existence of this requirement raises a larger question of whether investigators or IRBs are the appropriate makers of this decision. Some would ask why the mother should not have sole authority to determine the degree of risk to which both she and her fetus may be exposed. Once again, U.S. abortion debates may have shaped the outlines of current laws.

Some have also asked whether the fetal-protective nature of current regulations does not evidence inherent discrimination and injustice toward women. It has been pointed out that some substances have the potential to affect the genetic components of sperm and, through this, the health of any resulting child. Yet current regulations to do not require investigators and IRBs to balance the health needs of fertile men involved in research against possible risks to their offspring.[12] It is also pointed out that current regulations have had the broad effect of reducing the amount of research done on women of childbearing age, preventing this group as a whole from benefiting from that research.[13]

Fetal Tissue Transplantation Research

The curative potential of fetal tissue was recognized as early as 1928 when fetal tissue was first transplanted into patients suffering from diabetes. More recently, fetal neural tissue has been used, with mixed results, in the treatment of Parkinson's disease and other neurological disorders as well as other conditions.[14] During the 1980s there was substantial controversy about the ethical permissibility of fetal tissue transplantation (FTT) research. Concerns focused on a possible linkage between this research and abortion. Abortion opponents feared that the prospect of FTT might serve as inducement for women to terminate pregnancies. This could occur if women were able to designate donors of the tissue or if women or abortion providers benefited financially or otherwise from donation. Debate centered on whether it is possible to remove these incentives and render consent to FTT research independent of the abortion decision. It should be noted that fetal tissue donation for research purposes, when no prospect of transplantation is involved, remains uncontroversial. Under most existing regulatory regimes, once a fetus is dead, its cells, tissues, organs or placental material may normally be used in research with the consent of the mother.

In the United States, the first Bush administration established the Human Fetal Tissue Transplantation Research Panel in 1988 to examine this issue. A majority of the panel concluded that federal funding of FTT research under strict guidelines is "acceptable public policy."[15] However, the Bush administration did not accept this recommendation, and federal funding of FTT was prohibited until 1993, when President Bill Clinton, in one of his first acts of office, issued an executive order permitting it. Congress later passed this order into law in the provisions of the National Institutes of Health (NIH) Revitalization Act of 1993.[16]

Over the past decade, a strong international consensus has emerged about some of the central conditions for good clinical practice regarding FTT. These include the following: (1) The decision to abort should not be influenced by the prospect of tissue transplantation; among other things, this means fetal tissue donors should not be permitted to designate tissue recipients. (2) Commercialization is not acceptable; neither donors nor clinicians should profit from the provision of fetal tissue. (3) Tissue may only be obtained from dead embryos or fetuses. (4) Informed consent should be obtained. (5) The decision to terminate the pregnancy must be made before consent for donating fetal tissue is solicited. And (6) experimental studies should be approved by a qualified ethics committee.[17]

Within this broad consensus, some important debates continue over details of implementation. One question is whether it is either necessary or desirable for there to be an intermediary organization between the woman donor and the clinical research team utilizing fetal tissue.[18] The worry here is that if clinical researchers become involved in the woman's care, they can experience a conflict of interest between their responsibilities to her and their research goals. Another question concerns the timing of the donation decision. After a woman has decided to terminate a pregnancy, should she be asked to consent to tissue donation before undergoing the abortion, or should this request be postponed until the abortion has been completed? Postponing the request until after an abortion helps ensure that the prospect of donating fetal tissue doesn't make the decision to abort more likely, but it presents the decision to the woman at a time when her reflective capacity may be impaired by the recent medical procedure or the use of anesthesia. A third question is whether FTT—if proved effective—should be exceptional, used only in the rarest of cases when alternatives are demonstrably unacceptable, or whether it should be developed for widespread use, including the possible creation of an extensive network of fetal tissue providers. This question is complicated by the fact that some alternatives to FTT, such as stem cell technologies, are only in the beginning phases of research, whereas other more developed alternatives, such as xenotransplants, pose considerable risks of their own, including the introduction of animal pathogens into the human population.

There are voices that entirely reject this international consensus. The Roman Catholic Church continues to oppose FTT research. In August 2000, Pope John Paul II told an International Congress of the Transplantation Society that the manipulation and destruction of nascent human life with a view to obtaining tissues or organs for transplantation is morally unacceptable.[17] In the Netherlands, the Lindeboom Institute, a conservative Protestant biomedical ethics organization, has argued that the *separation principle,* the idea that the decision to abort and the decision to donate fetal tissue can be compartmentalized, is a fiction. The institute argues that the mere knowledge that fetal material can be used for transplantation purposes could influence the decision of a woman who is trying to determine whether she will or will not continue a pregnancy.[17] Nevertheless, in the United States it appears that the restrictions put into effect by the NIH Revitalization Act of 1993 have eased fears even among many abortion opponents. One sign of this is the fact that although President George W. Bush questioned any use of tissues from aborted fetuses in transplantation research shortly after coming to office,[19] his administration has taken no further action to change the law permitting federal funding of this research.

Relevant provisions of the NIH Revitalization Act of 1993 evidence the struggle between the opposing sides of the U.S abortion debate.[16] On the one hand, the provisions reflect many features of the international consensus permitting FTT research. A woman donating human fetal tissue must sign a statement declaring that the tissue is being donated for therapeutic transplantation research, the donation is being made without any restriction regarding the identity of individuals who may be the recipients of transplanted tissue, and without her having been informed of the identity of those individuals who may be the recipients. The attending physician must sign a statement declaring that the tissue has been obtained in accord with the donor's signed statement and that full disclosure has been made to her of the attending physician's interest, if any, in the research to be conducted with the tissue. Other provisions of the act declare it unlawful for anyone to solicit, acquire, receive or transfer human fetal tissue for "valuable consideration" or as the result of a promise to the donating individual that the tissue will be transplanted into a recipient specified by such individual or a relative of the donating individual.

On the other hand, some provisions of the act represent concessions to antiabortion sentiment in the United States. The attending physician's statement must declare that no alteration of the timing, method, or procedures used to terminate the pregnancy was made solely for the purposes of obtaining the tissue. This provision is not present in some other national regulations governing fetal tissue transplantation. Another provision requires the disclosure to all downstream researchers or tissue recipients that the tissue is from an aborted fetus. The assumption here is that such individuals have the right to learn about the source of the tissue and to decline its use. If we consider that fetal tissue obtained from abortions has been used without comment in biomedical research for decades, as in the development of vaccines for rubella, rabies, and polio,[20] we can see that the increasing polarization around the abortion issue has shaped U.S. law and policy on FTT research.

Human Embryo Research

Despite the heated nature of current debates about the use of human embryos in biomedical research and therapy, the ex utero human embryo did not emerge as a subject of research until the late 1970s. Some preliminary work on fertilizing human eggs ex utero had been done in the mid-1940s by Rock and Menkin,[21] but public debate about embryo research began in earnest in 1978 with the birth in Oldham and General District Hospital in the north of England of Louise Brown, the world's first "test tube" baby. For the first time in history, human embryos could be created outside the womb, cultured, studied during their earliest

phases of growth, and then returned to the womb for gestation and birth. Not only did the development of in vitro fertilization (IVF) make the early ex utero embryo a possible research "subject," but the rapid growth of infertility medicine created a demand for more successful and less risky infertility treatments. This intensified the demand for embryo research.[22]

In 1975, the U.S. Congress created an ethics advisory board (EAB) in the Department of Health, Education, and Welfare (now the Department of Health and Human Services) to recommend and apply guidelines for federally funded research in this area. The EAB took up its work in 1978 and after months of study, discussions, and public hearings, issued a report in May 1979 recommending support for a broad range of research using human embryos.[23] The report made no distinction between embryos created for research purposes and embryos remaining from infertility treatments. In endorsing the deliberate fertilization of eggs for research purposes, the EAB acknowledged a practice that had been employed by Edwards and Steptoe and others in the early development of IVF.[24] These pioneering researchers believed that in creating artificial reproductive technologies, it is scientifically and morally imperative to create and study embryos for research before transferring them to a womb.

The EAB's deliberations and its report stirred enormous controversy, including letter writing campaigns by conservative religious groups, and no action was ever taken on the report. When the EAB's charter expired in 1980, its membership was not renewed and no funding was provided. Because U.S. law required that any research in this area supported by the NIH or other federal agencies be reviewed by the EAB, the result was a de facto moratorium on federal support for embryo research during the administrations of Presidents Ronald Reagan and George H. W. Bush. Research continued, however, in the private sector.

In the United Kingdom, events took a different turn. A commission chaired by Dame Mary Warnock issued a report in 1984 recommending government permission and support for IVF and embryo research.[25] This resulted in the creation of a voluntary licensing authority that oversaw infertility clinics and IVF research projects in the United Kingdom. In 1990, Parliament passed the Human Fertilisation and Embryology Act.[26] This led the following year to the establishment of the Human Fertilisation and Embryology Authority (HFEA), an official government agency brought into being to provide oversight and guidance for clinical and research programs in infertility medicine. In its current activities, the HFEA oversees and licenses all clinical infertility programs in the United Kingdom as well as research on human embryos. British regulations are the most comprehensive concerning embryo research and among the most permissive in the world. Embryo research is permitted for a wide variety of reasons, including the following: to promote advances in the treatment of infertility; to increase knowledge about the causes of congenital disease and miscarriages; to develop more effective techniques of contraception and methods for detecting the presence of gene or chromosome abnormalities in embryos before implantation; to increase knowledge about the development of embryos; and to increase knowledge about serious disease or to enable such knowledge to be applied in the development of treatments to combat serious disease.[27] In the pursuit of these goals, British regulations permit the creation of embryos for research purposes and, more recently, cloned embryos for therapeutic cloning research. During this same period, Australian researchers were also able to conduct some embryo research using a feature of Australian regulations that permitted research before the occurrence of syngamy.[2]

In June 1993, the NIH Revitalization Act nullified the requirement for EAB approval of federal funding for infertility and embryo research projects. The NIH was free to respond to the backlog of research proposals it had received. Before approving any of them, however, NIH administrators felt they needed guidelines to instruct members of IRBs. These developments led to formation of the Human Embryo Research Panel, a 19-member multidisciplinary group that issued a report in late 1994 recommending a substantial program of federal support for human embryo research and establishing guidelines for the conduct of that research.[28] The most controversial of these was a recommendation for the deliberate creation of embryos for research purposes under specified circumstances.

Within hours of the acceptance of the Human Embryo Research Panel's report by the advisory committee to the director of the NIH, President Clinton issued an executive order rejecting this recommendation. Events soon prevented implementation of any of the other recommendations. Over the next two years, a newly elected conservative Congress sought to reverse most Clinton administration reproductive health initiatives. In this vein, Congress passed the Dickey-Wicker Amendment, raising to the level of law what had been a de facto ban on federal funding for human embryo research before the onset of the Clinton administration and extending the ban to research on parthenotes and embryos produced by cloning. Thus, although extensive manipulations of human embryos and the introduction of new clinical therapies have gone on in hundreds of private clinics in the United States over the last quarter of a century, human embryo research has not been funded by federal research agencies. Nor have there been federal regulations or ethical oversight of such research. This is in contrast to Great Britain, where the HFEA code of practice applies to both public and private research. In 2004, the President's Council on Bioethics, an entity created by the administration of George W. Bush, considered recommending increased federal regulation of infertility medicine generally. However, because Bush himself was on record as opposing embryo research, patient-advocate groups and clinicians who believe that federal regulations could lead to increased restrictions on clinical activities did not greet this idea favorably, and in its final report the Council backed away from recommending significant legal restrictions.[29]

The prolonged absence of federal support for human embryo research in the United States, a country with approximately 400 infertility programs, the largest of any nation, has had many unfortunate consequences. It has slowed progress in our understanding of the causes of birth defects and miscarriages. The relegation of research to privately funded clinics lacking sufficient resources for large or multicenter studies has contributed to the inefficiency and high cost of IVF.[30] Because of the reliance on stimulatory drugs for ovulation induction, thousands of women are exposed to medications whose long-term impacts on health remain uncertain.[31,32] The absence of research and federal oversight has also led to the introduction of new procedures, such as intracytoplasmic sperm injection (ICSI), without sufficient preliminary studies of their long-term safety for the children brought into being by them.[33,34] Inefficient procedures already play a large role in the epidemic of premature births associated with current infertility treatments.[35]

Behind the heated political debates that have stalled federal involvement in this area are major moral disagreements. The principal matter of controversy concerns the moral status of the early human embryo. Unlike fetal research, in which the welfare of women and the children to which they might give birth complicates matters, embryo research unavoidably poses the question of how much protection we should give to nascent human life. In these debates, two main positions have emerged. The first, strongly associated with the views of conservative religious groups, holds that human life deserves full moral protection from conception onward. This places the earliest embryo on a plane of equality with children and adults and rules out embryo research that is not medically to the benefit of the embryo under study. It forbids the deliberate creation and destruction of embryos for research purposes, and it also tends to oppose the creation of supernumerary embryos in infertility medicine to increase the chances of a pregnancy.[36,37]

Some who hold this view maintain that the genome represents a defining feature of the human being, the possession of which justifies according an entity the strictest protections.[36] Others draw less on the matter of genetic identity and stress the potential of human life even at the earliest stage of development as a sufficient reason to extend full moral protection.[38] Still others argue that there is no better "marker point" for human protections than conception. To choose later developmental events, they say, opens the way to making subjective judgments that put all human beings at risk.[39] Discussions by Roman Catholic moral theorists and statements by Roman Catholic leaders, which have been influential in shaping U.S. and European policy, incorporate elements of all of these views. Although the Catholic Church has not yet taken a formal position on when an individual human life begins, it insists that because of the possibility that an individual human soul may be present from conception, the embryo must be treated from that time as a human being meriting all protections.[40]

Opposing this position is a range of views that can be termed *gradualist* or *developmental*. These take various forms. Some stress the moral importance of qualities like sentience, brain activity, the presence of substantial bodily form, or the ability to survive independently of the mother (viability). Still others emphasize not one but a plurality of considerations that, taken together, compel us to extend protections.[28,41] What all of these views have in common is the conclusion that the moral weight of the embryo or fetus is not established once and for all, but increases over the course of a pregnancy as additional morally significant features make their appearance. Those holding these views may disagree about the precise protections that should be afforded at each stage, but they tend to agree that the early embryo has reduced moral status. Lacking differentiated cells and organs, bodily form, sentience, or cerebral activity, it has few of the features that elicit moral regard. Most who hold this view are willing to permit significant embryo research, including research that destroys the embryo, up to 14 days of development. At about this time, the "primitive streak" appears amidst the undifferentiated cells of the embryo's inner cell mass. This establishes the cranial-caudal (head-to-tail) and left-right body axes. In the following week gastrulation occurs, with the emergence of three discreet germ layers or tissue types, and formation of the neural tube begins. Because morally significant developmental events cannot be ruled out beyond the 14-day point, this has become the focus of an international consensus among those who support embryo research as the point beyond which research should not be allowed.

For those holding this position, other qualities of the embryo call into question any characterization of it as a protectable human individual. One is the early embryo's very high natural mortality. Although estimates differ, it is likely that at least 50% of all conceptuses stop growing within the first few days of development and pass, often unnoticed, out of the woman's body.[42,43] This high rate of natural mortality limits the force of claims about the embryo's developmental potential. Also noteworthy is the early embryo's unusual genetic character. Each of the blastomeres, or cells that compose the embryo, is totipotent (capable of giving rise to an entire organism). In some experiments this characteristic has been exploited to produce multiple embryos by dividing a single embryo and providing an artificial protective coating to replace the natural zona pellucida.[44] When this phenomenon occurs naturally in vivo it leads to the birth of monozygotic (identical) twins or triplets. This raises the question of whether the early embryo is not better described as a *community* of organisms rather than as a single individual. It sometimes also happens that two genetically distinct early embryos fuse. Because intracellular signaling drives body formation, the result is a single individual possessing cell populations from two distinct genetic lineages. Recent clinical reports describe such chimeric individuals.[45,46] All these possibilities run counter to the claims of those who maintain that personal identity overlaps with genomic identity and that the human individual begins at conception. They also pose significant metaphysical difficulties for religious views that assert the presence of a "human soul" at conception.[47–49] For if the start of spiritual individuality (ensoulment) occurs at this time, how can we explain the later appearance of souls in twinning or the disappearance of souls in embryo fusion? The uncertainty of the embryo's genetic uniqueness strengthens the view of those who emphasize the moral importance of the formation of the primitive streak at about 14 days development. Only then, with cellular differentiation rendering twinning or embryo fusion no longer possible, can we speak of the presence of a discrete individual organism.

These two opposing views on the status of the early embryo account for much, but not all, of the disagreement over the permissibility of human embryo research. In addition, some commentators believe that although the early embryo may not have features that render it an object of moral concern, abusing or destroying it can nevertheless threaten our respect for more mature forms of human life. Those holding this view stress the importance of the embryo as a symbol of human vulnerability and worth. This position has played a role in debates about the moral appropriateness of creating embryos for research purposes only.[50] Some opponents of such research have asked whether the deliberate creation of an embryo for use in research, followed by its destruction before the 14-day limit, violates at least the spirit of the Kantian maxim that individuals are not to be used as a "means only" for the betterment of others. Others fear the development of a vast commercial market in which human embryos are created, distributed, and used for morally trivial purposes, such as the testing of cosmetic products.[51,52] Such uses, they maintain, would reduce our respect for human life. Still others are prepared to allow the deliberate creation of supernumerary embryos for the purposes of establishing a pregnancy, but oppose doing so for research purposes. In the former case, they argue, the parents' reproductive intent sufficiently outweighs any negative symbolic implications.[53]

Many who share the view that the embryo has little intrinsic weight are not persuaded by these arguments. The NIH Human Embryo Research Panel took the view that "although the preimplantation human embryo warrants serious moral consideration as a developing form of human life, it does not have the same moral status as an infant or child."[28] On this basis, the panel endorsed the creation of embryos for research when two conditions were met: (1) "when the research by its very nature cannot otherwise be validly conducted"; and (2) "when a compelling case can be made that this is necessary for the validity of a study that is potentially of outstanding scientific and therapeutic value."[28] An example of the former is research whose endpoint is fertilization, such as studies of in vitro oocyte maturation followed by fertilization. Such research could lead to far safer fertility procedures and would greatly expand the supply of human eggs for clinical and research purposes. Examples of the latter are studies of the effects of powerful ovulation-inducing drugs on eggs and embryos in order to better establish the risks for the women exposed to, or the children produced by, the administration of these drugs. Although one member of the panel dissented from this recommendation, the others did not agree that symbolic concerns outweighed the possibility of clear therapeutic benefit. It has been noted that many couples using infertility procedures routinely create more embryos than can be transferred to a womb. As a result, approximately 400,000 frozen embryos now exist in the United States.[54] To those who remain unpersuaded by the symbolic arguments, it is not clear why such activities for reproductive purposes are acceptable, whereas life- and health-preserving biomedical research is not.[55]

The creation of embryos for research purposes remains one of the most controversial issues in human embryo research. The Human Embryo Research Panel's recommendation for federal funding of such research was never implemented. In Europe in 1996, following a lengthy process of deliberation, the Council of Europe approved a "Convention for the Protection of Human Rights and the Dignity of the Human Being" (see Chapter 17). Article 18.2 of this convention prohibits the creation of embryos for research purposes.[56] However, Britain has not ratified this convention and provisions of the Human Fertilisation and Embryology Act, as noted, permit the creation of embryos in vitro for research purposes.[23]

Whenever human embryo research is permitted or contemplated, questions arise regarding its conduct. These include questions about the norms governing gamete and embryo donation. In general, there is a consensus that all progenitors of reproductive materials used in embryo research must consent to its use and be informed of the specific purposes of a research program. This creates difficulties in the use of some embryos created by anonymous sperm donation and has occasioned debate about whether such embryos may ever be used.[24] It also raises the question of whether it is permissible to use in research oocytes harvested from aborted fetuses or oocytes that are procured from women after their death and that have been donated (without the woman's explicit consent) by family members. Although such donations of other bodily tissues are routine in many research areas, the sensitive nature of reproductive materials, and the fact that they can involve a new human life, justify adhering to the strictest standards of informed consent by donors. The selling of gametes or embryos is also normally prohibited, although compensation of women for the time and inconvenience involved in egg donation is sometimes allowed.[57] Finally, there is a strong presumption against the creation of human-animal chimeras or the transfer of human embryos to animal wombs for incubation.

New technological developments can sometimes challenge these guidelines. For example, how are we to assess the use of nuclear transfer with animal oocytes and human nuclear DNA to produce embryonic stem cells?[58] Although this runs counter to the view that it is wrong to create animal-human chimeras, the possible efficiency of this procedure and the promise that it may reduce the need for human eggs makes it scientifically and ethically attractive.

Stem Cells and Therapeutic Cloning

In its 1994 report, the Human Embryo Research Panel took note of the fact that it might be possible in the future to develop human embryonic stem cell (hESC) lines. These cells are undifferentiated, pluripotent (able to produce any cell or tissue type in the body), and theoretically capable of proliferating indefinitely in culture (self-renewing). Once techniques for growing and redifferentiating such cells are developed, stem cell lines may be used to replace damaged cardiac tissue following a heart attack, or repair now irreversible spinal cord injuries. Parkinson's disease and diabetes are on the long list of conditions that might be cured by the ability to produce new bodily tissues. Basing its discussion on information available from over a decade of mouse stem cell research, the Human Embryo Research Panel supported permitting the use of embryos remaining from infertility procedures ("spare" embryos) for the purpose of creating hESC lines. However, because of the remoteness of this prospect in 1994, it did not recommend the deliberate creation of embryos for this purpose.

Just four years later, in 1998, hESC research became a reality when James Thomson of the University of Wisconsin published a report documenting the creation of several hESC lines from donated spare embryos.[59] At almost the same time, a Johns Hopkins team headed by John Gearhart reported development of a human embryonic germ cell (hEG) line derived from the gonadal tissues of aborted fetuses.[60] Neither Thomson nor Gearhart relied on federal funding for the research. Concerned that he might run afoul of the prohibition of federal funding for embryo research, Thomson set up a separate laboratory to keep his work apart from other, federally funded activities at the university. Although Gearhart's work was legally eligible for federal funding under provisions of the NIH Revitalization Act that permit fetal tissue transplantation research, his team chose to use private funding rather than dealing with sensitive NIH administrators.

These developments once again moved human embryo research to the forefront of ethical and political debate. Supporters of human embryonic stem call research maintain that it holds out enormous medical promise.[61,62] Opponents argue that it is morally offensive and that "adult" stem cells, the somewhat differentiated progenitor cells that reside in all our bodies and that furnish replacement blood, bone, skin or other tissues, might be able to accomplish these purposes without requiring the use of human embryos.[63] In reply, defenders of hESC research point to the biological limitations of adult stem cells, including their absence in many tissues and their uncertain plasticity or proliferative ability.[64] These limitations, defenders of hESC research maintain, justify keeping both lines of inquiry open and providing generous federal support for continued research on both cell types. Ongoing studies support the claim that adult stem cells may have therapeutic potential but also show that many questions regarding their plasticity and proliferative ability remain unanswered.[65,66]

In December 1999, the NIH issued draft guidelines specifying the conditions and restrictions under which it would support research using hESCs. These guidelines rested on an NIH-solicited legal opinion that hESCs are not themselves "embryos" within the meaning of the Dickey-Wicker amendment, and that research "utilizing" but not deriving them from human embryos did not constitute research violating Dickey-Wicker's ban on "research in which a human embryo or embryos are destroyed." This use-versus-derivation distinction was subject to criticism by both friends and opponents of federally funded stem cell research. In September 1999, the Clinton-era National Bioethics Advisory Commission (NBAC) issued a report, "Ethical Issues in Human Stem Cell Research," that chose not to rely on the NIH's use-versus-derivation distinction. Instead, the NBAC recommended that Congress pass an exception to existing legislation that would allow both the derivation and use of stem cells from embryos remaining after infertility treatments.[61]

Following a period of public comment, the NIH proposed roughly similar guidelines on August 25, 2000.[67] These guidelines embodied the prohibition in Clinton's December 1994 intervention against any research using embryos that are deliberately created for research purposes. They specified that research on stem cells derived from embryos could be conducted "only if the cells were derived (without federal funds) from human embryos that were created for the purposes of fertility treatment and were in excess of the clinical need of the individuals seeking such treatment." In addition they adapted to this issue the logic of existing fetal tissue transplantation regulations. They specified that "no inducements, monetary or otherwise, [may be] offered for the donation of human embryos for research purposes." Research had to maintain "a clear separation between the decision to create embryos for fertility treatment and the decision to donate human embryos in excess of clinical need for research purposes to derive pluripotent stem cells." To ensure this separation, and to provide time for decision, only frozen embryos could be used as a stem cell source. Researchers or investigators proposing to derive or utilize human embryonic stem cells in research were to have no role in securing spare embryos for the research, and the attending physician for fertility treatment and the researcher were not to be one and the same person. The NIH guidelines would have permitted payment for cell lines using federal funding so long as payment did "not exceed the reasonable costs associated with the transportation, processing, preservation, quality control and storage of the stem cells." As is true for fetal tissue for transplantation, the NIH guidelines would have required that donation of human embryos be made "without any restriction or direction regarding the individual(s) who may be the recipients of transplantation of the cells derived from the embryo." Consent for such research would have to include statements acknowledging these restrictions and informing donors that donated embryos would not survive the human stem cell derivation process and would in no case be transferred to a woman's uterus.

Despite the considerable thought that went into the NIH guidelines, they never went into effect (although features of the donor consent portions of the guidelines have been incorporated in recent regulations).[68] During the 2000 election campaign, candidate George W. Bush spoke out against human embryo and hESC research. Following his election, it was widely anticipated that he would bar federal support for this research and perhaps try to extend this ban to research in the private sector. However, following months of lobbying by patient advocacy and biotechnology groups, on August 9, 2001, the president announced a more moderate position in a prime time televised statement. Federal funds would be made available for research using hESC lines that had been brought into being before that date. Justifying his decision, the president described these lines as those on which "the life and death decision has already been made."[69]

In the period since this announcement, NIH support for embryo research has moved at a slow pace. Although the NIH initially stated that there were at least 60 lines in existence that would qualify for funding, nearly five years later, in the winter of 2006, only 22 lines had been sufficiently characterized and freed of ownership restrictions to be made available for use by federally funded researchers.[68] Recent studies have also confirmed that all the lines authorized for NIH-funded research were contaminated with mouse molecules that were likely to cause rejection or disease if the cells were used in human transplantation.[70] Outside the United States, in countries like Sweden, Israel, and Great Britain, in which embryo research is less restricted, the development and banking of hESC lines have proceeded more rapidly.[71]

Further intensifying these U.S. debates is the emergence of private sector and overseas research on therapeutic cloning.[72,73] This employs somatic cell nuclear transfer technology to produce an embryo for stem cell purposes. In this procedure, a body cell (somatic cell) is taken from one individual and is inserted into an egg from which the nucleus has been removed. Following electrical or chemical stimulation, this reconstructed *nuclear transfer unit* begins to divide and develop as would a fertilized egg. Instead of being transferred to a womb, as in the case of reproductive cloning, the resulting embryo is disaggregated to make a pluripotent and immortalized hESC line.[74] The donor of the somatic cell used in this process can then receive a transplant of these tissues. Because most of the DNA in these tissues is from the somatic cell donor, they would presumably be genetically compatible, avoiding the problem of tissue rejection that is present in the use of immunologically unrelated hESC tissues. Because this research involves the creation and destruction of what Dickey-Wicker defines as an *embryo,* it is ineligible for federal funding. However, following a favorable report by Britain's Chief Medical Officer's Expert Group[75] and the intervention of Parliament, such research is now permitted in Great Britain. In 2004 and 2005, Korean researchers, led by veterinarian Woo Suk Hwang, reported dramatic advances in therapeutic cloning research, but these reports were later attributed to fraudulent data. This episode caused considerable distress in the stem cell and therapeutic cloning research communities.[76,77]

Those who defend this research emphasize not only possible medical benefits but also its contribution to our understanding of the process of the genetic reprogramming of cells. In the words of the British Expert Group report, therapeutic cloning may prove to be "transitional research" that will be replaced, as knowledge grows, by the reprogramming of adult cells and the direct production of replacement tissues from an individual's own cells.[75]

Opponents of this research raise many objections. They see it as involving the same issues as the deliberate creation and destruction of human embryos. They believe that the application of

nuclear transfer technologies to human cells will hasten the day when someone will attempt reproductive cloning, which they regard as inherently offensive. Based on these objections, bills were introduced in the U.S. Congress and Senate to ban all forms of cloning research in both the private and public sectors. Although the House of Representatives passed such legislation twice, by 2006 the Senate had not followed suit. One consequence of this was that bills that would ban only reproductive cloning, and for which there was much wider support, were sidelined. The same has happened at the international level. Despite opposition by Great Britain and some other traditional European supporters, the Bush administration repeatedly sought to have the U.N. General Assembly ban all types of cloning research.[78] In March 2005, the U.N. approved a "Declaration on Human Cloning" that urged member states to ban all forms of cloning, including therapeutic cloning.[79]

If we ask why U.S. conservatives invested so much energy and political capital in this issue, we are returned to the issue of human embryo research. Although opposition to cloning plays some role here, a review of the wording of bills to ban therapeutic cloning supports the conclusion that they very much represent an effort to embody in legislation the view that human life is sacred from conception onward. For example, a bill introduced in the New Hampshire legislature to ban all forms of cloning contains the statement, "all human embryos are simultaneously human beings."[80]

Benefiting From Evil

The preceding discussion reveals the sharp moral debates and political controversies that have been provoked by research involving the human embryo and fetus. It is unlikely that these debates will end anytime soon. It is also unlikely that fetal and embryo research, including stem cell and therapeutic cloning research, will be stopped. By 2006, California and several other U.S. states authorized and, in some cases, provided funding for both stem cell and therapeutic cloning research.[81] Even if opponents of this research prevail in some political jurisdictions, research will go on elsewhere, as it has already begun to do.[82,83] If that research is successful in producing stem cell lines or similar materials derived from human embryos or fetuses, clinical researchers and patients who oppose embryo research will have to answer a difficult moral question: When, if ever, is it permissible to derive benefit from the fruits of morally objectionable activities? Can a devout Roman Catholic neurologist, who believes that abortion is morally evil, participate in research that uses fetal tissues to alleviate symptoms in Parkinson's patients? Can the parents of a diabetic child who believe that life begins at conception ethically consent to the use of pancreatic cells developed from embryonic stem cells?

In the past, the question of benefiting from evil has been addressed somewhat indirectly in Roman Catholic moral theology under the heading "cooperation with evil."[84] It has also arisen previously in bioethics in connection with the utilization of the findings of Nazi biomedical research[85,86] (see Chapter 2). But it is likely to grow more common if fetal and embryo research yield valuable tissues and medical therapies. That we sometimes regard it as permissible to benefit from deeds we morally oppose is illustrated by the stem cell debate. Although President Bush was criticized by some of his conservative supporters for authorizing the use of existing stem cell lines, many others defended his decision as a legitimate effort to derive some good from a bad situation. Germany's Law for the Protection of Embryos makes it a criminal offense to injure or destroy embryos in research. Nevertheless, on January 1, 2002, the German Bundestag passed a law permitting the use of stem cell lines created outside Germany before that date.[87] These recommendations show that even those holding very conservative positions on the issue of embryo destruction are sometimes prepared to accept benefit from practices they oppose. Throughout the course of the stem cell debate, many individuals otherwise uncomfortable with the destruction of embryos for research purposes were prepared to go beyond President Bush's position and permit the creation of some new hESC lines from spare embryos. They reasoned that because these embryos were unquestionably slated for destruction, it would be better if they could be used to treat disease rather than merely being discarded.[88]

Benefiting from evil normally strikes us as wrong for at least several important reasons. One is an emotional aversion to being associated with evil deeds. This aversion is highly subjective. What repels one individual—for example, the use of data from unethical research—may not bother another. A second consideration is more objective and amenable to reasoned assessment. This is the concern that profiting from wrongful deeds will encourage their repetition in the future. This can occur when wrongdoers are rewarded (through payments or other valuable concessions) by those they benefit. This consideration partly explains laws that criminalize the receipt of stolen property. Or it can occur, even if the wrongdoer is not rewarded, when the acceptance of benefit somehow legitimizes the kind of conduct at issue. This may explain our discomfort about the use of Nazi research data. In doing so, we send to all researchers the unfortunate message that even heinous research can be partly redeemed through its value.[89]

If this brief analysis is correct, researchers, clinicians, and patients who oppose fetal tissue and stem cell research will not necessarily have to forswear use of tissues derived from that research. However, to conscientiously use these materials, they will have to provide convincing negative answers to the following questions: Will my use of these materials directly reward those who produce them? Will it in any way legitimize these activities and encourage their repetition? Am I morally compromised in my own and others' eyes by my association with activities to which I object? Those asking these questions will have to give careful attention to the actual causal connections between willingness to benefit and the possible encouragement of wrongful deeds. In some cases, even a modest willingness to benefit may subtly legitimize and thereby encourage wrongdoing (as conservative critics of President Bush's stem cell policy contend). In other cases, despite first appearances, a willingness to benefit may have surprisingly little connection with encouragement. Some who defend the use of spare embryos for stem cell research point out that the many thousands of frozen embryos will almost certainly be destroyed. Nothing that clinicians or patients do with regard to the use of tissues derived from these embryos will change that. Hence, they conclude, it cannot reasonably be said that the downstream use of cells derived from such embryos actually encourages embryo destruction.[89]

Conclusion

In retrospect, we can see that the moral issue of "benefiting from evil" has been a central theme in much ethical and policy discussion of fetal and embryo research. The earliest debates over fetal tissue transplantation (FTT) revolved around the question of whether regulations could be elaborated that would prevent FTT from becoming an encouragement to abortion. Working in the context of Dickey-Wicker's legal prohibition of funding for embryo destruction, the NIH sought to find a way of avoiding federal involvement in embryo destruction while facilitating the downstream use of cells derived from embryos in its August 25, 2000, guidelines on pluripotent embryonic stem cells. Even President George W. Bush's permission for some forms of research on previously destroyed embryos represents a moral position-taking on the question of what might or might not encourage the further destruction of nascent life.[8] Ongoing debates over the use of spare embryos versus those created for research are also partly driven by a concern to avoid direct involvement in morally controversial behavior.

The importance of this theme reveals how intractable the debates are over fetal and embryo research. Although bioethicists (the present author included) cherish the hope that more penetrating reasoning can resolve some of the vexing questions of moral status that fuel these debates, it is unlikely that the disagreements will soon go away. They are rooted in well-developed moral perspectives and deeply held religious views.

Progress in these debates will be slow. It will occur, in part, as a result of scientific or medical advances. For example, research that demonstrates the value of hESC therapies will certainly influence public opinion. Conversely, if adult stem cells demonstrate their value, appeals to use embryonic or fetal tissues may grow less urgent. Progress in resolving our disagreements will also require careful thinking about strategies for accommodating widely different perspectives. The distinction between active involvement in deeds one opposes and allowable benefiting from those deeds is one such strategy. It affords more flexible responses to controversial biomedical developments by making it possible for individuals to modulate their response. There is also room for new thinking about how to draw the line between strongly held personal moral convictions and appropriate public policy. If we cannot reach consensus on our moral conclusions about controversial research, perhaps we can agree on when those conclusions need not be embodied in laws or regulations. The separation of personal morality from public policy is a timeworn, but often overlooked solution to unbridgeable moral divisions.

References

1. Department of Health and Human Services, National Institutes of Health, and Office for Human Research Protections. The Common Rule, Title 45 (Public Welfare), Code of Federal Regulations, Part 46 (Protection of Human Subjects). [Online] June 23, 2005. Available: http://www.hhs.gov/ohrp/humansubjects/guidance/45cfr46.htm.
2. Tauer CA. Embryo research. In: Post SG, ed. *Encyclopedia of Bioethics*, 3rd ed. New York, N.Y.: Macmillan Reference; 2004:712–22.
3. Gratton B, for the European Group on Ethics in Science and New Technologies to the European Commission. *Survey on the National Regulations in the European Union Regarding Research on Human*

Embryos. Brussels, Belgium: European Union; 2002:17. [Online] July, 2002. Available: http://ec.europa.eu/european_group_ethics/publications/docs/nat_reg_en.pdf.

4. Kiessling AA. In the stem-cell debate, new concepts need new words. [letter] *Nature* 2001;413:453.

5. Cibelli JB, Grant KA, Chapman KB, et al. Parthenogenetic stem cells in nonhuman primates. *Science* 2002;295:819.

6. Rohn WG. Seven days of creation: The inside story of a human cloning experiment. *Wired* 2004;12(10):120–9.

7. U.S. Congress. The Dickey-Wicker Amendment; Sec.128 of the Balanced Budget Downpayment Act, I, Pub. L. No. 104–99, 104th Congress, 110 Stat. 26, Jan. 26, 1996. [Online] Available: http://frwebgate.access.gpo.gov/cgi-bin/getdoc.cgi?dbname=104_cong_public_laws&docid=f:pub199.104.

8. President's Council on Bioethics. *Monitoring Stem Cell Research*. Washington, D.C.: President's Council on Bioethics; 2004. [Online] January 2004. Available: http://www.bioethics.gov/reports/stemcell/pcbe_final_version_monitoring_stem_cell_research.pdf.

9. Buckle S, Dawson K, Singer P. The syngamy debate: When precisely does a human life begin? In: Singer P, Kuhse H, Buckle S, Dawson K, Kasimba P, eds. *Embryo Experimentation: Ethical Legal and Social Issues*. Cambridge, England: Cambridge University Press; 1990:213–25.

10. Green RM. Research involving fetuses and in vitro fertilization. In: Amdur RJ, Bankert EA, eds. *Institutional Review Board: Management and Function*. Sudbury, Mass.: Jones and Bartlett Publishers; 2002:373–9.

11. Office of the Secretary, Department of Health, Education, and Welfare. Minimum Criteria Identifying the Viable Fetus. *Federal Register* 1975;40(154):33552.

12. Merton V. The exclusion of pregnant, pregnable, and once-pregnable people (a.k.a. women) from biomedical research. *American Journal of Law and Medicine* 1993;19:369–451.

13. Charo RA. Protecting us to death: Women, pregnancy and clinical trials. *Saint Louis University Law Journal* 1993;38:135–81.

14. Freed CR, et al. Transplantation of embryonic dopamine neurons for severe Parkinson's disease. *New England Journal of Medicine* 2001;344:710–9.

15. Consultants to the Advisory Committee to the Director, National Institutes of Health. *Report of the Human Fetal Tissue Transplantation Research Panel*. Washington, D.C.: NIH; 1988.

16. U.S. Congress. National Institutes of Health Revitalization Act of 1993. Pub. L. No. 103–43, 103rd Congress, 1st Session, June 10, 1993.

17. Berghmans RLP, de Wert G, Boer GJ, for the European Commission BIOMED Project. *Ethical Guidance on the Use of Human, Embryonic and Fetal Tissue Transplantation: Final Report (Part B)*. Brussels, Belgium: EC BIOMED Project; 2002. [Online] December 2002. Available: http://ec.europa.eu/research/biosociety/pdf/bmh4_ct98_3928_partb.pdf.

18. Polkinghorne J, for Her Majesty's Government. *Review of the Guidance on the Research Use of Fetuses and Fetal Material* (The Polkinghorne Report). London, England: Her Majesty's Stationery Office; 1989.

19. Weiss R. Fetal cell research funds are at risk; scientists fear curbs over abortion. *Washington Post* January 26, 2001:A03.

20. Maher DP. Vaccines, abortion, and moral coherence. *The National Catholic Bioethics Quarterly* 2002;2:51–67. [Online] Available: http://www.immunize.org/concerns/maher.pdf.

21. Rock J, Menkin MF. In vitro fertilization and cleavage of human ovarian eggs. *Science* 1944;100:105–7.

22. Green RM. *The Human Embryo Research Debates: Bioethics in the Vortex of Controversy*. New York, N.Y.: Oxford University Press; 2001.

23. Ethics Advisory Board, Department of Health, Education and Welfare. HEW Support of Research Involving Human In Vitro Fertilization and Embryo Transfer: Report and Conclusions. *Federal Register* 1979;44(118):35033–58.

24. Edwards R, Steptoe P. *A Matter of Life*. New York, N.Y.: William Morrow and Company; 1980:92–4.

25. Warnock M. *A Question of Life: The Warnock Report on Fertilisation and Embryology*. Oxford, England: Basil Blackwell; 1985.

26. Human Fertilisation and Embryology Act 1990 (c. 37). [Online] Available: http://www.hmso.gov.uk/acts/acts1990/Ukpga_19900037_en_1.htm.

27. Human Fertilisation and Embryology Authority. *Code of Practice*, 6th ed., Section 10.2, p. 92. [Online] Available: http://www.hfea.gov.uk/cps/rde/xbcr/SID-3F57D79B-43E09108/hfea/Code_of_Practice_Sixth_Edition_-_final.pdf.

28. Ad Hoc Group of Consultants to the Advisory Committee to the Director, National Institutes of Health. *Report of the Human Embryo Research Panel, Vol. 1*. Bethesda, Md.; 1994. [Online] Available: http://ospp.od.nih.gov/pdf/volume1_revised.pdf.

29. President's Council on Bioethics. *Reproduction and Responsibility: The Regulation of New Biotechnologies*. Washington, D.C.: President's Council on Bioethics; 2004. [Online] March, 2004. Available: http://www.bioethics.gov/reports/reproductionandresponsibility/_pcbe_final_reproduction_and_responsibility.pdf.

30. Neumann PJ, et al. The cost of a successful delivery with in vitro fertilization. *New England Journal of Medicine* 1994;331:239–43.

31. Rossing MA, et al. Ovarian tumors in a cohort or infertile women. *New England Journal of Medicine* 1994;331:771–6.

32. Rebar R. American Society for Reproductive Medicine (ASRM) statement on risk of cancer associated with fertility drugs. [Online] January 24, 2002. Available: http://www.inciid.org/article.php?cat=&id=146.

33. Powell K. Seeds of doubt. *Nature* 2003;422:656–8.

34. Kovalesky G, Rinaudo P, Coutifaris C. Do assisted reproductive technologies cause adverse fetal outcomes? *Fertility and Sterility* 2003;79:1270–2.

35. Jones HW, Schnorr JA. Multiple pregnancies: a call for action. *Fertility and Sterility* 2001;75:11–7.

36. Sacred Congregation for the Doctrine of the Faith. *Donum Vitae (The Gift of Life): Instruction on Respect for Human Life in Its Origin and the Dignity of Procreation: Replies to Certain Questions of the Day*. Vatican City, Italy: The Vatican; 1987. [Online] Available: http://www.nccbuscc.org/prolife/tdocs/donumvitae.htm.

37. Pontifical Academy for Life. *Declaration on the Production and the Scientific and Therapeutic Use of Human Embryonic Stem Cells*. Vatican City, Italy: The Vatican; 2000. [Online] August 25, 2000. Available: http://www.vatican.va/roman_curia/pontifical_academies/acdlife/documents/rc_pa_acdlife_doc_20000824_cellule-staminali_en.html.

38. Noonan JT. *The Morality of Abortion*. Cambridge, Mass.: Harvard University Press; 1970.

39. Doerflinger RM. Ditching religion and reality. *The American Journal of Bioethics* 2002;2.1:31–2.

40. Tauer CA. The tradition of probabilism and the moral status of the early embryo. *Theological Studies* 1984;45:3–33.

41. Warren MA. *Moral Status: Obligations to Persons and Other Living Things*. New York, N.Y.: Oxford University Press; 1997.

42. Wilcox AJ, et al. Incidence of early loss of pregnancy. *New England Journal of Medicine* 1988;319:189–94.

43. Norwitz ER, et al. Implantation and the survival of early pregnancy. *New England Journal of Medicine* 2001;345:1400–8.

44. Massey JB, et al. Blastomere separation: Potential for human investigation. *Assisted Reproduction Reviews* 1994;4:50–9.

45. Van Steirteghem AC. Outcomes of assisted reproductive technology. *New England Journal of Medicine* 1998;338:194–5.

46. Ainsworth C. The stranger within. *New Scientist* 2003;180:34.

47. Ford NM. *When Did I Begin? Conception of the Human Individual in History, Philosophy and Science*. Cambridge, England: Cambridge University Press; 1988.

48. Shannon T, Wolter AB. Reflections on the moral status of the pre-embryo. *Theological Studies* 1990;51:603–26.

49. Mauron A. Is the genome the secular equivalent of the soul? *Science* 2001;291:831–2.

50. Ryan M. Creating embryos for research: On weighing symbolic costs. In: Lauritzen P, ed. *Cloning and the Future of Human Embryo Research*. New York, N.Y.: Oxford University Press; 2001:50–66.

51. Holland S. Contested commodities at both ends of life: Buying and selling gametes, embryos, and body tissues. *Kennedy Institute of Ethics Journal* 2001;11:263–84.

52. Lauritzen P. Appendix G. Report on the ethics of stem cell research. In: President's Council on Bioethics. *Monitoring Stem Cell Research*. Washington, D.C.: President's Council on Bioethics; 2004:237–72. [Online] January, 2004. Available: http://www.bioethics.gov/reports/stemcell/pcbe_final_version_monitoring_stem_cell_research.pdf.

53. Annas GJ, Caplan A, Elias S. The politics of human-embryo research—Avoiding ethical gridlock. *New England Journal of Medicine* 1996;334:1329–32.

54. Weiss R. 400,000 human embryos frozen in U.S. Number at fertility clinics is far greater than previous estimates, survey finds. *Washington Post* May 8, 2003:A10.

55. Davis D. Embryos created for research purposes. *Kennedy Institute of Ethics Journal* 1995;5:343–54.

56. Council of Europe. *Convention for the Protection of Human Rights and Dignity of the Human Being With Regard to the Application of Biology and Medicine: Convention on Human Rights and Biomedicine*. Strasbourg, France: Council of Europe; November 1996; opened for signature, April 4, 1997, Oviedo, Spain. [Online] Available: http://conventions.coe.int/Treaty/EN/Treaties/Html/164.htm.

57. Committee on Guidelines for Human Embryonic Stem Cell Research, National Research Council and Institute of Medicine. *Guidelines for Human Embryonic Stem Cell Research*. Washington, D.C.: National Academies Press; 2005.

58. Chen Y, et al. Embryonic stem cells generated by nuclear transfer of human somatic nuclei into rabbit oocytes. *Cell Research* 2003;13:251–64.

59. Thomson JA, et al. Embryonic stem cell lines derived from human blastocysts. *Science* 1998;282:1145–7.

60. Shamblott MJ, et al. Derivation of pluripotential stem cells from cultured human primordial germ cells. *Proceedings of the National Academy of Science* 1998;95:13726–31.

61. National Bioethics Advisory Commission. *Ethical Issues in Human Stem Cell Research*. Rockville, Md.: NBAC; 1999. [Online] September 1999. Available: http://www.bioethics.gov/reports/past_commissions/nbac_stemce111.pdf.

62. Committee on the Biological and Biomedical Applications of Stem Cell Research, National Academy of Sciences. *Stem Cells and the Future of Regenerative Medicine*. Washington, D.C.: National Academy Press; 2002.

63. Doerflinger R. The ethics of funding embryonic stem cell research: A Catholic viewpoint. *Kennedy Institute of Ethics Journal* 1999;9:137–50.

64. Vogel G. Stem cell policy: Can adult stem cells suffice? *Science* 2001;292:1820–2.

65. Quesenberry PJ, Abedi M, Aliotta J, et al. Stem cell plasticity: An overview. *Blood Cells, Molecules, and Diseases* 2004;32:1–4.

66. Constans A. Another chapter in going from blood to brain. *The Scientist* 2005;19(Nov.7):20–21.

67. National Institutes of Health, Department of Health and Human Services. Guidelines for Research Using Human Pluripotent Stem Cells.

Federal Register 2000;65(166):51975–81. [correction: *Federal Register* 2000;65(225):69951.] [Online] August 25, 2000. Available: http://frwebgate3.access.gpo.gov/cgi-bin/waisgate.cgi?WAISdocID=69304331869+1+0+0&WAISaction=retrieve.

68. National Institutes of Health. Stem Cell information: The official National Institutes of Health resource for stem cell research, frequently asked questions. [Online] Available: http://stemcells.nih.gov/info/faqs.asp.

69. President's Statement on Funding Stem Cell Research. *New York Times* August 9, 2001.

70. Ebert J. Human stem cells trigger immune attack. news@nature.com. [Online] January 24, 2005. Available: http://www.nature.com/news/2005/050124/pf/050124-1_pf.html.

71. Adam D. Britain banks on embryonic stem cells to gain competitive edge. *Nature* 2002;416:3–4.

72. Cibelli J, Lanza RP, West MD. The first human cloned embryo. *Scientific American* January 2002:44–51.

73. Vogel G. Scientists take step toward therapeutic cloning. *Science* 2004;303:937–8.

74. Lanza RP. The ethical validity of using nuclear transfer in human transplantation. *JAMA* 2000;284:3175–9.

75. Chief Medical Officer's Expert Group, Department of Health, United Kingdom. *Stem Cell Research: Medical Progress With Responsibility*. London, England: Department of Health; 2000. [Online] June, 2000. Available: http://www.lucacoscioni.it/cms/documenti/donaldson_eng.pdf.

76. Chong S, Normile D. How young Korean researchers helped unearth a scandal. *Science* 2006;311:24–5.

77. Couzin J. And how the problems eluded peer reviewers and editors. *Science* 2006;311:23–4.

78. Lynch C. U.S. may push cloning ban next year. *Washington Post* December 10, 2003:A24.

79. Lynch C. U.N. backs human cloning ban. *Washington Post* March 9, 2005:A15.

80. New Hampshire, H.B. 1464-FN (2002). "An Act Prohibiting Human Cloning in New Hampshire."

81. Wade N. California maps strategy for its $3 billion stem cell project. *New York Times* October 11, 2005.

82. Normile D, Mann CC. Cell Biology: Asia jockeys for stem cell lead. *Science* 2005;307:662–3.

83. Holden C. U.S. states offer Asia stiff competition. *Science* 2005;307:662–3

84. Smith RE. The principle of cooperation in catholic thought. In: Cataldo PJ, Moraczewski AS, eds. *The Fetal Tissue Issue: Medical and Ethical Aspects*. Braintree, Mass.: Pope John Center; 1994:81–92.

85. Post SG. The echo of Nuremberg: Nazi data and ethics. *Journal of Medical Ethics* 1991;7:42–4.

86. Segal NL. Twin research at Auschwitz-Birkenau: Implications for the use of Nazi data today. In: Caplan AL, ed. *When Medicine Went Mad: Bioethics and the Holocaust*. Totowa, N.J.: Humana Press; 1992:281–99.

87. Heinemann T, Ludger H. Principles of ethical decision making regarding stem cell research in German. *Bioethics* 2002;16:530–43.

88. Outka G. The ethics of human stem cell research. *Kennedy Institute of Ethics Journal* 2002;12:175–213.

89. Green RM. Benefiting from "evil": An incipient moral problem in human stem cell research. *Bioethics* 2002;16:544–56.

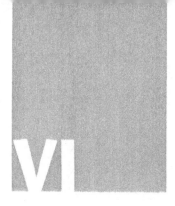

VI

Risk-Benefit Assessments

David Wendler   Franklin G. Miller

Risk-Benefit Analysis and the Net Risks Test

The goal of clinical research is to develop scientific knowledge that can guide the improvement of medical care for future patients. A central concern in research ethics is to protect participants from exploitation in the course of this socially valuable activity. To avoid exploitation, the risks to which research participants are exposed must be reasonable in relation to anticipated benefits.[1] This requirement raises a host of difficult questions. Must the potential clinical benefits to participants outweigh the risks they face? Or is it ethically acceptable to expose participants to some risks for the benefit of society? Assuming it is ethical to expose participants to some risks for the benefit of society, are there limits on the level of these risks? And if there are such limits, to what extent do they vary depending upon the participants in question, whether they can consent or not, whether they are children or not?

Developing answers to these questions is critical to protecting research participants from exploitation. In addition, implementing the answers in practice requires a method by which institutional review boards (IRBs) can assess the risks of research participation. For example, many guidelines allow individuals who are unable to consent to be enrolled in research that does not offer them the potential for clinical benefit provided the risks are minimal or, in some cases, a minor increase over minimal risk. To implement this safeguard, IRBs need a way to determine when research offers the potential for clinical benefit and to what extent the risks of research participation exceed its potential for clinical benefit. Unfortunately, as the U.S. National Bioethics Advisory Commission (NBAC) notes, "current regulations do not further elaborate how risks and potential benefits are to be assessed, and little additional guidance is available to IRBs."[2]

The NBAC, as well as numerous commentators, endorses what we will call "dual-track" risk assessment.[2-5] Dual-track assessment stipulates that IRBs should evaluate research risks using the widely accepted *components analysis*. That is, IRBs should evaluate the risks and benefits of individual interventions or procedures included in a research study, rather than simply conducting an overall risk/benefit assessment of the entire study. The distinctive feature of dual-track assessment is that it divides research interventions into two different categories with different risk standards, based on the distinction between therapeutic and nontherapeutic interventions. However, no clear definition exists for this distinction, and the use of different ethical standards appears unjustified. As a result, dual-track assessment provides IRBs with confusing guidance and has the potential to block valuable research that poses acceptable risks. Once it is recognized that the ethics of clinical research differ fundamentally from the ethics of medical care, the rationale for dual-track assessment is undermined.

Other guidelines, including the U.S. federal regulations for pediatric research, rely on the distinction between interventions that offer participants a *prospect of direct benefit* and those that do not. This distinction avoids the serious shortcomings of reliance on the distinction between therapeutic and nontherapeutic research. Unfortunately, this distinction also conflates research and clinical care, raising the need for a more appropriate method for assessing the risks of clinical research in particular. This chapter describes one alternative, the *net risks* test, and argues that this test offers a better approach for protecting research participants from excessive risks while allowing appropriate research.

Background

The research studies in which individuals participate often include a number of different interventions and procedures. To assess the risks of research participation, IRBs need a method for assessing the risks of these procedures and interventions. In particular, IRBs must assess each intervention or procedure to ensure that the risks to participants are not excessive and are justified by either the prospect of clinical benefits to the participants or by the social value of the knowledge to be gained from the research.

To consider one example, guidelines for clinical research must protect individuals who are unable to provide informed consent. One possibility, exemplified by the Nuremberg Code's stipulation that informed consent is "essential" to ethical research, would be to exclude these individuals from all research.[6] However, this approach would block important research that needs to enroll individuals who cannot consent, including some research on dementia and severe psychiatric disorders, as well as emergency research and research with children.[7] This approach would also prevent individuals from participating in research that may benefit them and research that poses only minimal risk.

Recent guidelines attempt to avoid these shortcomings, yet still protect individuals who cannot consent by allowing them to participate in clinical research provided additional safeguards are in place. In particular, most guidelines allow these individuals to be enrolled in research that does not offer the potential for clinical benefit when the risks are sufficiently low.[4,8-16] To implement this safeguard, and to protect individuals who cannot consent from excessive risks, IRBs need a way to distinguish between research interventions that offer participants a compensating potential for clinical benefit from those that do not offer such potential for benefit.

To assess the risks of research interventions, IRBs cannot simply assess the absolute risk level posed by each intervention. Even serious risks may be ethically acceptable when the research intervention offers participants a compensating potential for clinical benefit. For example, many Phase III treatments pose serious risks to participants. Yet such risks seem prima facie acceptable when there is persuasive evidence that the experimental treatment offers a compensating potential for clinical benefit. The risks of a purely research biopsy, in contrast, are ethically worrisome because the intervention does not offer participants a compensating potential for clinical benefit. This difference suggests IRBs need a method that allows them to assess whether the risks of undergoing a given research intervention exceed its potential for clinical benefit. For simplicity, we refer to the risks of undergoing an intervention that exceed its potential for clinical benefit as the *net risks* of undergoing that intervention.

IRBs should begin to assess the risk-benefit profile of research interventions by first ensuring that there is good reason to include the intervention in the study in question. Unnecessary interventions should be eliminated at this point in the review process. IRBs should then enhance the benefits of the intervention and minimize its risks, consistent with sound research design. For example, investigators can eliminate initial screening procedures, such as blood draws, scans, or biopsies, when the necessary information can be obtained by consulting the results of procedures the participants have recently undergone as part of their standard medical care. Similarly, the benefits of a research intervention might be enhanced by providing research participants with results of the intervention that are relevant to their clinical care. Once it has been determined that there is good reason to include a given intervention, and the benefits of the intervention have been enhanced and its risks reduced, IRBs need a method for assessing the acceptability of the risks of the intervention.

There is no regulatory consensus regarding whether there should be a limit on the net research risks to which competent adults may be exposed. The U.S. federal regulations, for example, do not mandate any such limits. Hence, in principle at least, competent adults may be exposed to serious net research risks as long as the societal value of the knowledge to be gained justifies the risks to which they are exposed. A noteworthy exception is the fifth requirement from the Nuremberg Code, which prohibits research when there is "a prior reason to believe that death or disabling injury will occur."[6] We are not aware of any data that reveals whether IRBs ever allow competent adults to be exposed to very serious net risks for the benefit of society. In our experience, IRBs tend to be very reluctant to allow even competent adults to be exposed to substantially more than minor net risks for the benefit of society.

Research regulations around the world agree that individuals who are unable to provide their own informed consent should be enrolled in research only when the net risks are "minimal" or, at most, a "minor increase" over minimal. Here again, the Nuremberg Code is a noteworthy exception, stating that research participants' informed consent is "essential" to ethical research, seeming to imply that it is unacceptable to enroll in any research individuals who are unable to provide informed consent.

Many regulations define *minimal* risks based on the risks of daily life. Using this standard, for example, children may be exposed to research interventions or procedures only when the net risks are no greater than the risks children face in daily life.

Dual-Track Assessment

To assess the risks of research interventions and procedures, some commentators and guidelines direct IRBs to place the interventions into two different categories, typically labeled *therapeutic* and *nontherapeutic* interventions (see Figure 47.1). Proponents of this approach sometimes call it *components analysis*. In the present chapter, we reserve this term for the widely accepted approach of evaluating the risks of the individual interventions and procedures that make up a given study. This approach is designed to ensure that the risks of one intervention in a given study are not justified by the potential clinical benefits offered by another intervention in the same study. That is, this method is intended to address what has been called the "fallacy of the package deal."

Components analysis understood in this sense does not offer a particular, substantive method for assessing the risks of the individual interventions and procedures. It does not say, for example, that IRBs should evaluate all the interventions using the same ethical standard, or whether IRBs should first divide the interventions into categories and then use different standards for evaluating the risks posed by the interventions in those categories. The method under consideration in the present section, endorsed by NBAC and other groups, does prescribe such a method. It directs IRBs to divide research interventions into two different categories and then apply different standards to the two categories. Given that the distinctive feature of this method is the recommendation that IRBs divide research interventions into two categories, we will refer

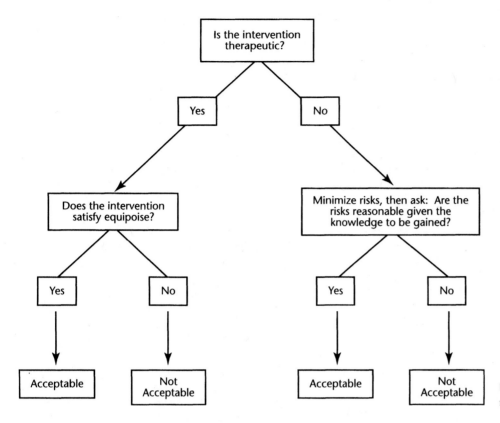

Figure 47.1. Dual-Track Assessment of Individual Interventions

to this substantive approach to assessing the individual interventions and procedures that make up a given study as *dual-track* assessment.

Under dual-track assessment, IRBs may approve interventions that are categorized as *therapeutic* only when they satisfy clinical equipoise. Clinical equipoise involves an assessment of whether the risk-benefit profile of a research treatment is at least as favorable as the risk-benefit profile of the clinically available alternative treatments.[17] If it is, the research treatment satisfies the requirements of clinical equipoise; if the risk-benefit profile of the research treatment is less favorable by any margin than the risk-benefit profile of the available alternative treatments, it fails to satisfy the demands of clinical equipoise.

Although intuitively appealing and widely accepted as a necessary ethical requirement for clinical trials, clinical equipoise presents serious theoretical and practical problems.[18] At the same time, the equipoise standard represents an essential aspect of risk-benefit assessment for clinical research, which needs to be recognized even if the dual-track approach is rejected. This aspect is the need to undertake a comparative analysis that examines the risks and benefits of research interventions for participants in comparison with the risks and benefits of interventions that would be appropriate for them in the context of medical care. The point of this comparison is not to insist that the risk-benefit profiles of research interventions must be the same as those in clinical practice, but to provide a benchmark for determining when interventions pose net risks to participants—risks that are not matched by clinical benefits to them.

One might wonder why there ever would be reason to conduct a study to evaluate an intervention when there was compelling evidence at the outset of the trial that the intervention has a less favorable risk-benefit ratio than the existing clinical options. Why spend the time and money, and why expose research participants to risks, in order to test an intervention that the evidence suggests is not as good as the interventions that are currently being used in clinical practice? In fact, there are a number of reasons why one might want to evaluate such interventions.

To take one example, the existing treatment may be so expensive that few patients are able to afford it. Or, in countries that provide health care to all individuals the existing treatment might be so expensive that it precludes the national health system from offering other important treatments. In this context, it could make sense for the national health plan to test a new intervention that would be significantly cheaper, even when it is known that the new treatment is likely to be somewhat less efficacious or have somewhat greater side effects than the existing treatment. In this case, it may be vital to assess how much less efficacious or how much greater the side effects of the new medication are, with the assumption that a slight increase in some side effects (say, transient nausea) may be deemed acceptable in return for a dramatic decrease in cost and other benefits for the health-care system.

The fact that a research treatment offers a less favorable risk-benefit ratio than the available alternatives, as determined by the equipoise standard, highlights the fact that the intervention poses net risks to participants. Hence, IRBs need to assess the net risks to ensure that they are not excessive. That is, the IRB needs to ensure that the risk-benefit profile of the research intervention is not excessively less favorable than the risk-benefit profile of the standard treatment alternatives. Dual-track assessment assumes that satisfying clinical equipoise is an ethical requirement, such that a research treatment that offers a less favorable risk-benefit ratio than the clinically available alternatives is unethical in all cases.[18]

Hence, dual-track assessment prohibits IRBs from approving interventions that are categorized as therapeutic when they are not in participants' medical interests, even if the social value to be gained from the procedures is very important and the net risks to participants are very low.

In contrast, dual-track assessment allows IRBs to approve interventions that are categorized as nontherapeutic even when they are not in participants' medical interests, such as blood draws to measure study outcomes. Unlike therapeutic interventions, dual-track assessment allows the net risks of nontherapeutic interventions to be justified by the social value to be gained by including them in the study.

Concerns With Dual-Track Assessment

Unnecessary Use of Two Ethical Standards

The central goal of assessing the risks of research interventions is to ensure that they do not expose participants to excessive risks. To make this determination, dual-track assessment directs IRBs first to divide the interventions under review into two different categories. Although this process adds complexity to IRBs' risk assessments, proponents of dual-track assessment fail to explain why the use of two different categories is necessary to protect research participants.

One hypothesis to explain the need for a dual-track assessment is the conviction that participants receiving treatment interventions should not be knowingly exposed to greater risks than they would be in receiving treatment for their condition in the context of medical care. However, in view of the goal of clinical research—to produce generalizable knowledge, not to provide optimal or standard medical treatment—it is difficult to see why this conviction should be presumed as an ethical requirement. Furthermore, commentators agree that it is ethically acceptable to expose participants to some level of risks from research interventions that are not justified by the prospect of medical benefits to them, such as a blood draw or lumbar puncture to measure study outcomes in a randomized trial. If it is acceptable to expose participants to net risks in the case of these interventions, why should it not be acceptable to do so in the case of treatment interventions (or placebo controls) provided the study has important social value? Nor is it clear that this dual-track approach is needed to protect research participants from excessive risks. There does not seem to be any reason to think that the net risks of "therapeutic" interventions are ethically more or less worrisome than the net risks of "nontherapeutic" interventions. Without an explanation of why the net risks of these two types of interventions have different ethical status, the dual-track approach appears arbitrarily to add complexity without increasing protection. A better approach would be to identify a method that assesses the net risks of all research interventions using the same ethical standard.

Lack of a Clear Definition

Some commentators define nontherapeutic interventions as ones *designed* to "achieve beneficial results for the public."[19] Because all research is designed to benefit the public, this definition has the potential to categorize all research interventions as nontherapeu-

tic. Hence, the risks of all interventions might have to be justified by their social value alone. Using this definition, then, dual-track assessment would have the potential to inadvertently prohibit research interventions whose risks are justified by their potential clinical benefits *to participants*.

Others distinguish between therapeutic and nontherapeutic interventions based on the intentions of the investigators. The NBAC adopts this approach at least with respect to nontherapeutic interventions, stating that interventions qualify as nontherapeutic when "their sole intent is to answer the research question(s)."[2] Unfortunately, investigators often have mixed intentions, aiming to benefit both participants and society. Even in research with healthy volunteers, researchers often attempt to benefit participants, for example, informing them of any research findings that might be of clinical significance. Hence, this definition fails to provide IRBs with a clear method to distinguish between therapeutic and nontherapeutic interventions.

Finally, some proponents of the dual-track approach appeal to the concept of *therapeutic warrant*, defining interventions as therapeutic when they are "administered with evidence sufficient to justify the belief that they may benefit research subjects." The therapeutic warrant approach then defines interventions as nontherapeutic provided they are "administered solely for the purpose of answering the scientific question."[5]

By defining nontherapeutic interventions based on the *purpose* of administering them, this definition seems to appeal either to research design or investigator intention. As a result, this definition fails to avoid the problems mentioned previously: All research interventions are designed to answer scientific questions, and investigators typically have multiple intentions when administering research interventions.

Second, defining therapeutic interventions as those that *may* benefit participants has the potential to create further confusion. Many research interventions offer an often very low chance of benefit to participants. For example, radiological scans done in healthy volunteers for research purposes seem to offer a paradigm example of a nontherapeutic intervention. Yet data provide compelling evidence that research scans conducted in healthy volunteers offer a very low chance of identifying an undiagnosed and treatable brain tumor, a very important clinical benefit.[20] Hence, this definition may cause IRBs to categorize essentially all research interventions as therapeutic.

Third, the two clauses that make up the therapeutic warrant definition are not mutually exclusive. To take one example, an intervention may be administered for scientific purposes, even when there is evidence that the intervention may benefit the participants. Thus, it seems that many interventions would qualify as both therapeutic and nontherapeutic, a problematic result given that the dual-track approach applies different requirements to therapeutic and nontherapeutic interventions. Specifically, therapeutic interventions must satisfy the requirement of clinical equipoise, whereas nontherapeutic interventions do not have to satisfy this requirement. Dual-track assessment provides IRBs with no guidance on how to assess interventions that qualify as both therapeutic and nontherapeutic.

Lack of Familiarity

Many research regulations make no mention of the therapeutic/nontherapeutic distinction. For example, the U.S. federal regulations for pediatric research refer to interventions that offer participants a *prospect of direct benefit*. To implement the dual-track approach, IRBs would have to reconcile a method that relies on the distinction between therapeutic and nontherapeutic interventions with regulations that do not include this distinction. In particular, IRBs would have to synthesize the concept of prospect of direct benefit which focuses on the impact of research on participants with the therapeutic/nontherapeutic distinction, which, depending on one's preferred definition, seems to focus on investigators' intentions or the design of individual interventions.

Arbitrary Judgments

Dual-track assessment allows IRBs to approve nontherapeutic interventions that are not in participants' medical interests, provided the net risks are sufficiently low and the knowledge to be gained justifies the risks. In contrast, dual-track assessment prohibits IRBs from approving therapeutic interventions that are not in participants' medical interests, even when the net risks are just as low or even lower, and the knowledge to be gained justifies the risks.

For example, to assess the pathophysiology of depression, investigators sometimes need to perform brain scans and other noninvasive procedures on persons diagnosed with depression who are not taking medication. The primary risk of such studies is the delay in receiving standard medically indicated treatment while individuals are on the study. Dual-track assessment allows such studies when they involve only nontherapeutic interventions. In contrast, dual-track assessment would not allow the very same

individuals to enroll in a clinical trial evaluating an experimental treatment for depression that included a nontreatment arm, even when the length of time off treatment, the risks, and the social value of the study are equivalent to those of the nontherapeutic, pathophysiology study.

This difference in judgment seems ethically arbitrary. In particular, it is not justified by the primary goal of risk assessment, namely, protecting participants from excessive risks. If it is acceptable to expose competent adults to these risks, then both studies seem acceptable. Conversely, if one thinks that it is ethically unacceptable to expose individuals to these risks for the benefit of society, both studies would be unacceptable. There does not seem to be any justification for claiming that IRBs should be allowed to approve the one type of study, but not the other, based on the distinction between therapeutic and nontherapeutic interventions.

Prospect of Direct Benefit Standard

Commentators have recognized that the therapeutic/nontherapeutic distinction is unclear, and that relying on it fails to offer adequate protection to research participants. As a result, many commentators and guidelines have rejected the therapeutic/nontherapeutic distinction. In its place, some guidelines rely on the prospect of direct benefit standard. For example, the U.S. National Commission for the Protection of Human Subjects of Biomedical and Behavioral Research endorsed, and current U.S. federal regulations have adopted, the prospect of direct benefit standard[21,22] (see Figure 47.2). The International Conference on

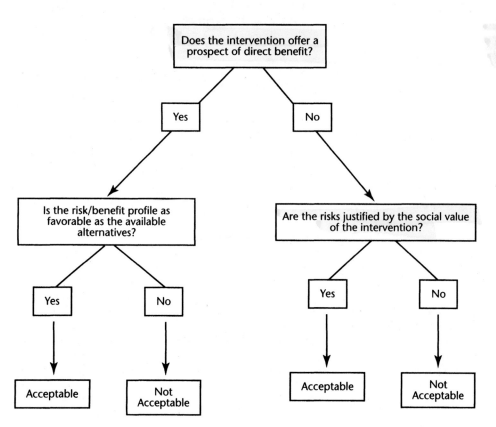

Figure 47.2. Prospect of Direct Benefit Assessment of Individual Interventions

Harmonisation of Technical Requirements for Registration of Pharmaceuticals for Human Use (ICH)[23] and the French Parliament[24] have done so as well. This standard mandates additional safeguards for research that does not offer participants sufficient prospect of direct benefit. By focusing on the impact that research has on participants, this approach provides better protection than the therapeutic/nontherapeutic distinction. Yet this standard still fails to provide sufficient protection.

The prospect of direct benefit standard focuses on the potential that research interventions offer for clinical benefit, rather than the risks they pose to participants. In general, this is problematic because it suggests that the ethical acceptability of clinical research depends upon whether it offers the potential for clinical benefit to participants. Although potential for clinical benefit is obviously a virtue, it is not required for the ethical acceptability of clinical research interventions. Rather research interventions are justified when they offer the potential for sufficient social value and do not expose participants to excessive risks. To make this determination, IRBs need a method that focuses on whether research interventions pose excessive risks.

More important, a requirement that IRBs may approve interventions only when the potential for direct benefit justifies the risks, and the risk-benefit profile is at least as favorable as the available alternatives, conflates the ethical standards for clinical research with the ethical standards for clinical care. Clinicians decide whether to offer patients a given intervention or treatment based on whether its potential clinical benefit justifies the risks. In the context of clinical care, interventions that do not offer patients sufficient potential for clinical benefit are unjustified.

Research interventions, in contrast, are justified when they offer important social value, and do not pose excessive risks.[26,27] For example, a research blood draw that offers no potential for clinical benefit may be justified when the risks are very low, and the intervention has the potential to yield information with important social value. Similarly, giving participants a research treatment that offers a less favorable risk-benefit ratio than an available clinical alternative may nonetheless be ethical provided the research has important social value and the research treatment has only a slightly less favorable risk-benefit ratio.

The focus on the potential for clinical benefit has led some commentators to miss the fact that both types of interventions—the research blood draw and the somewhat less favorable research treatment—may be ethically acceptable when the information to be gained is important and the net risks to participants are not excessive. As mentioned previously, this mistake is exemplified by the erroneous claim that clinical equipoise is a strict ethical requirement on clinical treatment trials. Focusing on the net risks of research interventions and procedures, as opposed to the prospect of direct benefit that they offer participants, reveals that the ethical acceptability of all research interventions depends on the same ethical standard: Are the risks excessive given the potential for participant and societal benefit?

This line of reasoning reveals that the prospect of direct benefit standard may lead to a mistake similar to that made by the dual-track assessment. As we have seen, dual-track assessment uses different standards for evaluating the ethical acceptability of research interventions depending upon whether the IRB categorizes the intervention as therapeutic or nontherapeutic. Specifically, nontherapeutic procedures may pose some net risks. Under dual-track assessment, therapeutic procedures are unethical if they pose any net risks, even when the level of risk is the same or less than the level of risk that would be deemed ethically acceptable for a nontherapeutic procedure.

Reliance on the prospect of direct benefit standard can cause similar errors. Specifically, directing IRBs to first assess whether research interventions offer a prospect of direct benefit ultimately leads to the need for two different assessments. The IRBs first must determine whether the intervention offers a prospect for direct benefit. However, as mentioned previously, interventions that do not offer a prospect of direct benefit may nonetheless be ethically acceptable provided the risks are sufficiently low and the interventions offer the potential for social value. Hence, IRBs then need to ask whether interventions that do not offer a prospect of direct benefit pose excessive risks. This process of dividing research interventions into two types leads to different standards for the two types of interventions.

This potential for instituting two different standards in practice is perhaps best exemplified by the U.S. federal regulations for pediatric research. As mentioned previously, these regulations allow children to be exposed to interventions that do not offer a prospect of direct benefit when the risks are minimal or, in some cases, involve only a minor increase over minimal risk. In contrast, the regulations allow IRBs to approve interventions that offer a prospect of direct benefit only when the potential benefits justify the risks and the risk-benefit profile is at least as favorable as that of the available alternatives.

These requirements on prospect of direct benefit interventions imply that IRBs may not approve an intervention that offers a prospect of direct benefit and also has a slightly less favorable risk-benefit ratio than the available alternatives, even when the net risks do not exceed minimal. Previously, we considered the possibility that public health officials might want to test an intervention that data suggest has a slightly less favorable risk-benefit ratio than established treatments, when the treatment costs significantly less than the existing treatments. Testing of this intervention might have vital social value and play an important role in ensuring adequate health care for everyone. In addition, imagine that the new treatment has the same efficacy as the established treatment, and a similar risk profile, except for a slightly higher risk of transient nausea. Presumably, children face a risk of transient nausea in their daily lives. Hence, the net risks of the new intervention may well be judged to be minimal by the IRB. In that case, the U.S. federal regulations would allow the IRB to approve the intervention if it did not offer a prospect of direct benefit. However, if the intervention does offer a prospect of direct benefit, then under the U.S. regulations it cannot be approved by an IRB because its risk-benefit profile is less favorable than the risk-benefit profile of some available alternatives. This double standard, similar to what we saw with respect to dual-track assessment, seems unjustified. In particular, this difference in assessment cannot be justified on the grounds that the one intervention, but not the other poses excessive risks to children.

This example highlights the fact that any approach to risk assessment that divides interventions and procedures into two categories based on whether they offer the research participants undergoing them a chance of clinical benefit is likely to end up establishing the same kind of unjustified double standard that plagues the dual-track approach. Once an intervention is categorized as offering the potential for clinical benefit, then the almost inevitable next step is to assume that those interventions, but not the interventions that fail to offer a prospect of direct benefit, are acceptable only when they do not conflict with participants' clinical interests. In the end, then, this approach ends up conflating research and clinical care.

One might address this concern by revising the standards that apply to interventions that offer the prospect of direct benefit. Specifically, guidelines could stipulate that such interventions either must offer a compensating potential for direct benefit or the net risks of the intervention must be sufficiently low. This approach would address the problematic imposition of different ethical standards for the two kinds of interventions. However, all interventions would be judged based on whether the net risks were sufficiently low. On that approach, there would be no reason to distinguish between the different types of interventions. This suggests that IRBs need a single standard that focuses on the net risks of the interventions and procedures to which research participants are exposed.

The Net Risks Test

To ensure that research participants are not exposed to excessive risks, IRBs should minimize the risks and burdens of all interventions included in the study under review, consistent with sound scientific design. IRBs then need a method that allows them to assess the ethical acceptability of the remaining risks and burdens to participants. In particular, IRBs need a method to ensure that research interventions do not pose excessive net risks.

There are at least two scenarios in which research interventions pose net risks to participants. Most obviously, research interventions pose net risks to participants when the risks of the interventions exceed their potential clinical benefits. For example, a blood draw that offers participants no potential for benefit poses net research risks, represented by all the risks that participants face from the blood draw. In addition, research interventions that have a favorable profile of potential clinical benefits to risks nonetheless pose net research risks when their risk-benefit profile is less favorable to participants than the risk-benefit profile of one or more of the available alternatives.

To better understand the etiology of certain diseases, investigators sometimes use older generation drugs that have different mechanisms of action than current treatments. Typically, the potential clinical benefits of older drugs exceed their risks. Administration of the older treatment nonetheless would pose net research risks if participants were precluded from receiving the newer treatment that offers a more favorable risk-benefit profile compared to the older generation intervention. For example, the older and current treatments may offer similar potential benefits, but the current treatment may have a slightly lower incidence of one side effect, such as nausea. In this case, participation in the research study would pose net risks to participants represented by the increased incidence of nausea on the older drug as compared to the current treatment.

Whether the risks of studies that involve administration of older generation treatments are acceptable depends on whether the risks are minimized, the net risks to participants are sufficiently low, and the value of the research justifies the net risks. To make this determination, IRBs need a method that focuses on the risks participants face and ensures that IRBs assess the two potential sources of net research risks. The net risks test, divided into the following three steps, provides such a method (see Figure 47.3).

1. Identify the Net Risk Interventions

The IRB first should identify the individual interventions included in the study under review. The IRB should assess the risk-benefit profile of each intervention by comparing its risks to the potential clinical benefits for participants. The IRB should then assess the risk-benefit profile of the available alternatives to each intervention, which, in some cases, may be no intervention at all, and then compare the risk-benefit profile for participants of each research intervention to the risk-benefit profiles of the available alternatives.

When the risk-benefit profile of the research intervention is at least as favorable for participants as the available alternatives, including not undergoing the intervention at all, it poses no net risks. Conversely, research interventions that offer participants a less favorable risk-benefit ratio than one or more of the available alternatives, including not undergoing the intervention at all, pose net risks. The magnitude of the net risks is a function of the extent to which the intervention presents increased risks or decreased potential benefits, compared to the available alternatives.

A study might provide an experimental treatment that is believed to have a risk-benefit profile equivalent to the standard of care, followed by a research PET scan. The treatment poses no net risks because its risk-benefit profile is considered as favorable for participants as the available alternative of standard of care. The PET scan, in contrast, poses net research risks from the use of low-dose radiation because it offers a negative risk-benefit profile to participants, compared to the alternative of not undergoing the intervention at all.

2. Assess the Net Risk Interventions

The IRB next should ensure that the risks of each intervention that poses net risks are not excessive and are justified by the social value of the knowledge to be gained by the intervention's use in the study. For example, the IRB should determine that the risks posed by the research PET scan are not excessive, and that these risks are justified by the information to be obtained by having participants undergo the PET scan.

3. Assess the Net Cumulative Risks

As the Institute of Medicine (IOM) warned in a 2004 study, limiting IRB assessment to the risk-benefit profile of individual interventions ignores the possibility that "research may involve several different procedures that may involve minimal risk or burden individually, but that may present more than minimal risk when considered collectively."[29] The finding that a single MRI and a single blood draw each pose minor risks fails to assess whether inclusion of a series of these procedures in a single study poses excessive risks. To address this concern, IRBs should calculate the cumulative net risks of all the interventions in the study, and ensure that, taken together, the cumulative net risks are not excessive.

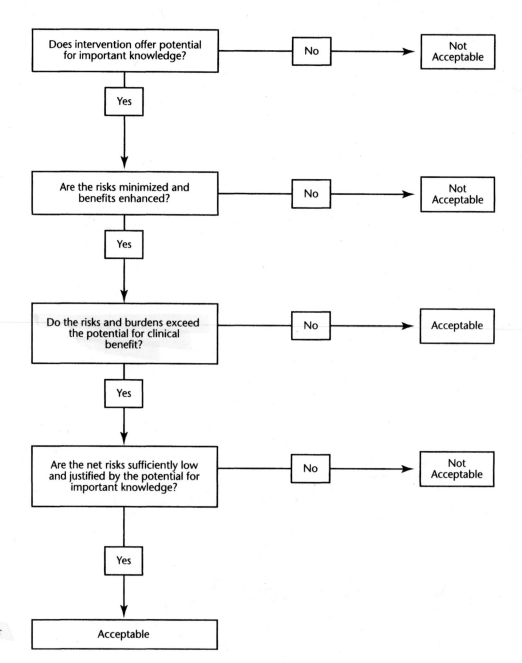

Figure 47.3. Net Risks Test for Individual Interventions

How should IRBs determine whether the net risks of individual interventions and the net cumulative risks of research studies are excessive? It is widely agreed that vulnerable research participants, such as children and adults who are unable to consent, should not be exposed to net risks that exceed a minor increase over minimal risk. In contrast, there is a lack of consensus over whether there should be a priori limits on the risks to which capacitated adults may be exposed for the benefit of society. For example, should capacitated adults be able to consent to enroll in a study that poses serious net risks to them, but offers the potential for profound social benefit, such as finding a cure for malaria? It seems that allowing such research raises the potential for serious abuses of research participants. This potential for abuse seems

especially grave given data on the extent to which research participants often fail to understand the nature of their research participation, including the risks, absence of direct benefits, and right to withdraw.

Conversely, precluding such research in all cases seems inconsistent with other contexts in which we sometimes allow capacitated adults to face serious risks for the benefit of society, such as firefighting and military service. Future research should address the questions of whether there should be a limit on the net risks to which capacitated adults may be exposed in the context of clinical research; if so, how this limit should be defined; and what safeguards, such as stringent assessment of informed consent, would be necessary to conduct high net risk research.

The net risks test is similar to the standard clinical assessment used by physicians to determine whether a given intervention is in patients' clinical interests. Both assessments evaluate the risk-benefit profile of the intervention in question compared to that of available alternatives. This similarity suggests that the net risks test should be more familiar to clinicians than the prospect of direct benefit standard. Granting this similarity, it is important to emphasize that, unlike the clinical setting, some net risks can be justified in the research setting. That is, the ethical standard for clinical medicine requires that the potential for clinical benefit justifies the risks of the intervention in question. In contrast, the ethical standard for clinical research is whether the net risks to participants, if any, are not excessive and are justified by the social value of conducting the research. Accordingly, risk-benefit assessment in clinical research is both similar to, but significantly different from, risk-benefit assessment in medical care.

Some might worry that the similarity between the net risks test and standard clinical judgment might foster the so-called therapeutic misconception, increasing the chances that patients fail to recognize the difference between clinical care and clinical research.[30] However, by focusing on the risks to participants and whether those risks are excessive in the effort to generate socially valuable knowledge, the net risks test seems to have less potential to foster the therapeutic misconception than would an approach that stipulates a distinctive standard for evaluating therapeutic interventions or that focuses on the extent to which research may benefit participants.

For example, the prospect of direct benefit standard seems to evaluate research participation based on the extent to which it offers clinical benefit to participants. If this message gets conveyed to research participants and investigators, they may confuse research with clinical care. Although the net risks test is not intended for use by research participants, if it is communicated to participants to explain the rationale for research interventions, it would be less likely to promote a therapeutic misconception than either the dual-track assessment or the direct benefits standard. In other words, it seems less likely that participants will confuse research with clinical care when told that the research in question poses a low level of net risks. This potential seems much greater if participants are informed that the intervention offers a prospect for direct benefit. The dual-track assessment seems even more worrisome in this regard. It is not difficult to imagine that research participants might confuse research with clinical care once told that the intervention being tested in the study was categorized by the IRB as therapeutic.

In the research setting, there often are few data available to make risk-benefit assessments. Recognizing this, IRBs will have to use their judgment to implement the net risks test, and they should err on the side of caution. When there are insufficient data to determine whether research participation poses risks in excess of the potential for clinical benefit, the IRB should mandate additional safeguards. Occasionally, the net risks test may reveal that research enrollment poses net risks, or greater net risks, to some eligible participants but not others. In these cases, IRBs might repeat the net risks test for individual participants at the time of research enrollment. On this approach, the IRB could require additional safeguards for only the individuals who face net risks or greater net risks. This individual level, or subgroup, assessment may be appropriate when little is known about the experimental intervention or when the intervention poses high risks. Assessment of the study population as a whole is likely to be sufficient when the research poses few risks, or when the inclusion criteria are sufficiently narrow to ensure that participation does not pose net risks to those who are eligible to participate.

The Net Risks Test and Phase I Studies

To exemplify the net risks test, consider the assessment of Phase I studies—a controversial research design. IRBs reviewing Phase I studies should minimize risks by eliminating duplicative procedures and assessing whether the same information could be gained using less risky procedures. The IRBs then should identify the net risk interventions and compare their risk-benefit profile to the risk-benefit profile of the available alternatives, including the alternative of not undergoing the intervention.

This assessment is very similar to the assessment used by many research regulations. For example, the U.S federal regulations require IRBs to compare the risk-benefit profile of the intervention under study to the risk-benefit profile of the available alternatives, including not undergoing the intervention at all when reviewing pediatric research interventions that offer a prospect of direct benefit (45 CFR 46.405).[1] To assess individual interventions that offer children a prospect of direct benefit, the federal regulations instruct IRBs to assess whether (a) the risk is justified by the anticipated benefit to the participants, and (b) the relation of the anticipated benefit to the risk is at least as favorable to the participants as that presented by available alternative approaches.

This assessment is essentially identical to the first two steps in the net risks test: Identify the risk-benefit profile of individual interventions and then compare them to the risk-benefit profile of the available alternatives. Notice that both approaches involve IRBs directly assessing the risk-benefit profile of research interventions rather than first dividing all interventions into two different categories as recommended by dual-track assessment. The similarity between the net risks test and the guidance offered by research regulations suggests that the net risks test, unlike dual-track assessment, should be relatively familiar to IRBs.

For Phase I studies in healthy volunteers, the preferred alternative would be not enrolling in the research at all. Hence, the net risks of the experimental agent, and the net risks of the other included interventions, such as blood draws, would be all the risks that these interventions pose to healthy volunteers. In this case, the IRB should approve the individual interventions only when the net risks to participants of each intervention are not excessive and are justified by the social value to be gained by inclusion of that intervention in the study.

For Phase I agents tested in patients, the IRB should determine the risk-benefit profile of all the interventions for participants, including administration of the tested agent, and then compare the risk-benefit profile of each intervention to the available alternatives. When other treatments are available, the Phase I agent should be compared to them. In the absence of treatment alternatives, this assessment should compare the risk-benefit profile of the Phase I agent to receiving palliative care or to no treatment at all. The IRB should approve each intervention only when the net risks it poses to participants, if any, are not excessive. Finally, the IRB should assess the net cumulative risks of the study, ensuring that they are not excessive and are justified by the social value of the study.

Conclusion

Dual-track assessment, endorsed by NBAC and other commentators and groups, directs IRBs to assess the risks of research interventions by first dividing the interventions under review into two categories, *therapeutic* and *nontherapeutic*. This approach complicates the process of risk assessment without adding any protection for research participants. In addition, confusion over the definitions of therapeutic and nontherapeutic interventions suggests that the dual-track method will be difficult to implement.

Guidelines that instruct IRBs to determine whether research interventions offer a prospect of direct benefit address these concerns, but seem to conflate ethical standards for research with ethical standards for clinical care. The net risks test avoids this conflation by focusing on the extent to which research interventions pose net risks, thus offering a practical method, based on familiar clinical judgments, for assessing research interventions. The net risks test, unlike dual-track assessment, also focuses IRB attention on the central challenge for protecting research participants, namely, whether they face excessive risks, thereby providing clearer guidance to IRBs and more appropriate protection for research participants.

Disclaimer

The opinions expressed are the authors' own. They do not represent any position or policy of the National Institutes of Health, Public Health Service, or Department of Health and Human Services.

References

1. Department of Health and Human Services, National Institutes of Health, and Office for Human Research Protections. The Common Rule, Title 45 (Public Welfare), Code of Federal Regulations, Part 46 (Protection of Human Subjects). [Online] June 23, 2005. Available: http://www.hhs.gov/ohrp/humansubjects/guidance/45cfr46.htm.
2. National Bioethics Advisory Commission. *Ethical and Policy Issues in Research Involving Human Participants, Vol. I.* Bethesda, Md.: NBAC; 2001. [Online] August, 2001. Available: http://www.georgetown.edu/research/nrcbl/nbac/human/overv011.pdf.
3. Weijer C. The ethical analysis of risk. *Journal of Law, Medicine, and Ethics* 2000;28:344–61.
4. Karlawish JHT. Research involving cognitively impaired adults. *New England Journal of Medicine* 2003;348:1389–92.
5. Weijer C, Miller PB. When are research risks reasonable in relation to anticipated benefits? *Nature Medicine* 2004;10:570–3.
6. The Nuremberg Code. In: *Trials of War Criminals Before the Nuremberg Military Tribunals Under Control Council Law No. 10. Volume 2.* Washington, D.C.: U.S. Government Printing Office; 1949:181–2. [Online]. Available: http://ohsr.od.nih.gov/guidelines/nuremberg.html.
7. National Institutes of Health. Interim—Research involving individuals with questionable capacity to consent: Points to consider. *Biological Psychiatry* 1999;46:1014–6.
8. Kim SYH, Caine ED, Currier GW, Leibovici A, Ryan JM. Assessing the competence of persons with Alzheimer's disease in providing informed consent for participation in research. *American Journal of Psychiatry* 2001;158:712–7.
9. National Bioethics Advisory Commission. *Research Involving Persons With Mental Disorders That May Affect Decisionmaking Capacity, Vol. I.* Rockville, Md.: NBAC; 1998. [Online] December 1998. Available: http://www.georgetown.edu/research/nrcbl/nbac/capacity/TOC.htm.
10. New York State Department of Health Advisory Work Group on Human Subjects Research Involving the Protected Classes. *Recommendations on the Oversight of Human Subjects Research Involving the Protected Classes.* Albany, N.Y.: State of New York Department of Health; 1998. [Online] August 2002. Available: http://purl.org/net/nysl/nysdocs/49377072.
11. Attorney General's Working Group. *Final Report on Research Involving Decisionally Incapacitated Subjects.* Baltimore, Md.: Office of the Maryland Attorney General, 1998.
12. United Kingdom Medical Research Council. *The Ethical Conduct of Research on the Mentally Incapacitated.* [Online] December 1991 (reprinted August 1993). Available: http://www.mrc.ac.uk/pdf-ethics-mental.pdf.
13. Canadian Institutes of Health Research, the Natural Sciences and Engineering Research Council, and the Social Sciences and Humanities Research Council. *Tri-Council Policy Statement: Ethical Conduct for Research Involving Humans.* [Online] 1998 (with 2000, 2002, and 2005 amendments). Available: http://www.pre.ethics.gc.ca/english/policystatement/policystatement.cfm.
14. Visser HK. Nontherapeutic research in the EU with adults incapable of giving consent? *Lancet* 2001;357:818–9.
15. Dresser R. Mentally disabled research subjects: The enduring policy issues. *JAMA* 1996;276:67–72.
16. Wendler D, Prasad K. Core safeguards for clinical research with adults who are unable to consent. *Annals of Internal Medicine* 2001;135:514–23.
17. Freedman B. Equipoise and the ethics of clinical research. *New England Journal of Medicine* 1987;317:141–5.
18. Miller FG, Brody H. A critique of clinical equipoise. *Hastings Center Report* 2003;33(3):19–28.
19. *Grimes* v. *Kennedy Krieger Institute, Inc.*, 782 A.2d 807 (Md. Ct. of App. 2001, reconsideration denied, Oct. 11, 2001).
20. Katzman GL, Dagher AP, Patronas NJ. Incidental findings on brain magnetic resonance imaging from 1000 asymptomatic volunteers. *JAMA* 1999;282:36–9.
21. Food and Drug Administration, Department of Health and Human Services. Title 21 (Food and Drugs), Code of Federal Regulation, Part 50.24: Exception from informed consent requirements for emergency research. [Online] April 1, 2006. Available: http://a257.g.akamaitech.net/7/257/2422/10apr20061500/edocket.access.gpo.gov/cfr_2006/aprqtr/21cfr50.24.htm.
22. Department of Health and Human Services, National Institutes of Health, and Office for Human Research Protections. The Common Rule, Title 45 (Public Welfare), Code of Federal Regulations, Part 46 (Protection of Human Subjects); Subpart D—Additional Protections for Children Involved as Subjects in Research. [Online] June 23, 2005. Available: http://www.hhs.gov/ohrp/humansubjects/guidance/45cfr46.htm#subpartd.
23. International Conference on Harmonisation of Technical Requirements for Registration of Pharmaceuticals for Human Use. *The ICH Harmonised Tripartite Guideline—Guideline for Good Clinical Practice.* Geneva, Switzerland: ICH; 1996. [Online] Available: http://www.ich.org/LOB/media/MEDIA482.pdf.
24. Berlin I, Gorelick DA. The French law on "Protection of Persons Undergoing Biomedical Research": Implications for the U.S. *Journal of Law, Medicine, and Ethics* 2003;31:434–41.

25. Shah S, Whittle A, Wilfond B, Gensler G, Wendler D. How do IRBs apply the federal risk and benefit standards for pediatric research? *JAMA* 2004;291:476–82.

26. DeCastro LD. Exploitation in the use of human subjects for medical experimentation. *Bioethics* 1995;9:259–68.

27. Emanuel E, Wendler D, Grady C. What makes clinical research ethical? *JAMA* 2000;283:2701–11.

28. Levine RJ. Uncertainty in clinical research. *Law, Medicine, and Health Care* 1988;16:174–82.

29. Institute of Medicine. *Ethical Conduct of Clinical Research Involving Children.* Washington, D.C.: National Academies Press; 2004.

30. Appelbaum PS, Roth CH, Lidz CW, Benson P, Winslade W. False hopes and best data: Consent to research and the therapeutic misconception. *Hastings Center Report* 1987;17(2):20–4.

Nancy M. P. King   Larry R. Churchill

48

Assessing and Comparing Potential Benefits and Risks of Harm

I. Overview

Assessment of potential benefits and risks of harm is an essential component of the scientific and ethical evaluation of clinical research, for three fundamental reasons. First, it is essential to determining whether a line of research has scientific validity and scientific/social value.[1] It is the task of the institutional review board (IRB) to examine both the scientific validity of proposed research (whether the research has the potential to produce generalizable knowledge), and also its scientific and social value (whether the intervention being studied has the potential to eventually become a treatment for patients with the disease or condition of interest).

Second, assessment of potential benefits and risks of harm helps to protect research participants by ensuring that the risks of harm to which they will be exposed are minimized and are reasonable under the circumstances, and also by ensuring that the research is able to produce results justifying the use of humans (because it is exploitation to ask people to participate in research that is poorly designed or otherwise cannot contribute to generalizable knowledge that has social or scientific value). In some types of research with children and other potentially vulnerable people, this assessment may even require the potential for medical benefit to the participants (see discussion of decisionally incapable subjects, later in this chapter).

Finally, assessment of potential benefits and risks of harm helps to facilitate potential participants' informed decisions about research participation. Information about the potential benefits and risks of harm in a clinical trial helps potential participants to determine whether the balance between potential benefits and risks of harm makes sense for each of them individually.

Regardless of whether individuals participate out of altruism, desire for personal benefit, or both, their informed choices alone cannot morally justify the conduct of research. Individual decisions about research participation cannot even be considered unless the IRB has already made a favorable comparison of potential benefits and risks of harm for the study as a whole. This is true even if individuals' views of the balance of potential benefits and risks of harm are different from the IRB's perspective on the study. Both a favorable assessment of potential benefits and risks of harm and the participant's informed choice are necessary conditions of ethically sound research, but neither is sufficient, and the former is both logically and chronologically prior to the latter.

Assessment of potential benefits and risks of harm is thus an essential part of the ethical evaluation of all clinical research. Moreover, in any properly conducted clinical trial, the task of assessment of potential benefits and risks of harm falls to many individuals and entities, each making independent judgments: not only potential participants and IRBs, but also investigators, sponsors, and data and safety monitoring committees, among others. Although the IRB has the ultimate authority to permit or preclude research based on its assessment of a clinical trial's potential benefits and risks of harm, assessments by others—in particular by sponsors and investigators—serve both to guide the IRB and to promote the conduct of thoughtful and responsible research. Research should not even be submitted to an IRB for consideration if the investigator or sponsor is not confident of its validity and value. Further, having all of these parties make their own independent assessments of the risk of harm/potential for benefit ratio is one means of fulfilling the responsibility to minimize harms.

Existing guidance on assessing and comparing risks of harm and potential benefits is largely oriented toward Phase III randomized controlled trials (RCTs), thereby failing to address much that IRBs and others need to consider when reviewing both early-phase clinical research and clinical trials that do not fit into classical phase designs. This chapter addresses those often-neglected considerations.

We first provide a brief typology and discussion of terminology used in assessing and comparing potential benefits and risks of harm in research. Next we offer a brief overview of how several key clinical research guidance documents from around the globe address assessment and balancing of potential benefits and risks of harm. Then we consider some ongoing controversies about assessment of risks of harm and potential benefits; and finally, we address some special issues, circumstances, and concerns in assessing and balancing potential benefits and risks of harm outside the RCT context.

II. Harms and Benefits: A Typology

The previous chapter addresses risks of harm comprehensively; in this typology we attend more closely to potential benefit. Potential benefits in clinical research fall into two broad categories: *benefits to participants* (that is, benefits from study participation) and *benefits to society* (that is, future benefits from research results). Benefits to participants are further divided into two types: *direct benefits* from receipt of the experimental intervention, and *inclusion benefits* (also called collateral or indirect benefits), which result from participating in a study regardless of whether the participant receives the experimental intervention. Inclusion benefits encompass such diverse items as free goods or services provided as an enrollment incentive; diagnostic testing and standard treatments provided on-study at no cost to participants; the opportunity to be monitored closely by disease experts; and hypothesized psychological benefits to patient-participants from "doing everything possible."[2]

Notably, direct benefits—arguably the benefits of greatest interest to potential participants—are by definition uncertain to materialize. However, some (but not all) types of inclusion benefits may be certain, whereas others are uncertain, and still others may be considered either benefits or harms, depending on how they are experienced by particular participants.

Potential harms to participants may similarly be divided into harms from the experimental intervention and harms from study participation regardless of whether the participant receives the experimental intervention. Potential harms from study interventions (experimental or otherwise) in clinical trials are often called side effects or adverse effects. And as with benefits, although the harms of greatest interest and concern are uncertain to occur, some harms (also sometimes referred to as discomforts or burdens) are inevitable. For example, drawing blood or obtaining a bone marrow specimen always causes discomfort, and making extra trips to the hospital for the purposes of study participation is always at least somewhat burdensome.

Both potential benefits and risks of harm should always be examined and characterized, to the extent possible, according to their nature, magnitude (size and duration), and likelihood. This kind of characterization is quite familiar to IRBs and investigators when it comes to risks of harm, and less familiar for potential benefits; however, it is equally important for both sides of the harm-benefit balance.[3]

III. Balancing Risks of Harm and Potential Benefits: Existing Guidance and Its Limits

Essentially every clinical research guidance document in existence, whether local, national, or international in scope, addresses the assessment and comparison of risks of harm and potential benefits. However, few go beyond general assertions that there should be a favorable balance between the two. We have chosen to closely examine a cluster of U.S. guidance documents, which are meant to be understood together, and one set of international clinical research guidelines that consider risks of harm and potential benefits in somewhat more depth than most. The reader is also referred to those chapters in this volume that discuss these and other guidance documents in detail.

Common Rule

The federal Common Rule governing research with humans conducted in connection with institutions receiving federal funding provides simple but far from straightforward guidance to IRBs in balancing risks of harm and potential benefits (see Chapter 15). The IRB's task is described as determining that "[r]isks to subjects are reasonable in relation to anticipated benefits, if any, to subjects, and the importance of the knowledge that may reasonably be expected to result. . . . The IRB should not consider possible long-range effects of applying knowledge gained in the research (for example, the possible effects of the research on public policy) as among those research risks that fall within the purview of their responsibility."[4]

There are four key things to note here. First, the inclusion of "if any" signals clearly that, generally speaking, potential benefit to participants is *not required* to justify the conduct of research—not even when participants are patients with the disease or condition of interest. Instead, balancing risks of harm and potential benefits requires a more complex judgment. Second, the meaning of the critical balancing term "reasonable" is completely undefined. Third, the Common Rule directs IRBs to consider the long-range potential benefits from research but specifically to exclude consideration of "possible long-range effects of applying knowledge gained in the research . . . as among . . . research risks." It might be thought that the reason for including potential future benefits to society in the calculation, while excluding long-term risks of harm from societal application of research data, is because long-range hazards are difficult to predict. Yet given the amount of attention paid to risks of harm generally, and the paucity of definition and precision in defining potential benefits, it is likely that long-range risks of harm are no more, and possibly less, speculative than future potential benefits. It is thus more likely that this asymmetry signals the inherent support of clinical research that is structured into the U.S. regulatory system. The Common Rule is not neutral; instead, the Rule as a whole, and the assessment and balancing of risks of harm and potential benefits in particular, is designed to promote clinical research while protecting participants.

This asymmetry in the consideration of long-term potential benefits and risks of harm has been challenged by IRBs faced with review of research whose results seem likely to lead to misuse.

Perhaps the most familiar example is when group harm seems likely to follow from the promulgation of research results, as has happened in some genetic research in which populations have been stigmatized by association with disfavored genetic conditions. For example, some genetic mutations, like BRCA in breast cancer, have been labeled "Jewish genes." However, it can be argued that even though the IRB is precluded from disapproving research on the basis of the probable misuse of its results, there are either other grounds for disapproving such research (e.g., the IRB could require modifications in design or dissemination calculated to reduce the likelihood of misuse of results) or other avenues of disapproval (e.g., the institution could choose not to permit the research as failing to reflect local values, or other legal avenues could be employed to limit such research based on societal assessments of potential harms, such as federal funding bans or legislative prohibitions of certain categories of research).

Finally, it should be noted that the two types of potential benefits named in the Common Rule—benefits to participants and "the importance of the knowledge that may reasonably be expected to result"—are quite distinct. Not only do they apply to different individuals and groups, but they may be very different in kind—for example, the knowledge gained might be (in fact, often is) negative knowledge, that is, knowledge that further development of a particular intervention is *not* a viable line of research. It is important to remember that benefit to society from the knowledge that may reasonably be expected to result from the research has priority over potential benefit to participants, in that potential benefit to society is necessary to justify research, and potential benefit to participants generally is of secondary importance. Moreover, it may be technically difficult to combine both types of potential benefits for the purpose of weighing them against risks of harm.

Belmont Report

The Belmont Report[5] is intended to elaborate the moral and conceptual foundations of the Common Rule (see Chapter 14). It goes beyond the Common Rule in setting forth an extensive discussion of the assessment of risks of harm and potential benefits. This discussion begins with a reminder that *risk* and *benefit* are not parallel terms, and that what is really being assessed is both the probability and the magnitude of various "possible harms and anticipated benefits." It continues with explicit instructions about the "systematic assessment of risks and benefits":

It is commonly said that benefits and risks must be "balanced" and shown to be "in a favorable ratio." The metaphorical character of these terms draws attention to the difficulty of making precise judgments. Only on rare occasions will quantitative techniques be available for the scrutiny of research protocols. However, the idea of systematic, nonarbitrary analysis of risks and benefits should be emulated insofar as possible. This ideal requires those making decisions about the justifiability of research to be thorough in the accumulation and assessment of information about all aspects of the research, and to consider alternatives systematically. This procedure renders the assessment of research more rigorous and precise, while making communication between review board members and investigators less subject to mis-

interpretation, misinformation and conflicting judgments. Thus, there should first be a determination of the validity of the presuppositions of the research; then the nature, probability and magnitude of risk should be distinguished with as much clarity as possible. The method of ascertaining risks should be explicit, especially where there is no alternative to the use of such vague categories as small or slight risk. It should also be determined whether an investigator's estimates of the probability of harm or benefits are reasonable, as judged by known facts or other available studies.

Belmont goes on to discuss further how risks of harm and potential benefits should be balanced, stating that "the risks and benefits affecting the immediate research subject will normally carry special weight," but adding that "interests other than those of the subject may on some occasions be sufficient by themselves to justify the risks involved in the research, so long as the subjects' rights have been protected." Some harms can never be justified, all significant risks of serious harm must have unassailable justification, and risks of harm should always be minimized. Finally, Belmont says, "Relevant risks and benefits must be thoroughly arrayed in documents and procedures used in the informed consent process."

One key implication of Belmont's discussion of the "metaphorical character" of the assessment and comparison of risks of harm and potential benefits has to do with reproducibility. Should the calculation of risks of harm and potential benefits be such that any IRB that is doing its work correctly ought to come to the same conclusion about a given clinical trial? That is, should the outcome of the calculation be reproducible? Certainly that is what sponsors and investigators in multicenter trials would prefer. However, Belmont's discussion seems instead oriented toward reproducibility of the calculation *procedure* rather than the *product*. The focus is on transparency—on explicit communication about how, and on what information, the assessment is made, so that investigators and IRBs can understand each other's reasoning and so that the model of reasoning about risks of harm and potential benefits can be recapitulated by the IRB in all its assessments.

Reproducibility of process seems more useful—and more possible—than reproducibility of outcome in such a dynamic and contingent enterprise,[6] but it does pose especially difficult questions for multicenter trials. It is therefore worth considering whether it is necessary to expand the typology of benefits and harms, as suggested earlier, and to develop further guidance for IRBs about the principles and information to be employed in the assessment and comparison process.

IRB Guidebook

The IRB Guidebook, produced by the Office for Protection from Research Risks (now the Office for Human Research Protections in the Department of Health and Human Services) also addresses the lack of parallelism in discussion of "risks and benefits," but adds a distinction between two meanings of *risk*. It states that risks can refer either to the chances that individuals are willing to take to attain a desired goal, or to the conditions that make a situation dangerous. "The IRB is responsible for evaluating risk only in the second sense"—that is, the IRB's task is to determine "whether the anticipated benefit, either of new knowledge or of improved health for the research subjects, justifies inviting any person to undertake the risks."[7] Key here is the recognition that a favorable assessment of risks of harm and potential benefits justifies the invitation to potential participants, which is logically and chronologically prior to the participant's informed decision about whether to undertake the risk in the first sense. The IRB is not to determine whether potential participants would judge the risk "worth it"; instead, the IRB is to judge whether the invitation is justified. The invitation may be justified even if no one decides that the risk is worth taking; similarly, many potential participants may be willing to take a risk that is deemed unreasonable by the IRB.

Thus, the Guidebook emphasizes that IRBs should be "sensitive to the different feelings individuals may have about risks and benefits," noting, for example that having the option of surgery instead of chronic medication might be viewed by some as a risk of harm and by others as a chance of benefit, and that some possible harms may loom larger to some potential participants than to others.

The Guidebook places somewhat more emphasis than Belmont on the contingent, nontechnical character of the assessment of risks of harm and potential benefits, stressing that "it is a judgment that often depends upon prevailing community standards and subjective determinations," such that "different IRBs may arrive at different assessments." It emphasizes the need for careful case-by-case determination that depends not only on currently available knowledge "but also on the degree of confidence about this knowledge."

Although the Guidebook acknowledges that different IRBs may assess and balance risks of harm and potential benefits differently, and that "IRB members should remember that their appraisals of risks and benefits are also subjective," it does not hold that IRBs should be free to use different standards altogether for assessing and balancing risks of harm and potential benefits. IRBs' assessments cannot be subjective in the same sense that someone's choices in weighing risks of harm and potential benefits are subjective. A participant's appraisal can be idiosyncratic or even arbitrary, as long as it is informed, whereas an IRB's cannot. Although there are no rules—or appropriate appeals mechanisms—to judge how participants should weigh risks of harm and potential benefits, for clinical research in the United States, the Common Rule, the Belmont Report, and the Guidebook do provide rules and procedures for IRBs' assessments. Nonetheless, some research has shown that American IRBs do indeed vary, perhaps excessively, in the standards they apply, even to the extent of approving only research that offers the possibility of direct medical benefit to participants.[8]

The Guidebook, like Belmont, distinguishes sharply between research that "involves the use of interventions that have the intent and reasonable probability of providing benefit for the individual subjects" (apparently synonymous with interventions "expected [or anticipated] to provide direct benefit to the subjects") and research that "only involves procedures performed for research purposes" (i.e., "solely to obtain generalizable knowledge"). The clarity and validity of that sharp distinction has been questioned for a variety of reasons, most notably by Robert Levine.[9–11] From the perspective of this discussion, there are two reasons to discredit it. First, the distinction is irrelevant because the same assessment of potential benefits and risks of harm must be made in either case. Second, the distinction is insidious because it gives rise

to an almost overwhelming temptation—for investigators, IRBs, and participants alike—to exaggerate the potential for direct benefit when research is deemed to have "therapeutic intent." Therapeutic intent is likely to be imputed whenever the participant is a patient with the disease or condition of interest, and/or a member of a "vulnerable" group, such as minors, pregnant women, or persons lacking decision-making capacity, to whose research participation more stringent regulations apply.[3,12–16]

It is controversial to characterize any clinical research enrolling patients with the disease or condition of interest as participants—even Phase I research—as not offering the potential for direct benefit. Because the ultimate goal of a line of clinical research is that the experimental intervention becomes a treatment, from which, therefore, patient-participants could theoretically benefit if all hopes about the experimental intervention are realized, IRB members often argue that it is acceptable for participants and investigators to believe and use some modest benefit language in all clinical trials. Nonetheless, it is highly problematic to characterize the tested intervention as having genuine potential for benefit under all such circumstances. Essentially, this conflates the theoretical possibility of some direct benefit with benefit at a future time from the hoped-for results.

A realistic potential for direct benefit is simply missing from the classic Phase I design, as the experimental intervention will not be assessed for benefit until Phase II. Moreover, the capacity of an experimental intervention to offer direct benefit in a Phase I trial is extremely limited at best, both by virtue of early-phase trial design and because most interventions do not become successful treatments—that is, few get as far as Phase II, let alone Phase III.

The *therapeutic misconception*—a misunderstanding of the essential difference between research and treatment, or an unrealistic overexpectation of direct benefit from research[13,17]—is nonetheless pervasive, and its persistence is attributable in part to the origins of codes and principles of research ethics. Belmont, the Common Rule, the Declaration of Helsinki, and other guidance documents tend to see research ethics as derivative of medical ethics; similarly, common law principles of liability in clinical research have been derived from medical malpractice principles developed in the treatment context. This underlying treatment orientation deflects attention from some central issues and problems, including not only the therapeutic misconception (see Chapter 58) but also confusion about the nature of research roles and relationships.[18]

CIOMS

Most other guidance documents addressing clinical research, many of which are discussed elsewhere in this volume, address the balancing of risks of harm and potential benefits with little if any detail beyond that offered by the Belmont Report and the IRB Guidebook. Examples include the Council of Europe's Additional Protocol to the Convention on Human Rights and Biomedicine, concerning biomedical research (see Chapter 17); Canada's Tri-Council Policy Statement: Ethical Conduct for Research Involving Humans;[19] and the Declaration of Helsinki (see Chapter 13).

One exception is the Council for International Organizations of Medical Sciences' (CIOMS') International Ethical Guidelines for Biomedical Research Involving Human Subjects (see Chapter 16).

Building on the Declaration of Helsinki's close identification of medical research with medical practice, CIOMS' Guideline 8 specifies differences in balancing risks of harm and potential benefits according to whether the experimental intervention does or does not "hold out the prospect of direct diagnostic, therapeutic or preventive benefit for the individual subject."[20]

Given the practice orientation of both Helsinki and CIOMS, it is not surprising that interventions that hold out the prospect of direct benefit are addressed first in Guideline 8. These interventions "must be justified by the expectation that they will be at least as advantageous to the individual subject, in the light of foreseeable risks and benefits, as any available alternative." This apparently high benefit threshold is confirmed in the Commentary on Guideline 8, which restates it thus: "Beneficial interventions are justified as they are in medical practice by the expectation that they will be at least as advantageous to the individuals concerned, in the light of both risks and benefits, as any available alternative."

The phrase "as they are in medical practice" makes clear that what CIOMS considers a prospect of direct benefit has a direct referent in the evidence supporting an established diagnostic, therapeutic, or preventive intervention. However, it is difficult to argue that any investigational intervention could meet such a standard. Even the prospect of benefit presented by interventions being studied in Phase III trials can at best be said to be a matter of equipoise (that is, the possibility that an unproven intervention is as effective as standard treatment) rather than expectation (that is, a judgment based on evidence sufficient to consider a new intervention an effective treatment). It is all the more difficult to make credible any such expectation in early-phase research, regardless of how few or inadequate the alternatives might be. And although the Guideline appears to acknowledge the imperfection of the parallel between research interventions and practice by using scare quotes, the balancing of risks of harm and potential benefits conspicuously omits benefit to society: "Risks of such 'beneficial' interventions or procedures must be justified in relation to expected benefits to the individual subject."

In stark contrast, interventions not holding out the prospect of direct benefit for participants "must be justified in relation to the expected benefits to society (generalizable knowledge)." That is, "risks . . . must be reasonable in relation to the importance of the knowledge to be gained."

The questions thus left unanswered by CIOMS are easy to articulate, but difficult to resolve: Is the dichotomy between these two types of interventions as great and complete as presented? If so, where should the line be drawn between them? The Commentary attempts to clarify the distinction by referring to the purpose of the research: "Biomedical research often employs a variety of interventions of which some hold out the prospect of direct therapeutic benefit (beneficial interventions) and others are administered solely to answer the research question (non-beneficial interventions)." However, the research question in clinical trials testing experimental interventions in participants who are also patients with the disease or condition of interest is usually "Does the intervention in fact hold out the prospect of direct benefit?" That question can only be answered by a demonstration that some percentage of participants does in fact experience the hypothesized benefit. Thus, distinguishing between the potential for benefit on the one hand and the research question on the other hand does not seem to work when participants are also patients and the intervention is being tested for its therapeutic potential, except

perhaps by categorizing only those interventions being studied in Phase III trials as holding out the prospect of direct benefit. Although CIOMS attempts to sidestep Belmont's false dichotomy between *therapeutic* and *nontherapeutic* research by applying the dichotomy instead to individual interventions within a given clinical trial, this maneuver does not succeed in addressing the core problem of evaluating the potential for direct benefit of an experimental intervention.

IV. Comparing and Balancing Risks of Harm and Potential Benefits: Ongoing Debates

Weighing potential benefits to participants and society together against risks of harm to participants reinforces a favorable view of research with humans. In the IRB's assessment, potential benefits to society must be combined in some way with potential benefits to participants and then weighed against risks of harm; but because benefits to participants and benefits to society differ in fundamental ways, some IRBs and investigators have understandable difficulty in considering both categories of benefit.

Benefit to society is synonymous with contribution to generalizable knowledge. Negative study findings (to be distinguished from the absence of findings) have social/scientific value comparable to that of positive findings. Notably, benefit to society is a necessary finding for any and all research with human participants to go forward, but benefit to participants is not—even in clinical research enrolling patients with the disease or condition of interest (except sometimes when participants lack decision-making capacity, and/or belong to groups considered vulnerable in the clinical research context; see discussion in Section V.C below ("First-Participant Issues" [page 522]) and in Chapters 43–45).

Yet overprotectiveness toward potential participants should be avoided when evaluating research that offers no prospect of direct benefit.[7,21,22] Such research can indeed provide an appropriate balance of risks of harm and potential benefits, and should not be disapproved solely because no direct benefits are reasonably possible. Should the IRB consider the balance of risks of harm and potential benefits inadequate, the IRB should require investigators to further reduce the risks of harm, or should determine that the research as designed is too risky to pursue, rather than attempting to increase potential benefits to participants. When clinical research poses significant risks of harm to participants, however, there is controversy about the appropriate response. Out of reluctance to expose any research participants to risks of harm without the possibility of direct benefit, some IRBs may be tempted to ensure that potential benefits to participants be found sufficient to balance those risks of harm; this may invite the therapeutic misconception or the addition of overly influential inclusion benefits. Other IRBs may focus on whether potential participants would be willing to enroll in the trial, out of altruism, self-interest, or both, and model their assessments thereon, which runs the risk of conflating the IRB's assessment with the participant's decision making.

Determining what counts as an appropriate balancing of risks of harm and potential benefits is one of the most important but least developed areas in research ethics.[21,23] The limited available literature is largely focused on RCTs, and many important aspects of the assessment and balancing of risks of harm and potential benefits in early-phase trials and nonstandard designs remain inadequately addressed. Several key issues are briefly surveyed below.

Should Balancing Risks of Harm and Potential Benefits in Clinical Research Be Comparable to Balancing Them in Medical Practice?

One obvious starting point for determining whether a particular balance of risks of harm and potential benefits is reasonable is to compare it to what is considered standard treatment for the disease or condition of interest. Agrawal and Emanuel,[23] in addressing this issue for Phase I oncology trials, endorse setting standards for clinical research "based on socially acceptable determinations of risk-benefit ratios already used for cancer treatments," using the risks of harm-potential benefit ratios for chemotherapeutic agents approved by the Food and Drug Administration (FDA) as examples. They provide numerous examples of agents with considerable toxicities and low probabilities of engendering partial or complete tumor responses of significant duration. They eloquently describe the frequent lack of connection between tumor response of any duration and prolongation of survival or improvement in quality of life. And they argue further that "[f]or patients in whom all standard therapeutic interventions have failed, a slight chance of therapeutic benefit is not unreasonable." Thus, they maintain that if an experimental intervention in an early-phase trial holds out the potential for a balance of risks of harm and potential benefits comparable to that of an approved standard treatment, the balance of potential benefits to risks of harm for that research is acceptable; moreover, if no standard treatments are available or all have failed, a less favorable ratio of risks of harm to potential benefits is likely to be acceptable to patient-participants, and thus should be acceptable to IRBs.

Although these arguments appear compelling, there are several important countervailing arguments to consider, which make equating the balance of risks of harm and potential benefits in research with that in the treatment context potentially problematic.

1. In the research context, benefit to society is always a factor in the balancing of potential benefits and risks of harm, but it is never a factor in the balancing of potential benefits and risks of harm in treatment. Thus it is conceivable that when risks of harm and potential benefits are balanced in research, the potential benefits *to participants* might be considerably lower than would be acceptable in treatment. Indeed, benefits to participants might even be nonexistent. The benefits in the calculus could be primarily or exclusively benefits to society. If the calculus for treatment is a starting point, it still must be remembered that treatment and research are different enterprises, with different primary goals.

2. Moreover, precisely because research and treatment are different, even when the balance of risks of harm and potential benefits in a clinical trial appears identical to that of an accepted treatment for the disease or condition of interest, it cannot be identical. It is essential to remember that any balancing of risks of harm and potential benefits for an experimental intervention is unproven, and that a goal of the research is to determine whether the anticipated harms and benefits in fact materialize; that is, proving the hypothesized balance of risks of harm and potential benefits is a research goal. A proven ratio of potential benefits and risks of harm necessarily carries more significance for clinicians and patients than the same ratio in a clinical trial can or should carry for investigators and IRBs. (Potential participants may, however, have understandable difficulty in applying either to themselves, because no matter what the odds and no matter how well the odds are known, a given harm or benefit is always either going to happen or not to a given individual.)

3. Finally, Agrawal and Emanuel rightly point out that what makes a ratio of risks of harm to potential benefits acceptable in a clinical trial depends on the whole range of standard and accepted treatments for the disease or condition of interest, as well as on the experience of the population of potential participants and the alternatives genuinely available to them. Yet they fail to acknowledge that every time a new treatment becomes accepted, the availability of that new treatment option changes the overall ratio of potential benefits and risks of harm for each existing treatment. Thus, in reality the availability of more effective or less harmful or even cheaper treatments could make previously acceptable alternatives no longer acceptable. Using FDA approval as a yardstick is therefore potentially misleading. The FDA imprimatur is rarely withdrawn simply because the overall balance of potential benefits and risks of harm has become less favorable by comparison with newer, more effective or less toxic alternatives, but certainly the decision-making process engaged in by physicians and patients will change as the range of available treatments changes. What is reasonable to offer to patients may become unreasonable, even though still FDA-approved. Similarly, what is reasonable to offer to potential participants should change with context—not only as different alternatives become available, but also with different participant populations.

In the clinical trial setting, then, the IRB's determination of whether a given balance of risks of harm and potential benefits is reasonable must be exquisitely contextual. It has to depend on a comparison of the balance offered by the experimental intervention with the balances offered by the available alternatives. But the IRB's determination is fundamentally one of reasonableness. From the standpoint of both ethics and design, what potential participants deem acceptable should not control the IRB's determination of what is reasonable. Even when patient-participants are prepared to undertake risks of considerable harm, the IRB must make an independent assessment of whether the risks of harm and potential benefits are reasonable and whether risks of harm can be further reduced. The IRB's role in making this assessment, independently of what potential participants might wish to risk, is not paternalism toward potential participants, but rather fulfillment of the duty to let only sound and reasonable research go forward in the first instance. It is true that potential participants' willingness to accept an apparently excessive risk of harm, or an exceedingly low likelihood of direct benefit, may reflect an especially complex contextual picture of disease burden and a paucity of meaningful alternatives, and in that respect may influence the IRB's determination of reasonableness under the circumstances. But participants' willingness to accept high risk should not replace the IRB's judgment.

Should Inclusion Benefits Be Balanced Along With Potential Direct Benefits Against Risks of Harm?

Importantly, the preceding discussion focuses on the balance between risks of harm to participants and potential direct benefits to participants from the experimental intervention. Inclusion benefits derive from trial participation rather than from the experimental intervention. The concept of inclusion benefits is specific to the context of clinical trials, and a key characteristic of most inclusion benefits is that they are in the control of the investigator. However, some inclusion benefits in some studies— namely, the psychological benefits for some seriously ill participants that can come from seeking out every potential benefit, no matter how small or unlikely, especially when all standard treatments have failed them—are analogous to the psychological benefits that comparable patients may gain from trying every available treatment, proven or innovative. Some other inclusion benefits are exclusive to research, such as the psychological benefit of altruism—that is, the benefit from knowing that one is contributing to generalizable knowledge, or the hope that one's experience can help patients in the future. Should these and other inclusion benefits—including benefits in investigators' control, such as obtaining desired experimental interventions, standard interventions and approved agents, or monitoring and diagnostic testing, for free or at reduced cost; or the increased attention and support that can accompany research participation in comparison with standard treatments or palliative interventions—be included in the calculus of risks of harm and potential benefits?

Agrawal and Emanuel, and Horng et al., both add inclusion benefits to the calculus.[23–25] Indeed, they eloquently describe inclusion benefits and their importance. But their discussion of inclusion benefits simply and unwittingly conflates them with direct benefits. It's not that simple, for several reasons.

1. Inclusion benefits are usually largely within the investigator's control—they can be "designed into" a study—and thus could be employed, problematically, to add weight to the benefit side of the balance, in ways that at best might draw attention away from minimizing risks of harm and at worst could unduly influence potential participants in favor of participation despite the risks of harm. (For similar reasons, payment to participants is generally not counted as a benefit: It would be too easy to skew the risks of harm/potential benefits calculus by offering to pay participants more in an attempt to offset concern about excessive risks of harm.)

Thus, to count inclusion benefits, which often are within the control of the investigator, in the balance of risks of harm and potential benefits could improperly tempt investigators to "jack up" potential benefits to participants in order to outweigh significant potential harms. The morally preferable course of action is instead to minimize harms, to the maximum feasible extent. Minimizing harms is a fundamental duty of investigators and IRBs. Even in trials with a very favorable risk of harm/potential benefit ratio, investigators and oversight bodies should work to minimize harms out of a core duty of nonmaleficence. In addition, as a practical matter, to focus on increasing potential benefits may distract from requiring investigators to make an articulate argument about potential harms and how they may be minimized.

The possibility that inclusion benefits may serve as undue inducements to participation for participants is most likely to be of concern when potential participants have limited access to necessary medical care, and that medical care is offered as an inclusion benefit. To give just one example, in much HIV/AIDS research, standard treatments are often offered free as an inclusion benefit in studies that add experimental medications to standard regimens. (By contrast, in most oncology research, standard treatment is not provided free; the participant's health insurer is expected to pay for it.) Thus, in some studies, inclusion benefits must be evaluated

very carefully by IRBs, to ensure that their provision does not substitute for appropriate risk minimization.

2. Some key inclusion benefits—especially the often-postulated "patients do better on study"—may pose especially problematic justice issues. Providing participants with more extensive and intensive individualized attention than they would normally receive as patients, including more study visits, greater support in disease management, and close relationships with investigators and study coordinators, permits investigators to hold out high-quality care as a quid pro quo of research participation, and to allow or excuse deterioration in access to and quality of off-study treatment. This is a significant ethical problem for the health-care system, especially as both reimbursement for treatment and contact time with patients shrink and the conduct of clinical trials grows more remunerative by comparison. It is likewise a problem of particular import for the uninsured and underinsured, who may increasingly seek participation in research as a means of obtaining treatment.

Of course, clinical investigators understandably wish to provide excellent care to participants. Moreover, they have clear duties as investigators to protect participants from harm by designing and following safe and reasonable inclusion/exclusion criteria and stopping rules, both for individual participants and for the study as a whole. These duties may be meaningfully discharged without regard to inclusion benefits. It is, however, increasingly true that in the current health-care system, investigators often perceive that the research environment enables them to feel as though they are being better caregivers for their research participants than for their patients, able to take more time and pay closer attention to their participants as people.[26] This unfortunate and poignant truth is in fact another reason to exclude inclusion benefits from the calculus, not a reason to include them. The case for excluding inclusion benefits is further strengthened by evidence that being on study results in no better outcomes for participants than for patients receiving treatment for the same conditions off study.[27]

3. A complicating factor is the equivocal character of many inclusion benefits. Whether some inclusion benefits are in fact benefits rather than burdens is in the eye of the beholder. Thus, even if the above arguments are not barriers to the consideration of inclusion benefits in the calculus, it is still imperative to consider whether they are benefits to all potential participants. If they do not have this universal character, they cannot be effectively added to the balance. Direct benefits are clearly benefits to participants; even if they do not materialize, their beneficial nature is clear. This is true of some inclusion benefits, but by no means is it true of all. More tests, closer monitoring, more attention, and more study visits all could be viewed as beneficial or could be viewed as burdens. Some participants may consider extra monitoring and study visits to be excessively time-consuming or intrusive, whereas others may welcome the attention. Additional monitoring and diagnostic testing may provide valuable new health information for participants, or it may give rise to alarming false-positive results that cause unnecessary anxiety and incur additional costs, because they have to then be further investigated. Some seriously ill participants may indeed garner psychological benefits from believing they are doing "everything possible" to fight their own disease, or from contributing to knowledge that may be used to help future patients. But other participants may not find these possibilities important or valuable for themselves in research. Encouraging or validating a "do everything possible" attitude may also turn out to be very costly in terms of quality of life for those who are severely

or terminally ill, insofar as participation in a study can be incompatible with good palliative care.

Whether particular inclusion benefits are in fact perceived as benefits by participants is one question. But when the answer could be either yes or no, whether a particular factor can be characterized as an inclusion benefit by investigators, weighed in the calculus by IRBs, and offered as such in the consent form and process is a very different question. The possibility that some research requirements may be viewed as either benefits or burdens can be discussed in the consent form and process, but should preclude their being considered inclusion benefits.

V. Risks of Harm and Potential Benefits in Special Types of Clinical Research

Early-Phase Trials (Classic and Nonclassic Designs)

Most characterizations of direct benefit in clinical research lack specificity.[8] This is not surprising; a similar lack of specificity about the nature, magnitude, and duration of potential benefits also characterizes much discussion of standard treatments in clinical medicine. Treatments are, generally speaking, supportable by evidence or clinical experience, whether or not that evidence or experience is communicated to the patient. And when research interventions are compared with standard treatments in randomized Phase III trials, it can plausibly be argued that potential benefits from the experimental intervention are implicitly described, at least to a limited extent, by the comparison itself—that is, by the existence of clinical equipoise.

For early-phase clinical trials, however, potential benefits merit further attention. Indeed, it may be morally necessary to describe potential direct benefits more thoroughly in early-phase trials, in particular to explain the limits of knowledge about potential benefits and the limited expectations of direct benefit that are reasonable therein. This additional specificity could assist patient-participants, investigators, and IRBs in preserving clarity about the distinctions between research and treatment, the goals of research, and the mixed and multiple goals of early-phase clinical trials.[29,30] What remains entirely unaddressed is whether there should be a minimum threshold standard for potential direct benefit (that is to say, a minimal magnitude and likelihood of a particular potential benefit) that must be met in order for a clinical trial to be reasonably said to hold out the prospect of direct benefit for participants.[2,3]

The balance of risks of harm and potential benefits in early-phase trials is somewhat different from that in Phase III RCTs. The classic Phase I study design, derived from drug studies, enrolls healthy volunteers in a cautious dose escalation format in order to make an initial determination of the side effect profile and to find the *maximum tolerated dose* (MTD)—that is, a dose beyond which the side effects and risks of harm are deemed excessive. In a changing research environment, this classic design is becoming less common, for many reasons. One primary reason is that new pharmaceuticals and biologics have substantially different modes of physiological action than ordinary pharmaceuticals, so that the dose-response relationship is often not linear, making MTDs both unreachable and potentially irrelevant. Assessing risks of harm is similarly affected by the use of nonclassic trial designs in early-phase trials. Although later-phase trials are better positioned to

predict harms by virtue of accumulated experience and constant dosing, if classic dose escalation designs are not employed in early-phase trials, then toxicities may be more difficult to predict. MTDs may not be reached, or they may be reached unpredictably or under unusual circumstances. Uncertain and unknown risks of harm may be more likely, or of more concern, when experience in humans is more limited.

The different modes of action of some new drugs can also make using healthy volunteers problematic, either because the side effects and risks of harm are deemed excessive for healthy participants, or because the physiological effects, whether harmful or beneficial, cannot be adequately assessed in participants who do not have the disease or condition of interest. Thus, many Phase I studies of otherwise classic design enroll patients with the disease or condition of interest. This poses interesting challenges in assessment of potential benefits to participants.

When patient-participants are enrolled in even the earliest human studies, the possibility of direct benefit arises, albeit in the most theoretical sense, simply because those with the disease or condition of interest are the intended beneficiaries of the future treatment, and therefore, if the experimental intervention functioned precisely as hoped, some direct benefit could in theory be possible for some earliest participants. Is this enough to reasonably anticipate direct benefit in the earliest studies? Is the reasonableness of the expectation increased if the design is changed—perhaps to start at a dose level expected on the basis of preclinical studies to have an efficacy-predictive effect?[31]

In Phase III RCTs, questions about the nature, magnitude, and likelihood of direct benefit to participants are usually addressed in terms of clinical equipoise—that is, by considering whether there is enough evidence of an appropriate balance of risks of harm with potential benefits to go forward with the research, without having so much evidence of a favorable balance that further research application of the intervention under study appears unjustified. A sizable literature on equipoise has been developed, and will not be rehearsed here (see Chapter 24). Here it is simply worth noting that applying the concept of clinical equipoise to early-phase research, although tempting, might obscure the need for careful attention to whether potential benefit is reasonably to be anticipated.

Freedman's definition of equipoise was designed to support research in which disturbing equipoise means determining whether a research intervention will become a treatment.[32,33] This equipoise is defined in terms of Phase III RCTs comparing an unproven intervention to a proven one (or to a placebo). It seems clear that this equipoise was not intended to apply to earlier-phase trials, in which disturbing equipoise does not result in a determination that an intervention has or has not become a treatment.

Essentially, the results of early-phase trials determine whether an intervention will progress to the next stage of research—or not. Thus, in a classic Phase I study, the relevant community of investigators must be sufficiently divided about the safety of a new intervention to support going forward with research to demonstrate or disprove that it can be tolerated by humans. Then, a classic Phase II study might seek data supporting the intervention's capacity to produce some evidence of direct benefit—enough to move forward to definitive assessment in a Phase III trial.

Investigators base their optimism and desire to go forward with clinical research at all stages on promising preclinical and prior clinical data. Yet going forward with research does not mean treating patients—it means continuing research until the research itself shows (or definitively fails to show) that the intervention has been proven to be a treatment. Each phase of clinical research demonstrates the tension between belief in the promise of a research intervention and scientific skepticism about what is as yet unproven.

Because clinical equipoise is so closely associated with Phase III RCTs, applying the concept in order to assess and balance the risks of harm and potential benefits in early-phase research is unlikely to be helpful. Instead, it could improperly strengthen the therapeutic misconception in early-phase trials, because equipoise has been traditionally and exclusively associated with issues of direct benefit. Further consideration is needed of the balancing of risks of harm and potential benefits in early-phase trials, and of the amount and nature of the evidence required to advance to the next phase, but this balancing ought not to overemphasize potential benefit when the participants, like all participants in classic Phase III RCTs, are also patients.

Surrogate Endpoints and Direct Benefit

Addressing questions about what expectations of benefit are reasonable in early-phase research requires careful consideration of the significance of surrogate efficacy endpoints (SEs). This is so because in early-phase research, SEs are commonly described as[2] or assumed to constitute[23,24,41] direct medical benefits for participants who are also patients. Just as in Phase III trials, SEs are often routinely measured in early-phase trials and used as statistically predictive stand-ins for desired clinical outcomes. The most common example is, not surprisingly, from oncology trials, in which tumor shrinkage stands in for prolongation of survival. It is also commonly recognized that the connection between tumor shrinkage and living longer can be extremely tenuous at best.[23]

Complicating the use of SEs in early-phase trials are two factors. First, the design and very short duration of the earliest trials generally work to attenuate the connection between SEs and clinical benefit even further. Much more significantly, the postulated relationship is meaningful in the first place only if it has been validated. That is, for traditional cancer chemotherapeutic agents, tumor shrinkage has been shown over time and in many studies to be reasonably predictive of increased survival by a measurable amount. However, tumor shrinkage resulting from agents with different biological action, if not similarly shown related to improved survival, cannot and should not be thought of as predictive of any clinical benefit at all.[33–40] As a result, even when an early-phase trial (whether Phase I, I/II, or, as is traditional, Phase II) seeks to measure an SE, the meaning of that endpoint is questionable and contested. It is nowhere near as simple as offering an SE as a potential direct benefit to participants. Indeed, it is likely that most SEs measured in early-phase trials have no meaningful relationship to clinical benefit. Without persuasive justification, based not only on theory but also on preclinical and prior and related clinical evidence, SEs in early-phase trials probably should not be included in the calculus of potential benefits and risks of harm. This position is a better reflection of the reality of early-phase clinical trials than is the current habit of generally treating SEs as direct benefits.

Although this degree of caution about SEs may seem extreme in light of persisting public and policy confidence in the promise of research, it is borne out by the scientific warrant for early-phase trials, which, as noted earlier, is distinct from that of RCTs. Because trial endpoints are often "translated" into potential benefits for participants who are patients, it is appropriate to reemphasize that the goals and endpoints of early phase clinical trials should translate very differently from those in Phase III studies, in order to promote clearer understanding of and reasonable expectations about direct benefit. Early-phase trials are characteristically different from RCTs in their designs, sample sizes, durations, and goals. These differences may be modified by nonclassic designs and new types of investigational agents, but it is far from clear that such modifications can significantly affect the nature, magnitude, or likelihood of direct benefit to trial participants.

First-Participant Issues

Who should be the first participants in early-phase trials, and how should participant choice affect assessment of risks of harm and potential benefits? From a trial design standpoint, a balance necessarily exists between minimizing potential harms to participants and maximizing the value of the knowledge to be gained from them. This balance is especially critical in early-phase trials, as minimizing harms is often most feasible in healthy volunteers, but the knowledge gained from enrollment of healthy participants may be minimal, irrelevant, or difficult to translate into the next phase of study.[3]

When participants with the disease or condition of interest are used, it is important to determine whether their role in the trial is like or unlike the role of a healthy volunteer. For example, in the gene transfer trial in which Jesse Gelsinger died, his role was similar to that of a healthy volunteer (see Chapter 10). Enrolling the sickest participants first—in that trial, enrolling newborns in the midst of a disease crisis—would have made it extremely difficult to distinguish the risks of harm from the gene transfer from the effects of the disease itself, lowering the value of the knowledge to be gained from the research. Thus, choice of participant can profoundly affect the assessment of risks of harm and potential benefits in a trial, including not only risks of harm and potential benefits to participants but potential benefit to society as well.

Seriously ill people, even those who are clearly dying, are enrolled in all phases and types of research. Assessing and weighing risks of harm and potential benefits for seriously ill participants is especially problematic. Investigators, IRBs, and potential participants may be tempted to assume that direct benefit is more likely when participants are very ill, when all standard treatments have failed, and when no standard treatments exist or no validated treatments are in use—as is often the case in emergency and critical care settings (see Chapter 27).

George Annas has argued that seriously ill and dying people should not be enrolled in clinical research.[42] Although it is commonly reasoned that patients for whom nothing has worked have "nothing to lose," he rightly points out that even patient-participants who are close to death always have something to lose from research participation. Possible harms include not only loss of the time expended on research visits that could have been spent with family and friends, but also toxic effects from the experimental intervention. Certainly it might be argued that the risk of death might be valued differently by potential participants with different prognoses, and might be least alarming to those who are dying. But how potential participants might evaluate a risk of harm is, again, a question that may be asked only *after* the risks of harm have been minimized and the appropriateness of the balance of risks of harm and potential benefits has been established for a given clinical trial. More generally, the idea that anyone can confidently calculate the value of another person's losses, including the loss of life, is troubling and should be avoided. We might be tempted here to state as a truism that the death of a 25-year-old healthy volunteer in a research project is a greater tragedy than the death of an 85-year-old with metastatic cancer in a clinical trial. But to do so would be to rely totally on quantitative measures of value.

Assessing risks of harm and potential benefits in research with seriously ill participants is often complicated by the existence of "partial" alternatives, that is, accepted treatments that are only partially effective, provide only symptomatic relief, are extremely burdensome, drastic, or disfiguring, or are otherwise undesirable in comparison to the promise of a new type of therapy. Comparing the potential benefits of an unproven intervention that is hoped to become a curative treatment to proven treatments that are partial or symptomatic only is a complex process. Gene transfer for X-linked severe combined immune deficiency (X-SCID) provides a provocative illustration of the difficulty. This serious genetic immune deficiency, popularly known as "bubble boy disease," can be managed in a variety of ways, including bone marrow or stem cell transplantation. Children with perfect matches can essentially be cured by a successful transplant. Children for whom only a partial match can be found can experience partial reconstitution of their immune systems, but with important residual immune deficiencies. Genetic intervention appears able to accomplish a significant reconstitution of the child's immune system, with little information as yet about whether and to what extent the beneficial effect can persist over time. And it is now known to carry a significant risk of insertional oncogenesis resulting in leukemia. In an attempt to balance this complex mix of potential harms, benefits, and alternatives, the Recombinant DNA Advisory Committee has recommended that only X-SCID children who do not have an identical or haploidentical transplant match, or whose transplant has failed, should be enrolled in gene transfer clinical trials.[43]

Decisionally Incapable Subjects

Many children and at least some seriously ill patients may lack decision-making capacity. When the decisional capacity of potential subjects is impaired, if they are to be enrolled in clinical research at all, protections must be instituted to ensure that they are not disadvantaged by the need to rely on substituted decision makers. Protections generally focus on limiting their research participation to studies with particular balances of risks of harm and potential benefits—in particular, to studies in which only minimal risks of harm are posed, or to studies thought to hold out a reasonable prospect of direct benefit. The central problem of this chapter—what constitutes a reasonable prospect of direct benefit, especially from the experimental intervention—is the same in these special contexts as it is in clinical trials generally. However, when research cannot go forward unless a reasonable prospect of direct benefit is identified, the temptation to find such a benefit is great—as is the temptation to set a very low, easy-to-meet threshold of reasonableness, regardless of the available alternatives to research participation. It is essential to interpret and apply such

specialized assessments of risks of harm and potential benefit cautiously, in order to protect participants from the temptation to overestimate potential benefits to ensure that important but risky research goes forward.

Genetic Research

Genetic research is discussed in detail in Chapter 29. We mention it here only to note that all types of genetic research potentially pose a particular challenge for assessing and balancing risks of harm and potential benefits, because genetic research often carries special risks of harm to participants, often without corresponding benefits. The collection of genetic information, including DNA samples, is often added to clinical trials. The collection and use of such information, as well as the maintenance of databases containing it, has privacy implications for participants, and can also adversely affect individual participants' sense of identity, self-esteem, and future life prospects, through common popular misunderstanding of the power of genetics, such as *genetic essentialism* (we are nothing more than our genes) and *genetic determinism* (our fate is determined by our genes). In addition to this overestimation of the importance and predictive power of genes in human health and welfare, it is also common to use genetic material and information to identify putative connections between genes and physical or behavioral characteristics in the absence of strategies for treating, preventing, or ameliorating the diseases or conditions so identified.

Genetic research also has the power to pose risks of harm to secondary participants,[44] and can also potentially stigmatize entire groups, such as ethnic, geographic, or religious communities.[45] As a result, IRBs are placed in the difficult position of needing to carefully consider how the balance of risks of harm and potential benefits for a particular study is affected by its genetic character, or by the addition of a genetic information-gathering component—which may have far-reaching social, familial, or economic ramifications for the participants.

Moreover, given that misconceptions about genetics are often widely repeated in both the popular and scientific press, IRBs must also determine whether *erroneous* beliefs about genetic illnesses or testing in research contexts constitute harms. For example, insurance companies and employers can still discriminate against persons who participate in genetics research, even if their reasons for discrimination are without scientific merit. The history of discrimination based on genetic misinformation in the United States, and in Europe, is extensive, and IRBs would be negligent to ignore this special risk of harm.

It is worthy of note that the risks of harm posed by research to secondary participants and nonparticipants are not unique to genetic research. Many clinical trials that include the collection of data through medical records, surveys, and questionnaires may implicate secondary participants. Similarly, many types of clinical research have the capacity to place third parties at risk of harm. Early gene transfer clinical trials often required participants to agree to remain in isolation until it was certain that they could no longer shed genetically altered viruses, even if they decided to leave the trial. Yet many clinical trials not involving gene transfer could place others at risk in a variety of ways, ranging from the risk of contracting an unusual infection from an immunosuppressed study participant to the risk of being injured by a research participant whose driving skills have been impaired by an investigational drug. Generally speaking, risks of harm that are posed by exposure to the research participant should be addressed by the IRB as part of the task of risk minimization. However, the risks of harm that are posed to the participant and others by the acquisition and use of the research data themselves may in some cases be appropriately included in the risk of harm/potential benefit calculus.

Complementary and Alternative Medicine (CAM)

Roughly 40% of the U.S. population use CAM, and this number, especially for those who use herbal remedies, is on the rise.[46] The Dec. 30, 2003, move by the FDA advising consumers to stop using dietary supplements containing ephedra immediately and to remove ephedra from the market[47] signals a future in which CAM remedies, especially dietary supplements and herbal remedies, will be increasingly subjected to clinical trials.

Assessing and weighing risks of harm and potential benefits in research with complementary and alternative medicines can be especially challenging. CAM is essentially a negative designation—anything that is not allopathic medicine—and includes a dizzying array of practices, from chiropractic, acupuncture, traditional Chinese medicine, Reiki, massage, homeopathy, biofeedback, herbal remedies, and megavitamins to various forms of spiritual healing and intercessory prayer. These are variously *complementary* or *alternative*. Some, such as chiropractic, are already on the cusp of legitimacy, widely subject to licensing and accreditation laws, and often covered through insurance. For some, such as acupuncture for nausea secondary to chemotherapy, there is research available about safety and efficacy. For others, such as intercessory prayer to reduce hospital stays, it is difficult to see how to formulate a testable hypothesis (although some have tried). What is and is not CAM can be a function of scientific evidence, public acceptance, reimbursement by insurance, what physicians do, and so forth. None of these ways of defining and delineating CAM is the obvious or stand-alone criterion, and this makes questions about what should be researched all the more difficult.

Many CAM therapies claim to connect the physical and the metaphysical, or at least deal with health in a more holistic sense. Hence one of the key elements in assessing risks of harm and potential benefits is trying to factor in a notion of benefit that is broad and complex enough that a CAM therapy can be tested on grounds commensurate with its putative health claims. It is important to note than any such testing must be referenced to pluralistic medical and cultural norms, not simply to standard biomedical notions, in designing the research.[48] Moreover, for many CAM practices, the absence of standardization among practitioners, combined with imprecise measures of outcomes, makes the harm/benefit ratio more difficult to assess and thereby renders the informed consent process more vague and fragile. For example, many CAM therapies emphasize a concept of *wellness* that is more inclusive than typically found in outcomes research. Whether and how to incorporate this broad view of health into a notion of *benefit* in a clinical trial is a question of both epistemology and ethics. That is, understanding harm/benefit assessment in CAM research implicates both research methodology and the ends we value and seek to achieve through research.

Although IRBs should assess potential benefits and risks of harm in CAM research in much the same way as they do in investigations of allopathic interventions, expanded and sometimes novel notions of benefit will probably be needed to adequately assess research in this emerging area. It will be especially important for IRBs to have CAM practitioners as part of any review process when risks of harm and potential benefits are assessed.[49] It is important to recognize that the need to devise new understandings of direct benefit in this area is consistent with the need described elsewhere in this chapter to assess potential benefit with caution and circumspection. We lack a robust common vocabulary of potential benefit; in the current clinical research environment, which is characterized by fluidity and rapid change, development of that common vocabulary of concepts must likewise be both flexible and precise—a considerable but worthy challenge.

VI. Conclusions

How should IRBs compare risks of harm and potential benefits? Bearing in mind that the process of assessment and comparison should be transparent and reproducible,[22] but that the product—an IRB's actual determination for a given study—may reasonably vary among IRBs, there are several things that IRBs can do to improve the process.

First, IRBs should ensure that investigators provide them with the information they need in order to assess and compare risks of harm and potential benefits effectively.[50] Second, they should directly address the challenge of making more explicit comparisons of risks of harm with potential benefits that are both consistent and appropriately flexible. Third, this explicit consideration should include all relevant dimensions of both risks of harm and potential direct benefits—nature, magnitude, duration, and likelihood. Fourth, IRBs should consider carefully how to address inclusion benefits, both in particular clinical trials and as a matter of policy.

Finally, to emphasize the primary role of benefit to society in the balancing of potential benefits and risks of harm, especially in early-phase research, IRBs should consider establishing "no direct benefit" as a rebuttable presumption except in Phase III studies comparing experimental and standard interventions. In order to rebut the presumption, investigators would have to provide evidence from prior studies supporting the existence of a reasonable chance of direct benefit under the circumstances. Rebutting this presumption would require the IRB to discuss and determine what likelihood of potential direct benefit of a given nature and magnitude is reasonable for a particular clinical trial. In this way, the IRB's model of comparing potential benefits and risks of harm can be both consistent and context dependent.

How should investigators view their obligations to participants based on the assessment of risks of harm and potential benefits? Clinical investigators understandably and genuinely seek to serve the best interests of their patient-participants, too often without directly addressing essential differences between treatment and research. Just as the moral framework of clinical research is derived from clinical practice, clinical investigators enrolling patients as research participants seem generally to derive their role morality from clinical care. It seems clear that a more robust ethic of participant-centered care in research is needed, in order to structure a moral role for investigators that is based on acknowledging the societal goals of research, ensuring that harms and risks of harm to participants are minimized, and supporting the development of professional norms for care in research relationships with participants.

Such professional, participant-centered norms might go a long way toward reducing the temptation of researchers to feel that they are acting more like physicians by promoting research benefits that are only speculative or, at best, remote possibilities. Developing such a role morality could help to focus investigators' obligations on the appropriate design and conduct of clinical trials without promoting the therapeutic misconception, either among themselves or in research participants.[51–56]

References

1. Emanuel EJ, Wendler D, Grady C. What makes clinical research ethical? *JAMA* 2000;283:2701–11.
2. King NMP, Henderson GE, Churchill LR, Davis AM, Hull SC, Nelson DK, Parham-Vetter PC, Rothschild BB, Easter MM, Wilfond BS. Consent forms and the therapeutic misconception: The example of gene transfer research. *IRB: Ethics and Human Research* 2005;27(1):1–8.
3. King NMP. Defining and describing benefit appropriately in clinical trials. *Journal of Law, Medicine, and Ethics* 2000;28:332–43.
4. Department of Health and Human Services, National Institutes of Health, and Office for Human Research Protections. The Common Rule, Title 45 (Public Welfare), Code of Federal Regulations, Part 46 (Protection of Human Subjects). [Online] 23 June, 2005. Available: http://www.hhs.gov/ohrp/humansubjects/guidance/45cfr46.htm.
5. The National Commission for the Protection of Human Subjects of Biomedical and Behavioral Research. *The Belmont Report: Ethical Principles and Guidelines for the Protection of Human Subjects of Research.* Washington, D.C.: Department of Health, Education and Welfare; DHEW Publication OS 78-0012 1978. [Online] April 18, 1979. Available: http://www.hhs.gov/ohrp/humansubjects/guidance/belmont.htm.
6. Kimmelman J. Valuing risk: The ethical review of clinical trial safety. *Kennedy Institute of Ethics Journal* 2004;14:369–93.
7. Department of Health and Human Services, Office for Health Research Protections. *Protecting Human Research Subjects: Institutional Review Board Guidebook.* Rockville, Md.: OHRP; 1993. [Online] Available: http://www.hhs.gov/ohrp/irb/irb_guidebook.htm.
8. Churchill LR, Nelson DK, King NMP, et al. Assessing benefits in clinical research: Why diversity in benefit assessment can be risky. *IRB: Ethics and Human Research* 2003;25(3):1–8.
9. Levine, R. Uncertainty in clinical research. *Law, Medicine and Health Care* 1988;16:174–82.
10. Levine R. The need to revise the Declaration of Helsinki. *New England Journal of Medicine* 1999;341:531–4.
11. Capron AM. Ethical and human rights issues in research on mental disorders that may affect decision-making capacity. *New England Journal of Medicine* 1999;340:1430–4.
12. Churchill LR, Collins ML, King NMP, Pemberton SG, Wailoo KA. Genetic research as therapy: Implications of "gene therapy" for informed consent. *Journal of Law, Medicine, and Ethics* 1998;26:38–47.
13. Appelbaum PS, Roth LH, Lidz C. The therapeutic misconception: Informed consent in psychiatric research. *International Journal of Law and Psychiatry* 1982;5:319–29.
14. Appelbaum PS, Roth LH, Lidz CW, Benson P, Winslade W. False hopes and best data: Consent to research and the therapeutic misconception. *Hastings Center Report* 1987;17(2):20–4.
15. Miller M. Phase I cancer trials: A collusion of misunderstanding. *Hastings Center Report* 2000;30(4):34–43.
16. Dresser R. The ubiquity and utility of the therapeutic misconception. *Social Philosophy and Policy* 2002;19:271–94.
17. Henderson GE, Easter MM, Zimmer C, et al. Therapeutic misconception in early phase gene transfer trials. *Social Science and Medicine* 2006;62:239–53.
18. Churchill LR. Physician-investigator, patient-subject: Exploring the logic and the tension. *Journal of Medicine and Philosophy* 1980; 5:215–24.
19. Canadian Institutes of Health Research, the Natural Sciences and Engineering Research Council, and the Social Sciences and Humanities Research Council. *Tri-Council Policy Statement: Ethical Conduct for Research Involving Humans.* [Online] 1998 (with 2000, 2002, and 2005 amendments). Available: http://www.pre.ethics.gc.ca/english/policystatement/policystatement.cfm.
20. Council for International Organizations of Medical Sciences in collaboration with the World Health Organization. *International Ethical Guidelines for Biomedical Research Involving Human Subjects.* Geneva, Switzerland: CIOMS and WHO; 2002. [Online] November 2002. Available: http://www.cioms.ch/frame_guidelines_nov_2002.htm.
21. Rajczi A. Making risk-benefit assessments of medical research protocols. *Journal of Law, Medicine, and Ethics* 2004;32:338–48.
22. London AJ. Does research ethics rest on a mistake? The common good, research risk and social justice. *American Journal of Bioethics* 2005;5:37–9.
23. Agrawal M, Emanuel EJ. Ethics of Phase 1 oncology studies: Reexamining the arguments and data. *JAMA* 2003;290:1075–82.
24. Horng S, Emanuel EJ, Wilfond B, Rackoff J, Martz K, Grady C. Descriptions of benefits and risks in consent forms for Phase 1 oncology trials. *New England Journal of Medicine* 2002;347:2134–40.
25. Horng S, Emanuel EJ, Wilfond B, Rackoff J, Martz K, Grady C. Authors Reply. *New England Journal of Medicine* 2003;348:1497.
26. Henderson GE, Davis AM, King NMP, et al. Uncertain benefit: Investigators' views and communications in early phase gene transfer trials. *Molecular Therapy* 2004;10:225–31.
27. Peppercorn JM, Weeks JC, Cook EF, Joffe S. Comparison of outcomes in cancer patients treated within and outside clinical trials: conceptual framework and structured review. *Lancet* 2004;363:263–70.
28. Miller FG, Rosenstein DL. The therapeutic orientation to clinical trials. *New England Journal of Medicine* 2003;348:1383–6.
29. Miller FG, Brody H. A critique of clinical equipoise: Therapeutic misconception in the ethics of clinical trials. *Hastings Center Report* 2003;33(3):19–28.
30. Brody B. *The Ethics of Biomedical Research: An International Perspective.* New York, N.Y.: Oxford University Press; 1998.
31. Freedman B. Equipoise and the ethics of clinical research. *New England Journal of Medicine* 1987;317:141–5.
32. Miller PB, Weijer C. Rehabilitating equipoise. *Kennedy Institute of Ethics Journal* 2003;13:93–118.
33. Von Hoff D, Turner J. Response rates, duration of response, and dose response effects in Phase 1 studies of antineoplastics. *Investigational New Drugs* 1991;9:115–22.
34. Smith TL, Lee JJ, Kantarjian HM, Legha SS, Raber MN. Design and results of Phase I cancer trials: 3 year experience at MD Anderson Cancer Center. *Journal of Clinical Oncology* 1996;14:287–95.
35. Decoster G, Stein G, Holdener EE. Responses and toxic deaths in Phase I clinical trials. *Annals of Oncology* 1990;1:175–81.
36. Fleming TR, DeMets DL. Surrogate end points in clinical trials: Are we being misled? *Annals of Internal Medicine* 1996;125:605–13.
37. Temple RJ. A regulatory authority's opinion about surrogate endpoints. In: Nimmo WS, Tucker GT, eds. *Clinical Measurement in Drug Evaluation.* New York, N.Y.: John Wiley & Sons; 1995:3–22.
38. Wagner JA. Overview of biomarkers and surrogate endpoints in drug development. *Disease Markers* 2002;18:41–6.
39. Colburn WA. Optimizing the use of biomarkers, surrogate endpoints, and clinical endpoints for more efficient drug development. *Journal of Clinical Pharmacology* 2000;40:1419–27.

40. Karlawish JHT. The search for a coherent language: The science and politics of drug testing and approval. *Ethics, Law, and Aging Review* 2002;8:39–56.

41. Horstmann E, McCabe MS, Grochow L, et al. Risks and benefits of Phase 1 oncology trials, 1991 through 2002. *New England Journal of Medicine* 2005;352:895–904.

42. Annas GJ. Questing for grails: Duplicity, betrayal and self-deception in postmodern medical research. *Journal of Contemporary Health Law and Policy* 1996;12:297–324.

43. National Institutes of Health. Conclusions and Recommendations of the NIH Recombinant DNA Advisory Committee Gene Transfer Safety Symposium: Current Perspectives on Gene Transfer for X-SCID. [Online] March 15, 2005. Available: http://www4.0d.nih.gov/oba/rac/SSMar05/index.htm.

44. Botkin J. Protecting the privacy of family members in survey and pedigree research. *JAMA* 2001;285:207–11.

45. Duster T. *Backdoor to Eugenics*. New York, N.Y.: Routledge; 1990.

46. Giordano J., et al. Blending the boundaries: Steps toward an integration of complimentary and alternative medicine into mainstream practice. *Journal of Alternative and Complementary Medicine* 2002;8:897–906.

47. U.S. Food and Drug Administration. FDA Announces Plans to Prohibit Sales of Dietary Supplements Containing Ephedra. [Online] December 30, 2003. Available: http://www.fda.gov/oc/initiatives/ephedra/december2003/.

48. Institute of Medicine. *Complementary and Alternative Medicine in the United States*. Washington, D.C.: The National Academies Press; 2005.

49. O'Connor B. Personal experience, popular epistemology, and complementary and alternative medicine research. In: Callahan D, ed. *The Role of Complementary and Alternative Medicine: Accommodating Pluralism*. Washington, D.C.: Georgetown University Press; 2002.

50. van Luijn HEM, Musschenga AW, Keus RB, Robinson WM, Aaronson NK. Assessment of the risk/benefit ratio of Phase II cancer clinical trials by institutional review board (IRB) members. *Annals of Oncology* 2002;13:1307–13.

51. Appelbaum PS. Commentary: Examining the ethics of human subjects research. *Kennedy Institute of Ethics Journal* 1996;6:283–7.

52. Katz J. Statement by individual committee member. In: Advisory Committee on Human Radiation Experiments. *Final Report of the Advisory Committee on Human Radiation Experiments*. New York, N.Y.: Oxford University Press; 1996:543–8.

53. Miller FH. Trusting doctors: Tricky business when it comes to clinical research. *Boston University Law Review* 2001;81:423–43.

54. Daugherty C, Ratain MJ, Grochowski E, et al. Perceptions of cancer patients and their physicians involved in Phase I trials. *Journal of Clinical Oncology* 1995;13:1062–72.

55. Joffe S, Weeks JC. Views of American oncologists about the purposes of clinical trials. *Journal of the National Cancer Institute* 2002;94:1847–53.

56. Dresser R. *When Science Offers Salvation*. New York, N.Y.: Oxford University Press; 2000.

Sumeeta Varma   David Wendler

49

Risk-Benefit Assessment in Pediatric Research

Without clinical research on pediatric illnesses and medical inter-ventions, children might receive dangerous or ineffective treat-ments. Yet society also has an obligation to protect children from excessive risks and foster their development, which could be threatened by enrolling them in research studies. Guidelines for pediatric research are needed to balance these aims, taking into account the fact that most children are not able to give informed consent.

Clinical research may offer some prospect of clinical benefit to the children who enroll in it. For example, in a study comparing two asthma treatments, the participating children may experience relief of their asthma symptoms as a result of being in the study. In such cases, if the potential for clinical benefit is great enough and the risks low enough, exposing participating children to the risks seems justified. Guidelines around the world reflect this view, allowing children to be enrolled in clinical research when it offers a potential for clinical benefit that compensates for the risks, and the risk-benefit profile of the research is at least as favorable as the available alternatives.

These guidelines raise the question of which benefits should be considered in this risk-benefit analysis. Clinical research may offer a prospect of *direct* benefit, such as improved health as a result of the study interventions; it also may offer *indirect* bene-fits to participants, such as payment, the opportunity to learn about the research process, or personal satisfaction from con-tributing to the research. Most commentators argue that research review boards should consider only clinical benefits from research procedures—but not any benefits from added services that are unnecessary for research purposes—when making risk-benefit

assessments.[1] Similarly, official guidelines for institutional review boards (IRBs) in the United States specify that payments for research participation should not be considered benefits to subjects.[2]

Very little work has been done to clarify precisely which types of benefits may be used to justify the risks of research, and more work in this area is needed. However, the present chapter focuses on research studies that do not offer participants any potential for clinical benefit. This type of research raises significant ethi-cal concern and has been the subject of ongoing debate.[3–9] Some commentators argue that research with children is inherently unethical when it does not offer them a compensating potential for clinical benefit. Paul Ramsey and Richard McCormick debated this question over the span of a decade, in one of the most fa-mous debates in research ethics. McCormick offered a number of arguments in support of such research,[10,11] including the claim that children would consent to it if they could, whereas Ramsey provided forceful objections to each of McCormick's proffered defenses.[12,13]

The theoretical debate over the ethical acceptability of pedi-atric research that does not offer a compensating potential for clinical benefit continues. In practice, almost all guidelines around the world now allow such research, provided the risks are suffi-ciently low. This was not always the case, however. For example, the German guidelines of 1931 prohibit "non-therapeutic" re-search with children no matter how low the risks.[14] Similarly, the Nuremberg Code, promulgated by the judges at the war crimes trial of the Nazi doctors following World War II, stipulates that informed consent of the subject is essential to ethical research, thereby seeming to prohibit all pediatric research.[15]

Research that does not offer the potential for clinical benefit is necessary to improve pediatric medicine. As a result, guidelines that prohibit such research may have enormous social costs. Caldwell and colleagues note that without trial-based data on therapies' specific effects in children, "clinicians, families and policy-makers are forced to extrapolate from results of studies in adults. This extrapolation is often inappropriate because children have a different range of diseases and metabolize medications differently, resulting in responses to treatment that are unpredictably different to adults."[16]

To take a specific example, when investigators wanted to determine whether the combination of lopinavir and ritonavir was safe and effective for children with HIV, they first needed to determine a safe dose that could be used in subsequent toxicity and efficacy trials. To make this determination, investigators gave children single doses of the combination to assess which dose levels they would tolerate. These studies, necessary preludes to future efficacy studies, did not offer the participating children any chance for medical benefit, and posed some risks to them. Similarly, the initial toxicity studies of the Dryvax smallpox vaccine, which were needed prior to future efficacy studies of the vaccine, posed risks to participants but did not offer them a prospect of direct benefit.[17]

Our historic reluctance to conduct such research on children appears to continue. It is estimated that approximately 75% of drugs prescribed for children lack adequate testing in children.[18] As a result, physicians often prescribe medications for children that have not been proven safe and effective for them.[16] To protect children from unsafe and ineffective medications, society needs to conduct and support pediatric research, including those necessary studies that do not have the prospect for direct benefit to participants.[19,20] At the same time, society has an obligation to ensure that the risks to which children in these studies are exposed are not excessive. To achieve an appropriate balance between allowing important research studies to proceed and protecting the children who participate in them, most research guidelines around the world rely on the concept of *minimal* risk to regulate pediatric research without a prospect of clinical benefit.

The concept of minimal risk is used to regulate a range of research studies. The Indian Council of Medical Research and the South African Medical Research Council guidelines use the minimal risk standard to determine when research may be conducted with a waiver of informed consent.[21] Other guidelines, including Nepal's guidelines for health research,[22] use the minimal risk standard to assess research with prisoners, whereas those from Uganda use the minimal risk standard to define allowable non-beneficial research involving fetuses.[23]

The use of a single standard for this range of studies has obvious practical virtues, requiring investigators, institutions, funders, and IRBs to learn only one standard in order to assess a wide range of research. However, the reliance on the concept of minimal risk raises the question of whether this or any other single standard provides the correct risk threshold for these myriad kinds of studies. For present purposes, we focus here on clarifying and assessing the minimal risk standard as it applies to pediatric research that does not offer participating children a compensating potential for clinical benefit. Although this analysis may be helpful for assessing the use of minimal risk in other contexts, we leave that analysis for another time.

Interpretation of the Minimal Risk Standard

Most research regulations, including those issued by the Council of Europe,[24] the Council for International Organizations of Medical Sciences (CIOMS),[25] the United States,[26] Australia,[27] Canada,[28] South Africa[29] and Uganda,[23] define minimal risks based on the risks of daily life. For example, at 45 CFR 46.102(i), the U.S. federal regulations define minimal risks as risks that are "not greater in and of themselves than those ordinarily encountered in daily life or during the performance of routine physical or psychological examinations or tests."[26]

This definition might be interpreted in several ways, depending upon which children's lives are used as the standard for assessing research risks. The *procedural* interpretation regards the "risks children ordinarily encounter in daily life or during the performance of routine examinations or tests" as referring to the activities children encounter in daily life, such as walking to school or taking paper-and-pencil tests. On the procedural interpretation, research interventions that children do not ordinarily encounter in daily life, such as PET scans, necessarily qualify as greater than minimal risk. This interpretation might be thought to be bolstered by the statement in the U.S. regulations that in order to approve research that poses more than minimal risk without a prospect of direct benefit, IRBs must consider whether the intervention in question "presents experiences to subjects that are reasonably commensurate with those inherent in their actual or expected" situations (45 CFR 46.406).[26] However, there are good reasons to think this interpretation is misguided.

First, section 406 of the U.S. regulations addresses a different category of research, namely, interventions that pose greater than minimal risk. The specific requirements of section 406 assume that the research has already been assessed with respect to the minimal risk standard. Thus, the requirement of commensurability with children's experience is not relevant to the interpretation of the minimal risk standard, but rather an additional constraint applied to research that has already failed to meet that standard. Further, in explaining its inclusion of this requirement, the National Commission for the Protection of Human Subjects of Biomedical and Behavioral Research—whose work led to the U.S. regulations—stated explicitly that it was intended as only one safeguard to ensure that research, even if posing greater than minimal risk, was not too psychologically distressing for the pediatric participants. Here the National Commission made clear that this requirement was not relevant to determining whether research poses minimal risk, but rather was an added safeguard on research that poses greater than minimal risk. The commissioners wrote:

> The requirement of commensurability of experience should assist children who can assent to make a knowledgeable decision about their participation in the research. . . . More generally, commensurability is intended to assure that participation in research will be closer to the ordinary experience of the subjects.[30]

In addition to helping children make an informed assent decision, the National Commission recognized that when a research procedure is unfamiliar to children, its psychological risks may increase. For example, children who undergo a PET scan for the first time may face a greater chance of experiencing stress or nervousness than they would if the procedure were familiar. Yet psychological considerations do not exhaust the types of risks that research participation poses to children. Even children who are very familiar with a research procedure may face risks from radiation and other sources. For this reason, contrary to the procedural interpretation, most regulatory definitions of minimal risk are based on the level of risk, not the kinds of activities, children ordinarily encounter in daily life. Using this approach, whether hypnosis poses greater than minimal risk depends on whether the risks are greater than the level of risks children encounter in daily life, not on whether children ordinarily undergo hypnosis.

The *relative* interpretation regards the "risks children ordinarily encounter in daily life or during the performance of routine examinations or tests" as referring to the level of risks ordinarily encountered in daily life by the particular children who will be enrolled in the research. This interpretation would allow researchers to expose children who face greater risks in daily life to greater risks in research, even when the research does not offer them a prospect of clinical benefit. Children who live in violent neighborhoods, or who face greater than average environmental health hazards, could thereby be exposed to greater research risks simply because they face greater risks in their daily lives. This result seems unjust, a kind of societally induced double jeopardy.

To avoid taking advantage of some children's unfortunate circumstances in this way, most commentators endorse the *objective* interpretation of the minimal risk standard. This interpretation regards the "risks children ordinarily encounter in daily life or during the performance of routine examinations or tests" as referring to the level of risks ordinarily encountered in daily life by average, healthy children.[31] In the words of a recent Institute of Medicine report, the minimal risk standard should be interpreted based on the level of "harms or discomfort that average, healthy, normal children may encounter in their daily lives or experience in routine physical or psychological examinations or tests."[19]

The risks that average, healthy children face in daily life vary enormously between countries. The risks currently faced by average, healthy Sudanese and Iraqi children are substantially higher than the risks faced by children in Norway or Costa Rica. Thus, although the objective interpretation blocks investigators from exploiting those children who face especially dangerous circumstances compared to other children in the same country, it does not prevent investigators from exploiting average, healthy children who live in especially dangerous countries. To address this concern, the South African guidelines limit the definition of minimal risks even further, to the risks of daily life for average, healthy children who live in *stable* societies.

Although the objective interpretation of the minimal risk standard appears to be appropriate in most cases, it does not seem to work in all cases, suggesting that it should be used as a default that allows for some exceptions rather than a strict requirement. One possible exception to the objective interpretation involves children's participation in research as bone marrow donors. In some cases, research studies may use a bone marrow procurement procedure that is different from that which donors would face in the clinical setting. In such cases, all the risks of donation would count as research risks, and the reviewing IRB may determine that these risks exceed the risks in daily life for average, healthy children. It follows on the objective interpretation of the minimal risk standard that these studies would necessarily qualify as greater

than minimal risk. This seems a counterintuitive result in cases in which the risks of the research procurement *replace* the risks of the standard procurement, and the research risks are equivalent to or lower than the risks of the standard procurement. In these cases, the research risks seem acceptable if the risks of the clinical donation are acceptable. To achieve this result in practice, it seems IRBs will have to appeal to the relative standard for minimal risk, concluding that the procurement risks are no greater than the risks that pediatric donors would face otherwise.

This example illustrates an appropriate exception to use of the objective standard for minimal risks, one that may apply to other protocols meeting the same criteria. In general, IRBs may use a relative standard—basing decisions on whether research risks are greater than the risks the specific children face in daily life—when (1) the risks the children face in daily life are considered acceptable by society and (2) the research risks replace the risks in the children's daily lives. Transplant research involving substantially different procurement procedures meets these conditions when the risks of research donation replace and are no greater than the risks of a standard donation.

Recognizing that there may be some exceptions, the objective interpretation appears to provide the appropriate standard in most cases. To determine whether the existing definition of minimal risk provides adequate protection, it is important to determine how IRBs apply this definition in practice. Do IRBs apply the minimal risk standard in ways that allow appropriate research, while protecting children from excessive risks? Or do IRBs apply this standard in ways that block valuable and appropriate research and/or have the potential to expose children to excessively risky research?

Implementation of the Minimal Risk Standard

A survey of the chairpersons of 188 IRBs responsible for reviewing and approving pediatric research in the United States provides some data on how IRBs apply the minimal risk standard under the *risks of daily life* definition.[32] In this survey, the chairpersons were asked to categorize eight common research procedures as "minimal risk, a minor increase over minimal risk, or more than a minor increase over minimal risk when done in healthy 11-year-olds for research purposes only."

A single 10 cc blood draw by venipuncture was the only procedure categorized as minimal risk by a majority (81%) of IRB chairpersons. Electromyography (EMG) was categorized as minimal or a minor increase over minimal risk by 53%, but as more than a minor increase over minimal risk, and hence too risky for IRB approval without a prospect of clinical benefit to the participants, by 41% of IRB chairpersons. Allergy skin testing was categorized as minimal risk by 23%, a minor increase over minimal risk by 43%, and more than a minor increase over minimal risk, hence too risky for IRB approval without a prospect of clinical benefit to participating children, by 27% of respondents. A single dose of a drug that had a 1/100,000 chance of death but no other side effects was categorized as minimal risk by 7%, a minor increase over minimal risk by 30%, but more than a minor increase over minimal risk by a majority (59%) of chairpersons.

This survey found that IRB chairpersons are significantly more likely to categorize a lumbar puncture (LP) without conscious sedation as minimal risk when performed in sick children who had numerous LPs in the past, than when the same LP is performed in healthy children. This finding suggests that some chairpersons may be applying the minimal risk standard based on the risks in the daily lives of specific groups of children. Hence, it appears that at least some IRBs may be using the relative interpretation of the risks of daily life standard, even in cases in which its use does not seem justified. Further research will be needed to assess this possibility.

These data also suggest that IRBs may be implementing the minimal risk standard inappropriately in other cases as well. The U.S. regulations define *minimal* risk as the risk of harm or discomfort "ordinarily encountered in daily life or during the performance of routine physical or psychological examinations or tests." Yet, 70% of the IRB chairpersons categorized allergy skin testing as more than minimal risk, despite the fact that it is a routine physical test.

IRB chairpersons' categorizations of research procedures varied widely. Overall, 27% of IRB chairpersons categorized allergy skin testing as too risky for IRB approval without a prospect of clinical benefit to the participating children, whereas 66% deemed it safe enough for IRB approval without a prospect of clinical benefit. Similarly, 59% would prohibit a pharmacokinetic study with a 1 in 100,000 risk of death as excessively risky, yet 37% would permit such a study as posing minimal risk or a minor increase over minimal risk. Although 19% of chairpersons considered a confidential survey of sexual activity to be too risky for IRB approval, 73% deemed it approvable by an IRB.

This variation seems unjustified. How can 37% of IRB chairpersons determine that the risks of a pharmacokinetic study are similar to the risks children face in daily life, whereas 59% determine that the same risks significantly exceed the risks children face in daily life? This level of variation raises concern that some IRBs may be categorizing overly risky procedures as only minimal risk, or other IRBs may be prohibiting minimal risk research based on the mistaken belief that the procedures pose greater risks than the federal regulations allow.

These data do not determine whether the risks of specific research procedures in fact are greater or less than the risks children face in daily life. Hence, these data do not determine which risk assessments are consistent with the risks of daily life standard in each case. However, the importance of protecting children from excessive risks while still allowing appropriate research suggests that errors in either direction are ethically troubling and need to be addressed.

The variation in IRB chairpersons' risk assessments may trace, in part, to the fact that IRBs are responsible for assessing the risks of pediatric research but often do not have complete data on the risks posed to children, especially nonphysical risks. For example, the variation in chairpersons' categorization of the risks of allergy skin testing may result from uncertainty over whether allergy skin testing poses more than a minimal risk of *anxiety* in children.

Implementation Without Empirical Data

Although the risks of daily life standard has been in effect in the United States for nearly 25 years, and data have been collected on the riskiness of some particular activities, no comprehensive empirical assessment of the risks average, healthy children ordinarily

encounter in daily life exists. Absent empirical data, IRB members must rely on their own perceptions to assess whether research risks exceed the range of risks that average, healthy children ordinarily encounter in daily life. Unfortunately, extensive psychological research demonstrates that individuals make systematic errors when they assess risks based on their own perceptions.[33–36] Individuals focus on characteristics of activities that do not correlate directly with the activities' risk level, including familiarity with the activity, perceived level of control over the activity, and reversibility of the activity's potential harms. They consistently judge less familiar activities, as well as activities over which the participants seem to exert less control, such as snowboarding, to be riskier.[37] For this reason, flying in commercial airplanes is commonly perceived to be riskier than driving in a car.

Given these systematic biases, IRB members who rely on personal perception rather than empirical data may end up rejecting low-risk studies when they involve unfamiliar procedures, while approving studies that pose excessive risks when they involve familiar procedures. To avoid these mistakes, it is imperative to empirically quantify the risks average, healthy children ordinarily encounter in daily life and during the performance of routine examinations and tests. Gathering these data also would provide an opportunity to assess the ethical appropriateness of the risks of daily life definition of minimal risk.

The Risks of Daily Life and Routine Examinations

Average, healthy children in stable societies encounter a range of risks in daily life, from the risks of reading a book to playing soccer, from taking a bath to riding in a car. To qualify as minimal, where within this range of risks encountered in daily life by average, healthy children must research risks fall? Most regulations define minimal risks as risks that do not exceed the risks children encounter in daily life. To make this determination, IRBs must assess whether research risks exceed the upper end of the range of risks children face in daily life.

Estimates of the level of risks average, healthy children in the United States ordinarily encounter in daily life can be developed by combining data from the Centers for Disease Control and Prevention's National Center for Injury Prevention and Control,[38] the National Highway Traffic Safety Administration,[39,40] American Sports Data, Inc.,[41] and other databases.

Mortality Risks

Riding in a car appears to pose the greatest risk of death for average, healthy children in the United States (see Table 49.1). For every million car trips taken by children aged 0–14 years, approximately 0.06 will die—that is, the risk of death is approximately 0.06 per million trips. The average risk of dying from a car trip for 15- to 19-year-olds is approximately 0.4 deaths per million trips. This average combines the mortality risks of riskier, but still ordinary, car trips with car trips that pose less than average mortality risks. The upper end of the range of mortality risks ordinarily encountered by average, healthy children can be estimated by identifying common factors that increase the risks of traveling by car. Young drivers increase the risk of dying on a car trip 2.0-fold.[39] Similarly, driving on rural highways increases the risk of

Table 49.1

Physical Risks in the Daily Lives of Average, Health Children[a]

| Harm | Activity | Risks per Million Instances of the Activity | | | | |
		< 1 yr	1–4 yrs	5–9 yrs	10–14 yrs	15–19 yrs
Deaths	Average car trip[b]	0.06	0.06	0.06	0.06	0.4
	Riskier car trip[c]	0.6	0.6	0.6	0.6	4.0
	Bathing/swimming[d]	0.05	0.08	0.02	0.02	0.04
Hospitalization	Average car trip	0.3	0.5	0.8	1.0	3.0
	Bathing/swimming	0.2	0.3	0.04	0.03	0.01
Emergency room visit	Average car trip		8.0	13.0	18.0	32.0
	Bathing/swimming	0.3	0.3	0.06	0.04	0.03

[a]Number of children in each age cohort (millions): < 1 yr = 4; 1–4 yrs = 16; 5–9 yrs = 20; 10–14 yrs = 21; 15–19 yrs = 20. [b]To determine the average risk of mortality from a single car trip, we assumed an average of 2 car trips per day and divided the annual risk of mortality by 365 days. [c]To estimate the risk of morality from a riskier but ordinary car trip we calculated the extent to which the combination of a young driver (2-fold increase in risk), rural highways (2.6-fold increase in risk), and wet conditions (1.8-fold increase in risk) increases the risk of mortality of an average car trip. [d]Estimate assumes an average of 1 exposure per day to bathing, swimming, or another water activity.

Data adapted from Centers for Disease Control and Prevention's National Center for Injury Prevention and Control, and the National Highway Traffic Safety Administration.[38–40]

dying on a car trip 2.6-fold.[40] Finally, driving in wet conditions increases the risk of dying on a car trip 1.8-fold.[40]

Although car trips that include all three factors are riskier than average, these trips nonetheless seem ordinary for average, healthy children. Reasonable parents who live in the country routinely allow their teenage children to drive in the rain. Thus, combining these three factors provides one estimate for the upper end of the range of mortality risks ordinarily encountered by average, healthy children. Specifically, these data suggest that the upper end of the range of mortality risks is approximately 10 times the risk of mortality of the average car trip, or approximately 0.6 deaths per million trips for children aged birth–14, and approximately 4.0 deaths per million trips for children aged 15–19.

Morbidity Risks

Participation in sports appears to be the activity that poses the greatest risk of injury for average, healthy children in the United States (see Table 49.2).[41] For every million times individuals in the United States play basketball, approximately 1,900 will be injured in some way, of whom approximately 180 will break bones, 160 will require surgery, and 58 will be permanently disabled. For every million times individuals play American football, approximately 3,800 (1 in 250) will be injured in some way, approximately 910 of whom will break bones, 270 will require surgery, and 42 will be permanently disabled (approximately 1 in 20,000). Because the data for sports injuries include all participants over the age of 6 years, it is difficult to estimate the extent of any age effects in these data. For younger children in the United States, bathing and swimming pose the highest risk of morbidity (see Table 49.1).

Psychological Risks

IRBs should consider all the risks that research participation poses to children, not just the physical risks. Although research participation typically does not pose economic or social risks to children,

it can pose psychological risks. No systematic data are available on the psychological risks children face from ordinary activities of daily life, such as riding on a roller coaster. However, a series of studies in thousands of healthy children in the United States found that approximately 27% of healthy children "sometimes" feel scared or afraid in daily life, and 26% "sometimes" worry about what will happen to them.[42] In addition, 3% of healthy children "often" or "always" feel scared or afraid, and 7% of healthy children "often" or "always" worry about what will happen to them. Although the data do not characterize the severity of these psychological harms, they do suggest that feeling scared or anxious is an ordinary experience for many average, healthy children in the United States.

Risks of Routine Clinical Examinations

Existing data reveal that routine examinations and tests pose very low risks to children. Routine clinical measurements of height and weight pose no risks; routine psychological tests pose no physical risks and very low risks of anxiety or distress. Routine clinical blood drawing poses small risks of transient pain, anxiety, and minor hematomas.[43] The only risk of serious harm from blood drawing is syncope (fainting), with approximately 375 of every million blood draws leading to syncope.[44] Syncope is also the only risk of serious harm from allergy skin testing, with approximately 1,625 of every million individuals who undergo allergy skin testing experiencing syncope.[45] These data reveal that as long as children are seated and antiseptic methods are used, blood drawing and allergy skin testing pose only small risks of pain and anxiety to children.

Limitations of the Data

Because the risks of many ordinary activities have not been systematically assessed, the extant data likely underestimate the risks of daily life. In addition, the extant data on many morbidity risks include both children and adults; the risks to children may be

Table 49.2

Physical Risks From Sports in the Daily Lives of Average, Healthy Children[a]

Sport	Risks per Million Instances of Participation				
	Total Injuries	Permanent Disability	Total Level IV Injuries[b]	Surgeries	Broken Bones
Football	3,800	42	500	270	910
Soccer	2,400	38	300	N/A	N/A
Basketball	1,900	58	300	160	180
Cheerleading	1,700	N/A	100	N/A	N/A
Baseball	1,400	60	300	120	30
Skateboarding	800	N/A	200	20	170

[a]Data are for all individuals over 6 years of age. [b]Level IV injures are those that resulted in emergency room treatment, overnight hospital stay, surgery or ongoing physical therapy, and that prevented participation in sports for at least one month. N/A = Not available

Data adapted from American Sports Data, Inc. *Comprehensive Study of Sports Injuries in the U.S.* (Hartsdale, N.Y.: American Sports Data, Inc. 2002).[41]

higher or lower than these figures. These data were gathered from U.S. sources, and even among stable societies there may be some variation in the incidence of injury from activities of daily life; for example, driving conditions may differ, as may the popularity of some activities such as particular sports. Finally, the data provide only approximate risk estimates. This uncertainty should not pose a serious obstacle to implementing the minimal risk standard in practice, however. IRBs rarely have precise estimates of the risks of research interventions. Hence, IRBs must make general comparisons between the estimates of the risks of daily life and the estimates of the risks of research procedures.

Cumulative Risks of Daily Life

Serially assessing the risks of individual research procedures fails to take into account the possibility that "research may involve several different procedures that may involve minimal risk or burden individually, but that may present more than minimal risk when considered collectively."[4] One way to address this possibility would be to compare the cumulative risks of all the non-beneficial procedures or interventions in a given study to the cumulative level of risks that average, healthy children ordinarily encounter during a similar time span in daily life (see Table 49.3). To determine whether the cumulative risks of a protocol that lasts eight hours and requires one overnight stay qualify as minimal

under the risks of daily life definition, IRBs could assess whether these cumulative risks exceed the upper end of the range of cumulative risks that average, healthy children ordinarily encounter in approximately one day.

The upper end of the range of ordinary, daily cumulative risks in the United States might be defined by (1) one roundtrip car ride with risks at the upper end of the range of ordinary mortality risks, (2) one instance of bathing, and (3) one episode of playing on a playground for children birth–4 years old or one instance of playing basketball for children 5–19 years old. Adding these risks together implies that, with respect to cumulative mortality risks, research studies qualify as minimal risk when the mortality risks participants face per day of participation are not greater than approximately 1.5 in a million for children 1–14 years old and approximately 10 in a million for children 15–19 years old (see Table 49.3).

Implications of the Risk Data

Data reveal that the ordinary activities of daily life, which are the basis of many definitions of minimal risk, pose up to a 1 in 250 risk of injury and a 4 in a million risk of death to average, healthy children in the United States. These findings are surprising. They suggest that the risks of daily life definition of minimal risk has the potential to expose children to significantly greater risks than most IRBs assume are allowable, and greater risks than many

Table 49.3

Cumulative Risks in the Daily Lives of Average, Healthy Children[a]

Age	Risks per Million Children per Day				
	<1 yr	1–4 yrs	5–9 yrs	10–14 yrs	15–19 yrs
Deaths	0.5	1.5	1.4	1.4	10
Hospitalizations	0.0	1.3	1.7	2.1	6.0
Emergency room visits	0.4	16.4	26.0	36.1	64

[a]The cumulative risks healthy children face in an average day is calculated based on the risks of one "riskier" roundtrip in a car, one instance of bathing, and one instance of playing on a playground for children 1–4 years or participating in basketball for children 5–19 years.

commentators regard as acceptable.[19] These data reveal that, under the objective interpretation of the risks of daily life definition, research *procedures* that pose up to a 1 in 250 risk of injury qualify as minimal risk. Similarly, nonbeneficial research *studies* that pose up to a cumulative daily mortality risk of 1 in 100,000 for children 15–19 years old qualify as minimal risk under this interpretation.

Using Data to Apply the Minimal Risk Standard

Research procedures sometimes pose the same types of risks that children face in daily life, such as a risk of death, thus allowing IRBs to compare the two risks directly. To determine whether these procedures pose greater than minimal risk, IRBs can directly compare the likelihood that children will die from undergoing the procedure to the likelihood children will die as a result of the ordinary activities of daily life, such as riding in a car.

In other cases, research interventions pose different types of risks than do the activities of daily life. Pediatric research participants may face a risk of airway abrasion from bronchoscopy; daily life for average, healthy children involves essentially no risk of airway abrasion. Hence, direct comparison would suggest that bronchoscopy necessarily qualifies as greater than minimal risk, no matter how low the chance of abrasion and how minor the abrasion. This result seems counterintuitive. If techniques advance to the point at which bronchoscopy poses a 1 in a million risk of airway abrasion and no other risks, it would seem less risky than a car ride that poses a 1 in a million risk of death. To avoid this counterintuitive result, IRBs must assess whether the level of risks is comparable to or exceeds the level of risks children face in daily life.

Although comparing risks of different types is conceptually complex, parents make these assessments every day. To decide how their children get to school, parents assess whether, taking into account both likelihood and magnitude, the risk of skin abrasions and broken bones from riding a bicycle is more serious or worrisome than the risk of injury or death from riding the bus. Applying this approach to research interventions requires a method for comparing the seriousness of research risks to the seriousness of the risks of daily life.[46] This approach could be clarified by using a systematic method, such as the comparative analysis method described below, to implement the minimal risk standard.

The Magnitude of Harms and Seriousness of Risks

Risk represents the probability that an individual will experience a particular harm. The seriousness of a risk is a function of the magnitude of the possible harm, together with the likelihood of experiencing that harm. For example, the seriousness of the risk of breaking a bone while riding a bicycle depends on the magnitude of the possible break, and the likelihood that riding will lead to a broken bone.

Harms can be understood as experiences that set back an individual's interests: A broken bone sets back individuals' interest in normal physical functioning; pain sets back individuals' interest in avoiding unpleasant experiences.[47] The magnitude of a given harm is a function of the extent to which, taking into account both degree and duration, it sets back an individual's in-

terests. A cramp lasting a few minutes represents a minor setback to one's interests; amputation of a leg represents a severe setback.

The potential harms that children face in daily life can be categorized into at least five levels of magnitude, as presented in Table 49.4: (1) negligible harms involve minor and fleeting setbacks, such as mild, transitory pain—average, healthy children almost inevitably experience negligible harms as a result of the ordinary activities of daily life, such as playing sports; (2) minor harms involve setbacks of slightly greater degree or duration, such as mild pain that lasts a day, or moderate nausea that lasts a few hours—the symptoms associated with the common cold, such as mild fatigue and aches lasting a few days, represent a minor harm that average, healthy children may experience in daily life; (3) moderate harms involve setbacks of moderate degree or duration—bone fractures are a moderate harm that average, healthy children face from the activities of daily life, such as playing basketball; (4) severe harms involve setbacks whose degree or duration goes beyond moderate, such as permanent disability as the result of playing baseball; and (5) catastrophic harms involve complete setbacks to one's interests, such as death or complete paralysis. Although this typology focuses on physical risks, it could be extended to include the other types of risks that research poses to children, including social and psychological risks.

The comparative analysis method would apply this typology to determine whether a research procedure is minimal risk. There are several steps an IRB using this method would carry out: The IRB would first identify the potential harms of undergoing the intervention and categorize the harms by magnitude into one of the five levels. For example, the IRB might find that airway abrasion due to bronchoscopy qualifies as a mild or a moderate harm. Then, the IRB would determine the likelihood of experiencing the harm from the research procedure, such as the likelihood of airway

Table 49.4

Harms of Daily Life Stratified by Severity

Level	Examples	Likelihood Faced in Daily Life Activities
Negligible	1. Transient pain 2. Transient nausea 3. Transient anxiety 4. Bruising 5. Superficial lacerations	Essentially 100%
Minor	1. Sustained nausea 2. Headache for a day 3. Small scar 4. Temporary claustrophobia	About 30,000 per million[a]
Moderate	1. Wrist fracture 2. Laceration requiring sutures	About 200 per million[b]
Severe	1. Hearing loss 2. Pulmonary fibrosis 3. Kidney failure	About 60 per million[c]
Catastrophic	1. Death 2. Persistent vegetative state	About 1 per million[d]

[a]Child's daily risk of contracting the common cold, generally due to contact with others in school/day care and other routine activities.[62] [b]Risk of breaking a bone from playing soccer;[8] [c]Risk of injury leading to permanent disability from playing baseball.[8] [d]Risk of death from riding in the car.[8]

abrasion as a result of undergoing research bronchoscopy. To carry this analysis out, IRBs must have access to the available empirical data on the risks of the intervention under review. In the absence of published data, this approach may require investigators to collect data on clinicians' experience with the intervention. Next, the IRB would compare the likelihood of experiencing the harm due to the research intervention to the likelihood that average, healthy children will experience a harm of the same magnitude from the ordinary activities of daily life. For example, the likelihood of airway abrasion due to bronchoscopy would be compared to the likelihood of mild or moderate harm in daily life. If the likelihood of the research-related harm is greater, the procedure in question is greater than minimal risk; if not, the procedure qualifies as no greater than minimal risk. Because risk data represent uncertain point or range estimates, with accompanying confidence intervals, IRB members may have to use their judgment to determine whether two risk estimates are effectively equivalent. In cases of uncertainty, IRBs should err on the side of caution, categorizing interventions as greater than minimal risk.

Applying Comparative Analysis in Practice

Section 407 of the U.S. regulations allows the Secretary of the Department of Health and Human Services to approve pediatric studies that the reviewing IRB deems to have important value, but which pose risks too high for IRB approval.[48,49] As of August 2005, 17 research proposals had been submitted to the Office for Human Research Protections (OHRP) for consideration under these provisions.[50] To clarify the application of the comparative analysis method to research proposals, drawing on the real life examples provided by the protocols submitted for so-called 407 review, the following three cases demonstrate different circumstances in which the framework may need to be applied.

Case 1

The first study proposed to enroll healthy children aged 8–11. Although the study involved a number of procedures, concern focused on the intravenous glucose tolerance tests (IVGTTs), which the reviewing IRB judged to pose greater than minimal risk.

In theory, IVGTT poses several possible harms: bruising and infection at the IV site, nausea and potential hypoglycemia leading to lightheadedness, and/or syncope. Yet IRBs should not attempt to categorize research interventions based simply on the harms that in theory are possible. The fact that an intervention might pose a risk of death does not establish that in practice it poses that risk.

At the time, there were no data in the medical literature detailing the likelihood of any of these adverse effects from IVGTT in children. However, IVGTTs have been performed in thousands of healthy children. The Diabetes Prevention Trial has performed 7,903 IVGTTs at sites across North America. Of these, 4,372 were performed in individuals less than 15 years of age, and 3,531 were performed in individuals 15 years of age or older. No serious adverse events were reported for any of these tests.[51] Extra monitoring for adverse events in 1,333 of the tests found only two cases of suspected hypoglycemia, both of which resolved with food. At another site, an investigator reports conducting over 200

euglycemic-insulin clamp tests in children with no side effects.[52] A third site systematically assessed the risk of hypoglycemia from frequently sampled IVGTT in 210 overweight Hispanic children. Hypoglycemia (plasma glucose less than 50 mg/dl) occurred in one child, who did not experience any symptoms.[53]

This experience suggests IVGTT poses approximately a 1 in 3,000 risk of hypoglycemia, which resolves with food. Given the potential for greater than negligible reactions, hypoglycemia due to IVGTT might be categorized as a minor harm, worse than transient mild pain but not as bad as a bone fracture. Assuming that this is the only documented harm of IVGTT in the research setting, whether this procedure qualifies as minimal risk depends on whether the likelihood of this reaction exceeds the likelihood average, healthy children will experience a minor harm in daily life. The fact that the activities of daily life pose approximately a 30 per 1,000 chance of experiencing a minor harm suggests IVGTT poses no greater than minimal risk (see Table 49.1).

Case 2

A second study involved administration of a single 10 mg oral dose of dextroamphetamine to healthy children between the ages of 9 and 18. The IRB categorized this intervention as more than minimal risk because it might increase the chances that participants see drug use as nonhazardous, thus increasing participants' likelihood of future drug abuse. There are no data on the chances that a single 10 mg oral dose of dextroamphetamine will increase future drug abuse in a healthy child. In the absence of data, IRBs should make a more general comparison between the risks of the research procedure and the risks of daily life.

In the absence of empirical data, IRBs sometimes will be able to compare the chance of harm posed by the intervention to the chance that children will experience the same harm in daily life. For example, performance-enhancing and recreational use of other stimulants (especially caffeine) is widely promoted to children— for example, in sports drinks.[54] It seems unlikely that a single 10 mg oral dose of amphetamine in a research setting would validate stimulant use more than the messages children are exposed to in daily life. This suggests that the drug abuse potential, although it exists, does not exceed the risks of drug abuse that children face from the activities of daily life, such as watching television and reading advertisements. This analysis suggests the study poses no greater than minimal risk.

In other cases, research participation will present unknown risks that are unlike the risks children face in daily life. In these cases, IRBs might ask whether reasonable parents would be more concerned by the prospect of their children facing the risks of the research intervention or facing the risks of the same magnitude of harm in daily life. For example, assuming future drug abuse represents a severe harm, would a reasonable parent be more concerned about the risk of future drug abuse from one dose of dextroamphetamine, or the approximately 60 in a million risk of permanent disability associated with playing a game of baseball? (See Table 49.4.) If reasonable parents would be more concerned by the risk children face in daily life, or if they would be indifferent between the two risks, the research intervention qualifies as minimal risk. When it is unclear which option would more concern reasonable parents, IRBs should err on the side of caution and categorize the intervention as greater than minimal risk.

Case 3

A third study aimed to test the efficacy of diluted smallpox vaccine in 2- to 5-year-olds. The smallpox vaccine, Dryvax, has been used in the past, and data have been collected on adverse events associated with it. According to the manufacturer's package insert for the vaccine, many types of adverse events—ranging from widespread rashes to death—have been reported in children aged 1–4 and 5–19. One of these adverse events is generalized vaccinia, a disseminated rash that is usually self-limited, but which the investigators described as a major systemic reaction and stated would lead to hospitalization.[55] It seems, then, that generalized vaccinia could be classified as a moderate harm, worse than a common cold, but less severe than permanent disability due to a sports injury (see Table 49.4). According to the vaccine manufacturer, the rate of generalized vaccinia is 233 per million in 1- to 4-year-olds.[56] (Although a national study found much lower rates of generalized vaccinia, the methods of that study underreported many mild and moderate complications. The rates given in the package insert are based on smaller studies using survey methods that better capture these complications.) This is not effectively different from the approximately 200 per million rate of moderate harm children face in activities of daily life, making administration of this vaccine minimal risk.

These three examples demonstrate the application of comparative analysis, a systematic method for implementing the risks of daily life definition of minimal risk, in a variety of situations. Analysis of the risk level of research interventions is most straightforward when empirical data on risks have been collected and are available, as in the example of the smallpox vaccine trial. When data on the risks of a research intervention have not been previously published, as in the IVGTT example, prior clinical and research experience with the procedure can still provide useful information. Even when empirical data on a research risk are completely unavailable, as in the case of the dextroamphetamine study, a systematic method for applying the risks of daily life standard can still help clarify the categorization of an intervention as minimal risk or greater than minimal risk.

Policy Alternatives to the Risks of Daily Life Standard

Research regulations include multiple safeguards to protect pediatric research participants from excessive risks. IRBs may reject individual research procedures, parents may decline to enroll their children in research, even when it satisfies the minimal risk standard, and children deemed capable of providing assent may refuse to participate in research that does not offer them a compensating prospect of benefit. Granting the importance of IRB, parental, and participant judgment, society has an independent obligation to ensure that medical advances are not won at the cost of exploiting pediatric research participants. To discharge this obligation, society must establish a sound standard for determining what constitutes minimal risk in the context of nonbeneficial pediatric research.

The data on the risks that children in the United States face in daily life and the research risks that IRBs in practice classify as greater than minimal risk suggest that the risks of daily life defi-

nition of minimal risk may be inappropriate. In light of the findings that the current definition categorizes as minimal risk research procedures that pose a 1 in 250 chance of injury to children, and that IRBs seem in practice to be more conservative than this, it may be that the current minimal risk standard allows excessive risks in some cases. These findings should be regarded as providing context for a discussion about what levels of risk without direct clinical benefits to participants are ethically acceptable in pediatric research, and what policy standard might ensure that the risks of pediatric research do not exceed this level. Some possible alternatives to the risks of daily life standard are described below to provide context for this discussion.

The *Reasonable Parent* Standard

The risks children are actually exposed to may be an inappropriate standard for determining the risks children should be exposed to in research. Some of the risks children currently face may be at socially unacceptable levels, or children may be exposed to certain risks only because parents and others are unaware of the dangers. To address these concerns, some commentators have endorsed defining minimal risk in terms of those risks that a "reasonable" parent would intentionally expose their children to.[5,57] Ross and Nelson state this definition of minimal risk as follows: "The probability and magnitude of physical or psychological harm is no more than that to which it is appropriate for a scrupulous parent to intentionally expose a child for educational purposes in family life situations."[57] This definition is useful in that it specifies a perspective from which investigators and IRBs ought to approach risk thresholds in pediatric research. In particular, it specifies that the nature and purpose of a minimal risk threshold should be to allow only research that scrupulous parents could reasonably enroll their children in. However, it leaves open the question of the standard by which a hypothetical parent qualifies as "scrupulous." Hence, this definition requires further interpretation before it can be implemented.

The *Routine Examinations* Standard

The present data reveal that the risks children face from the activities of daily life are much greater than the risks they face from routine examinations and tests. With this in mind, one might try to limit the risks allowed by the minimal risk standard by defining minimal risk based solely on the risks of "routine physical or psychological examinations or tests."[58,59] Some existing guidelines take this approach; the CIOMS guidelines stipulate that children and other vulnerable groups should be subject to nonbeneficial research procedures only when the risks do not exceed "those associated with routine medical and psychological examinations of such persons."[25]

The risks of routine examinations are justified by the potential benefit to the children who undergo them. Hence, it is not clear why this standard might be appropriate for assessing the risks of research that does not offer participants a prospect of clinical benefit. Recognizing this theoretical concern, what level of risks would this standard allow in practice?

The *Bright Futures* health guidelines, endorsed by the American Academy of Pediatrics, recommend that healthy children be assessed for height, weight, head circumference, vision, and hearing.[60] The only invasive examination recommended for healthy children is a single heel stick at birth to screen for metabolic disorders. Whether infants receive even a single blood draw for lead analysis depends on whether their exposure is deemed greater than normal. Thus, in practice, the routine examinations standard would be extremely restrictive, categorizing all procedures beyond a single heel stick as greater than minimal risk.

The *De Minimis* Standard

Psychologically, reasonable individuals often ignore the risks of daily life—those we assume by living, moving around, and going about our daily routine—when the risks are sufficiently low. This practice suggests that it may be acceptable to expose children to research risks provided they do not exceed the negligible risks we ignore in our daily lives.[1,6] This de minimis standard differs from the current risks of daily life standard because we ignore some risks of daily life, but not others. Parents typically ignore the risks involved in taking their child for a ride in the car; they often are painfully aware of the risks their children face while playing football.

Individuals tend to be less willing to accept risks that are explicitly brought to their attention, such as research risks outlined in a protocol or consent form. Future assessment of the de minimis standard should assess the ethical significance of this difference in our attitudes toward risks depending on our awareness of them. If explicitly stating a risk on a consent form alters an individual's ability to ignore or accept it, is this difference purely psychological or is it relevant to an ethical assessment of the risk in question?

The *Community Risk* Standard

Reasonable parents routinely expose their children to a risk of death on car trips to benefit their parents, siblings, and neighbors. Society accepts and even endorses this practice, provided the risks are not too great, because children derive important benefit from being part of a healthy and caring family. Children similarly gain tremendous benefits from living in a society that provides access to health care, clean water, and safe and effective medications and vaccines. One might argue that a price of living in such a society is that children are sometimes exposed to research risks for the benefit of other society members. Provided the risks are not too great, and the research is important, this practice seems acceptable in the same way that it is acceptable to expose children to risks for the benefit of others in family life.

Future research on the community risk standard should assess whether it is acceptable to expose pediatric research participants to the same, or somewhat lower, levels of risk compared to the risks children may be exposed to in the context of family life. May children be exposed to the same level of risks in order to benefit unrelated others as they are to benefit siblings and neighbors? Or should the risk threshold in the context of research be somewhat lower than it is in family and community life?

The *Charitable Participation* Standard

Many of the risks of daily life are deemed acceptable because the attendant activities offer children the potential for personal benefit. Parents allow their children to play basketball not because they consider the risks inherently acceptable, but because children are thought to benefit directly from participation in team sports. In contrast, nonbeneficial research, by definition, does not offer participants a compensating potential for direct benefit. Its risks are justified by the potential to benefit others. Viewed in this way, nonbeneficial pediatric research involves a kind of charitable activity, exposing children to risks for the benefit of unrelated others.

This comparison suggests that it may make sense to develop a minimal risk standard based on risks to which children may be exposed in daily life for the benefit of others. Specifically, are the research risks greater than the level of risk society deems acceptable for children in the context of activities that benefit unrelated others? Many widely respected organizations, including the Red Cross and Habitat for Humanity, have established charitable programs for children.[61] And parents often instruct their children to engage in activities that pose some risks to them for the benefit of others, such as shoveling the sidewalks and mowing the lawns of infirm neighbors.

Future research on the charitable participation standard should assess the appropriateness of the analogy between nonbeneficial research and charitable activities that society deems acceptable for children. Are these activities sufficiently similar that the risks of the latter provide a useful guide for assessing the ethical acceptability of the risks of the former? Or are there important differences between the two activities that undermine this approach?

Conclusion

Although it is understandably troubling to expose children, who cannot provide informed consent, to research risks without a compensating prospect of clinical benefit, almost all countries and international bodies recognize that such research is essential to provide children as a group with appropriate medical treatment. Guidelines have been written to ensure that the risks children face in research are not excessive, often relying on the concept of minimal risk to provide the threshold for acceptable risks in pediatric research that does not offer participants direct clinical benefits.

Minimal risk, in turn, has generally been defined in terms of the risks children face in daily life. The widely endorsed objective interpretation of this definition holds that minimal risks are those that do not exceed the level of risks that average, healthy children ordinarily face in daily life. Implementation of the minimal risk standard, however, may not consistently conform with this definition. IRBs must often implement the minimal risk standard without concrete data on either the risks of research procedures or the risks children face in daily life.

Data exist that can be used to estimate the level of risks children face in daily life. Systematically implementing the risks of daily life definition of minimal risk requires IRBs to identify risks of harm posed by research procedures, determine their magnitude and likelihood as specifically as possible, and compare these to the magnitude and likelihood of potential harm posed by activities of daily life. Assessment of research risks under this definition is clearest when empirical data on the risks of research procedures and risks of daily life are available and used, though the general framework still applies in the absence of data.

Analysis of IRB chairs' classification of research procedures suggests that IRBs may frequently classify as greater than minimal risk procedures that in fact are not riskier than the activities of daily life. This could be due simply to the frequent lack of empirical data available to IRBs and to the fact that data indicate the risks of daily life are higher than many assume. But it may also point to a conceptual error in using the risks of daily life to define minimal risk. Several other standards have been proposed, and it may be that one of these would better capture when exposing children to risk is ethically acceptable, or would better ensure that pediatric research is not excessively risky.

Disclaimer

The opinions expressed are the authors' own. They do not reflect any position or policy of the National Institutes of Health, Public Health Service, or Department of Health and Human Services.

References

1. King NMP. Defining and describing benefit appropriately in clinical trials. *Journal of Law, Medicine, and Ethics* 2000;28:332–43.
2. Department of Health and Human Services, Office for Health Research Protections. *Protecting Human Research Subjects: Institutional Review Board Guidebook*. Rockville, Md.: OHRP; 1993:3–8. [Online] Available: http://www.hhs.gov/ohrp/irb/irb_guidebook.htm.
3. May W. Experimenting on human subjects. *Linacre Quarterly* 1976;43:73–84.
4. Bartholome W. The ethics of non-therapeutic clinical research on children. In: National Commission for the Protection of Human Subjects of Biomedical and Behavioral Research. *Appendix to Report and Recommendations: Research Involving Children*. Washington, D.C.: U.S. Government Printing Office; 1977:3.1–3.22.
5. Ackerman TF. Moral duties of parents and nontherapeutic clinical research procedures involving children. *Bioethics Quarterly* 1980;2:94–111.
6. Kopelman L. When is the risk minimal enough for children to be research subjects? In: Kopelman LM, Moskop JC, eds. *Children and Health Care: Moral and Social Issues*. Boston, Mass.: Kluwer; 1989: 89–99.
7. Koocher GP, Keith-Spiegel P. Scientific issues in psychosocial and educational research with children. In: Grodin MA, Glantz LH, eds. *Children as Research Subjects: Science, Ethics and Law*. New York, N.Y.: Oxford University Press; 1994:47–80.
8. Brock DW. Ethical issues in exposing children to risks in research. In: Grodin MA, Glantz LH, eds. *Children as Research Subjects: Science, Ethics and Law*. New York, N.Y.: Oxford University Press; 1994: 81–101.
9. Ackerman TF. Nontherapeutic research procedures involving children with cancer. *Journal of Pediatric Oncology Nursing* 1994;11: 134–6.
10. McCormick RA. Proxy consent in the experimental situation. *Perspectives in Biology and Medicine* 1974;18:2–20.
11. McCormick RA. Experimentation in children: Sharing in sociality. *Hastings Center Report* 1976;6(6):41–6.
12. Ramsey P. The enforcement of morals: Nontherapeutic research on children: A reply to Richard McCormick. *Hastings Center Report* 1976;6(4):21–30.
13. Ramsey P. Children as research subjects: A reply. *Hastings Center Report* 1977;7(2):40–2.
14. 1931 German Guidelines on human experimentation (Circular of the Reich Minister of the Interior. Guidelines for New Therapy and Human Experimentation; Feb. 28, 1931). *International Digest of Health Legislation* 1980;31:408–11.
15. The Nuremberg Code. In: *Trials of War Criminals Before the Nuremberg Military Tribunals Under Control Council Law No. 10, Volume 2*. Washington, D.C.: U.S. Government Printing Office; 1949:181–2. [Online]. Available: http://www.hhs.gov/ohrp/references/nurcode .htm.
16. Caldwell PHY, Murphy SB, Butow PH, Craig JC. Clinical trials in children. *Lancet* 2004;364:803–11.
17. Office of Public Health and Science, Food and Drug Administration, Department of Health and Human Services. Solicitation of Public Review and Comment on Research Protocol: A Multicenter, Randomized Dose Response Study of the Safety, Clinical and Immune Response of Dryvax Administered to Children 2 to 5 Years of Age; Notice. *Federal Register* 2002;67(211):66403–4.
18. Roberts R, Rodriquez W, Murphy D, Crescenzi T. Pediatric drug labeling: Improving the safety and efficacy of pediatric therapies. *JAMA* 2003;290:905–11.
19. Institute of Medicine. *Ethical Conduct of Clinical Research Involving Children*. Washington, D.C.: National Academies Press; 2004.
20. Kauffman RE. Clinical trials in children. *Paediatric Drugs* 2000; 2:411–8.
21. Indian Council on Medical Research. *Ethical Guidelines for Biomedical Research on Human Subjects*. New Delhi, India: Indian Council on Medical Research; 2000. [Online] Available: http://icmr.nic.in/ ethical.pdf.
22. Nepal Health Research Council. *National Ethical Guidelines for Health Research in Nepal*. 2001. Kathmandu, Nepal: Nepal Health Research Council; 2001. [Online] Available: http://www.nhrc.org.np/ guidelines/nhrc_ethicalguidelines_2001.pdf.
23. Uganda National Council of Science and Technology (UNCST). *Guidelines for the Conduct of Health Research Involving Human Subjects in Uganda*. Kampala, Uganda: UNCST; 1998.
24. Council of Europe. *Convention for the Protection of Human Rights and Dignity of the Human Being With Regard to the Application of Biology and Medicine: Convention on Human Rights and Biomedicine*. [Online] 4 April 1997. Available: http://conventions.coe.int/treaty/en/ treaties/html/164.htm.
25. Council for International Organizations of Medical Sciences, in collaboration with the World Health Organization. *International Ethical Guidelines for Biomedical Research Involving Human Subjects*. Geneva, Switzerland: CIOMS and WHO; 2002: Commentary on Guideline 13. [Online] November 2002. Available: http://www.cioms.ch/frame _guidelines_nov_2002.htm.
26. Department of Health and Human Services, National Institutes of Health, and Office for Human Research Protections. The Common Rule, Title 45 (Public Welfare), Code of Federal Regulations, Part 46 (Protection of Human Subjects). [Online] June 23, 2005. Available: http://www.hhs.gov/ohrp/humansubjects/guidance/ 45cfr46.htm.
27. Australian Health Ethics Committee *National Statement on Ethical Conduct on Research Involving Humans*. *[Online]* 1999. Available: http://www.nhmrc.gov.au/ethics/human/conduct/guidelines/ index.htm.
28. Canadian Institutes of Health Research, the Natural Sciences and Engineering Research Council, and the Social Sciences and Humanities Research Council. *Tri-Council Policy Statement: Ethical Conduct for Research Involving Humans*. [Online] 1998 (with 2000, 2002, and 2005 amendments). Available: http://www.pre.ethics.gc.ca/ english/policystatement/policystatement.cfm.
29. South African Medical Research Council. *Guidelines on Ethics for Medical Research: General Principles*. [Online] Available: http://www .sahealthinfo.org/ethics/ethicsbook1.pdf.
30. National Commission for the Protection of Human Subjects of Biomedical and Behavioral Research. *Report and Recommendations: Research Involving Children*. Washington, D.C.: U.S. Government Printing

Office; 1977. [Online] Available: http://www.bioethics.gov/reports/past_commissions/Research_involving_children.pdf.

31. National Human Research Protections Advisory Committee. *Report From NHRPAC: Clarifying Specific Portion of 45 CFR 46 Subpart D That Governs Children's Research.* [Online] 2002. Available: http://ctep.cancer.gov/forms/nhrpac16.pdf.

32. Shah S, et al. How do institutional review boards apply the federal risk and benefit standards for pediatric research? *JAMA* 2004; 291:476–82.

33. Tversky A, Kahneman D. The framing of decisions and the rationality of choice. *Science* 1981;211:453–8.

34. Slovic P. Perception of risk. *Science* 1987;236:280–5.

35. Weinstein N. Optimistic biases about personal risks. *Science* 1989;246:1232–3.

36. Sandman PM. Responding to Community Outrage: Strategies for Effective Risk Communication. Fairfax, Va.: American Industrial Hygiene Association; 1993.

37. Tversky A, Kahneman D. Judgments under uncertainty: Heuristics and biases. *Science* 1974;185:1124–31.

38. National Center for Injury Prevention and Control, Centers for Disease Control and Prevention. Web-Based Injury Statistics Query and Reporting System (WISQARS™). [Online] Available: http://www.cdc.gov/ncipc/wisqars/.

39. National Center for Statistics and Analysis, National Highway Traffic Safety Administration, Department of Transportation. *Traffic Safety Facts: 2003 Data—Young Drivers.* Washington, D.C.: Department of Transportation; 2003. [Online] Available: http://www-nrd.nhtsa.dot.gov/pdf/nrd-30/NCSA/TSF2003/809774.pdf.

40. National Center for Statistics and Analysis, National Highway Traffic Safety Administration, Department of Transportation. *Traffic Safety Facts 2002: A Compilation of Motor Vehicle Crash Data From the Fatality Analysis Reporting System and the General Estimates System.* Washington, D.C.: Department of Transportation; 2004. [Online] January, 2004. Available: http://www-nrd.nhtsa.dot.gov/pdf/nrd-30/NCSA/TSFAnn/TSF2002Final.pdf.

41. American Sports Data, Inc. *A Comprehensive Study of Sports Injuries in the U.S.* Hartsdale, N.Y.: American Sports Data, Inc.; 2002. [Online] Available: http://www.americansportsdata.com/sports_injury1.asp.

42. Varni JW, Burwinkle TM, Seid M, Skarr D. The PedsQL™ 4.0 as a pediatric population health measure: Feasibility, reliability, and validity. *Ambulatory Pediatrics* 2003;3:329–41.

43. Galena HJ. Complications occurring during diagnostic venipuncture. *Journal of Family Practice* 1992;34:582–4.

44. Trouern-Trend JJ, Cable RG, Badon SJ, Newman GH, Popovsky MA. A case-controlled study of vasovagal reactions in blood donors. *Transfusion* 1999;39:316–20.

45. Turkeltaub PC, Gergen PJ. The risk of adverse reactions from percutaneous prick-puncture allergen skin testing, venipuncture, and body measurements: Data from the second National Health and Nutrition Examination Survey 1976–80 (NHANES II). *Journal of Allergy and Clinical Immunology* 1989;84:886–90.

46. Nicholson RH. *Medical Research With Children.* New York, N.Y.: Oxford University Press; 1986:40–60.

47. Feinberg J. *Harm to Others: The Moral Limits of the Criminal Law, Vol. 1.* New York, N.Y.: Oxford University Press; 1984: chapter 1.

48. Department of Health and Human Services, National Institutes of Health, and Office for Human Research Protections. The Common Rule, Title 45 (Public Welfare), Code of Federal Regulations, Part 46 (Protection of Human Subjects), Subpart D. [Online] June 23, 2005. Available: http://www.hhs.gov/ohrp/humansubjects/guidance/45cfr46.htm#subpartd.

49. Ross LF. Convening a 407 panel for research not otherwise approvable: "Precursors to diabetes in Japanese American youth" as a case study. *Kennedy Institute of Ethics Journal* 2004;14:165–86.

50. Kevin Prohaska, Office of Human Research Protections, personal communication.

51. Jay Skyler, personal communication.

52. Silva Arslanian, personal communication.

53. Cruz ML, Weigensberg MJ, Bergman RN, Goran MI. Frequently sampled IV glucose tolerance test in overweight Hispanic children and risk of hypoglycemia. Unpublished manuscript.

54. Wilson D. A sports drink for children is jangling some nerves. *New York Times* September 25, 2005:A1.

55. Centers for Disease Control and Prevention. Adverse reactions following smallpox vaccination. Smallpox Fact Sheet—Information for Clinicians. [Online] 2004. Available: http://www.bt.cdc.gov/agent/smallpox/vaccination/reactions-vacc-clinic.asp.

56. Wyeth Laboratories Inc. Smallpox Vaccine: Dryvax. 1989. Package insert.

57. Nelson RM, Ross LF. In defense of a single standard of research risk for all children. *Journal of Pediatrics* 2005;147:565–6.

58. Kopelman LM. Minimal risk as an international ethical standard in research. *Journal of Medicine and Philosophy* 2004;29:351–78.

59. Resnik DB. Eliminating the daily risks standard from the definition of minimal risk. *Journal of Medical Ethics* 2005;31:35–8.

60. Green M, Palfrey JS, eds. *Bright Futures: Guidelines for Health Supervision of Infants, Children, and Adolescents,* 2nd ed., rev. Arlington, Va.: National Center for Education in Maternal and Child Health. [Online] 2002. Available: http://brightfutures.aap.org/web/healthCareProfessionalstoolsAndResources.asp.

61. Habitat for Humanity. Campus Chapters and Youth Programs. [Online] Available: http://www.habitat.org/ccyp/youth_programs/default.aspx.

62. National Institute of Allergy and Infectious Disease, National Institutes of Health. *The Common Cold, NIAID Fact Sheets.* Bethesda, Md.: NIAID; 2004.

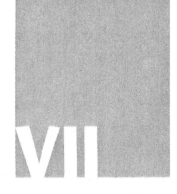

VII

Independent Review and Oversight

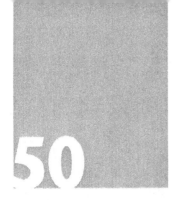

Charles R. McCarthy

The Origins and Policies That Govern Institutional Review Boards

Major turning points in history are often recognized only in hindsight. One example of a significant historical change that went almost unnoticed at the time is the statement made by James A. Shannon, director of the National Institutes of Health (NIH), before the National Advisory Health Council (NAHC) on September 28, 1965.

The NAHC had been created in 1930 to deal with a budget crisis faced by what was then a single, small federal agency called the National Institute of Health. Senator Joseph Randell, backed by Surgeon General Lewis R. Thompson, introduced sweeping legislation to authorize the National Institute of Health to carry out research that would address "all the ills that flesh is heir to." In direct contrast, Senator Joseph M. Neely proposed sharply focused legislation to direct the spending of all federal medical research dollars onto a single program to overcome cancer in all its many forms.[1]

The Randell bill was modified and enacted. It is now compacted into Section 301 of the Public Health Service Act as amended.[2] It grants the NIH authority to fund research into virtually any area that may be associated with human health or disease. Although the Neely bill failed in 1930, the concept of a concentrated research effort directed or targeted at one or several diseases remained alive in the Congress, and in the public mind. In succeeding decades, the Congress has enacted legislation targeted at virtually all major diseases and conditions—judged in terms of their impact on society as measured by morbidity and mortality. The plethora of institutes that make up the NIH, each dedicated to one or several diseases or disease clusters, is due in part to the concept of targeted research articulated by Neely. In 1930 the contest between those who supported the Randell con-

cept, which came to be known as *investigator-initiated research,* based on perceived scientific opportunities, and those who supported *targeted research* directed at public need as measured by morbidity and mortality data, created a tension that continues to the present time. In 1930 the debate threatened to stalemate the budget process and jeopardize the fragile existence of the NIH.

Congress addressed the Randell-Neely tension by a procedural compromise. It recommended creation of the NAHC—a standing committee of nonfederal advisers to establish or approve policies for both the surgeon general of the Public Health Service (PHS) and the director of the NIH (the research arm of the PHS) on a broad range of issues. As far back as 1902, the NIH had utilized ad hoc public advisory committees. But the creation of the NAHC marked the beginning of ongoing participation by nongovernment advisers in the formulation of national health research policies. The NAHC eventually evolved into a two-tiered peer review system consisting of initial review groups (IRGs—often called *study sections*) charged with assigning priority scores based on the perceived scientific merit of grant applications, and national advisory councils or boards to pass judgment on proposed research in the light of its expected social utility.[1]

When Shannon testified in September 1965, he brought to the attention of the NAHC a complex long-standing problem of medical ethics that had not previously been addressed at a policy level by any federal agency. Fragmentary stenographic notes of the NAHC meeting attribute the following statement to him:

> [R]esearch involving [humans] departs from the conventional patient-physician relationship where the patient's good has been substituted for by the need to develop new

knowledge. . . . [The] physician is no longer in the same relationship that he is in the conventional medical setting and indeed may not be in a position to develop a purely or wholly objective assessment of the . . . ethical act which he proposes to perform. [The PHS has] a dual responsibility. One is a minor one of keeping the Government out of trouble . . . but really the major one is . . . to try to encourage the flourishing of sound clinical investigation rather than discouraging it. I am searching for some way of creating a more profound sense of an institutional awareness of the importance of this aspect of the problem without tying [investigators] down and immobilizing them in their capabilities.[3]

Shannon was seeking a policy applicable to all research involving human subjects funded by the NIH. He wanted the policy to contrast and distinguish the relationship between research investigators and their subjects from the relationship between physicians and their patients. He identified several interrelated questions, which he put to the NAHC. First, how could the NIH make physicians aware that when they are functioning as research investigators, their responsibilities to subjects differ from their responsibilities to patients? Second, how could the ethics of research be incorporated into a workable public policy that would both protect the NIH from public criticism and protect subjects from physical or moral harms, without unduly restricting investigators?

Shannon knew that medical schools and science programs of his day provided little formal training in medical ethics.[4] The dictum *Primum non nocere* ("First, do no harm") and the Hippocratic tradition of respecting the privacy of patients were conveyed by way of mentors, role models, and institutional traditions. Ethical guidance pertaining to the conduct of research involving human subjects was virtually unmentioned in the training given to medical students. At the time that Shannon met with the NAHC, responsibility for the ethical conduct of medical research was left to the untutored consciences of physician/investigators who had little formal training in ethics and whose behavior was shaped and guided by the social customs of the time. Albert Jonsen, for example, describes the ethics training in the following words:

For doctors, medical ethics was incarnate in their behavior and social character and in the social arrangements that sustained the solidarity, respectability, and educated competence of the profession. There were ethical battles to be fought such as those against quackery, but there were few ethical dilemmas about the doctor's duties.[4]

Shannon presented to the NAHC a draft resolution that recommended that the protocol design of an investigator proposing to conduct research involving humans be submitted to the judgment of "peers" to provide an independent determination of the risks and expected benefits of research, and to assure maximum protection for the rights and welfare of those enrolled in each study.

The 1965 NAHC meeting marks the first time that what was later termed the *therapeutic misconception*—confusion of the investigator/subject relationship with the physician/patient relationship—was addressed at the level of national policy. Perhaps even more startling is the fact that Shannon recommended that nonfederal advisers—Shannon called them *"peer reviewers,"*

but that terminology was soon discarded because the reviewers were not, strictly speaking, peers of the investigator—should exercise ethical oversight of federally funded research involving humans.

The policy that Shannon recommended was borrowed in part from a policy pertaining to normal research volunteers that had been implemented in 1953 when the NIH Clinical Center opened its doors. Shannon recognized, of course, that the review of protocols for scientific merit was already an established practice at the federal level. The new policy called for review of protocols for ethical integrity to be conducted at the local level by panels composed of both experts and nonexperts at the site where the research was to be conducted.

By calling for review by impartial observers, Shannon was reversing two traditions that had been in place at the NIH for more than 25 years. The first tradition held that the physician in charge of the research is the best qualified person to make the judgment of what is in the best interests of research subjects. The second held that nonscientists, that is, *laypersons,* were not qualified to pass judgment on the ethical aspects of medical research. To understand the dramatic difference between what Shannon was proposing and the prevailing practices and attitudes of the time, we need to consider a few historical facts.

David Rothman tells us the following:

Until World War II, the research enterprise was typically small-scale and intimate, guided by an ethic consistent with community expectations. Most research was a cottage industry: a few physicians, working alone, carried out experiments on themselves, their families, and their immediate neighbors. Moreover, the research was almost always therapeutic in intent, that is, the subjects stood to benefit directly if experiments were successful. Under these circumstances the ethics of human investigation did not command much attention.[5]

Rothman acknowledges that there were some notable exceptions to the state of affairs described above. What he fails to emphasize is that in the period leading up to World War II the NIH extramural programs, though small by today's standards, were gradually expanding. Many NIH research scientists, whether intramural or extramural, were not conducting innovative therapy intended to benefit their families, their patients, or their neighbors. They were conducting more fundamental research intended to explore the causes of disease, the workings and interrelationships of complex organ systems, and distinctions between normal and abnormal bodily functions. Therapeutic benefit was seldom a characteristic of such research projects.

In addition to the changes in the kinds of research projects that were pursued, changes on the issue of informed consent also emerged after World War II. Prior to this time, although a few research investigators sought informed consent from subjects, most investigators gave little if any information to their subjects concerning the purposes and risks associated with research studies. Concern for the rights and welfare of research subjects was left in the hand, or more precisely, in the conscience of the research investigator. Although a handful of investigators recognized and respected the rights of research subjects, a majority of investigators were unaware of these rights and saw little difference in ethical responsibility between functioning as a physician and functioning as a research investigator.[6]

Ruth Faden and Tom Beauchamp note the following:

"Informed consent" first appeared as an issue in American medicine in the late 1950s and early 1960s. Prior to this period, we have not been able to locate a single substantial discussion in the medical literature of consent and patient authorization. For example, from 1930 to 1956 we were able to find only nine articles published on issues of consent in American medical literature.[7]

After World War II, as Rothman notes, there was a fundamental change in medical ethics and its importance. He dates the change a little earlier than do Faden and Beauchamp, but both sources agree that a national awakening to ethical concerns in research, particularly the issue of informed consent, came after World War II. According to Rothman,

The transforming event in the conduct of human experimentation in the United States, the moment when it lost its intimate and directly therapeutic character, was World War II. Between 1941 and 1945 practically every aspect of American research with human subjects changed.[5]

Faden and Beauchamp date the transformation later than does Rothman. They write,

Shortly after the middle of the twentieth century a major transformation occurred. The influential forces and documents in ethics and policy began to take on *external* roots. Sometimes these external influences were greeted as an unwanted alien force on medicine; but in other quarters of medicine they were greeted with open admiration.[7]

It was against this changing backdrop—changes both in kinds of research projects and in the appreciation of ethical issues in medical research—that the new NIH Clinical Center commenced functioning in 1953. At that time, most NIH investigators conducting research involving humans still thought of themselves as medical practitioners. Clinical Center officials argued that it would be an unjustified intrusion into the doctor-patient relationship to allow any administrative body to interfere with the relationship between physician/investigators and their research subjects/patients.[3] Nevertheless, even those who held this view recognized that this argument could not be made with respect to *normal volunteers*—that is, healthy people who volunteered to serve as research subjects.

During World War II, it was customary for the NIH to enlist conscientious objectors to serve as normal controls in medical research. Many investigators regarded conscientious objectors as being equivalent to military draftees. Were it not for conscientious objection to war, these investigators reasoned, such persons would have been serving in the military anyway. And this view had implications for how investigators thought of research volunteers. As Rothman notes,

Researchers [believed that they] were no more obliged to obtain the permission of their subjects than the selective service was to obtain the permission of civilians to become soldiers. One part of the war machine conscripted a soldier, another part conscripted an experimental subject, and the same principles held for both.[5]

Long after the war ended, this attitude on the part of principal investigators persisted. Reasons why it continued are not hard to find. In 1941, President Franklin D. Roosevelt established the Office of Scientific Research and Development (OSRD) to conduct research to address a wide variety of health issues occasioned by or pertinent to the war. OSRD in turn created the Committee on Medical Research (CMR), which selected some 600 medical research projects to be conducted at 135 institutions across the country. After the war, in a political coup that catapulted the NIH to the forefront of domestic agencies, the research portfolio of the OSRD was transferred in its entirety to the NIH. In some cases, OSRD investigators also moved to the NIH to continue their work in the intramural program. Others moved to institutions in which CMR-initiated research was now conducted with NIH funds. NIH administrators admired the accomplishments of CMR during the war, and they admired the energetic and efficient manner in which the research results were obtained, published, and applied. Many NIH administrators adopted the aggressive "can do" CMR attitude. They believed that the CMR approach to research served the country well during the war, and they were eager to use the same techniques in peacetime.

The Growth of the NIH

From 1944 until 1958, federally funded medical research expanded at a furious rate. A health lobby headed by Mary Lasker and sympathetic heads of important Senate and House Appropriation Committees (Senator Lister Hill and Representative John Fogarty), produced an ever-increasing flow of research dollars. The NIH budget rose from less than $1 million in 1944 to nearly $1 billion by the end of the 1950s. In some years, the NIH research budget increased by as much as 100% over the previous year. Frankel says that prior to World War II, medicine was viewed as the art of healing the sick and comforting the dying; after the war, medicine was viewed as the conquering of diseases and the promotion of health.[3]

In the face of unprecedented expansion of the medical research budget during the 1950s, NIH staff persons were preoccupied with locating and training research investigators to conduct research. The NIH Clinical Center operated a two-year program of training for research fellows, whose time at the NIH counted as military service, exempting them from the draft. The "doctor draft" provided training for hundreds of physician/investigators who formed the backbone of the expanding research effort throughout the country. The NIH fellowship program was supplemented by research training grants (made mostly to Ph.D. scientists) developed to match the supply of investigators to the increasing torrent of research dollars. Although training grants offered sophisticated scientific mentorship to new investigators, they provided virtually no education in research ethics.

A notable exception to the lack of research ethics policy occurred in the NIH intramural research program shortly after the Clinical Center opened in 1953. Following World War II, normal volunteers for intramural research at the NIH were recruited from small colleges located in the nearby District of Columbia, Maryland, and Virginia. Only persons judged to be in good health were accepted as normal volunteers. Exposing healthy volunteers to risks from research interventions designed to develop knowledge pertaining to conditions and diseases the volunteers did not have was a major departure from acceptable medical practice. The practice of using normal volunteers was patently inconsistent with the

Table 50.1
Development of Federal Protections for Human Subjects of Research

Date	Event
1798	U.S. Congress creates the Marine Hospital Service for sick and disabled seamen. Signed into law by President John Adams.
1887	Congress authorizes the conduct of medical research at the Marine Hospital. This one-room laboratory, directed by Joseph Kinyoun, will evolve into the National Institutes of Health (NIH).
1902	The Marine Hospital Laboratory is redesignated as the Public Health and Marine Hospital Service, which is reorganized into the Public Health Service (PHS) 10 years later.
1918	Chamberlain-Kahn Act expands the size of the PHS, directs it to study venereal diseases, and creates a commissioned corps under the direction of a surgeon general empowered to make grants-in-aid of research. Twenty-five institutions receive the first grants-in-aid.
1930	Congress gives the NIH broad authority and creates the National Advisory Health Council (NAHC) to advise the surgeon general on grants-in-aid (including contracts), considering both scientific opportunities and the social utility of research.
1942–45	Conscientious objectors who are exempted from the draft in World War II are required to serve as healthy "volunteers" for research at the NIH and awardee institutions.
1953	NIH opens the Clinical Center, later called the Warren G. Magnuson Clinical Center, the largest and most advanced biomedical research center in the world. The Clinical Center issues the first public policy for the protection of human research subjects, entitled *Group Consideration of Clinical Research Procedures Deviating From Accepted Medical Practice or Involving Unusual Hazards,* and requires peer oversight of research involving healthy volunteers. Philippe Cardon, deputy director of the NIH Clinical Center, is careful to explain the risk of the research and to elicit volunteers' informed consent. Although patient/subjects are often at much higher levels of risk than healthy volunteers, the oversight policy extends only to healthy volunteers.
1954–58	Saul Krugman conducts hepatitis studies in the Willowbrook State School for severely retarded children (see Chapter 7).
1956	Chester M. Southam and Emanuel Mandel conduct experiments at the Jewish Chronic Disease Hospital, injecting live cancer cells into elderly, indigent subjects without review of the research or consent from the subjects (see Chapter 6).
1959	Senator Estes Kefauver initiates hearings on the cost of products regulated by the FDA. In 1961, following reports of the thalidomide disaster in Europe and Canada, the hearings focus on protection of human subjects involved in testing of FDA-regulated products.
1961	Congress enacts the Kefauver-Harris amendments to the Food, Drug and Cosmetic Act, including a requirement for informed consent of subjects involved in the testing of FDA-regulated products.
1960–63	A three-year study by the Boston University Law-Medicine Research Institute concludes that only 16 PHS awardee institutions have policies for the protection of the rights and welfare of human research subjects, and in no case is an institutional policy satisfactory.
1963	NIH Director James Shannon creates the Robert B. Livingstone Committee to evaluate practices in institutions funded by the NIH and to recommend improvements. The Livingstone Committee reports that as research expands and becomes more complex, the risks to subjects will become greater, but it makes no formal recommendations.
1965	Shannon tells the NAHC that many research investigators confuse the role of principal investigator with the role of physician. He proposes the first federal policy for the protection of human subjects, calling for panels composed of both experts and non-experts to review research protocols for ethical integrity.
1966	In an article in the *New England Journal of Medicine,* Henry K. Beecher brands as unethical 22 research projects published in refereed journals. This article provides unexpected and powerful support for the establishment of ethics review panels, which initially are called *institutional review committees.*
1971	Donald S. Chalkley publishes the Yellow Book, an extension of the PHS policy to all research involving human subjects supported by any agency within the Department of Health Education and Welfare (DHEW).
1972	Senator Edward M. Kennedy begins a three-year series of hearings on human-subject research, including psychosurgery, whole-body radiation, forced sterilization of retarded women, a study of the contraceptive Depo-Provera in which some sexually active women were given placebo without their knowledge, and the Tuskegee Syphilis Study of the natural course of syphilis, during which treatment for the disease was withheld from impoverished black men in Alabama (see Chapter 8).
1972	NIH Director Robert Q. Marston calls for a broad study of the ethics of research involving human subjects. He appoints Ronald Lamont-Havers to create a task force to consider protections for many categories of vulnerable subjects.
1974	The National Research Act calls for the creation of the National Commission for the Protection of Human Subjects of Biomedical and Behavioral Research. The National Commission meets on a monthly schedule for the next four years, completing 16 studies and making about 125 recommendations for the protection of human subjects (see Chapter 14).
1981	DHEW Secretary Patricia Harris signs a federal regulation implementing virtually all the recommendations of the National Commission. Many of the recommendations are incorporated into revised regulations issued by the FDA.
1991	After a seven-year effort, 16 federal departments and agencies that conduct or support research involving human subjects adopt the Common Rule, a package of regulations virtually identical to the Department of Health and Human Services Regulations for the Protection of Human Subjects.

Hippocratic tradition. After considerable discussion, in 1953 the NIH Clinical Center issued a policy to protect the rights and well-being of normal research volunteers.

The policy, entitled Group Consideration of Clinical Research Procedures Deviating from Accepted Medical Practice or Involving Unusual Hazard,[8] required oversight of research involving normal volunteers by peers in the Clinical Center. Panels of reviewers were overseen by Philippe Cardon, deputy director of the NIH Clinical Center, who was careful to explain to the volunteers the risks of the research in which they were invited to participate, and to elicit their informed consent. Although patient/subjects were often placed at much higher levels of risk than normal volunteers, the oversight policy extended only to normal volunteers. The policy that Shannon recommended to the NAHC in 1965 borrowed and expanded the Clinical Center policy to all research subjects involved in both intramural and extramural research.

The Turbulent Decade of the 1960s

It was not until near the end of the 1950s that doubts concerning the beneficial results of research, and concern for the risks to research subjects and to society, began to surface in the public media. In 1959, Senator Estes Kefauver, chairman of the Senate Subcommittee on Antitrust and Monopoly, began a series of hearings concerned with the cost and availability of drugs. The hearings culminated in the 1962 Kefauver-Harris Amendments to the Food, Drug, and Cosmetic Act. Initially, the hearings were exclusively concerned with the economic aspects of drug production, distribution, and sale. Kefauver summoned pharmaceutical industry leaders to testify, and he demanded that pharmaceutical houses provide drugs to consumers at reasonable prices.

In 1961, while the Kefauver hearings were ongoing, the public media recognized that thalidomide—a drug administered to pregnant women in many countries as a sedative and to prevent morning sickness—was associated with limb anomalies in newborn infants. Thousands of infants whose mothers had used thalidomide were born without arms or legs. By 1961, a majority of U.S. homes had television sets, and televised images brought these tragedies into the living rooms of many thousands of Americans. Few of the birth defects occurred in the United States because the Food and Drug Administration (FDA) had not approved the drug. Nevertheless, the publicity given the tragic effects of thalidomide caused Kefauver to shift the focus of the hearings to the safety and efficacy of drugs. Senator Hubert H. Humphrey's Subcommittee on Reorganization and International Organization also held hearings on the thalidomide debacle. Frances Kelsey of the FDA was subsequently presented with a presidential medal because she had refused to grant FDA approval for marketing thalidomide in the United States. She based her refusal on the lack of animal research safety data.

Kefauver criticized the drug manufacturers' practice of providing experimental drugs to practicing physicians, who, in turn, treated their patients with the drugs. Patients were seldom informed that some of the drugs handed to them by their physicians were still experimental. Patients were unaware that they were sometimes used as de facto research subjects. The Kefauver bill was further amended to require FDA to certify that new drugs are both safe and efficacious. When the Kefauver-Harris bill was brought to the floor of the Senate, Senator Jacob Javits proposed an amendment—which became law—requiring that research subjects provide informed consent prior to their participation in any FDA-regulated study. Several years passed before the FDA learned how to implement the 1962 amendments. Nevertheless the Javits provision marked the first time that any sort of protection for human research participants was included in a federal statute.[3]

In the years following the thalidomide uproar, a cascade of alleged research abuses came to the attention of the media and the public. A number of research projects that had involved children were challenged as unethical. The most notable of these was the so-called Willowbrook State School study of the 1950s, in which severely retarded children were infected with a strain of hepatitis virus[4] (see Chapter 7). Similarly, failure by Chester Southam and Emanuel Mandel at the Sloan-Kettering Institute for Cancer Research and the Jewish Chronic Disease Hospital to obtain consent for the administration of live cancer cells to elderly, indigent patients in New York received critical newspaper headlines and eventually led to a condemnation by the New York State Board of Regents in 1965[3] (see Chapter 6).

Shannon, who had never accepted the view that regulation of research was an intrusion into the doctor-patient relationship, grew more and more restive about the absence of a policy governing the ethics of research. Although the peer review system for scientific merit was steadily growing more sophisticated, a policy for the protection of human research subjects had not even been articulated, much less implemented. It was this worry that prompted Shannon's recommendation to the NAHC that the extant NIH policy for normal volunteers be expanded to cover all subjects involved in both intramural and extramural research.

The Boston University Study

In 1960, encouraged or perhaps even directed by Shannon, the NIH made a three-year "grant" (today it would be classified as a contract) to the Boston University Law-Medicine Research Institute to conduct a study of ethical, legal, and moral issues associated with the practice of clinical research in the United States.[3] The Boston group conducted a survey that indicated that only 16 U.S. institutions used consent forms or documents, and only 2 had policy guidance for research involving humans. The group forwarded its report, including the survey, to the NIH in 1963.

Shannon acknowledged that he sought a policy to protect the rights of research subjects because he felt that failure to do so would jeopardize the medical research enterprise in the United States—an enterprise that after World War II was centered in the NIH. He believed that protection of the rights of subjects was essential to the development of the NIH mission. He was particularly upset when he learned that a U.S. surgeon, without prior consultation or approval from the NIH or anyone in his institution, transplanted a baboon's kidney into a human being. The patient died within minutes. The surgeon called his action "research."[9]

The Livingston Committee

The results of the Boston University Study, the publicity given to alleged research abuses, and discussions with the FDA—including discussions about how to implement the Javits amendment to the

Kefauver-Harris Act—prompted Shannon to appoint an NIH committee under the leadership of Robert B. Livingston to address these problems. The Livingston Report reached several conclusions:

> [A]s the number of investigators, subjects, and institutions engaged in clinical research increases, and as the nature of the risks . . . changes according to the extension of research into new areas, a mounting concern is expressed over the possible repercussions of untoward events which are increasingly likely to occur, and which may occur in an unfavorable pattern of [sic] context. . . . The NIH is not in a position to shape the educational foundations of medical ethics. . . . In our view, it would add to existing insecurities if the NIH were to assume an exclusive or authoritative position concerning the definitions of ethical boundaries or conditions necessary for clinical research.[10]

Shannon was in full agreement with the report's warning of increasingly frequent untoward events; but he found "wholly unsatisfactory" the report's conclusion that the NIH should set no ethical boundaries. He argued that the NIH was well within its authority to require institutions to meet ethical standards as a condition of receiving support for research involving humans. Following receipt of the Livingston report, Shannon forwarded four recommendations to the NAHC:

1. A professional group should . . . formulate a statement of principles relating to the moral and ethical aspects of clinical investigations.
2. There is a need for more factual information regarding actual research practices.
3. The NIH should consider providing advice concerning ethical problems, and risk-reducing practices.
4. Research grant documentation relating to clinical investigations using human subjects should be identified for special consideration throughout the PHS-NIH review process.[3]

Policy and Procedure Order #129, February 8, 1966

Following Shannon's presentation in September 1965, the NAHC deliberated for several months and then issued Policy and Procedure Order #129 (PPO #129) on February 8, 1966. The policy required awardee institutions to

> provide prior review of the judgment of the principal investigator . . . by a committee of his institutional associates. This review should assure an independent determination: (1) of the rights and welfare of the individual or individuals involved, (2) of the appropriateness of the methods used to determine informed consent, and (3) of the risks and potential medical benefits of the investigation.[3]

The slow pace of implementation of PPO #129 contrasted sharply with the energy that senior NIH officials had devoted to having it approved by the NAHC. Within months of its promulgation, Surgeon General William H. Stewart ruled that PPO #129 applied both to clinical research and to behavioral and social science research involving humans conducted or supported by any agency within the PHS. The policy was also extended to those enrolled in projects conducted under research training grants. PPO #129 required each awardee institution, domestic or foreign,

to submit an Assurance of Compliance with each application for funding. These documents, at least in theory, were to be completed and signed before any PHS project involving human subjects could begin. Had the requirement of PPO #129 been strictly enforced, federal research involving humans would have slowed to a crawl or come to a standstill. Neither the PHS nor the NIH had made provision for a well-staffed office to implement the requirements of the policy.

The Role of the Institutional Relations Branch

Shannon assigned the task of administering PPO #129 to the institutional relations branch within the Division of Research Grants (DRG-IRB). This tiny office, which included only four professional employees with experience in the peer review system, had many other duties besides implementation of PPO #129. Staff members could give only part of their time to implementing the new policy. Staff from the DRG-IRB traveled to institutions and negotiated the required assurance documents with these institutions. Each assurance was tailored to accommodate the organizational framework of each institution. This process could often take up to a week. Before long it became clear that the policy would never be implemented if this snail-like process remained unchanged.

The NIH, by far the largest agency in the PHS, soon altered its interpretation of the policy. For the most part, general assurances replaced single project assurances. Thus an institution could negotiate one assurance document that covered all research involving human subjects for a period of three to five years. Model assurances were developed and the policy was clarified. Surgeon General Stewart, in the face of fierce protests by nonmedical researchers, made clear that the new policy also applied to behavioral and social science research involving human subjects. The policy was amended, clarified, and reissued in July 1966, in 1967, and again in 1969. The FDA found that it could implement the Javits amendment by "piggybacking" onto the institutional review committees (IRCs) established in accord with PPO #129.

Donald S. Chalkley, director of the DRG-IRB, said,

> To many it was an entirely new and strange concept. The PHS provided few guidelines. . . . Institutions were permitted to review proposals [protocols] any time prior to their actual acceptance. Understandably many institutions followed the practice of reviewing only after the actual awarding of a grant. While this was an administrative advantage for the institution as well as the investigator, it was a cause for concern among NIH officials.[3]

PPO #129 received unexpected support from the 1966 publication of an influential article written by Henry K. Beecher in the *New England Journal of Medicine*.[11] Beecher identified 22 studies published in refereed journals that contained serious ethical flaws. Because of Beecher's exalted reputation among his peers, the article was considered to be entirely credible. Although other criticisms of research ethics had been published, the Beecher article seemed to have greater impact than any of the others. The article was a stinging rebuke to those who still considered research to be beyond the purview of committees because such committees were an intrusion into the doctor-patient relationship.

Within the PHS, the duties of the surgeon general's office were divided. The surgeon general continued to issue annual reports on the health of the nation and to exercise command over the Public Health Service Corps, but the line of authority from the Secretary of the Department of Health, Education, and Welfare (DHEW) to the agencies within the PHS ran through the assistant secretary for health (ASH), not through the surgeon general. In 1970 Philip Lee, a veteran health policy official, was assigned to the position of ASH. Lee quickly realized that PPO #129 needed clarification and improved implementation. He appointed Eugene A. Confrey to chair a task force to review and revise PPO #129. Among other statements, the task force issued the following recommendation:

> The primary duty of institutional committees was to protect the rights and welfare of human subjects. In doing so, the committee was to concern itself with the appropriateness and adequacy of efforts to obtain informed consent from subjects; weigh the risks to subjects against the potential benefits to subjects or the importance of the knowledge to be gained.[12]

The assertion that research could be justified by the "importance of the knowledge to be gained" constituted an important addition to PPO #129. It made possible the conduct of research that did not hold out the prospect of direct benefit to research subjects.[1]

The Yellow Book

Ernest Allen, director of the DHEW Division of Grants Administration Policy, recognized that the DHEW was supporting research involving human subjects with funds provided by agencies within the DHEW but outside the PHS. He therefore recommended that the policy be extended to cover all research involving humans conducted or supported by any agency within the DHEW. Donald S. Chalkley, special assistant to the director, DRG, was assigned to direct the DRG-IRB. In 1970, Confrey asked Chalkley to redraft the PPO #129.

In 1971, Chalkley published a DHEW-wide version of the policy in pamphlet form with a bright yellow cover. It was known thereafter as the *Yellow Book*. The document included the clearest version of the policy published up to that time. The Yellow Book also added commentary to help institutions understand and comply with each of its provisions.

The policy had matured to the point at which most awardee institutions considered it both workable and acceptable. Clinical investigators grudgingly accepted its requirements, and brought their studies into compliance. Nevertheless, implementation was far from ideal. Some institutions included ambiguous language in their assurance documents that provided enforcement loopholes. Almost all institutions understaffed the offices charged with implementing the policy, and only a few offered the staff training necessary to provide support for IRCs. Nevertheless, government staff learned by experience, and institutional staff members began to provide improved assistance to principal investigators and to IRCs. Many institutional staff members learned how to comply with the policy by networking with one another.

Chalkley wrote hundreds of longhand letters to heads of institutions urging them to comply, criticizing their shortcomings, and exhorting them to take their responsibility to protect human subjects seriously. Because Chalkley's letters often contained sarcasm and stinging criticism, Charles R. McCarthy, chief of the legislative development branch in the NIH's Division of Legislative

Analysis [and author of this chapter], was assigned by Associate Director Ronald Lamont-Havers to edit Chalkley's letters.

Senate Health Subcommittee Hearings and the Tuskegee Study

In 1971, Senator Edward M. Kennedy became chairman of the Health Subcommittee of the Senate Labor and Public Welfare Committee. He initiated a series of hearings spaced at intervals of three or four months. Many of the hearings dealt with research issues. Kennedy made no secret of the fact that he was accumulating evidence for the creation of a national commission to deal with health research. Kennedy held hearings on the following: contraception research, including the Depo-Provera study in which some women were given placebo instead of contraceptives without their knowledge; psychosurgery research involving frontal lobotomy; lethal whole-body radiation experiments to treat military cancer victims; and the need for a national agency or commission to oversee research in the United States. Among these hearings was one that considered S.J. Res. 75, a bill introduced by Senator Walter Mondale calling for a national commission on health, society, and science.[1]

The centerpiece of the Senate Health Subcommittee hearings turned out to be the Tuskegee Syphilis Study[13] (see Chapter 8). The hearings brought to public attention the PHS study that for 35 years had monitored the natural course of untreated syphilis in approximately 400 African American men who resided in Macon County, Alabama. Most of the men were illiterate, and most did not know they were research subjects. The infamous study had continued within the PHS since 1932. Initially, it was thought that not treating syphilis might be better for people who had the disease than the standard treatment with the heavy metals arsenic and mercury. But the study, which deprived subjects of all treatment for their disease, continued for more than 25 years after the discovery of penicillin, the drug of choice for treatment of syphilis. It continued for five years after promulgation of PPO #129 in 1966, and after review and approval by an IRC at the Tuskegee Institute (now University). At the time of the hearings, the study had been assigned to the Center for Disease Control (CDC, now the Centers for Disease Control and Prevention).

Portions of the hearings on the Tuskegee Study were televised. Monte DuVal, who was the ASH at that time in the Nixon administration, created a citizen's commission chaired by Jay Katz of Yale University to examine the study. DuVal ordered the PHS to take a posture of "anticipation" of legislative constraints on research rather than try to defend the Tuskegee Study. Upon receiving a recommendation from the Katz Committee, DuVal terminated the study. Senators Kennedy, Javits, Humphrey, John Sparkman, and Mondale introduced legislation intended to prevent research abuses. Representatives Edward Roybal and Paul Rogers introduced similar legislation in the House of Representatives. Kennedy and Rogers continued to hold hearings on the provisions in the bills that had been introduced.

In 1972, Robert Q. Marston, who succeeded Shannon as NIH director, renamed the DRG-IRB and transferred it to the Office of the Director, NIH. The new unit, still headed by Chalkley, was called the Office for Protection from Research Risks (OPRR). In that same year, Marston delivered a major address at the University of Virginia in which he called for a broad expansion of the

DHEW policy for the protection of human subjects. He assigned Ronald Lamont-Havers, associate NIH director for extramural affairs, to chair a PHS task force made up of a number of subcommittees dealing with research involving human fetuses, children, prisoners, cognitively impaired persons, and persons who were socially deprived. These subject categories came to be known as *vulnerable subjects* categories. In 1974, DHEW Secretary Caspar Weinberger, at Marston's suggestion, created a committee chaired by Seymour Perry to make recommendations for the compensation for research subjects injured in research process.

In the spring of 1974, congressional compromises led to the introduction of two bills, one in the Senate and one in the House of Representatives. Each included features of bills that been introduced in both houses of Congress. Kennedy's bill included a provision that would create a permanent government commission, patterned after the Securities and Exchange Commission, to oversee research. Rogers' bill called for a national advisory commission to make recommendations to the DHEW secretary. After considerable negotiation, Kennedy agreed to support the commission set forth in the Rogers bill. As a condition of this agreement, Kennedy insisted that the DHEW policy for the protection of human subjects be upgraded and reissued as a federal regulation. The DHEW, preferring to deal with a temporary advisory commission rather than with a permanent oversight agency, quickly formed a drafting committee that included Charles U. Lowe, Jane Fullerton, and Charles R. McCarthy. Richard Riseberg, a young attorney in the DHEW Office of General Counsel provided legal advice concerning provisions of the Administrative Procedures Act. Because the NIH had never before issued regulations, no one on the committee had any experience in producing regulations. Nevertheless, under pressure from Kennedy, the committee hurriedly drafted regulations for the protection of human subjects based primarily on Chalkley's Yellow Book. In its rush to placate Kennedy, the DHEW waived the usual clearance requirements and the Regulations for the Protection of Human Subjects (45 CFR 46, Subpart A) were published on May 30, 1974.[14] This version of the regulations had a number of flaws, but it sufficed to advance the protection of human subjects until such time as the National Commission could complete its work and the regulations could be carefully revised in the light of the Commission's findings and recommendations.

The publication of the regulations cleared the way for Rogers and Kennedy to agree to support an advisory commission for the protection of human subjects. One of the duties of the commission would be to measure the impact of research on society, as requested by Mondale. A study of psychosurgery supported by Roybal (who called psychosurgery "murder of the mind") was included, and in response to false rumors that the NIH was conducting research on living human fetuses, Representative Angelo Roncallo added a ban on fetal research. Rogers later persuaded him to accept a temporary moratorium on fetal research until the new commission could issue recommendations. Rogers and his staff drafted a new bill that included enough features of each of these initiatives to forge a compromise. The DHEW, in response to a request from Rogers for technical assistance, directed Charles R. McCarthy to draft a list of responsibilities that would be assigned to the new commission. McCarthy's draft of duties remained unchanged in the final version of the bill. The Rogers bill used a new term—*institutional review board (IRB)*—for the first time. The term *IRB* replaced *institutional review committee (IRC)*, the term that had

been in vogue since the passage of the Kefauver-Harris amendments to the Food, Drug, and Cosmetic Act in 1962.

Meanwhile, subcommittees of the Lamont-Havers task force were busy drafting pieces of what was intended to be a major report on the protection of human research subjects. Before this report could be finished, however, Congress enacted the National Research Act (PL 93–348), and President Nixon signed it into law on July 12, 1974. Title II of the Act addressed protection of human subjects. Foremost among its provisions was the creation of the National Commission for the Protection of Human Subjects of Biomedical and Behavioral Research (National Commission). The PHS turned over the drafts of the Lamont-Havers task force to the new commission.

The National Commission for the Protection of Human Subjects of Biomedical and Behavioral Research

Beginning in December 1974, the National Commission met for two days of each month, with rare exceptions, for the next four years. In 1975 it issued a report on fetal research that called for regulations allowing fetal research under stringent conditions.[15] In succeeding years it published reports on research involving prisoners, children, and those institutionalized as mentally infirm, as well as a report on IRBs. Perhaps its most important contribution was the report entitled *Ethical Principles and Guidelines for the Protection of Human Subjects*. This was popularly called the Belmont Report, named after the conference center in Maryland where it was conceived.[16] The Belmont Report identified and applied three overarching principles of research ethics: (1) respect for persons, (2) beneficence, and (3) justice. These principles were explained in simple but eloquent language, presented as guiding norms under which all research involving human subjects should be conducted. They provided a guide for the decisions of IRBs and a framework for the drafting of future regulations (see Chapter 14). The findings, reports, and recommendations of the National Commission were, for the most part, polished and carefully presented. Each new report was published by the OPRR in the *Federal Register*.

National Commission reports and recommendations were similar in many respects to those made by in the Lamont-Havers task force. However, National Commission reports differed in several important ways. First, they were thoroughly researched and their findings were meticulously documented. Second, they included many scholarly background documents that provided depth and credibility seldom associated with reports of federal advisory bodies. Third, because they were drafted in public hearings, they enjoyed support of the public—who were given an opportunity to testify at nearly every meeting—and of the press, which was allowed to be present for all of their deliberations.

During the four-year period when the National Commission was at work, the OPRR was also making significant progress. It finally managed to negotiate acceptable assurances with all of the research institutions that were supported by the DHEW. These assurances extended the regulations not only to subjects participating in DHEW-funded research but to all human subjects involved in research conducted within each institution.

In 1975, following the National Commission's report on fetal research, the OPRR issued Subpart B of the regulations to address research involving pregnant women and human fetuses. In 1977 OPRR Director Chalkley suffered a major stroke and retired from federal service. In 1978 the OPRR published Subpart C, entitled "Additional Protections Pertaining to Biomedical and Behavioral Research Involving Prisoners as Subjects." This report had been nearly completed before Chalkley retired. In September 1978, McCarthy was selected as the new director of the OPRR. He was assigned several additional duties, including staff director of the DHEW Secretary's Ethics Advisory Board and chair of the PHS drafting committee to incorporate recommendations of the National Commission into regulatory form."

The National Research Act contained what has come to be known as a *forcing clause.* This was a requirement that the DHEW secretary must either accept and implement the recommendations of the National Commission or publish in the *Federal Register* the reasons for not accepting them. Because few cabinet officers are ever willing to reject findings of a highly respected ethics commission, virtually all of the National Commission's suggestions (approximately 125) were accepted. The drafting committee worked for nearly two years to incorporate each of the commission's recommendations into a new version of 45 CFR 46 Subpart A, preparing a comprehensive regulation that would reflect the Belmont Principles and both the letter and spirit of the National Commission's work. The drafting committee considered about 1,500 public comments on the National Commission reports and proposed regulations.

In November 1980, Ronald Reagan was elected president of the United States. In the course of his campaign, Reagan had threatened to repeal all federal regulations. OPRR officials felt sure that he would not literally carry out that threat, but Reagan's transition team advised them that it might be very difficult to get regulations for the protection of human subjects published after he took office. The OPRR submitted Subpart A of the revised regulation to Health and Human Services Secretary Patricia Harris for final approval soon after the election. (The DHEW had been transformed into the Department of Health and Human Services, DHHS, earlier in 1980, when a separate Department of Education was created.) Harris's office called for a number of minor revisions and ordered a new preamble to be drafted. The regulations were returned to the OPRR for revision on January 16, 1981. The OPRR worked around the clock for several days, before it was finally able to secure approval from Harris on January 19, only a few hours before she left office.

The President's Commission and the Common Rule

After the National Commission disbanded, a new advisory body, the President's Commission for the Study of Ethical Problems in Medicine and Biomedical and Behavioral Research (President's Commission), was created. During its first year, the new commission operated on money that had been set aside for use by the Secretary's Ethics Advisory Board. Consequently, the ethics board was disbanded at the end of the Carter administration in January 1981. Much of the energy of the President's Commission was directed, not at research, but at problems in the health-care delivery system of the United States. However, the President's Commission issued two reports and one major directive concerning research involving humans. The Commission praised the DHHS "Regulations for the Protection of Human Subjects" and recommended

that all federal departments and agencies that conduct or support research involving human subjects should follow a Common Rule modeled after them.

The task of persuading 16 federal departments and agencies to follow the same regulations and to coordinate their efforts with the White House Office of Science and Technology, the Office of Management and Budget, and the State Department (for research conducted outside the United States) was assigned to the OPRR. It proved to be very difficult for two reasons: (1) Departments and agencies felt that regulations should be geared to specific programs operated within each department or agency, not to general standards designed for a vast array of programs across the government; and (2) turnover in departments and agencies meant that agreements had to be renegotiated whenever new appointees assumed senior positions in the agency or department. Joan P. Porter, special assistant to the director of the OPRR, worked tirelessly under direction of the OPRR director to fulfill the commission's recommendation. It took nearly 10 years to gain simultaneous agreement from all of the affected departments and agencies. The Common Rule was promulgated June 18, 1991[17] (see Chapter 15).

After 14 years, McCarthy retired as the OPRR's director. During his tenure, he also was staff director of the DHEW Secretary's Ethics Advisory Board, serving as liaison to two national commissions and implementing their recommendations, completing the assurance process for all institutions that receive funding from the DHEW, and publishing the Common Rule. (He also chaired the committee that issued a new policy for humane care and use of laboratory animals.) McCarthy emphasized education. When he was liaising with the staff of Congressman Rogers on the legislation that became the National Research Act, he had inserted a clause in the legislation that required the DHEW to conduct education as well as enforce compliance with the regulations governing research involving human subjects. His calendars show that during his tenure, OPRR personnel participated in at least 187 educational programs concerning the protection of human research participants. He strongly encouraged a fledgling organization called Public Responsibility in Medicine and Research (PRIM&R) to conduct workshops and educational events pertaining to the protection of human subjects. PRIM&R steadily improved the quality and breadth of its programs and underwent steady growth. Gradually the research community in the United States and in other research-intensive countries came to understand and carry out their responsibilities to human research subjects under rules that had been fashioned by the DHEW and honed by the National Commission.

Gary Ellis was named director of the OPRR in the fall of 1992. He emphasized conducting site visits and inspections to assure strict compliance with the regulations. He stressed improved record keeping and he often said, "If there is not a written record, it didn't happen." Under his aggressive leadership, the OPRR suspended the assurances of compliance of more than 13 domestic research institutions between 1992 and 2000. Until the suspension of an institution's assurance document was lifted, no research involving human subjects could be undertaken in that institution. Each suspension affected large numbers of personnel in the affected institutions, and also affected many of the institutes of the NIH, the PHS, and other funding agencies.

Ellis and many others contended that because the OPRR was regulating research funded by the NIH, the location of the OPRR within the NIH constituted a potential (and occasionally an actual) conflict of interest. He sought to have the OPRR transferred to the Office of the Secretary in order to avoid conflict or the appearance of conflict of interest. The assurance suspensions and the desire to move the OPRR to the level of the secretary, DHHS, made Ellis a controversial figure within the entire human research community.

When 45 CFR 46 was promulgated in 1981, most research projects were conducted under awards made to a single investigator in a single institution. Gradually the NIH and other funding agencies decreased the number of grants made to single institutions and increased the number of awards made multiple institutions. In the decade of the 1990s, awards often were made to a consortium of institutions conducting projects under the same protocol. Adjustments had to be made in the oversight process to avoid unnecessary duplication of review while protecting human subjects. Some institutions utilized central IRBs and commercial IRBs to address the problem.

The OPRR under Ellis's leadership moved from communication via regular mail and telephone to electronic mail, documentation, and record keeping. Guidance was published on the Internet rather than mailed to each awardee institution. New kinds of filing systems were created. Foreign institutions could communicate as swiftly and easily as domestic ones. Complex questions of how to apply the rules to institutions outside the United States involved diplomacy. Adjusting and adapting to these realities characterized Ellis' time in the OPRR.

In 2000, acting on recommendations from the National Bioethics Advisory Commission (NBAC), the DHHS moved the OPRR out of the NIH and placed it in the Office of the DHHS Secretary. The relocated office was called the Office for Human Research Protections (OHRP). In September 2000, Greg Koski, a Harvard University physician, was selected to be the new director. Koski worked closely with the Institute of Medicine within the National Academies of Science and with PRIM&R. He strongly endorsed creation of a nongovernment accrediting agency to assist research institutions to remain in full compliance with the Common Rule. He played an important role in persuading the Association of American Medical Colleges and other professional health organizations to join with PRIM&R in funding an independent, private accrediting agency to certify the adequacy of institutional research protection programs. By 2006, that organization, the Association for Accreditation of Human Research Protection Programs (AAHRPP), had announced full accreditation for approximately 43 institutions, and well over 100 institutions were seeking accreditation. Accreditation is seen as a mark of excellence and appears to be the wave of the future. Moreover, it offers institutions the opportunity to evaluate their programs from time to time, to make sure that they are in compliance with regulations and that human research participants are well protected.

In January 2003, Bernard Schwetz was named acting director of OHRP, and a year later, he was named director. Schwetz again stressed the need for education of a growing and changing research community. He emphasized the need for human research protection programs including, but extending well beyond, IRBs. Schwetz also offered the services of OHRP as an aid to institutions rather than an enforcer of regulations. He increased the number of "not for cause" site visits, in which OHRP representatives offer assistance to institutions to improve their programs rather than cite them for noncompliance. OHRP published a number of documents on the Internet to assist institutions to interpret and apply the regulations. Schwetz also created the Secretary's Advisory Committee on Human Research Protections (SACHRP) to provide outside advice on how best to provide protections for human research subjects.

In the meantime, the funding of both clinical and behavioral-social science research steadily increased. The need for protection of the rights and welfare of human subjects has grown apace. As stem cell research, genetic research, and proteomics research have expanded the traditional areas of research involving human subjects, so will the need for vigilant oversight need to change.

Growth With Continuity

From James Shannon's 1965 testimony to the National Advisory Health Council until the present time, progress has been made in protecting human research participants. The insights that Shannon presented to the NAHC found expression in PPO #129. Each expression of policy and each new regulation has included all of the best characteristics of the past. Progress in recognizing the rights and welfare of human research participants has been captured in each succeeding set of regulations. Progress in the understanding and application of sound research ethics has taken place in both domestic and the foreign settings. IRBs are established in more than 80 nations worldwide. They have become more insightful and sophisticated in conducting review and oversight of research protocols involving human subjects. Clinical investigators and behavioral and social scientists have come to know, understand, and apply the rules to their own research protocols. Administrators have come to understand that the regulations require institutions to train and oversee their personnel so that those enrolled in research will receive the protection that they are owed. Although the protection of human subjects has expanded in countless ways, IRBS continue to stand at the center of the program.

With the advent of funding for multicenter research involving humans, a single phrase in the 1981 version of the regulations has become extremely important. Section 46.111(a)(6) authorizes IRBs to make adequate provision for monitoring the data collected to ensure the safety of research participants. That clause provided for the creation of data and safety monitoring boards (DSMBs) to monitor the data collected in trials involving many sites (see Chapter 53). The DSMB has become a major and often essential tool in protecting human research participants in multicenter trials. The OHRP now faces the challenge of finding an efficient method of coordinating the work of IRBs and DSMBs.

The IRB has served the United States and many other countries well. It is here to stay. But unless it is considered to be an evolving and expanding mechanism, adapting to the problems of each period of history, it is in danger of becoming fossilized and ineffective. Administrators, research investigators, ethicists, regulators, Congress, and the general public bear the responsibility of creating mechanisms and methods for the IRB to continue to protect human research participants in a manner that is demanded by the highest principles of ethics.

References

1. McCarthy CR. Research policy, biomedical. In: Reich WT, ed. *Encyclopedia of Bioethics*. New York, N.Y.: The Free Press; 1978:1492–8.
2. U.S. Congress. Public Health Service Act. Title 42 (Public Health and Welfare), United States Code, Chapter 6A (Public Health Service).

[Online] January 5, 1999. Available: http://www.fda.gov/opacom/laws/phsvcact/phsvcact.htm.

3. Frankel MS. *Public Policy Making for Biomedical Research: The Case of Human Experimentation*. Ph.D. dissertation, Department of Political Science, George Washington University; 1976.

4. Jonsen AR. *The Birth of Bioethics*. New York, N.Y.: Oxford University Press; 1998.

5. Rothman DJ. *Strangers at the Bedside*. New York, N.Y.: Basic Books; 1991.

6. Personal communications with Donald S. Fredrickson, former director, NIH; Robert Gordon, former director of the NIH Clinical Center; and Philippe Cardon, former deputy director of the NIH Clinical Center.

7. Faden RR, Beauchamp TL, with King NMP. *A History and Theory of Informed Consent*. New York, N.Y.: Oxford University Press; 1986.

8. National Institutes of Health. Group Consideration and Informed Consent in Intramural Clinical Research at the NIH. Policy and Communication Bulletin (Clinical Center Medical Administrative Series No. 75–5), July 14, 1975.

9. Starzl TE, Marchioro TL, Peters GN, et al. Renal heterotransplantation from baboon to man: Experience with 6 cases. *Transplantation* 1964;12:752–76.

10. Livingston RB. Memorandum to the Director, NIH: Moral and Ethical Aspects of Clinical Investigation, February 20, 1964.

11. Beecher HK. Ethics and clinical research. *New England Journal of Medicine* 1966:274:1354–60.

12. Confrey EA. PHS grant-supported research with human subjects. *Public Health Reports* 1968;83:127–33.

13. Jones JH. *Bad Blood: The Tuskegee Syphilis Experiment*. New York, N.Y.: The Free Press; 1981.

14. Office of the Secretary, Department of Health, Education, and Welfare. 45 CFR 46: Protection of Human Subjects. *Federal Register* 1974;39(105):18913–20.

15. The National Commission for the Protection of Human Subjects of Biomedical and Behavioral Research. *Research on the Fetus: Report and Recommendations*. DHEW publication No. (OS) 76–127. Washington, D.C.: DHEW; 1975 [Online] Available: http://www.bioethics.gov/reports/past_commissions/research_fetus.pdf.

16. The National Commission for the Protection of Human Subjects of Biomedical and Behavioral Research. *The Belmont Report: Ethical Principles and Guidelines for the Protection of Human Subjects of Research*. Washington, D.C.: Department of Health, Education and Welfare; DHEW Publication OS 78–0012 1978. [Online] April 18, 1979. Available: http://www.hhs.gov/ohrp/humansubjects/guidance/belmont.htm.

17. Office of Science and Technology Policy. Federal Policy for the Protection of Human Subjects; Final Rule. *Federal Register* 1991;56(117):28002–32.

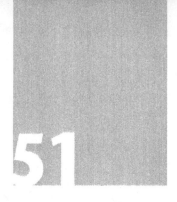

Angela J. Bowen

Models of Institutional Review Board Function

History

Many models of the institutional review board (IRB) have developed in the United States and other countries as awareness has increased within the research community that a need for such oversight bodies existed.[1] The Nuremberg Code and the Declaration of Helsinki both called upon other institutional structures, such as medical associations and legal systems, to oversee ethical behavior in both medical practice and research. The Declaration of Helsinki promoted physicians' awareness of their traditional responsibilities to patients, regardless of pressures to do otherwise. Research at that time was less a concern than were the practice of medicine and adherence to the traditional ethical standards of professional behavior.

In 1962, an amendment to the federal Food, Drug and Cosmetic Act required all new medicines marketed in the United States to have research showing them to be effective as well as safe for their intended use.[2] This amendment changed the research landscape dramatically. The Food and Drug Administration (FDA) began the process of bringing drugs already on the market back into testing to assess their safety and efficacy. This new requirement necessitated the commitment of vast sums of money to the research community by pharmaceutical manufacturers.

During the 1960s, the National Institutes of Health (NIH) was also rapidly growing. Hundreds of eager young researchers trained at the NIH migrated to medical schools across the United States to conduct research. It was a time of great energy in medical research and a time of great trust from the community at large that there would be public benefit from these research efforts. Patients were eager to enroll as participants in this new enterprise of medical research.

All of this activity caused James Shannon, then director of the NIH, to worry about the oversight of such things as scientific integrity and the maintenance of professional standards in research. He quietly implemented a requirement that scientists receiving federal funds should have an oversight committee composed of "peers" that would review and approve a research proposal prior to its implementation. Because virtually all federal funding went to universities and large medical centers, these institutions founded research review panels, often called "investigator judgment committees."

Shannon was also concerned about revelations of abuses in clinical research, including the Jewish Chronic Disease Hospital Study and the cases reported by Henry Beecher[3] (see Chapters 6 and 7). The policy of peer review proposed by Shannon was incorporated in the 1966 "Statement of Policy" by Surgeon General William H. Stewart and was aimed at the protection of research participants. But the initial committees formed in response to this policy were not focused on research protections, except for poor science or protocol design. No enforcement was designed into Stewart's guidance, and it was widely ignored.[4]

During this same era, William H. Masters and Virginia E. Johnson published their book *Human Sexual Response*,[5] in which they reported on a series of experiments they had conducted between 1959 and 1964 at Washington University in St. Louis. These studies recorded the many physiologic responses to sexual stimulation. Volunteers were recruited from the community and included commercial sex workers and other paid volunteers. Although the book was a scholarly work aimed at the medical profession, Washington University was profoundly embarrassed because it had not been aware that the work was being conducted in its facility. The work was widely covered by the lay press and much unwanted publicity ensued. Inevitably "wronged spouses" surfaced in the courts and the publicity continued well into the 1970s.[6] The book became a best seller.

This was a key event in raising institutional consciousness that protections needed to be developed for institutions themselves. Many institutions began to take precautions to prevent similar surprises from their own researchers. The committees established to do this work were similar to the investigator judgment committees, but their sole function was protection of the institution. No concern for the research participants was evidenced.

During the mid-1970s, following disclosure of the Tuskegee syphilis experiment (see Chapter 8), the Department of Health, Education and Welfare (now the Department of Health and Human Services, DHHS) promulgated regulations directed toward the protection of those who were institutionalized, regulations that prohibited their participation without an oversight mechanism in place.[7] Responsibility for forming oversight committees, called *institutional review boards,* was left with the institution, and an oversight body was established within NIH—the Office for Protection from Research Risks, now the Office for Human Research Protections (OHRP) within DHHS. This body had oversight of the NIH IRBs as well as all federally funded research. Nongovernmental institutions filed a promissory letter with the DHHS promising adherence to the guidance documents. It was a collegial system, without active enforcement, until the mid-1990s, when a more active approach began under the leadership of Gary Ellis. Widespread noncompliance was immediately apparent.

In the meantime, the pharmaceutical industry had set up a network of clinical investigators that were located in small hospitals, clinics, and private physician practices. Much, if not most, of this research was in support of medicinal compounds that were in development or of compounds already on the market and targeted by the FDA as requiring further documentation of safety and/or efficacy. At first these clinical investigators were not required either by the FDA, DHHS, or their institutions to have oversight for this work. It is of interest that some of these investigators set up, or caused to be set up, their own oversight committees, which were also called IRBs. Such committees were then converted to independent IRBs, not associated with a particular institution, when FDA regulations requiring them (21 CFR 50 & 56) were promulgated in 1981.[8,9] A federal policy for the protection of human participants was enacted at this time and is known as the Common Rule (45 CFR 46 Subpart A).[10] Government agencies had the option to adopt this rule or not. It was subsequently adopted by 17 agencies including DHHS.

Other countries with both government funding for research and a research-based pharmaceutical industry also have developed systems for the purpose of protecting research participants. Countries without either industry or U.S. government funding remain less developed in the protection of research participants. Much privately funded research remains exempt from enforceable oversight. As research has become increasingly competitive and the U.S. public less trusting of the research enterprise, there is more outreach by U.S. companies and universities to developing countries. There is concomitantly more interest in developing systems for protection of research participants in these nations.[11] Systems vary, but tend to be loosely patterned after the current U.S. models.

Research Review Systems in the United States

It is apparent from this brief historical overview how the U.S. system has become so diverse. The national tendency toward institutional autonomy reinforces the preference for local decision making over a central oversight model. The current U.S. models can be roughly categorized into institutional, independent, and private. These are similar in many respects but differ in a few fundamental areas.

Government Agencies

The 17 agencies of the federal government that have accepted the Common Rule have some kind of ethics review process directed to human participant protection. These agencies are as diverse as the Department of Defense, the Department of Agriculture, and the Agency for International Development. These committees are usually composed of agency employees and an outside member. This structure permits direct knowledge of both the research focus and the principal investigator and maximizes local knowledge and control. Any special considerations such as national security, confidentiality of materials, or even the title of the research can be closely held.

Such a structure could be worrisome if special care is not given to the protection of the employee members. For example, if research conducted by higher ranking employees of the agency is reviewed by lower ranking employees, the potential for coercion or the fear of coercion is a concern. Lower ranking employees might fear reprisal by those of higher rank. This concern could be ameliorated by careful selection of IRB members and strict institutional reinforcement of independent decision making by the IRB. A more effective measure might be to increase the number of outside members who will bring different perspectives to better balance that of agency members.

The IRB is generally accountable to the director of the agency, but they are also accountable to the FDA, in the case of regulated drugs or devices, and the OHRP for federally funded projects. Funding for the IRB comes directly from each agency's budget.

National Institutes of Health

There are 14 separate IRBs within the NIH. Each of the larger institutes maintains its own IRB to oversee intramural research with humans. Members are chosen from the staff of the institute and are supplemented by at least one public member. Each IRB is required to have a member with training in bioethics. Their workloads are variable and each is staffed separately. Each is funded by its own institute, which in turn is funded by congressional appropriations. Each IRB is accountable to the clinical director of the institute and ultimately to the NIH deputy director for intramural research. These IRBs are also accountable to the FDA and the OHRP.

The National Cancer Institute (NCI) formed a central IRB in 2000, then divided this into two panels in 2004—one covering treatment of adults and the other covering treatment of children.[12,13] The plan was that the central IRB would review all multicenter cancer protocols and that local IRBs would have the option of accepting this review. The adult-oriented NCI-CIRB has been meeting monthly since January 2001, whereas the NCI

Pediatric CIRB began meeting in November 2004. This has received only modest acceptance to date; institutions have generally preferred to conduct local review. These boards are responsible to the NCI, FDA, and OHRP. Funding is provided by the NCI.

Military Hospitals

These entities operate under the Department of Defense, which has adopted the Common Rule. Their IRB structure is similar to that of other governmental agencies, and the concerns are much the same. The strong military culture of rank recognition and esprit de corps may impair individual autonomy in decision making even more than in other governmental agencies. Special attention to internal conflicts of interest is necessary in these situations. In addition, outside or community members often are retired military. Accountability is to the commanding officer of the hospital, and to the FDA and the OHRP. Funding is through the Department of Defense.

States

Most states have a dedicated state IRB that reviews research done in or by state agencies, state prisons, and state hospitals. For many years research in state institutions for the mentally ill and in prison systems has been discouraged except when direct benefit to the participant is expected. These situations place an uncommonly heavy burden on IRB members. Prisons, in particular, have unique cultures and processes permitting coercive actions to occur that would not exist within a free population. Special knowledge of prison systems and greater awareness of these extraordinary responsibilities by all review board members is important.

Social and behavioral research is commonly reviewed through these state IRBs when it is to be conducted in state-run institutions. Members are usually chosen from the various state agencies. There may or may not be a member from the community. Accountability is to the Department of Social and Health Services (DSHS) in some states and to the governor of the state in others. These IRBs are also subject to oversight by the FDA when regulated drugs, devices, or biologics are involved and to the OHRP when federal funding applies. State IRBs may be subject to state regulations in addition to the federal regulations.[14] Funding usually comes from the state's general fund.

Academic Institutions

All U.S. academic institutions that conduct federally funded research hold either a multiple project assurance (MPA) agreement with DHHS or a federalwide assurance (FWA) agreement. These agreements bind academic institutions to uphold the regulations of both the OHRP and the FDA. Academic institutions consequently structure their IRBs according to the guidelines and regulations promulgated by these regulatory bodies.

Members are chosen from the faculty, often by conscription, and are supplemented with the traditional outside or community member (or members). The different schools within the university (nursing, pharmacy, medicine, etc.) are usually represented by one or more members. Few academic institutions have more than one community member. Transparency would be increased if wider

community representation existed. Community members can provide a powerful bond between the institution and the nonacademic community. This can be especially useful to the institution when complex and socially sensitive research is being conducted or if a research tragedy occurs.

Many universities with active research programs have multiple panels or IRBs. These committees operate as parts of a whole, following common standard operating procedures and policies. They are often coordinated through an executive policy committee (EPC) composed of the various panel chairs and others. Through this committee, the panel chairs agree on the common policies under which all panels operate. This lends a modicum of consistency to the process.

Some universities contract with independent IRBs to supplement or replace one or more of the internal panels. The outside IRB may operate as one of several panels or, in some situations, as the sole IRB. Under these conditions, the independent panel reports to the institution and adheres to previously agreed upon institutional policies. These panels extend capacity of the in-house panels and can provide relief from internal conflicts of interest that institutions commonly face when university-owned intellectual property is the subject of the research.

Universities sometimes collaborate to form a conjoint committee that reviews research from any member institution. Such joint review boards have been formed in New York, Tennessee, and the Midwest.[15,16] Members are chosen from the faculties of each member institution. Resolution of issues such as liability, insurance, and interinstitutional rivalries has been problematic.[17,18] Member institutions contribute funding from industry grants and other sources.

Accountability of these IRBs varies at the institutional level but all are accountable to the usual regulatory authorities. University IRBs usually report to the dean for research, the vice provost, or some other highly placed administrator of the institution. Accountability is therefore to the institution and through it to the federal regulatory authorities.

Institutionally based IRBs account for the bulk of the 3,000 to 5,000 IRBs said to exist in the United States. Funding is provided indirectly through funds from governmental sources and grants or fees from the pharmaceutical and medical device industries.

Independent or Fee-for-Service Review Boards

These review boards are usually operated under a corporate structure and are otherwise unassociated with a research institution. They take many forms, but all are subject to FDA oversight and some also to OHRP oversight. Board members may be employees of the corporation—and if so, must be supplemented by at least one outside or community member—but some boards are composed entirely of nonaffiliated community members. Like their institutional counterparts, they must have standard operating procedures and policies and are subject to audit by the regulatory authorities.

Much of the research reviewed by these boards is related to new drug and device development, so they are primarily funded by pharmaceutical or device manufacturers through a fee for service. This is thought to be one of the primary areas in which conflicts of interest may be problematic.[19] Wide client diversity can ameliorate this potential conflict, because less economic dependence on a single client could lessen the impact of pressure from a client to approve research. A second area of concern is the presence of stockholders on the review board. OHRP prohibits this practice for review of federally funded research. The presence of equity owners as board members is generally unacceptable. However, these review boards are remarkably free from many other conflicts that plague institutionally based IRBs. It is noteworthy that two of the first three review boards to receive full accreditation from the Association for the Accreditation of Human Research Protection Programs[20] were independent boards.

Independent review boards are accountable to the chief executive officer of their companies and through them to the usual regulatory authorities. Their funding comes from the corporation, which is generally supported by a fee for service collected from clients.

Hospitals

This category includes both small and large hospitals and clinics where research is conducted. These facilities are numerous but their research, with a few notable exceptions, is small in volume. Hospital-based IRBs are often challenged by inadequate volume to maintain the interest and experience of their board members. Funding may also be problematic, because hospitals rarely have large federal grants as a source of indirect funds.

IRB members are usually chosen from the medical staff and serve as a condition of staff privileges. There is rarely a dedicated staff on such review boards. Rather, staff is usually appropriated from other positions. These review boards usually have a solid knowledge of the local context and may surpass all other models in firsthand knowledge of the investigator and of community attitudes. This may be an especially important benefit when investigator diligence is in question. However, conflicts of various kinds may abound. Accountability is either to the president of the medical staff or the hospital administrator. Of these, the president of the medical staff is usually preferable to physician-investigators, but the hospital administrator controls the funds available for the review board. In the case of large multispecialty clinics and managed care organizations, there may be a vice president for operations or administration as the final authority.

These review boards are also accountable to the FDA and sometimes to the OHRP—for example, if there are large oncology practices located in an area where NCI studies are conducted. Funding, if any, is usually provided from general funds of the institution.

Private

This category is quite diverse and includes both for-profit and not-for-profit entities. The reporting structures are quite different and the review boards may not be subject to the same regulatory oversight as conventional boards unless the research involves regulated articles, in which case the FDA is the regulatory authority. The OHRP is rarely involved with these review boards because the research they review does not commonly have federal funding. This category includes companies that maintain in-house boards to review research conducted only within their facilities. Examples of such research include a pharmaceutical company with a dedi-

cated Phase I facility, or a device manufacturer that needs to evaluate a reported malfunction of a marketed device.

These facilities often recruit employees as research participants for these studies. If the product is not regulated by the FDA, it may fall outside the guidelines and regulations requiring research review. The company may nevertheless want IRB review for its own corporate oversight. These situations usually occur in companies with regulated products. The review board members tend to be employees without an outside member. They are responsible to the director of compliance or some other officer in midmanagement. Funding comes from corporate sources.

There are many small private foundations that receive funds from other private foundations. If their research projects fall outside the federal regulatory arena—that is, if the projects are neither federally funded nor aimed at winning federal regulatory approval—they may be totally unregulated. In these circumstances, if an IRB exists it may be the only oversight for the research, and it would be dependent upon the trustees of the foundation for authority to restrict certain behaviors. Therefore, unless the foundation is committed to the mission of human participant protection, the IRB is unlikely to prevail if the investigator resists its oversight recommendations.

Frequently, a small panel is set up to review the research of a single investigator or a small sponsor. These panels may be composed according to federal regulations and are generally responsible to the FDA. They are rarely attached to an institution and they tend to employ a fee-for-service funding model. Many examples of this model exist in and around the small device community.

Discussion of the U.S. System

It is apparent that U.S. IRBs can take many forms. Virtually all review committees in the United States conform to the regulations of the OHRP and the FDA. These regulations set minimum standards but are subject to much variation. Review boards most commonly have more than the five members required by the regulations, and it is not uncommon for IRBs to have 18, 20, or, in one case, 36 members. In the case of the 36-member board, it is necessary to have 19 members present for the entire meeting—an impractical and unusual event.

The common rationale for a large number of members is broad representation of the institutional departments and the availability of multiple medical specialties. Such IRBs frequently have trouble gaining a quorum and are often cited on audit for making decisions without a quorum. A better practice is to have fewer members who are faithful attendees and to have a broad roster of alternate members who can be called for special expertise when needed. The use of consulting, nonvoting members is acceptable when additional expertise is needed. It is probably not wise or practical to attempt complete coverage of all needs within the voting membership of the panel.

Research Review in Other Nations

When U.S. investigators conduct research in another country, a local board may review that research. These research ethics committees, as they are often called, may follow guidance from the World Health Organization (WHO),[11] the Council for International

Organizations of Medical Sciences (CIOMS)[21] or the International Conference on Harmonisation (ICH).[22] There are strong similarities among these various guidance documents; all were loosely based on U.S. regulations, and various members of the U.S. human participant protection community assisted in their development. The goal was to have as much common ground with U.S. regulations as possible and still include representation of the local cultures. However, these boards may not conform to all U.S. regulations and consequently may be supplemented with additional review by a U.S. IRB.

Canada adheres to ICH guidelines and to its own Tri-Council Policy Statement.[23] Most European countries have adopted the ICH model, although France and Germany have added unique local requirements. Both countries require research sponsors to provide insurance to cover research-related injuries. France also requires review by a French board.

It is important to recognize, however, that research ethics committees in most countries provide only recommendations and thus do not have the same authority as U.S. IRBs. United States boards have the authority to stop research by withdrawing approval or suspending the investigator. No such authority is vested in review committees in most other countries. Likewise, there may be little or no enforcement of research ethics committee review standards, committee composition, or operating procedures. In most cases, guidance emanating from the review board is strictly advisory to the investigator, who may choose to disregard it. If we have learned anything from a quarter century of experience, it is that regulatory enforcement is necessary for the protection of human research participants.

The Scandinavian countries use central committees and regional review. Review is generally limited to the initial protocol without continuing oversight. Regulatory oversight is limited. Denmark's system is unique in that its membership is composed entirely of nonscientists.

Many developing countries also have adopted either the CIOMS or ICH guidelines. Usually each government makes amendments to these international guidelines to better represent the local culture. Rarely do they meet the requirements of the U.S. FDA, but they are nonetheless valuable adjuncts to U.S. review of international research. Dual review—by a U.S.-based IRB in addition to the local review—is often conducted if the research has a U.S. sponsor.

The United Kingdom began with only local, institutionally based IRBs. That system resulted in lack of timeliness and consistency. Complaints from investigators and sponsors led to the establishment of regional boards. Local boards were then able to accept the review provided by the regional board or to conduct their own additional review. This process led to even greater delays because most local boards did not accept the central review. Local review is still dominant in the United Kingdom.[24,25]

Many Asian countries are making rapid progress in meeting both international and U.S. standards. Thailand, for example, has an aggressive program of IRB member training and is evaluating performance of review committees through a nonregulatory process. Taiwan, Korea, Malaysia, and the Peoples' Republic of China are all moving to codify regulations similar to those in the United States. It is likely that regulatory oversight may be adopted in these countries because they are on a path of harmonization with the U.S. FDA.

Singapore began with a single, state-run IRB model that reviewed all research conducted there. Most clinical trials conducted in Singapore are ultimately subjected to U.S. FDA review for drug or device approval. Singapore authorities are currently redeveloping their system to an institutional model, in which IRBs are based at individual research institutions.

Form and Function of IRBs

Until recently, there had been little in the way of systematic study of IRB models. Although public interest in the ethical review of medical research began in the 1970s, interest in the process and procedures of ethical review was not apparent until the late 1990s. As injuries occurring during the research process became front-page fare in the nation's newspapers and recruitment for study participants became more aggressive, Congress prompted the General Accounting Office (now the Government Accountability Office, GAO) to study the regulation of clinical research in 1996.[26] This was followed by a thorough assessment by the DHHS Office of the Inspector General (OIG) in 1998–2000.[1,27–29] Interviewing many IRB members, OIG investigators produced a survey that contains the most objective information available on the form and function of the various kinds of ethics review boards that exist in the United States. Recommendations for improvement of the system followed.[30]

In its reports, the OIG catalogued perceived flaws in the system and in 1998 it recommended remedial actions. In 2000 the secretary of the DHHS commissioned the Institute of Medicine (IOM) to thoroughly study the problem and to make consensus-based recommendations. This report was issued in 2002 and represents an attempt by the scientific and medical communities to inform and shape any remedial action.[31]

The initial part of the IOM report focused on accreditation. The IOM panel's interest stimulated two national bodies, the National Committee for Quality Assurance (NCQA)[32] and the Association for the Accreditation of Human Research Protection Programs (AAHRPP),[20] to set up systems of accreditation for the nation's system of human subjects protection. So tepid was the response that only three IRBs were accredited during the first year, all by the AAHRPP. The NCQA later joined forces with the Joint Commission on Accreditation of Healthcare Organizations[33] to form the Partnership for Human Research Protections. However, this effort was subsequently abandoned—the Partnership for Human Research Protections was dissolved Nov. 15, 2005—leaving the AAHRPP as the sole accreditation body.

The IOM attempted to assess what the effect of the accreditation process would be on the performance of the national system and concluded that the process would be helpful in extending their resources and would improve consistency between IRBs. Many others believe the process and attendant public notice will be beneficial to human participant protection. In 2006, approximately 200 institutions were said to be undergoing the preliminary self-assessment process as a prelude to accreditation.

The IOM encouraged the adoption of systems that had been shown to work in practice and to follow that with continuous quality improvement. These recommendations are as close to consensus as we have come in the development of a standard approach to the IRB function. The IOM rightly stressed the importance of an institutional culture that facilitates ethical behavior by the IRB members, clinical investigators, and other study personnel. The IOM report outlined four specific conditions that should exist: accountability, resources, ethics education, and transparency in process.

Accountability

It is apparent that the structure of the parent organization is important and that leadership is vital. The responsibility for functional human participant protection systems rests at the highest level of the institution, and this is true whether the institution is a university, a government, a hospital, or a corporation. The lines of authority should be clearly drawn, and each member of the human participant protection systems team should know his or her responsibilities and authority within the institution. IRBs are accountable to the volunteer research participants whose interests they represent. IRBs are also accountable to the institution that has entrusted them to provide the protections that the institution has assured the OHRP will be provided. In a way, they are also accountable to the investigators whose research they review. This level of accountability involves fairness in review, confidentiality of documents, adherence to federal regulations, and full disclosure to the prospective research participant in the consent document. Under FDA regulations, it is the investigator's responsibility to assure that the IRB is compliant with the FDA regulations, whereas under OHRP regulations, it is the institution's responsibility to assure IRB compliance. This is one of several areas in the regulations in which there are differences between the OHRP and FDA regulations.

Resources

Both the GAO and the OIG reports lamented the lack of resources provided to IRBs to do their work. Resource allocation usually comes from the top of an organization. Without resources, the very best IRB will soon founder. Adequate resources should include provision for well-trained staff members to assist the IRB in assembling materials for review. Staff should provide assistance with follow-up and tracking of approved protocols including, but not limited to, adverse events. United States regulations require at least annual review of approved research, but much research would benefit from more frequent scrutiny. Electronic systems can be used to perform tracking tasks and, if properly validated, much of the regulatory documentation as well.

Ethics Education

Many observers of the human participant protection process have cited inadequate research ethics training among those involved in research and its review. Certainly this training should be a part of the early preparation of career researchers and should be in depth. There has been a lack of national attention to structured systems for the production of well-trained clinical investigators. On-the-job training has too often replaced the structured research fellowships so common in earlier years. Pharmaceutical and device companies have recruited as clinical investigators many internists and family physicians who may or may not have been adequately prepared for conducting clinical research. A more structured approach to investigator training would be beneficial to the research enterprise. The University of Rochester implemented such a program to provide formalized training in the fundamentals of protocol writing, statistics, and regulatory adherence in the late 1990s. Completion of this core curriculum was required prior to beginning research activity. With wide acceptance, this kind of program could be a prerequisite for engaging in clinical investigation.

Bioethics has been a buzzword in research for over a quarter of a century and yet it has only recently been integrated into biomedical and behavioral medicine curricula. Regrettably, many premedical programs no longer require fundamental training in ethics, humanities, and history. It is therefore necessary to offer remedial training during the busy years of medical education. Most researchers will benefit from additional training in ethics, especially as it relates to research, early in their training. Solid programs in medical ethics should be in place and required for practicing physicians as well as researchers. Many supplemental courses are offered online.[34-45] NIH-funded researchers are required to complete a bioethics primer prior to receiving funding.

Many IRB members will not be scientifically trained and may lack even a basic knowledge of bioethics. It is incumbent on institutions to provide training for IRB members prior to board participation. A program of continuing education for members should be ongoing. There are many resources available, both web-based and in written format, that can provide training materials for members. Such training is recognized as best practice but not yet widely adopted.

Transparency

Transparency in the conduct of research is no longer optional. Research participants must be aware of the protocol and their role in its execution. The institution must cultivate and maintain an open interaction with the local community about research activities and the process of human participant protection. Key to this latter point is the importance of community members on the IRB. These members serve as a powerful conduit to the community, both to provide insight to the institution and to carry awareness of the research process to the local community. They will serve the institution well in times of tragedy or public relations debacles by providing an "outsider's" verification of the university processes. They also help scientific members of the IRB recognize problems in understanding consent documents, because scientists are often unaware that consent form language can be difficult and not readily comprehensible. Active lay members can correct this problem if allowed to participate as equals in the discussion. Both the OIG report and the IOM recommendations stress the need for greater numbers of nonaffiliated IRB members on the grounds that nonaffiliated, lay members provide greater transparency. Both recommended that 25 percent of panel members be nonaffiliated. Western IRB, a large independent organization, has traditionally constructed entire review boards of community members.[34]

Placing nonaffiliated, lay members on IRBs requires a structured training process to ensure that members are knowledgeable about the regulatory and ethical basis of the work, their responsibility to human participants, and the process of clinical research. These members provide important balance for institutional conflicts of interest. The institution should provide indemnification for legal liability because IRB members are sometimes named as defendants in lawsuits. The shift to more community members is vitally important to the success of any human participant protection program, because such members more fully represent research participants in their knowledge base and attitudes toward research risk and benefit.

Conclusion

It will be apparent to the reader that there are many models of IRBs and that structure can foster good decision making or perpetuate poor decision making. Identifying where hidden conflicts may exist or may arise will permit selection of a model that best fits the need. Strict accountability of all participants, adequate resource allocation, good educational programs, transparency in deliberations, and fierce independence in decision making by review board members will serve us all well.

References

1. Office of Inspector General, Department of Health and Human Services. *Institutional Review Boards: The Emergence of Independent Boards.* OEI-01–97–00192. Washington, D.C.: DHHS; 1998. [Online] June 1998. Available: http://oig.hhs.gov/oei/reports/oei-01–97–00192.pdf.

2. U.S. Congress. Kefauver-Harris Drug Amendments of 1962, Pub. L. No. 87–781, 76 Stat 780, 87th Congress (codified in scattered sections of 21 U.S.C.), October 10, 1962.

3. Faden RR, Beauchamp TL, with King NMP. *A History and Theory of Informed Consent.* New York, N.Y.: Oxford University Press; 1986:205–15.

4. Rothman DJ. *Strangers at the Bedside: A History of How Law and Bioethics Transformed Medical Decision Making.* New York, N.Y.: Basic Books; 1992:85–94.

5. Masters WH, Johnson VE. *Human Sexual Response.* Philadelphia, Penn.: Lippincott, Williams & Wilkins; 1966.

6. *New York Times* Aug. 26, 1970:20.

7. Office of the Secretary, Department of Health, Education, and Welfare. 45 CFR 46: Protection of Human Subjects. *Federal Register* 1974; 39(105):18913–20.

8. Department of Health and Human Services, Food and Drug Administration. Title 21 (Food and Drugs), Code of Federal Regulations, Part 50 (Protection of Human Subjects). [Online] April 1, 2006. Available: http://www.access.gpo.gov/nara/cfr/waisidx_06/21cfr50_06.html.

9. Department of Health and Human Services, Food and Drug Administration. Title 21 (Food and Drugs), Code of Federal Regulations, Part 56 (Institutional Review Boards). [Online] April 1, 2006. Available: http://www.access.gpo.gov/nara/cfr/waisidx_06/21cfr56_06.html.

10. Department of Health and Human Services, National Institutes of Health, and Office for Human Research Protections. The Common Rule, Title 45 (Public Welfare), Code of Federal Regulations, Part 46 (Protection of Human Subjects). [Online] June 23, 2005. Available: http://www.hhs.gov/ohrp/humansubjects/guidance/45cfr46.htm.

11. World Health Organization. *Operational Guidelines for Ethics Committees That Review Biomedical Research.* Geneva, Switzerland: WHO; 2000. [Online] Available: http://www.who.int/tdr/publications/publications/pdf/ethics.pdf.

12. Christian MC, Goldberg JL, Killen J, et al. A central institutional review board for multi-institutional trials. *New England Journal of Medicine* 2002;346:1405–8.

13. National Cancer Institute, in consultation with OHRP. The Central Institutional Review Board Initiative. [Online] Available: http://www.ncicirb.org/.

14. Serio JC, Tichner JB Jr., Dilley ME. *State-by-State Clinical Trial Requirements Reference Guide.* Centreville, Va.: Barnett Educational Services; 2004.

15. Forster D. Independent institutional review boards. *Seton Hall Law Review* 2002;32:513–23.

16. Scharke CC. Memorandum to Assurance Branch Staff: Update—Suitability of a Designated Institutional Review Board (IRB). [Online] February 4, 1997. Available: http://www.hhs.gov/ohrp/humansubjects/guidance/ind-irb.htm.

17. Loh ED. AAMC Survey: Use of Centralized Institutional Review Boards. Presentation to the Institute of Medicine Clinical Research Roundtable, Washington, D.C.; June 26, 2003.

18. Koski G, Aungst J, Kupersmith J, Getz K, Rimoin D. Cooperative research ethics review boards: A win-win solution? *IRB: Ethics and Human Research* 2005;27(3):1–7.

19. Lemmens T, Freedman B. Ethics review for sale? Conflict of interest and commercial research review boards. *Milbank Quarterly* 2000; 78:547–84.

20. Association for the Accreditation of Human Research Protection Programs, Inc. [Online] Available: http://www.aahrpp.org/.

21. Council for International Organizations of Medical Sciences in collaboration with the World Health Organization. *International Ethical Guidelines for Biomedical Research Involving Human Subjects.* Geneva, Switzerland: CIOMS and WHO; 2002. [Online] November 2002. Available: http://www.cioms.ch/frame_guidelines_nov_2002.htm.

22. International Conference on Harmonisation of Technical Requirements for Registration of Pharmaceuticals for Human Use. *The ICH Harmonised Tripartite Guideline—Guideline for Good Clinical Practice.* Geneva: ICH; 1996. [Online] Available: http://www.ich.org/LOB/media/MEDIA482.pdf.

23. Canadian Institutes of Health Research, the Natural Sciences and Engineering Research Council, and the Social Sciences and Humanities Research Council. *Tri-Council Policy Statement: Ethical Conduct for Research Involving Humans.* [Online] 1998 (with 2000, 2002, and 2005 amendments). Available: http://www.pre.ethics.gc.ca/english/policystatement/policystatement.cfm.

24. Tully J, Ninis N, Booy R, Viner R. The new system of review by multicentre research ethics committees: Prospective study. *British Medical Journal* 2003;320:1179–82.

25. Wood A, Grady C, Emanuel EJ. Regional ethics organizations for protection of human research participants. *Nature Medicine* 2004;10: 1283–8.

26. General Accounting Office. *Scientific Research: Continued Vigilance Critical to Protecting Human Subjects.* GAO/HEHS-96–72. Washington, D.C.: GAO; 1996. [Online] March 1996. Available: http://www.gao.gov/archive/1996/he96072.pdf.

27. Office of Inspector General, Department of Health and Human Services. *Institutional Review Boards: Their Role in Reviewing Approved Research.* OEI-01–97–00190. Washington, D.C.: DHHS; 1998. [Online] June 1998. Available: http://oig.hhs.gov/oei/reports/oei-01–97–00190.pdf.

28. Office of Inspector General, Department of Health and Human Services. *Institutional Review Boards: Promising Approaches.* OEI-01–91–00191. Washington, D.C.: DHHS; 1998. [Online] June 1998. Available: http://oig.hhs.gov/oei/reports/oei-01–97–00191.pdf.

29. Office of Inspector General, Department of Health and Human Services. *Institutional Review Boards: A Time for Reform.* OEI-01–97–00193. Washington, D.C.: DHHS; 1998. [Online] June 1998. Available: http://oig.hhs.gov/oei/reports/oei-01–97–00193.pdf.

30. Office of Inspector General, Department of Health and Human Services. *Protecting Human Research Subject—Status of Recommendations.* OEI-01–97–00197. Washington, D.C.: DHHS; 2000. [Online] April 2000. Available: http://oig.hhs.gov/oei/reports/oei-01–97–00197.pdf.

31. Institute of Medicine. *Responsible Research: A Systems Approach to Protecting Research Participants.* Washington, D.C.: National Academies Press; 2002.

32. National Committee for Quality Assurance. [Online] Available: http://www.ncqa.org/.

33. Joint Commission on Accreditation of Healthcare Organizations. [Online] Available: http://www.jcaho.org/.

34. Western Institutional Review Board. Olympia, Wash. [Online] Available: http://www.wirb.com.

35. National Cancer Institute. Human Participant Protections Education for Research Teams. [Online] Available: http://cme.cancer.gov/clinicaltrials/learning/humanparticipant-protections.asp.

36. National Institutes of Health. Protecting Human Subjects. [Online] Available: http://ohsr.od.nih.gov/cbt/.

37. Office of Research Administration, University of California, Irvine. On-Line UCI Research Tutorials. [Online] Available: http://tutorials.rgs.uci.edu/.

38. University of Minnesota. Informed Consent. [Online] Available: http://www.research.umn.edu/consent/.

39. Indiana University. Education on the Protection of Human Research Participants. [Online] Available: http://www.indiana.edu/~rcr/.

40. Indiana University, South Bend. Education Requirement for Researchers Using Human Subjects. [Online] Available: http://www.iusb.edu/~sbres/irb/test.html.

41. Jaeb Center for Health Research. Tampa, Fl. Investigator Education for the Protection of Human Research Subjects With HIPAA Privacy Rule Component. [Online] Available: http://ethics.jaeb.org.

42. Brookhaven National Laboratory. Ethics and Research. [Online] Available: http://training.bnl.gov/course/Ethics/index/frame.htm.

43. University of California, Los Angeles. UCLA Online Training: Protection Human Research Subjects Training and Certification for Medical and Social-Behavioral Sciences. [Online] Available: http://training.arc.ucla.edu.

44. Office for Health Research Protections, DHHS. Human Subject Assurance Training. [Online] Available: http://ohrp-ed.od.nih.gov/.

45. San Diego State University, Graduate and Research Affairs. Human Subjects Tutorial. [Online] Available: http://gra.sdsu.edu/irb/tutorial/.

Marjorie A. Speers

Evaluating the Effectiveness of Institutional Review Boards

Everyone who is part of the research enterprise—investigators, institution officials, government agencies, sponsors, and institutional review boards (IRBs)—has an idea about the way IRBs are supposed to function. Although there is no agreed upon set of criteria to measure the function of IRBs, there is consensus that IRBs do not function as well as interested parties would like.[1-5] Complaints overshadow compliments of the IRB: It takes a long time to get a protocol approved; IRBs that review the same multisite protocol require different changes at least to the consent document; IRBs miss issues important to research participant protection or regulatory compliance; IRBs cannot function as they aspire to because they lack sufficient resources; there is no institutional support of the IRB process; and so on. Rarely do we hear positive things about IRBs, such as that an IRB identified several important deficiencies in the protocols, or an IRB's review led to a better designed research study, or an IRB identified risks that the investigators had not considered, or that investigators are glad the IRB is there to help keep them out of regulatory trouble. Yet when an IRB functions well, it not only enhances the protection of research participants but also supports investigators in their research endeavors, both of which contribute to the public's trust in the research enterprise.[6,7]

Definition of the IRB

The idea of having committees to review research dates back to the 1960s, when the then director of the National Institutes of Health (NIH), James Shannon, required independent review of research by a committee of the investigator's "institutional associates," but offered virtually no guidance on the content of the review.[8] A couple of years later, and in response to debates about the Willowbrook State School experiments, the NIH developed further guidance for review committees, in the form of its so-called Yellow Book,[9] and finally codified the requirements for review committees in regulations in 1974.[10] These research review committees became known as institutional review boards (see Chapters 7 and 50).

The name of these review boards reveals how the research community thinks about them. Although IRBs are charged with determining the ethical justifiability of a proposed research study, some critics have argued that calling them institutional review boards indicates they are designed to protect the institution, not the prospective research participants. The risk-averse behavior of IRBs observed in recent years, and the upsurge of atrociously long and complicated consent documents, give support to the ultimately incorrect belief that IRBs function primarily to protect institutions.

Additionally, the term *institutional* reflects an intention that the locus of review should be at the institution conducting the research. This concept was reinforced by the National Commission for the Protection of Human Subjects of Biomedical and Behavioral Research, which argued that the local institution was in the best position to know the investigators and the community from which prospective research participants would be enrolled into studies[5] (see Chapter 14). The commissioners did not consider the inherent conflict of interest that IRBs would have between protecting research participants and protecting the institution. Only recently has this difference between single institution and central IRBs been raised.

Composition and Responsibilities of the IRB

The functions of the IRB are defined in the U.S. federal regulations for the protection of research participants at Title 45 Code of Federal Regulation Part 46 (known as 45 CFR 46), for the Department of Health and Human Services (DHHS),[11] and at Title 21 Code of Federal Regulations Parts 50 and 56, for the Food and Drug Administration (FDA).[12] (Further citations of the regulations will refer only to those of the DHHS.)

Composition

Whereas function generally relates to what an entity does, here it is also relevant to define function in terms of structure, because the composition of an IRB is assumed to directly affect the quality of the ethical analysis it performs. For example, it would be difficult for an IRB to properly consider the needs and perspectives of adults with impaired decision making if there were no one on the IRB with expertise or experience with this group.

The federal regulations at 45 CFR 46.107(a) require that "at least five members with varying backgrounds to promote complete and adequate review of research of research activities commonly conducted by the institution" sit on the IRB.[11] The role of the IRB is indirectly defined in the regulations: The IRB should be constituted in such a way as to promote the respect for its advice and counsel in safeguarding the rights and welfare of research participants (45 CFR 46.107(a)).[11] Although the regulators offered no definition of *respect,* it appears that they intended the IRB to have a form of legitimacy in the eyes of the institution and from the community. The IRB derives legitimacy within the institution by being sufficiently qualified through the experience and expertise of its members and legitimacy in the community through its diversity—including consideration of race, gender, and cultural background—and sensitivity to community attitudes. The regulations go on to require that no IRB consist of all men or all women, and that IRBs have at least one member whose primary concerns are in scientific areas, at least one member whose primary concerns are in nonscientific areas, and at least one member who is not otherwise affiliated with the institution (this requirement extends to immediate family members; 45 CFR 46.107(b)(c)(d)).[11] Finally, no IRB member who has conflicting interest may participate in the initial or continuing review of a proposed study, except to provide information requested by the remaining IRB members (45 CFR 46.107(c)).[11] A quorum for the IRB to conduct its business does not require that members unaffiliated with the institution be present (45 CFR 46.108(b)).[11] Further, there is no requirement that a layperson who represents the community from which the research participants are drawn, serve on the IRB. In the end, it rests upon the IRB and institution to compose a properly constituted board that will provide a meaningful review of the ethics of each research study.

Assuming the regulatory requirements pertaining to composition have moral relevance and relate to measuring the effectiveness of IRBs in protecting research participants, potential measures for evaluating whether IRBs represent the perspectives of the community are the number and presence at meetings of nonscientists, individuals who represent prospective research participants, and unaffiliated members, as well as the presence at IRB meetings of members who have expertise about certain populations such as children, adults with decision-making impairments, or other vul-

nerabilities that might subject individuals to undue influence when such research is reviewed. More refined measures would include whether such individuals participate in IRB deliberations or are selected as primary or secondary reviewers. Another measure is whether conflicts of interest are disclosed, and if so, whether members with conflicting interests leave the room during deliberations and voting.

Responsibilities

What IRBs must do is defined in the U.S. federal regulations and by the Office for Human Research Protections in DHHS (OHRP, formerly the Office for Protection from Research Risks in NIH), the FDA, institutions, and by the IRBs themselves. Tables 52.1 and 52.2 list typical IRB responsibilities. In Table 52.1, responsibilities are separated into two columns to distinguish those that are required under U.S. regulations and those that have been delegated to the IRBs, de facto, by agency guidance. According to the federal regulations (45 CFR 46.109, 46.110, and 46.111),[11] the business of the IRB is to conduct initial and continuing review of research. The review may be conducted by the full board or by using the expedited procedure, in which the IRB chair or a designee who is an experienced IRB member reviews the protocol.

The federal regulations are silent on who has the responsibility to decide whether an activity is research involving participants. This responsibility is generally shared between the IRB and investigators when on a daily basis investigators decide whether an activity is research involving human-subject participants or something else, such as patient care, quality assurance, or program evaluation. However, when an investigator is unclear, the IRB generally has the authority to make a final decision.

Once an activity is determined to be research involving participants, it is generally a responsibility of the IRB to determine whether the research qualifies as exempt from the federal regulations, and therefore, exempt from review by the IRB. Although the regulations do not state that this is the responsibility of IRBs, the responsibility is often delegated to the IRB because guidance from OHRP states that investigators should not make such determinations.[13]

Table 52.2 describes federal regulatory requirements of institutions. These responsibilities are generally delegated to the IRB. In addition to carrying out their primary function of research review, IRBs have a number of other tasks. Institutions that receive federal funding must have an assurance of compliance, now known as a federalwide assurance—a document in which the institution pledges to follow the federal regulations for protecting research

Table 52.1

Requirements in Federal Regulations Versus Those by OHRP

Requirements in Federal Regulations	Requirements by OHRP
• Initial review and approval of research	• Research determinations
• Primary reviewer systems	• Exemption determinations
• Expedited procedures for review	• Relevant materials for review
• Informed consent	
• Notification of investigators	
• Continuing review	
• Records retention	

Table 52.2

Federal Requirements of Organizations That Are Often
Imposed on IRBs

- Assurance of compliance
- IRB roster
- Procedures the IRB will follow for conducting initial and continuing review of research and reporting its findings to the investigator and the institution
- Procedures for determining which projects require review more frequently than annually
- Procedures for prompt reporting of unanticipated problems involving risk to subjects or others
- Procedures for prompt reporting of serious or continuing noncompliance
- Procedures for prompt reporting of suspensions and terminations
- Procedures for verification by a third party of no material changes since the last IRB review

participants in federally funded research.[14] The IRB office is generally responsible for completing the document, keeping it current, and filing it with OHRP. As part of the assurance, IRBs must supply copies of their rosters complete with information about board members.[15]

IRBs also are delegated responsibility for developing the procedures they will follow when conducting initial and continuing review of research, determining when research studies require more frequent than annual continuing review, and reporting their findings and actions to investigators and the institution. At 45 CFR 46.103(5),[11] the federal regulations require that institutions have written procedures for promptly reporting unanticipated problems involving risk to participants or others, serious or continuing noncompliance, and suspensions and terminations. These three requirements are more complex than it might appear. Recently, OHRP released draft guidance on one of these requirements—defining and reporting unanticipated problems involving risk to participants or others.[16] Each requires not only a definition of the time frame for reporting and to whom results should be reported, but also a definition of each type of event, the process for determining whether the event is legitimate, the actions the IRBs might take, and more.

An additional responsibility rarely noticed in the regulations at 45 CFR 46.103(4)[11] is that the institution must develop procedures describing the circumstances under which verification by a third party of no material changes since the last IRB review is required. IRBs have added all these functions to their duties.

The movement toward delegating institutional responsibilities to the IRB makes sense because these responsibilities are germane to the IRB's primary function. Many institutions and IRBs did not have written policies and procedures for these functions until recently. Beginning in the 1990s, OPRR (now OHRP) restricted or suspended assurances of compliance because institutions either lacked these procedures or had ones that were less than fully developed.[5,17] It is only within the past several years that many institutions have developed these procedures. Current OHRP determination letters indicate that some IRBs are still in need of developing these procedures.[18–21]

Finally, other responsibilities are sometimes added to the IRB's portfolio of responsibilities. These responsibilities do not exist in

the principal research regulations but have been promulgated through DHHS Final Guidance and NIH Guidance regarding disclosure and management of investigator conflicts of interest (COI) and education of investigators. With respect to managing COI of investigators, many institutions have separate COI committees. DHHS recommends that there should be communication between the IRB and the institutional COI committee. IRBs should see the determinations of the COI committee and review conflicts to ensure that they do not adversely affect the protection of research participants.[21]

It was not until 2001 that any type of education in participants' rights was required of investigators. At that time, NIH made it mandatory for all grant applications that principal investigators and research staff were certified to have received training in research participant protections.[22] The implementation of this requirement generally falls to the IRB or to the research oversight office within the institution. Although this is a positive step toward enhancing the knowledge of investigators, it requires that IRBs develop (or adapt) an educational training program for investigators, monitor training, and issue certificates. Surprisingly, there is still no regulatory requirement for IRB chairs, members, or staff. Nevertheless, it appears from numerous institutional web sites that IRBs offer training to members and staff.

The propensity to place more and more responsibilities on IRBs continues. Legislation introduced in Congress in 2004 and 2005 proposed that IRBs act as the principal site for monitoring clinical trial registration.[23,24] Were these bills passed by Congress and signed into law, IRBs would have to certify that certain clinical trials, as defined in the legislation, are registered in a clinical trials registry operated by the NIH before the IRB could approve the protocol. The relevance of this responsibility to the IRBs' primary function of ethics review is unclear. Moreover, it would be an unnecessary burden for IRBs that should lie with sponsors or the lead investigator.

In summary, the functions and responsibilities of the IRB are prescribed in federal regulations governing the protection of research participants. Although IRBs' primary function is to conduct an ethics review of the proposed research study, they have many additional functions. In recent years, there has been a trend to identify the IRB as the centerpiece for protecting research participants, placing all responsibilities for protection with the IRB regardless of whether this is a strategically effective decision for human research protection. This trend is being reversed somewhat by institutions adopting the framework of a human research protection program whereby they define the roles of the organization, investigators, research staff, and the IRB—and in which more often than not they recognize the obligations of other entities for protecting research participants. This is particularly the case with investigator and institutional conflict of interest and management of noncompliance.[1,25]

Measures to Assess IRB Effectiveness

Although the function of IRBs has been at the forefront of discussions about the protection of research participants, few studies have examined their effectiveness. Attention was drawn to IRBs in the late 1990s when the U.S. General Accounting Office (now the Government Accountability Office) and the Office of Inspector General in DHHS released many reports that described IRBs as overwhelmed and overworked, understaffed, and not appropriately composed to review research studies.[26-34]

Several studies have documented inconsistencies among IRBs in the time it takes to review a study,[35] in the number and types of revisions required by the IRB,[35-43] and in the approval of research involving children.[39,44,45] Although concluding that IRBs are inconsistent and add burden to the oversight system, none has differentiated between legitimate inconsistency due to the differences in the local setting or in state law and inconsistency that results from lack of knowledge of the federal regulations, inexperience, or risk-averse behavior. These studies are nonetheless important because they make clear why investigators are often frustrated with the IRB process.

Given the paucity of studies that have examined effectiveness of IRBs, I propose five general categories of potential measures of IRB effectiveness. The first two—protection of participants and compliance—stem from the federal regulations that govern IRBs. The next three—efficiency, investigator satisfaction, and sponsor satisfaction—derive from any user-based system.

Protection of Research Participants

Simple, cost-effective measures of participant protection can be evaluated using information found in protocol files and minutes of IRB meetings. The Belmont Report[46] and the federal research regulations lead us to look at four general types of protection to be measured and assessed: informed consent, including recruitment methods; risks and potential benefits; selection of research participants; and additional protections for those who are deemed vulnerable.

Informed Consent

Much attention is paid to the consent process and to its documentation, with an unfortunately greater emphasis placed on the latter.[5,47] This misplaced emphasis is, in part, driven by the federal regulations that strictly require a written, signed consent document, as opposed to the generic requirements of a consent process. The consent process should provide sufficient opportunity for a potential participant to consider whether to participate in the research, should minimize coercion; should provide information in an understandable language; and it should include no exculpatory language. Further, when OHRP cites IRBs for informed consent violations, the citations have been based on findings from the documentation, rather than the process (see any OHRP determination letter citing informed consent violations as an example).[17,18]

Although many have argued for a better understanding of the consent process and some research has been funded in this area,[48] the conclusion of the few studies that have been conducted appears to be that it is extremely difficult to measure whether participants understand the parameters of the protocol in which they are being asked to enroll.[49] It is also unclear whether individuals make truly voluntary decisions to participate in research (see Chapter 59).

Measures that document that there was a consent process and that individuals agreed to participate in a study would provide some evidence that participants are protected. These would include documentation that a consent process was reviewed and approved by the IRB, including all the required elements of disclosure, and evidence that the IRB had considered whether any additional disclosure elements were appropriate for inclusion. When there is no consent process, there should be documentation that the IRB has approved a waiver according to the criteria in the federal regulations. When the IRB approves alterations to the consent process it should do so according to the federal regulatory criteria.

Other measures might be appropriate in special circumstances, such as the use of translators to administer consent, translated consent documents when the prospective study population includes non-English speakers, and the use of assent when children or adults with diminished decision-making capacity are involved in the research.

Risks and Potential Benefits

IRBs are required to assess the risks and potential benefits of a proposed study. This includes the risks and potential benefits for the prospective participants, as well as the value of the knowledge expected to be gained from the research. IRBs must also determine that risks are minimized and that they are reasonable in relation to the potential benefits. The federal regulations specify two criteria for determining that risks are minimized: (1) The research involves procedures that are consistent with sound research design and do not unnecessarily expose participants to risk; and (2) the research uses procedures already being performed on participants for diagnostic or treatment purposes. Unfortunately, however, the federal regulations provide almost no guidance on how IRBs should determine that risks are reasonable in relation to potential benefits. Some have proposed models for making such a determination, but few IRBs seem to follow an identifiable model.[5,50,51]

Measures used to assess IRB effectiveness might include documentation that the IRB asks about and considers risks involved in the research, including nonphysical risks, and that it evaluates the relationship between risks and potential benefits—in particular, that it evaluates risks versus the importance of the knowledge that would be gained from the study and versus the potential for direct benefit to research participants.

Selection of Research Participants

The U.S. federal regulations stipulate that the selection of participants must be equitable (45 CFR 46.111(3)).[11] In making this assessment, IRBs need to take into account the purpose of the research, the setting in which the research will occur, and the recruitment of individuals who are especially vulnerable to undue influence or coercion, such as children or adults with impaired decision-making capability.[52,53] At the level of the individual study, protection could be measured by determining whether the IRB considered the characteristics of the study population in terms of the purpose and the location of the research. As a protection issue, participant selection should ensure that the burdens and benefits of research are fairly distributed across populations. Protection could thus be measured by looking at whether the same community groups or hospital patients are recruited repeatedly for different research studies.

The criterion for determining equity in the selection of research participants is not straightforward because of the differences between an individual investigator-initiated study conducted once and at one site, an individual investigator-initiated study conducted either multiple times or in multiple settings, and a sponsor-initiated, multisite clinical trial.[54] Whereas equity judgments might seem clear in the most simple study design—an individual investigator-initiated study at one site—the clarity blurs as the study design becomes more complicated. For example, in a multisite clinical trial involving hundreds of sites, the overall selection of participants across all recruitment sites might be equitable: Individuals are selected from a large cross-section of society including adult men and women and all races/ethnicities. However, at an individual site, participants might be from only one racial, ethnic or gender group, or from one social class stratum. In such cases, equity at the local level would not exist, even though it might be achieved for the study as a whole.

Protection of Vulnerable Individuals

Vulnerability as defined by the federal regulations refers to individuals who are subject to undue influence or coercion to initiate or continue participation in a research study. Several groups are considered to be vulnerable: pregnant women and fetuses, children, prisoners, persons with mental disabilities, economically disadvantaged persons, and educationally disadvantaged persons. Additional regulatory protections exist, though not consistently, for pregnant women and fetuses (Subpart B), prisoners (Subpart C), and children (Subpart D) in the DHHS regulations.[11] Both the FDA and the Department of Education have codified Subpart D into their regulations for protecting research participants. And although the Department of Justice has additional regulations for research involving prisoners, they are different from those issued by DHHS. Although the regulations of the different governmental agencies generally provide similar protections, there are subtle differences requiring IRBs to be knowledgeable about the regulations that apply when a research study is subject to various regulations. For the other categories of vulnerable persons, the IRB is left to its own wisdom to ensure that additional protections are provided.

Additional protections generally fall into three distinct categories:

1. Vulnerable individuals should not be enrolled in research unless it is necessary. If the research can be carried out using those who are not vulnerable, then this should be done.
2. Additional regulatory requirements not relating to informed consent apply to such research. For example, when research involves pregnant women, IRBs must determine that when scientifically appropriate, studies involving pregnant non-human animals or studies with nonpregnant women have been conducted and provide data for assessing potential risks to pregnant women and fetuses. As another example, IRBs can approve research involving prisoners or children only when it falls into one of the permissible categories of research (see Subpart C for research involving prisoners and Subpart D for research involving children).[11] In addition, when carrying out research involving prisoners, IRBs must make certain protocol-specific determinations pertaining to payments, parole, and other factors in order to satisfy the demand for increased protections for prisoners.
3. Additional consent requirements are imposed. Children should provide assent in addition to parents giving their permission, 45 CFR 46.408(a); and adults with impaired decision-making capacity should also provide assent and a

legally authorized representative must give consent, 45 CFR 46.116.[11]

Documentation of these additional protections can be found in protocol files, minutes of IRB meetings, or in the IRB's policies and procedures (e.g., its definition of a legally authorized representative and statements about whether the institution conducts research involving vulnerable populations).

The systematic exclusion of vulnerable populations is not necessarily the measure of a well-functioning IRB. IRBs that routinely exclude children or prisoners because the regulatory requirements are too burdensome or that do so out of ignorance do not operate in the best interests of research participants. This issue was hotly debated in 2000 and 2001 at the time of the reauthorization of the pediatric studies provision in the FDA Modernization and Accountability Act, leading the FDA to adopt Subpart D of the DHHS regulations, the additional protections for children involved in research.[55,56]

Regulatory Compliance

The United States is one of the few countries that enforces its protection system for research through regulations. Institutions must comply with the federal regulations. If they do not, they risk losing their federal funding, having their research programs suspended, or having the FDA reject data that are submitted in support of licensing an investigational drug or device. For this reason, institutions and sponsors define IRB effectiveness as operating consistently with federal regulatory requirements.

OHRP and FDA determine institutional compliance by evidence of policies and procedures and by documentation of specific requirements. The former follows directly from regulations that require institutions to have certain written policies and procedures, such as reporting policies and procedures for serious or continuing noncompliance, suspensions and terminations of IRB approval, and unanticipated problems involving risk to research participants or others.[19–21,57–59] Very few studies have examined the findings of OHRP or FDA audits and no study has created a regulatory compliance index or commented on degree of compliance. This is not surprising because audits, whether for cause or not for cause, do not review an institution's full set of policies and procedures.

There are two possibilities for measuring compliance. The first is through evidence that an institution has the required written procedures. The second is documentation that is required of certain IRB actions. This can usually be found in protocol files and IRB minutes. Documentation of specific requirements occurs, for example, when the IRB waives or alters the consent process and records protocol-specific findings in support of the criteria for waiver or alteration; or when it records protocol-specific findings to justify the category of permissible research when children or prisoners are involved.

An aggregate measure of compliance could be formed based on regulatory requirements. For example, an aggregate measure of at least 18 IRB functions could be developed from Tables 52.1 and 52.2. Such a measure could be more granular, increasing the number of items in the overall index, or more basic, concentrating only a few key regulatory functions.

The obligation to protect research participants and comply with the federal regulations extends beyond the IRB or institution to the investigator and research staff. Thus, an IRB's effectiveness is dependent upon investigators and research staff adhering to the terms of the IRB-approved protocol and any other conditions of approval. As part of implementing either of the two measurement categories mentioned above, an institution or IRB might include data from routine auditing of ongoing research. In the past few years, many institutions and IRBs have initiated auditing functions to ensure that protocols are followed, and they are likely to have readily assessable data.

Efficiency

It is unlikely that an IRB would be judged effective if its operation were not efficient. One factor that seems to matter is the time it takes to review and render a decision on a protocol. Anecdotal evidence suggests that review times in the range of one month are considered efficient. This implies that the IRB is meeting more than once per month. A period of approval of three months or longer is long, especially for review of industry-sponsored research. However, time to approval is highly dependent upon factors outside the control of the IRB, such as the time it takes an investigator to respond to an IRB's review of a protocol. A more accurate measure of IRB efficiency would be the amount of time from receipt of protocol until initial review.

Other measures of efficiency are the use of the expedited procedure for review of research involving no more than minimal risk, use of exemptions for research that qualifies, and use of other review mechanisms such as subcommittees, scientific review committees, or prereview by IRB staff to reduce times for review.

Investigator Satisfaction With IRBs

The U.S. system of protection is based on trust and goodwill by all involved. The system works because all parties at least tacitly agree to follow the rules. IRBs not only require the support of their institutions, when they are institutionally based, but also depend upon the cooperation of investigators to be effective. No studies were identified that looked specifically at investigator satisfaction with the IRB process.

Key variables of concern to investigators are length of approval times, confidence that the IRB has the expertise to understand the proposed research, fairness of the IRB in conducting its reviews, and transparency of the review process.[5] Combining these variables into an outcome measure would enable researchers to determine investigator satisfaction. Further, investigators could be asked how satisfied they are with their IRBs.

Compliance with the IRB determinations and with the approved protocol is another potential measure of investigator satisfaction. To the extent that investigators perceive the IRB as fair and objective, it is more likely they will follow the protocol, the IRB's determinations, and the federal regulations.

Sponsor Satisfaction With IRBs

Sponsor satisfaction also provides a measure of IRB effectiveness. Sponsors have the ability to place research at sites where the IRB functions effectively and efficiently. Industry wants both. A quickly approved protocol that lacks appropriate protections for participants or is out of compliance with the regulations is harmful. Although no empirical studies were found that examined sponsor satisfaction with the IRB process, sponsor satisfaction can

be assessed by variables such as approval time and regulatory compliance.

Responsibility for Measuring the Effectiveness of the IRB

Like most responsibilities of oversight, ensuring the effectiveness of the IRB is a shared responsibility. Many parties have a vested interest in IRBs performing effectively, beginning with those who participate in research as subjects and extending to IRBs themselves, investigators and research staff, institutions, sponsors, and federal regulatory agencies. The question of who audits or collects data on effectiveness seems less important than each party being interested in being held accountable for the IRB's efficiency and effectiveness.

In the past, and even today, IRBs argue that they do not want to be the "police." But auditing investigators and research staff by reviewing protocol files, or monitoring the consent process (as is permitted by the federal regulations), is not police work if done from a perspective of quality improvement. Likewise, investigators and research staff should not view monitoring or auditing as policing when the goal is to identify and fix what is not working.

At least three arguments favor having a third party rather than the IRB measure its own effectiveness. First, IRBs are already overworked, and inclusion of an auditing function would be another addition to their long list of responsibilities. Second, IRBs might not be objective about their effectiveness, especially their willingness to look internally for problems. And finally, the ultimate responsibility for an IRB rests with the institution. Thus, a third party, such as a compliance office within the institution, might be a better vehicle for assessing IRBs' effectiveness.

Through mechanisms like the accreditation that requires organizations to have activities in place to monitor the effectiveness of the human research protection program,[25] the quality assurance program offered by OHRP,[59] and the general movement toward greater accountability for universities supported by the professional organizations, such as the Association of American Universities and the Association of American Medical Colleges,[60–62] institutions are implementing audit or monitoring programs that include the function of the IRB.

Conclusion

I have suggested that the definition and measurement of IRB effectiveness derives from the regulatory requirements placed on IRBs and the service component of IRBs. The major indicators and potential measures are summarized in Table 52.3.

This chapter clearly points to the need for further research on the assessment of IRBs. After 30 years of experience with IRBs, we know embarrassingly little about how they function—what variables influence effectiveness or what variables increase or decrease efficiency. Government reports in the late 1990s highlighted many of the problems with the current IRB system. However, no reports have proposed measures to assess IRB performance. The Association for the Accreditation of Human Research Protection Programs (AAHRPP) was awarded a grant in 2003 from the Centers for Disease Control and Prevention to develop performance indicators and measures for evaluating the effectiveness of accreditation

Table 52.3

Indicators of IRB Effectiveness and Their Outcome Measures

Indicators of IRB Effectiveness	Outcome Measures
Composition of the IRB	• Number of nonscientists on the IRB • Presence of nonscientists at meetings • Number of members who represent the view of the participant • Presence of members who represent the view of vulnerable individuals • Management of conflict of interest in IRB members
IRB responsibilities	Protection of research participants • Informed consent • Analysis of risks and potential benefits • Selection of research participants • Protection of vulnerable individuals Regulatory compliance • Institutional compliance • IRB compliance • Investigator/research staff compliance
Efficiency	• Time to initial review after submission to IRB • Use of the expedited procedure • Use of exemptions • Use of other review mechanisms
Satisfaction with the IRB	• By investigators and research staff • By sponsors

in improving research protections.[63] To my knowledge, this is the only federally funded project to develop such measures. Although the grant is focused on accreditation, it is related to the subject at hand because accreditation standards examine IRB function as it relates to the protection of research participants and regulatory compliance. Pilot tests of potential indicators and measures were to be complete in 2005 with final indicators and measures disseminated in 2006. But this one endeavor is not enough, echoing the call of the Institute of Medicine and the DHHS Secretary's Advisory Committee on Human Research Protection that the oversight system for protecting those enrolled in research must be evaluated with changes based on data.[1,64]

Federal regulations provide a foundation from which measures of IRB function can be developed. Evaluations can easily be conducted locally or nationally using data that already exist in protocol files, minutes of IRB meetings, policies and procedures, or internal audits. For the other measures, surveys conducted either locally or nationally would suffice. However, evaluations of IRBs are unlikely until there is an agreed upon set of measures.

References

1. Committee on Assessing the System for Protecting Human Research Participants, Institute of Medicine. *Responsible Research: A Systems Approach to Protecting Research Participants.* Washington, D.C.: National Academies Press; 2002.
2. Research Revitalization Act of 2002. S. 3060, 107th Congress, 2002.
3. Human Subject Research Protection Act of 2002. H.R. 46907, 107th Congress, 2002.
4. Emanuel EJ, Wood A, Fleischman A, et al. Oversight of human participants research: Identifying problems to evaluate reform proposals. *Annals of Internal Medicine* 2004;141:282–91.
5. National Bioethics Advisory Commission. *Ethical and Policy Issues in Research Involving Human Participants.* Bethesda, Md.: NBAC; 2001. [Online] August 2001. Available: http://www.georgetown.edu/research/nrcbl/nbac/human/overv011.pdf.
6. Kelch RP. Maintaining the public trust in clinical research. *New England Journal of Medicine* 2002;346:285–7.
7. Shalala D. Protecting research subjects—What must be done. *New England Journal of Medicine* 2000;343:808–10.
8. Public Health Service. Clinical investigations using human subjects. In: *Final Report, Supplemental Volume I.* Washington, D.C.: U.S. Governmental Printing Office; 1966:475–76.
9. Department of Health, Education, and Welfare. *The Institutional Guide to DHEW Policy on Protection of Human Subjects.* Washington, D.C.: U.S. Governmental Printing Office; 1971.
10. Office of the Secretary, Department of Health, Education, and Welfare. 45 CFR 46: Protection of Human Subjects. *Federal Register* 1974;39(105):18913–20.
11. Department of Health and Human Services, National Institutes of Health, and Office for Human Research Protections. The Common Rule, Title 45 (Public Welfare), Code of Federal Regulations, Part 46 (Protection of Human Subjects). [Online] June 23, 2005. Available: http://www.hhs.gov/ohrp/humansubjects/guidance/45cfr46.htm.
12. Department of Health and Human Services, Food and Drug Administration. Title 21 (Food and Drugs), Code of Federal Regulations, Parts 50 (Protection of Human Subjects) and 56 (Institutional Review Boards). [Online] April 1, 2006. Available: http://www.gpo.gov/nara/cfr/waisidx_06/21cfrv1_06.html.
13. Division of Compliance Oversight, Office for Human Research Protections. OHRP Compliance Oversight Activities: Significant Findings and Concerns of Noncompliance. [Online] October 12, 2005. Available: http://www.hhs.gov/ohrp/compliance/findings.pdf.
14. Office for Human Research Protections. Assurances. [Online] Available: http://www.hhs.gov/ohrp/assurances/assurances_index.html.
15. Office for Human Research Protections. Update and Renewal of an IORG-IRB/IEC Registration. [Online] Available: http://www.hhs.gov/ohrp/humansubjects/assurance/renwirb.htm.
16. Office for Human Research Protections. DRAFT Guidance on Reporting and Reviewing Adverse Events and Unanticipated Problems Involving Risks to Subjects or Others. [Online] October 11, 2005. Available: http://www.hhs.gov/ohrp/requests/aerg.html.
17. Office for Human Research Protections. 2001 Determination Letters. [Online] Available: http://www.hhs.gov/ohrp/compliance/letters/2001.html.
18. Office for Human Research Protections. 2005 Determination Letters. [Online] Available: http://www.hhs.gov/ohrp/compliance/letters/2005.html.
19. Borror K, Carome M, McNeilly P, Weil C. A review of OHRP compliance oversight letters. *IRB: Ethics and Human Research* 2003;25(5):1–4.
20. Bramstedt KA, Kassimatis K. A study of warning letters issued to institutional review boards by the United States Food and Drug Administration. *Clinical and Investigative Medicine* 2004;27:316–23.
21. Department of Health and Human Services. Final Guidance Document: Financial Relationships and Interests in Research Involving Human Subjects: Guidance for Human Subject Protection. [Online] May 5, 2004. Available: http://www.hhs.gov/ohrp/humansubjects/finreltn/fguid.pdf.
22. National Institutes of Health. Required Education in the Protection of Human Research Participants. [Online] June 5, 2000 (Revised August 25, 2000). Available: http://grants.nih.gov/grants/guide/notice-files/NOT-OD-00-039.html.

23. Fair Access to Clinical Trials Act of 2005. S. 470, H.R. 3196. 109th Congress, 2005. [Online] Available: http://olpa.od.nih.gov/legislation/109/pendinglegislation/fact.asp.

24. Fair Access to Clinical Trials Act of 2004. S. 2933, H.R. 5252, 108th Congress, 2004. [Online] Available: http://olpa.od.nih.gov/tracking/house_bills/session2/hr-5252.asp.

25. Association for the Accreditation of Human Research Protection Programs, Inc. (AAHRPP). Standards and Principles. [Online] Available: http://www.aahrpp.org/www.aspx?PageID=21.

26. General Accounting Office. *Scientific Research: Continued Vigilance Critical to Protecting Human Subjects.* GAO/HEHS-96-72. Washington, D.C.: GAO, 1996. [Online] March, 1996. Available: http://www.gao.gov/archive/1996/he96072.pdf.

27. Office of Inspector General, Department of Health and Human Services. *FDA Oversight of Clinical Investigators* OEI-05-99-00350. Washington, D.C.: DHHS; 2000. [Online] June 2000. Available: http://oig.hhs.gov/oei/reports/oei-05-99-00350.pdf.

28. Office of Inspector General, Department of Health and Human Services. *Protecting Human Research Subject—Status of Recommendations.* OEI-01-97-00197. Washington, D.C.: DHHS; 2000. [Online] April 2000. Available: http://oig.hhs.gov/oei/reports/oei-01-97-00197.pdf.

29. Office of Inspector General, Department of Health and Human Services. *Recruiting Human Subjects: Pressures in Industry-Sponsored Clinical Research.* OEI-01-97-00195. Washington, D.C.: DHHS; 2000. [Online] June 2000. Available: http://oig.hhs.gov/oei/reports/oei-01-97-00195.pdf.

30. Office of Inspector General, Department of Health and Human Services. *Institutional Review Boards: A Time for Reform.* OEI-01-97-00193. Washington, D.C.: DHHS; 1998. [Online] June 1998. Available: http://oig.hhs.gov/oei/reports/oei-01-97-00193.pdf.

31. Office of Inspector General, Department of Health and Human Services. *Institutional Review Boards: The Emergence of Independent Boards.* OEI-01-97-00192. Washington, D.C.: DHHS; 1998. [Online] June, 1998. Available: http://oig.hhs.gov/oei/reports/oei-01-97-00192.pdf.

32. Office of Inspector General, Department of Health and Human Services. *Institutional Review Boards: Promising Approaches.* OEI-01-91-00191. Washington, D.C.: DHHS; 1998. [Online] June 1998. Available: http://oig.hhs.gov/oei/reports/oei-01-97-00191.pdf.

33. Office of Inspector General, Department of Health and Human Services. *Institutional Review Boards: Their Role in Reviewing Approved Research.* OEI-01-97-00190. Washington, D.C.: DHHS; 1998. [Online] June 1998. Available: http://oig.hhs.gov/oei/reports/oei-01-97-00190.pdf.

34. Office of Inspector General, Department of Health and Human Services. *Low-Volume Institutional Review Boards.* OEI-01-97-00194. Washington, D.C.: DHHS; 1998. [Online] October 1998. Available: http://oig.hhs.gov/oei/reports/oei-01-97-00194.pdf.

35. Larson E, Bratts T, Zwanziger J, Stone P. A survey of IRB process in 68 U.S. hospitals. *Journal of Nursing Scholarship* 2004;36(3):260-4.

36. Burman WE, Randall RR, Cohn DL, Schooley RT. Breaking the camel's back: Multicenter clinical trials and local institutional review boards. *Annals of Internal Medicine* 2001;134:152-7.

37. Burman W, Breese P, Weis S, et al. The effects of local review on informed consent documents from a multicenter clinical trials consortium. *Controlled Clinical Trials* 2003;24:245-55.

38. Kent G. Responses by four local research ethics committees to submitted proposals. *Journal of Medical Ethics* 1999;25:274-7.

39. McWilliams R, Hoover-Fong J, Hamosh A, et al. Problematic variation in local institutional review of a multicenter genetic epidemiology study. *JAMA* 2003;290:360-1.

40. Olsen DP, Mahrenholz D. IRB-identified ethical issues in nursing research. *Journal of Professional Nursing* 2000;16:140-8.

41. Sansone RA, McDonald S. Quality improvement with institutional review boards. *Quality Assurance Journal* 2004;8:258-61.

42. Sansone RA, McDonald S, Haley P, Sellbom M, Gaither GA. The stipulations of one institutional review board: A five year review. *Journal of Medical Ethics* 2004;30:308-10.

43. Silverman H, Chandros Hull S, Sugarman J. Variability among institutional review boards decisions within the context of a multicenter trial. *Critical Care Medicine* 2001;29:235-41.

44. Ross L. The need for consistency in 407 reviews. *Pediatrics* 2004; 114:901-2.

45. Whittle A, Shah S, Wilfond B, Gensler G, Wendler D. Institutional Review Board practices regarding assent in pediatric research. *Pediatrics* 2004;113:1747-52.

46. The National Commission for the Protection of Human Subjects of Biomedical and Behavioral Research. *The Belmont Report: Ethical Principles and Guidelines for the Protection of Human Subjects of Research.* Washington, D.C.: Department of Health, Education and Welfare; 1979. [Online] April 18, 1979. Available: http://www.hhs.gov/ohrp/humansubjects/guidance/belmont.htm.

47. Agre P, Campbell FA, Goldman BD, et al. Improving informed consent: The medium is not the message. *IRB: Ethics and Human Research* 2003;25(Suppl.5):S11-S19.

48. National Institutes of Health. Informed Consent in Research Involving Human Participants, RFA: OD-97-001. *NIH Guide,* Vol. 25, No. 32. [Online] September 27, 1996. Available: http://grants.nih.gov/grants/guide/rfa-files/RFA-OD-97-001.html.

49. Sachs GA, Houghman GW, Sugarman J, et al. Conducting empirical research on informed consent: Challenges and questions. *IRB: Ethics and Human Research* 2003;25(Suppl.5):S4-S10.

50. Churchill LR, Nelson, DK, Henderson GE, et al. Assessing benefits in clinical research: Why diversity in benefit assessment can be risky. *IRB: Ethics and Human Research* 2003;25(3):1-8.

51. Hamilton M. Some precision would be helpful. *IRB: Ethics and Human Research* 2004;26(5):19.

52. Nelson RM. Children as research subjects. In: Kahn JP, Mastroianni AC, Sugarman J, eds. *Beyond Consent: Seeking Justice in Research.* New York, N.Y.: Oxford University Press; 1998:47-66.

53. Brody BA. Research on the vulnerable sick. In: Kahn JP, Mastroianni AC, Sugarman J, eds. *Beyond Consent: Seeking Justice in Research.* New York, N.Y.: Oxford University Press; 1998:32-46.

54. Powers M. Theories of justice in the context of research. In: Kahn JP, Mastroianni AC, Sugarman J, eds. *Beyond Consent: Seeking Justice in Research.* New York, N.Y.: Oxford University Press; 1998:147-65.

55. Letter from Donald E. Cook, President, American Academy of Pediatrics to Dockets Management Branch (HFA-305), Food and Drug Administration, June 5, 2000. [Online] Available: http://www.fda.gov/ohrms/dockets/dailys/00/jun00/060700/c000008.pdf.

56. Department of Health And Human Services, Food and Drug Administration. Additional Safeguards for Children in Clinical Investigations of FDA-Regulated Products: Interim rule; opportunity for public comment. *Federal Register* 2001;66(79):20589-600. [Online] Available: http://www.fda.gov/ohrms/dockets/98fr/042401a.htm.

57. Letter from Greg Koski, Director, OHRP to OHRP staff regarding OHRP Compliance Oversight Procedures, December 4, 2000. [Online] Available: http://www.hhs.gov/ohrp/references/ohrpcomp.pdf.

58. Department of Health and Human Services, Food and Drug Administration. Guidance for Institutional Review Boards and Clinical Investigators: 1998 Update. [Online] Available: http://www.fda.gov/oc/ohrt/irbs/operations.html.

59. Office for Health Research Protections. Quality Assurance/Quality Improvement: A Guided Self-Assessment for Human Research Protection Programs. [Online] Available: http://www.hhs.gov/ohrp/qi.

60. Task Force on Research Accountability, Association of American Universities. *Report on Individual and Institutional Financial Conflict of*

Interest. Washington, D.C.: AAU; 2001. [Online] October, 2001. Available: http://www.aau.edu/research/COI.01.pdf.

61. Association of American Medical Colleges, Task Force on Financial Conflicts of Interest in Clinical Research. *Protecting Subjects, Preserving Trust, Promoting Progress: Policy and Guidelines for the Oversight of Individual Financial Interests in Human Subjects Research.* Washington, D.C.: AAMC, 2001. [Online] December, 2001. Available: http://www.aamc.org/research/coi/firstreport.pdf.

62. Association of American Medical Colleges, Task Force on Financial Conflicts of Interest in Clinical Research. *Protecting Subjects, Preserving Trust, Promoting Progress II: Principles and Recommendations for Oversight of an Institution's Financial Interests in Human Subjects Research.* Washington, D.C.: AAMC; 2002. [Online] October 2002. Available: http://www.aamc.org/research/coi/2002coireport.pdf.

63. Association for the Accreditation of Human Research Protection Programs, Inc. (AAHRPP). [Online] Available: http://www.aahrpp.org/.

64. Secretary's Advisory Committee on Human Research Protections (SACHRP). Final Accreditation Subcommittee Report, March 29, 2004. [Online] Available: http://www.hhs.gov/ohrp/sachrp/mtgings/mtg03–04/accredrpt_files/frame.htm.

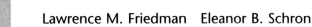

Lawrence M. Friedman Eleanor B. Schron

Data and Safety Monitoring Boards

Monitoring of Clinical Research Studies

All research studies involving people need ongoing oversight. For many, probably most, clinical research studies, this oversight is provided by the investigators, under the aegis of the local institution in which the research is being conducted, and with the oversight of the institutional review board (IRB) or its equivalent. Certain kinds of clinical research studies, though, might require different kinds of oversight. This oversight is not necessarily more intensive, but the features specific to the study might call for modifications in the oversight.

In particular, clinical trials that involve interventions (i.e., in which something is done to or administered to study participants) need different sorts of oversight or monitoring than do observational studies or surveys. Among the broad range of clinical trials, the phase of the trial, whether the trial is blinded (masked) or unblinded (open), and whether the trial is conducted at one or more than one site affect the kind of monitoring that is required. Also relevant is the nature of the study population and what sort of intervention is being administered to the participants. For example, studies involving participants who are at particularly high risk or procedures that carry exceptional risk would merit additional safeguards. Data and Safety Monitoring Boards (DSMBs)—which also go by other names such as data monitoring committees, safety monitoring committees, or safety and monitoring efficacy committees—can provide this additional monitoring. This chapter will discuss what monitoring of clinical studies by DSMBs entails, why it is done, what kinds of studies specifically require DSMBs, and how monitoring is done differently among different kinds of studies.

Single center, early phase clinical trials that do not involve particularly dangerous interventions, and that are uncontrolled (that is, trials that have no comparison group) or are not blinded, are often monitored by the investigators, with appropriate reporting to the IRBs. Sometimes, in order to avoid concerns about bias on the part of the investigator, another individual may be appointed to perform the monitoring function. What sorts of clinical trials require a DSMB? Several guidelines exist,[1–3] but the criteria are similar. In general, late-phase trials, especially those with an intervention that might produce adverse effects—such as drugs, devices, biologics, and surgical procedures—require DSMBs. It can be argued that potentially less harmful interventions, such as dietary changes or educational programs, should not need DSMBs. But even these interventions might cause possible psychological or emotional harm. Early-phase trials should also have DSMBs or other ongoing oversight independent of the investigator if the intervention and control groups are blinded to the investigator, or if the trials are multicenter, making it difficult for IRBs to provide the necessary monitoring, or involve study participants who need an extra layer of protection, or have interventions thought to convey extra risk such as gene transfer studies. (For a comprehensive, in-depth text on this topic, see Ellenberg, Fleming, and DeMets.[4])

History of DSMBs

One of the earliest studies with a DSMB was the Coronary Drug Project (CDP)[5] initiated by the National Heart Institute (now the National Heart, Lung, and Blood Institute, NHLBI) of the National Institutes of Health (NIH). The CDP was planned in the early

1960s, began enrolling participants in 1966, and ended in the mid-1970s. It was a multicenter trial testing the effects of several lipid-modifying drugs in people who had had a myocardial infarction. There were 53 clinics, a data coordinating center, a central laboratory, and an electrocardiogram reading center. The study organizers realized early in the trial that for participant safety reasons, accumulating data needed to be monitored regularly. An external Policy Board was established to provide study oversight and review outcome data. At first, accumulating outcome data were also provided to investigators.

Because multicenter trials were then quite new, in 1967 the National Heart Institute convened a committee of clinical research experts, the Heart Special Project Committee chaired by Bernard Greenberg, to make recommendations on the organizational structure and function of multicenter clinical studies.[6] Some of the recommendations of the *Greenberg Report* applied to monitoring:

> A Policy Board or Advisory Committee of senior scientists, experts in the field of the study but not data-contributing participants in it, is almost essential for a large complex cooperative project. . . . A mechanism must be developed for early termination if unusual circumstances dictate that a cooperative study should not be continued. Such action might be contemplated if the accumulated data answer the original question sooner than anticipated, if it is apparent that the study will not or cannot achieve its stated aims, or if scientific advances since initiation render continuation superfluous. This is obviously a difficult decision that must be based on careful analysis of past progress and future expectation. If the National Heart Institute must initiate such action, it must do so only with the advice and on the recommendation of consultants.

In line with the Greenberg Report recommendations, the CDP formed a Data and Safety Monitoring Committee in 1968 that regularly reviewed accumulating data. Investigators who enrolled or followed study participants were not members of this committee. However, it was far from independent. Members included staff from the coordinating center, other key central groups, and the sponsor. There were also several outside experts on the committee. Recommendations from this committee went to the Policy Board.[5]

After the CDP, the NHLBI modified its approach to monitoring committees. Perhaps most importantly, committees became more independent, with all voting members being separate from the study and the sponsor. With this change, it was no longer necessary to have a second oversight group, so most future NHLBI trials did not have an additional policy board.

In the 1970s and 1980s, other NIH institutes adopted the NHLBI model or variations on it.[7,8] One modification adopted first by the National Cancer Institute as part of its Cooperative Studies Program and by the Division of AIDS in the National Institute of Allergy and Infectious Diseases was to form DSMBs that monitored more than one trial.[9,10] In the 1990s, the NIH developed guidelines for the establishment of DSMBs. Most late-phase and many early-phase trials sponsored by NIH now include DSMBs. Other U.S. government sponsors of clinical trials, such as the Department of Veterans Affairs, routinely have monitoring committees. Industry, however, was slower to incorporate independent monitoring committees in its clinical trials. Only in recent years have they become fairly frequent. With the development of Food and Drug Administration (FDA) guidelines,[2] this trend will pro-

bably continue. Internationally, trends in the kinds of studies using DSMBs have been similar to those in the United States.[11]

More recently, the Issues in Data Monitoring and Interim Analysis of Trials (DAMOCLES) group[12] has surveyed monitoring committee practice.[13,14] One of its key recommendations was that more standard policies, including the use of structured charters, would aid in developing consistency in the kinds of trials employing DSMBs and in the management of monitoring committees.

Responsibilities and Functioning of the DSMB

The primary responsibility of a DSMB is to ensure, to the extent possible, that study participants are not unduly harmed. A second responsibility is to ensure the integrity of the clinical trial, so that valid data can be provided to the public and the medical community. These two responsibilities are not completely separate, but conflicts between them may arise. Examples of such conflicts are given later in the chapter.

The DSMB has several specific tasks. Before the study gets started, it reviews the study protocol. Generally, the review is not of the same depth as a scientific peer review. Rather, the DSMB considers whether the protocol is sufficiently well designed to answer the question being addressed by the trial. This includes factors such as the quality and safety of the intervention, participant eligibility criteria, outcome measure assessment, sample size, and the analysis plan. Are the safety measures adequate? Is there reasonable quality control? Before it agrees to spend months or years monitoring the trial, the DSMB needs to accept that the research question is important enough to put participants at risk of possible harm and that the trial has a sufficiently sound design to answer the question. The DSMB also reviews the consent form template. Each participating site will likely have an IRB (unless there is a "central" IRB) that will closely review the consent form. But a study-wide template is typically prepared so that the consent forms at all sites will contain the same key messages.

The DSMB must be comfortable with the monitoring plan that is proposed by the investigators. How often will the data be reviewed? What kinds of data will be reviewed? What criteria will be used to consider stopping the study ahead of schedule? Are there certain adverse events that must receive more intensive monitoring? The study should start to enroll participants only after the DSMB is comfortable with all of these factors.

A typical DSMB consists of from three to six or seven members, and occasionally more. The members have expertise in the particular field being studied, trial design, and biostatistics. Often, DSMBs include bioethicists and patient advocates. It is also essential that at least some of the members have prior experience in serving on DSMBs.

Independence of the DSMB is a major consideration. The members should not have a current or close connection with the investigators or with the sponsor. They need to be able to make objective judgments about the study. What constitutes independence is sometimes fuzzy. Can a member be from the same institution as one of the investigators? If yes, what about the same department? Can a member have been a past colleague or coauthored a paper with one of the investigators? Ideally, the more separate, the better. But if the best, most knowledgeable candidate is someone with some past connection, it may be appropriate to select expertise over complete independence.

Similar considerations arise involving financial conflict of interest. DSMB members should have no vested financial interest in the outcome of the trial. They should not hold stock in, be advisers to, or be on speakers' bureaus for the company that is manufacturing the product being tested. They also should not have connections with direct competitors of the manufacturer. But what about being an investigator in another study funded by that company? There may not be a clear answer to that question, so judgments may be needed.

Intellectual conflicts may be a more difficult problem. Those with expertise in the area will have conducted other studies or may be conducting other studies concurrent with the trial for which they are being proposed as DSMB members. They therefore have at least an intellectual interest in how the study turns out. As with independence, these sorts of interests should not prevent those who are most knowledgeable from serving on DSMBs. All potential conflicts should be disclosed to the sponsor and the other DSMB members and must be updated regularly.

The DSMB is usually appointed by the sponsor of the clinical trial, whether it is one of the NIH institutes, another government agency, or a pharmaceutical or device manufacturing company. Study investigators often provide input into the selection of members. The DSMB generally reports to and provides recommendations to the study sponsor. The nature of these reports and how any recommendations should be communicated to the sponsor and the investigators are matters of some debate, and will be considered later in the chapter.

A typical DSMB meeting consists of three sessions: open, closed, and executive. During the open session, study progress and "process" data for the study as a whole (not separated by treatment group) are reviewed. In addition to the DSMB members, this session may be attended by one or more investigators (usually including the chairperson of the trial), by staff from the group managing and analyzing the study data (often a data coordinating center), by one or more employees of the sponsor, and perhaps by someone from a regulatory agency. During the closed session, process, outcome, and other data broken down by treatment group are presented. Therefore, only those who should be aware of such data are present. This would include the biostatistician who presents the data and perhaps others from the data coordinating center and the sponsor. Again, this is an area of controversy and will be discussed later. The executive session is the time when the DSMB members can discuss what they wish in the absence of any other attendees, except perhaps for an executive secretary.

At the end of each DSMB meeting, recommendations (and they are recommendations, not decisions) are made. If the trial is proceeding well, the DSMB should clearly state that it thinks that the study should continue with the protocol unchanged. Other recommendations can consist of relatively minor items such as the need for clarification of data reports or forms; more serious matters such as modifications to the informed consent form or the protocol—for example, changes in eligibility criteria or in kind or frequency of assessment of biomarkers or outcome measures and adverse events; or major recommendations such as dropping a subgroup of participants, dropping an entire treatment arm, or completely ending the study ahead of schedule. Studies may be stopped early for five general reasons: (1) The intervention is more effective than originally thought, (2) there are unacceptable adverse events, (3) it is highly unlikely that additional data will alter a currently null result or provide other sufficiently important in-

formation if the study were to continue to its scheduled end, (4) the study is proceeding so poorly in terms of participant accrual or data quality or that no useful answer will likely be forthcoming, or (5) the question has been answered by external evidence that is reported while the trial is underway.

Typical Reports Reviewed by DSMBs

The typical report that the DSMB reviews contains several sorts of data. First, the report contains data regarding the conduct of the trial, or process data. That is, it has information showing how well the trial is doing in participant screening, accrual, and follow-up; performance of procedures and other measurements; quality control measures; and any problems such as inadvertent enrollment of ineligible participants or randomization mistakes. Second, it contains information on the kinds of participants who are being enrolled (i.e., baseline characteristics). Third, it has information about interim measures like biomarkers and other laboratory or imaging data, and measurements of adherence to the protocol. Fourth, it contains tables and figures showing the outcome measures at the time of the report. These are often accompanied by monitoring boundaries. Fifth, it includes reports of adverse events other than outcome or laboratory measures.

This chapter will not go into detail about monitoring boundaries. However, the basic concept is that repeated assessment of data, which is essential to protect study participants, can increase the type 1 error—the probability of incorrectly rejecting the null hypothesis. By convention, the type 1 error, or alpha, is often set at 5%. It will be 5%, however, only if the study data are analyzed just once, at the end of the trial. Examining the data once during the trial and again at the end would increase the probability of incorrectly rejecting the null hypothesis from 5% to about 8%.[15] If the null hypothesis is tested five times, the type 1 error would be 14% instead of 5%. Therefore, in order to maintain the type 1 error at the prespecified level, it is necessary to require more than simply finding a nominally statistically significant difference partway through the trial. If the protocol sets a two-sided alpha level of 0.05, a more extreme difference than the statistic nominally associated with that alpha level is required before the scheduled end of the study to declare that the trial has found a statistically significant result.

Monitoring boundaries are developed to assist the DSMB in deciding if an early result is truly statistically significant and to minimize the likelihood of a false positive result being found. Several kinds of monitoring boundaries have been used, but the most common ones all use quite extreme differences early in the trial, with less extreme differences near or at the scheduled end. The rationale for this is that early in the study, when only a small amount of data is available, the numbers are more unstable and likely to change, sometimes dramatically, as seen in one of the examples given later. It should be emphasized that because participant safety is paramount, monitoring boundaries are often asymmetric. That is, they require less evidence to stop a study early for harm than for benefit. For those interested, several references to development and interpretation of monitoring boundaries are provided.[16–20]

Reports for a DSMB are prepared by the data coordinating center or by an independent biostatistician. The frequency of the reports depends on the rate at which data are accumulating, but reports often are made every 6 or 12 months. Sometimes, in order to limit the problem of the type 1 error that is raised by interim looks at the data, some investigators and DSMBs prefer to see reports that contain outcome data less frequently than reports with adverse events and other data. Although this process has its advocates, it can impair the ability of the DSMB to do its job adequately. Almost always, recommendations to continue or stop a study or to change a protocol are based on judgment as to the balance of benefits and harms. Therefore, information about both is usually needed. Properly constructed monitoring boundaries can reduce concerns about frequent looks at outcome data.

Sometimes, because of serious adverse events, the DSMB may ask for interim or special reports. It is the obligation of the data coordinating center or biostatistician to provide whatever data are reasonably necessary for the DSMB to fulfill its responsibilities to study participants.

A different sort of concern when analyzing data is the so-called type 2 error. The type 2 error involves accepting the null hypothesis when in fact it is false. This kind of error is often due to a study that has inadequate power to detect what is thought to be a clinically meaningful difference between groups. From the perspective of the DSMB, type 2 errors are most important when a seemingly large difference between groups for an important outcome fails to reach statistical significance because the number of study participants or the number of events is too small. The DSMB needs to use its judgment in deciding whether the observed difference in, for example, an adverse event, is important or clinically significant, despite not reaching statistical significance. Table 53.1 summarizes the type 1 and type 2 errors.

Examples of Ethical Issues in DSMB Deliberations

The results of several DSMB deliberations have been published, and for those interested, a recent book contains almost 30 cases.[21] A few selected examples of DSMB deliberations are provided here.

Cardiac Arrhythmia Suppression Trial

The Cardiac Arrhythmia Suppression Trial[22] (CAST) was a placebo-controlled trial of three antiarrhythmic agents in people with heart disease and ventricular arrhythmias. The objective was to see if suppression of the ventricular arrhythmias would lead to a reduction in sudden cardiac death. Unfortunately, rather early in the trial, two of the three agents were found to cause an increase in both sudden death and total mortality.[23] Subsequently, the third agent was also shown to cause an increase in sudden death.[24]

When CAST was developed, it was designed as a one-sided test of hypothesis, with alpha = 0.05. The investigators did not envision that suppressing ventricular arrhythmias could possibly be harmful. The DSMB, when it reviewed the protocol at its first

meeting, asked that the design be modified. It remained a one-sided test, but with alpha = 0.025, and an advisory boundary for harm. This boundary for harm was set at the same level of significance as the boundary for benefit. It should also be noted that the DSMB decided to remain blinded to the identity of the treatment groups.

Differences in numbers of sudden deaths and deaths from all causes appeared early. However, the number of events was quite small, and the DSMB recommended that CAST continue and the identity of the groups continue to be withheld. Shortly after, however, the difference increased, and the DSMB was informed that the number of deaths was greater in the active treatment group, concentrated in two of the three antiarrhythmic drugs. The difference had crossed the advisory boundary for harm, which, as noted above, was symmetric with the boundary for benefit. The two drugs were discontinued and the trial was redesigned using only the remaining drug versus placebo. This time, the advisory boundary for harm was asymmetric, requiring less evidence for harm than for benefit to stop the study early. With time, the third drug also proved to be harmful and was discontinued.

Among the lessons of CAST were that the DSMB has to be prepared early and that harm, even though not anticipated, must be planned for. Also, there is usually little rationale for the DSMB to remain blinded to the identity of the treatment groups. But if it chooses to do so, in the name of objectivity, there needs to be a mechanism for unblinding whenever it becomes necessary.

It should also be noted that when the first two antiarrhythmic drug arms were stopped, CAST was essentially redesigned as a new study. The changes to the protocol, which included a new sample size, were sufficient in magnitude and scope that even though the relatively few participants who had originally been randomized to either the third drug or its placebo remained in the trial, it was considered a new trial. On the other hand, if the only sorts of changes that had occurred were those relating to modifications of eligibility criteria or frequency of assessment of outcome, they would not have likely been sufficient to start over as a new trial.

A more problematic situation is when there is a modest change in the intervention. In that case, a judgment must be made as to how similar the new intervention is to the old one, and whether the data from both can legitimately be combined.

Physicians' Health Study

The Physicians' Health Study[25,26] (PHS) was a factorial design (2 × 2), placebo-controlled trial of aspirin and beta carotene in healthy U.S. male physicians. The objectives were to see if aspirin reduced the incidence of cardiovascular mortality and if beta carotene reduced the incidence of cancer. The aspirin component of the PHS was stopped ahead of schedule for two main reasons. One, the incidence of cardiovascular mortality was very low, and it would have taken many more years than planned to reach the projected number of events. Two, there was a large, highly significant benefit for a secondary outcome, myocardial infarction, which was mainly nonfatal.

The DSMB considered whether stopping the aspirin study early for a beneficial finding in a secondary outcome was appropriate. Given the importance of the outcome and the remote likelihood of seeing anything for the primary outcome, the DSMB recommended to the principal investigator that the aspirin component end.

Table 53.1

Possible Decisions About the Null Hypothesis

Decision	Null Hypothesis	
	True	False
Accept null hypothesis	OK	Type 2 error
Reject null hypothesis	Type 1 error	OK

Breast Cancer Prevention Trial

The Breast Cancer Prevention Trial[27,28] (BCPT) was a placebo-controlled trial with the objective of evaluating if tamoxifen would reduce the incidence of breast cancer in women at high risk. The study was stopped ahead of schedule because the monitoring committee observed a large reduction in breast cancer in the tamoxifen group. A one-sided test of hypothesis, with alpha = 0.01, was used to determine benefit. A less extreme value was used for harm. Because tamoxifen was thought to have multiple effects in addition to the primary outcome of breast cancer, a global index incorporating several outcomes was also used to monitor the data.

A strong favorable trend for breast cancer appeared relatively early in the trial, as did the expected adverse trend for endometrial cancer. The monitoring committee, however, was concerned about an unexpected finding of ocular toxicity. As a result of this, all enrolled participants were provided with the information about ocular toxicity and asked to reconsent.[27]

The monitoring committee's recommendation to end the study occurred almost two years after the monitoring boundary for breast cancer had been crossed. The importance of getting sufficient information about adverse events with an intervention that would be used to prevent breast cancer in women who did not have it led to this delay.

Candesartan in Heart Failure Assessment of Reduction in Mortality and Morbidity Program

The Candesartan in Heart Failure Assessment of Reduction in Mortality and Morbidity[29,30] (CHARM) program consisted of three trials that compared candesartan against placebo in patients with heart failure. The primary outcome for each trial was cardiovascular death or hospitalization for heart failure; the primary outcome for the combined trials was death from all causes. The program continued to its scheduled end despite the fact that, early on, the monitoring committee had noted a large benefit with respect to overall mortality (see Table 53.2). Early results presented to the DSMB on March 27, 2000, were nominally statistically significant, with more than a 30% relative reduction in event rates. At the DSMB's March 1, 2001, meeting, the relative reduction was less, but the results had crossed the preestablished monitoring boundary. However, the results were not convincing for the primary outcome or for two of the three trials. In addition, DSMB members were concerned that early data might not be borne out by later data and that the results needed to be definitive in order to change medical practice. Therefore, the monitoring committee recommended continuing the trial. At the scheduled end of the trial, the results showed nowhere near the magnitude of benefit that had been observed earlier.

Trials of Antibiotic Treatment in Patients With Lyme Disease

Two trials of antibiotic treatment were conducted in patients with a history of Lyme disease[31] and persistent symptoms. The primary outcome for both trials was health-related quality of life. One trial, with seropositive patients, had a projected sample size of 194. This trial was designed to have 90% power to detect a 25% difference in the primary outcome between the antibiotic and placebo

Table 53.2
Deaths in the CHARM Program at Each Interim Analysis and at Study Closeout

Analysis Date	Overall Program		
	Candesartan Arm	Placebo Arm	P-value
August 9, 1999	8	4	0.3
March 27, 2000	76	123	0.0007
July 27, 2000	133	198	0.0002
March, 1, 2001	260	339	0.0006
August 9, 2001	337	474	0.0010
February 22, 2002	556	631	0.009
August 1, 2002	682	756	0.015
Final report**	886	945	0.055

Modified from Pocock S, et al.[30] and used with permission of publisher; ** final report on September 6, 2003, based on follow-up to March 31, 2003.

groups. A second trial, with seronegative patients, had a projected sample size of 66. This was designed to have 80% power to detect a 35% difference between the antibiotic and placebo groups.

When 129 patients had been enrolled (78 seropositive and 51 seronegative), of whom 107 had been followed for 180 days, the planned duration of the trials, the DSMB determined that there was only a 1.4% chance that the seropositive study would yield a significant difference between antibiotic and placebo, were the study to continue to its scheduled enrollment. Similarly, for the seronegative study, there was only a 4% chance of seeing a difference. Therefore, the DSMB recommended that both studies be stopped, because continuation in order to achieve the goal of showing benefit from antibiotic treatment would be futile. Although additional information about treatment might have been obtained if the trials had enrolled the full sample sizes, the DSMB needed to weigh the value of that information against the risks to study participants when there was little hope of demonstrating benefit from the intervention.

These examples demonstrate the inherent tensions, and at times conflicts, between the responsibilities of DSMBs to ensure the safety of the study participants and the goal of obtaining information important in the clinical management of patients and in the prevention of disease. DSMBs must weigh the benefits to society and to patients of continuing a trial against their duties to the study participants. Despite the general guideline that the safety of the participants is paramount, often, there is no clear "right answer," and vigorous discussions take place at DSMB meetings. If a study is stopped too soon, the wrong answer may be obtained and study participants will have volunteered without contributing to obtaining valid knowledge. These situations point out the need to have DSMBs made up of thoughtful members with different backgrounds and perspectives.

Unresolved Issues

As noted in several places in this chapter, unresolved or even controversial issues exist with regard to DSMBs. Some of these involve what might be considered aspects of real or perceived conflict of interest.

DSMB Reporting Practices

The DSMB is usually appointed and has its expenses paid by the sponsor of the trial. But the DSMB is responsible to more than just the sponsor. It is also responsible to the study investigators and, of course, to the study participants. Meeting minutes and recommendations are often provided to the sponsor, which then communicates the recommendations to the study investigators. One reason for not reporting directly to the investigators is that not all DSMB recommendations may be accepted by the sponsor. A second reason is that the sponsor may have other information that might cause it to question a recommendation. Third, there may not be unanimity among the DSMB members as to the recommendations; sometimes the DSMB deliberations are quite divisive. The sponsor then needs to make some decision, perhaps by convening an additional body. This happened in the Women's Health Initiative trial of estrogen.[32]

On the other hand, the investigators are closer than the sponsor to both the implementation of the protocol and the participants. Therefore, some clinical trial methodologists believe that direct communication between the DSMB and investigators would be more appropriate.[33] In addition, especially if the sponsor is a drug or device manufacturer, there may be strong financial reasons for it to accept or decline certain recommendations. Reporting directly to the investigators would reduce those pressures.

Regardless of to whom the DSMB reports, after each DSMB meeting a report needs to go to the IRBs. This report should not contain data that would unblind the study. However, it must mention the overall recommendation (continue or stop the trial); any recommended changes in protocol or informed consent, or other information that should be presented to the participants; and any adverse events not fully discussed during the consent process—for example, unexpected adverse events or any that are occurring more frequently or with greater severity than originally described.

On occasion, IRBs have refused to accept the judgment of the DSMBs and have asked to see the actual study data. It is important that the ground rules be established in advance, when the IRBs first review the protocols. IRBs need to accept that the DSMBs will perform their functions appropriately and that all necessary feedback will be provided. Some IRBs may not be willing to cede the responsibility of monitoring while still possibly being liable. If so, that needs to be understood at the beginning of a trial, not partway through. This whole area needs more discussion and clarification.

Access to Blinded Outcome Data

As noted above, various investigators and sponsor representatives may attend open sessions of the DSMB. Generally, in industry-sponsored trials, the sponsor is not present at the closed sessions, in which blinded data are presented. This is in line with FDA guidelines.[2] In many, if not most, NIH-sponsored trials, several institute staff are present and are routinely made aware of the blinded data. The arguments in favor of this practice are that NIH employees are responsible for public funds and must have full knowledge of the progress (including outcome data) of the trial in order to perform their duties. In addition, unlike employees of pharmaceutical or device manufacturers, they do not have direct

financial stakes in the results of the trial. The arguments against this practice are that any knowledge of outcome trends can bias the conduct of the trial. Protocol modifications often need to be made to enhance the feasibility of a trial, such as changes in eligibility criteria to improve accrual, or changes in outcome measures to increase power. If the sponsor is aware of the accumulating data, suspicion might arise that these changes were based on the blinded data, not simply on process data.[2]

The same argument applies to data coordinating center personnel. Some have proposed that there be a firewall between the biostatisticians who analyze, tabulate, and present the data to the DSMB and those who perform the daily management functions of the trial.[34–36] This would be accomplished either by a group completely separate from the data coordinating center or through a separate group at the center. The counterargument is that anything that impairs the ability of the DSMB to obtain the best information about the study is inappropriate. Using a biostatistician who is not completely familiar with the study protocol to present data to the DSMB might mean that some questions about the protocol could not be answered in a timely fashion. Complete independence of the DSMB and its management might not lead to optimal monitoring and safety of the study participants. When the two desirable goals of independence and safety are weighed against each other, safety must always win.

Control of Data by the Sponsor

Either the sponsor manages and analyzes the data and prepares the data tables for review by the DSMB or it arranges with another group to perform these functions. Some have argued that when the sponsor analyzes the data, there is an inherent conflict of interest. Whether this conflict is effectively managed by the use of a contractor is a matter of opinion. One can argue that even if the functions are contracted to another group, the contractor has an interest in satisfying the sponsor. Many would say that anything that distances the analysis functions from the sponsor is useful, if only for the sake of appearance. Ideally, accumulating data should be managed and analyzed by a group independent of the sponsor. In the end, however, one always has to rely on the integrity of the people doing the data analyses.

Confidentiality Issues

While a trial is ongoing, it is expected that all members of a DSMB will exercise caution to keep information about the trial confidential. That is, they are expected to refrain from discussing their deliberations and trends in data with anyone who is not already privy to that information. This bar includes discussions with study investigators as well as with investors. The only communications should be the official recommendations at the end of each meeting.

Instances of inappropriate discussions of ongoing trials with investors have occurred. Most reports cited study investigators, who generally would not know about trends in the data. But at least one report cited a DSMB member.[37] These actions on the part of DSMB members during a trial are completely inappropriate. It is less clear, however, whether confidentiality should apply after a trial ends. It is probably reasonable to maintain confidentiality until the main results have been presented and published. After that, as long as proprietary information is not disclosed, there may be good reasons for members of the DSMB to describe their experiences, with the goal of providing important guidance to future monitoring committees.

Disagreements Between DSMB and Sponsor or Investigator

On occasion, there may be disagreements between recommendations made by the DSMB, or by certain members, and actions taken or not taken by the sponsor or investigators. Most of these disagreements involve relatively minor protocol issues. More serious disagreements may revolve around management of adverse events and whether or not to stop a trial. Sometimes, the sponsor chooses to stop a trial earlier than scheduled, even when the DSMB has recommended continuing it. This may be done for scientific, ethical, or marketing reasons. The first two reasons can be legitimate, and the DSMB must acknowledge the right of the sponsor to do so. The last has rightly been harshly criticized.[38]

It is also a serious situation if the DSMB recommends early discontinuation of a trial and the sponsor or investigator wants to continue. An instance of this has been reported, due primarily to a lack of prior understanding of the responsibilities of each.[39] Because of safety concerns, the monitoring committee for a pilot study comparing various doses of candesartan, alone and in combination with enalapril, and against enalapril alone in patients with heart failure recommended early termination. After receiving the recommendation, reviewing the data, and noting that clear monitoring guidelines had not been established in advance, the lead investigators raised questions about the recommendation and asked to meet with the monitoring committee. When the monitoring committee rejected this, the investigators sought the opinion of another outside expert panel. This panel concluded that although there was lack of strong evidence of harm, the recommendation of the monitoring committee should be accepted. Therefore, the trial was discontinued. A clear charter for the DSMB, as advocated by the investigators in this trial[39] and by the DAMOCLES Group[13] would be helpful in similar situations.

Another kind of disagreement involves the interpretation of the data. In letters to the editor, two members of the DSMB for a trial of vitamin supplementation for retinitis pigmentosa challenged the investigators' conclusion that vitamin A was beneficial.[40–42] Regardless of the merits of each position, such squabbles are unfortunate. The DSMB can argue that it has lived with the data for considerable time (often years) and has a better understanding of the data than do the investigators, who may have seen the data for only a few weeks or months before they prepared their publication. The investigators can argue that they saw the final (and full) results, that they have a better appreciation of how to put them in the context of the entire area of research, and that data interpretation is their responsibility; they take either the plaudits or blame for the publication. One possible approach to minimizing such conflicts is for the DSMB to review draft presentations and publications. If the suggestions of the DSMB members are reasonable, most investigators would be appreciative of them. The DSMB members need to remember, though, that they are not the investigators or authors.

Sometimes, publications are inappropriately delayed (or never produced). It is particularly troublesome if serious adverse events were identified during the trial and, because of the lack of publication, are never made public. It is unclear what role or responsibility the DSMB has in such cases, and how it is to discharge that responsibility. This issue becomes particularly difficult if a confidentiality agreement has been signed that prevents DSMB members from disclosing information without the approval of the sponsor.

Conclusions

All clinical research studies must have monitoring procedures. For certain kinds of studies, generally late phase clinical trials, an external committee, such as a DSMB, is essential. DSMBs provide expert judgment and oversight independent of the investigator and the sponsor.

The procedures for how a DSMB will function, and how it will monitor the data and conduct of the study, must be established in advance. IRBs also must understand and be comfortable with the monitoring process before they approve the study protocol. Because some events, especially adverse events, can occur rapidly, the system for collecting, analyzing, and reviewing the study data needs to be in place early.

Monitoring boundaries and guidelines for deciding if and when a study should be stopped early are essential. But these are guidelines, not rules, and cannot replace judgment. Rigidity in the face of unexpected events serves neither the study nor the participants. Therefore, it is necessary to have experienced, thoughtful members of the DSMB. Independence is important, but it cannot come at the cost of doing the best job of safeguarding the study participants.

References

1. National Institutes of Health. NIH Policy for Data and Safety Monitoring. [Online] June 10, 1998. Available: http://grants.nih.gov/grants/guide/notice-files/not98–84.html.
2. Food and Drug Administration. Guidance for Clinical Trial Sponsors—Establishment and Operation of Clinical Trial Data Monitoring Committees. [Online] March 2006. Available: http://www.fda.gov/CBER/gdlns/clintrialdmc.pdf.
3. National Heart, Lung, and Blood Institute. Establishing Data and Safety Monitoring Boards (DSMBs) and Observational Study Monitoring Boards (OSMBs). [Online] October 30, 2001. Available: http://www.nhlbi.nih.gov/funding/policies/dsmb_est.htm.
4. Ellenberg SS, Fleming TR, DeMets DL. *Data Monitoring Committees in Clinical Trials: A Practical Perspective.* West Sussex, England: John Wiley & Sons; 2003.
5. Coronary Drug Project Research Group. The Coronary Drug Project: Design, methods, and baseline results. *Circulation* 1973;47:11–I50.
6. Heart Special Project Committee (Bernard G. Greenberg, Chairman). Organization, review, and administration of cooperative studies: A report from the Heart Special Project Committee to the National Advisory Heart Council, May 1967 (The Greenberg Report). *Controlled Clinical Trials* 1988;9:137–48.
7. Hawkins BS. Data monitoring committees for multicenter clinical trials sponsored by the National Institutes of Health. I. Roles and membership of data monitoring committees for trials sponsored by the National Eye Institute. *Controlled Clinical Trials* 1991;12:424–37.
8. Geller NL, Stylianou M. Practical issues in data monitoring of clinical trials: summary of responses to a questionnaire at NIH. *Statistics in Medicine* 1993;12:543–51.
9. George SL. A survey of monitoring practices in cancer clinical trials. *Statistics in Medicine* 1993;12:435–50.

10. DeMets DL, Fleming TR, Whitley RJ, et al. The data and safety monitoring board and acquired immune deficiency syndrome (AIDS) clinical trials. *Controlled Clinical Trials* 1995;16:408–21.

11. Buyse M. Interim analyses, stopping rules and data monitoring in clinical trials in Europe. *Statistics in Medicine* 1993;12:509–20.

12. DAMOCLES (Data Monitoring Committees: Lessons, Ethics and Statistics) Study Group. Issues in data monitoring and interim analysis of trials. [Online] Available: http://www.abdn.ac.uk/hsru/hta/damocles.shtml.

13. Clemens FJ, Elbourne DR, Darbyshire J, Pocock S, and the DAMOCLES group. Data monitoring in randomized controlled trials: Surveys of recent practice and policies. *Clinical Trials* 2005;2:22–33.

14. Sydes MR, Spiegelhalter DJ, Altman DG, Babiker AB, Parmar MKB, and the DAMOCLES group. Systematic review of Data Monitoring Committees in Randomised Controlled Trials. *Clinical Trials* 2004;1:60–79.

15. Armitage P, McPherson CK, Rowe BC. Repeated significance tests on accumulating data. *Journal of the Royal Statistical Society (Series A)* 1969;132:235–44.

16. Peto R, Pike MC, Armitage P, et al. Design and analysis of randomized clinical trials requiring prolonged observation of each patient. I. Introduction and design. *British Journal of Cancer* 1976;34:585–612.

17. O'Brien PC, Fleming TR. A multiple testing procedure for clinical trials. *Biometrics* 1979;35:549–56.

18. DeMets DL, Lan KKG. Interim analysis: The alpha spending function approach. *Statistics in Medicine* 1994;13:1341–52.

19. Whitehead J. *Design and Analysis of Sequential Clinical Trials.* New York, N.Y.: Halsted Press; 1983.

20. Friedman LM, Furberg CD, DeMets DL. *Fundamentals of Clinical Trials,* 3rd ed. New York, N.Y.: Springer-Verlag; 1998.

21. DeMets DL, Furberg CD, Friedman LM, eds. *Data Monitoring in Clinical Trials: A Case Studies Approach.* New York, N.Y.: Springer; 2006.

22. Friedman LM, Bristow JD, Hallstrom A, et al. Data monitoring in the cardiac arrhythmia suppression trial. *Online Journal of Current Clinical Trials* 1993; Doc. No. 79.

23. The Cardiac Arrhythmia Suppression Trial (CAST) Investigators. Preliminary report: Effect of encainide and flecainide on mortality in a randomized trial of arrhythmia suppression after myocardial infarction. *New England Journal of Medicine* 1989;321:406–12.

24. The Cardiac Arrhythmia Suppression Trial (CAST) II Investigators. Effect of the antiarrhythmic agent moricizine on survival after myocardial infarction. *New England Journal of Medicine* 1992;327:227–33.

25. Steering Committee of the Physicians' Health Study Research Group. Final report on the aspirin component of the ongoing Physicians' Health Study. *New England Journal of Medicine* 1989;321:129–35.

26. Cairns J, Cohen L, Colton T, et al. Issues in the early termination of the aspirin component of the Physicians' Health Study. Data Monitoring Board of the Physicians' Health Study. *Annals of Epidemiology* 1991;1:395–405.

27. Redmond CK, Costantino JP, Colton T. Challenges in monitoring the Breast Cancer Prevention Trial. In: DeMets DL, Furberg CD, Fried-man LM, eds. *Data Monitoring in Clinical Trials: A Case Studies Approach.* New York, N.Y.: Springer; 2006:118–35.

28. Fisher B, Costantino JP, Wickerham DL, et al. Tamoxifen for prevention of breast cancer: Report of the National Surgical Adjuvant Breast and Bowel Project P-1 Study. *Journal of the National Cancer Institute* 1998;90:1371–88.

29. Young JB, Dunlap ME, Pfeffer MA, et al. Mortality and morbidity reduction with Candesartan in patients with chronic heart failure and left ventricular systolic dysfunction: Results of the CHARM low-left ventricular ejection fraction trials. *Circulation* 2004;110:2618–26.

30. Pocock S, Wang D, Wilhelmsen L, Hennekens CH. The data monitoring experience in the Candesartan in Heart Failure Assessment of Reduction in Mortality and morbidity (CHARM) program. *American Heart Journal* 2005;149:939–43.

31. Klempner MS, Hu LT, Evans J, et al. Two controlled trials of antibiotic treatment in patients with persistent symptoms and a history of Lyme disease. *New England Journal of Medicine* 2001;345:85–92.

32. Wittes J, Barrett-Connor E, Braunwald E, Chesney M, Cohen HJ, DeMets D, Dunn L, Dwyer J, Heaney RP, Vogel V, Walters L, Yusuf S. Monitoring the randomized trials of the Women's Health Initiative: the experience of the Data and Safety Monitoring Board. *Clinical Trials* 2007;4:218–34.

33. Meinert CL. Clinical trials and treatment effects monitoring. *Controlled Clinical Trials* 1998;19:515–22.

34. Ellenberg SS, George SL. Should statisticians reporting to data monitoring committees be independent of the trial sponsor and leadership? *Statistics in Medicine* 2004;23:1503–5.

35. DeMets DL, Fleming TR. The independent statistician for data monitoring committees. *Statistics in Medicine* 2004;23:1513–7.

36. Fisher MR, Roecker EB, DeMets DL. The role of an independent statistical analysis center in the industry-modified National Institutes of Health model. *Drug Information Journal* 2001;35:115–29.

37. Timmerman L, Heath D. Drug researchers leak secrets to Wall St. *Seattle Times* August 7, 2005:A1.

38. Psaty BM, Rennie D. Stopping medical research to save money: A broken pact with researchers and patients. *JAMA* 2003;289:2128–31.

39. Pogue J, Yusuf S. Data monitoring in the randomized evaluation of strategies for left ventricular dysfunction pilot study: When reasonable people disagree. In: DeMets DL, Furberg CD, Friedman LM, eds. *Data Monitoring in Clinical Trials: A Case Studies Approach.* New York, N.Y.: Springer; 2006:330–6.

40. Berson EL, Rosner B, Sandberg MA, et al. Vitamin A supplementation for retinitis pigmentosa [authors' response]. *Archives of Ophthalmology* 1993;111:1463–5.

41. Marmor MF. A randomized trial of vitamin A and vitamin E supplementation for retinitis pigmentosa [letter to the editor]. *Archives of Ophthalmology* 1993;111:1460–1.

42. Norton EWD. A randomized trial of vitamin A and vitamin E supplementation for retinitis pigmentosa [letter to the editor]. *Archives of Ophthalmology* 1993;111:1460.

Robert Temple   Sara F. Goldkind

54

The Food and Drug Administration and Drug Development

Historic, Scientific, and Ethical Considerations

The regulation of drug development, especially human clinical trials and the evidence needed for drug marketing, has major implications for research ethics. Food and Drug Administration (FDA) oversight and direction derives from federal legislation—principally the Federal Food, Drug, and Cosmetic Act of 1938, as amended in 1962—from the regulations written under that law, and from FDA guidance and policy documents that interpret the law and regulations. In this chapter, we provide a historical review of those rules and policies, noting both their obvious ethical implications and some of the less apparent, but critically important, ethical aspects of drug regulation. Table 54.1, below, summarizes the important FDA milestones.

General History

The roots of the current FDA date back to 1867, when the Division of Chemistry, housed within the Department of Agriculture, was formed to investigate the adulteration of agricultural products. Harvey Washington Wiley, a chemist and physician, became the chief chemist in 1893 and focused his attention and efforts on chemically altered foods and food additives, and their impact on health, which he believed was a greater public health threat than fraudulent or misbranded drugs. The original Pure Food and Drug Act of 1906 was a response to revelations of false claims for adulterated and dangerous patent medicines. This statute, which is still operative today, prohibited the interstate and foreign commerce of adulterated and misbranded foods and drugs. The Division of Chemistry changed names and location repeatedly, be-

coming the FDA in 1930 and eventually coming to rest in the Department of Health and Human Services (DHHS).

The FDA's responsibility for drug regulation evolved substantially in the last century. Prior to 1938 its responsibility was minimal; it could try to attack fraudulent claims, but had a considerable burden of proof and little authority. Drugs could be marketed without any contact with the FDA. There was no requirement even for notification of intent to market and no required submission of evidence. Beginning in 1933 there were discussions about expanding FDA's standard-setting authority, but the result was a legislative standoff. Then, in 1937, an elixir formulation of a new sulfa antiinfective was marketed; its solvent, diethylene glycol, the active ingredient in antifreeze, was untested except for being smelled and tasted by the formulating chemist. More than 100 people, many of them children, died as a result of ingesting Elixir Sulfanilamide, and the Food, Drug, and Cosmetic Act of 1938 was passed in response to this catastrophe. The effects of the 1938 Act and subsequent regulatory and legal developments have been described at some length elsewhere.[1]

The Food, Drug, and Cosmetic Act of 1938 mandated profound changes in the drug regulation process. It required that drugs be tested for safety and shown to be safe for use and that they be labeled with adequate directions for safe use. Just as important was the new requirement for preclearance by the FDA. Anyone seeking to market a drug had to submit an application to the FDA, which could then reject it. There was no requirement for positive FDA action; the drug was approved if the FDA did not object. Preclearance was a giant step.

Although well armed with new authority, the FDA needed time and experience to develop its skills at evaluating drug safety.

The safety requirements placed into law in 1938 are identical to the current legal requirements—at least in the language of the underlying legislation—but there is a world of difference between current safety assessments and those of the 1940s, 1950s, and 1960s. For example, two drugs approved in the early 1950s, the antidepressant iproniazid (Marsilid) and the antituberculosis drug isoniazid (INH) were approved with no recognition of their serious hepatotoxicity, which would have been obvious in any reasonable clinical trial. Only after six years and hundreds of deaths was iproniazid removed from the market. Isoniazid was considered only mildly hepatotoxic until a prophylaxis study carried out in young Public Health Service officers revealed a 1/1000 mortality rate.[2] In contrast, since the 1990s, significant hepatotoxins have commonly been identified before marketing and, if not, are usually identified a relatively short time after marketing, as were bromfenac and troglitizone.

Although what might be called the "Age of Safety" had arrived in 1938, it started with no clear requirements as to what sort of studies manufacturers should conduct or what amount or type of data they would need to collect, no internal FDA standard procedures for reviewing the safety data provided, and no formal postmarketing safety surveillance. It was not understood that controlled trials often provided the most robust safety data, at least for common events. In 1938, the appropriate trials were rarely conducted. Ethical principles that might be applicable to research appear not to have been considered at this time, and the FDA did not really regulate the drug development process.

A critical expansion of FDA authority followed yet another medical disaster, commonly known as the thalidomide tragedy, in 1962. Thalidomide was developed as a sedative intended for use during pregnancy. Unfortunately, it causes phocomelia, a major teratogenic effect in which the long bones of the fetus's limbs fail to develop. Thalidomide was marketed in Western Europe, and thousands of babies were affected. But the drug never received U.S. approval for this use, thanks to the alertness of the FDA's medical reviewer, Frances Kelsey. The United States might therefore have been spared this disaster, but after the marketing application for thalidomide had been withdrawn from consideration in March 1962, the FDA found that about 1,100 physicians had received more than 2.5 million tablets of thalidomide and had dispensed them to almost 20,000 women, including 624 pregnant women, although information submitted to the FDA had indicated that only 40 to 50 doctors had been given the drug product.[3,4] Worse, as the manufacturer had not kept good distribution records, recall of the drug proved to be a near impossibility. The result was that some cases of phocomelia appeared in the United States, most of them after the abnormality's relationship to thalidomide was known. These terrible events spurred public support for stricter drug distribution controls by the FDA. Ultimately, in 1962, such controls were incorporated into the Kefauver-Harris Amendments to the Federal Food, Drug, and Cosmetic Act, cosponsored by Sen. Estes Kefauver (D-Tenn.) and Rep. Oren Harris (D-Ark.).[5]

But that is not all the 1962 amendments did. Although the requirement would seem to bear no relationship to the thalidomide disaster, the Kefauver-Harris Amendments required, for the first time, premarket demonstration of the effectiveness of a drug, in addition to the previously required evidence that the drug was safe for its intended use. Furthermore, the 1962 amendments required affirmative FDA approval before a drug could be marketed, radically altering the dynamic of the review process.

The law, at section 505(b)(1) of the Food, Drug, and Cosmetic Act, also required that an applicant provide the FDA with "full reports of investigations which have been made to show whether or not such drug is safe for use and whether such drug is effective in use."[6] Although full use of these data in FDA reviews took many years to develop, the "full reports" requirement made possible a kind of detailed review by the FDA that was previously impossible.

Moreover, the 1962 amendments added specific requirements related to human subject protection, most notably the requirement for informed consent. Congress thus identified the fundamental importance of consent before the appearance of the first version of the Declaration of Helsinki in 1964 (see Chapter 13). The law also provided an explicit expectation that the FDA would develop a process for the regulation of investigational drugs. The law, at sections 505(i)(1)(A)–(C) of the Food, Drug, and Cosmetic Act, offered only a few details of how to do this, saying that the Secretary of the Department of Health, Education, and Welfare (DHEW, predecessor of DHHS) should promulgate regulations to allow qualified experts to investigate the safety and effectiveness of drugs. Congress suggested that investigations be conditioned on the following:

1. Submission to the secretary of DHEW of preclinical tests (including tests on animals) adequate to justify the proposed human testing.
2. A signed agreement by each investigator that patients will be under his or her personal supervision or under the supervision of investigators responsible to him or her, and that he or she will not supply drugs to anyone else (a clear response to thalidomide).
3. Maintenance of such records and submission of such reports, of the results of the investigational use as the secretary of DHEW would need to evaluate the drug should an application be submitted.[6]

In addition to those suggestions, the law was explicit in saying that the regulations to be written had to provide that informed consent would be obtained.

Regulations written in response to this provision, generally codified at 21 CFR 312,[7] describe the investigational new drug (IND) application process, under which drugs in the United States must be studied. These regulations set forth the responsibilities of investigators and sponsors for the conduct of studies and for monitoring research participants, reporting adverse effects, and making a variety of reports to the FDA. In the Kefauver hearings, Congress had been strongly urged to require animal studies prior to human exposure, and by the end of the 1960s many of the now familiar animal testing requirements were in place. Animal carcinogenicity requirements were developed in the 1970s. Many of the preclinical study expectations were further refined in international safety guidelines developed under the auspices of the International Conference on Harmonization in the 1990s.[8] The preclinical requirements reflect the view that ethical research required testing for unacceptable toxicity in animals before exposing humans to a drug.

The new effectiveness requirement was the most recognized change created by the 1962 amendments. This change had no obvious connection to the thalidomide case. Where did it come from? Thalidomide probably put the Food, Drug, and Cosmetic Act in play, giving critics of existing law an opportunity to propose changes. There had been years of testimony before the Senate Subcommittee on Antitrust and Monopoly, headed by Kefauver, on the sorry state of data supporting the effectiveness of marketed drugs and the grossly inflated labeling claims that were common. The ground was therefore prepared for the subcommittee to propose an effectiveness requirement when the opportunity to amend the law arose. The specific new requirement in section 505(d)(5) was that the FDA could refuse to approve an application if "there is a lack of substantial evidence that the drug will have the effect it purports or is represented to have under the conditions of use prescribed, recommended, or suggested in the proposed labeling [of the drug]."[6]

The idea that effectiveness was relevant was not wholly novel. Congressional testimony by FDA Commissioner George Larrick in 1964 indicated that even before the 1962 amendments, the FDA was giving thought to a drug's value in deciding whether it was safe, at least in some cases involving life-threatening diseases.[9] But even if the FDA had wanted to be more concerned with effectiveness, the poor study designs used in the drug trials conducted in the 1940s and 1950s, especially the limited use of controlled trials, would have given the FDA little basis for an effectiveness assessment in most cases.

Moreover, although the 1962 amendments are known for promulgating the requirement, this requirement was not the most important change. More important was the way in which substantial evidence was to be obtained. The *substantial evidence* requirement was on its face not a high standard. In legal terms, the highest level of evidence is "beyond a reasonable doubt," the standard in criminal trials. A lower level of evidence is *preponderance*, which means a more than 50% probability, the standard typical in civil cases. *Substantial evidence* is a still lower level. But in an artful compromise, the law not only described the standard of evidence but also identified controlled clinical trials as the one acceptable source of that evidence. Thus, in section 505(d) of the Food, Drug, and Cosmetic Act, *substantial evidence* is said to mean the following:

> Evidence consisting of adequate and well-controlled investigations, including clinical investigations, by experts qualified by scientific training and experience to evaluate the effectiveness of the drug involved, on the basis of which it could fairly and responsibly be concluded by such experts that the drug will have the effect it purports or is represented to have under the conditions of use prescribed, recommended, or suggested in the labeling or proposed labeling thereof.[6]

Legislative history indicated that the use of the plural—investigations—was intended. The Food and Drug Administration Modernization Act of 1997,[10] however, explicitly recognized that the substantial evidence requirement can be satisfied by a single study in some cases (with "confirmatory evidence") and the FDA has developed guidance on this issue.[11]

The 1962 law thus set a relatively weak legal standard of evidence but stipulated that only the best-designed kind of study (indeed, more than one such study) could fulfill the standard, producing what is recognized today as a high standard for the evidence needed to support marketing approval. The promulgation of this standard, which influenced all drug studies intended to support marketing, has contributed greatly over the past 40 years to the fundamental change in the kind of data that is expected to support any effectiveness claim for a drug, device, or other intervention. It is the principal basis for evidence-based medicine. The adequate and well-controlled clinical trial became the evidentiary standard.

In enacting the law, Congress also recognized concerns that the standard not be so high that new drugs would be difficult to develop. The legislative history clearly stated that there was no relative effectiveness requirement. That is, a new drug need not be better than, or even as good as, available therapy, so long as it worked. Congress, in the legislative history of the 1962 amendments, sought to explain the balance it had tried to reach:

> The committee [Subcommittee on Antitrust and Monopoly of the Committee on the Judiciary] believes that this provision strikes a balance between the need for governmental control to assure that new drugs are not placed on the market until they have passed the relevant tests and the need to insure that governmental control does not become so rigid that the flow of new drugs to the market, and the incentive to undergo the expense involved in preparing them for the market, become stifled.[12]

Plainly, the balance reflected in the history is highly pertinent to current discussions of rapid availability of drugs for serious diseases with poor treatment options.

Since 1962 there have been substantial refinements of the broad requirements for adequate and well-controlled studies. The FDA wrote regulations in 1970 that for the first time described the characteristics required for such studies, a regulation that was somewhat modified in 1985 and is now codified at 21 CFR 314.126 ("Adequate and well-controlled studies").[13] The Adequate and well-controlled studies rule, however, was only an introduction to three decades of growing sophistication about study design and analysis—recognizing, for example, such issues as specifying in advance the outcomes and endpoints to be analyzed in a study, correcting analyses for multiplicity (that is, for examining more than one endpoint, considering subsets, etc.), accounting for all randomized patients,[14] performing intent to treat analyses, remaining blind to interim results of studies or using group-sequential methods, the problems of equivalence/non-inferiority studies,[15] and appropriate study designs for assessing dose-response. The increasing awareness of critical elements of study design was supported by substantial growth of medical and biostatistical staff at the FDA. This was matched, perhaps as a matter of necessity, by a vast increase in statistical support in the regulated industry. It became necessary to maintain industry and medical academic awareness of these matters, which was accomplished through guidance documents, industry-FDA meetings, great numbers of workshops and medical meetings, and public advisory committee meetings.

Beginning mainly in the 1980s, with the basic standards for evaluation of the safety and effectiveness of drugs well established, two important new themes began to draw public, FDA, and congressional attention: (1) assuring reasonably prompt availability of drugs, especially promising drugs for serious diseases without adequate treatment, and (2) individualization of treatment, especially for age, sex, and racial subsets of the population.

Availability of Therapeutics

Almost from the first passage of the 1962 amendments, concerns arose that drug development was slowing and that a *drug lag* had emerged.[16] It was fairly clear that, on average, drugs were entering the U.S. market later than they were available in Europe. This actually saved the United States some bad experiences. Drugs

Table 54.1

Important FDA Milestones

Date	Event	Impetus	Outcome
1867	Division of Chemistry formed (predecessor to FDA)	• Concerns about chemically altered foods and food additives	• FDA investigated adulteration of agricultural products
1906	Pure Food and Drug Act	• Revelations about adulterated and dangerous patent medicines	• Act prohibited interstate and foreign commerce of adulterated and misbranded foods and drugs
			• FDA received no information; had to develop its data for each case
1938	Federal Food, Drug, and Cosmetic Act	• Elixir Sulfanilamide disaster	• Required drugs to be tested for safety and shown to be safe for use as labeled
			• Required that a new drug application (NDA) must be submitted to FDA prior to drug marketing
1962	Kefauver-Harris Amendments to the Federal Food, Drug, and Cosmetic Act	• Thalidomide tragedy • Kefauver hearings on drug promotion and evidence	• Required explicit approval of NDA prior to marketing.
			• Required "substantial evidence of effectiveness," derived from adequate and well-controlled studies, as a condition of marketing
			• Required closer monitoring of drug investigations, control of distribution, and the informed consent of patients in trials
1992	Prescription Drug User Fee Act (PDUFA)	• Slower-than-desired action on NDAs	• Substantially increased FDA staff and improved timeliness of actions on NDAs
1997	Food and Drug Administration Modernization Act	• Interest in access and pediatric studies	• Allowed single study in some cases to provide substantial evidence of effectiveness
			• Encouraged early access to new drugs
			• Facilitated pediatric studies by allowing 6 months extension of patents

withdrawn in Europe for toxicity prior to any U.S. introduction included practolol, lidoflazine, perhexilene, Aminorex, and others. But delayed market entry of new therapeutics was not a desired FDA goal, nor was it defensible as a matter of policy. Since the late 1970s, a variety of legal, regulatory, and policy initiatives have sought to speed the development and approval of drugs that meet the standards specified by law. These initiatives are of long-standing, beginning in the 1970s and 1980s, predating the appearance of AIDS (to which the changes are sometimes attributed). They have been supported importantly in some cases by patient advocacy groups. The changes represent a clear evolution within the FDA from a perception of its role as wholly one of protection against unsafe or ineffective drugs to a role that also includes facilitation of the development of valuable agents.

This evolution within the FDA reinforced and coincided with changes in societal attitudes, with research moving from an activity perceived as risk-laden to one viewed as hope-laden. It could be said that the avoidance of harm was the FDA's and society's operating principle during the 1940s through the 1960s and even into the early 1970s. But the rapid growth of useful therapies led to a new focus on the attainment and availability of benefit, with continuing attention to drug safety.

A necessary step toward a more active FDA role in drug development was recognition that the FDA had an obligation to define its expectations and explain to manufacturers how they could provide the data needed for drug approval. In the 1960s, many reviewers believed that too much involvement by the FDA in

the development process would leave the agency "co-opted," unable to be appropriately neutral, analytical, and critical when the time came to review the data. But the cost of not describing its expectations, allowing inadequate studies to proceed without comment, and criticizing those studies only when they were submitted to support a drug application, came to be seen as unacceptable in terms of waste, avoidable delays in development, and inappropriate and possibly unethical exposure of research participants in trials of no value. The first major effort to end the FDA's relatively passive approach was the preparation of more than 30 clinical guidelines in the late 1970s, often with involvement of FDA advisory committees and public workshops. These guidelines described the FDA's expectations for study designs and data for various therapeutic classes such as antianginal drugs, antidepressants, and drugs for peptic ulcer disease.

Development of guidance for specific drug classes continues to the present day. Several other critical guidance documents help drug companies generate the data needed to document the effectiveness and safety of a drug and present the data in a reviewable form. These include the FDA's 1988 Guideline for the Format and Content of the Clinical and Statistical Sections of Drug Applications,[17] as well as guidelines promulgated by the International Conference on Harmonisation of Technical Requirements for Registration of Pharmaceuticals for Human Use (ICH) that deal with exposure to drugs and clinical safety (ICH E-1),[18] the structure and contents of study reports (ICH E-3),[19] the proper assessment of dose response (ICH E-4),[20] the use of statistical methods (ICH

E-9),[21] and the choice of control group (ICH E-10).[22] ICH E-10, apart from its scientific value, has been a crucial document in the debate over the use of placebo controls.

The second major change, also continuing to the present, was increasing willingness of the FDA to meet with drug sponsors at critical times in the development process to discuss the planned studies and the overall database intended to support approval. Recent estimates are that about 2,300 such meetings take place each year, during which FDA staff respond to questions regarding the sponsor's planned approach, analyze overall development plans and specific study designs, and offer views about what will be needed to support approval. That the industry finds these very helpful is indicated by a 70% increase in requests for such meetings between 2000 and 2006. There seems little doubt that the decline in drug approval times since 1990, although importantly the result of increased staff and timeliness goals arising from the Prescription Drug User Fee Act of 1992, also reflects the FDA's increasing willingness to make its expectations clear.

The third significant change was facilitating broad public access to the FDA's evaluations and policies, reflected in the initiation and subsequent growth of open FDA advisory committee meetings and the availability, after approval of a drug, of the FDA's scientific reviews and administrative records. The result is the sharing with drug developers and the interested public of a great deal of information about the FDA's current expectations for data and analyses.

A more direct effort to shorten the time taken to review and act on marketing applications was the Prescription Drug User Fee Act, passed by Congress in 1992, and reauthorized in 1997, by the Food and Drug Administration Modernization Act, in 2002, by the Public Health Security and Bioterrorism Preparedness and Response Act, and in 2007 by the Food and Drug Administration Amendments Act of 2007.[23] FDA review staff had grown little since the 1970s, even while the size and complexity of new drug applications had grown and the FDA's efforts to give advice during development had increased. The FDA contended, and Congress and industry agreed, that review times could not change materially, while maintaining review quality, without a significant increase in staff. To provide such an increase, fees were assessed for submission of applications, and the revenues were used to substantially enhance the FDA clinical review staff from about 90 clinical reviewers to well over 200 in 2006, with similar increases in other disciplines. The FDA agreed to time goals for completion of reviews and action on applications—initially 12 months, later reduced to 10 months, for *standard* applications, that is, for drugs that do not appear to offer a clinical advantage over available treatment, and six months for *priority* applications involving drugs that do appear to offer a therapeutic advantage. Although the agency did not agree to goals for approval time, which obviously would have represented an inappropriate "preference for yes," proponents of the user fee program expected that timely action would decrease the time from submission to approval—and it has done so, from approximately 27 months in 1990–92 to approximately 13 months in recent years. The most striking results are for priority drugs, with action times averaging about six months during the first half of the decade.

One of the most important additions to the FDA's ability to facilitate development of drugs for unmet needs was a process providing for accelerated approval. In 1992, the FDA promulgated the Accelerated Approval Rule (codified at Subpart H of 21 CFR 314),[13]

part of which was incorporated into the 1997 Food and Drug Administration Modernization Act. It allowed a drug for a serious or life-threatening disease without good treatment to be approved on the basis of a surrogate endpoint that was "reasonably likely" to lead to a clinical benefit, on condition that such clinical benefit be established on the basis of controlled clinical trials after marketing. A surrogate endpoint is "a laboratory measurement or physical sign that is used in therapeutic trials as a substitute for a clinically meaningful endpoint that is a direct measure of how a patient feels, functions, or survives and that is expected to predict the effect of the therapy."[24] Although nothing in the law bars reliance on surrogate endpoints, and surrogates such as blood pressure, hemoglobin A1c (used in diabetes), and lipid levels have long been used, the "reasonably likely" standard represented an explicitly weaker standard of evidence than those well-established surrogates. The evidence supporting the effect of the drug on the surrogate endpoint must meet the usual adequate and well-controlled studies standard. Accelerated approval has been used primarily for drugs to treat AIDS, using the surrogate endpoints CD_4 lymphocyte count and viral load, and cancer, using tumor response as the surrogate endpoint.

Making promising drugs available to patients even before they were approved for marketing was an additional step toward greater availability. This was not an entirely novel idea. In the 1970s and 1980s, many thousands of patients had received important new agents like nifedipine, for vasospastic angina, metoprolol, a cardioselective beta blocker, and amiodarone, an antiarrhythmic agent, under various arrangements before formal marketing approval. Concern with whether such extensive distribution, without changes in regulation, could legally represent *investigational use,* with the term's implication that the studies were intended to develop evidence to support marketing, led the FDA to propose in 1982 a regulation for the *treatment IND* or *treatment protocol,* now codified at 21 CFR 312.34.[7] The rule allowed wide distribution of a drug under the IND process for serious or life-threatening diseases without satisfactory treatment if the drug was under active development and there was sufficient evidence of effectiveness and safety—which is explicitly less than that needed for marketing approval—and if clinical studies to evaluate the drug's effectiveness and safety were ongoing or complete.

Made final in 1987, the Treatment IND Rule was thought by many to be a response to AIDS. However, it was originally proposed in 1982, when AIDS was not yet a well-described clinical entity and there were no promising therapeutic interventions for the disease. What the Treatment IND Rule tried to assure, in addition to the availability of a promising drug prior to its approval, was that the availability of such a drug would not be limited to patients whose physicians had inside knowledge, but would go to any patient with the condition to be treated. If the FDA finds that the expanded access under a treatment protocol is interfering with the conduct of the well-controlled studies needed to evaluate the drug's effectiveness, it can stop the treatment protocol.

Individualization of Treatment

Beginning in the early 1980s, there was growing recognition that responses of individual patients to drugs could be very different. The first differences to be well studied were pharmacokinetic differences. It had long been known that disorders of excretory function could lead to drug accumulation, and slow and fast acetylators of isoniazid and hydralazine were known, with adverse consequences to the slow acetylators. The 1980s and 1990s saw an enormous growth in understanding of metabolic pathways and individual differences in the activity of those pathways, including the potential for inhibition of those pathways by concomitant therapies (a kind of drug-drug interaction). The "poster child" for these interactions was the interaction of terfenidine, the first nonsedating antihistamine, with cytochrome P450 3A4 inhibitors such as ketoconazole. The inhibitors blocked metabolism of terfenidine to its active metabolite, resulting in substantial accumulation of the parent drug, which caused fatal torsades de pointes arrhythmias. Assessment of metabolism and interactions is now a routine part of all drug development.

Apart from individual pharmacokinetic differences, interest also grew in possible differences in clinical responses among demographic subgroups of the population, such as groups defined by gender, age, and race. Advocacy groups for women, the elderly, blacks, and children, and the medical community were instrumental in raising this interest. Beginning in 1982, the FDA developed a series of guidance documents and regulations that drew attention to these demographic subsets and called for appropriate analyses of potential differences in response among them. The FDA did not find that members of these groups had been excluded from trials,[25] as has sometimes been asserted, but did find that there had been no attempt to see whether responses differed by group.

In the revised new drug application (NDA) regulations of 1985, now codified at 21 CFR 314.50,[13] a novel requirement for integrated summaries of safety and effectiveness data specifically called for analyses of safety and effectiveness by subgroup, and identified pediatric or geriatric patients and those with renal failure. This did not really address the breadth of demographic groups of interest, however. Consequently, in the 1988 Guideline for the Format and Content of the Clinical and Statistical Sections of New Applications,[17] the FDA called for analyses of safety, effectiveness, and dose response by demographic subgroup—in particular, subgroups based on age, gender, and race—in both individual studies (if large enough) and in the integrated summaries. In 1998, the FDA went further, stating in 21 CFR 314.50, the regulation describing an NDA submission, that the overall analyses of effectiveness and safety had to examine effectiveness, dose response, and safety by age, gender, and racial subgroups. An application that lacked these analyses was thus incomplete and would not be reviewed.[13]

In 1989[26] and 1993,[25] respectively, the FDA published guidelines on studying the elderly and both genders. Neither guideline gave specific numbers or percentages of patients in the subgroup that needed to be included in studies but both urged attention to their inclusion and specifically called for analyses of data by subgroup. The 1993 *Federal Register* notice announcing the gender guidelines also specifically revoked previous guidance urging that women be excluded from Phase 1 and early Phase 2 trials until animal teratogenicity studies had been completed, an exclusion representing concern over reproductive toxicity.[25] Further, in 2000 the FDA ruled (21 CFR 312.42)[7] that it could stop any early IND study of a life-threatening disease if patients were excluded solely because of the risk of reproductive toxicity. The encouragement to include a diverse population and insistence on analyzing databases for possible demographic differences in drug response reflected the growing scientific appreciation of individual differences in responses to treatment. But it also reflected a view

that a manufacturer was responsible for collecting data that described effectiveness and safety in the larger relevant population, a view that reflects the ethical principles of beneficence and justice, not only for the subjects in trials but for the whole community.

Since the 1980s, the FDA has increased efforts to encourage studies that enroll children. In general, children represent a small market and studies in children pose potential ethical and logistic difficulties. Through the mid-1990s only about 25% of drugs widely used in children had been studied in them.[27] Since then, two principal approaches have been tried to correct this imbalance: requiring studies in children, and granting extended marketing exclusivity, that is, an additional period of protection from generic competition, to manufacturers that carry out the pediatric studies requested by the FDA.

The Food and Drug Administration Modernization Act of 1997 created a powerful stimulus to conduct pediatric drug trials.[10] It allowed manufacturers six months of additional market exclusivity, added to whatever patent or marketing protection the manufacturer already had, if the manufacturers conducted studies specifically requested by the FDA to evaluate the drug in children. The studies did not have to succeed—that is, to show effectiveness—but they needed to be scientifically sound and to study the indication in the manner outlined by the FDA. It was expected that studies would often lead to appropriate labeling of drugs for children. The exclusivity provision was later reauthorized in the Best Pharmaceuticals for Children Act of 2002,[28] and most recently in the Food and Drug Administration Amendments Act of 2007.[23] Conduct of the studies requested by the FDA under this Act is voluntary.

A 1998 regulation titled Pediatric Use Information, codified at 21 CFR 314.55,[13] generally referred to as the Pediatric Rule, required manufacturers submitting a marketing application to include information about the use of the drug in pediatric age groups unless the requirement was waived or deferred until the postmarketing period. The Pediatric Rule was enjoined in 2002 by a federal court, but many of its elements were reinstated in the Pediatric Research Equity Act of 2003, which mandates pediatric studies of certain drugs and biological products "if there is a new element to the application (e.g., indication, dosage form, route of administration, dosing regimen, or active ingredient) or if the innovator product represents a meaningful therapeutic benefit over existing therapies for treatment, diagnosis or prevention, or if there is a need for additional therapeutic options."[29]

One further issue relevant to research ethics should be noted: the use of data from studies conducted outside the United States and not under a U.S. IND. These studies would not have been conducted under the specific ethical rules applicable in the United States, yet rejecting them and causing unnecessary duplication of studies would be ethically problematic. In 1987 the FDA adopted a regulation, codified at 21 CFR 312.120 and entitled "Foreign clinical studies not conducted under an IND,"[7] that described the criteria for acceptance of such data. The rule said, among other things, that the studies had to be conducted in accordance with a specific version of the Declaration of Helsinki (at the time, the 1989 version) or the laws of the country in which the study was conducted, whichever "represents the greater protection of the individual." The primary goal of 21 CFR 312.120 was to make sure that foreign studies on which the FDA relied met appropriate ethical norms, but it was also critical to assure that they were scientifically valid. In 2004 the FDA proposed a modification of the rule to emphasize both ethical conduct and assurance of data quality, and to eliminate reference to the Declaration of Helsinki, a document for which the FDA has no responsibility and that, in its 2000 revision, had included several provisions at odds with FDA rules and guidance. The modification to the rule instead refers to Good Clinical Practice, such as practices described in the ICH Good Clinical Practice consolidated guideline,[8] (ICH E-6), which was adopted by the FDA in 1997, and which helps assure both ethical conduct of trials and a high level of data quality.

Overview: Dietary Supplements

By law, dietary supplements are classified as foods and are subject to requirements quite different from those that apply to drugs, a difference established by the Dietary Supplement Health and Education Act of 1994 (DSHEA).[30] The distinction is important because dietary supplements are often accompanied by claims about beneficial effects on the structure or function of the body; that is, they bear some of the same claims as drugs. Section 201(c)(1) of the Federal Food, Drug, and Cosmetic Act defines a drug as the following:

1. An article intended for use in diagnosis, cure, mitigation, treatment, or prevention of disease.
2. An article (other than food) intended to affect the structure or any function of the body.[6]

Dietary supplements are defined as products that, among other things, are intended for ingestion, are intended to supplement the diet, and that contain one or more of the following dietary ingredients: a vitamin, a mineral, an herb or other botanical, or an amino acid. Under DSHEA, a dietary supplement is subject to regulation—including premarket approval, evidence of safety, and substantial evidence of effectiveness—only if it is marketed as a treatment for disease. On the other hand, a supplement manufacturer can claim an effect on structure or function (such as "builds strong bones") on the basis of the manufacturer's own conclusions about the available evidence. The claim is not subject to prior FDA review, and there are no specified standards for reaching a conclusion about effectiveness.

Structure-function claims are subject to other requirements, however; they must be accompanied by a disclaimer noting that the FDA has not evaluated the claim and that the product is not intended to diagnose, treat, cure, or prevent any disease. Structure-function claims are also subject to a postmarket notification requirement. The FDA has issued a regulation, codified at 21 CFR 101.93, that distinguishes between "disease" claims and structure-function claims for dietary supplements.[31]

Dietary supplements must be safe, but there is no expressed standard for safety and, except for certain dietary supplements that contain a "new dietary ingredient" (a dietary ingredient not marketed in the United States before Oct. 15, 1994) that is not present in the food supply, no safety documentation is required. The FDA may declare dietary supplements unsafe via rulemaking if the scientific evidence is sufficient to prove adulteration under the legal standard established by DSHEA.

Not surprisingly, in the absence of a requirement for substantial evidence of effectiveness, dietary supplements at present fall largely outside the realm of adequate and well-controlled studies, at least with respect to structure-function claims. In recent years, however, the National Center for Complementary and Alternative Medicine, part of the NIH, and other groups have conducted randomized trials of such supplements in the treatment of disease, including trials of B vitamins for lowering homocysteine and reducing coronary events,[32] echinacea for mitigating upper respiratory infections,[33] saw palmetto for treating benign prostatic hypertrophy,[34] St. John's wort for treating depression,[35] and chondroitin sulfate and glucosamine[36] for treating arthritis. Most of these trials have failed to demonstrate effectiveness. As noted above, a dietary supplement becomes a drug if it is marketed to treat, mitigate, or cure a disease. Thus, for example, if saw palmetto were marketed to treat benign prostatic hypertrophy, the FDA would regulate it as a drug.

Ethical Issues

The FDA's regulatory authority clearly gives it the ability to implement and enforce ethical norms for research with humans. In addition, many of the FDA's broader activities in regulating drug investigation and approval have ethical implications pertaining to (1) protecting the clinical research participant, (2) providing access to treatments, and (3) effective drug development.

Protecting the Clinical Research Participant

FDA regulations require the informed consent of research participants, independent review of studies, and a favorable risk-benefit ratio of studies at their commencement and as they progress. The early regulation of clinical trials focused almost entirely on the need to protect participants from harm and from being misled or deceived. This is not surprising, given scandals such as the Tuskegee syphilis study[37] and other instances of abusive investigation[38] (see Chapters 6, 7, and 8). The protections built into the Federal Food, Drug, and Cosmetic Act and its regulations are straightforward and readily understood. The first law giving the FDA a significant role in monitoring investigational studies included a requirement for informed consent, reflecting early attention to the basic ethical principle of autonomy. The law also called for prior animal tests to justify human exposure and close personal supervision of studies by investigators. The FDA IND regulations at 21 CFR 312 focus heavily on sponsor and investigator responsibilities for detecting and reporting adverse effects of test drugs.[7] The FDA is authorized to stop ("hold") a study if subjects would be "exposed to an unreasonable and significant risk of illness or injury." The development of the requirement for review of every study by a group external to the interests of the investigators—that is, an institutional review board (IRB)—reflects a similar concern with subject protection, within the FDA and the government in general.

Informed Consent and Respect for Participants

The FDA's informed consent regulations, developed following enactment of the Kefauver-Harris amendments, initially tried to distinguish between therapeutic and nontherapeutic research, but by 1981 the regulations applied to all research studies and described the critical elements of consent. FDA regulations mandate that eight basic requirements delineated in 21 CFR 50.25, "Elements of informed consent," be part of consent in all FDA-regulated research.[39] These mirror requirements in §46.116 of the federal Common Rule[40] (see Chapter 15). The basic requirements are (1) a statement that the study involves research, (2) a description of any reasonably foreseeable risks, (3) a description of any benefits to the subject or others, (4) disclosure of alternatives to research participation, (5) a description of mechanisms to ensure confidentiality, (6) an explanation as to whether any compensation and medical treatments are available if injury occurs for research involving more than minimal risk, (7) the name of a contact person for questions about the research, and (8) a statement that one's participation in research is voluntary.

FDA regulations permit a legally authorized representative to give (or withhold) consent for those with decisional incapacity, but the regulations do not allow for the total exemption of the requirement of either informed consent or consent by a legally authorized representative except under two circumstances. One, codified at 21 CFR 50.23, allows research involving a person participating in a military operation, without informed consent, in emergency situations or with a presidential waiver when consent is not feasible and nonuse of the investigational drug is contrary to the interests of the person or national security.[39] The second, codified at 21 CFR 50.24, allows an exception to informed consent for emergency research in life-threatening situations in which the study subject is incapacitated and no one is available to provide valid consent.[39] This exception is accompanied by several protections, including community consultation, public disclosure, a required data monitoring committee, the prospect that the intervention may provide direct benefit to subjects, and a plan for obtaining informed consent from either the subject or a legally authorized representative as soon as possible.

Monitoring Patients: Maintaining a Favorable Risk-Benefit Ratio

In addition to requiring consent, rules for investigators and sponsors of clinical trials require continuous monitoring of adverse effects by the investigator and the sponsor, reporting of serious unexpected events to the FDA and all investigators by sponsors, and reporting to IRBs by investigators of unexpected problems. The investigators' brochures and consent forms are modified as needed. The FDA's review, which can incorporate information gleaned from related drugs, adds a layer of protection beyond that provided by the investigator and sponsor. The more general requirements under the IND process, enforced by the FDA, also protect research participants. Thus, the need for animal data prior to any human exposure, the requirement for longer animal studies to be carried out before the longer human studies, the conduct of studies on the reproductive systems of animals early in drug development, and the progression of human data from initial short studies involving just a few patients to longer, larger studies, all contribute to maintaining a favorable risk-benefit ratio in ongoing studies. A significant safety concern at the start of a trial or during it can lead the FDA to place a *clinical hold* on the study, preventing further exposure.

In addition, the FDA's Bioresearch Monitoring Program examines the conduct of investigators in carrying out their responsibilities, including obtaining valid informed consent, appropriately monitoring research participants in accordance with the protocol, and overseeing the activities of other's participating in the study under their direction.[41]

Independent Review

The need for review of a protocol by an independent body was an early ethical concern; it first appeared at the FDA in a rule proposed in 1969 that would have required peer-group committees to review studies of new drugs. Independent review was endorsed in the 1975 version of the Declaration of Helsinki. The FDA made several proposals in the 1970s, and by 1981 the current FDA regulations at 21 CFR 56, which describe the composition and activities of IRBs in detail, were codified.[42] Every drug trial conducted in the United States, including studies exempted from the need to file an IND, as per 21 CFR 312.2,[7] must have review by an IRB; foreign studies, to be accepted in support of an application, must have been reviewed by an independent research ethics committee. IRBs must avoid or minimize conflict of interest on the part of the members, must interact with the community—generally including representatives of the community on the IRB—and must assure the integrity of the research enterprise by providing independent review. In order for an IRB to approve a protocol, it must determine that risks to subjects are minimized and are reasonable in relation to the importance of the knowledge that the study may produce and the anticipated benefits, if any, to the research subjects. IRBs also evaluate the merits of the patient inclusion and exclusion criteria, for both their scientific and ethical justification.

Access to Treatments: Fair Subject Selection and Social Value

If concerns about autonomy and nonmaleficence reflect primarily a concern about possible harm to those participating in a trial, concerns about access to potentially important benefits of therapy arise principally from ethical concerns about beneficence and justice. Moreover, these concerns focus not primarily on the protection of individuals in a trial, but on ethical concerns related to the whole community or to particular subsets within that community. Just as the FDA evolved from an organization almost solely interested in subject protection, at least during the IND phase, to one concerned also with designing clinical programs that would efficiently assess the value of a drug so that it could become available for use by the community, the FDA and the community have recognized that the potential value of drugs raises ethical concerns about access, both to investigational agents and to marketed drugs, and about the fairness of participation in clinical studies.

This has led to two principal changes in attitude: (1) a desire for inclusion of a wider range of subjects in studies, reflecting both a concern about fairness of subject selection and about the broad applicability of results, and (2) a desire for greater and earlier access to investigational agents and, to some degree, to marketed drugs.

The recognition of potential differences among individuals or groups was accompanied by a strong belief that subject selection was unfair because women, the elderly, and blacks were being excluded from the clinical trials of new drugs. Apart from concern about possible exclusion from the direct benefits of being in the clinical studies, there was also concern that there would be inadequate knowledge about how to use new drugs properly in those groups once the drugs were marketed. In most cases, however, the FDA found that the groups had not been excluded but that there had been no attempt to analyze data for possible differences in response in demographic subsets of the population.[25] These analyses are now required, a clear manifestation of the view that failing to study how drugs work in the whole population is unjust and that it is the duty of the community to benefit the broad, not a narrow, population.

Demand for greater, and earlier, access to treatments is an unequivocal reflection of a belief in the potential benefits of those treatments. The principle of autonomy, or self-determination, is commonly invoked to support this demand, but it also reflects belief in the social value of research, in terms of both specific product development and attainment of generalizable knowledge. Although AIDS and cancer are the most conspicuous loci for the sense of urgency with respect to new treatments, similar feelings arise for neurological and other serious conditions for which few good treatment options exist. There are, however, persistent tensions between early access to investigational treatments in a study and early marketing of drugs, and the need for good data on the safety and effectiveness of a drug. Even people with a serious disease can be made worse by a toxic drug that has not been adequately evaluated, and no one is well served if a marketed drug proves ineffective, especially for a serious illness.

In the face of these tensions, drugs have been made available more quickly for serious illnesses with a more limited database than drugs for less serious illnesses, reflecting the greater risks that are acceptable when treating very serious diseases. Despite the increased speed of availability, FDA reviewers continue to pay attention to the need to develop the valid evidence of effectiveness and safety that is called for in law and that is also owed to the community.

Just as the Treatment IND process provides early access to drugs for serious illnesses that are still being studied, drugs for serious illnesses can also be marketed earlier than other drugs. The Accelerated Approval Rule allows the FDA to approve such a new drug based on the effect on a surrogate endpoint that is "reasonably likely" to predict a clinical benefit, even if it has not been fully demonstrated as predictive. As clearly stated in the rule, there are risks in this approach. A plausible effect on a surrogate may fail to predict benefit, and the drug may be harmful. The most striking example of this comes from the Cardiac Arrhythmia Suppression Trial (CAST) study.[43] Although the antiarrhythmics encainide and flecainide had never been approved for use after a heart attack—labeling specifically disclaimed any data on such use—the drugs were widely used in clinical practice after a heart attack to suppress the ventricular premature beats (VPBs) that were well known to predict an increased risk of sudden death. Suppression of the VPBs was, in most people's eyes, a plausible surrogate endpoint to use when trying to modify risk of death. The results of CAST were shocking. The drugs suppressed the VPBs dramatically, but more than doubled mortality among study subjects.

Despite the risk that drugs that are given accelerated approval might prove ineffective or even harmful, most accelerated approval drugs have been shown effective and none has had an adverse outcome, although some have not yet yielded demonstrable clinical benefit. The program is generally considered a valuable way to enhance the therapeutic armamentarium for treatment of life-threatening diseases with no good treatment.

In addition, the amount of safety data needed to support an application varies according to a sliding scale. Drugs with a major benefit in life-threatening and severely debilitating diseases can be approved with smaller safety databases. A detailed discussion of this issue is beyond the scope of this chapter; but in 21 CFR 312.80 (subpart E: Drugs Intended to Treat Life-threatening and Severely-debilitating Illnesses),[7] which addresses development of such drugs, the FDA offers to have meetings earlier in development than usual so that the first controlled trials (Phase 2) can be definitive and serve as the basis for approval. Approval after Phase 2 trials, not uncommon in oncology, plainly represents a smaller than usual safety database, but is nonetheless appropriate under the circumstances.

Assuring Scientific Validity

Although they may not be generally recognized as ethical issues, two other FDA activities constitute major contributions to the ethics of drug development—policing the scientific validity of the process and assuring the social value of the endeavor. The FDA also conducts much of its business in public, providing access to the detailed basis for its decisions, creating informative labeling for approved products, and considering significant problems at public advisory committee meetings. Through meetings, protocol reviews, guidance, and public availability of the basis for its decisions, the FDA endeavors to assure that human studies are at least potentially useful. The ethical obligation to provide such assurance is suggested, if not stated in so many words, in the various versions of the Declaration of Helsinki, all of which stress the need to base research on generally accepted scientific principles. A considerable part of the FDA's resources and efforts over the years has been devoted to providing this assurance. The result is that studies are designed rigorously and incorporate the best available medical and statistical advice.

Moreover, the FDA assures the public that marketed drugs are in fact effective for the uses claimed in the package insert, have been evaluated for safety by all tests *reasonably applicable* (the legal standard) and have been shown to be *safe,* meaning that their benefits outweigh their risks. Drugs—and in slightly different ways medical devices and biologic products—are thus treated differently from the vast array of other products sold to people. They must be evaluated and approved by the FDA before they can be sold. This is a requirement that is not generally discussed as a matter of ethics, except perhaps by Congress in passing the 1962 Kefauver-Harris amendments, but it is surely based on a perceived ethical obligation to have solid evidence to support the marketing of health-care products.

Over the years, in pursuit of its legal obligation, the FDA has developed methods and practices for reviewing the evidence submitted in support of applications and has provided extensive guidance to manufacturers on how to develop good evidence of effectiveness and safety. Its efforts on occasion result in published analyses of trials[14] or commentaries on important research practices,[44,45] but far more often lead to internal reviews (which are publicly available in many cases), letters to manufacturers, and advisory committee presentations.

The FDA certainly does not work alone in this effort. Drug manufacturers, academics, practicing physicians, and patients all make significant contributions to the agency's efforts at improving the design of studies and analysis of data. But there is no independent body that has comparable capability or resources for the close examination of clinical trial design and results. Journal peer reviewers, diligent and qualified as they are, rarely have the clinical trial protocol, much less the raw data for the study, in the manuscript they are reviewing. The FDA has full access to all such information.

The FDA's advice and the expectation of careful review of data has led over the years to a wide range of stimuli to best practices in study design and conduct in such areas as randomization, blinding, specification of study hypotheses and analyses, dealing with multiplicity, appropriate selection of the control group, examination of dose response, and examination of demographic and other baseline variables, and in general, to studies of high scientific quality that can answer the questions they are designed to examine. Assurance of study quality is not regularly recognized as an ethical question, but adequate scientific quality is an essential component of an ethical clinical trial.[46]

The entire purpose of biomedical research, conveyed in many guidelines, ethical frameworks, and the Declaration of Helsinki, is to improve therapy and understanding of disease, and poorly designed studies cannot do this. A subject participating in poorly designed studies is exposed to risk without the possibility of personal or societal benefit. Guideline 11 of the International Ethical Guidelines for Biomedical Research Involving Human Subjects, produced by the Council for International Organizations of Medical Sciences (CIOMS), speaks to this as well by stating that "a clinical trial cannot be justified ethically unless it is capable of producing scientifically reliable results." The guideline also notes that "a placebo-controlled trial is often much more likely than an active control to produce a scientifically reliable result."[47]

A recent well-publicized debate over a change in the Declaration of Helsinki illustrates the FDA's role in assuring the usefulness of clinical trials and the validity of evidence used to support new drugs. In 2000, the World Medical Association proposed this substantial modification of the Declaration of Helsinki, including paragraph 29:

> The benefits, risks, burdens and effectiveness of a new method should be tested against those of the best current prophylactic, diagnostic, and therapeutic methods. This does not exclude the use of placebo, or no treatment, in studies where no proven prophylactic, diagnostic, or therapeutic method exists.[48]

This paragraph essentially barred the use of placebo controls whenever there was existing therapy, even for conditions where a short period of nontreatment represented no risk at all of harm to the patient, such as in trials of mild analgesics, antimigraine drugs, antihistamines, anxiolytics, hypnotics, baldness treatments, or dermatologic treatments. This proposal was not accompanied by any rationale or ethical justification, and would have made it difficult or impossible to evaluate many treatments properly.

Just months before, FDA scientists had published two papers exploring both the ethics of placebo-controlled trials and the interpretive problems posed by the active-control noninferiority trials that are the alternative to placebo study design.[44,45] They had pointed out that there was no ethical basis for objecting to placebo when receiving it would not lead to harm and that active control trials are uninterpretable in evaluating many symptomatic conditions. In addition, in 2000 the International Conference on Harmonisation also noted these interpretative problems and enunciated a different ethical standard in a guidance document called "Choice of Control Group and Related Issues in Clinical Trials."[22] When there is no serious harm, the ICH said, it is "generally

considered ethical to ask patients to participate in a placebo-controlled trial, even if they may experience discomfort as a result," although patients must be given treatments that prevent serious harm—such as death or irreversible morbidity—if such treatments are available.[22]

Concerned that the Declaration of Helsinki's paragraph 29 would make it impossible to provide valid evidence of effectiveness for many classes of drugs, representatives of the FDA, the National Institutes of Health, the Department of Health and Human Services, many academics, and representatives of the World Medical Association participated in conferences and meetings that led to a *clarification* of paragraph 29 in 2001. The "clarified" paragraph said placebo-controlled trials may be ethically acceptable, even if there is effective therapy, under the following conditions:

1. Where for compelling and scientifically sound methodological reasons its use is necessary to determine the efficacy or safety of a [treatment], or
2. Where a prophylactic, diagnostic, or therapeutic method is being investigated for a minor condition and the patients who received placebo will not be subject to any additional risk of serious or irreversible harm.[48]

This resolved the apparent absolute ban on placebos but left remaining questions, notably the doubtful ethics of suggesting that when a placebo was needed for interpretability, known life-saving treatment could be omitted. That was surely not intended, and such a study would be considered unacceptable by the FDA and most others. There has generally been agreement with the FDA's and ICH's position on placebos.[49,50]

The unusually public FDA effort to preserve the option of using placebo controls when they were needed and when patients would not be harmed by their use was a visible part of the continuing effort by the FDA to assure that well-designed studies provide the evidence of effectiveness and safety the public and medical community expect and deserve.

Conclusion

Familiar ethical issues, such as autonomy and patient protection, are implicit in much of what the FDA does in the course of regulating the clinical studies that are necessary for product development. But the need to treat disease, especially when no good therapy exists, and the importance to physicians and patients of having reliable information introduce another set of ethical concerns that involve the methods used to assess treatments and the level and quality of evidence needed to support wide availability and marketing. By virtue of its responsibility and its concerns and interests, the FDA has been at the forefront of the development of effective methods of drug evaluation and the interpretation of results—two issues not always recognized as having ethical implications.

Disclaimer

This work represents the views of the authors and does not necessarily represent the views of the Food and Drug Administration or the Department of Health and Human Services.

References

1. Temple R. Development of drug law, regulations, and guidance in the United States. In: Munson PL, Mueller RA, Breese GR, eds. *Principles of Pharmacology: Basic Concepts and Clinical Applications.* New York, N.Y.: Chapman and Hall; 1994:1643–64.

2. Garibaldi RA, Drusin RE, Ferebee SH, Gregg MB. Isoniazid-associated hepatitis: Report of an outbreak. *American Review of Respiratory Disease* 1972;106:357–65.

3. Food and Drug Administration, Department of Health, Education, and Welfare. Obligations of Clinical Investigators of Regulated Articles: Proposed Establishment of Regulations. *Federal Register* 1978; 43(153):35210–36. [Online] August 8, 1978. Available: http://www.fda.gov/cder/Offices/DSI/federalRegister.pdf.

4. Interagency Drug Coordination, Committee on Government Operations, United States Senate, 89th Congress, 2nd Session. Report No. 1153, May 5, 1966.

5. U.S. Congress. Kefauver-Harris Drug Amendments of 1962, Pub. L. No. 87–781, 76 Stat 780, 87th Congress (codified in scattered sections of 21 U.S.C.), October 10, 1962.

6. U.S. Congress. Federal Food, Drug, and Cosmetic Act (codified in scattered sections of 21 U.S.C.; as amended through December 31, 2004). [Online] Available: http://www.fda.gov/opacom/laws/fdcact/fdctoc.htm.

7. Food and Drug Administration, Department of Health and Human Services. Title 21 (Food and Drugs), Code of Federal Regulations, Part 312 (Investigational New Drug Application). [Online] April 1, 2006. Available: http://www.access.gpo.gov/nara/cfr/waisidx_06/21cfr312_06.html.

8. International Conference on Harmonisation of Technical Requirements for Registration of Pharmaceuticals for Human Use. *E-6: ICH Harmonised Tripartite Guideline—Guideline for Good Clinical Practice.* [Online] June 10, 1996. Available: http://www.ich.org/LOB/media/MEDIA482.pdf.

9. Hutt PB, Merrill RA, eds. *Food and Drug Law, Cases and Materials,* 2nd ed. Westbury, N.Y.: The Foundation Press; 1991:522–3.

10. U.S. Congress. Food and Drug Administration Modernization Act of 1997, Pub. L. No. 105–115, 105th Congress, 1st Session (codified as amended in scattered sections of 21 U.S.C.). [Online] January 7, 1997. Available: http://www.fda.gov/cder/guidance/s830enr.txt.

11. Food and Drug Administration, Department of Health and Human Services. Guidance for industry: Providing clinical evidence of effectiveness for human drug and biological products. [Online] May 1998. Available: http://www.fda.gov/cder/guidance/1397fnl.pdf.

12. Hoffman JE. Administrative procedures of the Food and Drug Administration. In: Adams DG, Cooper RM, Khan JS, eds. *Fundamentals of Law and Regulation: An In-Depth Look at Therapeutic Products, Volume II.* Washington, D.C.: Food and Drug Law Institute; 1997: 13–53.

13. Food and Drug Administration, Department of Health and Human Services. Title 21 (Food and Drugs), Code of Federal Regulations, Part 314 (Applications for FDA Approval to Market a New Drug). [Online] April 1, 2006. Available: http://www.access.gpo.gov/nara/cfr/waisidx_06/21cfr314_06.html.

14. Temple R, Pledger G. Special report: The FDA's critique of the Anturane Reinfarction Trial. *New England Journal of Medicine* 1980; 303:1488–92.

15. Temple R. Difficulties in evaluating positive controlled trials. *Proceedings of the American Statistical Association* (Biopharmaceutical Section) 1983:1–7.

16. Wardell WM. Introduction of new therapeutic drugs in the United States and Great Britain: An international comparison. *Clinical Pharmacology and Therapeutics* 1973;14:773–90.

17. Food and Drug Administration, Department of Health and Human Services. Guideline for the format and content of the clinical and statistical sections of an application. [Online] July 1988. Available: http://www.fda.gov/cder/guidance/statnda.pdf.

18. International Conference on Harmonisation of Technical Requirements for Registration of Pharmaceuticals for Human Use. *E1: The Extent of Population Exposure to Assess Clinical Safety for Drugs Intended for Long-Term Treatment of Non-Life-Threatening Conditions.* [Online] October 27, 1994. Available: http://www.ich.org/LOB/media/MEDIA435.pdf.

19. International Conference on Harmonisation of Technical Requirements for Registration of Pharmaceuticals for Human Use. *E-3: Structure and Content of Clinical Study Reports.* [Online] November 30, 1995. Available: http://www.ich.org/LOB/media/MEDIA479.pdf.

20. International Conference on Harmonisation of Technical Requirements for Registration of Pharmaceuticals for Human Use. *E-4: Dose-Response Information to Support Drug Registration.* [Online] March 10, 1994. Available: http://www.ich.org/LOB/media/MEDIA480.pdf.

21. International Conference on Harmonisation of Technical Requirements for Registration of Pharmaceuticals for Human Use. *E-9: Statistical Principles for Clinical Trials.* [Online] February 5, 1998. Available: http://www.ich.org/LOB/media/MEDIA485.pdf.

22. International Conference on Harmonisation of Technical Requirements for Registration of Pharmaceuticals for Human Use. *E-10: Choice of Control Group and Related Issues in Clinical Trials.* [Online] July 20, 2000. Available: http://www.ich.org/LOB/media/MEDIA486.pdf.

23. Food and Drug Administration Amendments Act of 2007, Publ. L. No.110–85, 121 Stat. 823 (2007).

24. Food and Drug Administration, Department of Health and Human Services. New Drug, Antibiotic, and Biological Drug Product Regulations: Accelerated Approval; Proposed Rule. *Federal Register* 1992;57(73):13234–42.

25. Food and Drug Administration, Department of Health and Human Services. Guideline for the study and evaluation of gender differences in the clinical evaluation of drugs: Notice. *Federal Register* 1993; 58(139):39406–16.

26. Food and Drug Administration, Department of Health and Human Services. Guideline for the study of drugs likely to be used in the elderly. Rockville, Md.: FDA/Center for Drug Evaluation and Research; 1989.

27. Roberts R, Rodriguez W, Murphy D, Crescenzi T. Pediatric drug labeling: Improving the safety and efficacy of pediatric therapies. *JAMA* 2003;290:905–11.

28. U.S. Congress. Best Pharmaceuticals for Children Act, Pub. L. No. 107–109, S. 1789, 107th Congress, 1st Session (codified as amended in scattered sections of 21 U.S.C. and 42 U.S.C.). [Online] January 4, 2002. Available: http://www.fda.gov/opacom/laws/pharmkids/contents.html.

29. U.S. Congress. Pediatric Research Equity Act of 2003, Pub. L. No. 108–155, S. 650, 108th Congress, 1st Session. [Online] January 7, 2003. Available: http://www.fda.gov/cder/pediatric/S-650-PREA.pdf.

30. U.S. Congress. Dietary Supplement Health and Education Act of 1994, Pub. L. No. 103–417, 108 Stat. 4325, 103rd Congress, 2nd Session. [Online] October 25, 1994. Available: http://www.fda.gov/opacom/laws/dshea.html.

31. Food and Drug Administration, Department of Health and Human Services. Title 21 (Food and Drugs), Code of Federal Regulations, Part 101.93 (Food Labeling), Section 101.93 (Certain types of statements for dietary supplements). [Online] April 1, 2006. Available: http://www.access.gpo.gov/nara/cfr/waisidx_06/21cfr101_06.html.

32. The Heart Outcomes Prevention Evaluation (HOPE) 2 Investigators. Homocysteine lowering with folic acid and B vitamins in vascular disease. *New England Journal of Medicine* 2006;354:1567–77.

33. Barrett, BP, Brown RL, Loken K, et al. Treatment of the common cold with unrefined Echinacea: A randomized, double-blind, placebo-controlled trial. *Annals of Internal Medicine* 2002;137:939–46.

34. Bent S, Kane C, Shinohara K, et al. Saw palmetto for benign prostatic hyperplasia. *New England Journal of Medicine* 2006;354:557–66.

35. Hypericum Depression Trial Study Group. Effect of Hypericum perforatum (St John's Wort) in major depressive disorder: A randomized, controlled trial. *JAMA* 2002;287:1807–14.

36. Clegg DO, Reda DJ, Harris CL, et al. Glucosamine, chondroitin sulfate, and the two in combination for painful knee osteoarthritis. *New England Journal of Medicine* 2006;354:795–808.

37. Brandt AM. Racism and research: The case of the Tuskegee Syphilis Study. *Hastings Center Report* 1978;8(6):21–9.

38. Beecher HK. Ethics and clinical research. *New England Journal of Medicine* 1966;274:1354–60.

39. Food and Drug Administration, Department of Health and Human Services. Title 21 (Food and Drugs), Code of Federal Regulations, Part 50 (Protection of Human Subjects). [Online] April 1, 2006. Available: http://www.gpo.gov/nara/cfr/waisidx_06/21cfr50_06.html.

40. Department of Health and Human Services, National Institutes of Health, and Office for Human Research Protections. The Common Rule, Title 45 (Public Welfare), Code of Federal Regulations, Part 46 (Protection of Human Subjects). [Online] June 23, 2005. Available: http://www.hhs.gov/ohrp/humansubjects/guidance/45cfr46.htm.

41. Food and Drug Administration, Office of Regulatory Affairs, Department of Health and Human Services. FDA/ORA Bioresearch Monitoring information page. [Online] Available: http://www.fda.gov/ora/compliance_ref/bimo/default.htm.

42. Food and Drug Administration, Department of Health and Human Services. Title 21 (Food and Drugs), Code of Federal Regulations, Part 56 (Institutional Review Boards). [Online] April 1, 2006. Available: http://www.gpo.gov/nara/cfr/waisidx_06/21cfr56_06.html.

43. Echt DS, Liebson PR, Mitchell LB, et al., for the CAST Investigators. Mortality and morbidity in patients receiving encainide, flecainide, or placebo: The Cardiac Arrhythmia Suppression Trial. *New England Journal of Medicine* 1991;324:781–8.

44. Temple R, Ellenberg S. Placebo-controlled trials and active-control trials in the evaluation of new treatments. Part 1: Ethical and scientific issues. *Annals of Internal Medicine* 2000;133:455–63.

45. Ellenberg S, Temple R. Placebo-controlled trials and active-control trials in the evaluation of new treatments. Part 2: Practical issues and specific cases. *Annals of Internal Medicine* 2000;133:464–70.

46. Emanuel EJ, Wendler D, Grady C. What makes clinical research ethical? *JAMA* 2000;283:2701–11.

47. Council for International Organizations of Medical Sciences, in collaboration with the World Health Organization. *International Ethical Guidelines for Biomedical Research Involving Human Subjects.* Geneva, Switzerland: CIOMS and WHO; 2002. [Online] November 2002. Available: http://www.cioms.ch/frame_guidelines_nov_2002.htm.

48. World Medical Association. *Declaration of Helsinki: Ethical Principles for Medical Research Involving Human Subjects.* Tokyo, Japan: WMA; October 2004. [Online] 2004. Available: http://www.wma.net/e/policy/b3.htm.

49. Lewis JA, Jonsson B, Kreutz G, Sampaio C, van Zwieten-Boot B. Placebo-controlled trials and the Declaration of Helsinki. *Lancet* 2002;359:1337–40.

50. Emanuel EJ, Miller FG. Placebo-controlled trials—A middle ground. *New England Journal of Medicine* 2001;345:915–9.

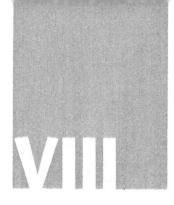

VIII

Informed Consent

Erika Blacksher   Jonathan D. Moreno

A History of Informed Consent in Clinical Research

This chapter traces the evolution of informed consent as a concept and practice in biomedical research, attending to the evolving content and justification of consent, and when possible, the actual consent practices of researchers. We include the predecessors of informed consent, some of which bear only a faint resemblance to the concept and practice as we understand them today. These precursors lack what are now considered essential features of informed consent, having evolved from mere acquiescence to become informed, comprehending, and voluntary. As there was no clear policy delineation between medical research and clinical care until perhaps the 1960s, we find that the evolution of informed consent doctrine occurred in both contexts and actually helped to distinguish these medical encounters.

The plasticity of informed consent can be attributed not only to the emergence of new medical sciences, diseases, and research contexts, but also, and more importantly for the purposes of this chapter, to the growing collective understanding of and demands for the ethical treatment of persons who participate in research. The assessments and distinctions we make among various conceptions of consent reflect a currently and commonly held normative account of informed consent. As such, our analysis tracks whether consent is informed, comprehending, voluntary, and justified on the basis of individual autonomy.[1]

These essential features of informed consent have been forged in response to two persistent themes in research with humans: the misrepresentation of research and the unfair selection of participants. Historically and currently, the research community often has faltered in its duty to present sufficient and clear information about the nature, purpose, risks of, and alternatives to research and to clearly distinguish research from clinical care. Because

medical research emerged within the conceptual parameters and physical settings of clinical practice, the task of distinguishing one from the other took researchers and onlookers more than a century. The distinction was not formally codified until the 1960s and not widely recognized until the early 1980s. Still, the tendency to present research as a form of therapy remains today. Informed consent doctrine also evolved in response to researchers' failures to ensure that participants had the capacity to decide, to fully understand the information presented, and to make truly voluntary decisions. Together these features of informed consent—full disclosure, comprehension, and voluntariness—are intended to promote the autonomy of potential participants, enabling them to make choices about research participation that align with their values and interests.

Our analysis traces the evolution of these ethical ideas more so than the reasons for their emergence and change. We point to the people, events, and movements related to or responsible for the turning points in this concept and practice in research with humans, but we do not attempt a detailed analysis of the larger societal forces within which these actors operated and activities took place. Changing conceptions of the individual and the civil rights movement, the reorganization of medicine and its delivery, and the emergence of new sciences and their accompanying power and prestige are important histories.[2] But these topics are beyond the scope of this chapter. This chapter also draws largely, though not exclusively, on U.S. cases and events. Much of the history of informed consent, especially in the research context, occurred in the United States, and the history in other countries often is unknown or as yet unwritten. Table 55.1 presents some important events in the evolution of the informed consent doctrine.

Table 55.1
Informed Consent Timeline

Date	Event
c. 400 B.C.	• Hippocratic texts, first set of Western writings about medical professional conduct, discusses truth telling, advises physicians to hide as much as possible from patients.
1260–1325	• Henri de Mondeville, surgeon and anatomy teacher, instructs physicians to compel obedience by threatening patients.
1724–1773	• John Gregory advocates public/patient education and honesty, but justified on basis of patient beneficence, not autonomy.
1746–1813	• Benjamin Rush, "American Hippocrates," advocates sharing information with patients, but does not advocate seeking consent or respecting patient decisions that diverge from those of the physician.
1767	• *Slater* v. *Baker and Stapleton* cited as first informed consent case but no direct or indirect line to modern legal doctrine.
1803	• Thomas Percival publishes landmark work that emphasizes physician virtues; basically upheld Hippocratic approach.
1847	• American Medical Association (AMA) establishes and issues first code of ethics based on Percival's work; enhanced physician authority.
1849	• Worthington Hooker publishes *Physician and Patient*, an uncompromising denunciation of deception in medicine. Had little impact on practice of medicine.
1874	• AMA condemns Cincinnati physician Robert Bartholow's experiments on dying patient, who he claimed gave "cheerful assent."
1884	• Reports of the anesthetic properties of cocaine fostered widespread self-experimentation among surgeons and medical students.
1886	• Boston physician Charles Francis Withington advocates that patient consent should be sought when studies involve risk and discomfort and offer no potential benefit.
1888	• Gynecologist James W. Etheridge advises colleagues that patient consent is essential for most difficult and risky procedures.
1891	• French and German physicians graft cancerous tissue onto cancer patients to see if it was contagious. Victor Cornil analyzed tissue grafted on by another surgeon; act denounced as "criminal."
	• Prussian government enacts regulation to insure that tuberculin would "in no case be used against the patient's will."
1897	• Giuseppe Sanarelli announces discovery of bacillus of yellow fever and maintained that he had produced yellow fever in five patients. Act is condemned as criminal by William Osler.
Turn of 20th century	• Growing number of lawsuits over unauthorized surgical procedures prompts increasing use of written consent forms, even though verbal and implicit consent remain legal.
1900	• Written contracts used in Walter Reed's yellow fever experiments.
	• Proposal for regulation of human experimentation (and animal cruelty) introduced in Washington, D.C., legislature, requiring disclosure of investigator's purpose and procedures and written consent in experiments with no potential benefit. Legislation fails.
1903	• Boston physician Richard Clarke Cabot reports study results showing that patients and families benefit from truth about prognosis.
1905	• *Mohr* v. *Williams*, court opinion uses language of "the free citizen's right to himself."
1906	• *Pratt* v. *Davis* opinion cites *Mohr* language.
1907	• William Osler's address to Congress of American Physicians and Surgeons proposes three criteria for human experimentation: (1) tried on animals, (2) absolutely safe, and (3) full consent.
1913	• *Rolater* ruling strengthens patient consent.
1914	• *Schloendorff* v. *Society of New York Hospital* produces Judge Cardoza's widely cited opinion: "Every human being of adult years and sound mind has a right to determine what shall be done with his own body; and a surgeon who performs an operation without his patient's consent commits and assault, for which he is liable in damages." Subsequent cases adopted self-determination as justification for informed consent.
	• Walter Cannon, chair of the Council for Defense of Medical Research, requests that research participant's consent be made a requirement of journal publication.
1916	• Cannon proposes uniform guidelines be developed for human experimentation. No agreement could be achieved.
	• Cannon publishes editorial in *JAMA* outlining ethics of experimentation on humans and recommends that the AMA adopt formal code explicitly recognizing patient consent. Idea rejected.
1925	• Army regulation to promote infectious disease research specifies that volunteers be used in experimental research.
1930–1956	• Only nine published articles on consent and patient authorization.
1931	• Germany issues world's first guidelines for human experimentation and innovative medical therapies; later deemed more adequate than Nuremberg Code.
	• Richard Clarke Cabot develops code of conduct for hospital physicians requiring patient consent.
1932	• U.S. Public Health Service begins Tuskegee Syphilis study (1932–1970).
	• U.S. Navy requires research volunteers to be "informed."

Table 55.1
(Continued)

Date	Event
1941	• John Bonner, 15-year-old black student in Washington, D.C., seriously harmed by experimental skin graft conducted without his or his parent's consent; court rules in favor of physician.
1943	• Secretary of Navy requires all research receive prior approval from secretary; Navy uses "waivers" in wartime experiments using prisoners and conscientious objectors.
1945	• International Military Tribunal to try Nazi physicians and other war criminals established.
1946	• AMA adopts first formal statement on human experimentation.
1947	• Atomic Energy Commission general manager, Carroll Wilson, uses language of "informed consent."
1948	• Trial of Nazi physicians produces 10-principle Nuremberg Code.
	• AMA's expert witness at Nuremberg trials, Andrew Ivy, publishes report on which Nuremburg Code is later partly based, in *JAMA*.
1950	• Atomic Energy Commission (AEC)–sponsored Oak Ridge Institute for Nuclear Studies (ORINS) research hospital institutes policy to advise incoming patients of experimental nature of procedures and requires signed consent forms.
1951	• Perhaps first ethics code for behavioral sciences; includes a strict consent requirement.
1952	• Pope Pius XII endorses principle of consent for both healthy volunteers and sick patients at First International Congress of Neuropathology.
1953	• Department of Defense, following proposal by Armed Forces Medical Policy Council, adopts Nuremberg Code for defensive research on atomic, biological, and chemical weapons.
	• Department of Health, Education and Welfare adopts policy on research for NIH's new hospital devoted to experimental work; includes detailed definition of informed consent.
	• American Psychological Association adopts ethics code that includes a strict consent requirement, which remained in tension with profession's routine use of deceit as a methodology.
	• Irwin Berg publishes article in *American Psychologist* arguing that research is unethical if informed consent not obtained.
1953–1954	• Army-sponsored, secret research carried out under supervision of Harvard's Henry Beecher in which hallucinogens given to uninformed healthy persons.
1954	• Willowbrook study begins.
1956	• AEC advises Los Alamos researchers to fully inform healthy research participants.
1957	• *Salgo* v. *Leland Stanford Jr. University Board of Trustees* ruling requires physicians to disclose all pertinent information, including risks and alternatives.
1958	• Veterans Administration's research program recognizes consent requirements for participants.
1959	• National Society for Medical Research acknowledges Nuremberg Code as Western world's guide to research.
	• Henry Beecher publishes "Experimentation in Man" in *JAMA*.
1960	• *Natanson* v. *Kline*.
1961–1962	• Law-Medicine Institute Study finds that few institutions have procedural guidelines governing research with humans.
1963–1966	• Jewish Chronic Disease Hospital study takes place.
	• Stanley Milgram's research becomes most controversial and instructive case on problems of deceit and consent in psychology.
	• U.S. Army issues formal regulations.
1961–1963	• Thalidomide tragedies in Europe prompt new FDA policy, which includes consent requirement.
1964	• World Medical Association adopts Declaration of Helsinki guidelines.
1965	• U.S. Air Force regulations clearly require voluntary and written informed consent from all research participants.
1966	• *Gray* v. *Grunnagle* ruling defines consent as necessarily "accompanied by deliberation" and issuing from quasi-contractual relationship.
	• Henry Beecher publishes article in the *New England Journal of Medicine* presenting 22 cases of research misconduct.
	• New FDA provisions produced based on Nuremburg Code and Declaration of Helsinki.
	• Public Health Service issues landmark policy requiring institutions receiving federal grant support from PHS to provide prior review to address (1) rights and welfare of participants, (2) methods to obtain informed consent from patients and healthy participants, and (3) balance of risks and benefits.
	• NIH Clinical Center updates guidelines, emphasizing informed consent requirements.
1967	• U.S. Navy's medical department manual clearly requires written consent, unclear whether it applies to patients.
1969	• *Berkey* v. *Anderson* ruling holds that withheld information constitutes deceit and that patient-physician relationship creates a duty of full disclosure.
	• U.S. Department of Health, Education and Welfare (DHEW, now Department of Health and Human Services [DHHS]) revises policy with thorough treatment of informed consent, addressing both substantive and procedural elements.
	• U.S. Navy requires written consent from both patients and healthy volunteers.

(continued)

Table 55.1

(*Continued*)

Date	Event
1970	• National Welfare Rights Organization drafts statement; genesis of patient's rights movement.
1971	• *The Institutional Guide to DHEW Policy on Protection of Human Subjects* (Yellow Book) expands requirements to all programs.
	• *Cooper v. Roberts* ruling fortifies informed consent doctrine.
	• Zimbardo's mock prison research study shifts attention to quality of consent.
1972	• *Canterbury v. Spence* ruling uses self-determination as primary justification for protecting patients' rights to decide.
	• *Cobbs v. Grant* and *Wilkinson v. Vesey* rulings hold that treatment decisions require reference to the patient's values.
	• Cook Commission adopts 10-principle code for behavioral research, half of which deal with disclosure and consent; deception in behavioral research still permitted.
	• *New York Times* exposes Tuskegee Syphilis study.
1973	• Tuskegee Syphilis study stopped.
1974	• DHEW converts policies into regulations and expands definition of informed consent.
	• *New York Times* exposes CIA experiments conducted on uninformed subjects.
1974–1978	• National Research Act creates National Commission for the Protection for Human Subjects of Biomedical and Behavioral Research.
	• American Hospital Association publishes patient bill of rights.
1975	• Church Committee and Rockefeller Commission investigate CIA experiments.
1975–1977	• Twenty-five states enact informed consent legislation (30 states by 1982).
1976	• President Gerald Ford issues executive order on intelligence activities prohibiting human experimentation with drugs, with strict informed consent standards. (Presidents Carter and Reagan expand to cover all research.)
1979	• National Commission publishes *Belmont Report.*
	• DHEW creates Ethical Advisory Board as recommended by National Commission.
1980	• *Truman v. Thomas* ruling requires duty to disclose even in cases of treatment refusal.
1980–1983	• President's Commission for the Study of Ethical Problems in Medicine and Biomedical and Behavioral Research publishes nine reports.
1981	• DHHS secretary signs regulations resulting from National Commission.
	• AMA Judicial Council publishes statement on patient rights and informed consent.
1982	• Study on physician attitudes finds that obtaining informed consent has become routine practice.
	• Council for International Organizations of Medical Sciences (CIOMS) issues draft guidelines for international research.
1986	• Congressional investigation of human radiation experiments yields "Markey Report."
1987	• *United States v. Stanley* is only U.S. Supreme Court case to address application of Nuremberg Code to experimentation conducted by United States.
1991	• Federal government issues Common Rule regulations.
	• CIOMS revises its international guidelines.
1993	• CIOMS and World Health Organization issue International Ethical Guidelines for Biomedical Research Involving Human Subjects and emphasize both individual consent and community review.
	• *Albuquerque Tribune* exposes U.S. government sponsorship of human radiation experiments.
1994	• President Bill Clinton creates Advisory Committee on Human Radiation Experiments.
1996	• Declaration of Helsinki revised.
1998	• Joint United Nations Programme on HIV/AIDS presents ethical guidelines to address ethical issues specific to HIV/AIDS in international context; informed consent important feature.
2000	• Declaration of Helsinki revised and informed consent requirements strengthened.

Prehistory: Voluntary Consent

The emergence of new sciences, technologies, and social structures during the 19th century ripened the practice of medicine for research on humans.[3] Once associated solely with the physician's role as healer and provider of care, medicine during the 1800s increasingly became associated with the physician's role as experimenter and collector of data. By the century's end, medical experimentation had redefined the practice and image of medicine in the United States and generated considerable agreement among members of the public and medical profession about the ethical criteria that should guide research.[3] The relative safety of untried treatments and procedures, the possibility of therapeutic benefit, and the voluntary consent of patients and participants were considered essential for ethical research.[3]

These ideas remain relevant 100 years later. They have undergone significant analysis, augmentation, and transformation as the result of focused, sustained discussion in the latter half of the

20th century. During the dawn of medical research, however, the formulation of ethical criteria did not benefit from focused discussion on how to protect the health and dignity of persons while enabling the advancement of medical science. Protagonists and antagonists were engaged in a battle over more basic questions about whether human experimentation should be permitted at all and whether participant consent was even necessary. Inchoate ethical criteria were often embedded in attacks on and defenses of physicians' nascent forays into medical research. "Hostile exchanges, extravagant accusations, and vehement denials eclipsed any candid public discussion of the moral problems posed by clinical and laboratory research," writes historian Susan Lederer.[3]

Many critics who sought to abolish this novel enterprise belonged to a movement to protect not only human beings, but also animals from medical experimentation. The antivivisection movement, formally organized in the United States in 1866 with the establishment of the American Society for the Prevention of Cruelty to Animals, was originally devoted solely to the abolition of animal experimentation, but grew to contain many factions and over time split into separate movements. A reformist faction came to view the inclusion of humans, particularly vulnerable groups such as children, as central to its mission. Lederer has argued that "American opposition to animal experimentation cannot be understood independently of the expectation . . . that unrestrained experimentation on animals would culminate in the scientific exploitation of vulnerable human beings."[3]

At stake in this debate were not only the lives and welfare of vulnerable persons, but also the goals of medicine. As growing numbers of physicians began to search for the underlying causes of human disease and to develop new techniques for diagnosis, treatment, and prevention, their attention shifted from the therapeutic needs of current patients to research that would serve future patients.[3] With this shift in the priorities of research-oriented physicians came a need for new norms. Physicians' traditional commitments to promote patient welfare and "at least do no harm" derived from the Hippocratic oath written around 400 B.C. With the advent of medical research, these commitments needed to be replaced with moral rules to guide interactions between clinical investigators and research participants.

During the latter decades of the 19th century there was general agreement that in principle patients should not be subjected to research that did not promise them benefit unless they were true volunteers. The absence of injury and willingness to self-experiment also worked to shield researchers from scrutiny. Experimentation that transgressed these ethical boundaries received sharp and certain criticism. Yet, clarity and certainty in principle yielded neither in clinician practice. None of the key terms was well analyzed. What constituted an experiment, whether research offered the possibility of benefit, when potentially beneficial research could be considered standard medical care, and what *volunteer* meant were questions mired in confusion and controversy. The issues were not academic; they had direct implications for the issue of consent. In general during this time, physician-researchers were not inclined to share their uncertainty with patient-participants. Research thought to offer potential benefits to patient-participants was often presented to patients as "medical therapy." Physicians had no duty to seek patient consent when providing therapy; on the contrary, they were considered to have a duty to hide potentially harmful information from patients. Physicians' professional ethics, from ancient Greece through much of the 20th century, required them to keep medical information from patients in the belief that doing so promoted the patients' welfare. This practice, called *benevolent deception,* justified not only withholding information from patients, but also lying, manipulation, and even threats.[1]

Physicians who advocated honesty with patients were the rare exception. Influenced by Enlightenment ideas, the 18th century Scottish physician John Gregory, for example, advocated public and patient education.[1] His student, Benjamin Rush, brought those ideas to the United States, where he encouraged physicians to share much information with patients, on the belief that free choice was a condition of good health.[1] Still, Rush did not advocate seeking the consent of patients nor honoring decisions that diverged from that of the physician. The authority of physicians still ruled the day.

The absolute authority of physicians was tempered only when the risks posed by experimental treatment were significant. The advice of U.S. gynecologist James W. Etheridge to colleagues in 1888 is illustrative. He emphasized the necessity of obtaining patient consent, without coercion, when procedures were difficult and dangerous, as was the case at the time with caesarean section.[3] But there was no expectation that patients be presented with information about the procedures, only that they "volunteer." The term *volunteer* not only lacked formal definition, but practice patterns surely deflated the practical force of this expectation among physicians and patients. Physician authoritarianism coupled with patients' general trust of physicians and medicine likely compelled many patients to comply with physician requests. Although patients could in principle decline participation, physician expectations ran high. Some viewed the fact of hospitalization as a license to experiment on patients.[3] This expectation was a function not only of physicians' professional ethics but of blatant prejudice. Hospitals during much of the 19th century served largely as custodial institutions for poor people who were sick and dying. Some physicians viewed patients' participation in research as appropriate repayment for the free care they received.

Although consent practices left much to be desired, 19th century ideas about consent standards were more rigorous. Insight into these ideas can be gained by examining attitudes toward the involvement of various kinds of people in research. The use of members of groups deemed incapable of understanding or volunteering for research was uniformly and swiftly criticized by antivivisectionists. Those deemed most vulnerable were children living in orphanages. Others considered vulnerable were persons with cognitive impairments, poor people, new mothers and their infants, prisoners, and soldiers. Although strident antivivisectionists included professional participants (those paid for their participation) among those vulnerable to coercion because of the inducement of compensation, others endorsed the practice of compensation for research participation.[3]

The participant pool that yields the most interesting insights into 19th century attitudes, however, is researchers' use of themselves. Today, cases of self-experimentation are reported occasionally, but it is an uncommon practice and there is no public expectation of it. During the 19th century, however, self-experimentation was a widely accepted and some believed obligatory practice. The reasons for its widespread acceptance were not analyzed or articulated explicitly at the time;[3] however, an analysis of self-experimentation yields a formula for consent that meets current standards. Researchers considering self-experimentation would know better than anyone the purpose of the research and the nature and degree of risks; they were best prepared to comprehend this information and speculate as to potential consequences; their self-administered inoculations and applications clearly demonstrated voluntariness; and this action was grounded in autonomy by furthering their interests and promoting their values. Self-experimentation was a radical act of "self-determination." Researchers' consent duties to other participants would not reach such high-bar standards until well into the 20th century.

A number of events at the turn of the 20th century, however, signaled the beginning of a shift in researchers' duties to participants. Instances of self-regulation, increased efforts by antivivisectionists to regulate human experimentation, and landmark court decisions regarding medical care began a shift in attention from a researcher's duty to obtain consent to the content and quality of consent. Proposed and implemented reforms addressed issues such as disclosure requirements, written consent forms (then usually called *contracts, releases,* or *waivers*), decision-making capacity, and fairness in participant selection, albeit all in cases of research with no intended benefits. Consent standards for potentially beneficial research would continue to languish in the shadows of the Hippocratic tradition of benevolent deception for decades to come.

In 1900, in what seems to be the first such case, researchers used written contracts with participants. The yellow fever research conducted in Cuba led by Walter Reed required potential participants (American soldiers and local workers) to sign written agreements that outlined the risks and benefits of participation (see Chapter 1). The agreement explained that exposure to yellow fever endangered participants' lives; it also implied that the chances of becoming infected on the island were great and that intentional infection would ensure access to the "greatest care and most skillful medical service."[3] Scholars suggest that the written contracts were flawed in several respects: They offered compensation excessive enough to exert undue pressure on potential participants; they overstated the inevitability of natural infection; and they understated the danger to life posed by yellow fever. Nonetheless they "marked a significant departure in the history of human experimentation,"[3] according to Lederer.

That same year, pressures to regulate human experimentation came from outside the medical profession. Antivivisectionists persuaded an ally in the U.S. Senate to propose a bill to regulate human experimentation. Jacob H. Gallinger, a physician and past surgeon general of New Hampshire, introduced a proposal to regulate research in the District of Columbia. Senate Bill 3424 addressed requirements for prior disclosure of the purpose of and procedures involved in research, written consent, and protection of vulnerable populations. The bill would have made it illegal to do research with a long list of people incapable of granting consent or those especially vulnerable to coercion.[3] The bill failed due to fierce and effective lobbying by the American Medical Association (AMA), which two years earlier had established a task force to track such legislative efforts.

The failed Senate bill and Walter Reed's yellow fever study are significant for several reasons. Prior to 1900 debate centered primarily on a researcher's duty to obtain consent in advance of experimentation. Reed's investigation and the Senate bill began to raise the bar by focusing on the content and quality of consent. To different degrees, they addressed the information to be disclosed

to potential participants. By requiring written consent, they also could be interpreted as efforts to convey the seriousness of research participation and to promote careful consideration among potential participants. Of course, sheer self-interest may also have been operative. As researchers became increasingly aware of cases in which physicians were successfully prosecuted for transgressing the bounds of ethical research, written contracts may have been seen as mechanisms for self-protection.

One such case was that of German bacteriologist Albert Neisser, who discovered the leprosy bacillus and gonococcus. His testing of a syphilis vaccine on three young girls and five female prostitutes, who were neither informed nor asked for their consent, resulted in Neisser's criminal prosecution and culminated in extensive German legislation.[3] In 1900, the German minister for religious, educational, and medical affairs issued a directive that required a "proper explanation of the possible negative consequences" of the experiment and that insisted that the person give his or her "unambiguous consent."[4] Despite all this, the directive "was not legally binding and little is known of its impact on human experimentation,"[4] according to Vollmann and Winau. Thirty-one years later, the Reich government issued detailed and formidable guidelines that distinguished between therapeutic and "nontherapeutic" research and required consent from participants. These guidelines were not annulled during the Nazi period in Germany but tragically had no deterrent effect on Nazi physicians during World War II[4] (see Chapter 2).

In the same period, a number of U.S. lawsuits over unauthorized surgical procedures, along with increasing use of hospitals by middle- and upper-class patients, sensitized surgeons to the need for more formalized consent records, even outside the research context.[4] Four court decisions within the first 14 years of the 20th century introduced important new ideas about the nature and justification of consent. The 1905 *Mohr v. Williams* (Minnesota Supreme Court), 1906 *Pratt v. Davis* (Illinois Supreme Court), 1913 *Rolater v. Strain* (Oklahoma Supreme Court), and 1914 *Schloendorff v. Society of New York Hospital* (New York Court of Appeals) cases are largely responsible for developing the basic features of informed consent to medical care in U.S. law.[1]

These cases were preceded by a 1767 English case, *Slater v. Baker and Stapleton*, often cited as the first medical consent case.[1] Although the patient's consent was at issue in this case, the judicial reasoning would in subsequent centuries be categorized as malpractice law.[1] Leading scholars claim there "is no direct, or even indirect, line between *Slater* and the modern legal doctrine" of informed consent.[1] The judicial reasoning in the U.S. cases, however, reveals a growing appreciation for the patient's decision-making process and right to self-determination. Together these court decisions raised expectations for physician disclosure, expanded patients' rights to specify the meaning and content of consent for particular procedures, and justified informed consent on grounds of patient autonomy.[1,5] Indeed, the court's language in *Schloendorff* would become the most widely quoted in the current informed consent literature.[1] Technically it was not a consent case, and the court neither found a violation of consent nor commented on consent requirements. Nonetheless, Justice Benjamin Cardozo's language became a classic statement for patient self-determination: "Every human being of adult years and sound mind has a right to determine what shall be done with his own body; and a surgeon who performs an operation without his patient's consent commits an assault, for which he is liable in damages."[1]

Two years later, the chair of the AMA's Council for the Defense of Medical Research used strikingly similar language in the context of research.

In 1916, Walter Bradford Cannon recommended uniform guidelines for human experimentation and published a sharply worded editorial in the *Journal of American Medical Association* in response to a young researcher's morally outrageous experimentation on six syphilitic, paretic patients at Pontiac State Hospital in Michigan. Cannon wrote, "There is no more primitive and fundamental right which any individual possesses than that of controlling the uses to which his own body is put. Mankind has struggled for centuries for the recognition of this right. Civilized society is based on the recognition of it. The lay public is perfectly clear about it."[6] Udo Wile's failure to obtain consent from the patients whose brains he punctured to determine the presence of active spirochetes, his use of a dental drill to do so, and his utter lack of contrition for doing either worked together to prompt even staunch defenders of medical research, such as Cannon, to propose uniform guidelines. Cannon's recommendation was not heeded by his American Medical Association (AMA) colleagues, who were preoccupied by the United States' entry into World War I. U.S. clinical investigators would continue to work without guidelines until 1946, when the AMA amended its code of ethics as part of its involvement in the prosecution of Nazi physicians for atrocities committed during World War II.

In the decades between the world wars, researchers would continue to struggle with the meaning of voluntary consent in principle and practice. A number of research activities set in motion during the 1930s came under scrutiny only decades later, including the notorious U.S. Public Health Service syphilis study involving poor African American men in Tuskegee, Ala., and the advent of radiation medicine, which led to the abuse of hospitalized patients and others.[2] During the 1930s, however, U.S. medical researchers experienced a reprieve from public scrutiny. The U.S. medical profession was held in unprecedented esteem in the first decades of the 20th century as the public began to become aware of and benefit directly from the fruits of medical research, such as the discovery of insulin and sulfa drugs.[3] People also became aware of increasing numbers of researchers who lost their lives by "going first." Novels popularized the yellow fever research led by Reed and memorialized the medical "heroes" and "martyrs" who lost their lives for the sake of research.[3] Although the antivivisectionists regained their momentum after World War I, their crusade against researchers' use of vulnerable groups did not persuade most Americans.[3] Indeed, as World War II approached and throughout the war effort, experimentation on those unable to consent was viewed by many Americans as no different than the military draft. The sentiment that all citizens needed to contribute to the war effort—whether against totalitarianism or disease—seemed to justify the use of vulnerable persons, even when their participation came "at great personal cost," according to Rothman.[7]

This positive attitude toward medical research persisted even after World War II, when Nazi physicians and administrators were indicted for horrific crimes committed on concentration camp inmates in the name of "medical science" (see Chapter 2). The 1947 judgment in the Nuremberg Doctors' Trial, *United States* v. *Karl Brandt et al.*, not only addressed the defendants' guilt or innocence, it produced 10 principles to guide ethically justifiable research. These 10 principles—the first of which is the absolute requirement to obtain the participant's voluntary consent—

make up what posterity has come to know as the Nuremberg Code (see Chapter 12). The Nuremberg Code defines consent as having four fundamental characteristics: voluntary, competent, informed, and comprehending.[1]

It appears the judges drew the 10 principles from two sources: a 22-page report prepared by physiologist Andrew Ivy, who had been appointed by the AMA to testify on medical ethics at the trial, and a memorandum written by their court-appointed expert, neurologist Leo Rosenberg. Ivy's report also was sent to the AMA's Judicial Council (the ethics group), which in December 1946 approved a distilled version of Ivy's rules and published them in *JAMA*.[8] This was the first time formal guidelines for research with humans were widely available to U.S. medical researchers; the guidelines required both voluntary consent and prior animal testing.

The consent provisions in both the AMA amendment and the Nuremberg Code seem to have been interpreted at the time as applying only to healthy volunteers, not patient-participants. Although transcripts from the trial suggest that Ivy viewed patients and healthy volunteers as morally equivalent for purposes of obtaining voluntary consent, and it is clear that Rosenberg did, this view did not find expression in Ivy's reports. "At that time, and for many years to come, patient trust and medical beneficence were viewed as the unshakable moral foundations on which meaningful interactions between professional healers and the sick should be built," according to the 1996 report of the Advisory Committee on Human Radiation Experiments.[9]

Despite the drama of the Nuremberg trials and the events leading up to them, the U.S. public remained relatively unaware of them. Departing from its watchdog role during the late 19th century, the press gave only limited coverage to the trials. Assuming that research with humans conducted in the United States occurred only with volunteers, most of the press viewed it approvingly. A small number of press accounts voiced concern about human experimentation taking place in the United States. Some accounts focused on experiments with volunteers; others on research with patients.[10]

Mainstream physicians who were aware of the Nuremberg trial and resulting code had varied reactions to them. Some physicians believed the code had no relevance to them or their work. Alienated by the gruesome nature of the experiments and settings in which they took place, these physicians viewed the Nuremberg Code as unnecessary for the ordinary physician. Others felt personally implicated by and compelled to follow these new standards, but unsure how to go about it in practice. Groundbreaking work by medical sociologist Renée Fox during the early 1950s, in which she followed the daily activities of physicians and patients in a metabolic research ward, suggests that physicians had difficulty translating the abstract norms into action guides for their work.[10] Isolated anecdotes and events throughout the 1950s suggest that some physicians did struggle to learn more about and comply with these new standards for clinical research, but they were a distinct minority.[10]

In the United States, the Nuremberg Code's greatest impact was felt within the defense establishment as it entered the cold war. The newly created civilian Atomic Energy Commission (AEC) and the Department of Defense (DoD) were planning for defense against atomic, biological, and chemical warfare and viewed research as essential to their plans. The national security establishment's discussion of the Nuremberg Code was discovered by the

Advisory Committee on Human Radiation Experiments (ACHRE), established in 1994 by President Bill Clinton in response to an *Albuquerque Tribune* series published the year before on human radiation experiments conducted by the federal government during the Cold War. Although some of the experiments had been the focus of a 1986 congressional investigation,[2] they did not catch the public's attention until journalist Eileen Welsome reconstructed the story of 17 plutonium injections of hospitalized patients in 1945. President Clinton tasked the ACHRE with unearthing the history of human radiation experiments conducted by the government and intentional releases of environmental radiation between 1944 and 1974, identifying ethical and scientific standards for evaluating these events, and making recommendations to prevent such activity in the future.

Early Signs of Change: Written Consent

The AEC developed rules for research with human participants that were progressive but not widely communicated or implemented. Yet they were the first known instance in which the term *informed consent* was used and the first time sick patients were included in the consent provisions. Created in January 1947 to oversee the nation's nuclear stockpile, the AEC had good reason to develop mechanisms to prevent abuses occurring during research with humans.[11] The AEC inherited the contracts and projects of the Manhattan Project, which included secretive and sensitive studies involving the injection of 17 hospitalized patients with plutonium. The AEC also would be the sole distributor of radioisotopes used in thousands of human radiation experiments and an equally rich source of funding for other research.

In preparation for this research and in light of the human experiments already conducted under the auspices of the Manhattan Project, AEC General Manager Carroll Wilson spelled out rules for research with humans in two separate and slightly different letters in April and November 1947. Both letters are significant for requiring consent from patient-participants. Wilson specified that the "patient give his complete and informed consent in writing."[11] Although he neither explained nor defined the meaning of informed consent, Wilson's union of the words *informed* and *consent* predated by a decade what scholars had thought to be its earliest use.[11]

The AEC had ample opportunity to disseminate Wilson's rules on human participant research, but largely failed to do so. Frequent requests came from researchers under contract with the AEC, and the AEC routinely disseminated educational and administrative materials for funding opportunities and radioisotope applicants. Although Wilson's research rules were not disseminated, the ideas contained in them penetrated at least one research setting. The AEC-sponsored Oak Ridge Institute for Nuclear Studies (ORINS), which opened in 1950, implemented a local process for informing patients of research risks. The process provided potential participants written information and required their signature to indicate they were "fully advised" about the "character and kind of treatment and care," which would be "for the most part experiments with no definite promise of improvement in my physical condition."[9]

During this same period, the DoD also faced ethical questions regarding the use of humans in atomic, biological, and chemical weapons research. Standards that would ultimately be signed into effect in February 1953, like the AEC policy, would both raise the bar for consent requirements and suffer from a lack of dissemination and implementation. The policy ultimately endorsed is notable for being the only instance of a U.S. agency (or any agency of any government) adopting the Nuremberg Code, an event that took place amid deep and widespread opposition among internal Pentagon advisory committees to regulations of any kind.[12] Concern about the DoD's legal authority to conduct atomic, biological, and chemical research on humans, however, forced the question. Still, the discussions that took place in internal Pentagon committees focused not on how such research should occur, the matter addressed by the Nuremberg Code, but rather on whether it should take place at all. Preoccupied with the wrong question, officials failed to address vitally important ones, such as the meaning of *volunteering* in the military context.[12]

Two years of discussions led to the conclusion that research with humans was unavoidable. Seeking input from other government agencies developing such research rules, the DoD involved the National Institutes of Health (NIH) in some of its policy deliberations. As the emerging leader in biomedical research, with plans to open a state-of-the-science research hospital, the NIH had started drafting human research rules. When the NIH Clinical Center opened in 1953, its policy required of all research participants, including patient-participants, "voluntary agreement based on informed understanding," and it required signed consent from some patient-participants involved in especially risky research.[9] One year later, signed consent forms were required of all healthy volunteers. Although the AEC's policy requiring consent from patient-participants predated this provision by six years, the NIH policy was a far clearer expression and endorsement of the requirement to obtain consent from patient-participants.

DoD policy would parallel the AEC and NIH Clinical Center policies. Eventually referred to the top-ranking medical advisory body in the Pentagon at the time, the Armed Forces Medical Policy Council (AFMPC), the matter received prompt attention from Stephen S. Jackson, who staffed the council and was an assistant to the Pentagon's general counsel. Jackson argued that the Nuremberg Code had international judicial sanction and should be adopted verbatim with the addition of a statement prohibiting the use of prisoners of war in research. Jackson's superior, Assistant Secretary for Manpower and Personnel Anna Rosenberg, the highest-ranking woman to serve in the defense establishment up to that time, added the requirement for written and witnessed consent. The AFMPC's proposal passed swiftly into policy when President Eisenhower's newly appointed secretary of defense, Charles E. Wilson, approved it shortly after taking office.

Had Wilson explored the level of support for the policy, he would have discovered support lacking among those who would have to implement it.[11] As Wilson signed the policy into effect, defense officials continued to debate whether regulations were necessary at all. Implementation was further complicated by the means used to communicate it: a top secret memo to the secretaries of the Army, Navy and Air Force. The memo remained classified until August 1975, although efforts were made to communicate its content down the chain of command. Levels of awareness varied, interpretations were inconsistent, and implementation sporadic throughout the 1950s and 1960s; however, by 1973, the Army, Navy, and Air Force had promulgated regulations that required written informed consent from both patient-participants and healthy volunteers.[9]

Opposition to formalizing and regulating consent standards was expressed not only by military and mainstream researchers but also by some critics of medical research, most notably Harvard physician and researcher Henry K. Beecher. A forceful and frequent critic of research abuses, Beecher also opposed rule-based regulations externally imposed on clinical researchers. His role in exempting Harvard researchers from the Army's newly endorsed Nuremberg rules in 1961 illustrates his persuasive power. When the assistant dean of Harvard Medical School, Joseph W. Gardella, expressed concern to his board about new rules that applied to their army medical research contracts, Beecher, in his capacity as a board member, crafted a statement of Harvard's principles for human research.[9] His statement not only served to exempt Harvard from the Army's rules but a later paper of his became one of the most influential articles in research ethics.[13]

Beecher faulted the Nuremberg Code on three grounds. First, he believed the Code's absolutist consent provision would prove problematic in practice; he like many medical researchers believed the complexities of some research would be too difficult to communicate to participants, especially those burdened by serious illness and disease. He also objected to the Code's requirement that research be neither "random" nor "unnecessary in nature." Beecher believed valuable medical tools and drugs, such as X-rays and penicillin, could be attributed to chance experimentation and that the phrase *unnecessary in nature* defied definition. Finally, and most importantly for Beecher, he believed that rules would not prevent research abuses.[9] In Beecher's view, unscrupulous researchers would conduct unethical research, regardless of rules prohibiting it. That pre-Nazi Germany in 1931 issued human participant research rules that now are described as more adequate than the Nuremberg Code makes his point in tragic terms.[1]

Beecher's suggested solution to research abuse was self-regulation by the "truly *responsible* investigator."[13] Physicians needed to be sensitized to the complexity of the moral problems in human research, but they should not be forced to comply with "rigid rules."[1] Beecher's faith in virtuous physician-researchers extended to participant consent. Beecher endorsed the necessity of obtaining consent but believed disclosure should vary in accordance with the type of research and the pool of participants. Like most physicians of his time, he did not believe researchers needed to fully disclose information to patient-participants who might benefit from the research. For Beecher, sick patients remained a "protected" class.

Beecher's influence was significant and, ironically, helped to promote the very regulatory regime he resisted. His identification of research abuses prompted the Public Health Service to commission a study of ethical and administrative practices of U.S. researchers and their institutions. The 1961 study, conducted by the Law-Medicine Research Institute at Boston University, found vast inconsistencies among institutions and concluded that "internal institutional regulation of research was generally insensitive and sporadic."[1] Moreover, transcripts revealed that status as a patient not only failed to protect people, but endangered them. Physician interviews portray attitudes and practice patterns disturbing not only by today's standards but also, no doubt, by those of Beecher in 1960. Physicians reported their discomfort with informing and seeking consent for research not intended to benefit patients and their ease with enrolling unconsenting patients in low-risk research; their view of patients as "rats from a laboratory" and their own status as "king or queen"; and their facility at pre-ssuring sick patients into participation and their expectation that indigent patients repay their debt through research participation.[9]

Meanwhile, physician practices in the clinical context were coming under intense scrutiny. The 1957 *Salgo v. Leland Stanford Jr. University Board of Trustees* ruling by a California appellate court continued to press consent standards in the direction of patient rights. Martin Salgo, who suffered permanent paralysis after undergoing translumbar aortography, sued his physician not only for medical negligence but also for failing to disclose the risk of paralysis. The court ruled in his favor and in its opinion used the term *informed consent*. The court held that Salgo had clearly consented to the procedure but without all the pertinent facts, which it ruled precluded his ability to make "an intelligent consent."[5] Although the phrase *informed consent* had been used a decade before in Carroll Wilson's 1947 memo to a handful of AEC contract researchers and medical advisors, *Salgo* put informed consent on the map for the mainstream U.S. medical community working in a clinical rather than a research context.

The court's explicit attention to the information on which a patient's decision is based bolstered the patient's right to make an autonomous choice. The court tempered this move toward patient autonomy with a step back toward physician paternalism: "[I]n discussing the element of risk a certain amount of discretion must be employed consistent with the full disclosure of facts necessary to an informed consent."[5] The court provided no analysis or explanation of the allowable *discretion*, leaving patient self-determination at the feet of physician judgment. As Jay Katz has noted of the ambiguity, "[T]he court did not appreciate the futility of its endeavors, for it gave an undefined task to a group that has had neither the experience with nor the commitment to patient self-determination."[5]

Great Scandals of the 1960s and 1970s

Deference to professional judgment, especially physician paternalism, imploded in the 1960s. A series of incendiary cases cast a bright light on researchers' struggle to balance the dual responsibilities of being both investigators and physicians. Congressional hearings, scholarly critiques, print and broadcast media coverage, and the public's outrage in response to these cases all led to significant reforms by the mid-1970s. For the first time, informed consent for research with humans was put before a public body for explicit discussion, analysis, and recommendation. The resulting reports and regulations would plant informed consent firmly in the ground of patient autonomy and would expand and elaborate on the meaning and the requirements of informed consent.

Tragic events surrounding the use of the sedative thalidomide set this reform process in motion. Thalidomide was approved for clinical use in Western Europe and was used extensively, especially in West Germany and Sweden, before its devastating effect on fetuses was identified. Although safe for pregnant women, the drug commonly caused fetuses to be born with missing or deformed limbs. The drug was considered experimental in the United States, yet physicians were given free samples by pharmaceutical companies and paid to collect patient data, a practice that led to some birth defects in newborn infants in the United States. Hearings held by Tennessee Senator Estes Kefauver, combined with television coverage and corresponding public outcry, helped to push the passage of the 1962 Kefauver-Harris amendments to the Food,

Drug, and Cosmetic Act, which among other conditions required patient consent when testing investigational drugs.

This was the first time in U.S. history that researchers were required to inform participants of a drug's experimental nature and obtain their written consent.[1] However, just as the *Salgo* ruling retreated from patient consent in deference to physician discretion, so, too, did the new Food and Drug Administration (FDA) policy. Physicians were not required to obtain consent when it was "not feasible" or was deemed not in the best interest of the patient.[1] The vaguely worded best interest clause and FDA Commissioner George P. Larrick's refusal to clarify it caused confusion for the next two years.

In 1966 the new FDA Commissioner, James Lee Goddard, appointed a small task force of FDA officials to study and settle the matter. The resulting policy drew heavily on the Nuremberg Code and the recently passed World Medical Association (WMA) policy regarding human experimentation, commonly known as the Declaration of Helsinki (see Chapter 13). Importantly, the FDA policy accepted wholesale the WMA's distinction between *therapeutic* and *nontherapeutic* research and its accompanying consent standards. The Declaration of Helsinki embraced the Nuremberg Code's absolute requirement for consent in nontherapeutic research, but qualified consent standards for therapeutic research. Continuing the traditions of benevolent deception and therapeutic privilege, the Declaration allowed physicians to determine whether or not consent was "consistent with patient psychology"[1] It also permitted third-party consent by a legal guardian for both types of research, another noteworthy deviation from the Nuremberg Code.

This FDA policy, which applied only to experimental drugs, devices, and biologics, was one among many factors that prompted NIH Director James Shannon's advocacy of formal controls on research with humans. As the director of the largest funder of U.S. human research, Shannon's commitment to formalizing human research rules was bolstered by unprecedented public and professional scrutiny, including the lackluster results of the Law-Medicine Research Institute's study; the 1963 attempt to transplant a chimpanzee kidney into a human at Tulane University; the WMA's 1964 adoption of the Declaration of Helsinki; Beecher's high-profile activism; and, in particular, a controversial study conducted on poor, elderly patients at the Jewish Chronic Disease Hospital (JCDH) in New York City, funded in part by the Public Health Service.

The research conducted at JCDH achieved notoriety not only for what the researchers did, but also for how they did it (see Chapter 6). Principal investigator Chester M. Southam of the Sloan-Kettering Cancer Research Institute had been studying the role of the body's immune system in cancer for a decade and persuaded JCDH's medical director, Emmanuel E. Mandel, to allow him to inject 22 indigent patients with live cancer cells. Although some patients were informed orally of their involvement in an experiment, neither their oral nor written consent was sought. The failure to obtain consent was not Southam's only transgression. He failed to disclose any information about the nature and risks of the research, a well-established responsibility by this time; he proceeded without review by the hospital's research committee and over the objections of three physicians; and he used frail, vulnerable patients in research obviously intended not to benefit them but to answer a scientific question. Despite these numerous and obvious infractions, the people and institutions responsible for

them went relatively unpunished. Both Southam and Mandel were originally censured and their medical licenses suspended, but subsequently they were put on probation for one year, still a remarkable punishment for the day.[9] Their respective institutions escaped untouched.

In response to this case, Shannon created a committee to study the issues and make recommendations. He appointed NIH's associate chief for program development, Robert Livingston, to lead the commission's work. The Livingston report, delivered one year later, recommended no changes in NIH policies and warned that policy reforms would thwart research progress and interfere with the physician-patient relationship. The report concluded that the NIH was "not in a position to shape the educational foundations of medical ethics, or even the clinical indoctrination of young investigators."[1] Disappointed but determined that NIH should play a pivotal role in ensuring responsible research, Shannon, joined by U.S. Surgeon General Luther Terry, in 1965 took his concerns to the National Advisory Health Council (NAHC), an advisory committee to the surgeon general of the Public Health Service. The NAHC affirmed their concerns and issued a statement that recommended PHS funding be given only to investigators willing to meet key ethical criteria, including obtaining the informed consent of participants.

The statement failed to define informed consent but led to the creation of landmark government regulations. In February 1966, the new surgeon general, William H. Stewart, accepted the NAHC recommendations and issued a policy that compelled PHS grantee institutions to provide prior committee review of proposed experiments and for the first time recognized patient-participants in the consent provisions. Specifically, the PHS policy required that independent review committees at grantee institutions address the following: (1) the rights and welfare of the individual(s) involved, (2) the appropriateness of methods to secure informed consent, and (3) the risks and potential medical benefits of the investigation.[9] The policy, like the statement that inspired it, failed to address the substantive content of informed consent, leaving its meaning and criteria to determination by local committees.[9]

A detailed, substantive account of informed consent was soon after provided by the NIH Clinical Center. The new policy required an oral explanation of the research, suited to participant's comprehension level; detailed disclosure regarding the nature, purpose, and risks of the study and procedures to be performed; and signed consent forms. The policy also addressed issues such as voluntariness and compliance with FDA policy. The policy has been described as the "most careful and comprehensive statement" on informed consent up to that point in U.S. history.[1]

Continued efforts to update the Department of Health, Education, and Welfare (DHEW) policy culminated in 1971 in *The Institutional Guide to DHEW Policy on Protection of Human Subjects,* better known as the Yellow Book because of the cover's color. The policy extended requirements to all DHEW programs and activities, provided detailed analyses of a number of issues, and retained the procedural requirement of committee peer review. Ironically, informed consent was both strengthened and weakened. The policy required that consent be obtained from both patients and healthy volunteers, or authorized representatives, after explaining the procedures; describing the risks, discomforts, benefits, and alternatives; offering to answer all questions; and ensuring that participants know they may withdraw consent and discontinue at any time.[1] However, the policy permitted consent to be either oral or written, obtained after research participation if a complete and prompt briefing was done, and in some cases to be considered implicit in the act of volunteering, if the nature and terms of the research were adequately advertised.[1] The policy's inadequacy would soon be illustrated.

Meanwhile, Beecher continued his activism and in 1965 he broke with professional protocol by taking his concerns to the press. Addressing a group of science journalists, Beecher presented 22 instances of ethically dubious human research. He pointed a finger at the nation's leading medical schools, university hospitals, the military, governmental institutes, industry, and even himself. His presentation was eventually published by the *New England Journal of Medicine* in June 1966 (after having been rejected by *JAMA*) and spurred several articles in popular magazines. The public's gaze now joined that of the U.S. government; when Willowbrook and Tuskegee caught light, all would be watching.

One of the studies Beecher cited in his article was conducted by New York University (NYU) researcher Saul Krugman at the Willowbrook State School for the Retarded on New York City's Staten Island (see Chapter 7). Willowbrook posed vexing questions about informed consent, research with children, and risk-benefit analysis. The institution housed children with severe mental and physical disabilities, most of whom had an IQ below 20 and many of whom were incontinent. According to Krugman, nearly all the children contracted a fecally borne, mild strain of hepatitis within 6 to 12 months of residency. Krugman and his team were highly regarded scientists, having identified hepatitis A and B in 1959. In their attempt to develop a prophylaxis, they deliberately infected some of the newly admitted children and cared for them in a well-equipped, well-staffed hepatitis unit, where the children were protected from exposure to other infectious diseases prevalent at the school. Only children whose parents consented were enrolled in the study, and wards of the state were never included. Moreover, the research received approval from Armed Forces Epidemiological Board and an NYU committee. The researchers' approach to seeking consent from the children's parents evolved over the years, as Willowbrook's population doubled from 3,000 to 6,000. Originally the researchers sought consent after conveying information about the research to parents through personal letter or interview; eventually they resorted to group discussions of the project.

The debate that surrounded this case, like so many before it, turned on assessments of *therapeutic benefit,* validity of consent, and the fair selection of participants. That the Willowbrook case involved institutionalized children with severe cognitive impairments made it all the more controversial. Research with children would not receive clarification and guidance until 1983, when the federal government adopted regulations based on the work of the nation's first federally appointed bioethics commission. Subpart D of these regulations permits children to be used in research with the assent of the child, if the child is capable of assent, and the permission of the parent(s) only after meeting certain risk requirements. For research involving possible benefit to the child, the risk must be " justified by the anticipated benefit to the subjects," and such research is acceptable only if "the relation of the anticipated benefit to the risk is at least as favorable to the subjects as that presented by available alternative approaches."[14] The requirement to obtain the assent of the child may be waived for research that holds out an important medical benefit to the child that can be received only in a research context.[14] Research not

presenting possible benefit must present "no greater than minimal risk." Moreover, participation in research involving more than minimal risk may be approved by the reviewing institutional review board (IRB) only if the risk "represents a minor increase over minimal risk, the procedures involved are commensurate with the general life experiences of subjects, and the research is likely to yield knowledge of 'vital importance' about the subjects' disorder or condition."[14] Riskier research may be approved only by the secretary of the Department of Health and Human Services (DHHS), following appropriate review.

Against the backdrop of such carefully articulated guidelines, one can fault the Willowbrook physicians on a number of counts. But at the time, the issues were far less clear. The physicians justified their research on grounds that they had obtained parental consent and offered the children the therapeutic benefits of "immunity," protection from other infections, and skilled medical care.[15] Critics, however, pointed out that the children might have become infected and developed immunity naturally, and that they were denied possibly protective doses of gamma globulin, thought by many to be an established and effective means of controlling viral hepatitis and shown to reduce the incidence of hepatitis by up to 85%. Critics also attacked the informed consent on procedural and substantive grounds.[15] The consent forms suggested the children would receive a vaccine; admissions to the special unit were expedited; when overcrowding precluded admission to the school, the hepatitis unit continued to accept children; and group meetings were characterized by financial and social pressure. The question of whether these severely retarded children possessed even limited capacity to assent to research was left untouched. This case continues to be debated and has become a paradigmatic research ethics case.

On the heels of Willowbrook came a case of blatant research abuse. The notorious 40-year Tuskegee syphilis study conducted by the U.S. Public Health Service (PHS) breached research rules well established not only in 1970 but even when the research began in 1932 (see Chapter 8). Poor African American men living in and around rural Tuskegee, Ala., were used by PHS researchers to study the natural history of syphilis. Originally designed as a six- to eight-month project, the study was extended for four decades. Some 400 syphilitic men and 200 nonsyphilitic men were induced to "participate" by being told they would receive free treatment for "bad blood," a term used in the community to describe many ailments but which the researchers assumed referred to syphilis. The researchers disclosed nothing about the research to these men nor sought their consent for participating in it. The men were not told that they had syphilis or that they would not benefit from participation. Their free treatment was limited to purely diagnostic procedures such as lumbar punctures. The research protocol was designed to impede their awareness of and access to available treatments, including penicillin, which was used in the treatment of syphilis by the late 1940s.

Despite many opportunities to halt the research, the syphilis study was not stopped until a 1972 front-page article in the *New York Times* caught public attention and stirred moral outrage. The DHEW established an ad hoc panel to review the study and the department's research rules, which found them inadequate across the board. The panel ordered the research stopped and recommended the establishment of a "permanent body with the authority to regulate *at least* all federally supported research involving human subjects."[1]

The panel's call for direct oversight of all federally funded research by an independent body with punitive authority was met with a compromise, delivered in the 1974 National Research Act. The Act established the National Commission for the Protection of Human Subjects of Biomedical and Behavioral Research, a four-year advisory body, in return for the DHEW's conversion of research policies into regulations applicable to the entire department.[9] The regulations required grantee institutions to establish IRBs and charged them with reviewing research proposals for safety and informed consent provisions. Informed consent requirements were made slightly more stringent, closing waiver and documentation loopholes, and all research, not just risky protocols, was required to undergo review. Still, the regulations did not apply to all federally funded research and suffered from ambiguities and unanswered questions that would become the work of the National Commission.

The National Commission was charged with developing and delivering recommendations to the DHEW Secretary. It produced seventeen reports and appendices, including the Belmont Report, which remains a touchstone for U.S. human participant research (see Chapters 14 and 19). The Commission made the first formal attempt to clearly state the ethical import of the distinction between medical research and medical practice and addressed many other issues including the role and function of IRBs, informed consent and third-party permission, and research involving vulnerable populations. Its extensive and detailed recommendations largely became U.S. government policy.[1]

Central among the Commission's tasks was the development of basic ethical principles that could become the basis of research oversight, especially research with vulnerable populations. The Commission created a framework of three principles, each of which was to guide and justify a key function of the IRB process: respect for persons, beneficence, and justice. These "Belmont principles" were proposed as ethical guides and justifications for informed consent provisions, risk-benefit analysis, and selection of participants.[16] The Commission's elaboration on the intent and function of respect for persons made respect for *autonomy* fundamental to informed consent. "[M]ore decisively than any previous publication in case law or research ethics, the Commission's volumes reflected the view that the underlying *principle and justification* of informed consent requirements, at least for autonomous persons, is a moral principle of respect for autonomy, and no other [emphasis in original]."[1]

The Commission's attention to informed consent produced an analysis of its content and criteria that remains standard. The Commission identified three necessary conditions for informed consent: information, comprehension, and voluntariness. These conditions were used to analyze consent for vulnerable classes of participants, such as children, prisoners, and institutionalized persons with cognitive impairments. The Commission devoted a report and two appendices to informed consent, but these volumes are so complex and detailed that their usefulness for IRBs has been questioned. However, they are among the most widely read sections of the Commission's many reports.

By the time the National Commission had completed its work in 1978, informed consent had currency in mainstream U.S. society. Scholars, courts, hospital board rooms, classrooms, and state legislatures were focused on patients' rights to make autonomous decisions about their health care. Commentary on informed consent flooded the medical literature.[1] Three 1972 court rulings left

no doubt about patients' right to make medical decisions based on their values and information a reasonable person, not a medical professional, would need to know. The following year the American Hospital Association published "A Patient's Bill of Rights," which included informed consent provisions. Between 1975 and 1977, 25 states enacted informed consent legislation.[1]

Revised AMA policy issued in 1981 cinched the place of informed consent in modern medicine. The AMA Code of Ethics had undergone numerous revisions since its creation in 1847, including a 1980 revision that acknowledged the physician's obligation to respect patients' rights. Not until the following year, however, did the AMA issue a policy explicitly addressing informed consent, using much of the language in one of the three landmark 1972 court decisions. The ruling by the U.S. Circuit Court for the District of Columbia in *Canterbury* v. *Spence* described consent as "the informed exercise of choice" based on "enough information to enable an intelligent choice."[17]

Post-Belmont

The National Commission's pioneering work largely became policy in 1981. The DHHS regulations were based on the National Commission's recommendations and influenced by a subsequent bioethics commission, the President's Commission for the Study of Ethical Problems in Medicine and Biomedical and Behavioral Research, which worked from 1980 to 1983. Established to address unresolved and new issues, the President's Commission stressed the importance of the informed consent recommendations to federal officials drafting the regulations.[1] The subsequent regulations provided in-depth guidance on informed consent, particularly disclosure requirements. In addition to disclosing the purpose and nature of the research, potential risks and benefits, and alternatives, researchers were now also obligated to provide an explanation and information about the confidentiality of records, compensation for injury and medical treatment, if necessary, and a contact for pertinent questions.[1] The new regulations also required researchers to disclose information discovered during the study that could influence someone's participation. The regulations applied to both biomedical and behavioral research, but they effectively exempted much of behavioral research by providing broad exceptions for research entailing minimal risk, such as interviews, surveys, or observational research.[1]

The President's Commission continued to prove its influence. Its recommendation that the regulations be adopted by all federal agencies led to the development of what has become known as the Common Rule (see Chapter 15). Adopted in 1991 by 16 federal departments and agencies, the rule details how research with humans should be reviewed and conducted and applies to research conducted by both governmental and, in some cases, nongovernmental agencies. Although all 16 federal agencies conduct research according to the Common Rule's requirements, the administrative structure of their oversight programs varies. Any institution that conducts clinical research must make assurances that protections will be provided and enforced in order to receive federal funding.

As in the prior DHEW and DHHS regulations, the IRB continues to serve as the key protective mechanism. IRBs have the authority to approve, disapprove, require modifications of, suspend, and oversee all human research conducted at the institution. Predominant among IRBs' numerous responsibilities is ensuring the adequacy of research protocols' informed consent provisions; however, several conditions must be met prior to considering the use of humans in research. The research must have scientific value; the research design must be sound and must achieve a reasonable balance of benefits to the participant and society over risks to the participant; and the use of humans must be absolutely necessary, and they must fairly selected.[15,18] Only after these conditions are met can an IRB consider an investigator's informed consent provisions. The rule specifies items that must be disclosed to potential participants and emphasizes that obtaining informed consent should be an ongoing "process" of communication between researcher and participant.[9] Ideally, the process entails an exchange of questions and answers that promotes the potential participant's ability to make a choice that aligns with his or her values and interests.

The Common Rule represents a significant achievement in many respects. It applies uniformly to all federally funded research, carries binding authority, and reflects the focused analysis and discussion of knowledgeable, dedicated members of diverse sectors of the society. The Common Rule also strives to achieve a balance of values central to U.S. society, the advancement of scientific and medical frontiers and the protection and promotion of human health and individual autonomy. Moreover, the Common Rule is fortified by a climate of heightened public and scholarly interest and scrutiny. The ethical principles of medical research are now the subject of ongoing articulation and refinement.

Still, significant gaps remain in the system of human participant protections, including informed consent provisions. Informed consent as a concept and practice was challenged by a number of scandals and new developments in the last decade of the 20th century. These scandals and developments reveal the difficulty of achieving informed consent, especially for the most vulnerable classes of participants, and even cast doubt on the adequacy of individual autonomy as an ideal.

The provision to potential participants of accurate, complete, and candid information about the purpose and risks of research continues to challenge the research community. Although significant energy and attention is now directed to the development and articulation of policy, and such policy is the subject of much public scrutiny, the actual practice patterns of researchers have proven more difficult to reform. The ACHRE's review of 125 research proposals attests to this difficulty. Together, the committee and an individual committee member's separate inquiry found in 1999 that consent forms were "flawed in morally significant respects, not merely because they are difficult to read but because they are uninformative or even misleading."[9] Specifically, consent forms often presented inadequate information about risks that might be significant to patients; lacked important information about alternative treatments and preliminary data gathered from earlier experiments; and used the language of *treatment* and *therapy* to describe research that *might* yield therapeutic benefit even though therapy was not its purpose.

Two cases that occurred in close proximity at the turn of the 21st century highlight the research community's reluctance to share risk information with potential participants. In September 1999, 18-year-old Jessie Gelsinger died four days after receiving an infusion of new genes as part of an experiment intended to determine whether this *gene therapy* might lead to a cure for an inherited liver disease, ornithine transcarbamylase deficiency (see Chapter 10). Among the many infractions committed by the

University of Pennsylvania researchers was their failure to reveal in the consent form the deaths of four monkeys subjected to higher levels of similar gene infusions; they also failed to notify the FDA of *adverse events* that occurred in participants in the study of which Gelsinger was a part.[19] The fact that Gelsinger was living a relatively healthy life, controlling his disease through medication and diet, made his enrollment in the study all the more controversial. Two years later, an asthma study with healthy volunteers at Johns Hopkins University resulted in the death of 24-year-old Ellen Roche. Like the gene therapy experiment, the study was cited for numerous infractions, including the failure to disclose risk information. The consent form failed to indicate that the drug being used to create symptoms similar to an asthma attack, hexamethonium, was not an approved medication but, rather, was intended to provoke a physiologic response.[20]

Such deficient consent practices may mislead many potential participants into research participation. But sick patients may be particularly vulnerable. Patients with poor prognoses who have exhausted their options for medical treatment may feel that they have no choice but to participate in research; yet they also may fail to understand that they are *in fact* participating in research.[9] A study of participants conducted by the ACHRE revealed that most patient-participants believed they would personally benefit from participation and that their physicians would not offer them opportunities that did not benefit them.[9]

These data stand in contrast, however, to a recent study of cancer patients in Phase I trials.[21] Over 70% of patients studied understood that they might not directly benefit from the intervention, even though they hoped they would. Researchers of this study concluded that patients who enrolled "provide adequate informed consent."[21]

Still, a 1999 report by the National Bioethics Advisory Commission (NBAC) on research involving persons with mental disorders that may affect decision-making capacity reaffirmed the ACHRE's findings. In addition, NBAC found that existing policy fails to adequately guide researchers and IRBs on the complex matter of determining a person's capacity for making decisions. Mental disorders can compromise decision-making capacity to varying degrees, and no consensus exists as to what degree of incapacity counts as a lack thereof.[22] NBAC made a number of recommendations, including that researchers indicate to IRBs who will conduct the assessment and which method they will use; NBAC also recommended the development of more specific guidance on the definition of decisional capacity and improved assessment procedures.[22]

Important questions about decision-making capacity also have been raised for another class of vulnerable persons: potential HIV vaccine research participants in sub-Saharan Africa. Some African scholars have argued that severe and persistent poverty confounds not only the ability to achieve the basic elements of informed consent but also decision-making capacity itself. Widespread illiteracy and language barriers may complicate disclosure requirements, and the offer of free medical care and pay may constitute undue pressure for people living in dire material circumstances. In addition, some scholars have suggested that the precondition of informed consent—competence—may itself be at risk for these potential participants. The effects of persistent and severe poverty, malnutrition, and illiteracy may render potential participants unable, or limited in their capacity, to understand the complexities of biomedical science.[23,24] This possibility is exacerbated by cultural beliefs about illness and causation that differ drastically from those of Western medical science; for example, the word *randomization* may not exist in some cultures.[25]

The aim of informed consent—to promote individual autonomy—has also been questioned in this research context. Many African cultures place more value on human collectives than on individuals.[23] In these cultures, family elders or community leaders may be viewed as appropriate decision makers for others on many issues, including research participation. Some have argued that both traditions—of individualism and collectivism—can be accommodated.[26] The most widely used international guidelines for human research, developed by the Council for International Organizations of Medical Sciences (CIOMS) in collaboration with the World Health Organization, stress the importance of obtaining *both* individual consent and community review and involvement.[27] (see Chapters 16) The "International Guidelines for Biomedical Research Involving Human Subjects," issued first in 1982 and revised in 1993 and 2002, emphasize community involvement in decisions about research design and participant participation but rely on the same principles specified in the Belmont Report to address the requirements of individual informed consent. Whether both the community and individual can or should be respected in the informed consent process is a matter of significant debate. Serious concerns exist about whether women's interests can be adequately protected in patriarchal societies.[28]

Conclusion

During the 100-plus years detailed here, significant strides have been made in articulating the conditions under which people may be invited to participate in research and the conditions under which they may be permitted to participate. Informed consent is a central criterion for research participation. In this chapter we have traced the history of informed consent, from its precursor forms of voluntary consent to current, more rigorous forms that require participants to volunteer on the basis of information and understanding. A series of U.S. commissions during the latter half of the 20th century have created numerous reports that detail and elaborate on the conditions and ethical justifications of informed consent. U.S. regulations, in turn, have created numerous mechanisms designed to promote the review of research protocols and the protection of humans involved in research.

Despite these advances, the system of research protections remains fragile. Informed consent, a cornerstone of all modern research ethics codes, has been challenged conceptually and practically. The research community and regulatory infrastructure too often have faltered in their duties to present potential participants with complete, clear, and candid information about the purpose and risks of research; to promote and ensure the understanding and voluntariness of participants' decisions; and to accurately assess the decision-making capacity of potential participants. All of these elements are essential to a truly autonomous decision, an ethical idea which itself has come under scrutiny as HIV research has been exported to societies that may not prize this moral norm.

As this chapter shows, the concept of informed consent in research involving humans has marched steadily toward the ideal of individual autonomy as an expression of respect for persons. Led by the United States, the criteria for informed consent have been designed not only to promote an individual's informed decision but to protect that decision from the interference or influence of others. Some contend that to impose this value on other cultures runs the risk of "ethical imperialism." But we believe the ethical goal of universal respect for persons—regardless of race, gender, caste, or tribe—remains a worthy one.

References

1. Faden RR, Beauchamp TL, with King NMP. *A History and Theory of Informed Consent.* New York, N.Y.: Oxford University Press; 1986.
2. Martensen R. If only it were so: Medical physics, U.S. human radiation experiments, and the Final Report of the President's advisory commission. *Medical Humanities Review* 1997;11:21–36.
3. Lederer SE. *Subjected to Science: Human Experimentation in America Before the Second World War.* Baltimore, Md.: The Johns Hopkins University Press; 1995.
4. Vollmann J, Winau R. Informed consent in human experimentation before the Nuremberg Code. *British Medical Journal* 1996;313: 1445–6.
5. Katz J. *The Silent World of Doctor and Patient.* New York, N.Y.: The Free Press; 1984.
6. Cannon WC. The right and wrong of making experiments on human beings. *JAMA* 1916;67:1372–3.
7. Rothman DJ. Ethics and human experimentation: Henry Beecher revisited. *New England Journal of Medicine* 1987;317:1195–9.
8. American Medical Association. Supplementary Report of the Judicial Counsel. *JAMA* 1946;132:1090.
9. Advisory Committee on Human Radiation Experiments. *Final Report of the Advisory Committee on Human Radiation Experiments.* New York, N.Y.: Oxford University Press; 1996.
10. Faden RR, Lederer SE, Moreno JD. U.S. medical researchers, the Nuremberg doctors trial, and the Nuremberg Code: A review of findings of the Advisory Committee on Human Radiation Experiments. *JAMA* 1996;276:1667–71.
11. Moreno JD, Lederer SE. Revising the history of cold war research ethics. *Kennedy Institute of Ethics Journal* 1996;6:223–7.
12. Moreno JD. "The only feasible means": The Pentagon's ambivalent relationship with the Nuremberg Code. *Hastings Center Report* 1996;26(5):11–9.
13. Beecher HK. Ethics and clinical research. *New England Journal of Medicine* 1966;274:1354–60.
14. Department of Health and Human Services, National Institutes of Health, and Office for Human Research Protections. The Common Rule, Title 45 (Public Welfare), Code of Federal Regulations, Part 46 (Protection of Human Subjects). [Online] June 23, 2005. Available: http://www.hhs.gov/ohrp/humansubjects/guidance/45cfr46 .htm.
15. Beauchamp TL, Childress JF. *Principles of Biomedical Ethics,* 5th ed. New York, N.Y.: Oxford University Press; 2001.
16. The National Commission for the Protection of Human Subjects of Biomedical and Behavioral Research. *The Belmont Report: Ethical Principles and Guidelines for the Protection of Human Subjects of Research.* Washington, D.C.: Department of Health, Education and Welfare; DHEW Publication OS 78-0012 1978. [Online] April 18, 1979. Available: http://www.hhs.gov/ohrp/humansubjects/guidance/ belmont.htm.
17. *Canterbury v. Spence,* 464 F.2d 772, (D.C. Cir. 1972), cert. denied, 409 U.S. 1064 (1972).
18. Miller F. Clinical research with healthy volunteers: An ethical framework. *Journal of Investigative Medicine* 2003;51(Suppl. 1):S2–S5.
19. Weiss R, Nelson D. Methods faulted in fatal gene therapy. *The Washington Post* December 8, 1999:A1.
20. Levine S. FDA cites flaws in Hopkins asthma study. *The Washington Post* July 3, 2001:B03.

21. Agrawal M, Emanuel EJ. Ethics of Phase 1 oncology studies. *JAMA* 2003;290:1075–82.

22. National Bioethics Advisory Commission. *Research Involving Persons With Mental Disorders That May Affect Decisionmaking Capacity, Vol. I.* Rockville, Md.: NBAC; 1998. [Online] December 1998. Available: http://www.georgetown.edu/research/nrcbl/nbac/capacity/TOC.htm.

23. Moodley K. HIV vaccine trial participation in South Africa: An ethical assessment. *Journal of Medicine and Philosophy* 2002;27:197–215.

24. van Niekerk AA. Moral and social complexities of AIDS in Africa. *Journal of Medicine and Philosophy* 2002;27:143–62.

25. De Zulueta P. Randomized placebo-controlled trials and HIV-infected pregnant women in developing countries: Ethical imperialism or unethical exploitation? *Bioethics* 2001;15:289–311.

26. Porter J. Informed consent issues in international research concerns. *Cambridge Quarterly of Healthcare Ethics* 1996;5:237–43.

27. Council for International Organizations of Medical Sciences in collaboration with the World Health Organization. *International Ethical Guidelines for Biomedical Research Involving Human Subjects.* Geneva, Switzerland: CIOMS and WHO; 2002. [Online] November 2002. Available: http://www.cioms.ch/frame_guidelines_nov_2002.htm.

28. IJsselmuiden CB, Faden RR. Research and informed consent in Africa—Another look. *New England Journal of Medicine* 1992;326:830–3.

Dan W. Brock

Philosophical Justifications of Informed Consent in Research

The rule that, with a few exceptions, research with humans should not take place without participants' informed consent is a settled ethical and legal principle.[1-7] This chapter explores the philosophical foundations of this principle. Exploring these foundations helps to clarify how the requirement of informed consent should be understood as well as what limits, if any, should be placed on its implementation. No such requirement exists for the use of things or nonhuman animals, such as microorganisms or mice. The simple explanation of the difference, of course, is that things and animals are not capable of giving informed consent, so it would not be possible to require it of them, whereas human beings or persons are so capable. But that tells us only why it is possible to require informed consent of human research participants, not why we should do so. Why can't people be used in research in the way that we use things? We have reason not to be wasteful of things and animals because they have instrumental and economic value to others, but that is a limitation on their use for the sake of other persons, not for the sake of the things or animals themselves.

What is it about human beings, or persons—I will use these interchangeably here—that gives them a moral status that things and animals do not have, specifically that requires their informed consent to take part in research? Some people will give a religious answer to this question, grounding persons' moral status in their special relationship to God, but public policy about the use of humans in research is not generally understood to have a religious foundation, or at least an exclusively religious foundation. Nor should public policy, which governs all citizens, be grounded in reasons that only have force within a particular religion that some citizens may reasonably reject. So we need a secular answer to the

question. Probably the most common answer is appeal to respect for persons or, similarly, respect for persons' autonomy, as a fundamental moral principle; respect for persons certainly is relevant to our question, but it leaves open what it is about persons that requires respect, and what respect requires in our treatment of persons in the context of research.[8,9]

Philosophical Conceptions

Philosophical conceptions of autonomy derive largely from the work of Immanuel Kant and are often highly abstract and not well suited to the role autonomy has come to play in bioethics and in the doctrine and practice of informed consent. Instead, we need a conception of autonomy that is empirically ascertainable and within the reach of ordinary persons, for the principle of respect applies to persons generally.[10-12]

Although other animals engage in goal-directed behavior guided by instinct and environment, only persons have the capacity to reflect on what kinds of beings they want to be, what kinds of activities they want to pursue, what kinds of lives they want to live. Persons have the capacity to form values, not just desires; indeed, persons sometimes find their values in conflict with their desires and can take steps, within limits, to bring their desires more into conformance with their values. Persons have the capacity to form, and act on, a conception of the good life. So our interest in autonomy is our interest in making significant decisions about our lives for ourselves and according to our own conceptions of a good life, and then to be free, at least within limits, to act on those decisions without interference from others. In this way, persons are self-directed agents, not just beings acted upon be external forces.

Each individual person has a life of his or her own to live, with the capacity to take control over and responsibility for directing that life. This is not to say, of course, that individuals are not deeply influenced by other persons and subject to many constraints and limitations in carrying out their life plans. But it is this capacity for self-governance, for autonomy or self-determination, that respect for persons requires us to respect.

The reason things may be used to suit people's purposes is because things have no interests, purposes, or values of their own. Persons, on the other hand, do have purposes, interests, and values of their own, and it is the capacity for these that a principle of respect for persons requires us to respect. Persons are what we can call normative agents. Even higher animals are not normative agents in this sense. For purposes of understanding the ethical basis of the requirement of informed consent, we need an understanding of when persons are making autonomous choices.[10] Choice implies selection from among alternatives, in this context in the simplest terms the choice whether or not to enroll in a particular research project. I shall argue that the three central requirements of informed consent—that the choice is informed, voluntary, and made by a competent person—can be understood as spelling out a conception of autonomous choice in the context of decisions about research participation. Respect for autonomy in this context then requires obtaining the informed consent of those who are competent, able to understand and make a voluntary choice, and are being invited to participate in the research.

Other Considerations

There are other moral considerations besides respecting autonomy that support the general practice of informed consent, although they do not support it as a universal requirement in the way that respect for persons and their autonomy does.[5] Respect for persons and their autonomy grounds a moral right not to be experimented on without one's consent. The other considerations are consequentialist—the good consequences that usually, but not in every instance, come from not experimenting on persons without their informed consent.

The first consideration rests on an assumption that individuals are generally, though of course not always, the best judges of their own interests, and so if they are left free to decide whether to participate in research projects they will generally do so when it serves their interests and values.

Second, public support for medical research rests on the belief that it is being conducted ethically; obtaining participants' informed consent is essential to sustain that belief. The lack of informed consent was one feature of notoriously unethical research like the Tuskegee experiment that created great public mistrust of medical research (see Chapter 8). Public support for medical research is of obvious importance for maintaining continued substantial public funding of research by government institutions like the National Institutes of Health, which is necessary for securing the continued public health benefits of that research. Public trust of the research enterprise is also important for maintaining public willingness to participate in research trials.

Third, informed consent encourages rational decision making by those contemplating research participation, and it also en-

courages self-scrutiny by investigators about the design and protections incorporated into the research. No doubt there are other examples of good consequences that come from the practice of securing consent from research participants, but the general point is that these examples hold in most, but not all, cases and so need to be supplemented by respect for autonomy in order to ground a universal requirement of informed consent.

Contrast of Therapy and Research

The goal of medical therapy is to improve the patient's medical condition. Yet even medical therapy should not proceed without patients' consent. In research, however, the primary goal is the production of generalizable knowledge, not the research participant's benefit, even if both researcher and participant may sometimes hope for or even expect benefit.[13] As a result, there is always an inherent conflict of goals between researchers and participants, a conflict between participants' typical goal of securing their well-being and the researchers' goal of producing knowledge. This is what gives special importance in the research context to the ethical injunction against using persons for the benefit of others without their consent; the goals of research always include at least in part the benefit of others, namely, those who stand to benefit as a result of the knowledge produced by the research.

Sometimes a distinction is made between therapeutic and nontherapeutic research, with the suggestion that this conflict of goals does not obtain in the context of therapeutic research, which is thought to have the goal of the participants' own clinical benefit. This is a mistake. Some research may have therapeutic components, but all research has the goal of producing generalizable knowledge, implying that the conflict of goals arises from the components of the research that serve research aims, rather than participants' therapeutic goals.

Research investigators often are also physicians who in other contexts function in a therapeutic role, and this can result in confusion about the different roles on the part of physician/investigators or others.[14] This confusion can be compounded when a potential research participant is also a patient—particularly if the participant is a patient of the investigator—and is considering entering a research trial in the hope of therapeutic benefit. In these cases, it is especially important that the potential participant understand how his or her relationship with the physician will be altered in the research context.

Elements of a Valid Informed Consent

Valid informed consent is typically understood to have three distinct components: Consent must be informed, voluntary, and given by a competent person. More specifically, what does each of these components require, and what obligations do they place on investigators?

Information

The requirement that consent be informed places a demand on the investigator to provide the appropriate information in an understandable form to each potential participant. Because the goal of this component is to enable people to make an informed decision about participation, the investigator also has a responsibility to invite and answer any questions that potential participants may have about the research. One difficult issue about this condition is how to decide what information should be provided.[5]

U.S. federal regulations specify what information is always legally required to be given to potential participants. This includes the following: a statement that the project is research, not therapy; the purposes of the research; a description of the research—in particular, what will happen to the participants; a description of foreseeable risks and discomforts, as well as benefits; appropriate alternatives, if any; the extent of confidentiality that can be expected; an explanation of any medical treatment available for injury and/or compensation for disability; a pledge that that participation is entirely voluntary and participants can withdraw at any time without loss of benefits to which they are otherwise entitled; and whom to contact for answers to questions.[15] This is the information that federal regulators have determined should always be included in the informed consent process and on the informed consent form. Other information may be appropriate in particular circumstances or for particular research projects.

Although this specifies the kinds of information that should be provided as part of the informed consent process, it leaves open how much detail should be provided, in particular details about the potential risks and benefits of participation. In the law, there are two principal legal standards that most states have adopted on this question, though they have generally been applied to medical therapy rather than research.[16,17] The so-called professional practice standard directs the investigator to provide the information that most other professionals would provide in similar circumstances. This standard has the obvious defect that it assumes professional practice is adequate, which may not always be the case. It implies that criticism of past practices—in which little or even no information was provided to patients or research participants—was unwarranted provided the practice in question was widely adopted. A widespread practice of providing little or no information would seem to be an additional reason to object to the practice, not a reason to regard it as ethically appropriate.

The other standard is the so-called reasonable person standard, which directs the investigator to provide the information that a reasonable person would want in order to make the decision in question. This standard provides less clear guidance than the professional practice standard, which allows examination of the actual practices of other professionals. Although the reasonable person standard lacks the defect just noted in the professional practice standard, it is not always clear what information a reasonable person would want, particularly with regard to the potential risks and benefits of the research. For example, would a reasonable person always want to know that research participation poses a risk of death, no matter how small or remote that risk? If not, how probable must the risk be before the reasonable person would want to be informed of its presence? This standard requires looking at the probability of particular risks and benefits—how common they are, as well as how serious or important they are—and uncertainty and controversy will remain about where to draw the line in particular cases.

It is common practice to spell out the risks of research projects in considerable detail. In part this is for protection against legal liability, not for ethical reasons. However, many investigators fail to spell out the potential benefits of research, including potentially therapeutic components, in comparable detail, and they fail to provide any basis for judging the probability of the benefits. Of course, in some medical research there is no expected benefit to participants, which should be clearly stated. In research with potential benefits to participants, however, one often finds little more than a statement to the effect that it is unknown what benefit, if any, participants will receive from the research. Because it is a nonvalidated therapy that is under investigation in clinical research—for example, in a clinical trial of a new oncology treatment—this statement is true. Moreover, it has the benefit of helping disabuse participants of the therapeutic misconception that the goal of the research is to benefit them.[18,19]

Nevertheless, merely stating that it is unknown whether participants will receive any benefit is insufficient to allow potential participants to make a rational decision about whether the potential risks of the research are warranted by its potential benefits. Certainly, in a Phase III clinical trial there will be some preliminary data from earlier Phase I and II trials, from animal studies, from studies of biologically related compounds, or from basic laboratory research to give some basis for assessing the potential for individual benefit. Some summary of these preliminary data should be provided to participants as part of the consent process to enable them to make a rational decision about whether to participate in the study.

In the context of medical therapy, a third subjective standard for what information informed consent requires is sometimes ethically defended: What would *this* person want to know in order to make a decision about therapy? This standard directs the physician to tailor the information provided to any known special concerns or interests of the patient in question. Because information to be provided to all participants on a consent form for a research project cannot be individualized in this way, it might seem that this standard is inapplicable in research. But the obligation of the investigator to answer any questions of the potential participant about the research allows for an appropriate individuation of information to the needs and concerns of individual persons in research, at least to the extent that they are or can be known.

This point illustrates the common mistake of confusing the consent form with the process of obtaining informed consent.[20] In medical therapy, an actual consent form is only sometimes required, and practice varies from institution to institution regarding when it is required, even though informed consent itself should always be obtained. In research with humans, on the other hand, a consent form is always required unless the institutional review board (IRB) has explicitly waived the requirement. The greater documentation and assurance that proper consent has taken place, which can be provided by a signed consent form, is justified by the conflict of goals that exists between investigator and participant in research that does not typically exist between physician and patient in medical therapy. However, a signed consent form is neither necessary nor sufficient for ethically valid consent. It is not necessary, as the practice of oral consent illustrates, so long as the appropriate process of obtaining consent has taken place; but a signed consent form is not sufficient if an appropriate informed consent process has not taken place, for example, because the form is not in a language or at a level that the person can understand. New information may be obtained after participants have enrolled in a research study, and the individuals' own preferences and values may evolve. Give these potential changes, informed consent should be understood as an ongoing process, both in therapy and research, not as the single event of signing a consent form.[21,22]

The practice and requirement of informed consent has come under considerable criticism, both in research and in other contexts, with most of the criticism focusing on whether participants can truly understand relevant information and make an informed choice whether to participate in the research.[23] For example, it has been argued that typical participants never have the scientific and medical training to understand the project as fully as the investigator who designed and is carrying out the research.[24] But this objection, like analogous objections to informed consent for medical treatment, misconstrues what people need to understand to make an informed decision. They do not need to understand the entire underlying scientific and medical basis of the research; rather, they need to know how their lives, and what is important to them in their lives, are likely to be affected, both positively and negatively, by participation in the research. If investigators carry out their responsibility to use their scientific and medical training and knowledge to convey this information to potential participants, then typical participants will be capable of understanding what they need to know to make an informed decision.

Other critics argue that participants can never be given complete information. Indeed, attempting to do so would result in information overload and confusion, not understanding. But we have already seen that appropriate standards for information to be provided do not require complete information in this sense. Under the reasonable person standard, for example, investigators should provide the information that reasonable people want to make the decision in question. The fact that provision of all information, even if possible in theory, would overwhelm individuals provides compelling reason to think that this is not the level of information desired by reasonable individuals.

Finally, critics point to studies showing a variety of significant misunderstandings that participants have about the research, such as the therapeutic misconception—failing to understand the difference between research and therapy—or the nature of randomization, and so forth.[25] These are serious concerns, and efforts should be made to reduce such misunderstandings, but comparable degrees of misunderstanding could probably be found in many decisions that individuals make in other areas of their lives, and those misunderstandings are not considered sufficient grounds for denying individuals the right to make those decisions for themselves.

Some have argued that although making relevant information available to participants may be necessary for valid consent, complete understanding of that information is not required.[26] They point to evidence of various limitations in both patients' and research participants' understanding, such as the therapeutic misconception about research, despite the consent having been accepted as valid.[22]

A distinction should be made here between, on the one hand, making relevant information available to participants in understandable form together with a process that enables them to ask questions and to clarify information, and, on the other hand, requiring a particular level of understanding of the information. Ethically valid informed consent requires the former but not the latter. To require no relevant misunderstandings would simply be impractical and incompatible with practice in a wide variety of other circumstances in which important decisions are made. Moreover, some participants may not wish to understand all or even much of the relevant information, for example, because they trust the researcher, or they may even waive their right to obtain the relevant information. This is compatible with ethically valid consent, even if for legal or policy reasons we may place limits on this kind of uninformed consent in research.

Voluntariness

A second condition for valid consent is that it be voluntary. This requirement places a responsibility on the investigator to ensure that participants' consent is in fact voluntary. Consent can be made involuntary in more than one way. The most obvious is when one is coerced to consent.[27] Coercion involves a threat that unless a person agrees to participate in the research, the coercer will make him or her worse off in some respect; a crude example would be a patient's physician threatening that unless the patient agrees to take part in a research project, the physician will not continue to provide therapeutic care. This kind of crude coercion from an investigator is no doubt rare. Nevertheless, patients may sometimes feel that their care will become worse if they do not accept their physician's invitation to participate in a research project, even if that is not true and their physician has done nothing to suggest it; physician-investigators need to make efforts to reassure patients that this is not the case in order to avoid inadvertent coercion. Coercion from family members is probably more common than from investigators and other health-care personnel, and can equally invalidate a person's consent.

In understanding coercion, it is important to distinguish it from warnings. A patient who has failed standard therapy may be told by his physician or others that his only chance of improvement is to participate in a clinical trial; if he does not do so, further decline or even death is likely. This does not constitute coercion to participate in the trial, but rather a warning of what can be expected if the patient does not participate. It is the disease that will make the patient's condition worse, not anything that the physician will do, which is why this is a warning and not a threat.

Some commentators consider it "coercion" if a patient is impelled by the disease to join a clinical trial, in particular when the intervention being studied has serious side effects but is the patient's only chance of preventing death or very serious harm.[28,29] Both alternatives are in a sense very bad choices with very bad features; the patient would much prefer not to be in the position of having to make such a choice. But that is not enough to make the choice coerced and to invalidate the patient's choice about trial participation. The fact that individuals sometimes are forced by circumstance or nature to make choices that they would much prefer not to have to make is not grounds for failing to respect the choices they make in such unfortunate circumstances. Were this not the case, we would regard all patients with life-threatening illnesses as deciding under conditions of coercion, thereby freeing us to disregard their choices.

Although coercion involves threats that arise from other persons, rather than from circumstance or nature, it can also come from social institutions.[30] Prior to the mid-1970s it was common to do much drug testing with prison populations. They were in a controlled environment, and they could be motivated to participate with relatively little financial compensation, because of their limited opportunities to earn money, or from the hope of securing an earlier release or better treatment while in prison. Largely due to the work of the National Commission for the Protection of

Human Subjects of Biomedical and Behavioral Research, this practice was essentially stopped, in part on the ground that any choice prisoners made to participate in research was likely coerced because of the total control of the prison environment. The rationale was that prisoners were so completely under the control of prison authorities that they would feel pressured to comply with those authorities' desire that they participate in the research. This reasoning could apply to individuals confined to other so-called total institutions, such as involuntarily committed mental patients.[31]

Manipulation of the choice by others is perhaps a more common form of involuntariness than coercion in the research context.[32] Yet it can sometimes be difficult to distinguish unethical manipulation from acceptable education or persuasion. Very roughly, manipulation means such practices as selective provision of information or playing on potential participants' fears. It is probably best understood as deliberately misinforming the potential participant (selective information) or as putting unwarranted pressure on the decision maker (playing on fears). In either case, it aims to have potential research participants make a choice they would not make if fully informed and choosing freely according to their own values. Like coercion, manipulation seeks to produce a choice that promotes the manipulator's good, or the manipulator's conception of the person's good, not the person's conception of his or her own good. In this respect, it is a clear violation of the person's autonomy.

There is controversy whether offers, not just threats, can sometimes be coercive.[33] Offers improve an individual's position by adding a new option that is better than the individual's existing options, while also leaving the previous options in place. Offers are generally not considered coercive or leading to involuntariness because they leave individuals with the option of remaining as they were before the offer. However, concerns arise when very substantial offers are made for research participation. Such offers may lead individuals, especially those in conditions of unjust deprivation, to accept excessive risks.[34,35] Offers to very poor participants of very large financial compensation or of otherwise unavailable medical care for participation in research carrying substantial risks or burdens can be exploitative of the participants' disadvantaged position; they are morally objectionable as exploitation, even if they are not coercive. This can be an especially troubling issue in some research carried out in very poor developing countries (see Chapters 20, 64–67).

Competence

The third requirement for ethically valid informed consent is that the participant be competent to give his or her consent.[36,37] Competence is a requirement for valid consent because without it, participants lack the reasoning capacities to arrive at a choice that fits their values and interests, even if relevant information has been made available and no involuntariness is present. Competence is part of what is necessary for autonomous choices. Strictly speaking, competence is a legal status, but it is also an ethical requirement and investigators, not the courts, make most determinations of competence for research participation, just as physicians do for therapy.[38] In general, adults are presumed to be competent to decide about participation in research unless determined otherwise. Children are presumed not to be competent to make that decision and so others, typically parents, must decide for them; in the case of older children, their assent to participation is typically required.[39]

Sometimes decision-making competence or incompetence will be a global property of a person; a normal adult should be competent to make any decision about research participation, and an individual who is comatose or suffering from advanced dementia will not be competent to make any such decisions. In borderline cases, however, in which there is some but not complete impairment of an individual's decision-making capacities, the individual may be competent to make some research participation decisions but not others. That is because both the complexity of different decisions, as well as the risks associated with participation, can vary greatly across different research projects. Moreover, a potential participant's decision-making capacities can vary substantially over time from fluctuations in his or her medical condition, the effects of medications, and other factors such as being moved to an unfamiliar setting. Investigators are responsible for attempting to maximize the potential participant's decision-making capacities, for example, by tapering or temporarily stopping medications, particularly if there may be significant potential benefits to the person from enrolling in the research.

What decision-making capacities are needed for competence? First are capacities for understanding and communication. Capacities for understanding relevant information are needed to permit an informed choice, and capacities for communication are needed both for the process of becoming informed and to communicate a choice once it has been made. Second are capacities for reasoning and deliberation. This will most often be "if/then" reasoning; if I do this, then that will happen. A part of deliberation is the capacity to entertain alternative courses of action simultaneously so that they can be compared and a choice made. Third is the possession of aims and values that can be used as the basis for selecting from among alternative courses of action. Of course, whether to participate in a particular research project may not fit within the potential participant's past experience and so it may not be decided by reference to preexisting aims and values; then what is needed is the capacity to decide what weight to give to relatively new aims, outcomes, and values.

The competence evaluation should focus on the exercise of these various capacities in the person's reasoning about whether to participate in the research project at hand, not simply on the outcome of that decision process—whether consent is given or refused.[40,41] That is, the competence evaluator should look for serious defects in the participant's decision-making process, not whether the participant has arrived at a decision that others consider correct, rational, or best. In the face of serious defects, of course, the first response should be to help the decision maker correct them; only if they prove uncorrectable can they serve as evidence for incompetence.

When there is some impairment of the person's decision-making capacities, but far from complete impairment, how should one determine whether the impairment is sufficient to render the individual incapable of making an informed choice?[42] The function of the competence assessment in the therapeutic context is to determine whether the patient will retain decision-making authority or instead if that authority will be transferred to a surrogate to decide for the patient. There are two principal values at stake for the patient in that determination: on the one hand, the interest in making treatment decisions for oneself when one is sufficiently able, and, on the other hand, protecting one's well-being when seriously impaired decision-making capacities may result in a choice harmful to oneself. These two values must often be balanced when a patient wishes to make the decision, but is making an apparently harmful choice. In particular, sometimes honoring an impaired refusal of consent for importantly beneficial treatment may be sufficiently harmful to the patient that he or she is correctly found incompetent to make the decision.

In the context of research participation, the interest in making the decision for oneself is essentially the same, but interest in the protection of well-being typically differs. In the case of research without benefit to the participant and with any significant risk, the interest in protection of well-being principally concerns not letting the individual participate in the research unless its risks are well understood. However, some medical conditions, such as some cancers, are often treated in a research context in which the patient's best hope of medical improvement lies in research participation. In this case, the patient may have a medical interest in participating in the trial, but refusal to participate does not necessarily demonstrate incompetence to decide, because the intervention being investigated is by definition of unproven medical benefit, with its potential risks also often not well established. In general, because benefits to the participant in research are either nonexistent or uncertain and unproven, there will rarely be a persuasive case for overriding a person's refusal to participate if that person is sufficiently able to understand the choice. Unlike in therapy, in which a patient's refusal of treatment may raise the question of competence to decide, in research the important competence evaluation will often be of a patient who consents to participate when there is significant or unknown risk in participation.

Conclusion

We are now in a better position to see how the specific requirements for informed consent for research participation spell out a conception of autonomous choice whether to do so. If the decision is not informed, the patient will be unable to reliably determine whether participating would serve his or her interests, aims, and values. If the choice is not voluntary, then the decision will serve someone else's interests, or someone else's conception of the patient's interests, not the patient's own conception of his or her interests. If the patient is not competent, he or she lacks the capacity to use the information to deliberate whether to participate in the research. Together, these three requirements provide reasonable assurance that the participant is exercising the capacity for autonomous choice and action when deciding whether to participate in research.

References

1. Faden RR, Beauchamp TL, with King NMP. *A History and Theory of Informed Consent.* New York, N.Y.: Oxford University Press; 1986.
2. *Canterbury v. Spence,* 464 F.2d 772 (D.C. Cir. 1972), cert. denied, 409 U.S. 1064 (1972).
3. *Natanson v. Kline,* 350 P.2d 1093, 1106 (Kan. 1960).
4. World Medical Association. *Declaration of Helsinki: Ethical Principles for Medical Research Involving Human Subjects.* Tokyo, Japan: WMA; October 2004. [Online] 2004. Available: http://www.wma.net/e/policy/b3.htm.
5. Levine RJ. *Ethics and Regulation of Clinical Research,* 2nd ed. New Haven, Conn.: Yale University Press; 1986.
6. Appelbaum PS, Lidz CW, Meisel A. *Informed Consent: Legal Theory and Clinical Practice.* New York, N.Y.: Oxford University Press; 1987.
7. The Nuremberg Code. In: *Trials of War Criminals Before the Nuremberg Military Tribunals Under Control Council Law No. 10, Volume 2.* Washington, D.C.: U.S. Government Printing Office; 1949:181–2. [Online] Available: http://www.hhs.gov/ohrp/references/nurcode.htm.
8. Beauchamp TL, Childress JF. *Principles of Biomedical Ethics,* 5th ed. New York, N.Y.: Oxford University Press; 2001.
9. The National Commission for the Protection of Human Subjects of Biomedical and Behavioral Research. *The Belmont Report: Ethical Principles and Guidelines for the Protection of Human Subjects of Research.* Washington, D.C.: Department of Health, Education and Welfare; DHEW Publication OS 78-0012 1978. 9. [Online] April 18, 1979. Available: http://www.hhs.gov/ohrp/humansubjects/guidance/belmont.htm.
10. Dworkin G. *The Theory and Practice of Autonomy.* New York, N.Y.: Cambridge University Press; 1988.
11. Haworth L. *Autonomy: An Essay in Philosophical Psychology and Ethics.* New Haven, Conn.: Yale University Press; 1986.
12. Schneider C. *The Practice of Autonomy: Patients, Doctors, and Medical Decisions.* New York, N.Y.: Oxford University Press; 1998.
13. Miller FG, Rosenstein DL. The therapeutic orientation to clinical trials. *New England Journal of Medicine* 2003;348:1383–6.
14. Brody H, Miller FG. The clinician-investigator: Unavoidable but manageable tension. *Kennedy Institute of Ethics Journal* 2003;13:329–46.
15. Department of Health and Human Services, National Institutes of Health, and Office for Human Research Protections. The Common Rule, Title 45 (Public Welfare), Code of Federal Regulations, Part 46 (Protection of Human Subjects). [Online] June 23, 2005. Available: http://www.hhs.gov/ohrp/humansubjects/guidance/45cfr46.htm.
16. Meisel A, Kuczewski M. Legal and ethical myths about informed consent. *Archives of Internal Medicine* 1996;156:2521–6.
17. Brock DW. Informed consent. In: Brock DW. *Life and Death: Philosophical Essays in Biomedical Ethics.* New York, N.Y.: Cambridge University Press; 1993:21–54.
18. Appelbaum PS, Roth LH, Lidz CW, et al. False hopes and best data: Consent to research and the therapeutic misconception. *Hastings Center Report* 1987;17(2):20–4.
19. Horng S, Grady C. Misunderstanding in clinical research subjects: Distinguishing the therapeutic misconception from the therapeutic misestimation. *IRB: Ethics and Human Research* 2003;25(1):11–6.
20. Wendler D, Rackoff J. Informed consent and respecting autonomy: What's a signature got to do with it? *IRB: Ethics and Human Research* 2001;23(3):1–4.
21. Davis TC, Holcombe RF, Berkel HJ, et al. Informed consent for clinical trials: A comparative study of standard versus simplified forms. *Journal of the National Cancer Institute* 1998;90:668–74.
22. Flory JH, Emanuel E. Interventions to improve participants understanding in informed consent for research. *JAMA* 2004;292:1593–1601.
23. Katz J. Informed consent—A fairy tale? Law's vision. *University of Pittsburgh Law Review* 1977;39(2):137–74.
24. Ingelfinger F. Informed (but uneducated) consent. *New England Journal of Medicine* 1972;287:465–6.
25. Wirshing DA, Wirshing WC, Marder SR, et al. Informed consent: Assessment of comprehension. *American Journal of Psychiatry* 1998;155:1508–11.
26. Sreenivasan G. Does informed consent to research require comprehension? *Lancet* 2003;362:2016–8.
27. Wertheimer A. *Coercion.* Princeton, N.J.: Princeton University Press; 1988.

28. Agrawal M. Voluntariness in clinical research at the end of life. *Journal of Pain and Symptom Management* 2003;25:S25–S32.

29. Bosk CL. Obtaining voluntary consent for research in desperately ill patients. *Medical Care* 2002;40(9 Suppl.):V64–V68.

30. Moser DJ, Arndt S, Kanz JE, et al. Coercion and informed consent in research involving prisoners. *Comprehensive Psychiatry* 2004; 45:1–9.

31. Singer R. Consent of the unfree: Medical experimentation and behavior modification in the closed institution. Part II. *Law and Human Behavior* 1977;1:101–62.

32. Klingman M, Culver CM. An analysis of interpersonal manipulation. *Journal of Medicine and Philosophy* 1992;17:173–97.

33. Feinberg J. *The Moral Limits of the Criminal Law, Vol. 3. Harm to Self.* New York, N.Y.: Oxford University Press; 1986.

34. Wilkinson M, Moore A. Inducement in research. *Bioethics* 1997;11:373–89.

35. Emanuel E. Ending concerns about undue inducement. *Journal of Law, Medicine, and Ethics* 2004;32:100–5.

36. White BC. *Competence to Consent.* Washington, D.C.: Georgetown University Press; 1994.

37. Buchanan AE, Brock DW. *Deciding for Others: The Ethics of Surrogate Decision Making.* New York, N.Y.: Cambridge University Press; 1989.

38. Berg JW, Appelbaum PS, Grisso T. Constructing competence: Formulating legal standards to make medical decisions. *Rutgers Law Review* 1996;48:348–96.

39. Grodin MA, Glantz LH, eds. *Children as Research Subjects: Science, Ethics and Law.* New York, N.Y.: Oxford University Press; 1994.

40. Grisso T, Appelbaum PS. *Assessing Competence to Consent: A Guide for Physicians and Other Health Professionals.* New York, N.Y.: Oxford University Press; 1998.

41. Moye J, Gurrera RJ, Karel MJ, et al. Empirical advances in the assessment of the capacity to consent to medical treatment: Clinical implications and research needs. *Clinical Psychology Review* 2006;26:1054–77.

42. Chen DT, Miller FG, Rosenstein DL. Enrolling decisionally impaired adults in clinical research. *Medical Care* 2002;40(9 Suppl.):V20–V9.

Alexander M. Capron

Legal and Regulatory Standards of Informed Consent in Research

Legal rules embodied in judicial decisions and in statutes and regulations are at the heart of modern bioethics, and nowhere more clearly than in research with humans. Of the basic ethical principles associated with clinical research, autonomy—in the guise of "informed consent"—is, in its origins as well as its content, the most legal. Whereas other aspects of bioethics, such as the principles of nonmaleficence and beneficence, can be traced to ancient medical texts as well as to the professional orientation of modern physicians, informed consent was first articulated in legal documents, and it has been further elaborated by judges, legislators, and regulators over many decades.

Besides being central, the law may also seem the most straightforward aspect of research ethics. Yet the role of law in research ethics is not simple, for several reasons. First, although the law has been a major stimulus for research ethics, in practice it does not always support the ethical norms it inspired. Second, the apparent primacy of autonomy and its legal handmaiden, informed consent, among bioethics principles is belied by the larger framework of ethics review of clinical research. Third, and most ironically, when applied with the greatest apparent rigor, the law—which can be a very blunt instrument—can impede the realization of the sorts of relationships and outcomes in clinical research most often endorsed by ethicists. In sum, the law of informed consent in research is a paradox enveloped in an enigma, though this reality is obscured by an outer wrapping of legal parchment.

This description could prompt several responses. The first might well be to give up on informed consent as a snare or a waste of effort. A better alternative, though one requiring greater effort and attention, would be to seek to recover what is valuable, indeed essential, in informed consent by recognizing the limitations of the

law and compensating for them. To illuminate the problems that need to be avoided, one must understand not only the current law of informed consent in research but also how it developed. This chapter therefore begins by examining the contribution various events and documents made to the contemporary legal regulation of research consent.

I. The Origins of the Law of Consent in Research

The roots of informed consent lie not in traditional medical ethics but in the law. To the extent that consent appeared in the norms laid down by medicine's early leaders, it was only by implication: Physicians needed the permission of sick persons to attend them in their homes. Yet, however willingly patients may have accepted their physicians' ministrations, this would not have been based on anything like what is now called informed consent. Even Plato, who favorably compared the doctors who cared for freemen with those who treated slaves without ever talking to their patients individually, still described the former as "instructing" the sick person, who was brought "under his persuasive influences."[1] Rather than reveal the nature of ailments or the therapeutic options, Hippocratic physicians were schooled to withhold information and to soothe their patients by distracting their attention from their illness or the risks of treatment. After all, what would a patient, ignorant of medical art and perhaps anxious and confused, be able to contribute to a medical decision?

Although research in the current sense was not a part of medicine until well into the 19th century, nothing in the writing of Hippocrates or his professional descendants suggests that informed consent was seen as any more necessary should a physician be performing an experiment rather than providing ordinary medical care. Physicians may have recognized that experiments are "perilous." But because each new patient might react differently to a customary remedy and the therapeutic armamentarium was limited, experiments were inevitable, and a physician's moral authority to proceed rested not on the patient's consent but on the well-meaning exercise of medical art. Even when later medical moralists, such as Moses Mamonides or Claude Bernard, recognized the risks that inhere in treating patients as means to advance scientific knowledge, they counseled their fellow practitioners to avoid this practice rather than suggesting that physicians involve patients as knowing and voluntary partners in its undertaking.

For a long time, this combination of physicians' beneficent intent and consent by implication (or lack of objection) was apparently accepted as the legal as well as the moral justification for both medical practice and experimentation. To appreciate the current law of consent for research, it is necessary to keep in mind not only the processes by which the law formally responded to research scandals and the claims of victims but also the development and limitations of the law of consent to treatment, which has shaped, and continues to shape, the assumptions of courts and regulators as well as the practices of physicians when they engage in research.

A. Battery

The law first began to move beyond its deference to physicians in the 18th century, in judicial decisions involving consent to surgery. Judges relied on ancient principles of battery law to hold that surgery, like any other "touching" of a person, could occur only with consent, the absence of which would render the intervention actionable at law despite the good intentions of the medical practitioner. By the beginning of the 20th century it was well established, as Judge Benjamin Cardozo memorably declared in *Schloendorff v. New York Hospital,* that "[e]very human being of adult years and sound mind has a right to determine what shall be done with his own body; and a surgeon who performs an operation without his patient's consent commits an assault, for which he is liable in damages."[2]

Applying the concepts emerging in contract law to the physician-patient relationship, courts also concluded that submitting to surgery could be presumed to signify agreement unless the patient, like any other party to a contract, "was the victim of false and fraudulent misrepresentation."[3] The result was a somewhat circumscribed affirmation of self-determination: Absent an emergency, surgery was battery if performed on a competent adult without consent, and consent would be invalid if obtained through misinformation or for an intervention other than the one performed. Plainly, this fell far short of requiring full disclosure of the information a patient would need to make an autonomous decision.

Although these rules about contractual breaches and battery arose in cases involving ordinary treatment, a third line of cases involving experimental treatment evolved (in line with the general movement of tort law) from strict liability to negligence. Judges initially took as self-evident that a doctor, no matter how skillful, who departs from "the known rule and usage" of his profession "to try an experiment" does so at his peril.[4] In time, however, liability

was narrowed to cases in "which a system of treatment has been followed for a long time, [so that] there should be no departure from it, unless the surgeon who does it is prepared to take the risk of establishing, by his success, the propriety and safety of his experiment." Otherwise, when "there is no established mode of treatment," a patient "must trust to the skill and experience of the surgeon he calls" and not complain of novel interventions, providing the usual rules for consent to treatment were met.[5]

For most of the past century, consent developed along separate tracks for treatment and for research. On their face, the rules for research were more explicit and extensive than those for treatment. Yet the rules on consent for research frequently did not have their intended effect on physicians' conduct, a failing that may be traced in part to the influence of physicians' view of their ordinary consent obligations; indeed, this influence seemed to extend beyond physicians' behavior to the formulation and application of the legal rules for medical research.

B. Government Regulation

Beginning in the middle of the 19th century, as physicians turned to scientific methods to develop their knowledge of disease, they increasingly used patients as subjects in studies unconnected with their medical conditions. A few researchers provided subjects formal contracts, most famously the board appointed in 1900 by the U.S. Army surgeon general to carry out studies on yellow fever in Cuba, under Major Walter Reed. The physicians on the board began by experimenting on themselves, but when one of them died, they decided to use U.S. servicemen and Hispanic laborers instead. To meet criticisms, especially in the Spanish-language press, Army officials drew up a formal contract (in Spanish and English versions), in which subjects agreed to allow themselves to be intentionally exposed to yellow fever, in exchange for gold worth the equivalent of six-months' pay, to be doubled if they became infected. Each subject (apparently thinking in the third person) had to acknowledge that he understood "that in the case of the development of yellow fever in him, he endangers his life to a certain extent but it being entirely impossible for him to avoid the infection during his stay on this island he prefers to take the chance of contracting it intentionally in the belief that he will receive . . . the greatest care and most skillful medical service."[6]

Most researchers in the second half of the 19th century and the early years of the 20th not only failed to describe risks accurately but engaged in experiments that fell into a category sometimes labeled *human vivisection.* Often using orphans, paupers, residents of mental institutions, or other marginalized persons as their subjects, these early researchers exposed them to a number of serious diseases, including gonorrhea and syphilis, resulting not merely in physical harm but sometimes in death. Although these shocking acts apparently did not lead to any disciplinary response in the medical community, they did prompt the first official regulation of research with human beings. In 1900, in response to reports in the general and medical press about such abuses, particularly in asylums and hospitals, the Prussian government issued a directive to the heads of clinics and similar establishments "absolutely prohibiting" medical interventions "for purposes other than diagnosis, therapy, and immunization" under any of the following conditions:

1. The person in question is a minor or is not fully competent on other grounds.
2. The person concerned has not declared unequivocally that he consents to the intervention.
3. The declaration has not been made on the basis of a proper explanation of the adverse consequences that may result from the intervention.[7]

In 1931, the German government expanded upon the Prussian regulations and even more clearly differentiated between "therapeutic experimentation and modes of treatment which serve the process of healing even though the effects and consequences cannot yet be adequately determined," which were permitted, and "human experimentation" that consists of "operations and modes of treatment . . . carried out for research purposes which are not therapeutic" and that were not to be carried out on incompetent or uninformed persons.[8]

It is striking that these regulations embodied several features that continue through the present day in many legal regimes. First, they established a stricter set of requirements for experiments using "normal volunteers" than so-called therapeutic research with patients. Second, the Prussian rules included three of what are still regarded as the four essential elements of valid consent for research participants: that participation in research requires unambiguous agreement of the person prior to the start of the study; that the agreement be based upon a clear statement of the risks involved; and that the person must be legally competent. (The only element not addressed is the *voluntariness* of the consent.)

Regrettably, the 1931 German guidelines also serve as a sober reminder that the existence of legal rules is not enough to produce ethical research, for they proved to be wholly ineffectual in protecting the thousands of victims of the depraved physicians and their assistants who carried out lethal experiments in German concentration camps during World War II. This lack of effect might be ascribed to the 1931 rules being mere guidelines without legal force, as some authorities contend,[9] though others maintain that the rules were German law with binding effect until the Third Reich's fall in 1945.[10] In any case, the rules were relied on by the prosecution's expert witnesses at the trial of the Nazi concentration camp doctors after the war as one basis for concluding that the defendants had violated established standards of medical ethics[11] (see Chapters 2 and 12).

C. The Nuremberg Code

In the Doctors' Trial, 23 Nazi experimenters were tried before a U.S. military tribunal sitting at Nuremberg in occupied Germany. In handing down judgment in August 1947, the court accepted the view of medical experts that "certain types of medical experiments on human beings, when kept within reasonably well-defined bounds, conform to the ethics of the medical profession generally" if "such experiments yield results for the good of society that are unprocurable by other methods or means of study." The "well-defined bounds" were spelled out in 10 "basic principles" that "must be observed in order to satisfy moral, ethical, and legal concepts."[12] The judges found that 16 defendants, having violated these principles, were guilty of war crimes and crimes against humanity. Although judicial holdings are usually known by the name of the case in which they appear, these 10 principles are

enshrined not as the ruling in *United States* v. *Karl Brandt* but as the Nuremberg Code. In addition to its historic origins, the Code's broad influence on and frequent citation in laws, regulations, and court decisions for the past six decades has made it the cornerstone of the law of medical research and especially of informed consent. "[A]lthough the field of international research ethics has evolved greatly over the past 40 years, its origins can always be traced back to the 10 principles first enunciated at the trial of the Nazi physicians."[13]

Several points in the Code concern what might be termed the scientific aspects of ethical research (a clear purpose, adequate preparation, qualified researchers), but "judicial concern" lay with those "so clearly related to matters legal that they assist . . . in determining criminal culpability."[12] Thus, the court focused on the exposure of subjects to excessive risk of death or grave injury and on the absence of informed consent. Indeed, the Code's first principle begins with the unequivocal declaration that "[t]he voluntary consent of the human subject is absolutely essential."[12] The Nuremberg court elaborated two elements of valid consent in line with existing common law doctrine and the prewar German law: The subject must "have legal capacity to give consent" and "should have sufficient knowledge and comprehension of the elements of the subject matter involved as to enable him to make an understanding and enlightened decision."[12] To this the court added that the subject must be "able to exercise free power of choice, without the intervention of any element of force, fraud, deceit, duress, over-reaching or other ulterior form of constraint or coercion."[12] (By rejecting defense claims that some or all of the experimental subjects had implicitly agreed to participate, the Nuremberg tribunal implicitly endorsed a fourth requirement, namely that subjects must unequivocally indicate their agreement before the research may begin.) Principle 1 also makes clear that the person initiating and directing an experiment has a "personal duty and responsibility which may not be delegated to another with impunity" to ascertain the quality of consent. Finally, in light of the horrible suffering of many subjects in the Nazi experiments, the court in Principle 9 added a new requirement, the right to withdraw consent, which has become an essential part of subsequent regulations: "During the course of the experiment the human subject should be at liberty to bring the experiment to an end if he has reached the physical or mental state where continuation of the experiment seems to him to be impossible."[12]

The Nuremberg Code moved the governance of research from domestic regulations to international human rights law. Article 5 of the Universal Declaration of Human Rights, adopted by the United Nations General Assembly in 1948 in the wake of the Nuremberg court's judgment, states, "No one shall be subjected . . . to cruel, inhuman or degrading treatment or punishment."[14] In 1966, the International Covenant on Civil and Political Rights explicated that this means that "[i]n particular, no one shall be subjected without his free consent to medical or scientific experimentation."[15] Many countries have incorporated this provision or its equivalent into their constitution[16-22] or public health legislation and regulation,[23-25] and regional organizations have based their rules on the same premises.[26] The violation of international human rights principles, specifically as embodied in the Nuremberg Code, has also been alleged as a basis for liability in one case which involved a trial of an antibiotic during an outbreak of meningitis, measles, and cholera among children in Kano, Nigeria.[27]

D. The Declaration of Helsinki

The Nuremberg Code is important as a legal and human rights document: "The Code remains a viable force. It squarely acknowledges the scientist's responsibility for the respect of human rights."[28] Yet despite its importance and its clear rules on subject's consent, the Nuremberg Code has had only an indirect effect on medical research because physician-investigators regard it as relevant only to the barbaric acts of war criminals rather than to what they do with, and hence say to, their patient-subjects. The World Medical Association (WMA), formed by national medical bodies after World War II to reassert the ethical foundations of the profession, formulated in 1948 a new Hippocratic Oath that asserted that "the health and life of my patient will be my first consideration." Shortly thereafter, the WMA began work on principles for medical research, but it was not until June 1964 in Helsinki, Finland, that it adopted its guide for physicians in clinical research. Although the Declaration of Helsinki reminded physicians that their acts must conform to the criminal, civil, and ethical rules of their own countries, it has itself assumed a large role in the legal regulation of research. This is the case where statutes or regulations explicitly incorporate or refer to the Declaration, as in the European Union (EU) clinical trials directive.[29] It is also true when research ethics committees use it as the standard to which researchers must adhere, with or without the expansion provided by the Council for International Organizations of Medical Sciences (CIOMS) in its *International Ethical Guidelines for Biomedical Research Involving Human Subjects,* first prepared in 1982 and revised in 1993 and 2002, to indicate how the ethical principles "set forth in the Declaration . . . could be effectively applied."[30]

Starting from the premise that "it is essential that the results of laboratory experiments be applied to human beings to further scientific knowledge and to help suffering humanity," the 1964 Declaration of Helsinki drew a "fundamental distinction" between clinical research with and without a therapeutic aim.[31] The second section, entitled "Clinical Research Combined With Professional Care," makes clear that the WMA meant to spell out physicians' responsibilities, not subjects' rights. In Section II, Article I, it proclaims that physicians "must be free" to use new measures, and the duty to obtain consent receives only a brief and qualified mention:

> If at all possible, consistent with patient psychology, the doctor should obtain the patient's freely given consent after the patient has been given a full explanation. In case of legal incapacity consent should also be procured from the legal guardian; in case of physical incapacity the permission of the legal guardian replaces that of the patient.[31]

The Declaration's treatment of research combined with clinical practice is a reminder of the significant influence that the often paternalistic norms of ordinary medical care have had on the legal regulation of consent in research. Frequently, no sharp line exists between research and clinical care; moreover, when research is conducted with patients, they remain in physicians' eyes patients and not merely subjects. It is thus not surprising that the Declaration should reflect norms that doctors find appropriate to the physician-patient relationship, and that this in turn should have shaped the thinking of the framers of the legal rules for consent in research.

In addressing "Non-Therapeutic Clinical Research," the Declaration followed both prewar law and the Nuremberg Code in mandating, in Sec. III, Arts. 3a and 2, that research "cannot be undertaken without [the subject's] free consent, after he has been fully informed" of "the nature, the purpose, and the risk of clinical research."[31] The Declaration echoed the Nuremberg Code in stating that the subject "should be in such a mental, physical, and legal state as to be able to exercise fully his power of choice" (while also noting the difficulty of safeguarding "personal integrity, especially if the subject is in a dependent relationship to the investigator") and "should be free to withdraw permission for research to continue"[31] (Sec. III, Arts. 3a, 4a, 4b). The Declaration went beyond prior law in requiring that "[c]onsent should as a rule be obtained in writing" and in allowing research on a legally incompetent subject provided "the consent of the legal guardian [is] procured" (Sec. III, Arts. 3c, 3a), an extension it did not explain.[31] These elements—competence; information about the nature, purpose, and risk of a study; voluntary consent in writing; the right to withdraw; and allowing guardians to consent to research on incompetent subjects—cover virtually all the important requirements found in contemporary law. One might say that in the years since, the law has merely elaborated the details.

Yet the Declaration has itself been revised five times since 1964 (most recently in 2000); these revisions reflect the influence of both critical analysis concerning the shortcomings of the original Declaration and the condemnation aimed at problematic research projects conducted despite the Declaration. For example, the document now requires disclosure of "sources of funding, any possible conflicts of interest, [and] institutional affiliations of the researcher."[32] Concern about subjects' dependency on researchers has been made more specific by requiring subjects to be assured that they may "abstain from participating, or may withdraw, at any time without reprisal." Moreover, according to paragraph 22, should the relationship of researcher and subject risk producing consent under duress, consent should be obtained instead "by a well-informed physician who is not engaged in the investigation and who is completely independent of this relationship."[32]

Most significantly, the latest revision of the Declaration turned the special treatment of "research combined with medical care" on its head: Rather than providing a license for physician-researchers to treat patient-subjects simply as patients—who could be enrolled in research based on no more disclosure than is "consistent with [their] psychology"—the Declaration now adds five special requirements for this category of research. (Two of these, which deal with placebo-controlled clinical trials and posttrial obligations to patients, have proven so controversial that the WMA has had to issue "notes of clarification" about them.) The evolution of the Declaration—which has become much longer and more detailed, and which now takes into account interests beyond those of practicing physicians—reflects the reality that in many parts of the world, this document, produced by a professional association, provides the de facto legal criteria for consent and other ethical requirements in research. Indeed, the U.S. Food and Drug Administration (FDA), which in 1975 first incorporated the original Declaration into its regulations for foreign clinical trials conducted without an investigational new drug application (IND), still relies on the Declaration's 1989 version as the standard to which investigators are held.[33] The Declaration has ceased being simply a short statement of *principles* or moral aspirations for physicians engaged in research.[34] Yet, although it may appear more regulatory, the Declaration still lacks the level of precision needed to guide investigators and research ethics committees.

II. The Procedural Aspects of Informed Consent Requirements

Greater specificity in the rules for research, including informed consent, is provided principally by national laws and regulations and related international documents such as the guideline on *good clinical practice* (GCP) issued by the major drug regulatory authorities through the International Conference on Harmonisation.[35] Even greater detail can be found in some of the rules adopted by research review bodies at an institutional (or regional or national) level; these rules take on the character of private law to the extent that these bodies have made commitments to regulators to follow them in reviewing research protocols submitted for their approval.

Among this welter of national and international regulations, two related sets of rules provide the basic legal framework for informed consent, the so-called Common Rule for research with human beings supported by most agencies of the U.S. federal government[36] and the research regulations of the U.S. FDA.[37] In what is surely the strangest example of global health governance, these rules, originating in a single country, have achieved influence worldwide because they encompass studies conducted or supported by the major research agencies of the U.S. government as well as those carried out with nonpublic funds (principally by biotech companies or drug or device manufacturers) with the intention of submitting the findings in an application for licensing approval by the FDA. The U.S. regulations achieve further reach because they have also directly influenced the law in other jurisdictions; for example, some provisions of the so-called Tri-Council Policy Statement, (TCPS) promulgated in 1998 by the three Canadian governmental agencies with primary responsibility for research with human beings, closely follow parts of the U.S. rules.[38]

The comprehensive requirements for research projects set forth in these rules include many regarding informed consent. The consent-related rules fall into three groups: those that speak to the procedural aspects of informed consent (Who must do what when?), those that apply to the substantive aspects (What is the content of valid consent?), and those that involve the administrative aspects (How is consent reviewed and approved?). The procedural aspects are addressed in this section, followed by the substantive and administrative aspects in sections III and IV, respectively.

A. Activities Falling Outside the Rules

Before getting to the question of who has to obtain consent, one must know which activities are excluded, or may be exempted, from the Common Rule and related regulations. According to 45 CFR §46.116[36] and 21 CFR §50.20,[37] the basic procedural requirement for research consent is clear: With a few exceptions, "no investigator may involve a human being as a subject in research . . . unless the investigator has obtained the legally effective informed consent of the subject or the subject's legally authorized representative." The threshold question is thus whether a "human subject" is "involved" in "research." When an ac-

tivity does not entail "systematic investigation, including research development, testing and evaluation, designed to develop or contribute to generalizable knowledge," it is not considered research (45 CFR §46.102).[36] This does not mean that informed consent is not required (for example, when a patient receives an innovative treatment outside a research protocol), merely that the relevant legal rules would be those applicable in the jurisdiction to therapy rather than to research.

Likewise, the term *human being* erects a threshold because it limits application of the Common Rule to a *living individual* about whom an investigator obtains either "(1) [d]ata through intervention or interaction with the individual, or (2) [i]dentifiable private information" without interacting with the person (45 CFR §46.102).[36] The study of dead people or of information that is already available to an investigator and is not private does not qualify as research with human subjects under the Common Rule, though its use may be regulated in other ways.

In addition to these threshold exclusions, a broader exemption exists for six categories of research with human subjects (other than research on prisoners) that need not follow the federal requirements, including those on informed consent (45 CFR §46.101(b)).[36] Three exemptions are for studies involving education, one covers federal research and demonstration projects, and one is for food studies. Only one relates to health research:

> (4) Research involving the collection or study of existing data, documents, records, pathological specimens, or diagnostic specimens, if these sources are publicly available or if the information is recorded by the investigator in such a manner that subjects cannot be identified, directly or through identifiers linked to the subjects.[36]

For most medical outcomes or health systems research, or for studies using human biological specimens not collected for research purposes, the relevant material is unlikely to be *publicly available*. Therefore, for an investigation using existing private records or specimens to be exempt from federal research rules, an investigator would need to record the information derived in an unlinked anonymous fashion. Many activities involving monitoring and evaluation (of quality, safety, comparative outcomes, etc.) can adhere to this limitation, but many other research uses of existing records and specimen collections cannot and would therefore not be exempt from the rules. When an activity is neither excluded nor exempted, however, an institutional review board (IRB) may waive or alter the requirements for informed consent in various circumstances, as discussed in Section D below("Waivers of Consent Requirements").

The exclusion or exemption of an activity implies that the activity does not involve any action that, in the regulators' view, could not ethically be performed without the consent of the people involved, because the effect of being excluded or exempted is to relieve the persons conducting the activity of the obligation to follow the rules, including the consent requirements. Nonetheless, the exemption of a project from federal review does not remove it from any other legal requirements in the jurisdiction, including review by an ethics committee or the obligation to obtain informed consent if specified by local law (45 CFR §46.101(b)).[36] Investigators and review committees must be familiar with those local rules, especially in collaborative research projects that will actually be carried out by researchers in other provinces or countries.

B. Form and Timing of Consent

The basic requirements of a "legally effective informed consent" for research are that it must be (a) prospective, (b) informed, and (c) voluntarily provided by (d) a person with the legal capacity to give it. Furthermore, the Canadian federal rules state a fifth requirement as typically do the statutes and regulations of other countries, namely, that (e) "evidence of free and informed consent . . . should ordinarily be obtained in writing," as stated in Art. 2.1.b of the Canadian TCPS.[38] Although this may seem principally a procedural matter—consent formally exists when the subject signs the form—having a written consent also has administrative and substantive aspects. As to the former, a consent form can be reviewed in advance by an IRB, and the easiest way to demonstrate to research monitors that subjects have consented is with signed consent forms. As to the latter, the act of signing the form can impress on prospective subjects that they are making a serious decision and, indeed, manifest the essential fact that there is a choice to be made.

The procedural issues largely concern the first and last characteristics of consent, namely, that it be prospective and in writing; the other three characteristics (adequate disclosure, voluntariness, and legal capacity) are better regarded as substantive matters, though the requirement of legal capacity to consent raises an issue that it is convenient to frame in procedural terms in the section below on who must obtain consent from whom: When and how may consent be obtained from someone other than the subject him- or herself?

1. Signed, Written Form

It is frequently stated (yet all too often forgotten) that consent is a process not an event. When the consent form—a mere record of the understanding reached at a certain point between an investigator and a subject concerning the latter's participation in a research project—is conflated with informed consent, the likelihood that genuine and legitimate consent has been given is greatly diminished. Yet it is understandable that this occurs for several reasons. First, those who are required to obtain "legally effective" consent typically have little orientation or training in their medical education to treat consent as a process. Second, the Common Rule, in line with other national regulations, requires at 45 CFR §46.117(a) that informed consent be documented "by the use of a written consent form approved by the IRB and signed by the subject" (or legal representative).[36] Such rules encourage the tendency of research ethics committees to focus on the consent form and related materials as the easiest means of satisfying themselves that a researcher will obtain valid consent; rarely do committees utilize any means of observing or evaluating the act of obtaining consent from prospective subjects. Third, this requirement simply reinforces the general sense among clinicians that the best protection against tort liability is a piece of paper that lists all possible risks and bears the future plaintiff's signature. The rules are quite explicit at 45 CFR §46.117(b)(2) that the consent form must either contain all the required information or state that all necessary elements have been presented orally, in which case "there shall be a witness to the oral presentation" who, along with the person obtaining consent, must sign a written summary, approved by the IRB, of what is to be said to subjects.[36]

The legal requirement that consent be documented on a form, or as a summary of material presented orally, has the beneficial effect of generating a document, a copy of which can be given to subjects, as is indeed required by the regulations at §46.117 (a) and (b).[36] This enables subjects to review the information (either alone or with their own physician or family and others) and, if the circumstances allow, to return to the researcher with questions. Even when an investigator has followed the injunction to "give . . . the subject . . . adequate opportunity to read [the form] before it is signed" (§46.117 (b)(1)),[36] the added chance to review the information later may prove useful and reassuring. Consent to research is, after all, a continuous process, not an event.

According to the U.S. rules, an IRB may waive the requirement of a signed consent form under two circumstances. The first involves research in which "the principal risk would be the potential harm resulting from a breach of confidentiality" and the only record linking the subject to the research would be the form itself. If the IRB grants the waiver, each subject must be presented with the option whether to dispense with the documentation; the subject's wishes govern. The second is research presenting "no more than minimal risk of harm to subjects" and involving only procedures for which written consent is not normally required outside of research (45 CFR §46.117(c)).[36] The latter standard is contextual, as it depends upon the expectations existing in ordinary care at that time and place. Such waivers apply only to the requirement of a signed consent document, not to the obligation to obtain consent; moreover, even when it grants a waiver, the IRB may still require that the investigator "provide subjects with a written statement regarding the research," just as investigators must give to a person signing a consent form a copy of the document or of the summary of the information that has been provided. The Canadian TCPS adds a third category in Art. 2.1.b that is especially relevant in international research: Written consent is not required where it "is culturally unacceptable,"[38] as, for example, when written documents are only used as a means for people to forfeit rights (such as signing away a property claim) or when putting one's signature on written document, rather than simply giving a handshake, implies distrust.

2. Prospective Consent

The origins of consent in tort law make clear the legal presumption that consent will be obtained in advance of an intervention, since any "touching" by a physician or scientist would be a battery had not the person already given permission. The presumption is also reflected in all contemporary regulations on consent. Sometimes it appears only indirectly, as in the Common Rule, which states that in order to approve research, an IRB must determine that (among other things) "informed consent will be sought from each *prospective* subject [emphasis added]" (§46.111 (4)).[36] Other times, as in §4.8.8 of the ICH-GCP guideline, the requirement is clear: "Prior to a subject's participation in the trial, the written consent form should be signed and personally dated by the subject or by the subject's legally acceptable representative, and by the person who conducted the informed consent discussion."[35]

One circumstance in which it is especially important to attend to the timing of consent is when researchers know that biological materials being taken for diagnostic or therapeutic purposes are going to be used (or stored for future use) in research. In such cases, according to Article 12 of the Council of Europe's 2006 recommendations, whenever possible, informed consent for that use should be sought before the materials are removed.[39] Furthermore, the time between the intervention and the use may be quite long; when personal data and/or samples are maintained for years in *biobanks* or other collections, it will often be impossible to predict the nature or purpose of studies for which the material would later be useful. Although informed consent ought to "be as specific as possible with regard to any foreseen research uses and the choices available in that respect," unless such consent is very broad (and hence of questionable ethical value), it will be necessary for researchers to make reasonable efforts to contact the person in order to obtain consent to use the materials beyond the scope of the original consent; failing that, according to the Council of Europe, research is limited to that which is essential or can be conducted with anonymized materials (Arts. 10, 22).[39]

The two major situations in which the obligation to obtain prior consent may be waived are certain studies involving observation or deception, in which case subjects must be *debriefed* afterward and retrospective consent sought then, and research on treatments for emergency patients whose condition renders them unable to consent, in which case subjects must be informed "at the earliest feasible opportunity of the subject's inclusion in the research, the details of the research and other information contained in the informed consent document" and "that he or she may discontinue . . . participation at any time without penalty or loss of benefits to which the subject is otherwise entitled" (21 CFR §50.24).[37] The requirements for waiving consent before commencing research in these circumstances, which vary among countries, are examined under "Waivers," below.

C. Who Must Obtain Consent From Whom

The world of contemporary research, and particularly clinical trials of pharmaceutical and biological products, poses many challenges to the Nuremberg Code's easy assumption that ethical research will involve an investigator personally obtaining consent from a person with the legal capacity to give it.

1. Person Obtaining Consent

Subsequent ethical and legal codes have accepted the position taken by the Nuremberg tribunal that the duty to obtain consent rests with the scientist conducting the study. The ICH-GCP Guideline even places the article "Informed Consent of Trial Subjects" in §4.8 of Section 4, which addresses the qualifications and conduct of the investigator.[35] Yet the Nuremberg Code's classification of the duty as nondelegable does not mean that the task of informing the subject and obtaining his or her consent cannot be carried out by someone else; for example, Article 3.2(b) of the EU clinical trials directive states that information should be disclosed to subjects "in a prior interview with the investigator or a member of the investigating team."[29] But being nondelegable, the obligation to ensure that the task is carried out correctly always remains the investigator's, so if fault arises, responsibility rests with the investigator.

2. Person Giving Consent or Authorizing Participation

All adults are presumed to be capable of giving consent for medical procedures, including the choice to participate in a clinical trial. Most of the legal rules on informed consent do not dig below this presumption but simply acknowledge that some potential subjects, such as children, are legally incapable of giving valid

consent, and that, as the EU clinical trials directive states, "other persons [are] incapable of giving consent, such as persons with dementia, psychiatric patients, etc." (Preamble, paras. 3, 4).[29] Although not well elaborated in most regulations, the question of potential subjects' capacity deserves careful attention.

Capacity to consent is not simply a matter of cognitive ability, though the ability to understand that one is being asked to be a subject in research with certain obligations and potential risks and benefits is essential. Capacity also signifies that one is able to exercise free choice; hence, in certain circumstances, such as a prison, a person might be said to lack situational capacity. The contextual nature of the capacity to consent—that is, it is specific to a particular person facing a particular decision under particular circumstances—means that, just as in treatment decisions, a person may not be capable of making certain decision but can make others, or may lack the capacity at one point and then regain it, and vice versa. Blanket exceptions are particularly suspect when aimed at psychiatric patients, since even involuntary hospitalization for psychiatric treatment does not necessarily involve a finding of lack of capacity to make medical decisions.

Care in deciding which subjects are incapable of giving valid consent is especially important because research regulations now generally allow surrogate decision makers to act for such persons. Although limitations may be placed on trials in this situation (e.g., the same results should not be obtainable from a study with consenting subjects; the results of the study must be of value directly to the subjects or the group from which the subjects are drawn), recourse to the person's *legal representative* underlines rather than removes the special vulnerability of those unable to consent for themselves. Whereas even a few decades ago, the legitimacy of any nonconsenting person being involved in a medical intervention not for his or her own direct benefit was strenuously debated, studies that entail "only minimal risk and minimal burden for the individual concerned" are now permitted, in accordance with Article 15.2.ii of the Council of Europe's Additional Protocol, with subjects who are unable to consent for themselves.[40] Indeed, some rules, such as Guideline 9 of the CIOMS guidelines, go further, both in explaining that in the context of research interventions that do not hold out the prospect of direct benefit, minimal risk means "no more likely and not greater than the risk attached to routine medical or psychological examination of such persons" (who may be routinely exposed to burdensome examinations), and in allowing "[s]light or minor increases above such risk . . . when there is an overriding scientific or medical rationale for such increases and when an ethical review committee has approved them."[30] Such an extension apparently rests on regarding such subjects as having an identity as members of a group (e.g., "the same age category or afflicted with the same disease or disorder or having the same condition," as Art. 15.2.i of the Council of Europe's Additional Protocol states),[40] and assuming that their identification with such a group justifies (to them, or at least to those making decisions on their behalf) the risks and burdens imposed on them.

It is common in the legal rules to describe legal representatives as giving "free and informed consent" for those incapable of consenting, as Art. 2.5 of Canada's TCPS does.[38] However, it would be preferable to restrict the term *consent* to people deciding for themselves and to say instead that a legal representative provides "authorization" (Art. 15.1.iv of the Additional Protocol)[40] or "permission" (45 CFR §46.402(c))[36] for the subject. Whatever the terminology, the rules consistently require that the legal representative be given the same information in the same (usually written) form that a consenting subject would receive, signify agreement in the same manner, and have the same authority over participation and withdrawal that a consenting subject would have. Finally, regulations commonly impose an obligation to make such disclosures to a subject incapable of giving consent as he or she would be able to understand. Some regulations, such as the U.S. Department of Health and Human Services' (DHHS') Additional Protections for Children Involved as Subjects in Research (known as Subpart D), specify that, in most cases, "adequate provisions" must be made for "soliciting the assent of . . . children" when "in the judgment of the IRB the children are capable of providing assent" (45 CFR §46.408(a)), "assent" being "a child's affirmative agreement to participate in research" (45 CFR §46.402).[36] Other legal provisions stipulate that persons without the capacity to consent may not be enrolled in research if they object, even with their legal representative's authorization (Additional Protocol, Art. 15.1.v).[40]

D. Waivers of Consent Requirements

A number of grounds for waiving informed consent requirements are now recognized in regulations: the impracticability of obtaining consent, the need to study new treatments for emergency patients, and the need to test new interventions against chemical, biological, and nuclear weapons among members of the armed forces who may be exposed to them.

1. Omitting Consent When Obtaining It Is Not Practicable

Under the U.S. rules, an IRB may waive or alter informed consent requirements on grounds of "impracticability" in two situations. The first is for a governmentally approved study of a "public benefit or service program" that "could not practically be carried out without the waiver" (45 CFR §46.116(c)).[36] The second occurs under the following conditions:

1. The research involves no more than minimal risk to the subjects;
2. The waiver or alteration will not adversely affect the rights and welfare of the subjects;
3. The research could not practically be carried out without the waiver or alteration; and
4. Whenever appropriate, the subjects will be provided with additional pertinent information after participation (45 CFR §46.116(d)).[36]

Although both of these exceptions start from the premise that research can be licit without informed consent when investigators would find it very difficult or unduly burdensome to obtain consent, the two exceptions differ in scope.

The first is narrow, being restricted to a type of research sometimes called a social policy experiment. The forgoing of informed consent here can be explained by the difference between the circumstances for which federal research rules were written—namely, biomedical experiments where drugs, surgery, or similar intervention could usually be used only with consent and where investigators enjoy no inherent privilege to enroll people in research absent their agreement—and social policy experiments where the approval of government officials serves a function simi-

lar to that of consent, since the interventions involved are usually ones that governments may alter without individuals' consent. Indeed, when approved by an appropriate federal official, studies of the latter sort are exempt not only from the consent rules but from all federal research review requirements (45 CFR §46.101(b)(5)).[36]

Though it rests on a similar premise, the second exception is potentially much broader, taking in any study involving "no more than minimal risk" so long as the alteration of consent "will not adversely affect the rights and welfare of the subjects." The latter clause seems to underline that in addition to physical risks, subjects should not be exposed to other injuries to their "rights and welfare," but the protection provided is rather ephemeral because allowing researchers to omit the usual requirement to obtain informed consent in and of itself deprives subjects of the basic right not to be placed in research without their prior consent.

Paragraph (4) connects the exception to social and behavioral science studies in which the claim that prior informed consent would be impracticable to the design of the study, such as when results could be invalidated if subjects were forewarned that their behavior (or particular aspects thereof) was being studied. In such cases, Paragraph (4) states that subjects can be provided "pertinent information after participation," which would involve either taking the subjects through a complete consent process if none had occurred or providing them with those facts that had been omitted from the consent process to disguise the true purpose of the study to which they had "consented." As noted by the Canadian TCPS—which in Article 2.1(c) permits an exception to prospective consent under virtually identical rules (save that it adds a further limitation, disallowing waiver when a therapeutic intervention is involved)—this "debriefing" should be "proportionate to the sensitivity of the issue," in order to underline the importance of adequate counseling of subjects when the deception concerns matters such as relationships involving trust or revelations of a very personal nature.[38] Regardless of the sensitivity of the topic, research protocols should usually ensure that once the debriefing has occurred, subjects who object to having been involved without prior informed consent can have all information collected from or about them removed from the research records or database.

The scope of the second exception is, however, much broader than merely deception or behavioral studies involving after-the-fact debriefing and consent. An IRB may base its finding of impracticability on the character of the material (such as closed medical files or biological samples from a large group of patients who may be very difficult to contact), provided that the IRB also documents the absence of more than minimal risk and the investigator ensures that information from the records or specimens will not be used in a manner that adversely affects the subjects' welfare. Thus, consent requirements may be waived for studies that do not qualify for exemption from IRB review under §46.101(b)(4) because they involve data linked to an identifiable person that are derived from existing private records or specimens.[36]

In exercising its authority to grant this exception, an IRB should be cautious about allowing consent to be waived in research that could lead to intellectual property (IP) rights involving findings based on the use of patients' records or specimens because the extent to which patients have any IP claim in such circumstances remains unsettled. In some recent cases, research review bodies have, for example, insisted that the holders of traditional knowledge used to produce a patentable invention must share in the IP rights or should at least derive some benefit from the exploitation of those rights. Yet at least one court has held that a person whose biological material had certain unusual qualities that made it useful in producing a patentable product did not have a claim on the IP rights for that product. Nevertheless, the court in *Moore v. Regents of University of California* held that patients are owed a duty of full disclosure, including the intention of the physicians involved to make use of material taken from patients in a research project that could yield intellectual property.[41] Therefore, in such circumstances, it would not seem possible for an IRB to certify that allowing research without prior informed consent would "not adversely affect the rights . . . of the subjects," since in the absence of consent, the patients would not even know that their records or specimens might contribute to the physician-researchers' IP claims.

2. Emergency Research Waiver

It is conventional law that consent is not needed to treat a patient who is unable to provide consent because of a medical condition that could cause death or grave impairment if not treated before the person regains the ability to consent and before authorization can be obtained from his or her surrogate decision maker. In such circumstances, an unproven treatment may be used if it offers the best potential outcome for the patient. For example, FDA rules at 21 CFR §50.23(a) allow the unconsented use of an investigational drug or device when a life-threatening situation necessitates the use and "no alternative method of approved or generally recognized therapy" is available "that provides an equal or greater likelihood of saving the life of the subject." The rules specify that these conditions must be certified not only by the investigator but also by a second, independent physician.[37]

The use of an intervention in a formal investigation of its efficacy for emergency patients (such as a randomized, placebo-controlled trial) is research, not treatment, and hence would not automatically qualify for the emergency exception. But, "in response to growing concerns that current regulations . . . are making high quality research in emergency circumstances difficult or impossible to carry out at a time when the need for such research is increasingly recognized," the Secretary of Health and Human Services in 1996 created "a narrow exception" to the requirements of informed consent (which are grounded in statute) for "a limited class of research activities."[42] Thus, under U.S. rules and those since adopted in a number of other countries, a research ethics committee may allow such a trial (provided certain conditions have been met) even if neither the consent of the patient-subject nor the authorization of his or her legal representative can be obtained within a predetermined time period (termed the *therapeutic window*). The law in some jurisdictions explicitly allows the use of an advance directive for research,[43] and the FDA rules at 21 CFR §50.24(a)(2)(iii) seem to have such a research advance directive in mind in specifying that advance consent be sought when it is feasible "to identify prospectively the individuals likely to become eligible for participation in the clinical investigation."[37] The most difficult cases arise when such prospective consent cannot be obtained.

The traditional ethical view, that physicians should intervene with nonconsenting patients only for therapeutic reasons, has eroded in recent decades. The most conservative view—that of the EU's clinical trial directive, preamble para. 4—now seems to be that patients should only be involved in research "when there are grounds for assuming that the direct benefit to the patient outweighs the risk,"[29] but in many cases, a more liberal exception is permitted, based on an essentially utilitarian justification. The FDA specifies at 21 CFR §50.24(a)(3) that such a trial may be approved when, based on "[a]ppropriate animal and other preclinical studies," the research ethics committee finds that "[r]isks associated with the investigation are reasonable in relation to what is known about the medical condition of the potential class of subjects, the risks and benefits of standard therapy, if any, and what is known about the risks and benefits of the proposed intervention or activity."[37] The Common Rule includes the same provisions for research not subject to FDA approval.

Given the inherently grave condition of emergency patients and the potential harm that could be caused by an experimental intervention, investigators and research ethics committees should be very wary about proceeding without consent. At least two conditions are essential. First, as the Council of Europe declared in Art. 19.2.i of its additional protocol on biomedical research, a waiver is acceptable only when "research of comparable effectiveness cannot be carried out on persons in non-emergency situations."[40] Second, as articulated in Article 2.8 of Canada's TCPS, such research should be allowed only when it "addresses the emergency needs of [the] individuals involved."[38] In other words, it is not permissible to conduct research under the waiver on a matter not related to the emergency (in contrast to a patient who could consent to being enrolled in a study unrelated to his or her disease or condition). Finally, when consent or legal authorization becomes feasible, it should be obtained. Under ICH-GCP provisions at §4.8.15, the subject or his or her legal representative "should be informed about the trial as soon as possible and consent to continue and other consent as appropriate should be requested."[35] A similar provision exists in the FDA regulations at 21 CFR §50.24(b), which stipulates that the person deciding should be told that he or she may "discontinue the subject's participation at any time without penalty or loss of benefits to which the subject is otherwise entitled."[37]

The leading regulatory systems respond in varied ways to the ethical dilemmas inherent in permitting research on emergency patients who cannot consent. The FDA rules require that an independent data monitoring committee be established to exercise oversight of the clinical investigation (21 CFR §50.24(a)(7)(v));[37] such a committee is supposed to have access to "unblinded" data on a regular basis, so that it can order a halt to any study whose continuation would be wrong. By contrast, the Council of Europe's Additional Protocol restricts the permissible risk by relying on the method typically used for research on children. It specifies in Art. 19.2.iv that emergency research that offers no direct benefit to the person concerned, but that may produce knowledge that might benefit that person or others "in the same category or . . . having the same condition," may be conducted without the subject's consent if it entails "minimal risk and minimal burden."[40]

The U.S. rules (both FDA and the Common Rule as modified by the HHS secretary's waiver) impose two "additional protections of [subjects'] rights and welfare," whose intent and actual dictates are not entirely clear. First, when unable to contact the patient's legally authorized representative, the investigator, in accordance with 21 CFR §50.24(a)(7)(v), must "commit" in the protocol, "if feasible, to attempting to contact within the therapeutic window the subject's family member who is not a legally authorized representative, and asking whether he or she objects to the subject's participation in the clinical investigation."[37] How a physician-investigator faced with an emergency would be able to track down family members who do not qualify as legal representatives is only the first problem with this requirement. Because the laws of most jurisdictions recognize a hierarchy of authority among next-of-kin, under which those lower down on the list gain authority only upon the unavailability of those more closely related to the individual, the basis for seeking out such a person is unclear. Why, for example, would it be appropriate to burden any relation of the patient that a researcher can find (the definition at 21 CFR §50.3(m) includes "any individual related by blood or affinity whose close association with the subject is the equivalent of a family relationship"[37]), much less a child or a person with mental impairments, with this responsibility? And what if more than one such person were located or came forward, especially if they disagreed?

Even more problematic is what weight an objection voiced by such a person should have. This portion of the consent-exception rule does not actually require an investigator to exclude a subject on the basis of the family member's objection, merely to "summarize efforts made to contact family members and make this information available to the IRB at the time of continuing review." At 21 CFR §50.24(b), the rule provides that the IRB must "ensure that there is a procedure to inform the subject, or if the subject remains incapacitated, a legally authorized representative of the subject, or if such a representative is not reasonably available, a family member, that he or she may discontinue the subject's participation."[37] Assuming this applies as well to the decision to enroll a subject, it suggests that the family member's views would be controlling; however, such an interpretation would not be consistent with ordinary legal standards for medical decision making by third parties, under which a family member's objection to the research would not be dispositive unless it also represented the choice the emergency patient would have made.

The second requirement in the U.S. exception for research on emergency patients involves a process of "consultation . . . with representatives of the communities in which the clinical investigation will be conducted and from which the subjects will be drawn" and public disclosure to such communities "of plans for the investigation and its risks and expected benefits" prior to its initiation (21 CFR §50.24(a)(7)(i and ii))."[37] Although the regulation requires this process, it does not make clear what the investigator, or the IRB (if it carries out the consultation "where appropriate," as stated in the regulation), should do. Is the consultation intended to be a means simply for disclosure or is it also supposed to provide information to the investigator and IRB about the acceptability of the proposed trial to the community? If most people in the community find the study acceptable, should this be regarded as a form of proxy consent? Conversely, if most object, should the study be cancelled, or at least moved to another locale? The regulation does not answer such questions but hints that the regulators intend consultation primarily to serve a *disclosure* rather than *veto* function, because they also place a similar *disclosure* requirement on researchers when the trial has been completed "to apprise the community and researchers of the study, including the demographic characteristics of the research population, and its results" (21 CFR §50.24(a)(7)(iii)).[37] Why public disclosure would be needed to apprise the researchers of the study is opaque.

The regulation's uncertainties manifest that its authors realized that waiving consent in emergency research is problematic; these uncertainties also make it necessary for IRBs to be especially thoughtful in setting the conditions for research projects in this field. The regulation is also unusual in providing that if an IRB determines that it cannot approve a clinical investigation, the IRB must document its findings and provide them to the clinical investigator and the sponsor, who must promptly disclose this information not only to the FDA but also to other "clinical investigators who are participating or are asked to participate in this or a substantially equivalent clinical investigation of the sponsor, and to other IRB's [sic] that have been, or are, asked to review this or a substantially equivalent investigation by that sponsor" (21 CFR §50.24(e)).[37]

3. Drug and Vaccine Research With Armed Forces Personnel

In response to fears about biological, chemical, and nuclear warfare attacks, the U.S. Food, Drug, and Cosmetic Act was amended several times in the 1990s to create a further exception, at 21 CFR §50.23(d)(1), to the usual informed consent requirements for "the administration of an investigational new drug to a member of the armed forces in connection with the member's participation in a particular military operation."[37] Under 10 U.S. Code §1107(f),[44] the president may waive the prior consent requirement (for a period up to one year) if the president determines in writing that obtaining consent is either not feasible or contrary to the best interests of the military member (in which case, the president must adhere to the usual FDA grounds for waiver in 21 USC §355(i)(4),[45] involving an immediate threat to the subject's life) or that obtaining consent would not be in the interests of national security.

In enacting the exception, Congress insisted on a high level of responsibility. The president's waiver must be initiated by a request from the secretary of defense that documents the substantial risk of an attack, the absence of a satisfactory medical alternative, the approval by a duly constituted IRB, the manner in which the intervention will take place, the ability of the Defense Department's record-keeping system to track the drug, its use and the medical follow-up, and that "conditioning use of the investigational new drug on the voluntary participation of each member could significantly risk the safety and health of any individual member who would decline its use, the safety of other military personnel, and the accomplishment of the military mission" (21 CFR §50.23(d)(1)(iv))."[37] Even when a waiver is granted and prior consent is not required, the disclosure requirements remain. Thus, according to 10 USC §1107(d), the armed forces member must still be provided with the following:

1. Clear notice that the drug being administered is an investigational new drug or a drug unapproved for its applied use.
2. The reasons why the investigational new drug or drug unapproved for its applied use is being administered.
3. Information regarding the possible side effects of the investigational new drug or drug unapproved for its applied use, including any known side effects possible as a result of the interaction of such drug with other drugs or treatments being administered to the members receiving such drug.[44]

Furthermore, the statute specifies that the secretary of HHS may require additional information, and FDA regulations have been issued, at 21 CFR §50.23(d)(1)(viii), which require that subjects be given "a specific written information sheet concerning the investigational new drug, the risks and benefits of its use, potential side effects, and other pertinent information about the appropriate use of the product."[37] In addition, the Department of Defense must "provide public notice as soon as practicable" in the *Federal Register* "describing each waiver of informed consent determination, a summary of the most updated scientific information on the products used, and other pertinent information," as required by 21 CFR §50.23(d)(1)(xvii).[37]

Although the exception might be thought of principally as a military matter, its relationship to clinical research can be seen in the requirement that the Department of Defense must document that it "is pursuing drug development, including a time line, and marketing approval with due diligence" (21 CFR §50.23(d)(1)(xi)).[37] In effect, the Department is being treated as legally equivalent to any other clinical trial sponsor, which would mean, at least in theory, that its reason for administering the drug or vaccine to the armed forces members should be the same as that of any sponsor of a *therapeutic research* project: to produce information needed for licensing the product (and potentially to benefit the subjects). Given the open-ended nature of the "national security" justification for dispensing with consent, and the fact that, with advance planning, the other circumstances for an unconsented trial could usually be avoided, this exception, like the others, rests on a utilitarian justification for proceeding without prior informed consent. Moreover, dispensing with consent is grounded neither on the burden to the researcher in disclosing information prior to the trial nor on any potential risk to the subjects in doing so but rather on the Defense Department's unwillingness to allow subjects to refuse to participate.

III. The Substantive Features of Valid Informed Consent

The essential requisites of a valid consent are that it be *informed* (which requires disclosure and comprehension) and *free* (which requires that the subject has acted voluntarily). The expectations for each aspect elaborated in the regulations are largely consistent between the Common Rule and the FDA, as well as the ICH-GCP guidelines and European regional requirements (see Table 57.1). These rules all pay much more attention to the disclosure requirements (which can more easily be enumerated and checked, at least on paper) than to the elements of comprehension and voluntariness.

A. Disclosure

Relevant U.S. regulations (namely, §46.116 of the Common Rule[36] and §50.20 of the FDA regulations[37]) specify 13 mandatory elements that must be disclosed to prospective subjects ("shall be provided to each subject") as well as six discretionary elements ("when appropriate . . . shall also be provided"); the elements of legally effective consent in the ICH-GCP guideline and the Canadian TCPS are substantially the same. The U.S. regulations permit an IRB to require that additional information "be given to subjects when in the IRB's judgment the information would meaningfully add to the protection of the rights and welfare of

subjects" (45 CFR §46.109(b)).[36] The regulations also specify one item that must not be part of informed consent, whether written or oral, namely "any exculpatory language through which the subject or the representative is made to waive or appear to waive any of the subject's legal rights, or releases or appears to release the investigator, the sponsor, the institution, or its agents for liability for negligence" (45 CFR §46.116),[36] and the ICH-GCP guideline contains nearly identical language in its section §4.8.4.[35]

Several things are notable about these lists, which are at once incomplete and overlong. On the one hand, the lists omit important topics that appear elsewhere, such as among the 26 points specified in Guideline 5 of the International Ethical Guidelines produced by CIOMS[30] to elaborate the 2000 version of the Declaration of Helsinki (see Table 57.2). Also not mentioned is information about issues that have come to the fore since the Common Rule was issued in 1991, such as what will happen with biological specimens collected in the research, or subjects' access to new medical products validated in the research, as well as other basic issues, such as the reasons the subject was selected to participate or potential conflicting interests of the investigator or institution. Some of these topics are covered in other guidance documents such as Article 2.4(e) of Canada's TCPS, which requires disclosure of "the possibility of commercialization of research findings, and the presence of any apparent or actual or potential conflict of interest on the part of researchers, their institutions or sponsors."[38] The importance of these topics can hardly be doubted, especially from the viewpoint of liability; allegations that undisclosed conflicting interests undermined the adequacy of informed consent have been made in several recent suits against research institutions, such as *Gelsinger v. University of Pennsylvania*, in which the family of an 18-year-old volunteer who died in a gene therapy study alleged lack of informed consent and misrepresentation[46] (see Chapter 10).

On the other hand, the Common Rule's list is so lengthy that a consent form that complied with it risks not being the sort of succinct document that a person of ordinary intelligence with an elementary education would be likely to understand. Thus, the legal requirements for disclosure may interfere with expectations for comprehension and even voluntariness.

Unfortunately, investigators and IRBs that hope to achieve truly free and knowing consent while meeting the legal requirements receive scant help from the manner in which the elements are presented in the regulations. The points mix together factual statements (e.g., "an explanation of whom to contact in the event of a research-related injury" or " . . . [whom to contact] for answers to pertinent questions about the research") with justifications (e.g., "an explanation of the purposes of the research"), and some things that are descriptions are called explanations (e.g., "an explanation of . . . the expected duration of the subject's participation").[36] Furthermore, the five points at 45 CFR §46.116(a)(1) that begin "a statement that . . . ," which would seem to amount to language prescribed for a consent form, are not presented separately nor are they all mandatory, including the statement that some risks may be unforeseeable, which pertains to all human actions.[36] (Similarly, another optional statement—that findings developed during the study will be provided to subjects if they might be relevant to the subjects' decision to continue—ought always be included, except, of course, when the study is not expected to produce any findings until after all subjects have taken part in the research.)

Table 57.1

Requirements, Process, and Ethical Basis for Legally Valid Consent to Research in Leading Rules Having Legal Effect

	Nuremberg Code[12] (by numbered principle)	Declaration of Helsinki (revised, 2000)[32] (by paragraph)	45 CFR Part 46[36] (by subsection number)	ICH-GCP Guideline[35] (by subsection number, within §4.8)
Norm for validity	"voluntary consent" (1)	"freely-given informed consent" (22)	"legally effective informed consent" (116)	"informed consent" (1)
Basis for norm	Ethics of the medical profession and basic principles to satisfy moral, ethical, and legal concepts	Declaration of Geneva, International Code of Medical Ethics; legal requirement may not reduce or eliminate protections set forth (9)	Belmont Report; for foreign research, guidelines consistent with 1989 Declaration of Helsinki, if they afford "at least equivalent" protections (101(h))	"ethical principles that have their origin in the Declaration of Helsinki" (1)
Use of subjects who lack capacity to consent (legally, physically, or mentally)	Only subjects who are "able to exercise free power of choice" (1)	Allowed with consent of legally authorized representative if necessary to promote health of affected group and cannot be done otherwise (24)	Legally authorized representative may provide consent (111(a)(4)); for research involving children, special procedures in Subpart D, including children's assent	Allowed with consent of legally acceptable representative if "therapeutic" or risks are low and objectives require using these subjects, who must be informed (12 and 14)
Disclosure	"sufficient knowledge and comprehension of the elements of the	"subjects must be . . . informed participants," (20) "adequately informed [on 8 topics]" (22)	"in seeking informed consent the following information shall be provided [8 required and 6 optional topics]" (116 (a) & (b))	"should fully inform of all pertinent aspects of the trial" (5); written information must "include explanations of 20 topics" (10)
Comprehension	subject matter involved [nature, duration, and purpose; method and means; inconveniences and hazards] as to enable . . . an understanding and enlightened decision" (1)	Consent should be obtained "after ensuring that the subject has understood the information" (22)	"language understandable to the subject" and "sufficient opportunity to consider whether or not to participate" (116)	"language used should be as non-technical as practical and should be understandable to the subject" (4.8.6); "ample time and opportunity to inquire about details of the trial and to decide"; and "all questions "should be answered to the satisfaction of the subject" (7)
Voluntariness	"able to exercise free power of choice, without the intervention of any element of force, fraud, deceit, duress, over-reaching or other ulterior form of constraint or coercion" (1)	"subjects must be volunteers" (20), may decline "without reprisal" (22). "If the subject is in a dependent relationship with the physician or may consent under duress" consent should "be obtained by a well-informed physician who is not engaged in the investigation and who is completely independent of this relationship" (23)	"circumstances . . . that minimize the possibility of coercion or undue influence" (116); tell subjects that participation is voluntary, with no penalty or loss of benefits for refusal (116(a)(8); added safeguards for "subjects likely to be vulnerable to coercion or undue influence, such as children, prisoners, pregnant women, mentally disabled persons, or economically or educationally disadvantaged persons" (111(b))	should not "coerce or unduly influence" subject to participate or to continue" (3)
Limitations on waiver of rights	[not specified]	[not specified]	No exculpatory language to waive/appear to waive or to release negligence (116)	No language to waive/appear to waive any rights or to release negligence (4)
Written vs. implicit consent	"an affirmative decision"	in writing, or "formally documented and witnessed" (22)	Document by written consent, unless that risks breach of confidentiality or consent not usual for procedures used (117(c))	"written consent form should be signed and personally dated by the subject" and "by person who conducted consent" (8)
Right to withdraw	"at liberty to bring the experiment to an end" (9)	"Subject should be informed of the right . . . to withdraw consent to participate at any time without reprisal." (22)	May "discontinue participation at any time without penalty or loss of benefits to which the subject is otherwise entitled" (116(a)(8))	May "withdraw from the trial, at any time, without penalty or loss of benefits to which the subject is otherwise entitled" (10(m))
Role of the IRB/REC	[no committee]	"consideration, comment, guidance, and where appropriate, approval" with "right to monitor ongoing trials" (13)	Require that information given to subjects meets regulations, plus any that would "meaningfully add" protection (109(b))	Prior to beginning trial, should have IRB's "written approval/favorable opinion of written informed consent form" (1)

Table 57.2

"Essential Information for Prospective Research Subjects"
That Does Not Appear in 45 CFR Part 46

Before requesting an individual's consent to participate in research, the
investigator must provide the following information, in language or
another form of communication that the individual can understand:

3. . . . an explanation of how the research differs from routine medical
care;

8. that subjects have the right of access to their data on demand, even if
these data lack immediate clinical utility . . .;

17. the sponsors of the research, the institutional affiliation of the
investigators, and the nature and sources of funding for the research;

21. whether the investigator is serving only as an investigator or as both
investigator and the subject's physician;

22. the extent of the investigator's responsibility to provide medical
services to the participant;

26. that an ethical review committee has approved or cleared the research
protocol.

From: Guideline 5, Council for International Organizations of Medical
Sciences (2002)[30]

Table 57.3 sorts the required elements into seven categories,
keyed not only to the U.S. requirements but to the ICH-GCP
guideline approved by the Committee for Proprietary Medical
Products (CPMP) of the European Agency for the Evaluation of
Medicinal Products (EMEA), which provides the standard for
clinical trials within, or whose data will be submitted to, the European Union. The purpose of the categorization in Table 57.3 is
to encourage thoughtful and creative use of the legal requirements
in the ethical review of research proposals and especially of the
informed consent process.

The consent process should be focused on what is most important: that the potential subject is being invited to participate in
a research project, the primary purpose of which is to produce
new knowledge about a particular topic (as stated by the Declaration of Helsinki and built into the definition of *research* in the
regulations); that this will involve being exposed to certain experimental interventions (including possible assignment to the control or placebo arm of the trial) and assuming certain responsibilities (that is, accepting burdens or limitations on one's life); that
the person does not have to participate; and that failing to do so
will not lead to loss of any existing alternative interventions the
person would otherwise receive. These aspects are better conveyed
when discussion of the first element under Orientation ("that the
study involves research") is used as an opportunity to explain
what *research* means, and further when the elements gathered
under Prediction do not lead to a mind-numbing recitation of
remotely probable harms but instead produce an honest statement of the (small) likelihood of benefit and the existence of
uncertainty.

Of course, for both ethical and liability reasons, it is important
that all risks that could be material to a decision be conveyed; the
suggestion in one Canadian judicial decision that all rare risks
be listed has fortunately not been picked up by other courts.[47] The
ICH-GCP guideline moves in the right direction by adding to the
statement about reasonably expected benefits that "[w]hen there is
no intended clinical benefit to the subject, the subject should be
made aware of this" (§4.8.10(h)).[35] But to comply with the spirit

of this rule, investigators and research ethics committees will need
to resist the temptation to omit this warning whenever even a
small possibility of benefit can be hypothesized. The regulations
should be read to avoid allowing the informed consent process to
add to the already great risk that subjects will agree to participate
under the influence of a *therapeutic misconception* (see Chapter 58).
Bluntly put, subjects should be "asked if they are willing to be
used as means to the ends of others."[48]

Several other points inherent in Table 57.3 bear mention.
"The approximate number of subjects involved in the study,"
which is optional under the U.S. rules (but required by the European), is placed under Orientation rather than Description because this fact can help to make clear to a potential subject what
kind of a trial is being proposed. Will few people be involved
because the intervention is at an early stage of investigation (such
as a Phase I trial) in which *benefit* is not an endpoint? Conversely,
are only very small effects expected at best, which requires a large
number of participants in order to produce statistically significant
results? Again, IRBs can use this element to stimulate those preparing informed consent materials to communicate what is truly
involved in enrolling in a trial.

At the center of the seven categories is Options. The use of this
term is intended to highlight that because the actual details of the
intervention will be controlled by the protocol, the choices available to people participating in a clinical trial are very different from
those available to patients in therapy. Thus, the two mandatory
elements gathered here—a description of available alternatives,
and assurance that no penalty will attach to declining to enroll or
deciding to withdraw—represent a very modest version of *free
choice*. Moreover, despite its inclusion in all sets of regulations, the
right to withdraw is not without controversy.[48] Especially in situations far removed from the horrors of the Nazi camps that
prompted the rule in the first place, a less absolute right may be
appropriate. For example, in the context of stored specimens in
research collections, the right to withdraw consent may mean
that the biological materials should be rendered anonymous
rather than removed from the repository, according to Article 15
of the Council of Europe's recent recommendations.[39] Perhaps
the greatest value to the right is the reassurance it provides to
subjects—even if few of them exercise it—that the choice to enroll
in a research project is not irrevocable; of course, if this leads
subjects not to weigh the choice carefully, that would, ironically,
detract from the process of informed decision making.

B. Comprehension

As already suggested, the other two substantive attributes of legally valid consent, comprehension and voluntariness, are deeply
dependent on what is disclosed to subjects and particularly on
how well the basic choice whether or not to participate in the
research project is presented. The other two elements are themselves important, however. Plainly, comprehension is essential for
truly informed consent, for the act of disclosure would otherwise
be pointless. As stated in the first principle of the Nuremberg
Code, the subject "should have sufficient knowledge and comprehension of the elements of the subject matter involved as to enable
him to make an understanding and enlightened decision."[12]

At a minimum, then, "the language used should be as non-
technical as practical and should be understandable to the subject," in the language of the ICH-GCP (§4.8.6).[35] This also means

Table 57.3

Information to Be Disclosed to Research Subjects Under U.S. Federal Regulations and European Community Rules (ICH-GCP)

Category	U.S. Mandatory Elements (EC Elements are essentially similar **except as indicated in boldface**) U.S. Discretionary Elements (EC Elements are essentially similar [but all are mandatory])	45 CFR §46.166/ 21 CFR §50.25	ICH-GCP §4.8.10
Orientation	"a statement that the study involves research"	(a)(1)	A
	"an explanation of the purposes of the research"	(a)(1)	b
	"identification of any procedures which are experimental"	(a)(1)	f
	"the trial treatment(s) and the probability for random assignment to each treatment"		c
	"the approximate number of subjects involved in the study"	(b)(6)	t
Description	"an explanation of . . . the expected duration of the subject's participation"	(a)(1)	S
	"a description of the procedures to be followed" ", **including all invasive procedures"**	(a)(1)	d
	"the subject's responsibilities"		e
	"the anticipated prorated payment, if any, to the subject for participating"		k
	"any additional costs to the subject that may result from participation in the research"	(b)(3)	l
Prediction	"a description of any reasonably foreseeable risks or discomforts to the subject"	(a)(2)	
	"and, when applicable, to an embryo, fetus or nursing infant"		g
	"a description of any benefits to the subject or to others which may reasonably be expected from the research"	(a)(3)	
	the reasonably expected benefits." **"When there is no intended clinical benefit to the subject, the subject should be made aware of this."**	(b)(1)	h
	"a statement that the particular treatment or procedure may involve risks to the subject (or to the embryo or fetus, if the subject is or may become pregnant) which are currently unforeseeable"		
	"anticipated circumstances under which the subject's participation may be terminated by the investigator without regard to the subject's consent"	(b)(2)	r
Options	"a disclosure of appropriate alternative procedures or courses of treatment, if any, that might be advantageous to the subject"	(a)(4)	I
	"a statement that participation is voluntary, refusal to participate will involve no penalty or loss of benefits to which the subject is otherwise entitled, and the subject may discontinue participation at any time without penalty or loss of benefits to which the subject is otherwise entitled"	(a)(8)	m
	"the consequences of a subject's decision to withdraw from the research and procedures for orderly termination of participation by the subject"	(b)(4)	
	"a statement that significant new findings developed during the course of the research which may relate to the subject's willingness to continue participation will be provided to the subject"	(b)(5)	p
Identification	"a statement describing the extent, if any, to which confidentiality of records identifying the subject will be maintained" [FDA: "and that notes the possibility that the Food and Drug Administration may inspect the records"]	(a)(5)	o
	"records identifying the subject will be kept confidential and, to the extent permitted by applicable laws . . . , will not be made publicly available. If the results of the trial are published, the subject's identity will remain confidential."		n
	[Direct access to study records by monitors, auditors, IEC/IRB, and regulatory authorities is authorized]		
Remediation	"for research involving more than minimal risk, an explanation as to whether any compensation and an explanation as to whether any medical treatments are available if injury occurs and, if so, what they consist of, or where further information may be obtained"	(a)(6) (a)(7)	J
	"an explanation . . . of whom to contact in the event of a research-related injury to the subject"		q
Questions	"an explanation of whom to contact for answers to pertinent questions about the research and research subjects' rights . . . "	(a)(7)	Q

that consent materials (including materials approved by the research ethics committee for soliciting subjects) need to be reliably translated into the language used by potential subjects when that differs from that of the investigator. (Back translation is a frequently used method for establishing reliability, but does not appear to be required in any statute or regulations.) More generally, in-

vestigators and research ethics committees should use some means to ensure that the reading level required to understand the consent form is appropriate for the group of potential subjects.

Section III (above) discussed the procedural requirement that consent must be sought from someone who has the capacity to give it; what is at issue now is whether that capacity has been used to comprehend the information provided. Regrettably, the legal regulations on informed consent provide little guidance about how comprehension should be achieved or ascertained. The Common Rule, at §46.109(e), provides that an IRB "shall have authority to observe or have a third party observe the consent process and the research," but this provision seems to be aimed at unusual research situations or at monitoring the conduct of researchers whose past conduct has raised questions about their reliability.[36] Given the burden that monitoring the process of obtaining consent would impose on IRB members or staff, it does not offer a routine means of ascertaining that subjects have understood the information provided.

Short of monitoring the consent process, the IRB can require that subjects be given an adequate opportunity to have any uncertainties cleared up. For example, §4.8.7 of the ICH-GCP guideline requires that before consent may be obtained, the investigator "should provide the subject or the subject's legally acceptable representative ample time and opportunity to inquire about details of the trial and to decide whether or not to participate," and all questions "should be answered to the satisfaction of the subject."[35] Especially in settings in which those in power are not usually questioned, special effort may be needed to encourage subjects to ask for clarification or raise doubts. Furthermore, to fulfill the obligation stated in Paragraph 22 of the Declaration of Helsinki to ensure "that the subject has understood the information," the person obtaining consent can be required to pose questions politely to prospective subjects about what they have been told and to exclude those whose answers indicate inadequate comprehension.[32] The discretion accorded to ethics committees in all the regulations is broad enough to enable them to impose such requirements.

C. Voluntariness

As boldly declared in the Nuremberg Code's opening words, "The voluntary consent of the human subject is absolutely essential."[12] Yet this criterion for valid consent is the most difficult to implement in practice because voluntariness is a state of the mind, whereas the law, which deals with externalities, is dependent on discerning the state of mind from outward signs and circumstances. The elements in the Nuremberg tribunal's litany—"force, fraud, deceit, duress, over-reaching or other ulterior form of constraint or coercion"—are not only inherently wrong as assaults on human dignity but are forbidden in the context of informed consent because they are used to produce a choice or action that their victim would otherwise not make. Yet, given the psychological overdetermination of most behavior, cases certainly arise, perhaps not infrequently, when the choice that a subject makes under pressure from someone else is nevertheless the same choice the person would have made absent that pressure. Nor is it always possible to use a choice itself to establish the voluntariness of an action because there is no one measure of which choices "make no sense" and hence hint at hidden coercion or undue inducement. For example, a choice that one person would reject as being insufficiently self-protective may represent another's rational and voluntary embrace of an altruistic goal. Indeed, to the extent that the compulsion to act comes from inside, not out, what are investigators (much less IRBs) to do? A compulsion that is strong enough to be apparent—for example, a manifest desire to engage in risky behavior despite repeatedly injuries—might not render an

act involuntary, since the choice might reflect the person's values and desires, though it could negate the presumption that the person has the capacity to make such decisions.

These difficulties do not mean that the legal rules on consent for research have ignored the requirement of voluntariness. In the main, besides repeating injunctions against investigators using coercion or undue influence (ICH-GCP §4.8.3),[35] the rules aim to protect persons who are vulnerable to having their free choice overridden. The problems in explaining when and why vulnerability arises are illustrated by the Common Rule's requirement at 45 CFR §46.111(b) that "additional safeguards [be] included in the study to protect the rights and welfare" of "subjects likely to be vulnerable to coercion or undue influence, such as children, prisoners, pregnant women, mentally disabled persons, or economically or educationally disadvantaged persons."[36] This lumping together of disparate groups does nothing to sort out the different meanings of vulnerability among them nor to help determine whether the circumstances of any particular person are inconsistent with the exercise of free choice about enrolling in a research project or what "additional safeguards" might thus be expected to be effective in restoring voluntariness.

Article 12 of the Council of Europe's Additional Protocol obliges signatory countries to have regulations under which ethics committees are expected to give "particular attention" to "vulnerable or dependent persons" in making sure that "no undue influence . . . will be exerted on persons to participate in research."[40] The accompanying Explanatory Report classifies subjects' vulnerability due to cognitive, situational, institutional, deferential, medical, economic, and social factors (Para. 69) but offers no particular means of overcoming the resulting effects on voluntariness, which may be at odds with the assumption behind the disclosure rules.[40] For example, it is commonplace, in response to concerns about conflicts of interest, to insist that subjects be told about any incentives the enrolling physician is receiving from the trial sponsor. Such information would certainly be relevant in reaching an independent evaluation of the merits of participating in a study, but the disclosure would not in itself enable patients who feel dependent on the enrolling physician to exercise such independence. Paragraph 23 of the Declaration of Helsinki tells physician-investigators to "be particularly cautious" when obtaining consent "if the subject is in a dependent relationship with the physician or may consent under duress."[32] To increase the subject's ability to exercise free choice, the ethics committee may insist that consent be obtained "by a well-informed physician who is not engaged in the investigation and who is completely independent of this relationship."[32]

Other legal rules exist to eliminate undue inducements and penalties as well as to overcome the effects of more subtle coercive forces. Policing the "rewards" given for trial participation poses a particularly difficult task. Cash payments are allowable; reimbursement of expenses and of direct losses (wages forgone or the like) being economically neutral are prima facie acceptable. Compensation for time or burden may, however, rise to a level at which, in the words of Paragraph 64 of the Additional Protocol's Explanatory Report, subjects would "accept a higher level of risk than would otherwise be the case."[40] This limit is, however, a matter of judgment and cannot be applied literally, because any payment—no matter how modest—may have the effect (and indeed the intent) of persuading some people to participate in research when they otherwise would not; because the rule is clearly meant to exclude only certain inducements to accept "a higher level of risk," ethics committees are left with the problematic task of applying their own sense of reasonableness (i.e., at what level a payment becomes an impermissible inducement to a subject to accept an unreasonable level of risk). Obviously, in judging inducements and penalties, familiarity with the circumstances of the potential subjects is necessary. Something as minor as bars of soap or transistor radio batteries might provide an undue inducement in a particular population, and the will of a feeble patient might be overborne by pressure to accept an experimental intervention where persons who are less weak would be able to refuse.

A circumstance that may involve both inducements and coercion is suggested by Subpart C of the U.S. DHHS research regulations ("Additional Protections Pertaining to Biomedical and Behavioral Research Involving Prisoners as Subjects"), which recognizes that "prisoners may be under constraints because of their incarceration which could affect their ability to make a truly voluntary and uncoerced decision whether or not to participate as subjects in research" (45 CFR §46.302).[36] Rather than focus principally on direct force, as might be expected in prisons, the regulation aims mostly at ensuring that the possible advantages to a prisoner from participating in research "compared to the general living conditions, medical care, quality of food, amenities and opportunity for earnings in prison" not be "of such a magnitude that his or her ability to weigh the risks of the research against the value of such advantages in the limited choice environment of the prison is impaired" (45 CFR §46.305(a)(2)).[36] The IRB has the burden of making sure that the advantages of participating in research are kept to a modest level.

The prospect that participation in research offers access to possible benefits (e.g., drugs or vaccines) not available outside the research setting is not unique to prisons, of course. In many clinical settings, either when no therapeutic alternatives exist or when those that do are unavailable to a prospective subject outside of a clinical trial, the notion of choice may seem rather hollow. Of course, the requirement, articulated in Paragraph 22 of the Declaration of Helsinki and repeated in many regulations, that subjects should be reassured that they may decline to participate in, or may withdraw from, a research project "without reprisal" is an essential ethical norm.[32] Yet its legalistic formulation in the Common Rule (45 CFR §46.166(a)(8))—"refusal to participate will involve no penalty or loss of benefits *to which the subject is otherwise entitled* [emphasis added]"[36]—which is echoed in the ICH-GCP guideline at §4.8.10(m),[35] is a reminder that the circumstances that make the offer of a place in a trial something that some subjects feel they cannot refuse often lie beyond a researcher's direct control. Furthermore, physicians as well as patients are subject to the pressures created by constrained resources, and a physician in a low-resource setting may well decide to take part in research because the physician has nothing else to offer patients. "From that perspective," as one such doctor has noted, "enrolling patients in a clinical trial will always look attractive, no matter how unethical that research may turn out to be."[49] It is very difficult for IRBs to affect this barrier to voluntariness except by refusing to allow trials to be conducted among populations that have no alternative treatments or diagnostic regimens available; sometimes, however, these are the very settings in which research to develop new medical products is the most needed.

IV. The Administrative Aspects of Informed Consent Requirements

In light of the important rules governing the process and substance of obtaining valid consent, the administrative aspects may seem of only secondary importance. Yet the obligation of institutions to operate an IRB if their faculty or staff conduct federally sponsored and/or regulated research is the core legal requirement established by the National Research Act of 1974 (Public Law 93–348, codified at 42 U.S.C. 289(a)),[50] upon which the entire regulatory structure rests. The responsibility of such committees for the research process, including informed consent, is now a standard feature in research regulation globally. The administrative features of informed consent law take the form of rules on preparation, submission, review, implementation, and monitoring.

A. Preparation

Although the responsibility to obtain informed consent rests with investigators—indeed, in the ICH-GCP guideline, the provisions on informed consent appear in Section 4, "Investigator"[35]—the rules describe consent forms in the passive voice, leaving unspoken who will prepare them. Whoever fulfills this role, the very formality of the requirements can stimulate careful reflection about what will occur in the research; the need to spell this out in the consent form and to be prepared to defend it before the ethics committee can generate self-reflection that benefits not only the consent process but even the design and execution of the research itself.[51]

In investigator-initiated research, it can be assumed that consent forms will be written by principal investigators and their associates, whereas in most clinical trials sponsors prepare them, along with the protocol and related materials. Sponsors' greater familiarity with regulatory requirements makes it easier for them to write consent materials that cover all the requirements, but their financial interest in having trials executed quickly raises the danger that the consent document may be subtly slanted. The ICH-GCP guideline insists that the "investigator's brochure" (a compilation of clinical and nonclinical data on the product being investigated, which is provided to researchers) present information "in a concise, simple, objective, balanced, and non-promotional form that enables a clinician, or potential investigator, to understand it and make his/her own unbiased risk-benefit assessment of the appropriateness of the proposed trial" (§7.1).[35] Although the research regulations all declare that consent forms must be nontechnical and understandable, none mandates objectivity and balance. (When reviewing consent forms, however, ethics committees should address potential bias and ensure that the forms are as evenhanded as possible; central to this is conveying that the activity involves an experiment, not a new treatment).

The person responsible for preparing the consent materials is also responsible for updating them. A promise to convey to subjects new findings from a trial that might affect their willingness to continue in the trial is a discretionary element in the federal rules (45 CFR §46.166(b)(5)).[36] By implication, the consent form for new subjects would need to be revised to reflect such information along with equally significant new information from other sources.

The ICH-GCP guideline, at §4.8.11, obliges investigators to provide existing subjects with such updated forms.[35]

B. Submission

The Common Rule specifies that each IRB shall have written procedures for its work; the manner in which informed consent materials will be submitted is left to such local rules. Greater specificity appears in newer regulations, such as the guidance provided in February 2006 on the documentation needed under the EU clinical trials directive, which explains what information on recruitment arrangements (§6.1.2.4) and the informed consent procedure (§6.1.2.5) must be included in an application to an ethics committee before commencing a clinical trial.[52] The application to the ethics committee must describe the procedure to provide information and obtain consent from the subjects—that is, who will give the information to potential subjects and when. The application also must provide the justification, and the procedures, for using legal representatives (such as for minors) and for relying on witnessed consent. The guidance document suggests the use of a "subject information leaflet," which may go beyond the information in a typical consent form and may contain, for example, instructions on proper storage, handling, use, and disposal of the drug being studied. Pursuant to the EU clinical trials directive, the guidance also requires, at §6.1.2.5, the submission of an informed consent form that contains at least three elements:

- Consent to participate in the trial
- Consent to make confidential personal information available (direct access) for quality control and quality assurance by relevant personnel from the sponsor, a nominated research organization on behalf of the sponsor, and inspection by the competent authorities/institutions assigned this task in the Member State or, if applicable, the Ethics Committee
- Consent to archive coded information, and for its transmission outside the Community if applicable[52]

C. Review

The central administrative procedure for informed consent is, of course, the research ethics committee's review of relevant materials, especially the consent form. The committee is responsible for making sure that all required information will be provided to subjects and all procedural elements (such as needed documentation) will be satisfied, and it may add more requirements (such as means of measuring subjects' comprehension) when doing so would, in the committee's judgment, "meaningfully add to the protection of the rights and welfare of subjects" (45 CFR §46.109 (b)).[36] The committee's authority to require modification in the informed consent materials or procedures is most frequently manifested in changes in the consent form (or leaflet). Once the committee is satisfied that the forms and process accord with the legal requirements, and it notifies the investigator that the proposed research has been approved, the research may commence. The investigator and the sponsor must retain documentation of this approval in their files.

The ethics committee has the responsibility to conduct continuing review of approved projects at appropriate intervals and the authority to require modifications in the protocol and/or consent form as indicated.

D. Implementation and Monitoring

Investigators and sponsors are responsible for implementing research protocols (including consent procedures) as approved by the ethics committee, except that they may make any changes urgently needed "to protect the subjects . . . against any immediate hazard to their health or safety"[53] and may terminate the trial if the risk of harm from continuing is too great, without breaching any duty owed to subjects, provided due care is exercised and the consent form explains this possibility.[54] If an investigator or sponsor believes that significant changes in the protocol are necessary after a trial has commenced, than according to Article 10(a) of the EU's clinical trial directive, the ethics committee must first be notified, must conduct a new review, and must decide whether to renew its approval, with such modifications in informed consent as are indicated under the circumstances.[29]

In addition, the regulations give IRBs the authority to monitor research, including the consent process. The drug approval laws provide that clinical trial monitors should be appointed by sponsors to verify that the rights and well-being of subjects are protected, that the data reported are accurate and complete, and that the trial is being conducted in compliance with the approved protocol and applicable regulations. Monitoring, which typically involves on-site inspection, includes ascertaining that informed consent was obtained in the manner approved by the ethics committee, through review of the files that investigators are required to maintain. Monitors submit written reports to sponsors in which they summarize major findings, including any deviations and deficiencies regarding subjects' consent and actions taken or needed. In addition to having monitors, sponsors are expected to conduct periodic independent audits of trials, which can also involve inspection of the records. When monitoring or auditing reveals problems, according to ICH-GCP the sponsor is responsible for ensuring compliance (§5.20.1) and, if necessary, for terminating an investigator's participation in the study (§5.20.2).[35]

V. Conclusion

The legal regulation of clinical research, including several essential elements of contemporary rules on informed consent, dates to the turn of the 20th century. The earliest legal standards arose in response to abuses of unconsenting subjects, just as the historic Nuremberg Code affirmed the basic rights of human beings in research in reaction to the Nazi concentration camp experiments. The formal protection of informed consent has waxed and waned over the six decades since Nuremberg. The text that gives the most limited scope to patient-subjects' choices, the Declaration of Helsinki, is routinely invoked as the guiding document by research ethics committees around the world that are formally committed to protecting subjects.

In its first principle, the Nuremberg Code proclaims autonomy—the authority of each person to make his or her own choices about serving as a research subject—to be the core of research ethics: The prior, voluntary, informed consent of research subjects is "absolutely essential." Yet, despite the apparent incorporation of this principle into laws and regulations, utility and beneficence have emerged as the dominant values, though this has been disguised by the attention lavished on the rituals of "informed consent." Given that the legal requirements that might actually ensure that people have made free and well-informed choices about whether to take part in research are quite weak, subjects remain relatively minor decision makers regarding the research enterprise, compared to sponsors, investigators, and review bodies.

If the principle of autonomy is imagined as a disk, it would be one that had been trimmed back substantially from the outer edge by regulations allowing research without the prior informed consent of many of the people being studied (see Figure 57.1). In some of these situations, such as research on minors or circumstances in which obtaining consent is not practicable, the IRB is supposed to ensure that research "involves no more than minimal risk to the subjects" (or a "minor increase" that is within the range experienced by the particular subjects in medical care). But other research studies—such as tests of emergency interventions, or clinical trials of drugs and vaccines on military personnel—are not limited to minimal risk, though the risks must be balanced by potential benefits. Equally important, though less obvious, the disk is also cut away from the center by the allocation to the IRB of the authority to decide which studies may be conducted on risk-benefit or other grounds. Such an exercise of judgment is not inherently problematic; indeed, it simply represents an independent body (the IRB) ensuring that investigators have fulfilled the long-recognized obligation of beneficence, itself a part of the

Nuremberg Code. But the result is to cut back the metaphorical disk to a relatively small ring around a large hole, because people other than the research subjects have weighed the potential harms and benefits and decided whether to proceed.

Subjects thus exercise their right of informed consent in only a limited range of remaining studies, in which their formal agreement is a necessary, albeit not sufficient, ground for the study to proceed. Prime among allowable studies are clinical trials in which the risk of the intervention is minimal, such as studies comparing standard therapy (or a placebo) to a minor variation on standard therapy or observational studies that produce data with personal identifiers. The ring also includes some studies that pose more than minimal risk, namely when seriously ill patients might derive a large benefit from the intervention being studied (though it excludes research that some potential subjects might be willing to undergo that in the judgment of an IRB would entail an unfavorable balance of risk and benefits).

To conclude that the legal rules on informed consent have, perhaps unintentionally, narrowed the range of research in which prior informed consent actually plays a role is not to deny the importance of autonomy as an ethical principle. Rather, to accept that consent operates in a narrow range of cases is to underline that an essential question needs always to be clearly posed to potential subjects: Do you understand what it means to participate in research and, if so, do you want to participate in this trial? If the needed attention to this question is absent—either because the decision to encounter a minor risk is treated as inconsequential or because the

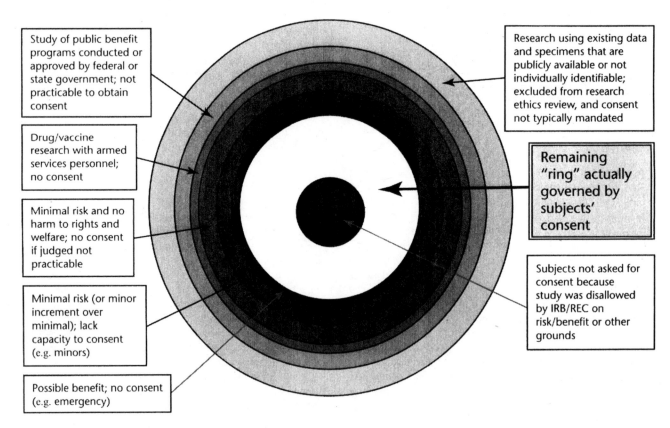

Figure 57.1. The Limited Scope for Informed Consent in Research: The "Autonomy Disk," Diminished From Within and Without

possibility that subjects might benefit leads all concerned to treat the research as *therapy*—then the listing of many other factors, as required by informed consent regulations around the world, will be of little significance. This is the paradox at the heart of research regulation. A system erected on a deep commitment to autonomy has evolved such that the law of informed consent provides little protection for the vital choice it is intended to protect.

An enigma remains, beyond the scope of this chapter: Is this problem inherent or only a result of having lost sight of the ethical starting point as the legal standards have been formulated and applied? The original 1964 Declaration of Helsinki claimed that the "responsibility for clinical research always remains with the research worker; it never falls on the subject, even after consent is obtained."[31] Does this embody a preference for protection over autonomy, or merely an insistence that the consent form should not be seen as a contract that relieves the researcher of liability for proceeding with unjustified research? It may be that informed consent is freighted with expectations generated by its use in the therapeutic context in which it can be a vehicle for open discussion between physician and patient to arrive at choices that aim to align individual preferences and values with interventions and outcomes. Given the dictates of research protocols, such expectations are unrealistic; for subjects, the "choice" is often nothing more than *à prendre ou à laisser* ("take it or leave it"). Thus, perhaps the more modest version of informed consent that is found in the laws regarding research should come as no surprise. Yet the legal rules are a floor, not a ceiling. It thus remains for investigators, sponsors, and research ethics committees to execute their respective responsibilities in a fashion that gives subjects the opportunity to make choices in as voluntary and understanding a manner as they are individually able. In particular, the formal requirements to disclose information can open the door for the investigator to share further information honestly, "answering questions and identifying unanswerable questions, appreciating doubts and respecting fears."[55]

References

1. Plato. *The Laws.* Taylor AE, trans. London, England: Dent & Sons Ltd.; 1943:104–5.
2. *Schloendorff* v. *New York Hospital,* 211 N.Y. 127, 105 N.E. 92 at 93 (1914).
3. *State* v. *Housekeeper,* 16 A. 382 (Md. 1889).
4. *Slater* v. *Baker and Stapleton,* C.B., 95 Eng. Rep. 860 (1767).
5. *Carpenter* v. *Blake,* 60 Barb. 488 (N.Y. Sup. Ct. 1871), reversed on other grounds, 50 N.Y. 696 (1872).
6. Bean WB. Walter Reed and the ordeal of human experiments. *Bulletin of the History of Medicine* 1977;51:75–92.
7. Capron AM. Human experimentation. In: Veatch R, ed. *Medical Ethics,* 2nd ed. Sudbury, Mass.: Jones and Bartlett Publishers; 1989:135–84, at 137.
8. Reichsgesundheitblatt 11, No. 10 (March 1931), pp. 174–5 (translated and reprinted in *International Digest of Health Legislation* 1980;31:408–11).
9. Howard-Jones N. Human experimentation in historical and ethical perspective. In: Bankowski Z, Howard-Jones N, eds. *Human Experimentation and Medical Ethics.* Geneva, Switzerland: CIOMS; 1982: 453–95.
10. Sass HM. Reichsrundschreiben 1931: Pre-Nuremberg German regulation concerning new therapy and human experimentation. *Journal of Medicine and Philosophy* 1983;8:99–111.
11. Grodin MA. Historical origins of the Nuremberg Code. In: Annas GJ, Grodin MA, eds. *The Nazi Doctors and the Nuremberg Code.* New York, N.Y.: Oxford University Press; 1992:121–44.
12. *United States* v. *Karl Brandt et al.,* Trials of War Criminals Before the Nuremberg Military Tribunals Under Control Council Law 10, Military Tribunal 1, Case 1, October 1946–April 1949, Vol. II. Washington, D.C.: Superintendent of Documents, U.S. Government Printing Office; 1950.
13. Perley S, Fluss SS, Bankowski Z, Simon F. The Nuremberg Code: An international overview. In: Annas GJ, Grodin MA, eds. *The Nazi Doctors and the Nuremberg Code.* New York, N.Y.: Oxford University Press; 1992:149–173, at 168.
14. United Nations General Assembly. Universal Declaration of Human Rights. Resolution 217A (III) of 10 December 1948. [Online] Available: http://www.un.org/Overview/rights.html.
15. United Nations General Assembly. International Covenant on Civil and Political Rights, Article 7. Resolution 2200A (XXI) of 16 December 1966; 23 March 1976, in accordance with Article 49.
16. Armenia. Constitution, Article 19 (adopted 9 July 1995).
17. Bulgaria. Constitution, Article 29(2) (adopted 13 July 1991).
18. Fiji. Constitution, Section 25 (2) (adopted 23 September 1988).
19. Lithuania. Constitution, Article 21 (4) (adopted 25 October 1992).
20. Oman. The Basic Law, Article 26 (promulgated by Crown Decree No. 101/96, 6 Nov. 1996).
21. Poland. Constitution of the Polish Republic, Ch. II, Sec. 31 (2 April 1997).
22. Ukraine. Constitution, Article 28 (adopted 28 June 1996).
23. Indonesia. Government Regulation of the Republic of Indonesia No. 39 of 1995, concerning health research and development, Ch. IV, Art. 8 (14 November 1995).
24. Peru. General Law No. 26842 of 9 July 1997, Sec. 15(d), El Peruano, No. 6232, pp. 151245–151252 (20 July 1997).
25. Turkey. Ministry of Health Regulations, Principle 5(e), Resmî Gazette, No. 23420, pp. 67–76 (1 August 1998).
26. Council of Europe. *Convention for the Protection of Human Rights and Dignity of the Human Being with regard to the Application of Biology and Medicine: Convention on Human Rights and Biomedicine,* Articles 5 and 16. Strasbourg, France: Council of Europe, November, 1996; opened for signature, April 4, 1997, Oviedo, Spain. [Online] Available: http://conventions.coe.int/Treaty/EN/Treaties/Html/164.htm.
27. *Abdullahi* v. *Pfizer Inc.,* 77 Fed. Appx. 48 (2nd Cir. 2003) (reversing and remanding the district court's dismissal on forum non conveniens grounds).
28. Bassiouni MC, Baffes TG, Evrard JT. An appraisal of human experimentation in international law and practice: The need for international regulation of human experimentation. *Journal of Criminal Law and Criminology* 1981;72:1587–1666, at 1642.
29. European Union. Directive 2001/20/EC of the European Parliament and of the Council of 4 April 2001 on the approximation of the laws, regulations and administrative provisions of the Member States relating to the implementation of good clinical practice in the conduct of clinical trials on medicinal products for human use. *Official Journal of the European Communities* 2001;L121:34–44. [Online] Available: http://europa.eu/eur-lex/pri/en/oj/dat/2001/1 _121/1 _12120010501en00340044.pdf.
30. Council for International Organizations of Medical Sciences, in collaboration with the World Health Organization. *International Ethical Guidelines for Biomedical Research Involving Human Subjects.* Geneva, Switzerland: CIOMS and WHO; 2002. [Online] November 2002. Available: http://www.cioms.ch/frame_guidelines_nov _2002.htm.
31. World Medical Association. *Code of Ethics of the World Medical Association: Declaration of Helsinki.* Helsinki, Finland: WMA; June 1964. *New England Journal of Medicine* 1964;271:473.

32. World Medical Association. *Declaration of Helsinki: Ethical Principles for Medical Research Involving Human Subjects.* Tokyo, Japan: WMA; October 2004. [Online] 2004. Available: http://www.wma.net/e/policy/b3.htm.

33. Food and Drug Administration, Department of Health and Human Services. Title 21 (Food and Drugs), Code of Federal Regulations, Part 312 (Investigational New Drug Application), Sec. 312.120 (Foreign clinical studies not conducted under an IND). [Online] April 1, 2006. Available: http://www.access.gpo.gov/nara/cfr/waisidx_06/21cfr312_06.html.

34. Report of a Workshop held at the Royal Society of Medicine, London. Revising the Declaration of Helsinki: A fresh start. *Bulletin of Medical Ethics* 1999;151:13–7.

35. International Conference on Harmonisation of Technical Requirements for Registration of Pharmaceuticals for Human Use. *The ICH Harmonised Tripartite Guideline—Guideline for Good Clinical Practice.* Geneva: ICH; 1996. [Online] Available: http://www.emea.eu.int/pdfs/human/ich/013595en.pdf.

36. Department of Health and Human Services, National Institutes of Health, and Office for Human Research Protections. The Common Rule, Title 45 (Public Welfare), Code of Federal Regulations, Part 46 (Protection of Human Subjects). [Online] June 23, 2005. Available: http://www.hhs.gov/ohrp/humansubjects/guidance/45cfr46.htm.

37. Food and Drug Administration, Department of Health and Human Services. Title 21 (Food and Drugs), Code of Federal Regulations, Part 50 (Protection of Human Subjects). [Online] April 1, 2006. Available: http://www.gpo.gov/nara/cfr/waisidx_06/21cfr50_06.html.

38. Canadian Institutes of Health Research, the Natural Sciences and Engineering Research Council of Canada, and the Social Sciences and Humanities Research Council of Canada. *Tri-Council Policy Statement: Ethical Conduct for Research Involving Humans.* [Online] 1998 (with 2000, 2002 and 2005 amendments). Available: http://www.pre.ethics.gc.ca/english/policystatement/policystatement.cfm.

39. Council of Europe. Recommendation Rec (2006) 4 of the Committee of Ministers to members states on research on biological materials of human origin, Appendix (Guidelines). Strasbourg, France: Council of Europe; March 15, 2006. [Online] Available: https://wcd.coe.int/ViewDoc.jsp?id=977859&BackColorInternet=9999CC&BackColorIntranet=FFBB55&BackColorLogged=FFAC75.

40. Council of Europe. *Additional Protocol to the Convention on Human Rights and Biomedicine Concerning Biomedical Research,* with Directorate General I, Legal Affairs, *Explanatory Report to the Additional Protocol to the Convention on Human Rights and Biomedicine Concerning Biomedical Research.* Strasbourg, France: Council of Europe; 2005. [Online]

41. Available: http://conventions.coe.int/treaty/en/Treaties/Html/195.htm.

42. *Moore* v. *Regents of University of California,* 793 P.2d 479 (Cal. 1990).

43. Department of Health and Human Services. 45 CFR Part 46: Waiver of Informed Consent Requirements in Certain Emergency Research; Waiver. *Federal Register* 1996;61(192):51531–3.

44. Newfoundland, Canada. The Advance Health Care Directives Act, §5(3)(a) (31 May 1995).

45. U.S. Congress. Title 10 (Armed Forces), Unites States Code, Chapter 55 (Medical and Dental Care), §1107. Notice of use of an investigational new drug or a drug unapproved for its applied use. [Online] Available: http://www.law.cornell.edu/uscode/html/uscode10/usc_sec_10_00001107—000-.html.

46. U.S. Congress. Title 21 (Food and Drugs), Unites States Code, Chapter 9 (Federal Food, Drug, and Cosmetic Act), §355. New drugs. [Online] Available: http://www.law.cornell.edu/uscode/html/uscode21/usc_sec_21_00000355—000-.html.

47. *Gelsinger* v. *Trustees of the University of Pennsylvania,* Phila. Cnty. Ct. of C.P., filed 18 September 2000.

48. *Weiss* v. *Solomon* [1989] A.Q. 312 (Sup. Ct.).

49. Levine RJ. *Ethics and Regulation of Clinical Research,* 2nd ed. New Haven, Conn.: Yale University Press; 1986.

50. Proceedings of a symposium. The Declaration of Helsinki: A symposium to review current proposals for change (quoting Jim Black). Victorian Institute of Forensic Medicine, August 30, 1999, Monash University, Melbourne, Australia.

51. U.S. Congress. Title 42 (Public Health and Welfare), Unites States Code, Chapter 6A (Public Health Service), §289. Institutional review boards; ethics guidance program. [Online] Available: http://www.law.cornell.edu/uscode/html/uscode42/usc_sec_42_00000289—000-.html.

52. Katz J, Capron A. *Catastrophic Diseases—Who Decides What?* New York, N.Y: Russell Sage Foundation; 1975.

53. European Commission, Enterprise and Industry Directorate-General. Detailed guidance on the application format and documentation to be submitted in an application for an Ethics Committee opinion on the clinical trial on medicinal products for human use, ENTR/CT2, Rev.1. Brussels, Belgium: EC; 2006.

54. United Kingdom. The Medicines for Human Use (Clinical Trials) Regulations 2004 (Statutory Instrument 2004 No. 1031), Art. 30(1). London, England: Her Majesty's Stationery Office, 2004. Available: http://www.opsi.gov.uk/si/si2004/20041031.htm#30.

55. *Suthers* v. *Amgen,* 372 F. Supp. 2d 416 (S.D.N.Y. 2005).

56. Katz J. The regulation of human research—Reflections and proposals. *Clinical Research* 1973;21:785–91.

Paul S. Appelbaum   Charles W. Lidz

58

The Therapeutic Misconception

In the early 1980s, in the course of conducting a study of informed consent in psychiatric research, we noticed an interesting phenomenon exemplified by the following case example.

A 25-year-old woman, who was participating in a randomized, double-blind, placebo-controlled study of two medications for borderline personality disorder, was interviewed shortly after consenting to enter the project. At the time of the interview she displayed no apparent psychiatric symptoms, and her intellectual ability seemed consistent with her history of having completed three years of college. Her understanding of the research was generally excellent. She recognized that the purpose of the research project was to find out which treatment worked best for the class of patients of which she was a member. She spontaneously described the three groups, including the placebo group, and indicated that assignment would be random. She understood that dosages would be adjusted according to blood levels, not her level of symptomatology, and that a double-blind would be used. When she was asked directly, however, how her medication would be selected, she said that she had no idea. She then added, "I hope it isn't by chance," and suggested that each subject would probably receive the medication he or she needed. Given the conflict between her earlier use of the word "random" and her current explanation, the issue was pursued. She was asked what her understanding of "random" was. Her definition was entirely appropriate: "By lottery, by chance, one patient who comes in gets one thing and the next patient gets the next thing." She then began to wonder out loud if this procedure were being used in the current study. Ultimately, she concluded that it was not.[1]

What is going on here? This was a well-educated, intelligent, asymptomatic patient in a clinical research trial who seemed to have an excellent understanding of the project to which she had just consented. When it came to applying that knowledge to her own situation, however, she was unable to do so. That is, though she appeared to understand in the abstract that the methods of this clinical trial, specifically randomization, meant that decisions about participants' treatment would not be made on the basis of an individualized judgment as to what would be best for them, she seemed unable to appreciate that this would also be true in her own case. As a result, it appeared probable that she had consented to research participation with a false assumption about the consequences of becoming a subject in this study, including the possibility that she might receive a placebo.

We dubbed this phenomenon the *therapeutic misconception* (TM), and defined it as the mistaken belief that decisions about one's treatment while a research subject would be made solely based on one's individual condition and needs.[1] Since publication of our initial paper and later article with more detailed data from our study,[2] TM has been recognized as a major obstacle to obtaining ethically valid consent in clinical research.[3–10] In this chapter, we review the tension between the ethics of clinical care and the ethics of research that lies at the core of TM, describe its probable origins among research subjects, provide an overview of TM's phenomenology, and suggest ways in which its prevalence might be reduced.

The Tension Between Clinical Ethics and Research Ethics

The ethics of clinical medicine are governed by what the legal philosopher Charles Fried referred to as the principle of *personal care*.[11] By this he meant that the dominant assumption among both physicians and their patients is that all decisions made by a physician will be intended to advance the patient's well-being. When a treatment is recommended for a patient, it will be chosen because the physician believes that it is the regimen most likely to cure the patient's illness or control the patient's symptoms, or because it is thought to offer the best available balance between the likelihood of effectiveness and magnitude and probability of side effects. In either event, it is the patient's interests that have primacy. There are some rare occasions, such as the imposition of quarantine, when physicians may make decisions that are contrary to their patients' interests or wishes; however, these are clearly departures from the norm and the long-standing debates about them are evidence of their exceptional nature.[12] Of course, there may be circumstances in which physicians fall short of fully embodying the ideal of personal care, as when treatment recommendations are made on the basis of the physician's financial interests or convenience, or as a manifestation of overt malevolence. That such situations occur, however, does not negate the normative force of the principle of personal care, on the basis of which these behaviors will be condemned as inappropriate deviations by both physicians and patients.

Note that adherence to the principle of personal care does not require that physicians be correct in their judgments as to how best to advance patients' interests. Their choices may be objectively wrong (i.e., existing data indicate another approach is more likely to be effective) or simply unsuccessful after the fact. Or, in the patient's particular situation, there may be no scientific reason to prefer one approach to another. In all of these cases, so long as the physician makes a decision based on what the physician reasonably believes is most likely to be in the patient's interests, the principle of personal care is vindicated.

As Fried points out, however, in a clinical research study "the care [participants] receive is not chosen exclusively on the basis of a concern for their individual well-being, but with regard to the success of the experimental design."[11] We have identified several aspects of research methodology that involve—to a greater or lesser extent—the sacrifice of personal care for the sake of protecting the integrity of the research data. These include randomization, double-blind procedures, placebos, protocols that restrict discretion in the administration of treatment, and limits on the use of adjunctive treatments.[2] We consider each in turn.

Randomized assignment to treatment conditions, common in research as a means of controlling bias in the allocation of subjects, undercuts the individualized determination of treatment needs that lies at the core of personal care. Some ethicists have argued that because randomization is used only when the treatment options are in clinical equipoise (i.e., there is no persuasive empirical evidence of an advantage for one over another in the patient population as a whole),[13] there is no sacrifice of personal care in these situations. However, even in the absence of agreement in the medical community regarding general preferences for treatment of a given condition, there may be important reasons to favor one over another for particular patients.[14] The treatments being compared may have a differing range or likelihood of side effects, about which patients might have clear preferences because of the differing impacts on their lives. It will not be a matter of indifference, for example, to an architectural draftsman whether he receives a medication that induces a tremor or a likely equally effective one with a different side-effect profile. When new treatments are being compared with standard approaches, there may again be reasons for particular persons to have decided preferences among those choices. It is precisely because potential subjects may have failed to obtain acceptable results with "treatment as usual" that they may decide to enroll in research. Patients may also have individual characteristics that suggest a better response to one treatment than another (e.g., a sibling who successfully responded to one treatment, but not to another). Even if none of these situations obtains, it is clear that patient/participants who believe that individualized choices are being made about the treatments they receive—witness the case described at the beginning of this chapter—have badly misconstrued the situation into which they are entering.

Given that treatment will be assigned randomly, the use of double-blind procedures, in which neither the treating physician nor the patient/participant knows which treatment is being administered, may not seem to involve a further compromise of personal care. But in fact, when blind to the treatment, the ability of the physician to monitor and respond to unwanted effects of the treatment, or to instruct the patient/participant in self-monitoring, may be reduced. Not knowing whether the patient/participant is receiving a medication that induces nausea, for example, cannot help but complicate the task of trying to decide whether one is dealing with a medication side effect or the first sign of a recurrent gastric ulcer. Even mechanisms to flag subjects in some way as participants in a blinded trial, which may have value in emergency situations, do not entirely diminish this risk. Moreover, the failure to appreciate that a double-blind is being used often reinforces patient/participants' misconception that treatment is being selected based on their individual needs.

Use of placebos provides one of the most striking contrasts between ordinary clinical and research settings. Because placebos' use in the treatment context often involves deception of the patient, they are rarely employed for clinical purposes.[15] However, they may have considerable utility in research as a means of establishing a baseline of spontaneous improvement or clarifying the impact of nonspecific factors, such as the increased attention that patient/participants may receive in a research clinic, against which the therapeutic effect of active treatments can be measured.[16] Placebo use has become a matter of controversy when even partially effective treatments exist,[17] although placebos may be scientifically appropriate depending on the circumstances of a particular clinical trial.[18] In any event, it should be clear that when placebos are used, they violate the usual assumption of personal care that the physician will select an active treatment intended to alleviate the patient's symptoms.

More subtle, perhaps, is the impact of fixed protocols for the administration of treatment. Many studies, for example, specify the dosage of a medication to be administered, the intervals (if any) that must pass before adjustments can be made, and the magnitude of these alterations. The extent of such restrictions can vary substantially across studies. Unless treatment is standardized in some way, however—except for purely observational studies—it will be difficult to know precisely which intervention has been tested or to replicate the research. In ordinary practice, of course, physicians routinely raise or lower the dose of a medication in response to side effects or to accelerate therapeutic response. When a physician loses the freedom to make such changes, the patient experiences the loss of some degree of personal care. Arguments that patients are often better treated by means of fixed protocols, because these eliminate the sometimes irrational variability in physicians' decision making, may be true on occasion, but in the context of research participation are largely beside the point. Whether such flexibility is ultimately to their benefit or not (and it is hard to see that it would not be beneficial whenever avoidance of side effects is the goal), patient/participants have lost the opportunity for an individualized decision to be made about whether and when to deviate from protocol-driven approaches to treatment.

Finally, when adjunctive treatments are limited or banned entirely, patient/participants lose another attribute of personal care that would ordinarily obtain in clinical settings. Such restrictions are not irrational from an investigator's perspective. Unless the treatment is limited to the intervention being tested, it will be impossible to know which aspect of care was responsible should a positive result be obtained. For example, although it is not uncommon for more than one antidepressant medication to be prescribed to a depressed patient who has not been responsive to a single treatment, allowing such concatenation of medications in a clinical trial of a new drug will preclude definitive assessment of that medication's effectiveness. Medications that alleviate side effects, or in some situations medications that treat other conditions, may be restricted because of the possibility that they will interfere with assessment of the therapeutic effect of the medication(s) being tested. For example, patient/participants in a clinical trial of a new sleep medication may not be allowed to take antihistamines for their allergies because of the possibility that the antihistamines will augment the sleep medication's effect. Once more, the difference between being in a research project and receiving ordinary clinical treatment may be significant.

To be clear, none of these approaches to research is necessarily illegitimate. Indeed, in many cases they will be critical to the conduct of a meaningful clinical trial. Designing a study without using methods that protect the integrity of the data may only serve to expose patient/participants to risk with no likelihood of a compensating incremental gain in knowledge. Any or all of the research methods that we have identified as diminishing personal care are acceptable when (1) they do not alter the risk/benefit ratio for patient/participants to a degree that makes experimentation with humans unacceptable, (2) they are scientifically necessary (or at least extremely helpful) to generate meaningful data, and (3) patient/participants have provided a valid informed consent for their use. It is the final condition of these three that is affected by the presence of TM. Whether TM by itself is sufficient to invalidate consent is considered below.

To summarize, the ethical tension inherent in most clinical trials arises from deviations from the principle of personal care that controls physicians' behavior in the ordinary clinical context. These practices should not be undertaken without the valid consent of patient/participants. When TM is present, however, such consent is impaired at best and may be effectively compromised. Hence, TM's importance as a major potential obstacle to informed consent in clinical research.

The Origins of the Therapeutic Misconception

Why might patient/participants manifest a TM? Although careful studies of the origins of the phenomenon remain to be performed, we believe two sets of causative factors play a role here. One reflects the preconceptions with which patients arrive in the clinical research setting, and the second results from the experiences they have in that setting itself.

Patient/participants bring concepts shaped by a lifetime of contact with medical professionals into the context in which they are asked to give consent for research participation. As a consequence of those interactions, they have learned that physicians are supposed to deliver personal care—though it is probable that they have never heard that term. Instead, they are likely to say, "My doctor will recommend whatever he or she thinks is best for me." Precisely that attitude is often carried into the setting of clinical research.

Although ethicists differentiate carefully between clinical and research settings, the differences may not be as clear to potential patient/participants. Referral to clinical trials often results from a visit to a physician (perhaps even one's personal physician) seeking help for a clinical problem, and the referral itself may be seen as a response to that request. When patient/participants meet the staff of a research project, they may find physicians and nurses in white coats or scrubs with stethoscopes slung around their necks—precisely the images they have always associated with ordinary treatment situations in which they have received personal care. Indeed, in some cases, it will be the patient/participants' own physicians who recruit them and carry out the research study. Far from being irrational for patient/participants to assume that their needs will have primacy in this new context, in many respects it would be rather odd if they did not.

Media coverage of the research enterprise may reinforce this tendency. News outlets often portray research efforts in terms that suggest research centers provide the best care—something that these institutions' own advertising frequently reinforces.[19] Hence, the findings of the Advisory Committee on Human Radiation Experiments, based on interviews with more than 500 former research participants, seem entirely natural: "Patient-subjects frequently expressed the belief that an intervention [e.g., research participation] would not be offered if it did not carry some promise of benefit; many certainly assumed that the intervention would not be offered if it posed significant risks."[4]

Investigators' behavior may also contribute to the development of TM. Research projects are often denoted by titles or acronyms that suggest that patient/participants will receive optimal care, such as "BEST," " MAGIC," "MIRACL," or "PROVED."[20] Newspaper and website advertising aimed at recruiting participants may emphasize clinical benefits while underplaying the potential costs of enrolling in a clinical trial. Mark Hochhauser has assembled a telling collection of such promotional material, including the following from a press release posted on the website of a major academic medical center: "Chosen for their interdisciplinary nature and potential benefits to patients, these programs range from fundamental investigations of the origin of disease to advanced clinical trials in which patients have access to the latest and most promising treatments." As Hochhauser notes, " 'Latest' and 'most promising' are not the same as effective," nor would potential patient/participants glean from this glowing description that they may receive a placebo or an older comparison drug, and that they will otherwise sacrifice the personal care they are being led to expect.[20]

Disclosures from research personnel themselves, whether written or verbal, may subtly or directly suggest to patient/participants an illusory adherence to personal care. Consent forms often avoid terms that directly indicate the experimental nature of the research endeavor, for example, referring to a "study medication" or a "new drug," rather than an "experimental medication," and avoiding "experiment" and even "research" in favor of "study," "project," or "clinical trial."[20] Patient/participants may have very different associations to each of these terms.[4] Consent forms may also be vague and misleading about the degree of likely benefit, as was the case in a recent large-scale study of gene-transfer research.[21] Even a study that concluded that consent forms in Phase I oncology trials were generally unobjectionable found that the experimental agent was referred to as "treatment" or "therapy" on 260 of 272 forms that were examined.[22] Verbal disclosures may fail to include discussion of those research methods that limit personal care, and may even underscore the therapeutic potential of a study in an overtly misleading way.[23–26]

These behaviors may stem in part from a desire to be as persuasive as possible in recruiting patient/participants, as well as from investigators' own reluctance to recognize the ways in which they are departing from clinical norms. One study of American oncologists who were queried about the purposes of clinical trials revealed that 13% to 38% of respondents in various oncologic subspecialties "believed that ensuring state-of-the-art therapy for trial participants, rather than improving the treatment of future cancer patients, is the main societal purpose of trials."[27] Indeed, discomfort with deviating from the interests of their patients has sometimes led researchers to subvert their own studies, for example by tampering with randomization procedures to obtain the treatment they think will be most helpful for their patients,[28,29] perhaps not a surprising phenomenon in a profession trained to place individual patients' interests first.

Even when investigators do their best to disclose to patient/participants the nature of the research and the ways it may differ from ordinary clinical care, impediments to communication may limit their effectiveness. Research terminology is foreign to many patients. In a study of participants drawn from the general population, Waggoner and Mayo found that 25% did not know what a placebo was, 83% could not define a *double-blind,* and 78% did not know the meaning of *random.*[30] A striking example of how confused patient/participants can become from research jargon that is routinely used by investigators and their staff comes from an interview that our research staff performed with a cancer patient who was recruited for a cancer chemotherapy trial in which she was informed that she would be assigned to one of the treatment "arms" of the study:

INTERVIEWER: What does the project involve? The research study? What does your participation involve?

SUBJECT: Well, they choose an arm . . . one arm [subject points to her arm] . . . for an operation . . . the other one for the IV. If they choose the arm for the operation . . . I mean for the IV, there's no operation involved.[31]

In fact, the patients in this study would in no case have received an operation, and would in either case have gotten intravenous chemotherapy. But the use of the term *arm* to mean treatment

group had left this patient totally confused as to the nature of the research project to which she had just consented.

It is worth noting that although the paradigmatic situation in which TM arises is a clinical trial—in which patient/participants have at least some opportunity to receive what may be effective treatment for their conditions—it may appear in even less probable venues. Wholly nontherapeutic research studies, such as investigations of pathophysiologic mechanisms underlying disease states, may be wrongly interpreted by participants as involving treatment and hence as holding the potential for therapeutic benefit. Somewhere along the lower end of the spectrum of potentially beneficial research are Phase I medication trials, which are intended to assess the tolerability and toxicity of experimental medications. Phase I trials of chemotherapeutics for cancer have been a particular focus of attention. Although the generally accepted data suggest that less than 5% of experimental cancer medications in Phase I trials are found to have any therapeutic benefits at all,[32] an overwhelming proportion of participants in several studies—as will be discussed below—have attributed to them therapeutic intent.

Phenomenology of the Therapeutic Misconception

Defining the Therapeutic Misconception

Before considering how TM is typically manifested, we need to offer a more detailed definition of the phenomenon. We suggested above that at its core TM involves a patient/participant's failure to recognize how personal care may be compromised by research procedures. Our research has led us to the conclusion that this core concept of TM can appear in two ways: (1) an incorrect belief that the patient/participant's individualized needs will determine assignment to treatment conditions or lead to modifications of the treatment regime (TM1) or (2) an unreasonable appraisal of the nature or likelihood of medical benefit from participation in the study, due to misperception of the nature of the research enterprise (TM2). In the case of TM2, the misconception relates to aspects of research involvement other than individualization of care.

We have already examined some of the ways in which an incorrect belief that treatment decisions will be based on individual needs may be evident, such as when patient/participants fail to grasp that the treatment they receive will be chosen at random, rather than on the basis of what the physician believes is most likely to be of benefit to them—an example of TM1. But some patient/participants manifest a broader misconception about the nature of the research enterprise itself, as it relates specifically to the likelihood of benefit from participation—TM2. An obvious example is when a person misinterprets a research project that has no therapeutic intent—for example, a study of the pathophysiology of migraine—as holding the prospect of personal benefit. Even in research that tests clinical interventions, however, patient/participants may fail to recognize that the research is being done precisely because of uncertainty as to whether a new treatment is effective (or is more effective than existing treatments), and hence may believe that their involvement is highly likely to be beneficial. Often this belief is linked to the previously noted conviction that a physician would not suggest enrollment unless it was very likely to be of benefit to everyone in the study and very unlikely to present any substantial degree of risk. Here, the misconception involves a misunderstanding of the very purpose of research rather than of a particular methodologic aspect precluding individualization of treatment.

Horng and Grady have recently attempted to draw some finer distinctions, differentiating TM from what they refer to as *therapeutic misestimation,* which occurs when "[t]he research subject underestimates risk, overestimates benefit, or both."[33] This category would appear to include both genuine manifestations of TM2 and misestimations that occur for other reasons, such as participants' difficulty understanding probability statements or the failure of investigators to disclose risks. When misestimation occurs as a result of a misconception of the nature of the research itself, we would include it within the definition of TM2.

Prevalence of the Therapeutic Misconception

TM was initially described as part of a study (led by Loren Roth) of informed consent in four psychiatric research projects.[1,2] Among the 88 patient/participants who were interviewed after consenting to participate in a clinical trial, 69% were unaware that their assignment to treatment interventions would be randomized and 40% explicitly said that treatment assignment would be made on the basis of their therapeutic needs. Forty-four percent of patient/participants failed to recognize that the use of placebos and nontreatment control groups meant that some who desired the experimental intervention would not receive it. And when explicitly asked, only 9% could identify a single way in which joining a protocol would restrict their options for treatment.

Some critics dismissed these data as displaying merely the expectable confusion that people with psychiatric disorders would naturally evidence. But they are consistent with data from a variety of areas of medicine suggesting that a desire for personal benefit is the major motive driving research participation, even in studies with little prospect of benefit.[34–37] A typical survey in a combined sample of patients and nonpatients showed that when asked why people in general should participate in research, 69% of respondents cited benefit to society, and only 5% cited benefits for participants themselves. But when asked why they might participate in a research project, 52% said they would do it to get the best medical care, and only 23% responded that they would participate to contribute to scientific knowledge.[34] Although the desire for medical benefit is not in itself an indication of TM, when it is manifest as an unreasonable belief in the likelihood of benefit—for example, because the research is understood as offering the opportunity to receive the latest treatments of proven efficacy—it may reflect TM2.

Moreover, studies exploring the attitudes of patient/participants in nonpsychiatric research come up with findings at least as striking as those from the original TM study. In a study of 144 patient/participants in Phase II and III cancer chemotherapy trials, the authors reported that "[d]espite statements in most consent forms that benefits could not be guaranteed, 43% of patients stated that they had no doubts at all about benefits from the treatment," a degree of certainty incompatible with the yet-to-be-demonstrated efficacy of the treatment being tested.[38] Even more remarkably, a study of 127 patients in four cancer chemotherapy protocols at the National Institutes of Health showed that despite being provided with contrary information, 100% of the patient/participants in Phase I studies described their protocols as having both treatment and research aims.[37] Another study of 144 Phase I cancer chemotherapy patient/participants found that 88% of them said that the goals of their current treatment were no different than in prior noninvestigational treatments, and not a single person mentioned altruistic reasons for participation.[39] A final study of 207 cancer patient/participants showed that 74% did not recognize that they might receive a nonstandard treatment, 63% did not understand the potential for incremental risk, 70% failed to grasp the unproven nature of the experimental treatment, and only 29% thought that trials are done mainly to benefit future patients.[40]

Nor are these kinds of findings limited to cancer chemotherapy trials. Researchers in England, looking at parental reactions to a randomized controlled trial of extracorporeal membrane oxygenation (ECMO) for severely ill neonates, found that in only 12 of 21 parent pairs was at least one parent aware of the randomization. Interestingly, after the fact, many of the parents explained their experiences in a way that resolved any cognitive dissonance, but without making reference to randomization. Parents of neonates who received the intervention tended to believe that all participants were treated with ECMO, whereas parents whose babies had not gotten ECMO explained that it turned out not to be indicated on clinical grounds.[41] This development of post-hoc explanations has been observed in other randomized studies.[42] One could summarize the literature as indicating that people frequently overestimate the benefits of entry into a study,[37–39] underestimate the risks,[40] are confused about how treatments will be assigned,[40,41,43,44] and generally tend to conflate research with ordinary treatment.[4,39,45]

Recently, in the first attempt to identify the prevalence of TM across a range of patient/participants and research studies, we interviewed 225 patient/participants from 44 clinical research studies that spanned the medical spectrum from oncology to cardiology to rheumatology.[31] Transcripts of interviews exploring participants' understanding of the studies to which they had just consented were scored for the presence of TM. Thirty-one percent of participants expressed inaccurate beliefs about the degree of individualization of their treatment (TM1), whereas 51% manifested an unreasonable belief in the nature or likelihood of benefit, given the methods of the study in which they were enrolled (TM2). A total of 62% of participants were judged to have TM on one or both of these bases. This finding of a substantial prevalence of TM is echoed in a study of participants in gene transfer trials, 74% of whom scored 10 or higher on a 15-point composite scale largely focused on TM2,[46] and in a study of those with schizophrenia and schizoaffective disorder, approximately two-thirds of whom showed at least some evidence of TM1 on a 6-item scale.[47]

Taken as a whole, then, the existing research indicates that TM is an extremely prevalent phenomenon among patient/participants.

Common Presentations of the Therapeutic Misconception

As suggested above, TM can be manifested in a number of ways. Some patient/participants evidence clear-cut beliefs that their treatment will be individualized for their particular needs (TM1). The examples we offer here are drawn from interviews with research participants in our previously mentioned study of TM.[31]

INTERVIEWER: Agree or disagree: Doctors are not allowed to choose the treatment I receive based on my needs?

PATIENT/PARTICIPANT: Um, disagree.

INTERVIEWER: So you think in the study they are allowed to pick which group you're going to be in?

PATIENT/PARTICIPANT: I think so.

Another example of TM1 is reflected in the response of a different patient/participant.

INTERVIEWER: [clarifying previous response] So [the choice of treatment] does depend on what each individual needs?

PATIENT/PARTICIPANT: I think so, yes. I think they do take into account what each person needs.

Unreasonable appraisal of benefit (TM2) can be seen in the following excerpt. In contrast to the examples above, which display the incorrect belief that treatment will be individualized for each person, this person's response reflects his apparent belief that there is a single "best" treatment, and that everyone in the study will be receiving it. Hence, although there is no individualization of treatment in the usual sense, this patient/participant believes that everyone who participates will end up with the best possible care.

INTERVIEWER: So do you think that they think that they are giving everyone the best treatment?

PATIENT/PARTICIPANT: I don't think they'd be in this if they didn't. You know it's just like being a doctor with a sign on the door. You know, they're healers.

The following person reflects not just a belief in her physician's therapeutic intentions, but firm certainty about her likelihood of benefiting from the study.

INTERVIEWER: Um, OK, what is the primary goal of the project, meaning is it gonna help people in the future or is it gonna help people in the project? Or a combination of both?

PATIENT/PARTICIPANT: Oh, I expect it to help me.

INTERVIEWER: Mhm.

PATIENT/PARTICIPANT: Um, I feel like I am already cured, but I expect it to make absolutely sure that I am.

In fact, the woman who gave this response had just entered a clinical trial comparing autologous peripheral stem cell transplantation with or without immunotherapy for Stage II–IV breast cancer. Defined as a "high risk" patient, not only was it unlikely that she was already cured, but there was no guarantee that she would even receive the experimental intervention (which, in any event, proved ineffective).

TM2 can also be seen when risks of participation apart from the risks of treatment per se are downplayed or discounted. In our study sample, we found that 24% of patient/participants reported no risks or disadvantages of any sort from participation in the trials to which they had consented; 3% reported disadvantages incidental to study participation such as having to drive further than they would if they were treated by their personal physicians; 14% noted the risks of treatment per se, which would have obtained even in non-research settings (e.g., the side effects associated with the control intervention); 46% cited risks of the experimental treatment (e.g., its side effects), but not risks or disadvantages associated with the study design; and only 13%

pointed to risks or disadvantages flowing from the design of the study itself (e.g., from randomization or a placebo arm).[48]

Although it would be simple to say that all patient/participants either clearly manifest TM or appear to grasp fully the implications of research participation, the reality is more complicated than that. Some people seem at times to appreciate what they have gotten into in entering a clinical research project, but at other times to voice beliefs consistent with TM. Consider this example from three different points in an interview of the same person.

Excerpt 1:

INTERVIEWER: Do you think they are giving everyone in the study the best possible treatment?

PATIENT/PARTICIPANT: Well, no. Not if they're giving one a placebo.

Excerpt 2:

INTERVIEWER: Agree or disagree: This study has not been designed primarily to help the people who participate.

PATIENT/PARTICIPANT: To help everybody.

Excerpt 3:

INTERVIEWER: Are they allowed to choose [the treatment] on what best suits your needs?

PATIENT/PARTICIPANT: I would hope so.

Whereas the first of these excerpts appears to reflect a recognition that some participants will receive an inactive treatment that represents something less than optimal care, by the time of the second excerpt, the person appears to be suggesting that the study design is intended to benefit everyone who participates in the clinical trial. And in the third excerpt, when asked directly about his own treatment, he appears to have put the possibility that he will be randomly assigned to placebo entirely out of his mind. The "now you see it, now you don't" presentation in this case is consistent with what we know about people's beliefs in general. It is not uncommon for us to hold contradictory views simultaneously, never fully resolving the conflict, with the contingencies of the moment determining the perspective to which we give voice. Because the concepts related to clinical research so challenge our usual views of the roles of physicians and the purpose of medical care, it is not surprising to see recognition of those concepts alternate in the minds of patient/participants with efforts to make the research setting conform to the usual presumptions of clinical care.

To these varying presentations of TM must be appended the acknowledgment that it is not always easy to know to what extent—if at all—TM has affected a person's decision making. This is especially true when evidence both for and against TM is present, as in the last example, but it may be true in other cases as well. There is a large literature on why people decide to enter clinical research studies, or to enroll their children or others incapable of making decisions for themselves. The results of these studies are not always consistent, with some showing that most participants are interested in personal benefit[39] and others suggesting that altruism, reflecting a desire to advance knowledge and thereby help others, plays a substantial role.[49] But many participants and surrogate decision makers in these studies offer multiple reasons for participation, with belief in benefit for patient/participants very often playing some role.[50,51] To the extent that this belief is unrealistic and reflective of TM, obvious concerns exist about the legitimacy of enrolling such patient/participants.

Studies of the prevalence of TM or certain aspects of it provide a rough upper limit for the percentage of research participants whose consent to enter the study may be problematic.

Characteristics Associated With the Presence of a Therapeutic Misconception

Prior to our recent study, there were only inferential data on those characteristics either of patient/participants or of the studies in which they were enrolled that may predispose to the development of TM. Our original TM study suggested that education and gender were related to understanding of disclosed information, although we did not determine their relationship to TM per se.[2] Roth and colleagues described a strong tendency for patient/participants to misinterpret research procedures as therapeutic, and found that overall understanding correlated with education and age; but they, too, did not explain the correlates of the misinterpretation they described.[52] A large body of research data indicates—not surprisingly—that education, occupation, and age predict understanding of consent disclosures in both treatment and research settings.[53] Although poor understanding is not the same as TM, it would not be unreasonable to hypothesize that these variables would correlate with TM as well.

A number of studies have demonstrated that illness severity affects understanding of information, and moreover, that the most severely ill patient/participants are most likely to attribute therapeutic goals to research aimed at other ends and in which the prospect of benefit is extremely remote, such as Phase I trials.[37,39,54] Of course, not every person who enters a Phase I trial because of hope of benefit is manifesting TM, which was not directly assessed in these studies; some subjects may realistically recognize a very low probability of positive impact but, having exhausted all other options, be willing to try a Phase I study as a last resort. But the attribution of therapeutic goals to the researchers creates a cognitive framework in which unreasonable assumptions about the likelihood of benefit (TM2) may flourish. Finally, researchers' disclosures to participants have been shown in several studies to be an important determinant of patient/participants' understanding, as well as of elements of TM.[24,25,55]

Our research found a number of characteristics of patient/participants to be associated with TM, using a combined measure of TM1 and TM2.[31] As in many studies of understanding of consent disclosures, these include lower levels of education and increased age. Greater pessimism about one's current health and more optimism about one's future health were also related to TM, as one might expect from studies suggesting that greater illness severity (here combined with hope for the future) makes people more likely to see research as designed to help them. Finally, based on data from the SF-36, a short questionnaire that measures health status, we showed that the worse one's self-described health and functional status, the greater one's likelihood of TM. However, we did not find a relationship between TM and race, gender, previous involvement in research, or having an occupation in higher education, health care, or research.

As far as study characteristics were concerned, higher rates of TM were observed in studies that exposed participants to the risk of death (as stated on their consent forms) and studies testing treatments (generally medications) for which alternatives approved by the Food and Drug Administration (FDA) were available outside the study. It is notable that none of the study methods that most compromise personal care—randomization, blinding of treating physicians, placebo controls—was significantly associated with the presence of TM.

How does one put these data together? Based on one large-scale study, the only systematic data that now exist, vulnerability to TM seems to be associated with factors that may limit patient/participants' understanding of studies and heighten their need to believe that entering a research study will be beneficial for them. The data on study characteristics underscore the influence of desperation on the part of patient/participants; studies that present a risk of death ordinarily involve only patients who are severely ill and for whom there are no other available treatment options. When an FDA-approved alternative exists, that fact may lead many to believe that they would not be asked to enter a study unless it was likely to offer benefit at least equivalent to ordinary treatment. Of course, these hypotheses, based as they are on data from a single study, require further examination and verification.

Effects of the Therapeutic Misconception on Enrollment, Retention, and Satisfaction

No data exist on the impact of TM on enrollment of patient/participants, their retention in studies, or their satisfaction at the conclusion of their involvement in clinical research. But each of these issues has been the target of speculation that is worthy of mention here. As far as recruitment is concerned, it is widely assumed that those with TM are more likely to agree to participate in clinical trials. As a corollary, investigators often express discomfort with suggestions that potential research participants should be disabused of TM for fear that this will negatively impact their ability to recruit participants for their studies. To be sure, the data indicating that many patient/participants join clinical trials out of a desire for personal benefit lend credibility to these beliefs. But to date no one has compared the prevalence of TM among patients who consent and those who refuse to enter clinical research studies. Nor do we know whether altruistic motives might become more prominent if unrealistic beliefs about personal benefit were dispelled.

The relationship between TM and retention in studies that extend beyond a single contact is similarly unexplored. However, we speculate that patient/participants who discover that they are not as likely to benefit as they thought at the outset—perhaps because they begin to appreciate that placebos are being used, or that assignment to treatment is random—may be more likely to drop out than they would have been if, at the time of recruitment, they had had a good grasp of the impact of the study on personal care. If this is correct, it may be that the putative advantage in recruiting patient/participants as a result of TM is somewhat mitigated by a deleterious impact on retention in longer-term studies, a potentially serious problem because dropouts represent wasted resources from the investigator's perspective and needless exposure to risk from the participant's viewpoint.

Lastly, there is the relationship between TM and satisfaction with the research experience to consider. Anecdotal reports indicate that some former research participants later feel themselves to have been "deceived" or "used" by investigators.[56–58] In part, this feeling appears to relate to their ultimate recognition that the personal care they expected to receive did not materialize. These feelings typically surface when the patient/participant experiences a poor outcome. One example comes from the case of a research participant who later filed suit against the investigators and their university. He contrasted his disappointment at the adverse consequences of study participation with his initial willingness to enter the study, "because I thought I was going to get the premier treatment, while they did a little research on the side."[56] Snowdon and colleagues similarly found that many parents interviewed after a clinical trial involving their neonates who were critically ill expressed anger about the use of randomization, especially those parents who had not grasped at the outset of the study that decisions about treatment would not be made on an individualized basis.[41] Feelings of anger at such treatment may generalize to the research enterprise as a whole and can fuel efforts to restrict research, limit research funding, or discourage enrollment in research projects.

Addressing the Therapeutic Misconception

Why Worry About the Therapeutic Misconception?

A necessary condition for deviating from medicine's usual adherence to the principle of personal care is the informed consent of the patient/participant or, for those without the legal capacity to consent on their own behalf, of an appropriate surrogate decision maker. (Research in emergency settings may constitute an exception to this generalization; in the United States, federal rules allow some studies of emergency care to be conducted without consent in circumstances in which consent from either patients or surrogates cannot be obtained in a timely fashion (see Chapter 27). To the extent that patients decide to enter research projects in the belief that they will receive personal care, we believe that it cannot be said that they appreciate the implications of their decision, and the validity of their consent is in question. But not everyone agrees that even flagrant examples of TM invalidate consent to research, and the argument that TM does not negate informed consent is worth considering.

Some of those who make this argument look to the legal doctrine of informed consent for support.[59] As the doctrine of informed consent to treatment was shaped by the courts, there was often a lack of clarity regarding whether physicians were required merely to disclose material information or whether patients must comprehend such disclosure for the ensuing consent to be valid.[60] At times, courts have expressed concern that a requirement for actual understanding might have the unintended result of denying medical care to patients who, for whatever reason, were unable to comprehend even adequate disclosures, and concerns about evidentiary difficulties may have shaped this approach as well. Thus, legal standards for consent may be weaker than ethical doctrines may demand. Echoing such precedents, Gopal Sreenivasan maintains that an accurate comprehension of the risk/benefit ratio of participation in clinical research ought not to be required for consent to be considered acceptable.[59] He suggests that the well-being of research participants can be adequately protected, even in the face of TM, by an independent judgment of an institutional review board (IRB) that the study in question has a favorable risk/benefit ratio. Moreover, requiring good appreciation of the consequences of involvement in a study might restrict entry to a small group of patient/participants, thus impeding the conduct of important research.

In considering this approach, we note first that the assumption that comprehension by patients should not be required in the treatment setting has been criticized as focusing unduly on ensuring decision making autonomy in a narrow sense (i.e., the right to say yes or no), while failing to protect a patient's interests in informed choice—the true goal of informed consent.[60] Nor would a requirement for actual understanding by patients necessarily preclude needed treatment; patients who are unable to comprehend the essential elements of disclosure, despite efforts to help them do so, are not likely to be competent to make decisions for themselves, and substitute decision-making mechanisms can be provided. Transposed into the research realm, the argument against requiring comprehension seems even more problematic. Whereas the presumption that treatment recommendations are being made in a patient's interests obtains in the treatment setting, no such blanket conclusion can be reached in clinical research. Thus, it seems even more important for consent to research to reflect an accurate assessment of the risks and benefits of participation by the prospective participant.

Sreenivasan's retort is that an objective body, an IRB, will have determined that the research project has a favorable risk/benefit ratio before a patient is asked to participate. Hence an independent judgment by each patient/participant is unnecessary.[59] But this reflects confusion about the particular tasks of IRBs and potential patient/participants. The IRB's role, in part, is to determine whether the net potential benefits exceed the potential risks. But the benefits that IRBs consider include societal benefits that may accrue as a result of the knowledge gained, thus allowing approval of projects in which there are likely to be little to no benefit for some or all of the participants. Each individual, in contrast, must decide whether the combination of possible personal benefit and altruistic contributions to the good of others warrants the risks associated with the research, including the risk, for those in a placebo-controlled study, of receiving no active treatment at all. Only the prospective participant can weight appropriately both the altruistic component of the benefit calculus and the salience of the potential risks to his or her unique situation. Moreover, because the inclination to self-sacrifice is not something that can be determined for others by a committee, prior IRB approval in no way removes the need for a meaningful judgment about participation by a potential participant. And the only way such a meaningful decision can be made is if the person is substantially free of the confusion embodied in TM.

It is of interest that both IRBs and investigators appear to be thinking increasingly along similar lines. In a growing number of higher risk protocols or studies involving populations with a greater prevalence of impaired decisional capacities, investigators are more frequently checking individuals' understanding and appreciation of the implications of participation prior to accepting their consent. Whether this practice impedes recruitment or just encourages better and more creative disclosure practices remains to be determined. But we believe that there is a growing consensus that, given its apparent prevalence, TM constitutes a major obstacle to genuine informed consent in research, and efforts to diminish or eliminate TM are clearly warranted. How might such a task be undertaken?

The Inadequacies of the Current Consent Process

Current consent practices, driven by concerns about legal liability and the sometimes obsessive focus of IRBs on the precise wording of consent forms, have evolved in a direction that complicates the task of neutralizing TM. Potential research participants are often given lengthy and highly detailed consent forms to read and assimilate. The forms, which in our experience can reach up to 20 single-spaced, typewritten pages and seem to get longer every year, recite with great precision the procedures to which patient/participants will be exposed, the risks they may face, and the possible benefits of participation, along with such items as whom to contact with questions and whether the costs of medical care will be covered should injuries occur. Risks are given particularly detailed exposition, even the minor risks of procedures such as drawing small amounts of blood or answering potentially embarrassing questionnaires. The dominant fear appears to be that some potential risk left unexplicated will materialize, leading to liability for the investigators, the institution, and perhaps for members of the IRB.[61]

As a result, patient/participants are often overloaded with information of varying degrees of importance. Frequently buried in this confusing mass of data is the very information that would help them grasp the substantial differences between clinical research and ordinary treatment. Somewhere in the midst of the form may appear an explanation of random assignment of treatment. Placebo use, double-blind procedures, and the limits placed on physicians' discretion by the protocol are also likely to be embedded in the depths of the form, but from a prospective participant's perspective, equally likely to be lost in the tangle of verbiage. Sometimes, of course, the information is framed so poorly or in such complex language that patient/participants are not likely to comprehend its significance even if they spot it. And sometimes the forms are subtly or overtly misleading, for example when experimental interventions or even placebos are referred to simply as *treatment,* or important risks of the study are omitted or downplayed. Even when investigators make a conscientious effort to explain these factors, however, the prevalent structure and length of consent forms greatly increase the risk that the information will go unnoticed or unappreciated.

Consent forms, of course, are not the only source of information for potential research participants. The recruitment process typically involves discussions with an investigator, research nurse, or research assistant who provides an overview of the study. This conversation may have a greater impact on the potential participant's understanding than anything written on the consent form. But the primary goal of these interactions is typically to persuade the patient to become a participant, and to the extent that focusing on the ways that research differs from ordinary clinical care is thought to dissuade patients from enrolling, there is an understandable tendency for research personnel not to emphasize these issues. Moreover, insofar as researchers themselves fail to recognize the ways in which research is not the same as clinical care, which appears to be surprisingly common,[27] they will be unable to discuss these matters clearly with potential participants,[62] as preliminary evidence suggests they often are.[63]

Dispelling the Therapeutic Misconception

Addressing TM in an effective way will require a multifaceted approach. The first step must involve the education of investigators and other research staff regarding the ethically significant differences between ordinary treatment and treatment in the context of clinical research. If this sounds simplistic or superfluous, our interactions with the clinical research community over

several decades suggest that it is neither. Perhaps because of physicians' habitual reliance on the ethical model in which they are trained—which emphasizes a dedication to patients' interests—it is extremely difficult for clinical investigators to see themselves as sacrificing those interests in any way for the sake of advancing scientific knowledge, no matter how important that knowledge may be. This tendency is reflected in the frequently heard assertion that clinical research is superior to ordinary treatment (despite data to the contrary),[64] because it provides closer monitoring by more experienced clinicians who are taking a more systematic approach to treatment. It may, in fact, be true that there are advantages to patients in participating in research projects, and those advantages are likely to be greater when the design of a project is less restrictive of physicians' discretion to act on patients' behalf. But to acknowledge this is in no way to diminish the ethically significant differences between the two situations. Unless researchers themselves recognize this discrepancy, they are likely to undercut through their communication with patient/participants whatever other efforts are made to dispel TM.

Investigators and others involved in recruiting participants can be trained to describe and underscore the differences between research and ordinary treatment in relatively simple ways. As we have suggested elsewhere,[60] unless patient/participants are educated about the reasons for deviations from personal care (e.g., the use of placebos), they are likely to reconstruct disclosures in a way that reinforces their preconceptions, such as the assumption that all participants will receive active treatment because no physician would permit a patient to go untreated. And data suggest that many lay people are unaware of the purpose of routine investigational procedures such as randomization.[65] Thus, as the investigator describes the purpose of the study and the procedures involved, he or she should emphasize the differences between research and clinical care and the reasons for them. For example, in describing placebo use, the investigator could say, "One-half of the people in this study will be selected by chance to receive sugar pills that are not intended to help the condition you have, in place of active medication. This is done so we can find out whether the medications are really effective, or if many people with your condition would get better even with no active medication at all." Once the differences are underscored, the remainder of the risks and benefits of participation can be disclosed.

Properly constructed consent forms have a role to play in this process as well. Consent forms ideally should be much shorter than they are today, because we have known for a long time that the more detail that is provided to potential participants, the less they assimilate.[66] Too many consent forms today spend pages detailing the intricacies of the study (for example, exactly what will happen at each visit over the next year, or precisely which blood tests will be drawn), when this level of minutiae is not likely to be meaningful to most patient/participants or materiale to their decisions whether to enter the study. This additional information could be offered in an informational pamphlet to those who enroll. A more effective consent form would again highlight the ways in which research diverges from the principles of personal care, emphasizing these items in bold print, or otherwise setting them off from the rest of the text. If multipage forms continue to be used—and we despair of persuading IRBs and investigators to abandon what we believe to be the illusory security of this approach—at the least they should be accompanied by one-page summaries that highlight the major issues, including, of course, the departures from personal care.

Because we know that disabusing potential participants of their preconceptions about research will not be an easy task, it makes sense to quiz them routinely about their understanding of the disclosures and their appreciation of the implications of becoming involved in a research project. Such brief questionnaires—currently in use by some investigators[67]—should include queries designed to probe for the presence of TM, in addition to ensuring that potential participants understand more basic issues such as the nature and purpose of the study, risks and benefits, and so forth. If a tendency toward viewing the project in therapeutic terms is detected, it should be addressed directly and effectively before the person is allowed to enter the study.

Higher risk studies, or studies that recruit particularly vulnerable groups, may call for additional measures to insure that TM has not compromised the consent of patient/participants. Our earlier work with Loren Roth demonstrated that an independent educator—in that study, a nurse not affiliated with any particular research project—could make a substantial difference in improving patient/participants' appreciation of TM-related issues, above and beyond the impact of disclosure by investigators.[2,24] Some researchers may resist such proposals, fearful that an independent person educating potential participants will dissuade them from entering the studies. But in studies in which the quality of the consent is crucial, IRBs may want to look to this mechanism to ensure that patient/participants are protected from the consequences of decisions based on false premises.

A final consideration relates to the compensation that is sometimes given to participants in clinical research, although this occurs more commonly in studies that provide no treatment, such as studies that require participants to complete questionnaires or undergo tests that are unlikely to contribute in any way to their care. Such compensation is often an issue of contention because of concern that financial rewards may unduly influence people to enter projects, running risks that they otherwise would not have accepted. It has been suggested, however, that paying patient/participants for their participation might be an extremely effective way of dispelling TM.[68,69] Payments are usually part of a two-way exchange of something of value. For patient/participants, who certainly are not paid by their physicians when they receive ordinary care, payments might have the salutary effect of concretizing the fact that they are surrendering something of worth—the wholly beneficent attention of their physicians—and are receiving compensation in return. Payments would have to be proportionate to the demands on patient/participants to reduce fears of undue influence,[8] but it is the symbolic value that is of greatest significance here.

We should stress that—apart from the previously mentioned use of a neutral educator—there are no systematic data to indicate whether any of these approaches to the problem of TM are likely to be effective. Given the importance of the issue to the legitimacy of clinical research, however, investigations of how TM may be diminished should be a matter of the highest importance in research ethics.

The Consequences of Addressing the Therapeutic Misconception

Although there will be benefits to attacking TM at its roots, there will be costs as well. The most significant benefit, of course, will be protection of the validity of informed consent in clinical research. It cannot seriously be maintained that patient/participants who view research merely as a form of "super" treatment have made a meaningful choice about participation. Yet, on their willingness to surrender the perquisites of ordinary care rests the legitimacy of the entire clinical research enterprise. If it is true that patient/participants and family members turn against the research enterprise as a whole when they discover after the fact the ways in which clinical research limits personal care, researchers' self-interest alone would seem to call for serious efforts to minimize the prevalence of TM.

In an intelligent discussion of what they refer to as "the therapeutic orientation to clinical research," Miller and Rosenstein point to other salutary effects of addressing TM for the field of research.[8] They contend that "the therapeutic orientation to research involving patients interferes with investigators' development of a sense of professional integrity." To the extent that researchers tolerate or even encourage TM among their patient/participants, and then act toward them—as they must—in ways inconsistent with patient/participants' expectations, the researchers are fostering an ethical dissonance in their profession. Behavior of this kind borders on deception and exploitation. No self-aware group of professionals can long tolerate such a situation without further corruption of their integrity.

If there are potent reasons to combat TM, we ought not to lose sight of the probable costs as well. It has been argued that reducing TM will strip patient/participants of hope.[70] Although we do not know whether this is true, false hope that leads to unwise choices about research participation hardly seems a boon to patients. Moreover, it is widely believed—though unproven—that recruitment to clinical trials will be adversely affected if potential participants recognize the sacrifices they are being asked to make. If true, and it may be, this could increase the cost and slow the pace of clinical research, perhaps delaying the introduction of new treatments that could be helpful to many patients. Of course, it may be that the effect on patients' willingness to enter trials will not be as great as feared—that is, that altruistic motivations may be more powerful than is commonly accepted. Even if some patients decide not to participate in research, however, that may be a cost that we must accept, unless we are willing to exploit vulnerable persons for what is presumed to be the greater good.[9] We suspect that most people, asked to make a choice, would favor a slower rate of medical progress in exchange for greater respect for the rights and interests of patients who may be asked to participate in clinical research.

References

1. Appelbaum PS, Roth LH, Lidz C. The therapeutic misconception: Informed consent in psychiatric research. *International Journal of Law and Psychiatry* 1982;5:319–29.
2. Appelbaum PS, Roth LH, Lidz CW, Benson P, Winslade W. False hopes and best data: Consent to research and the therapeutic misconception. *Hastings Center Report* 1987;17(2):20–4.
3. National Bioethics Advisory Commission. *Research Involving Persons With Mental Disorders That May Affect Decisionmaking Capacity,* Vol. I. Rockville, Md.: NBAC; 1998. [Online] December 1998. Available: http://www.georgetown.edu/research/nrcbl/nbac/capacity/TOC.htm.

4. Advisory Committee on Human Radiation Experiments. *Final Report of the Advisory Committee on Human Radiation Experiments.* New York: Oxford University Press; 1996.

5. Morin K, Rakatansky H, Riddick FA, et al. Managing conflicts of interest in the conduct of clinical trials. *JAMA* 2002;287:78–84.

6. Kahn JP, Mastroianni AC. Moving from compliance to conscience: Why we can and should improve on the ethics of clinical research. *Archives of Internal Medicine* 2001;161:925–8.

7. Wolf LE, Lo B. Ethical issues in clinical research: An issue for all internists. *American Journal of Medicine* 2000;109:82–5.

8. Miller FD, Rosenstein DL. The therapeutic orientation to clinical trials. *New England Journal of Medicine* 2003;348:1383–6.

9. Moreno J. Abandon all hope? The therapeutic misconception and informed consent. *Cancer Investigation* 2003;21:481–2.

10. Dresser R. The ubiquity and utility of the therapeutic misconception. *Social Philosophy and Policy* 2002;19:271–94.

11. Fried C. *Medical Experimentation: Personal Integrity and Social Policy.* Amsterdam, Holland: North Holland Publishing Company; 1974.

12. Beauchamp T, McCullough LB. *Medical Ethics: The Moral Responsibilities of the Physician.* Englewood Cliffs, N.J.: Prentice-Hall; 1984.

13. Freedman B. Equipoise and the ethics of clinical research. *New England Journal of Medicine* 1987;317:141–5.

14. Lilford RJ. Ethics of clinical trials from a Bayesian and decision analytic perspective: Whose equipoise is it anyway? *British Medical Journal* 2003;326:980–1.

15. Bok S. *Lying: Moral Choice in Pubic and Private Life.* New York, N.Y.: Vintage Books; 1978.

16. Temple R, Ellenberg SS. Placebo-controlled trials and active-controlled trials in the evaluation of new treatments. Part 1: Ethical and scientific issues. *Annals of Internal Medicine* 2000;133:455–63.

17. Kaptchuk TJ. Powerful placebo: The dark side of the randomized controlled trial. *Lancet* 1998;351:1722–5.

18. Carpenter W, Appelbaum PS, Levine R. The Declaration of Helsinki and clinical trials: A focus on placebo-controlled trials in schizophrenia. *American Journal of Psychiatry* 2003;160:356–62.

19. Hochhauser M. Is "therapeutic misconception" being used to recruit subjects? *ARENA Newsletter* 2003;16(2):5–7.

20. Hochhauser M. "Therapeutic misconception" and "recruiting doublespeak" in the informed consent process. *IRB: Ethics and Human Research* 2002;24(1):11–2.

21. King NMP, Henderson GE, Churchill LR, et al. Consent forms and the therapeutic misconception: The example of gene transfer research. *IRB: Ethics and Human Research* 2005;27(1):1–8.

22. Horng S, Emanuel E, Wilfond B, Rackoff J, Martz K, Grady C. Descriptions of benefits and risks in consent forms for Phase 1 oncology trials. *New England Journal of Medicine* 2002;347:2134–40.

23. Benson PR, Roth LH, Winslade WJ. Informed consent in psychiatric research: Preliminary findings from an ongoing investigation. *Social Science and Medicine* 1985;20:1331–41.

24. Benson PR, Roth LH, Appelbaum PS, Lidz CW, Winslade W. Information disclosure, subject understanding, and informed consent in psychiatric research. *Law and Human Behavior* 1988;12:455–75.

25. Simes RJ, Tattersall MHN, Coates AS, et al. Randomised comparison of procedures for obtaining informed consent in clinical trials of treatment for cancer. *British Medical Journal* 1986;293:1065–8.

26. Sankar P. Communication and miscommunication in informed consent to research. *Medical Anthropology Quarterly* 2004;18:429–46.

27. Joffe S, Weeks JC. Views of American oncologists about the purposes of clinical trials. *Journal of the National Cancer Institute* 2002;94:1847–53.

28. Taylor KM, Margolese RG, Soskolne CL. Physicians' reasons for not entering eligible patients in a randomized clinical trial of surgery for breast cancer. *New England Journal of Medicine* 1984;310:1363–7.

29. Schulz KF. Subverting randomization in controlled trials. *JAMA* 1995;274:1456–8.

30. Waggoner WC, Mayo DM. Who understands? A survey of 25 words or phrases commonly used in proposed clinical research consent forms. *IRB: A Review of Human Subjects Research* 1995;17(1):6–9.

31. Appelbaum PS, Lidz CW, Grisso T. Therapeutic misconception in clinical research: Frequency and risk factors. *IRB: Ethics and Human Research* 2004;26(2):1–8. [Correction and clarification, 2004; 26(5):18.]

32. Daugherty CK. Impact of therapeutic research on informed consent and the ethics of clinical trials: A medical oncology perspective. *Journal of Clinical Oncology* 1999;17:1601–17.

33. Horng S, Grady C. Misunderstanding in clinical research: Distinguishing therapeutic misconception, therapeutic misestimation, and therapeutic optimism. *IRB: Ethics and Human Research* 2003;25(1):11–6.

34. Cassileth BR, Lusk EJ, Miller DS, Hurwitz S. Attitudes toward clinical trials among patients and the public. *JAMA* 1982;248:968–70.

35. Gallo C, Perrone F, De Placido G, Giusti C. Informed versus randomised consent to clinical trials. *Lancet* 1995;346:1060–4.

36. Gotay CC. Accrual to cancer clinical trials: Directions from the research literature. *Social Science and Medicine* 1991; 26:569–77.

37. Schaeffer MH, Krantz DS, Wichman A, Masur H, Reed E, Vinicky J. The impact of disease severity on the informed consent process in clinical research. *American Journal of Medicine* 1996;100:261–8.

38. Penman DT, Holland JC, Bahna GF, et al. Informed consent for investigational chemotherapy: Patients' and physicians' perceptions. *Journal of Clinical Oncology* 1984;2:849–55.

39. Daugherty CK, Banik DM, Janish L, Ratain M. Quantitative analysis of ethical issues in Phase I trials: A survey interview study of 144 advanced cancer patients. *IRB: A Review of Human Subjects Research* 2000;22(3):6–14.

40. Joffe S, Cook EF, Clearly PD, Clark JW, Weeks J. Quality of informed consent in cancer clinical trials: A cross-sectional survey. *Lancet* 2001;358:1772–7.

41. Snowdon C, Garcia J, Elbourne D. Making sense of randomization: Responses of parents of critically ill babies to random allocation of treatment in a clinical trial. *Social Science and Medicine* 1997;45:1337–55.

42. Featherstone K, Donovan JL. Random allocation or allocation at random? Patients' perspectives of participation in a randomized controlled trial. *British Medical Journal* 1998;317:1177–80.

43. Featherstone K, Donovan JL. "Why don't they just tell me straight, why allocate it?" The struggle to make sense of participating in a randomized controlled trial. *Social Science and Medicine* 2002;55:709–19.

44. Vitiello B, Aman MG, Scahill L, et al. Research knowledge among parents of children participating in a randomized clinical trial. *Journal of the American Academy of Child and Adolescent Psychiatry* 2005;44:145–9.

45. Cox K. Informed consent and decision-making: Patients' experiences of the process of recruitment to Phase I and II anti-cancer drug trials. *Patient Education and Counseling* 2002;46:31–8.

46. Henderson GE, Easter MM, Zimmer C, et al. Therapeutic misconception in early phase gene transfer trials. *Social Science and Medicine* 2006;62:239–53.

47. Dunn LB, Palmer BW, Keehan M, Jeste DV, Appelbaum PS. Assessment of therapeutic misconception in older schizophrenia patients with a brief instrument. *American Journal of Psychiatry* 2006;163:500–6.

48. Lidz CW, Appelbaum PS, Grisso T, Renaud M. Therapeutic misconception and the appreciation of risks in clinical trials. *Social Science and Medicine* 2004;58:1689–97.

49. Agrawal M, Emanuel EJ. Ethics of Phase 1 oncology studies: Reexamining the arguments and data. *JAMA* 2003;290:1075–82.

50. Mastwyk M, Ritchie CW, LoGiudice D, Sullivan KA, Macfarlane S. Carer impressions of participation in Alzheimer's disease clinical trials: What are their hopes? And is it worth it? *International Psychogeriatrics* 2002;14:39–45.

51. Rothmeier JD, Lasley MV, Shapiro GG. Factors influencing parental consent in pediatric clinical research. *Pediatrics* 2003;111: 1037–41.

52. Roth LH, Lidz CW, Meisel A, et al. Competency to decide about treatment or research: An overview of some empirical data. *International Journal of Law and Psychiatry* 1982;5:29–50.

53. Raich PC, Plomer KD, Coyne CA. Literacy, comprehension, and informed consent in clinical research. *Cancer Investigation* 2001;19: 437–45.

54. Daugherty CK, Ratain MJ, Grochowski E, et al. Perceptions of cancer patients and their physicians involved in Phase I trials. *Journal of Clinical Oncology* 1995;13:1062–72.

55. Aaronson NK, Visser-Pol E, Leenhouts GHMW, et al. Telephone-based nursing intervention improves the effectiveness of the informed consent process in cancer clinical trials. *Journal of Clinical Oncology* 1996;4:984–96.

56. Hilts P. Agency faults a UCLA study for suffering of mental patients. *New York Times* March 10, 1994:A-1.

57. Hassner V. What is ethical? What is not? Where do you draw the line? *Journal of the California Alliance for the Mentally Ill* 1994;5(1):4–5.

58. Otto MA. ALLHAT team sued for death of subject; lack of informed consent, negligence cited. *Medical Research Law and Policy Report* (Bureau of National Affairs). July 16, 2003.

59. Sreenivasan G. Does informed consent to research require comprehension? *Lancet* 2003;362:2016–8.

60. Berg JW, Appelbaum PS, Lidz CW, Parker L. *Informed Consent: Legal Theory and Clinical Practice,* 2nd ed. New York, N.Y.: Oxford University Press; 2001.

61. Mello MM, Studdert DM, Brennan TA. The rise of litigation in human subjects research. *Annals of Internal Medicine* 2003;139:40–5.

62. Miller FG, Brody H. A critique of clinical equipoise: Therapeutic misconception in the ethics of clinical trials. *Hastings Center Report* 2003;33(3):19–28.

63. Robinson EJ, Kerr C, Stevens A, et al. Lay conceptions of the ethical and scientific justifications for random allocation in clinical trials. *Social Science and Medicine* 2004;58:811–24.

64. Peppercorn JM, Weeks JC, Cook EF, Joffe S. Comparison of outcomes in cancer patients treated within and outside clinical trials: Conceptual framework and structured review. *Lancet* 2004;363:263–70.

65. Brown RF, Butow PN, Ellis P, Boyle F, Tattersall MHN. Seeking informed consent to cancer clinical trials: Describing current practice. *Social Science and Medicine* 2004;58:2445–57.

66. Epstein LC, Lasagna L. Obtaining informed consent—Form or substance. *Archives of Internal Medicine* 1969;123:682–8.

67. DeRenzo EG, Conley RR, Love R. Assessment of capacity to give consent to research participation: State of the art and beyond. *Journal of Health Care Law and Policy* 1998;1:66–87.

68. Dickert N, Grady C. What's the price of a research subject? *New England Journal of Medicine* 1999;341:198–203.

69. Dunn LB, Gordon NE. Improving informed consent and enhancing recruitment for research by understanding economic behavior. *JAMA* 2005;293:609–12.

70. Weinfurt KP, Sulmasy DP, Schulman KA, Meropol NJ. Patient expectations of benefit from Phase I clinical trials: Linguistic considerations in diagnosing a therapeutic misconception. *Theoretical Medicine and Bioethics* 2003;24:329–44.

James H. Flory   David Wendler   Ezekiel J. Emanuel

59

Empirical Issues in Informed Consent for Research

In theory and practice, informed consent is considered a require-ment of ethical clinical research. Since the late 19th century it has been a recognized ethical goal that people not only decide freely whether to participate in clinical research, but decide with an un-derstanding of the relevant facts. This requirement helps to protect the autonomy of research participants and avert serious research abuses.

This simple doctrine—that consent should be not just vol-untary but informed—has proven difficult to realize in practice. The data show that research participants can have significant mis-conceptions about the nature of research even when researchers diligently follow consent procedures required by regulation. Truly informing research participants is very hard, and therefore the goal of truly informed consent poses serious challenges in policy and ethics. To help to address these challenges, we consider three relevant empirical questions: How well do participants under-stand their research participation? Is there any way to predict who will have the most trouble understanding? And which interven-tions might improve participants' understanding?

Methodological Issues in Empirical Research on Informed Consent

Numerous studies have quantitatively measured participants' understanding using interviews and questionnaires. These studies tend to focus on how well participants understand the elements of informed consent as described in U.S. federal regulations. In par-ticular, most studies have focused on how well participants grasp the purpose of research, their right to withdraw, the nature of study procedures, the use of randomization, risks, and benefits. The accelerating pace of research on informed consent means that there is a great deal of work to draw on. Because new studies are being completed on a regular basis, even a comprehensive review will be outdated before it is complete.

Furthermore, the heterogeneity of the data that have already been collected poses a challenge for any review. The studies we examine take place in many different settings, from tests of new drugs on dying cancer patients in Chicago to studies of maternal iron supplementation in Bangladesh. Such diversity compels cau-tion in comparing the results of different studies.

The studies also vary in methodology and quality. The studies use different questions to assess participants' understanding, making direct comparison of the results difficult. There is also little doubt that the quality of data collection varies from study to study: there are many methodological pitfalls in empirical in-formed consent research (see Table 59.1). In particular, some stu-dies have less ambiguous, more carefully validated questions than do others.

Timing of data collection is also important. Some studies administer questions within a few hours after the informed con-sent process, whereas others wait days, weeks, or even months. Early data collection is preferable in this case because it captures understanding at the time participants are making their enroll-ment decision. Studies that wait longer end up measuring reten-tion of information as much as understanding at the time of de-cision making.

Due to variability in setting, methodology, and quality, there is no way to integrate all of these data sources to create definitive, meta-analyzed conclusions. Nor is there any reason to assume that

Table 59.1

Common Problems in Empirical Studies of Informed Consent

	Problem	*Possible Solution*
Timing: Many studies use mailed questionnaires, so that participants don't have their understanding assessed until weeks after the consent process.	Delayed data collection makes it hard to distinguish understanding from retention.	Interview participants immediately after they give consent.
Questions about purpose: "Is the purpose of the study to determine which malaria drugs are most effective for children?"	This question doesn't show whether participants understand that a study could require extra risks and procedures that make it different from standard clinical care.	Additional question to resolve the ambiguity: "Will the study require that my child have more blood draws and other procedures than she would need just for her medical care?"
Questions about voluntariness: "Are you free to withdraw from the study at any time?"	This question doesn't clarify whether the participant needs a doctor's permission. This question also does not clarify whether there will be consequences if a participant withdraws. Nor does it clarify whether the participant feels constrained to stay in a study because of external circumstances, as opposed to coercion by researchers.	A change in wording and two additional questions: "Are you free to withdraw from the study whenever you want, even without a doctor's permission?" "If you withdraw from the study, will doctors still give you the same health care you had access to before the study started?" "If you were not in this study, would you be able to find and afford enough medical care?"
Questions about prospect of benefit: "How likely is it that you will receive medical benefit from participating in this trial?"	This question cannot distinguish optimism from mistaken beliefs about the chances of benefit.	Add a question that requests the objective assessment of chances, rather than a subjective (potentially hopeful) statement: "How many patients do the doctors expect to benefit from this experimental treatment? Fewer than 1 in 10, about half, or greater than 9 in 10?"

observations from one particular study generalize to different settings. Given this uncertainty, we proceed cautiously, focusing on observations that have been reproduced several times and in different settings.

Understanding the Purpose of Research

Empirical data on research participants' understanding of study purpose is typical of the data on participants' understanding in general (see Table 59.2). These data suggest that participants' understanding varies considerably from study to study but in general is relatively poor. At the encouraging end, a study of parents enrolling their children in a trial of malaria drugs in Uganda found that 80% of parents knew that the study purpose was "determining which malaria drugs are most effective for children."[1] In a rather different setting, a survey of people enrolled in oncology research in Boston found that 75% of participants agreed with the statement that "the main reason cancer clinical trials are done is to improve the treatment of future cancer patients."[2] But much of the data reflects poorer understanding. A study that focused on Phase I oncology research participants in Chicago found that only 27% could correctly describe the purpose of the research as dose finding/toxicity determination.[3] In rural Bangladesh, half of the women in a study of iron supplements thought that participation in research was part of routine health care.[4]

These numbers, and similar data from other studies, provide a glimpse at the state of understanding in research studies across the world. Generalizing from data like this must be done cautiously, but we can at least note that the percentage of participants who

seem to understand the purpose of the studies in which they participate varies a great deal from study to study. It is rare for all participants to understand a study's purpose and common for fewer than 75% to understand it. In addition, there is no consistent evidence that people from poor nations understand less than those from affluent countries.[5]

But the data are more difficult to interpret than they at first appear. In most of the examples given above, there is a more complicated story to tell. In the Uganda study, most parents knew that the study was meant to answer a scientific question about which malaria drugs are most effective for children.[1] But in contrast to the high rate of correct responses to the purpose question, only 19% of these parents realized that different children in the study were being assigned to different treatments. Did these parents understand that the design of the study meant doctors would be unable to make treatment decisions based on what was deemed best for the child?

The Boston oncology study addressed this point more directly, asking whether participants agreed that the study was designed primarily to benefit future patients.[2] The statement that a study is designed primarily to benefit future patients is a truism of research ethics, and one's first reaction is concern about the 25% of participants who didn't agree with it. Yet that 25% were in good company: Only a minority of health-care providers (46%) agreed with this statement when they were given the same survey. Were providers more poorly informed than the participants they recruited? A more likely explanation is that in much of oncology research, the care participants receive on-protocol is arguably better than they would receive off-protocol, and it is reasonable to think of the protocol as partly or even primarily intended to benefit its

Table 59.2

Selected Studies Evaluating Understanding of Purpose

Study	Context	Measure of Understanding	Responding Correctly	Comments
Pace (2005)[1]	A pediatric trial of malaria drugs in Uganda. Interviews with parents.	Chose "determining which malaria drugs are most effective for children" on a multiple-choice question.	80%	
Fitzgerald (2002)[48]	Study of HIV-1 transmission in Haiti. Questionnaires given to participants.	Correctly answered a true/false question on study purpose.	33%	
Joffe (2001)[2]	Phases I, II, and III oncology studies in United States. Questionnaires mailed to participants.	Agreed with statement that "the main reason cancer clinical trials are done is to improve the treatment of future cancer patients."	75%	46% of health-care providers also agreed with this statement. Questions were answered a median of 16 days after consent to trials.
		Disagreed with the statement "All treatments and procedures in my clinical trial are standard for my type of cancer."	48%	
Lynoe (2001)[4]	Study of maternal iron supplementation in Bangladesh. Interviews with participants.	Answered NO to the question "Did you get the impression that participation was only part of routine health care?"	47%	
Daugherty (2000)[3]	Phase I oncology studies in United States. Interviews with participants.	Said that purpose of study was "dose finding/toxicity determination."	27%	Subjects were interviewed within one week of beginning of oncology study. 61% stated erroneously that purpose of study was to determine the efficacy of the cancer drug; 8% agreed with both statements.
Van Stuijvenberg (1998)[22]	Pediatric study of ibuprofen to prevent febrile seizures, in Netherlands. Questionnaire mailed to parents.	Were able to correctly state the purpose of the study in their own words.	53% gave completely correct answer. 35% gave a partially correct answer.	Questionnaire sent to parents at home, so presumably some delay between consent and consent study.
Daugherty (1995)[15]	Phase I oncology studies in Chicago. Interviews with participants.	In interview, described purpose as dealing with dose determination or tolerability.	33%	52% expressed the erroneous belief that the purpose was to determine response/benefit from treatment.
Howard (1981)[19]	Study of beta-blockers in post-MI patients in the United States. Interviews with participants.	In interview, demonstrated knowledge that they were in research.	90%	Average delay of four months between consent and interview.
		In interview, demonstrated good understanding of study purpose.	80%	
Taub (1981)[25]	Study of comprehension and memory in the elderly, in the United States. Questionnaire given to participants.	Correctly identified purpose of study on multiple-choice question.	71%	Participants could refer to consent form while answering questions.

own participants. How is one to be sure that the remaining 25% of participants were really ill-informed about the study's purpose?

In the study of Phase I oncology research participants, researchers asked a more specific question about the scientific question addressed by the study. Only a third of participants correctly identified dose finding and toxicity as the purpose of this protocol; 61% of participants believed that the purpose of the study was to evaluate the efficacy of the cancer drug. How far wrong were these participants, and did their confusion make their consent invalid? Another way to view this data is to observe that nearly 90% of participants in this study realized they were in research: Is this good news, or should we focus on the bad news that most of them failed to make the further distinction between screening for safety and screening for efficacy?

The point of these examples is that the purpose of a research study is a surprisingly complex article of information. One can understand it at different levels, from the simple appreciation that a study is meant to create scientific knowledge to more detailed knowledge of the type of knowledge in question and the specific scientific issues involved. Even the most superficial levels of understanding can be murky with ambiguity. Although concern over the therapeutic misconception has led many theorists into the habit of thinking that studies are not meant to provide optimal medical care, the fact is that many studies have a dual effect, both generating scientific information and providing superior care for participants. This is especially true in settings in which individuals have little or no access to standard medical care.

Many questions about study purpose assume participants should recognize that the researchers' purpose is to create generalizable knowledge, and that anyone who fails to answer in this way fails to understand. But the fact that researchers' purpose is to create generalizable knowledge does not exclude the possibility that they also intend to benefit those who enroll in the research. Investigators at some sites may participate in the research with the primary purpose of helping their own patients. And, of course, many individuals enroll in research with the explicit purpose of receiving treatment. Therefore, questions about intentions and purpose can have more than one right answer.

Moreover, it is not always clear that understanding of the purpose of the research is necessary for a valid informed consent—at least, not for every study. Imagine participants who enroll in a Phase II treatment study of a new medication for a disease without any currently effective treatment. How important is it for participants to recognize that the purpose of the study is not to treat them per se, but to create generalizable knowledge on the efficacy of treating groups of patients?[6]

Understanding Voluntariness

Whereas study purpose is a complex topic, voluntariness stands out at first as simple. The topic has its complexities, but there is no fundamental ambiguity: Participants should be free to refuse research participation and to withdraw from research without pressure or coercion. This right to withdraw should be understood by 100% of participants. Against such simplicity, it is striking how many people do not fully appreciate that their participation in research is voluntary (see Table 59.3). In general, studies have shown that most but by no means all participants were aware that

they did not have to join a study and that they had the right to withdraw from it. In some cases, however, the percentage of participants aware of these rights was below 50%.[4]

Studies that delved deeper into the right to withdraw revealed that in many cases, participants' understanding is worse than it first appears. In one case, 65% of parents knew they had the right to withdraw their children from research, but only 17% knew they could exercise that right at any time. Essentially, they thought that they had the right to withdraw as long as investigators said that they could.[1] In another case, 91% of parents knew that they had the right to withdraw their children from research, but 25% of them still felt obligated to continue their participation.[7] In a third case, although 93% of participants thought they were free to quit a perinatal HIV transmission study, only 2% believed that the hospital would allow them to quit. In addition, 32% felt their care would be compromised if they did not participate.[8] In each of these cases, the initial impression that participants understood their rights is complicated by aspects of the responses that suggest participation may be less free than first appeared.

It is difficult to know for certain what these participants were thinking, but several possibilities present themselves. A relatively benign possibility is that participants were quite aware of the right to withdraw, yet felt they had to continue to participate because of external factors, as opposed to pressure from researchers. For example, they might feel that the study was the best or only way for them to get needed medical care.[9] This possibility does not imply poor informed consent, coercion, or inappropriate pressure from researchers.

A second possibility is that participants thought the right-to-withdraw language is an empty promise. This is illustrated by those who thought they were free to quit at any time as long as investigators gave permission. A variation is illustrated by those who thought they were free to quit but that there would be adverse consequences to their medical care. This reveals confusion about the nature of the right to withdraw that has a parallel in everyday life: I have the right to say unflattering things about my boss; even so, there will be some unpleasant consequences if I exercise this right. Without specific information to the contrary, research participants may assume that the right to withdraw does not protect them from negative consequences if they exercise this right.

Thus it turns out that voluntariness is in its own way a complicated concept. There are different degrees of freedom. Research participants should have the highest degree of freedom, namely, the ability to refuse or quit a study whenever they want, with the knowledge that doing so will not compromise their routine medical care. Accordingly, investigators need to offer this freedom and should take care to communicate it fully. Investigators and regulators should also be careful not to mistake participants who feel obliged to participate by external circumstances, like the severity of their illness or limited options, for participants who feel that they are being coerced or inappropriately pressured by researchers. The fact that individuals feel compelled to enroll in research due to the severity of their illness, and the absence of alternative treatments, does not necessarily undermine the validity of their informed consent, any more than patients' experiencing respiratory distress undermines the validity of their consent to intubation.[10,11] The data do not always clearly distinguish pressure from one's illness from more ethically worrisome pressure, especially pressure from the research investigators.

Table 59.3

Selected Studies Evaluating Understanding of Voluntariness

Study	Context	Measure of Understanding	Responding Correctly	Comments
Pace (2005)[1]	A pediatric trial of malaria drugs in Uganda. Interviews with parents.	Understood right to withdraw.	65%	
		Understood could withdraw at any time.	17%	
		Understood that could have refused to enroll.	41%	
Fitzgerald (2002)[48]	Study of HIV-1 transmission in Haiti. Questionnaires given to participants.	Correctly answered two true/false questions on voluntariness.	47%	
Joffe (2001)[2]	Phases I, II, and III oncology studies in United States. Questionnaires mailed to participants.	Understood right to decline enrollment.	99%	Questions were asked a median of 16 days after consent to trials.
		Understood right to withdraw.	90%	
Lynoe (2001)[4]	Study of maternal iron supplementation in Bangladesh. Interviews with participants.	Answered YES to the question "Did you know that after giving consent you were free to withdraw from participation at any point in time?"	48%	87% of women answered YES to the question "Did you get the impression that participation might mean such great advantages that it was difficult to say no?"
		Answered YES to the question "Did you know that you were free to abstain from participation?"	65%	
Hietanen (2000)[16]	Study of adjuvant therapy for breast cancer in Finland. Questionnaires mailed to participants.	Reported feeling free to decide about their participation independently.	85%	11-month delay between consent and informed consent study.
Abdool Karim (1998)[8]	Study of perinatal HIV transmission in South Africa. Questionnaires given to participants.	Understood were free to quit.	93%	32% believed their care would be compromised if they quit the study.
		Understood hospital would allow them to quit.	2%	
Van Stuijvenberg (1998)[22]	Pediatric study of ibuprofen to prevent febrile seizures, in the Netherlands. Questionnaire mailed to parents.	Parents understood right to withdraw.	91%	25% of parents felt obliged to participate.
Schaeffer (1996)[18]	Various studies at the NIH, in the United States. Questionnaires given to patients.	Understood right to withdraw.	Variable: over 90%	
Taub (1981)[25]	Study of comprehension and memory in the elderly, in the United States. Questionnaires given to patients.	Correctly answered multiple-choice question about freedom to withdraw.	76%	Participants could refer to consent form while answering questions.
Bergler (1980)[20]	Study comparing hypertension medications, in the United States. Questionnaires given to patients.	Understood were free to withdraw at any time and still receive best available treatment.	77%	Study was done within two hours of consent procedure. At three months, retention of this information was 61%.

Understanding Protocol Design and Randomization

Research on how well participants understand protocol design almost invariably focuses on randomization and placebo control (see Table 59.4). Although there are exceptions, the majority of studies show that fewer than half of participants understand these issues. There is far less evidence on how well participants understand prosaic but important details like whether a study drug is oral or injected, or the length and frequency of clinic visits they need to make as part of their participation. The limited available data suggest that investigators may do a good job communicating this information, yet still fail to get the concept of randomization across to participants.

Table 59.4

Selected Studies Evaluating Understanding of Protocol Design and Randomization

Study	Context	Measure of Understanding	Responding Correctly	Comments
Pace (2005)[1]	A pediatric trial of malaria drugs in Uganda. Interviews with parents.	Understood there would be 7 clinic visits.	78%	
		Understood children would be taking oral drugs.	79%	
		Understood children would be assigned to different treatments.	19%	
		Understood children would be assigned treatment at random.	7%	
		Understood that blood samples would be taken.	98%	
		Could name one or more side effects of study drugs.	18%	
		Understood biological samples could be used for future research.	52%	
Kodish (2004)[12]	Pediatric leukemia trials in the United States. Interviews with parents.	In interview, expressed understanding of randomization.	50%	Parents were interviewed within 48 hours of consent meeting.
Appelbaum (2004)[14]	Variety of clinical studies at academic medical centers in the United States. Interviews with participants.	Did NOT express inaccurate beliefs in individualization of their treatment.	69%	
Hietanen (2000)[16]	Study of adjuvant therapy for breast cancer in Finland. Questionnaires mailed to participants.	Understood that they would be randomized.	23%	11-month delay between informed consent and interview.
Van Stuijvenberg (1998)[22]	Pediatric study of ibuprofen to prevent febrile seizures, in the Netherlands. Questionnaire mailed to parents.	Understood the child had a 50% chance of being assigned to placebo.	88%	
		Understood that treatment would be allocated randomly.	50%	
Howard (1981)[19]	Study of beta-blockers in post-MI patients in the United States. Interviews with participants.	Demonstrated understanding of placebo control.	89%	Average delay of four months between consent and interview.
		Demonstrated understanding of randomization.	72%	
Taub (1981)[25]	Study of comprehension and memory in the elderly, in the United States. Questionnaires given to patients.	Correctly identified length of session.	78%	Participants could refer to consent form while answering questions.
		Correctly identified the type of tests being used.	40%	
Bergler (1980)[20]	Study comparing hypertension medications, in the United States. Questionnaires given to patients.	Understood that trial would last one year.	64%	Two hours after consent procedure; at three months, understanding was unchanged.
		Understood that trial was double-blind.	64%	At three months, understanding had fallen to 46%.

The malaria study in Uganda offers a detailed example of this point.[1] Of those participating, 78% knew that they would have to make seven clinic visits in the course of the study, 79% knew their children would be taking drugs orally, and 98% knew that the study involved blood samples. Only 19% knew that children were being assigned to different treatments, and only 7% went further to understand that assignment would be random.

What is one to make of such a striking shift, from the majority of patients understanding practical details of the protocol to a tiny minority understanding randomization? There are several possible explanations. First, randomization may simply be a hard concept to understand. Few studies assess whether most people fail to grasp randomization due to the therapeutic misconception, as opposed to simple confusion about a complicated concept. Another possibility might be that participants must understand practical details in order to comply with the protocol, so investigators and participants find it easier to focus on them. Finally, investigators might gloss over the subject of randomization. Against this possibility, one study in which consent procedures were videotaped and compared against participants' later understanding found that understanding of randomization continued to be poor even when investigators devoted significant time to explaining it.[12]

Table 59.5

Selected Studies Evaluating Understanding of Risks and Benefits

Study	Context	Measure of Understanding	Responding Correctly	Comments
Appelbaum (2004)[14]	Variety of clinical studies at academic medical centers in the United States. Interviews with participants.	Did NOT express an unreasonable belief in nature of likelihood of benefit.	49%	
Joffe (2001)[2]	Phases I, II, and III oncology studies in United States. Questionnaires mailed to participants.	Disagreed with statement that "the treatment being researched in my clinical trial has been proven to be the best treatment for my type of cancer."	30%	Questions were asked a median of 16 days after consent to trials.
		Disagreed with statement that "all the treatments and procedures in my clinical trial are standard for my type of cancer."	26%	
Daugherty (2000)[3]	Phase I oncology studies in United States. Interviews with participants.	Knew fatigue and GI symptoms possible side effect.	71%	Subjects were interviewed within one week of beginning of oncology study.
		Knew hair loss possible side effect.	48%	
		Knew neutropenia possible side effect.	29%	90% of participants expected medical benefit.
Daugherty (1995)[15]	Phase I oncology studies in Chicago. Interviews with participants.	22% of participants expected to receive treatment benefit; 70% expected to receive psychological benefit.		
Van Stuijvenberg (1998)[22]	Pediatric study of ibuprofen to prevent febrile seizures, in the Netherlands. Questionnaire mailed to parents.	Awareness of possible negative side effects.	40%	
Miller (1994)[21]	Trial of analgesics in United States. Interviews with participants.	Could recall any of the 12 potential side effects.	52%	Interview within 60 days of consent.
Penman (1984)[13]	Phases II and III oncology studies in United States. Interviews with participants.	Were able to list more than 3 side effects.	31%	43% of participants agreed with the statement that they had no doubts at all about benefits from the trial.
		Knew nausea was a side effect.	99%	
		Knew hair loss was a side effect.	65%	
		Knew risk of decreased WBC and infection.	23%	One- to three-week delay between consent and informed consent study.
Bergler (1980)[20]	Study comparing hypertension medications, in the United States. Questionnaires given to patients.	Aware of both side effects.	28%	After three months, only one participant (4%) recalled both side effects, whereas an additional 70% could recall 1.
		Aware of 1 side effect.	44%	

Understanding of Risks and Benefits

The literature approaches understanding of risks and benefits in two ways (see Table 59.5). The broad approach asks research participants how much they expect to benefit from or be harmed by their study participation. Here, the literature suggests that research participants tend to be quite optimistic, possibly unreasonably so, about their potential to benefit from research participation. The narrow approach assesses how well participants remember specific details about the risks and benefits of their trial. The data here show that participants have difficulty absorbing and retaining lists of potential adverse events, but occasionally have good retention of particular facts.[2,3,13–22]

There are several examples of what seems to be excessive optimism. In one survey, 43% of patients stated that they had no

doubts at all about benefits from a treatment even though most of their consent forms stated that no benefit could be assured.[13] A study specifically designed to identify the prevalence of unreasonable optimism reported that 51 percent of participants expressed an unreasonable belief in the likelihood of benefit.[14] It seems reasonable to expect that many research participants will tend to overestimate the likelihood that they will benefit. In spite of these results, it is hard to determine whether this is a widespread problem or not. At least in oncology, it is clear that some participants can be realistic. In one example, only 22% of participants thought they would receive benefit in a Phase I trial.[15] The rest of the participants appeared to have faced up to a difficult reality. It is hard to be sure whether understanding was a problem among the 22% who thought they would benefit. A key issue in communication of risk and benefit is the difficulty of distinguishing a patient who is mistaken about the prospect of benefit from one who is simply hopeful and prefers to make positive statements about the future.[17] Confusion implies inadequate informed consent; hope does not.

Given this ambiguity about the meaning of broad expressions of optimism or pessimism, the narrow approach of seeing how many facts about risks and benefits participants are able to absorb has obvious appeal. Studies taking this approach make it clear that retaining long lists of possible adverse events is difficult for participants.[13,15,20,21] In one oncology study, only a minority of participants were able to remember three side effects within one to three weeks of receiving that information. Although most participants were aware of the risk of vomiting or nausea, only 20% to 30% were aware of more abstract risks, like lowered white cell counts.[13] In another study looking at retention of information for up to 60 days after informed consent, only about half of participants could recall even 1 of 12 side effects. In a study looking at recall of two side effects from heart-failure drugs, only 28% of participants could name both side effects shortly after the study was explained to them, although an additional 44% could name one.[20]

These data raise a question as to whether it is reasonable to expect research participants to benefit from long lists of potential adverse events, when it is clearly difficult to remember more than a few side effects. A telling example from the literature is a study of hospital employees who were asked to consider joining a sham protocol in which they would take an experimental drug. Employees were randomized to one of three consent forms for this trial. Each consent form described the side effect profile of the sham experimental drug in a different level of detail, and in each case the profile was an accurate description of the potential side effects of aspirin. Employees given the most detailed description grossly overestimated the risk of taking the drug; those given the brief description formed a much more accurate conception of the drug's risk even though they had less raw information to work with.[23]

These data suggest investigators should be careful about encouraging too much optimism in research participants. They also indicate that expecting participants to recall a laundry list of risks is unrealistic, and they cast doubt on the utility of loading consent forms with long lists of side effects.

The Effect of Demographics on Understanding

Several demographic factors have been shown to be associated with better understanding in informed consent. The literature offers strong evidence that better education is associated with better understanding. A more limited evidence base indicates that advancing age (over 50) and mental illness are risk factors for low understanding. Other basic demographic characteristics, including sex, minority status, and income, have not been consistently linked with poor understanding. Importantly, there is no evidence that participants from poor countries understand less well than participants from industrialized nations.

At least 13 studies have showed that higher education and reading levels are significantly associated with increased overall understanding scores.[12,15,24–35] Frequently these differences are striking. In a study of parents who were considering pediatric leukemia trials for their children, 7% of parents with less than a

high school education understood randomization, whereas 78% of parents who were college graduates understood it ($p < .001$).[12] Another study of advanced cancer patients enrolling in Phase I trials found that 69% of college graduates correctly stated the purpose of Phase I trials as a determination of dose toxicity, whereas only 26% of noncollege graduates were right about this ($p = .002$).[15] The relationship between education and understanding is robust across many settings and studies, and it is strong enough to be of major practical significance.

Increased age was associated with significantly lower understanding in five studies that enrolled participants with mean age older than 50 years (all $p < .05$).[24,27,28,32,33] However, two other studies have reported no association between understanding and age.[34,35] In addition, mental illness, particularly schizophrenia, has been associated with lower understanding in four studies that compared mentally ill research participants with healthy or medically ill volunteers (all $p < .05$).[31,35–37]

A review article comparing informed consent in research in poor countries to that in affluent democracies found no evidence that participants from the poor countries understood less.[5] In light of generally lower levels of education in poorer countries, this is a surprising finding. One possibility is that international studies might have more heavily monitored and effective consent processes than is the norm in industrialized countries. It is worth noting that saying understanding in poor countries is as good as it is in developed countries is not the same as saying it is good on an absolute scale.

Interventions to Improve Understanding

Helping research participants understand better is a challenge. An extensive and growing literature has tested diverse approaches. At least 42 trials have compared the understanding of research participants who had undergone a standard informed consent process with the understanding of those who had received an intervention to improve their understanding. Unfortunately, no clearly effective solutions have emerged.

Interventions that have been tested can be categorized into five groups: (1) multimedia, including computer-based informed consent; (2) enhanced consent form; (3) extended discussion; (4) test/feedback; and (5) miscellaneous. Overall, 12 trials tested multimedia interventions, using computer or video technology in place of,[35,38–40] or in addition to,[31,40–42] the usual written informed consent form. A further 15 trials evaluated consent forms with modified content, writing style, format, or length.[23,24,27–29,33,37,39,40,43–47] Five trials of extended discussion evaluated interventions in which a member of the study team or a neutral educator scheduled additional time to discuss the disclosed information with research participants.[30–32,34,48] These interventions ranged from a 30-minute telephone conversation with a nurse[32] to multiple counseling sessions lasting up to 2 hours.[48] Another five trials evaluated test/feedback interventions, in which research participants were quizzed about the information disclosed to them and were given a review of questions that they answered incorrectly.[25,26,37,49,50] Five trials of miscellaneous interventions were not readily comparable with any of the other interventions that were tested.[36–37,40,50,51] For example, one trial put research participants through a weeklong tryout period for the procedures in the protocol before asking for consent.[51]

The studies can be compared on the basis of whether a trial employed randomization, whether the trial evaluated real or simulated informed consent processes, the number of participants in the trial, and whether the trial was published in a peer-reviewed journal. Simulated trials, which asked volunteers to consider a hypothetical or sham decision to enroll in research, were less realistic, hence potentially less relevant to actual clinical trials, than those comparing two real informed consent processes. Overall, peer-reviewed randomized trials in a real setting with relatively large enrollment have the greatest validity but are rare: Only eight trials met this standard and had enrollment of over 100 people.[30,32,33,39,43,49]

A minority of studies attempted to assess the effect of interventions on research participants' satisfaction and accrual. Studies that assessed satisfaction simply asked participants to rate their satisfaction. Studies in a real setting measured accrual directly; studies of simulated consent processes asked participants either to make a hypothetical decision or to rate their willingness to enroll.

The Effectiveness of Interventions

Overall, 12 trials of multimedia interventions revealed that such interventions often failed to improve research participants' understanding[31,35,38–42] (see Table 59.6). One published trial showed a statistically significant improvement in understanding using a computerized presentation of information.[35] The population for this trial was primarily patients with mental illness, with a few healthy volunteers. In addition, two unpublished trials reportedly produced increases in understanding, one from a video presentation and the other from a computerized presentation;[40] but the significance of these results is difficult to assess prior to complete analysis, peer review, and publication of the data. None of the other nine trials reported a significant improvement in understanding, although two trials of video interventions that showed no increase in understanding immediately after disclosure did show improved retention of information weeks later.[41,42]

Of the 15 trials with enhanced consent forms, 6 studies showed significant gains in understanding[23,29,44–47] whereas 9 did not[24,27,28,37,39,40,43,45] (see Table 59.7). The nine negative studies included four of five more rigorous randomized controlled trials of real consent processes.[27,28,33,39] Of the 6 studies that showed significant gains, 5 evaluated simulated consent processes with no discussion of the information in the consent form; the consent form was the only means used to disclose information to participants.[23,29,45–47] Because in most real consent processes research participants receive some information through discussion, the effect of improvements to the consent form is likely to be larger in such a hypothetical scenario than in a real research context.

When modifying consent forms, investigators used four basic strategies: reducing the length of the form; revising the content of the form to make it more comprehensible and readable; improving formatting through the use of techniques like larger font size and italics; and adding graphics. The data do not indicate that any of these approaches is more successful than the other approaches. But the one randomized controlled trial in a real setting to show a significant improvement used a dramatically shortened form, from four pages to two.[44] This reduction in length was accomplished by removing standard but irrelevant information on risk.

Extended discussion between study staff and research participants resulted in statistically significant increases in understanding in three of five trials[32,34,48] (see Table 59.8). Both negative trials showed trends toward improved understanding ($p = .054$ and $p = .08$, respectively).[30,31] Three of the trials in this category have questionable validity due to their small sample sizes and nonrandomized designs.[31,34,48]

The test/feedback approach, in which participants were evaluated for understanding and then given additional explanation if their understanding was inadequate, had significant impact (all $p < .05$) in all five trials that evaluated this approach[25,26,37,49,50] (see Table 59.9). But each study in this category measured the outcome using the same questionnaire that was used in the test/feedback intervention itself. This is a serious methodological flaw because any improvement in the test score could reflect rote memorization of the answers to questions rather than increases in real understanding.

Among the five miscellaneous interventions, two were combinations of more common approaches (see Table 59.10). One trial compared a standard consent process with a process enhanced by a combination of extended discussion time, additional written information, and simple teaching aids.[50] A second trial used extended discussion time and teaching aids that included computerized presentation.[36] Both trials simulated a consent process and resulted in significant gains to understanding. A one-week tryout period in which research participants underwent some protocol procedures before deciding whether to give consent was also associated with a significant improvement in understanding.[51] Two other trials did not show a significant increase in understanding.[37,40]

Actual accrual to real protocols, or stated willingness to join simulated protocols, were secondary outcomes for 12 trials. Two multimedia trials[38,42] and one enhanced consent form trial[23] noted significantly higher willingness to join for the intervention group, although the other trials noted no statistically significant difference.[29,32,41,44,45,50] No trial documented statistically significant reduction in accrual or willingness to join due to an intervention.

Two enhanced consent form trials that asked research participants to rate their satisfaction with the disclosure processes found that participants were more satisfied with the enhanced form than with the control form.[33,43] Two more trials, which had an enhanced consent form and a computerized presentation, found that the intervention and control groups reported comparable satisfaction.[38,44] The only other trial to measure satisfaction found that an extended discussion intervention was viewed as "worthwhile" or "very worthwhile" by 89% of patients.[32]

Overall, these data indicate that multimedia and enhanced consent form interventions do not consistently improve research participants' understanding. Person-to-person interactions, especially the extended discussion interventions, may be more effective in improving understanding.

This review suggests several conclusions and recommendations for policy and future research. First, although multimedia interventions may have the potential to improve understanding, this potential has not been realized in practice. Of 12 trials, only 1 published and 2 unpublished trials of such interventions have documented an improvement in understanding among research participants.[35,40] Most participants in the published trial were mentally ill, suggesting that multimedia intervention might be helpful for that population. In addition, two trials that used video

Table 59.6
Results of Trials of Video and Computer Multimedia Interventions

Author/Publication Status	Intervention	Population	Scenario	Methodology	Sample Size	Understanding Scores		P value
						Control	Intervention	
Dunn (2002)[35]	PowerPoint presentation replaces consent form	Psychiatric outpatients and normal volunteers	Real	Randomized	99	85	91	.014
Kass (unpublished)[40]	Supplementary touch-screen presentation on oncology clinical research	Oncology patients	Real	Randomized	87	Significant improvement reported		
Mintz (unpublished)[40]	Supplementary video encouraging participant involvement in decision-making	Psychiatric patients	Real	Randomized	37	Significant improvement reported		
Benson (1988)[31]	Supplementary video prepared by investigator	Psychiatric patients	Real	Nonrandom	44	51	54	NS
Benson (1988)[31]	Revised version of supplementary video	Psychiatric patients	Real	Nonrandom	44	51	58	NS
Llewellyn-Thomas (1995)[38]	Interactive computer program replaces consent form	Oncology patients	Simulated	Randomized	100	81	79	NS
Fureman (1997)[41]	Supplementary video in question and answer format	Injecting drug users	Simulated	Randomized	186	81	80	>0.10*
Weston (1997)[42]	Supplementary 10-minute video	Pregnant women	Simulated	Randomized	90	91	95	NS*
Agre (2003)[39]	Video replaces consent form	Patients and normal volunteers	Real	Randomized	221	68	73	NS
Agre (2003)[39]	Computer presentation replaces consent form	Patients and normal volunteers	Real	Randomized	209	68	66	NS
Campbell (unpublished)[40]	PowerPoint presentation replaces consent form	Parents of pediatric research participants	Simulated	Randomized	No significant improvement reported			
Campbell (unpublished)[40]	Narrated video replaces consent form	Parents of pediatric research participants	Simulated	Randomized	No significant improvement reported			

*A significant increase in retention of information weeks later was reported; hence, this intervention was shown to improve memory, though not comprehension at the time of disclosure; NS = not significant.

Table 59.7

Results of Trials of Enhanced Consent Form Interventions

Author	Intervention	Population	Scenario	Methodology	Sample Size	Understanding Score		
						Control	Intervention	P value
Epstein (1969)[23]	Less detailed description of drug side effects	Hospital employees	Simulated	Randomized	44	45*	67	.001
Young (1990)[29]	Readability improved from 16th to 6th grade level	Normal volunteers	Simulated	Nonrandom	666	64	67	.005
Rogers (1998)[44]	Less unnecessary information, signing indicated "opt-out" rather than "opt-in"	Recent mothers	Real	Randomized	44	30	47	.02
Bjorn (1999)[45]	Shorter sentences, less technical language, text rearranged into subsections	Normal volunteers	Simulated	Randomized	135	Significant improvement reported		.05
Murphy (1999)[46]	Less redundant material, text reorganized, simpler writing, graphics, focus groups	HIV high-risk group	Simulated	Randomized	141	70	83	.0001
Dresden (2001)[47]	Less unnecessary information, simpler vocabulary, bullets, larger font, other formatting	Asthma patients	Simulated	Randomized	100	72	88	.0001
Taub (1980)[24]	Readability improved from 12th grade to 6th–7th grade level	Elderly volunteers	Real	Nonrandom	56	No improvement reported[§]		
Taub (1986)[27]	Readability improved from college to 7th grade level, shorter sentences, less technical or unnecessary language	Cardiac patients	Real	Randomized	188	71	74	NS
Taub (1987)[28]	Readability improved from college to 7th grade level	Elderly volunteers	Real	Randomized	235	68	70	NS
Davis (1998)[43]	Revised with patient input, readability improved from college to 7th grade level, shortened, booklet format, graphics	Patients and normal volunteers	Simulated	Randomized	183	56	58	NS
Bjorn (1999)[45]	Shorter sentences, less technical language, text rearranged into subsections	Normal volunteers	Simulated	Randomized	100	No improvement reported		
Stiles (2001)[37]	Different fonts, bold and italicized text, focus groups	Mentally ill and normal volunteers	Simulated	Randomized	227	81	81	NS
Agre (2003)[39]	Form put into booklet format, summary sections added	Patients and normal volunteers	Real	Randomized	221	68	70	NS
Coyne (2003)[33]	Readability improved from college to 7th grade level, less technical language, simpler paragraphs, question–and–answer format, treatment calendar, larger font, more white space	Oncology patients	Real	Randomized	207	69	72	.21
Campbell (unpublished)[40]	More white space, bold headings, photographs, figures	Parents of pediatric participants	Simulated	Randomized	No significant improvement reported			

*This trial tested three consent forms; the longest consent form yielded the lowest understanding, but was so verbose as to be unrealistic for a control and is not shown here; § understanding was measured two to three weeks after information disclosure.

Table 59.8

Results of Trials of Extended Informed Consent Discussion Interventions

Author	Intervention	Population	Scenario	Methodology	Sample Size	Understanding Scores		P value
						Control	Intervention	
Aaronson (1996)[32]	Semistructured phone conversation with oncology nurse, lasting about 30 minutes	Oncology patients	Real	Randomized	180	66	83	.001
Kucia (2000)[34]	Detailed repetition of clinical trial information	Cardiac patients	Real	Longitudinal	20	52	68	.0005
Fitzgerald (2002)[48]	Three meetings with a counselor, lasting up to 40 minutes each	Haitians at risk for HIV	Real	Nonrandom	45	73	93	.0001
Benson (1988)[31]	Extra meeting with independent educator	Psychiatric patients	Real	Nonrandom	43	51	67	.054
Tindall (1994)[30]	Extra meeting to discuss trial with research participant's enrolling physician	HIV patients	Real	Randomized	113	60	63	.079*

*This trial was designed with a significance threshold of $p = .1$ to avoid a risk of false-negative results. Therefore by the standards of this trial, the results were positive; but by the standards applied to other trials in this review, the results are nonsignificant.

Table 59.9

Results of Trials of Test/Feedback Interventions

Author	Intervention	Population	Scenario	Methodology	Sample Size	Understanding Scores		P value
						Control	Intervention	
Taub (1981)[25]	Research participants were given an 8-question test and received brief feedback on incorrect answers. Total time for intervention was 15 minutes or less.	Elderly volunteers	Real	Randomized	87	37	52	.01*
Taub (1983)[26]	Research participants were given an 11-question test up to 3 times, and received brief feedback on incorrect answers.	Elderly volunteers	Real	Longitudinal	100	69	89	.01
Wirshing (1998)[49]	Research participants were tested and received brief feedback on incorrect answers until they were able to score 100%, then reevaluated for understanding 7 days later.	Psychiatric patients	Real	Longitudinal	49	Significant improvement reported[¥]		.02
Stiles (2001)[37]	Research participants were tested up to 3 times with a quiz and received brief feedback on incorrect answers.	Mentally ill and normal volunteers	Simulated	Randomized	111	82	97	.001
Coletti (2003)[50]	Deficiencies in participant knowledge identified with questionnaires and discussed with research participants. Three such meetings occurred at 6-month intervals.	At risk for HIV	Simulated	Longitudinal	3908	55	69[§]	.05

*Understanding was measured two to three weeks after information disclosure; ¥ significance based on evaluation seven days after test/feedback intervention compared to initial evaluation; § final understanding score is after two sessions of feedback with 12 months between *control* and *intervention* values.

Table 59.10

Results of Trials of Miscellaneous Interventions

Author	Intervention	Population	Scenario	Methodology	Sample Size	Understanding Scores		P value
						Control	Intervention	
Rikkert (1997)[51]	Week long tryout before consent	Elderly patients	Real	Longitudinal	50	55	70	.001
Carpenter (2000)[36]	Extended discussion, computerized presentation, and other simple teaching aids such as a flip chart	Mentally ill	Simulated	Longitudinal	20	32	71	.001
Coletti (2003)[50]	Extended discussion, additional pamphlet, and other teaching aids	At-risk for HIV	Simulated	Randomized	4,572	55	70	.05
Stiles (2001)[37]	Neutral facilitator present at research participant's meeting with investigator	Mentally ill and normal volunteers	Simulated	Randomized	227	82	81	NS
Merz (unpublished)[40]	Educational vignettes included with consent information	Apheresis patients	Simulated	Randomized	206	Unpublished: no increase in understanding reported		

technology, which did not find an increase in understanding, did establish an increase in retention of disclosed information.[41,42] If this result were further verified, video technology might be useful as a tool for improving retention of information.

The lack of consistent improvement in understanding due to video and computer technology may seem surprising, partly because previous studies have suggested that multimedia interventions increase patients' understanding in routine medical care.[52,53] This disparity may result from the fact that in research, the informed consent process is already formalized through federal regulations that require a written consent form. Video-based and computer-based interventions may not add much to this relatively thorough disclosure process. Indeed, in previous studies, when a decision aid was compared with standard medical care, increases in understanding were quite large; but when a more elaborate decision aid was compared with a simple one, increases were small.[54] In the same way, multimedia interventions could be much better than nothing but not necessarily better than the disclosure processes already common in clinical research.

Second, the data indicate that enhanced consent forms do not typically yield significant increases in understanding. Although enhanced consent forms seemed to have a significant effect in several trials, most of these trials simulated the consent process unrealistically; they included no discussion, only a reading of the form. In such a setting, the form becomes the participant's only source of information and this exaggerates the impact of changes in the form. The one realistic trial that showed an effect suggests that shortening forms by removing unnecessary standardized content appears to improve understanding.[44]

Third, limited evidence suggests that more person-to-person contact, rather than videos or paper forms, may be the best way to improve understanding. The most promising model is that advanced by Neil Aaronson and his colleagues, in which a nurse made 30-minute phone calls to participants at home and went through a semiscripted conversation with them.[32] One purpose of this conversation was to ask questions to find out how much

participants understood and to review key topics with them. The 10 trials of extended discussion and test/feedback interventions provide preliminary support for a hypothesis that in-person human contact tends to be more successful in improving understanding than relying on tools like consent forms and multimedia interventions.[25,26,30–32,34,37,48–50] Extended one-on-one interaction with another person may offer more opportunity for active engagement and responsiveness to the individual needs of the research participant. This hypothesis would support the idea that informed consent is more than just the action of reading a form and signing it. It is better thought of as a process, ideally a dialogue, that takes place over time and largely depends on interactions between humans.

Fourth, lower educational attainment, mental illness, and perhaps advanced age are associated with lower understanding. Indeed, the differences in understanding between well-educated and less well-educated individuals outweigh any improvement in understanding from the various interventions. These results may reflect poorer test-taking skills among less educated research participants, causing them to score lower on tests of understanding even when their understanding is actually adequate. It may also indicate that these interventions are still not effective for individuals with less education and that disclosure processes need to be more appropriate for individuals with lower cognitive skills.

Recommendations for Improving Informed Consent

For clinical investigators who seek to better inform participants in their clinical trials, these data support several conclusions.

Using a standard consent process and adding an extra meeting with a qualified person has the best evidential support. There is no evidence that this person needs to be an investigating physician; it might be ideal to use a nurse or outside educator to reduce the risk that a physician with vested interest in the study might unduly influence the research participant's decision. If resources are limited, researchers should consider targeting interventions to at-risk groups: Less well-educated, mentally ill, and possibly elderly populations. Further studies of extended discussion would be useful, particularly if they collected data to define how much extra time is helpful and what aspects of the interaction are most effective at improving understanding.

Multimedia interventions are not a reliably good investment for improving understanding, being expensive and time-consuming to produce without dependable positive effect. There may be effective ways of using multimedia interventions, but the burden is on investigators to show that this approach really helps research participants. Investigators who invest in multimedia should do research to confirm that its use is actually improving understanding.

Investing additional effort in consent forms is unlikely to have a large effect on understanding, although some evidence suggests that brevity and the elimination of irrelevant boilerplate information improves research participants' understanding.

A randomized controlled trial is needed to determine the effectiveness of test/feedback interventions that avoid the rote-memorization methodological problem. The test/feedback approach is intriguing, but research on it must be rigorous in order to show that it is really enhancing understanding, not just improving the participants' ability to parrot the correct answers to standard questions.

Future studies should avoid simulated consent processes because such simulations are often unrealistic. For instance, in evaluating improved consent forms, research results would be much more persuasive if they came from a real consent process in which the form assumed its usual role as only part of the consent process.

Finally, there is no reason to think that research participants will be dissatisfied with interventions to improve understanding or that interventions will diminish accrual.

Conclusion

This chapter synthesizes the empirical literature on informed consent to answer the following questions: How much do research participants understand? Do some participants understand more than others? How can understanding be improved?

The reason for asking these relatively simple questions is to help answer more complicated ethical and policy questions. Were this not primarily an empirical review, we might dwell further on questions such as the following: Are research participants well enough informed that their participation is ethical? What should investigators do to improve understanding? Hopefully the evidence accumulated here will be useful to anyone who wants to explore these questions in greater depth.

These are important questions for anyone involved in research, partly because researchers are as tightly bound by regulations as they are by financial and technical concerns. Research must have a satisfactory consent process for a conscientious institutional review board (IRB) to approve it. But nobody knows for certain what is and is not a satisfactory consent process. There is no evidence on what steps are necessary to achieve a given level of understanding in a given population. There is no way to show whether an IRB's demands are reasonable; there is no way to show whether an investigator's efforts to inform potential participants are adequate.

IRBs lack consistent standards to apply, investigators have no reliable tools to achieve informed consent, and it is not clear that participants are adequately protected by a system of informed consent that is flying blind.

This situation is dangerous. It retards valuable research and consumes the time of IRB members and investigators in unproductive debates lacking valid answers. Particularly in international research, in which everyone struggles with the challenge of communicating information to people from a different culture, this process can be a major logistical barrier. Meanwhile, inadequately informed research participants are less able to protect themselves either from exploitation or from the inherent risks of research.

We propose that participants will be safer and regulatory processes will run more smoothly if informed consent can become an evidence-based discipline. At this point, it is essentially never evidence-based. The information summarized here is still insufficient to design a consent process to achieve any given goal. But we now have testable hypotheses, and we can identify the further research needed to develop a reliable set of ways to help research participants understand. If this research is conducted, we can hope that the demands of IRBs and the capabilities of investigators will become closely matched, and that the volunteers who make research possible will more often be well enough informed to be true partners, rather than passive subjects.

Disclaimer

The opinions expressed are the authors' own. They do not reflect any position or policy of the National Institutes of Health, Public Health Service, or Department of Health and Human Services.

References

1. Pace C, et al. Quality of parental consent in a Ugandan malaria study. *American Journal of Public Health* 2005;95:1184–9.
2. Joffe S, et al. Quality of informed consent in cancer clinical trials: A cross-sectional survey. *Lancet* 2001;348:1772–7.
3. Daugherty CK, et al. Quantitative analysis of ethical issues in Phase I trials: A survey interview study of 144 advanced cancer patients. *IRB: Ethics and Human Research* 2000;22(3):6–14.
4. Lynoe N, et al. Obtaining informed consent in Bangladesh. *New England Journal of Medicine* 2001;344:460–1.
5. Pace C, Grady C, Emanuel E. What we don't know about informed consent. SciDev.Net [Online] August 28, 2003. Available: http://www.scidev.net/content/opinions/eng/what-we-dont-know-about-informed-consent.cfm.
6. Sreenivasan G. Does informed consent to research require comprehension? *Lancet* 2003;362:2016–8.
7. van Stuijvenberg M, et al. Informed consent, parental awareness, and reasons for participating in a randomised controlled trial. *Archives of Disease in Childhood* 1998;79:120–5.
8. Abdool Karim Q, Abdool Karim S, Coovadia H, Susser M. Informed consent for HIV testing in a South African hospital: Is it truly informed and truly voluntary? *American Journal of Public Health* 1998;388:637–40.
9. Pace C, Emanuel EJ, Chuenyam T, et al. The quality of informed consent in a clinical research study in Thailand. *IRB: Ethics and Human Research* 2005;27(1):9–17.

10. Hawkins JS, Emanuel EJ. Clarifying confusions about coercion. *Hastings Center Report* 2005;35(5):16–9.

11. Wertheimer A. *Coercion.* Princeton, N.J.: Princeton University Press; 1987.

12. Kodish E, Eder M, Noll RB, et al. Communication of randomization in childhood leukemia trials. *JAMA* 2004;291:470–5.

13. Penman DT, Holland JC, Bahna GF, et al. Informed consent for investigational chemotherapy: Patients' and physicians' perceptions. *Journal of Clinical Oncology* 1984;2:849–55.

14. Appelbaum PS, Lidz CW, Grisso T. Therapeutic misconception in clinical research: Frequency and risk factors. *IRB: Ethics and Human Research* 2004;26(2):1–8.

15. Daugherty C, Ratain MJ, Grochowski E, et al. Perceptions of cancer patients and their physicians involved in Phase I trials. *Journal of Clinical Oncology* 1995;13:1062–72. [Erratum in: *Journal of Clinical Oncology* 1995;13:2476.]

16. Hietanen P, Aro AR, Holli K, Absetz P. Information and communication in the context of a clinical trial. *European Journal of Cancer* 2000;36:2096–104.

17. Horng S, Grady C. Misunderstanding in clinical research: Distinguishing therapeutic misconception, therapeutic misestimation, and therapeutic optimism. *IRB: Ethics and Human Research* 2003;25(1):11–6.

18. Schaeffer MH, Krantz DS, Wichman A, Masur H, Reed E, Vinicky JK. The impact of disease severity on the informed consent process in clinical research. *American Journal of Medicine* 1996;100:261–8.

19. Howard JM, DeMets D. How informed is informed consent: The BHAT experience. *Controlled Clinical Trials* 1981;2:287–303.

20. Bergler JH, Pennington AC, Metcalfe M, Freis ED. Informed consent: How much does the patient understand? *Clinical Pharmacology and Therapeutics* 1980;27:435–40.

21. Miller C, Searight HR, Grable D, et al. Comprehension and recall of the informational content of the informed consent document: An evaluation of 168 patients in a controlled clinical trial. *Journal of Clinical Research and Drug Development* 1994;8:237–48.

22. van Stuijvenberg M, Suur MH, de Vos S, et al. Informed consent, parental awareness, and reasons for participating in a randomised controlled study. *Archives of Disease in Childhood* 1998;79:120–5.

23. Epstein LC, Lasagna L. Obtaining informed consent: Form or substance. *Archives of Internal Medicine* 1969;123:682–8.

24. Taub HA. Informed consent, memory and age. *Gerontologist* 1980;20:686–90.

25. Taub HA, Kline GE, Baker MT. The elderly and informed consent: Effects of vocabulary level and corrected feedback. *Experimental Aging Research* 1981;7:137–46.

26. Taub HA, Baker MT. The effect of repeated testing upon comprehension of informed consent materials by elderly volunteers. *Experimental Aging Research* 1983;9:135–8.

27. Taub HA, Baker MT, Sturr JF. Informed consent for research: Effects of readability, patient age, and education. *Journal of the American Geriatrics Society* 1986;34:601–6.

28. Taub HA, Baker MT, Kline GE, Sturr JF. Comprehension of informed consent information by young-old through old-old volunteers. *Experimental Aging Research* 1987;13:173–8.

29. Young DR, Hooker DT, Freeberg FE. Informed consent documents: Increasing comprehension by reducing reading level. *IRB: A Review of Human Subjects Research* 1990;12(3):1–5.

30. Tindall B, Forde S, Ross MW, et al. Effects of two formats of informed consent on knowledge amongst persons with advanced HIV disease in a clinical trial of didanosine. *Patient Education and Counseling* 1994;24:261–6.

31. Benson PR, Roth LH, Appelbaum PS, Lidz CW, Winslade WJ. Information disclosure, subject understanding, and informed consent in psychiatric research. *Law and Human Behavior* 1988;12:455–75.

32. Aaronson NK, Visser-Pol E, Leenhouts GH, et al. Telephone-based nursing intervention improves the effectiveness of the informed consent process in cancer clinical trials. *Journal of Clinical Oncology* 1996;14:984–96.

33. Coyne CA, Xu R, Raich P, et al. Randomized, controlled trial of an easy-to-read informed consent statement for clinical trial participation: A study of the Eastern Cooperative Oncology Group. *Journal of Clinical Oncology* 2003;21:836–42.

34. Kucia AM, Horowitz JD. Is informed consent to clinical trials an "upside selective" process in acute coronary syndromes? *American Heart Journal* 2000;140:94–7.

35. Dunn LB, Lindamer LA, Palmer BW, et al. Improving understanding of research consent in middle-aged and elderly patients with psychotic disorders. *American Journal of Geriatric Psychiatry* 2002;10:142–50.

36. Carpenter WT Jr, Gold JM, Lahti AC, et al. Decisional capacity for informed consent in schizophrenia research. *Archives of General Psychiatry* 2000;57:533–8.

37. Stiles PG, Poythress NG, Hall A, Falkenbach D, Williams R. Improving understanding of research consent disclosures among persons with mental illness. *Psychiatric Services* 2001;52:780–5.

38. Llewellyn-Thomas HA, Thiel EC, Sem FW, Woermke DE. Presenting clinical trial information: A comparison of methods. *Patient Education and Counseling* 1995;25:97–107.

39. Agre P, Rapkin B. Improving informed consent: A comparison of four consent tools. *IRB: Ethics and Human Research* 2003;25(6):1–7.

40. Agre P, Campbell FA, Goldman BD, et al. Improving informed consent: the medium is not the message. *IRB: Ethics and Human Research* 2003;25(Suppl 5):S11–S19.

41. Fureman I, Meyers K, McLellan AT, Metzger D, Woody G. Evaluation of a video-supplement to informed consent: Injection drug users and preventive HIV vaccine efficacy trials. *AIDS Education and Prevention* 1997;9:330–41.

42. Weston J, Hannah M, Downes J. Evaluating the benefits of a patient information video during the informed consent process. *Patient Education and Counseling* 1997;30:239–45.

43. Davis TC, Holcombe RF, Berkel HJ, Pramanik S, Divers SG. Informed consent for clinical trials: A comparative study of standard versus simplified forms. *Journal of the National Cancer Institute* 1998;90: 668–74.

44. Rogers CG, Tyson JE, Kennedy KA, Broyles RS, Hickman JF. Conventional consent with opting in versus simplified consent with opting out: An exploratory trial for studies that do not increase patient risk. *Journal of Pediatrics* 1998;132:606–11.

45. Bjorn E, Rossel P, Holm S. Can the written information to research subjects be improved: An empirical study. *Journal of Medical Ethics* 1999;25:263–7.

46. Murphy DA, O'Keefe ZH, Kaufman AH. Improving comprehension and recall of information for an HIV vaccine trial among women at risk for HIV: Reading level simplification and inclusion of pictures to illustrate key concepts. *AIDS Education and Prevention* 1999;11:389–99.

47. Dresden GM, Levitt MA. Modifying a standard industry clinical trial consent form improves patient information retention as part of the informed consent process. *Academic Emergency Medicine* 2001;8: 246–52.

48. Fitzgerald DW, Marotte C, Verdier RI, et al. Comprehension during informed consent in a less-developed country. *Lancet* 2002;360: 1301–2.

49. Wirshing DA, Wirshing WC, Marder SR, et al. Informed consent: Assessment of comprehension. *American Journal of Psychiatry* 1998;155:1508–11.

50. Coletti AS, Heagerty P, Sheon AR, et al. Randomized, controlled evaluation of a prototype informed consent process for HIV vaccine efficacy trials. *Journal of Acquired Immune Deficiency Syndromes* 2003;32:161–9.

51. Rikkert MG, van den Bercken JH, ten Have HA, Hoefnagels WH. Experienced consent in geriatrics research: a new method to optimize the capacity to consent in frail elderly subjects. *Journal of Medical Ethics* 1997;23:271–6.

52. Agre P, Kurtz RC, Krauss BJ. A randomized trial using videotape to present consent information for colonoscopy. *Gastrointestinal Endoscopy* 1994;40:271–6.

53. Mason V, McEwan A, Walker D, Barrett S, James D. The use of video information in obtaining consent for female sterilisation: A randomised study. *BJOG* 2003;110:1062–71.

54. O'Connor AM, Stacey D, Entwistle V, et al. Decision aids for people facing health treatment or screening decisions [Cochrane Review]. In: *Cochrane Library, Issue 1*. Chichester, England: John Wiley & Sons; 2004.

David Wendler

The Assent Requirement in Pediatric Research

Jimmy, a bright, energetic, and confident 8-year-old, suffered from a serious inborn immune deficiency characterized by a disorder in white cell function. Jimmy spent a significant percentage of his life in the hospital, fighting off obscure infections. Given the rarity of his disease, Jimmy also spent a good deal of time enrolled in clinical research aimed at understanding his condition and immune function in general.

In the spring of 1999, investigators developed a protocol to obtain white cells from individuals with Jimmy's disease. The investigators believed that studying the cells in the laboratory might provide information about the specific white cell deficiency that characterizes the disease and, perhaps, might yield important insights into immune function in general. Several factors made Jimmy an especially good candidate for the procedure. He had undergone similar procedures in the past and had never experienced any ill effects. In addition, Jimmy had a rare genetic variant of the disease that was little understood.

Jimmy's parents strongly supported his participation in the study. They had already lost one child to the disease and were committed to understanding it better. Because the study investigator did not want to pressure Jimmy into agreeing, she asked a bioethics consultant to explain the procedure to Jimmy and solicit his agreement. The consultant met with Jimmy, accompanied by his primary nurse. The consultant explained that the procedure would involve placing two needles in Jimmy's arms and would require that he sit relatively still, in a reclining chair, for approximately 30 minutes.

The consultant also explained that the procedure posed very low risks to Jimmy, apart from a remote possibility of some blood loss if the tubing became clogged. The investigators proposed to

use a topical anesthetic, which would reduce and might fully eliminate the pain associated with the initial needle sticks. Jimmy related that he remembered undergoing a similar procedure, and stated that the procedure had not bothered him and had caused him no anxiety. Indeed, Jimmy explained that he enjoyed the time he spent undergoing the procedure because the nurses had brought in a television and played one of Jimmy's favorite videos.

By the end of the 45-minute discussion, it was clear to both the consultant and the nurse that Jimmy understood the procedure and was not afraid or made anxious by the prospect of undergoing it. Based on several years of caring for Jimmy, the nurse assured the consultant that Jimmy made his views clear when he did not want to undergo a particular procedure. Indeed, after Jimmy was told that the procedure would not help him, and that he could refuse to undergo it, he quickly refused. To explain his refusal, he pointed out that the procedure would not help him and said he would rather spend the 30 minutes required to undergo the procedure playing basketball in the hospital hallway.

Two days later, Jimmy's mother asked the bioethics consultant to meet with him again regarding the procedure. The previous day, Jimmy's 14-year-old sister, who suffered from the same disease, had undergone the procedure and told Jimmy that it was easy, and that he should do it. The sister explained that the procedure was not painful or difficult, that Jimmy could watch videos while undergoing it, and that his participation would help the doctors learn more about their terrible disease.

Jimmy worshiped his sister, and his mother assumed that the sister's report was likely to influence him. The consultant agreed, and met with Jimmy alone in his room. The consultant again explained the procedure, and again explained that the doctors thought Jimmy's participation would be helpful to the study. The consultant also again explained that the decision was up to Jimmy and that he could refuse, even though his parents and sister supported his participation. With very little hesitation, Jimmy again declined, explaining that the procedure would not help him. He stated his second refusal in almost identical terms, expressing surprise that the consultant seemed unable to understand that playing basketball is more fun that sitting in a chair with needles in one's arms. Based on Jimmy's refusal, the procedure was not performed.

Everyone agrees that, with some exceptions, parents or legal guardians should give permission for their children to be involved in research. The question of assent for pediatric research participation asks whether children's prospective agreement should be solicited in addition to their parents' permission. In requiring Jimmy's assent, were the investigators showing appropriate respect for him, or inappropriately treating a child as if he were an adult? Does appropriate respect imply that children should be asked to provide prospective assent? If so, should all children be asked to give assent, or only some subset of children? At a practical level, how should the assent requirement be implemented? And what is the appropriate approach for children who are not being asked to assent?

The Regulatory Landscape

Most research ethics guidelines allow children to be enrolled in research studies that do not offer them a prospect of direct benefit only when their parents or legal guardians give permission. Many guidelines, including those from the Council for International Organizations of Medical Sciences (CIOMS),[1] South Africa,[2] and the United States,[3] also require the assent—defined as "positive agreement"—of children who are capable of providing it. Specifically, most regulations require the assent of children when the research does not offer them a compensating potential for clinical benefit. Most regulations either do not require children's assent when research does offer a compensating potential for clinical benefit or allow the reviewing IRB to waive the requirement when the research offers such potential for clinical benefit. The Ugandan guidelines, for example, allow children to be enrolled in nonbeneficial research only when "adequate provisions have been made for the solicitation of the children's assent."[4] Similarly, the Indian Council on Medical Research guidelines require that the "assent of the child should be obtained to the extent of the child's capabilities."[5] The U.S. regulations require the assent of children capable of providing it in all cases. However, the U.S. regulations, at 45 CFR 46.408, allow IRBs to waive this requirement when the research offers the "prospect of direct benefit that is important to the health or well-being of the children and is available only in the context of the research."[3] These regulations also allow IRBs to waive the requirement for assent in cases that qualify for waiver of informed consent, such as minimal risk research when obtaining consent is not practicable.[3]

Most commenters regard the assent requirement as an important protection for children in the context of clinical research that does not offer them a compensating potential for clinical benefit.[6] But it is unclear *which* children are capable of assent, and research ethics guidelines provide little guidance in this regard. The U.S. federal regulations, for example, specify only that the

determination of which children are capable of assent should take into account the children's "ages, maturity, and psychological state."[3] This guidance leaves many questions unanswered. Which aspects of children's age, maturity, and psychological state should investigators take into account when determining whether they are capable of assent? Is the ability to nod one's head sufficient? Must children understand certain aspects of their research participation? And, if so, which ones?

Several commentators argue that, as a general rule that admits of exceptions, children become capable of assent at the age of 7. The American Academy of Pediatrics and the U.S. National Commission for the Protection of Human Subjects of Biomedical and Behavioral Research (hereafter, National Commission) have taken a similar stance.[7,8] This view traces to the centuries-old "Rule of Sevens."[9]

The Rule of Sevens states roughly that children under the age of 7 do not have the capacity necessary to make their own decisions; children 7–14 years of age are presumed not to have this capacity until proven otherwise in individual cases; and children over age 14 are presumed to have the capacity to make their own decisions and lead their own lives, unless proven otherwise. The fact that age 7 has been regarded, for hundreds of years at least, as an important threshold for the purposes of making decisions may explain why a number of commentators have endorsed it as the age of assent. That is, historic precedent may have been viewed by commentators, either consciously or not, as an additional argument in favor of adopting this threshold, providing reason to prefer age 7 over, say, age 6 or age 10. Alternatively, one may argue that the prior acceptance of the Rule of Sevens had a more pernicious effect, biasing commentators in favor of this age threshold to the extent that it was endorsed without sufficient analysis.

It is worth noting, however, that the assumption that children are capable of assenting to research participation by age 7 is inconsistent with the Rule of Sevens. Strict application of the Rule of Sevens would classify children between ages 7–14 as incapable of providing assent, unless proven otherwise. In addition, a 2004 survey of the chairpersons of 188 IRBs revealed great variation in practice in the United States. Specifically, only 20% of U.S. IRBs used the age 7 cutoff, 9% used age 5 or 6, and 18% used an age between 8 and 12.[10] In addition, 54% of U.S. IRBs left the decision of which children are capable of assent to the judgment of the investigators in charge of a given study.

These data on implementation point to the need for systematic analysis of the rationale for the assent requirement. Is such variation appropriate? Should individual IRBs, or even individual investigators, make their own decisions about which children are capable of assent? Or should there be a consistent threshold across IRBs and across studies?

Appealing to Family Practice to Set a Threshold

Some commentators argue that the debate over the appropriate age threshold for assent should be informed by data on how families engage their children in decision making outside the research context.[11] Specifically, at what age do parents allow their children to make various decisions? Gathering this information would provide background on the types of decisions that children are allowed to make in their daily lives. This information would have important practical implications, clarifying the ages at which children make decisions in other contexts and thereby revealing how familiar children and families might be with different age thresholds for assent, and how they might react to these thresholds. Similarly, it would be useful to gather data on the ages at which children's agreement is required for decisions outside of the research context. Is children's assent required for them to serve as a bone marrow donor for a sibling, for instance? At what age are children allowed to decide they no longer want to go to school, or to go on family vacations?

Families presumably involve their children in decision making to different degrees, and the extent to which they do so varies by the decision in question and diverse cultural and social norms. Hence, without further argument, this view seems to imply that no substantive regulatory stance should be adopted. Instead, the regulations should state simply that the research should be presented to the family and that the family should be asked to decide whether the child will be enrolled, using whatever decision-making process the family relies on outside of the research context. Under this approach, parents who do not involve their children in day-to-day decisions would decide on their own; families that decide together would do so in the research setting as well; and any parents who defer completely to their children would also be able to do so in the research setting.

In contrast, one might endorse the view that there should be no assent requirement at all. First, one might argue that, by definition, children are individuals who are legally not able to make their own decisions. Therefore, children should not be asked to make their own decisions regarding research participation. This view might be supported by the claim that it is consistent with respect for families.[12] Children are dependent on their parents, and parents are responsible for their children. In general, society allows parents to decide how to involve their own children in decision making. We allow parents to determine whether their children get to decide when they go to bed, or what they wear to school. On these issues, we do not legislate standards for all families to follow.

It is true that there is value to allowing families to decide how to run their respective lives and society should interfere with families only when there is good reason to do so. However, the policy of granting families a sphere within which they are allowed to make their own decisions without societal interference does not imply that whatever families do, and however they decide to engage their children in the decision-making process, is acceptable. Rather, it reflects the fact that unless the matter is sufficiently important, interfering is not justified, even when families may be treating their children inappropriately.

Furthermore, the practice of allowing families wide discretion in choosing their own decision-making styles does not apply directly to the research setting. Research involves exposing children to risks for the benefit of society at large. Thus, in this setting, society has a greater responsibility to ensure the proper treatment of children. In this setting, society cannot grant that some families may be making mistakes in whether and when they allow their child a say, but justify noninterference on the ground that noninterference promotes other goods that are not outweighed by minor mistakes. In the research setting, society is already involved and already responsible for ensuring that proper practices are followed. The practices that society allows families to pursue in their private sphere apply to research only if there is independent reason to think that they are appropriate to that setting; the fact that families rely on these practices in their own lives does not settle the matter. Instead, we need to determine what constitutes an appropriate practice in the research setting. We need to figure out why requiring assent is important, and how important it is compared to other values, such as allowing families to make their own decisions. And we need to determine how assent practice is relevant to the nature of the research context. The fact that parents are allowed to disrespect their own children in their own homes does not imply that I am obliged to allow the same parents to disrespect their children in my home. At that point, others become involved and their interests and obligations become relevant to the moral calculation. The fact that the ethical concerns of the research team often get short shrift in research ethic literature does not make them less important or relevant. For example, the fact that parents treat their children one way at home does not necessarily entail that research nurses should be party to such treatment in the research setting.

Arguments for Assent

The U.S. federal regulations governing research with humans are based on the recommendations of the National Commission in the late 1970s. Therefore, to identify the rationale behind the assent requirement as it is expressed in the U.S. regulations, the National Commission's recommendations provide a good starting place. The National Commission's consideration of pediatric assent began with the principle of respect for subject autonomy: Individuals who can understand and shape their lives should be allowed to decide whether to enroll in research based on their own conception of a flourishing life. Conversely, individuals who cannot understand the proposed research cannot make an autonomous decision. They cannot decide whether research enrollment, or one of the available alternatives, would further their conception of a flourishing life.

The autonomy rationale implies that the threshold for assent should be fixed at the age at which most children become capable of making their own research decisions. Although one often thinks of respect for autonomy as applying to adults only, the National Commission recognized that individuals do not suddenly develop the capacity to make their own decisions at age 18. An individual's capacity develops over time, and many children are able to make their own decisions before they reach the legal age of adulthood.[13]

To make an autonomous decision regarding research enrollment, potential research participants must be able to understand the study in question and their own medical and personal situations, and to make a voluntary decision whether to participate on this basis. To understand the study in question, potential participants must understand the "elements of informed consent": the study's purpose, risks, potential benefits, requirements, procedures, and alternatives.[14] Potential participants must also appreciate how the elements of informed consent pertain to their own circumstances. Recognition that the capacity to make research decisions requires individuals to understand and appreciate all the elements of informed consent suggests one way to identify the age at which children develop this capacity, namely, identify the age at which children come to understand and appreciate the *final*—that is to say, the last to develop—element of informed consent.

Appreciation and the Purpose of Nonbeneficial Research

Children first understand concrete facts about the world and later come to understand more abstract facts. This suggests that the age at which children understand and appreciate the more abstract elements of informed consent provides an approximation of the age at which they should be able to make their own research decisions. Perhaps the most abstract element of informed consent is the *purpose* of research for which children's assent is required, namely, nonbeneficial research that is intended to develop generalizable knowledge that might help future patients.

The capacity to decide whether to enroll in nonbeneficial research requires children to understand and appreciate the potential to be altruistic, that is, the possibility of taking on risks and burdens to help others. Again, children do not have to be motivated to help others; they need only to understand this possibility. Children who do not understand the concept of altruism cannot decide for themselves whether helping others by enrolling in nonbeneficial research would further their conception of a flourishing life. They cannot decide whether the moral reasons to help others outweigh the risks of the research. Therefore, the autonomy rationale suggests that the assent threshold should be fixed at the age when (most) children develop the concept of altruism.

The Concept of Altruism

The term *altruism* is often used to describe those who are motivated to help others. Empirical studies of altruism tend to focus on helping behavior, often labeled *pro-social* behavior, independent of why individuals behave in this way.[15] Because these studies do not assess individuals' motivations for acting, they provide only limited evidence regarding when children develop the concept of altruism. The fact that children behave in a helping way at this or that age does not establish that they possess the concept of altruism at that age; it depends on why they act in this way.

The current data on prosocial behavior describe a roughly U-shaped function between age and altruistic behavior.[16–18] Starting at approximately age 2, many children will help others who are present and experiencing visible distress—for instance, offering a toy to a crying baby.[19–21] By age 5, most children will respond to the needs of individuals who are not within the child's circle of intimates. For example, a number of studies have found that many 5-year-olds will contribute to charity.[22] Finally, children's helping behavior appears to drop off after age 5, before increasing linearly starting around age 10.

Because of the inherent difficulties in assessing the motivations underlying individual behavior, it is not surprising that very few studies have assessed why children help others at various ages. Given this paucity of data, any recommendations must be tentative and subject to revision in light of future data. With this caveat in mind, the existing data suggest that most children younger than 10–12 years old behave altruistically for nonaltruistic reasons. They help others because they expect to be rewarded, to comply with the request of an adult, or because they feel bound by unwritten social rules.[23,24] These data suggest that most children under age 10 do not possess the concept of altruism.

At some point after age 10, most children begin to understand that there are moral reasons to help others, independent of the

possibility of reward or punishment.[25] For example, in a longitudinal study of children 5–16 years of age, Eisenberg and colleagues found that adolescents begin to understand and develop the ability to act from moral motivations at 11–12 years of age.[26] That is, they begin to understand that there are moral reasons to help others, even when doing so is not required and may place burdens on them.

It is important to distinguish this argument from the claim that potential research participants must be *motivated* to help others. The difference here is roughly the difference between acting altruistically versus understanding the concept of altruism. The claim that people must understand the concept of altruism in order to understand the purpose of nonbeneficial research, and hence to give informed consent, does not imply that they must be motivated to help others. Similarly, the claim that participants must understand the potential benefits of the research does not imply that they must enroll because they want access to those benefits.

These data suggest that most children cannot appreciate that the potential to help others provides a reason to enroll in nonbeneficial research until 10–14 years of age. Therefore, to the extent that the assent requirement is based on the principle of respect for autonomy, the age threshold for assent should be fixed somewhere in the range of 10–14 years. Before endorsing an age threshold within this range, however, one should consider whether there are any nonautonomy based reasons to support an earlier threshold. Are there reasons to require children's assent for nonbeneficial research before they develop the capacity to make their own enrollment decisions?

Other Arguments

The National Commission argued that investigators should obtain children's assent at age 7, not out of respect for their autonomy, but to help teach them to become autonomous. Effectively teaching children to become responsible and autonomous adults involves asking them to make decisions they are capable of making. For this reason, parents typically begin with fairly minor decisions and proceed, as children mature, to more important decisions. For instance, parents often begin by allowing children 5–8 years of age to help decide what to wear, or how to decorate their bedrooms. At what age should the decision to participate in nonbeneficial research be added to this teaching process?

Asking children to decide whether to enroll in research before they can understand and appreciate the elements of informed consent is ill-suited to teaching them to become good decision makers. For instance, a child who can understand the risks or potential benefits of research, but not both, is unlikely to make a decision that promotes their interests. Similar concerns arise when investigators ask for children's assent for nonbeneficial research before they can recognize that there are moral reasons to help others. From the child's perspective, asking children whether they want to enroll in nonbeneficial research before they have developed the concept of altruism amounts to asking them to accept burdens and risks for no reason. To the extent the children respond in a rational way, they will refuse, simply because they do not understand that there are reasons to agree.

Of course, parents and investigators may encourage reluctant children, and such encouragement may influence children to agree to enroll in nonbeneficial research. Nonetheless, this approach is unlikely to teach children to make decisions that promote their interests. It is more likely to teach them to doubt the judgment of adults, or simply to follow the advice of others, even when the advice makes no sense from their point of view. This analysis suggests that the importance of teaching children to become effective decision makers supports the proposal to fix the assent threshold at the age when (most) children are able to understand and appreciate the elements of informed consent.

In some places, the National Commission argued that assent should be required as a way to respect the ability of children 7 years of age or older to make "decisions concerning their activities." Does the ability to understand *some* aspects of research participation, and to make a decision on that basis, provide an independent reason to require children's assent for nonbeneficial research?

One might argue that the principle of respect implies that we should obtain children's assent even before they are able to make autonomous decisions. It is not clear, however, whether the principle of respect alone has substantive implications. Respect for persons tells one, roughly, to treat others in the way they deserve or ought to be treated. The principle of respect for persons itself does not tell one specifically how to treat them. To determine how one ought to treat a given individual—which is a necessary prelude to determining whether a particular behavior toward the individual is consistent with respect—one needs to know more about the individual in question. To take an example from the research ethics literature, there is ongoing debate about the conditions under which it is ethically appropriate to conduct research on the dead. Everyone agrees that we should respect the dead, yet appeal to a principle of respect does not settle the issue. We need to know whether research on the dead is consistent with appropriate respect. We cannot answer that question by analyzing the principle of respect. We need to understand something about corpses, including the relationship that the corpse bears to the previously living person.

Similarly, the principle of respect for persons tells us to treat children as they ought to be treated. Whether asking children to make research decisions is integral to respecting them is a further question. Should investigators solicit children's assent at the point at which they can nod their heads? when they can understand at least one aspect of research participation? when they can understand several aspects of research participation? If so, which ones? when they can understand all the elements of informed consent? or only when they become emancipated from their parents? The principle of respect for persons, although obviously relevant and important, does not answer this question. Rather, the principle of respect for persons implies only that investigators should solicit children's assent at the ages at which it is appropriate to do so, and not before. But this is the very question that the appeal to the principle of respect for persons is intended to answer in the first place.

The Existing Data

It is important to emphasize that the existing data are scanty with respect to those aspects of human development that are relevant to assent for research. Thus, only tentative conclusions will be possible, and these conclusions will be subject to revision as further data appear.

With that caveat in mind, the existing data suggest that children cannot understand many aspects of research participation until at least age 10. For instance, Ondrusek and colleagues found that children under age 9 do not understand most aspects of research participation.[27] At the same time, children over age 7 can understand some elements of informed consent.[28,29] For instance, Susman, Dorn, and Fletcher found that a majority of children involved in research understand the research's potential benefits and duration, what participation requires of them, and that they have an option to ask questions.[30]

The ability to understand and make decisions develops gradually, and children as young as 2 years old can understand some rudimentary aspects of research participation, such as the fact that it requires them to leave home, or allow strangers to touch them. Hence, the claim that children's assent should be required once they can understand any aspect of research participation, and express a choice on that basis, implies that the threshold for assent should be lowered to the age at which most children first understand at least one aspect of research participation, likely around 2 years of age.

What reason might justify requiring investigators to obtain the affirmative agreement of children as young as 2 years old? We have seen that respect for persons implies that investigators should obtain children's assent starting sometime in the range of age 10–14. Of course, respect for persons is not the only reason why it might be important for investigators to obtain children's assent. In particular, it is also important to consider the relevance of the principle of nonmaleficence to this issue.

The Role of Nonmaleficence

The principle of nonmaleficence applies to individuals of all ages, whether they are autonomous or not. This principle implies that children should not be required to participate in nonbeneficial research that is more than minimally distressing. In many cases, children will not know whether research participation will be distressing until they experience it. Thus, requiring children to make a prospective decision whether to enroll does not offer an effective mechanism to protect them from harm, particularly because children may be reluctant to go back on agreements with, or promises to, doctors. Children may also find it positively distressing to be asked to make decisions about research they cannot understand. Hence, the principle of nonmaleficence does not seem to support, and in some cases may conflict with, a requirement to ask children to decide whether to enroll in nonbeneficial research before they are able to understand the research in question.

Supporters may respond that the principle of beneficence, as distinct from the principle of nonmaleficence, implies that investigators should obtain children's assent at the point that they understand some aspects of the research in question. More research is needed to assess what impact asking young children to make research decisions has on them. In principle, however, there is no reason to think that asking individuals who cannot fully understand to make their own decisions will further their welfare. This is supported by the fact that children may find it distressing to have to make prospective enrollment decisions, especially for research their parents support, but for which they can find no reasons to enroll. Furthermore, asking children to make decisions they cannot understand conflicts with teaching them to become good decision makers.

Once children are enrolled in research, they will be in a good position to assess whether it is causing them distress. And because most children who experience distress will communicate this verbally or through body movements, the principle of nonmaleficence supports adoption of a dissent requirement: The dissent of all children should be respected in the context of research that does not offer them a compensating potential for clinical benefit.[31–33] Although this dissent requirement is not explicit in many regulations, including the U.S. federal regulations, it is included in some national regulations. For example, the Tanzania guidelines for research with humans stipulate that researchers "must recognize when a child is very upset by a procedure and accept that as genuine dissent from their being involved."[34]

Although the importance of a dissent requirement seems clear, it may not always be clear in practice, because a child's statements and behavior do not always reflect actual distress. For instance, an infant may cry in the absence of distressing stimuli. Nevertheless, children's participation in nonbeneficial research should be halted and reassessed at any indication that the child is experiencing more than minimal distress. The first question to ask is whether the signals from the child reflect actual distress. With respect to very young children, this judgment may require input from parents who are familiar with the behavior of their children. To err on the side of protecting children, unclear signals should always be regarded as reflecting underlying distress.

Because children's distress may be the result of nonessential aspects of their research participation, a dissent requirement need not stipulate that children must be removed from research at the first sign of dissent or distress. Instead, investigators and parents should attempt to identify and address the source of distress. Simple reassurance, a short pause, or a minor modification in the procedure may be sufficient to eliminate the distress. However, indications of more than minimal distress that cannot be alleviated should always be respected in nonbeneficial research.

Although some children may express apparent dissent in the absence of underlying distress, others may experience significant distress without expressing dissent. To address this concern, children participating in nonbeneficial research should be explicitly told to inform the investigators or nurses if they experience any distress. In addition, everyone involved in pediatric research should be trained to monitor children for signs of distress the children cannot or are unwilling to communicate.[7]

Setting an Age Threshold

The present analysis suggests that children should be asked to provide assent at the age at which they have the capacity to understand the nature of the research study in question. Because human development occurs at different rates, there will no single age at which all children develop the ability to understand. Some children will develop this ability at a relatively young age, whereas others will not develop this ability until much later. Thus, one possibility would be to require investigators to assess individual children to determine whether they have the capacity necessary to give assent. Investigators could then solicit assent on an individual basis, from the time that specific individuals develop the necessary capacities.

This approach has obvious virtues in terms of tailoring one's practice to the abilities of individual children, thereby ensuring sufficient respect for all children in this regard. At the same time, assessing each child's capacity is likely to require a good deal of resources for any study that involves more than just a few children. This is especially true given the fact that no one has developed an instrument that would allow such an assessment. Some instruments have been developed for the purposes of assessing adults' capacity to give consent, but these would have to be modified for evaluating children. In particular, these instruments typically assume that adults are able to understand the purpose of nonbeneficial research and do not assess this understanding directly. Adapting the instruments for this purpose would likely be difficult in practice. Further research is needed. In particular, it will be important to develop ways to assess understanding and determine how much time and resources they require.

At least until such research has been conducted, investigators will have to rely on more general thresholds. The use of general thresholds in the face of a continuum of age development and the absence of assessment tools is common in other areas. No one thinks that all people suddenly become capable of drinking alcohol responsibly at age 21 and that all adolescents suddenly develop the abilities necessary to vote responsibly at age 18. We recognize that children develop these abilities at different ages. Nonetheless, as opposed to theorizing about particular individuals, society endorses a general threshold, recognizing that whatever threshold is chosen will be too low for some and too high for others.

Current data suggest that most children come to appreciate what is likely the *final* element of informed consent—the ability to understand the possibility that nonbeneficial research may help others—sometime between ages 10 and 14. A plausible decision procedure in the face of insufficient data is to select the option that minimizes the potential resulting harms. The primary risk of choosing the lowest age in the range for the assent threshold is that children who are not autonomous will be asked to make their own research enrollment decisions. Conversely, the primary risk of choosing the highest age in the range is that investigators will fail to respect the autonomy of those children who develop the ability to make their own research decisions at an earlier age. Choosing intermediate ages involves balancing these two risks to varying degrees. How should we choose among these options?

It is important to improve medical treatments for children. Requiring the assent of children who are incapable of understanding the moral importance of helping others may carry significant costs if many children decline to participate based on a failure to appreciate these reasons. On the other hand, failing to allow children to make their own research decisions, if they are capable of doing so, carries the moral harm of failing to respect their autonomy. This is also an important concern: It would deny some children the chance to make a fully informed, altruistic decision to participate in the research. It would deny some other children the right to make a fully informed decision not to participate. However, to the extent that this failure is limited to the research context, it will be a relatively isolated event. Moreover, adoption of a dissent requirement will ensure that children who are upset at being enrolled will be able to control their fate by dissenting. The addition of this protection, together with the importance of improving medical treatments for children, supports choosing age 14, the highest age in the range, as the threshold.

To implement the dissent requirement with children who are unable to provide assent, investigators should explain what they are proposing to do, emphasize that the child's parents gave their permission, and tell the child to inform the investigator if he or she has any questions or experiences any distress. Under a dissent requirement, the investigators would then proceed with the research procedure without asking for the child's positive agreement, while carefully monitoring him or her for any signs of dissent or distress.

IRBs often mandate that researchers inform children about their prospective research participation by means of an assent form. Given this practice, fixing the assent threshold at age 14 may inadvertently result in younger children not receiving any information about their research participation. Yet very young children often want to know what is going to happen to them, and they find it reassuring to know how long their participation will last and where they will stay. To address this concern, IRBs might develop information sheets for children who are not able to give assent.

The fact that some children are not able to provide assent to research enrollment does not imply that they should be left out of all research decisions. Research participation often involves many small decisions—when to get medications, what clothes to wear, which elevator to take—that children can make and often enjoy making. The principle of beneficence suggests that children should be allowed to make these decisions when possible. The principle of beneficence also implies that investigators and IRBs should work to make research participation as enjoyable and beneficial for children as possible. To take one example, children may benefit from age-appropriate explanations of the science behind the research and the procedures it involves.

Some might argue that the present proposal that children become capable of assent at the point at which they are able to understand this decision confuses assent with consent. This issue is an important one, but deserves its own treatment. The fact that children can understand as well as adults at age 14, say, does not immediately imply that they should be able to make their own research decisions without parental input. Specifically, future research should consider whether being a dependent member of a family implies that parents should still have a say in their children's participation in research, especially nonbeneficial research, even when the children are capable of making an autonomous decision.

Practical Implications

Given that a dissent requirement allows children to veto their parents' decision to enroll them in nonbeneficial research, what is the difference between requiring children to make an affirmative decision versus respecting their dissent? The possibly subtle difference between these two requirements may explain why the drafters of the federal regulations adopted the National Commission's proposed assent requirement, but not its proposed dissent requirement. The drafters of the federal regulations may have assumed that adoption of the assent requirement was tantamount to requiring investigators to respect children's dissent.

In practice, there are three important differences between requiring assent and respecting dissent. First, respect for dissent does not imply that investigators should ask children to make a prospective decision on whether to participate in a given research study. A dissent requirement allows children to stop their research participation; it does not allow them to prevent their initial enrollment. An assent requirement, in contrast, requires that children make a prospective decision and lets children block their research enrollment. Second, an assent requirement alone does not require investigators to respect the dissent of children who are unable to provide assent. For this reason, it is important to adopt a dissent requirement in addition to an assent requirement. Third, asking children to make their own affirmative decisions puts them in the position of having to assess the options and prospectively choose the best course of action for themselves. When they cannot understand the research in question, requiring children to make this decision puts them in the position of having to choose (or reject) a course that their parents endorse but they cannot understand.

A dissent requirement places children who cannot understand the elements of informed consent in a very different position. Under a dissent requirement, children are not required to understand the research and make their own prospective decisions. Instead, they simply react to how the research is affecting them and indicate any distress they experience.

Assent and the Necessity Requirement

It is widely agreed that investigators should not enroll individuals who are unable to consent in research that could just as well be carried out by enrolling individuals who are able to consent. Should a similar *necessity* requirement be applied to research with children who are able to assent? That is, should investigators be allowed to conduct research with children who are unable to assent only when they cannot conduct the research equally well with children who are able to consent? The National Commission endorsed a variation of this requirement, stating that investigators should always enroll older children in research before enrolling younger children. This suggests, for instance, that in the process of testing drugs on children, investigators should first assess drugs in older children and only then move on to testing them in younger children.

The relevance of a necessity requirement for research with children seems to depend in large part on the basis one uses for determining which children are capable of assent. For example, if one simply uses the age of 7 as the threshold for assent, it is not clear what reason there might be to prefer the enrollment of children just under this threshold to children who have recently turned 8. To be sure, any requirement that prefers the enrollment of older children over younger children makes sense in that such a requirement generally will favor children who are more mature and better able to understand. Although this seems an important result, the inclusion of the age of assent does not seem to be doing any independent work here. Instead, this threshold simply forces investigators to prefer older children, a preference which could be stated equally well without any mention of the age of assent.

In contrast, with a threshold of age 14, the age of assent gets set at the age at which most children are able to understand the essential elements of informed consent. This threshold provides a clear reason to prefer the enrollment of children who are capable of assent to the enrollment of children who are not so capable. As with the necessity requirement as it is applied to adults, there are good reasons to prefer the enrollment of those who are able to understand over those who are not able to understand.

Conclusion

What, then, is the most appropriate way for investigators and IRBs to handle cases like that of Jimmy, described at the beginning of this chapter? Some commentators who emphasize the importance of respect for persons seem to assume that respect requires that individuals be asked to make their own decisions in all cases. Endorsement of such a view suggests that Jimmy's case was handled appropriately, even though he was not able to understand crucial elements of the decision in question. Indeed, this view seems to imply that children should be treated as competent and autonomous decision makers from the time they are able to make any decisions at all. Most commentators, however, do not take the principle of respect for persons so far that they argue that children should be able to veto their enrollment in research that offers them a prospect of direct benefit. We do allow competent adults to veto such participation. Those who appeal to the principle of respect for persons need to explain why, if that principle requires children as young as 3 or 4 to give assent to nonbeneficial research, it does not have the same implications for beneficial research.

Other commentators suggest that assent requirements should be patterned on the ways in which families engage their children in decision making outside of the research context. Although these data seem relevant, it is not clear that families' current practices are necessarily the appropriate ones. It may rather be that society simply tolerates the practices of some families on the ground that interference would be too costly, not on the ground that the practice is appropriate. In addition, I have argued that the context of research is fundamentally different. Research with humans involves exposing some individuals to risks for the benefit of society. For this reason, society needs to identify the correct policy in the context of research.

I have argued that children should be required to provide their assent at the point at which they are capable of understanding the research in question. Given the paucity of current data on the development of human understanding, any recommendations in this regard must be considered very tentative and subject to future modification. Accepting that caveat, the existing data suggest that children should be asked for their assent at the age of 14.

Importantly, this proposal does not confuse the child's assent with informed consent that is necessary for the research to proceed. The fact that individuals can understand the essential elements of consent at age 14 implies, on the current view, that their assent should be solicited. However, one might further argue that at that point, children should be able to provide their own consent, independent of their parents, rendering the question of assent moot. Although this view sounds plausible, and may be correct in many cases, it does not immediately follow. The fact that children continue to live in families may provide sufficient reason to require the parents' permission, in some cases at least, even after the children have adequate understanding. At any rate, that is a distinct issue that requires its own consideration.

Finally, the view endorsed here implies that the treatment of Jimmy, although consistent with U.S. regulations and a good deal of the existing literature on pediatric assent, was mistaken. The approach inappropriately treated Jimmy as being able to make his own decisions. Instead, after obtaining the parents' permission, the investigators should have explained the procedure to Jimmy and answered any questions he might have had. The investigators should then have gone ahead while monitoring him for any signs of distress or dissent. If this procedure turned out like his previous ones, the investigators would have obtained the cells for their studies and Jimmy would have lost only some free time. If the procedure had caused any more than minimal distress to Jimmy, it could have been stopped at that point. If the source of the distress could not be eliminated, the procedure should have been terminated at that point.

Disclaimer

The opinions expressed are the author's own. They do not represent any position or policy of the National Institutes of Health, Public Health Service, or Department of Health and Human Services.

References

1. Council for International Organizations of Medical Sciences in collaboration with the World Health Organization. *International Ethical Guidelines for Biomedical Research Involving Human Subjects.* Geneva, Switzerland: CIOMS and WHO; 2002. [Online] November 2002. Available: http://www.cioms.ch/frame_guidelines_nov_2002.htm.
2. South African Medical Research Council. *Guidelines on Ethics for Medical Research: General Principles.* [Online] Available: http://www.sahealthinfo.org/ethics/ethicsbook1.pdf.
3. Department of Health and Human Services, National Institutes of Health, and Office for Human Research Protections. The Common Rule, Title 45 (Public Welfare), Code of Federal Regulations, Part 46 (Protection of Human Subjects). [Online] June 23, 2005. Available: http://www.hhs.gov/ohrp/humansubjects/guidance/45cfr46.htm.
4. Uganda National Council of Science and Technology (UNCST). *Guidelines for the Conduct of Health Research Involving Human Subjects in Uganda.* Kampala, Uganda: UNCST; 1998.
5. Indian Council on Medical Research. *Ethical Guidelines for Biomedical Research on Human Subjects.* New Delhi, India: Indian Council on Medical Research; 2000. [Online] Available: http://icmr.nic.in/ethical.pdf.
6. Kodish E. Informed consent for pediatric research: Is it really possible? *Journal of Pediatrics* 2003;42:89–90.
7. American Academy of Pediatrics, Committee on Bioethics. Informed consent, parental permission, and assent in pediatric practice. *Pediatrics* 1995;95:314–7.
8. The National Commission for the Protection of Human Subjects of Biomedical and Behavioral Research. *Research Involving Children: Report and Recommendations.* Washington D.C.: U.S. Government Printing Office; 1977. [Online] Available: http://www.bioethics.gov/reports/past_commissions/Research_involving_children.pdf.
9. Blackstone's Commentaries on the Laws of England, Book IV, Chapter 2, "Of the persons capable of committing crimes." [Online] Available: http://www.lonang.com/exlibris/blackstone/bla-402.htm#fn1u.
10. Shah S, Whittle A, Wilfond B, Gensler G, Wendler D. How do IRBs apply the federal risk and benefit standards for pediatric research? *JAMA* 2004;291:476–82.
11. Joffe S. Rethink "affirmative agreement," but abandon "assent." *American Journal of Bioethics* 2003;3(4):9–11.
12. Ross LF. *Children, Families, and Health Care Decision-Making.* New York, N.Y.: Oxford University Press; 1998.
13. Bartholome WG. Informed consent, parental permission, and assent in pediatric practice. *Pediatrics* 1995;96:981–2.
14. Berg JW, Appelbaum PS, Lidz CW, Parker LS. *Informed Consent: Legal Theory and Clinical Practice.* New York, N.Y.: Oxford University Press; 1991.

15. Chou KL. Effects of age, gender and participation in volunteer activities on the altruistic behavior of Chinese adolescents. *Journal of Genetic Psychology* 1998;59:195–201.

16. Grunberg NE, Maycock VA, Anthony BJ. Material altruism in children. *Basic and Applied Social Psychology* 1985;6:1–11.

17. Harbaugh WT, Krause K. Children's contribution in public good experiments: The development of altruistic and free-riding behavior. *Economic Inquiry* 2000;38:95–109.

18. Underwood B, Moore B. Perspective-taking and altruism. *Psychological Bulletin* 1982;91:143–73.

19. Zahn-Waxler C, Radke-Yarrow M, Wagner E. Development of concern for others. *Developmental Psychology* 1992;28:126–36.

20. Thompson C, Barresi J, Moore C. The development of future-oriented prudence and altruism in preschoolers. *Cognitive Development* 1997;12:199–212.

21. Eisenberg N, Fabes R, Miller PA, Shell R, Shea L, May-Plumlee T. Preschoolers' vicarious emotional responding and their situational and dispositional prosocial behavior. *Merrill-Palmer Quarterly* 1990;36:507–29.

22. Rai SN, Gupta MD. Donating behavior as a function of age, culture and outcome feedback conditions. *Psycho-Lingua* 1996;26:105–10.

23. Raviv A, Bar-Tal D, Lewis-Levin. Motivations for donation behavior by boys of three different ages. *Child Development* 1980;51:610–3.

24. Rouch Cl, Hudson LM. Quantitative versus qualitative dimensions of prosocial development: Age-related contributors to children's donating behavior. *Child Study Journal* 1985;15:157–65.

25. Leikin S. Minors' assent, consent, or dissent to medical research. *IRB: A Review of Human Subjects Research* 1993;15(2):1–7.

26. Eisenberg N, Miller PA, Shell R, McNalley S, Shea C. Prosocial development in adolescence: A longitudinal study. *Developmental Psychology* 1991;27:849–57.

27. Ondrusek N, Abramovitch R, Pencharz P, Koren G. Empirical examination of the ability of children to consent to clinical research. *Journal of Medical Ethics* 1998;24:158–65.

28. Weithorn L, Campbell S. The competency of children and adolescents to make informed decisions. *Child Development* 1982;53:1589–98.

29. Lew C, Lewis M, Ifekwunique M. Informed consent by children and participation in an influenza vaccine trial. *American Journal of Public Health* 1978;68:1079–82.

30. Susman EJ, Dorn LD, Fletcher JC. Participation in biomedical research: The consent process as viewed by children, adolescents, young adults, and physicians. *Journal of Pediatrics* 1992;121:547–52.

31. Ackerman TF. Fooling ourselves with child autonomy and assent in nontherapeutic clinical research. *Clinical Research* 1979;27:345–8.

32. Ackerman TF. Moral duties of parents and nontherapeutic clinical research procedures in children. *Bioethics Quarterly* 1980;2:94–111.

33. United Kingdom Medical Research Council. *Medical Research Involving Children*. [Online] 2004. Available: http://www.mrc.ac.uk/pdf-ethics_guide_children.pdf.

34. Tanzania Health Research Forum. *Guidelines on Ethics for Health Research in Tanzania*. Dar es Salaam, Tanzania: 2001, reprinted in 2004.

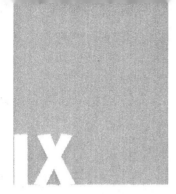

Respect for Human Research Participants

James G. Hodge Jr.   Lawrence O. Gostin

Confidentiality

Protecting the confidentiality of individually identifiable health information that is acquired, used, disclosed, or stored in the design, performance, or analysis of human subjects research is essential to respecting the dignity and privacy of human subjects participating in clinical research. Theories of confidentiality and privacy of identifiable health data are featured in the earliest conceptions of medical ethics. These theories are replicated in research ethics that evolved in the latter half of the twentieth century. Research ethics have consistently reflected a strong respect for the autonomy of individuals participating in research studies by protecting identifiable health data used in conducting research studies. Legal requirements at the international, federal, and state levels specifically address confidentiality protections in human subjects research and other settings.

These protections are not only theoretically, legally, and ethically grounded, they are critically important for practical reasons. Without adherence to principles of confidentiality, researchers may engage in, and individuals may fear, misuses of health data. Breaches of confidentiality involving human subjects in clinical research can lead individuals to avoid future participation in research studies. Unwarranted disclosures of identifiable health data can cause direct and indirect harm to individuals who are the subjects of such data, or to vulnerable groups of which they are members. Protecting data confidentiality, in sum, is essential to conducting human subjects research.

Most researchers understand the principle of confidentiality protections in human subjects research. They agree with the need to respect the private nature of research participants' health and other data, to avoid disclosures of such data without individual authorization, and to safeguard data to avoid unintended releases

or nonapproved uses. Yet, what does it really mean to respect the confidentiality of human research subjects' health data? Protecting confidentiality, in theory, is easy; in practice, however, it is complex and fraught with essential trade-offs. Modern principles—grounded in law, such as the U.S. Common Rule; in international agreements on human rights, such as the United Nations Universal Declaration of Human Rights; and in biomedical ethics—seek to clarify the scope of confidentiality and its applications in human subjects research. These principles provide a collective series of guideposts and norms that set formal, structural requirements for protecting individual (and group) confidentiality. This chapter seeks to explain the historical and modern understandings of confidentiality protections through an assessment of the ethical, legal, and policy issues, as well as their implications for the design and performance of clinical research involving humans.

History

The history of confidentiality is intrinsically tied to the history of medical ethics. "Requirements of confidentiality appear as early as the Hippocratic Oath,"[1] and are featured in virtually every code of medical ethics since. An adherent to the Hippocratic oath vows, "What I may see or hear in the course of the treatment or even outside of the treatment in regard to the life of men, which on no account one must spread abroad, I will keep to myself, holding such things shameful to be spoken about."[2] Early origins of medical confidentiality demonstrated the dual needs of medical practitioners to promote the welfare of their patients and to sanctify the role of physicians through ethical and increasingly legal practices that sought to restrict uses of identifiable data.[3] Restricting physicians' use and disclosure of patient health data, though unpopular as applied to some research and public health uses, was justified as protecting patients from unwarranted, and potentially damaging, exchanges of health data. Nineteenth-century codes of medical ethics articulated this theme of self-restriction by medical practitioners. The American Medical Association Code of 1847, based on Percival's code from Britain, followed the tradition of the Hippocratic oath and imposed on physicians an "obligation of secrecy," which required that physicians should divulge "no infirmity or disposition or flaw of character observed during professional attendance . . . except when he is imperatively required to do so."[4]

Even these early, basic statements of medical confidentiality, however, were qualified by the fundamental premise that individual privacy is not absolute. Confidentiality protections of individually identifiable health data must be balanced with communal or other needs for disclosure. Government may need routine access to identifiable health data to promote the public's health, prevent emergencies, investigate criminal actors, or protect individuals from known harms. Justifications for breaching individual expectations of confidentiality have also traditionally included disclosures to researchers. Public and private sector entities have asserted strong claims to identifiable health data to perform clinical and health services research. The need to balance individual and communal interests in health data, explained further below, is one of the key challenges in health information privacy.

By the beginning of the 20th century, ethical conceptions of medical confidentiality were featured more prominently in laws of medicine and practice. One of the primary tenets of individual autonomy in research with humans, informed consent, found meaning beyond consenting to the risks and benefits of the research itself. Informed consent also came to be applied to research participants' authorization to acquire, use, and disclose their identifiable health data as part of research activities.[5] This application of informed consent has been clarified through legal principles. Courts have imposed legal duties of medical confidentiality for decades. After Warren and Brandeis persuasively articulated individual rights to privacy in their famous article *The Right to Privacy*,[6] lawmakers and policy makers focused on privacy as a legal and ethical norm worthy of significant additional protections. Ethicists justified strong respect for data confidentiality through utilitarian and normative principles. Utilitarian arguments centered on the value of confidentiality in facilitating honest communication between doctor and patient, or health researcher and subject. Expectations of privacy allow patients to feel comfortable in divulging personal information that is often needed for accurate diagnosis and treatment. Unauthorized uses or disclosures may subject individuals to embarrassment, social stigma, and discrimination, which consequently impact their health and interfere with the physician's ability to render effective medical care.

The principle of respect for autonomy, a foundational norm in bioethical discourse, contributed to a restructured conception of privacy and its incumbent rights, especially in research settings. Addressing the horrors of medical experimentation during World War II, the Nuremberg Code affirmatively stated the preconditions for, and the condition of, autonomy in the context of medical research[7] (see Chapter 12). In the United States, the Belmont Report, addressing ethical requirements for human subjects research, clarified principles of autonomy: "To respect autonomy is to give weight to autonomous persons' considered opinions and choices, while refraining from obstructing their actions, unless they are clearly detrimental to others"[8] (see Chapter 14). Modern bioethicists defend health information privacy on grounds of respect for persons. According to this reasoning, competent adults have full moral authority to make their own decisions about their physical and mental well-being.[1] Informational privacy enhances individual autonomy by allowing individuals control over identifiable health information. By exercising control, individuals can limit disclosures to persons of their choosing, deciding in effect which disclosures are worth the potential risk of having sensitive information in the possession of various actors.

As they were formalized in ethical and legal discourse, principles of confidentiality evolved to reflect changing conceptions on the proper balance between individual privacy and communal needs for health data. A model social welfare act devised by the U.S. National Social Welfare Assembly in 1958, for example, proposed a balance favoring access to confidential data for research purposes:

> Research by its very nature, often must have access to original material. . . . [Consequently,] undisguised case records may be made available for studies and research activities which seek to advance social work objectives if they are carried out under direction that assures protection of case information.[9]

Over the latter half of the century, however, the powerful rise of autonomy and its concurrent tenet of informed consent reshaped this balance between individual privacy and communal uses of health data for research uses. The World Medical Association's Declaration of Helsinki, which has provided international ethical guidance for human subjects research since 1964, specifically mentions the need to respect subjects' privacy through data confidentiality protections (paragraphs 10 and 21[10]; see Chapter 13). In 2002, the Council for International Organizations of Medical Sciences (CIOMS), in collaboration with the World Health Organization (WHO), noted in its International Ethical Guidelines for Biomedical Research Involving Human Subjects that researchers "must establish secure safeguards of the confidentiality of subjects' research data. Subjects should be told the limits, legal or other, to the investigators' ability to safeguard confidentiality and the possible consequences of breaches of confidentiality"[11] (see Chapter 16). The increasing development of longitudinal electronic health records and their prospective linkage through a national electronic health information infrastructure have heightened individual concerns about the potential for widespread data sharing and unwarranted uses, including unauthorized research. The result is broader requirements for individual authorization for all acquisitions, uses, and disclosures of identifiable health data for research purposes, except in specific circumstances, as noted in sections below.

Core Concepts

Confidentiality, as an ethical and legal principle, is often bundled with conceptions of privacy and security. People tend to think of these concepts interchangeably. They are, however, ethically and legally distinct. *Privacy*, in the context of health care and research, refers broadly to an individual's right to control identifiable health information. (This conception may be contrasted with U.S. constitutional notions of privacy that protect an individual's bodily integrity or interest in making certain types of intimate decisions.) Legal privacy interests, such as those provided in the U.S. Privacy Rule issued under the 1996 Health Insurance Portability and Accountability Act (HIPAA),[12,13] support individual rights to inspect, copy, and amend health data, to limit the acquisitions and uses of health data, and to demand an accounting of disclosures. Additional fair information practices expressed through legal and ethical norms also stem from broad conceptions of privacy. Whereas privacy represents an individual right, confidentiality is the corresponding duty to protect this right. *Confidentiality* comprises those legal and ethical duties that arise in specific relationships, such as doctor/patient or researcher/subject. A physician or researcher's duty to maintain confidentiality, which invokes the "secrecy" aspect of privacy, is one mechanism to protect the individual's broader privacy interests, which also include the individual's right to access or correct his or her own information. *Security* refers to technological or administrative safeguards or tools to protect identifiable health information from unwarranted access or disclosure. Although researchers may work hard to keep confidential the data that they acquire, use, and disclose, privacy breaches can occur if they fail to maintain adequate security protections. These distinct terms are accurately linked in the following statement: "If the *security* safeguards in an automated system fail or are compromised, a breach of *confidentiality* can occur and the *privacy* of data subjects can be invaded [emphasis added]."[14]

Ethical and legal norms of privacy and confidentiality impose standards on the relationship between researchers and their subjects and set requirements for the acquisition, use, and disclosure of identifiable health data for clinical research purposes. In the United States, human subjects research that is conducted or supported by a federal department or agency must comply with a set of regulations designed to protect human subjects—the Federal Policy for the Protection of Human Subjects, known as the "Common Rule"[15] (see Chapter 15). Among other requirements, one of the conditions for approval of research proposals by institutional review boards (IRBs) is that "[w]hen appropriate, there are adequate provisions to protect the privacy of subjects and to maintain the confidentiality of data" (§46.111(a)(7)).[15] Furthermore, the Common Rule requires, in most cases, that investigators obtain the informed consent of research participants, which must include "[a] statement describing the extent, if any, to which confidentiality of records identifying the subject will be maintained" (§46.116(a)(5)).[15]

Federal and state research protections like the Common Rule stipulate the need to protect privacy and confidentiality, but significant gaps in the protection of data of research subjects remain. These laws typically only apply to research conducted or funded by the government, and not to private sector research, although the Common Rule has been widely adopted by private research entities in the United States.[16] The Common Rule also has gaps. It exempts from complying with the full requirements of the regulations several categories of research, including the collection or study of existing data, documents, records, pathological specimens, or diagnostic specimens, if these sources are publicly available or if the data are not individually identifiable (§46.102(b)(4)).[15] Genetic databases are especially problematic because they may be deemed

nonidentifiable even though technological methods can increasingly link genomic data to individuals. Moreover, the Common Rule (1) does not require confidentiality protections in all cases, (2) allows investigators to dispense with protections so long as subjects provide informed consent, (3) fails to explicate further uses of research data, and (4) allows for expedited reviews of several types of research proposals.[16] As a result, considerable variation in IRB reviews leads to inconsistent protection of research participants' privacy.

For example, an investigator may disclose personal data to other researchers for related or nonrelated purposes without violating the Common Rule. If the data are in a format that cannot reasonably identify or be matched with other available information to identify an individual, such disclosures are completely exempt from the Common Rule and the HIPAA Privacy Rule. As a policy matter, the Common Rule allows data to be exchanged like a commodity, without limits, provided they are nonidentifiable. But research participants still may feel that their privacy has been infringed, even if they cannot be personally identified. By itself, the Common Rule thus provides minimal and insufficient protections for the privacy of research subjects' information.[17]

Myriad additional protections are found in U.S. federal and state health information privacy laws, although many commentators view these protections as insufficient to fully protect the privacy of digitized health data within an ever-growing national electronic health information infrastructure. Under Section 242m(d)—a.k.a. section 308(d)—of the U.S. Public Health Service Act,[18] identifiable health information collected by federal public health agencies cannot be used for any purpose other than that for which it was supplied, unless the agency or person has consented. However, under Section 241(d) of the same Act,[18] the Department of Health and Human Services (DHHS) can issue Certificates of Confidentiality that protect research participants from legally compelled, nonconsensual disclosures of any identifiable information, including health data, to persons not connected with the research. This protection is generally sought by researchers for sensitive health data, such as genetic information or data related to sexual practices, to encourage subjects to participate or to provide accurate or complete data. This protection is not limited to federally supported research.[19] IRBs reviewing research proposals regularly recommend that the researcher obtain a Certificate of Confidentiality as part of the IRB approval for the study.

Informed consent requirements, assurances, and Certificates of Confidentiality offer opportunities for respecting the private nature of health data, but collectively lack clarity as to what is ethically and legally required to protect individual privacy. Protecting data privacy is more than an aspirational goal. Fundamental principles of privacy require that responsible persons take action, or avoid mistakes, to ensure that data are kept confidential. The HIPAA Privacy Rule seeks to specify these requirements. Promulgated by DHHS in 2002 and codified at 45 CFR 160[12] and 164,[13] the Privacy Rule provides the first systematic national health information privacy protections in the United States. It governs "covered entities," which include health insurers and health plans, health-care clearinghouses, and health-care providers that conduct transactions electronically, as well as their business associates (§160.103).[12] Notably, covered entities do not include clinical researchers unless they are performing "covered functions" while conducting research. Covered functions are services that assimilate the functions of covered entities. Thus, if a researcher provides clinical care to humans during the course of a study, and bills or conducts other standard transactions electronically for these services, the researcher may be required to adhere to the Privacy Rule. Even if a researcher is not performing covered functions, the Privacy Rule may still affect clinical research activities by limiting the flow of health data from covered entities to researchers.

The Privacy Rule protects most individually identifiable health information created or received in any form by covered entities (§160.103).[12] Protected health information includes individually identifiable data that relate to the past, present, or future physical or mental health or condition of a person, or the provision or payment of health care to a person (§164.501).[13] But protected health information does not include nonidentifiable health information or de-identified data—health statistics or other aggregate data that do not or cannot identify individuals (§164.514(a)(b)).[13] Covered entities, their business associates, and those providing covered functions are responsible for establishing and adhering to a series of privacy protections related to protected health information that reflect modern ethical norms. These include (1) providing notice to individuals regarding their privacy rights and how their protected health information is used or disclosed (§164.520),[13] (2) adopting and implementing internal privacy policies and procedures (§164.530),[13] (3) training employees to understand privacy policies and procedures (§164.530(b)(1)),[13] (4) designating persons who are internally responsible for implementing privacy policies and procedures (§164.530(a)(1)),[13] (5) establishing appropriate administrative, technical, and physical safeguards to protect the privacy of protected health information (§164.530(c)(1)),[13] and (6) helping patients exercise their rights under the Privacy Rule to inspect and request corrections or amendments to their protected health information, or to seek an accounting of certain disclosures (§§164.524, 164.526).[13]

As with any privacy law or policy, the Privacy Rule balances individual and communal interests, most notably through its disclosure provisions. In general, a covered entity may not disclose protected health information without individual written authorization, subject to a series of exceptions (§164.508(a)(1)).[13] Among these exceptions are some disclosures for research. Both the Privacy Rule and the Common Rule define research as "a systematic investigation, including research development, testing, and evaluation, designed to develop or contribute to generalizable knowledge."[13,15] Covered entities can disclose protected health information to others for research without individual authorization, but only under certain limited instances.[13,20] These are the following:

1. *IRB or Privacy Board Approval of Waiver of Written Authorization.* A covered entity may disclose protected health information for research purposes without written authorization if an IRB or a privacy board (a specialized institutional board authorized by the Privacy Rule and constituted of noninterested members with the professional competency to review the effects of research on individual privacy interests, including at least one person who is not affiliated with the covered entity) waives the requirement, based on three criteria: (1) The use or disclosure of protected health information must involve no more than a minimal risk to individual privacy, based on the existence of an adequate plan to protect identifiers from improper use and to destroy the identifiers

at the earliest opportunity, along with written assurances that the data will not be reused or disclosed to any other nonauthorized person or entity; (2) the research could not practicably be conducted without the waiver; and (3) the research could not practicably be conducted without access to and use of protected health information (§164.512(i)(1)(i)).[13] These criteria are very similar to the requirements for waiving informed consent under the Common Rule.[21]

2. *Preparatory to Research.* A researcher can review protected information to design a research study or assess its feasibility without written authorizations, if the researcher represents to the covered entity that the disclosure is needed to prepare a research protocol or for similar purposes preparatory to research, that the protected health information will not be removed from the covered entity, and that the protected health information is necessary for the research (§164.512(i)(1)(ii)).[13]

3. *Research Using Decedents' Protected Health Information.* A researcher may acquire protected information about deceased individuals if the researcher represents to the covered entity that the disclosure is solely for research on decedents' information, that the information is necessary for the research, and, if requested, provides documentation of the death of the individuals about whom information is being sought (§164.512(i)(1)(iii)).[13]

4. *Limited Data Sets With a Data Use Agreement.* A covered entity may disclose a limited data set of protected health information if it obtains a data use agreement from the researcher assuring that the data will only be used or disclosed for the limited purposes authorized by the agreement (§164.514(e)).[13] Limited data sets exclude specified individual identifiers from the health data disclosed. Data use agreements establish permitted uses and disclosures of the limited data set by the recipient consistent with the purposes of the research.

Thus, the Privacy Rule typically requires advance, written authorization of each individual whose identifiable health data are acquired or used in research, unless a researcher can obtain a waiver of authorization, is performing activities preparatory to research, is using decedents' health information, is willing to work with stripped data in a limited data set, or uses nonidentifiable data. Though similar requirements may arise under the Common Rule, the Privacy Rule's protections extend farther. The Privacy Rule applies to virtually all producers of identifiable health data in public or private sectors. Its ability to impose disclosure restrictions on covered entities for research purposes may enhance individual privacy interests, but it has also led to some deleterious results. Covered entities complain that the Privacy Rule's requirements place financial, time, and human resources burdens on them. Facing the costly need to secure specific written authorization for many acquisitions of health data, some researchers have abandoned or curtailed their research plans.[22] Some types of research may be particularly hampered by Privacy Rule requirements because they cannot utilize nonidentifiable data. For example, a study to assess determinants of cancer or other chronic diseases may collect a wide array of information from the review of hospital records including other diagnoses, birth dates, place of residence, family history, DNA, and environmental or behavioral factors over several years. Identifiers are essential to follow-up with participants throughout the study.

To circumvent the Privacy Rule in other cases, activities that have previously been considered human subjects research may increasingly be categorized by investigators and IRBs as public health practice activities. For example, if research is classified as a program evaluation, a quality improvement exercise, public health surveillance, or an epidemiological investigation, disclosures may be allowed under Privacy Rule without written authorization, and the Common Rule would not apply. Although it is difficult to disguise a clinical trial involving living human subjects as one of these public health activities, some research activities involving only data or biological samples can more closely resemble nonresearch public health activities. The Privacy Rule allows more liberal data exchanges for public health purposes, therefore providing incentives for classifying data uses as public health activities.[23]

Ethical Issues

Despite its risks, there is little doubt as to the importance of clinical research in the modern health and public health systems. Biomedical research on the determinants, prevalence, prevention, and treatment of diseases and injuries advances clinical care and the public's health.[24] Expansive electronic health care databases can facilitate research studies.[25] Small- and large-scale clinical trials offer opportunities to uncover promising new treatments, to study the safety and efficacy of pharmaceuticals and vaccines, or to improve the quality of health-care services. These studies, however, require the exchange of enormous amounts of health information related to health outcomes, existing conditions, and individual behaviors and characteristics.

The quintessential ethical question bridging historic and current confidentiality protections is how to properly balance individual privacy interests and communal research needs.[3] It is a debate that requires difficult choices and trade-offs. If societal restrictions on the use of identifiable health data are too severe, research may be curtailed. If sensitive health data are too easily acquired, used, or disclosed, individual privacy is threatened. People will then avoid some clinical care and research studies, again hampering research.

Some commentators believe that modern privacy protections go too far in protecting data confidentiality, threatening the accuracy and use of health information for medical research. Privacy protections that allow consumers to restrict the flow of their data through requirements for informed consent or advance authorization may hinder the collection of comprehensive and accurate information that may benefit health consumers.[26] Congress and some state legislatures, for example, have attempted to protect the privacy of genetic information by giving individuals proprietary interests in their genetic information.[27] Vested with property rights, individuals could seek even greater control over how these data are used, including for clinical research.

Other privacy laws that require specific written authorization of research subjects in many cases, such as the HIPAA Privacy Rule, can stymie clinical research while offering few benefits for research participants.[28] Responding to public pressure for rigorous privacy protection, Minnesota enacted legislation in the late 1990s that restricts access to medical records for research purposes. The law requires advance, written informed consent of patients for health records to be used for medical research. After the law was implemented, the Mayo Clinic in Minneapolis reported that 96% of patients contacted for the purposes of ob-

taining informed consent agreed to allow their medical information to be released to researchers. This response rate suggests that most people receiving medical care are willing to allow their information to be used for medical research and that the Minnesota provisions are unnecessary.[29]

Policy Implications

The ethical and legal debate concerning appropriate acquisition, use, and disclosure of identifiable health data for clinical research is not over. Significant policy choices must still be made as the environment for information practices continues to evolve from paper-based records to electronic, from mostly local sources of data to regional, national, and international health databases, and from societal perspectives that focus on the autonomy of the individual to a focus on the protection of communal health. We suggest that rules for balancing private and public interests in identifiable health data should go beyond the conception of individual autonomy as a dominating factor.[30] Privacy interests should be maximized when they matter most to the individual. Communal interests in the exchange of identifiable health data should be maximized when they are likely to achieve the greatest public good. For example, population-based registries of genetic data are critical to assessing the clinical validity and usefulness of new genetic tests.[31] Thus, where the potential for public benefit is high and the risk of harm to individuals is low, health data should be usable for communal purposes. Privacy rules should not be so arduous and inflexible that they significantly impede, for example, clinical research or public health surveillance that is necessary to promote the community's health. Provided that the data are used only for the public good and that the potential for harmful disclosures is negligible—because researchers respect the confidentiality of the data in their possession—there are ethically sound and practical reasons for permitting data sharing.

If, however, identifiable data are used or disclosed in ways that are unlikely to achieve a strong public benefit (such as testing a protocol that has already been shown to be ineffective), or if the personal risks are high (if, for example, the data may be used to discriminate against high-risk individuals in employment or insurance), individual interests in autonomy should prevail. Disclosure of identifiable health data to family, friends, neighbors, employers, insurers, or others can cause stigma, embarrassment, and discrimination. Such unauthorized disclosures can lead to a loss of patient trust in health care and research professionals, as well as other potential harms. Consequently, when the public benefits are negligible and individual privacy risks are high, release of information without the patient's consent should be prohibited.

Like the Privacy Rule, this framework rejects the use of enhanced legal or ethical protections for exceptional or sensitive health data. Absent an overriding public benefit, all individually identifiable health data warrant privacy protections. Correspondingly, acquisition, use, or disclosure of health information for important public purposes would be permitted without specific informed consent provided that (1) uses are restricted to the purposes for which the data are collected, and (2) subsequent disclosures for other purposes are prohibited without authorization by the individual involved. Acquisition, use, or disclosure of health information that can lead to harm would be subject to strict privacy protections. Although adherence to this balancing test may entail some diminution in current conceptions of autonomy, it offers individuals greater benefits from the communal goods offered by clinical research, public health, and other enterprises.

Study Design Implications

The modern ethical and legal frameworks for protecting confidentiality in the performance of clinical research have several implications for the ethical design of research studies. Investigators may have to adhere to national privacy standards in the performance of clinical care activities as part of the study itself if they are a covered entity or otherwise performing covered functions. For any study involving the acquisition, use, or disclosure of identifiable health data, investigators must be able to build confidentiality protections into their study design. These protections include sufficient language within informed consent documents to specify the nature of confidentiality protections. Alternatively, investigators may seek to acquire health data without either informed consent under the Common Rule or written authorization under the Privacy Rule, pursuant to a waiver under these laws and similar state protections. To do so, however, they generally must demonstrate that the use or disclosure of protected health information involves no more than a minimal risk to individuals or their privacy, consistent with suitable, written plans for protecting data confidentiality, and that the research could not practicably be conducted without the waiver or access to identifiable health data. Other exceptions apply as discussed above.

Collectively, these exceptions are meant to set a high standard for the unauthorized access, use, or disclosure of identifiable health data. By default, investigators must be cognizant of the need to seek full informed consent and written authorization from research participants prior to the use of their identifiable health data for research purposes. This requires development of sound, IRB-approved consent documents that spell out in detail the confidentiality protections inherent in the study design and implementation.

Of course, investigators can always use nonidentifiable health information for any research purpose without advance consent or authorization. Ethical and legal norms almost universally allow researchers, or anyone for that matter, to exchange nonidentifiable health data. Under existing standards of what constitutes nonidentifiable health data within the Privacy Rule and the Common Rule, however, these data may be so stripped of helpful information as to be unusable. Nonidentifiable data under the Privacy Rule, for example, are aggregate health statistics or any other collection of health information that does not—or cannot when coupled with other accessible information—identify the individuals to whom it pertains. Realistically, researchers need identifiable data to perform meaningful research, and thus must be prepared to adhere to ethical, legal, and societal expectations of confidentiality that accompany these data.

Unresolved Ethical Issues and Data Requirements

Considerable ethical debate remains over several important questions, including the scope of confidentiality protections, the treatment of group privacy interests, and the difference between research and public health activities.

The Scope of Confidentiality Protections

At the macro level, the proper balance between individual privacy interests and communal needs for data is still unresolved. Uncertainty also exists on a micro level as to the extent of privacy protections needed for research data. Current legal frameworks give investigators substantial discretion to design appropriate protections, allow individuals to dispense with these protections through informed consent, and limit the responsibility of those supplying health data, such as covered entities under HIPAA, to assessing the legality and ethicality of the initial disclosure of data to researchers. There is still no uniform approach as to how to protect the privacy of health data used by clinical researchers. What has yet to be proposed is a data use policy that attaches privacy protections to health data no matter what its use, disclosure, or setting. The Privacy Rule goes far in applying legal and ethical privacy standards to most entities that produce or transmit identifiable health data, but its protections do not fully carry over to research settings. Covered entities are not responsible per se for what happens to health data in the possession of researchers. Researchers who are not performing covered functions do not have to adhere to the Privacy Rule.

Perhaps some flexibility in data confidentiality practices is necessary, given the breadth of clinical research applications and significant variance in health data. Do we as a society need to protect the confidentiality of mental health records or genetic data used in research to the same extent as clinical indicators of heart disease? Many may respond, "No," although the trend in privacy discourse is to attempt to protect all health data in particular settings uniformly. Participants in nonexempted research studies have the ability to determine their comfort level with confidentiality protections through informed consent requirements. Still, a vast amount of research does not require specific informed consent, nor does everyone who participates in research studies know or understand the nature of confidentiality protections. Principles of justice suggest a need to equalize privacy protections across the spectrum of research data uses.

Group Privacy Interests

Justice also requires an examination of privacy interests of individuals in clinical research, not merely as research participants, but also as members of vulnerable groups whose interests may be affected by the results of the study. Since the early 1990s, public and private researchers have increasingly targeted communities or other definable groups for clinical research into the etiology, especially genetic factors, of multiple diseases and conditions.[32,33] Communities selected for genetic research include specific ethnic groups such as the Kahnawake Mohawks in Canada,[34] religious groups such as the Amish, disease groups such as people with Huntington's disease or diabetes, and even entire nations with homogeneous populations, such as Iceland.[35] Genetic research among targeted groups offers significant individual (clinical) and societal (public health) benefits by revealing propensities for genetic diseases among segments of the population. For example, particular genetic mutations predisposing to breast or ovarian cancer have been identified through studies involving Ashkenazi Jews.[36] With knowledge of these propensities, members of this group may seek individualized genetic testing, and, if positive, utilize environmental or clinical interventions to potentially avoid the onset of disease.

The proliferation of group genetic research, however, raises questions as to whether other members of identifiable groups, in addition to those who choose to participate in group research studies, are entitled to some level of control over research activities to protect themselves from stigmatization, discrimination, or other negative consequences. Nonparticipatory group members may have ethical claims, similar to privacy interests that might justify requiring informed consent. Some scholars suggest that these interests are more appropriately framed in terms of justice;[37] others disagree on the need for group protections through consent.[38] The fundamental interests of nonparticipating community members regarding information produced through group research studies may lie in control over how information is used or disclosed through group research.

Acknowledging the need for group privacy protections is simple; protecting nonparticipatory members of groups without significantly infringing on the rights of others is complicated. What level of control should group members have over potential or actual information produced from genetic studies? Who should speak for identifiable groups—group leaders, activists, experts, or laypersons? For that matter, who constitutes an identifiable group entitled to privacy protections? Although some legal and ethical scholars, researchers, and human rights committees have proposed that group privacy protections are based on a principle of "respect for communities,"[39] formal protections are largely nonexistent. Additional discussions are needed to determine when, or whether, investigators have an ethical or legal obligation to respect group privacy interests in the performance of some clinical studies.

Distinguishing Research and Public Health Practice

One of the core premises of confidentiality protections under any standard of law or ethics is that disclosures or uses for research purposes should be made under clearly defined standards. Practical application of this premise, however, is seriously flawed due to the absence of specific legal distinctions and uncertainty over how to distinguish research and nonresearch. The Common Rule and the Privacy Rule systematically require investigators and data handlers to distinguish human subjects research activities from clinical care and public health practice. Yet, neither rule provides meaningful guidance on what distinguishes research from other activities, particularly public health practice, that often resemble research. Legislators, policy makers, scholars, ethicists, researchers, IRB members, and public health practitioners struggle to draw these distinctions, resulting in confusion, inconsistent applications, and potential breaches of confidentiality arising from poor, improper, and even unethical decisions. It is unethical, for example, to systematically collect identifiable health data under the guise of a public health purpose, only to use the data for human subjects research. Yet, this scenario is entirely possible under the Privacy Rule, as discussed above.

Other scenarios may not be unethical, but may still pose challenges to practitioners assessing the legal requirements for their

activity. For example, an acute epidemiological investigation of airline passengers possibly exposed to the SARS virus may be viewed as a quintessential public health activity necessary to protect their and their contacts' health. Yet if the investigation continues to collect data from asymptomatic passengers after incubation periods have expired, the data collection serves no health purpose for those individuals, though it may help public health officials assess important characteristics about the disease. Public health practitioners at the federal, state, and local levels have struggled with these and other examples to determine whether their activities are public health practice or research (see Chapter 31).

We and others have attempted to provide improved guidance on the need to make clearer distinctions between human subjects research and public health practice activities.[23] Researchers, practitioners, IRB board members, and others, for example, may confuse public health surveillance activities and human subjects research in which both activities involve the systematic acquisition and use of identifiable health data for laudable communal purposes. We propose a two-stage framework for classifying these activities. The first stage draws on key assumptions and foundations of public health practice and research to distinguish these activities in relatively easy cases by reviewing those parameters that are exclusive to each activity. Eliciting essential characteristics, or foundations, of public health practice and research helps separate the easy and hard cases, and eliminates some cases altogether from further need for classification. Essential characteristics of public health practice (i.e., the collection and analysis of identifiable health data by a public health authority for the purpose of protecting the health of a particular community, in which the benefits and risks are primarily designed to accrue to the participating community), include the following:

- Specific legal authorization for conducting the activity as public health practice at the federal, state, or local level.
- A governmental duty to perform the activity to protect the public's health.
- Direct performance or oversight by a governmental public health authority (or its authorized partner) and accountability to the public for its performance.
- Involvement of people who did not specifically volunteer to participate (i.e., they did not provide informed consent).
- Adherence to principles of public health ethics that focus on populations while respecting the dignity and rights of individuals.

Essential characteristics of human subjects research (i.e., the collection and analysis of identifiable health data for the purpose of generating knowledge that will benefit those beyond the participating community who bear the risks of participation) include the following:

- The subjects of the research are living individuals.
- Identifiable private health information is gathered and produced.
- Research subjects participate voluntarily, or participate with the consent of a guardian, absent a waiver of informed consent.
- The researchers adhere to principles of bioethics that focus on the interests of individuals while balancing the communal value of research.

These characteristics help distinguish public health practice from research in many of the easy cases. For example, a public health reporting requirement may be specifically authorized via legislation or administrative regulation. Laws may require the public health agency to perform the activity to protect the public's health. Some states, like New York, clarify by statute that epidemiological investigations or other common public health practices are not human subjects research.[40] These activities are public health practice so long as their design and implementation do not cross over to the realm of research. As well, if an activity may lawfully require the nonvoluntary compliance of autonomous individuals, it is likely not classifiable as research because voluntary consent is a foundation of research. Only through the waiver of the consent requirement—which requires regulatory approval—may persons participate in human subject research without providing specific informed consent. Furthermore, if an activity is designed as research but does not involve identifiable health data about living individuals, it should not be included in this analysis because it does not implicate the Privacy Rule.

The second stage of analysis introduces and explains enhanced principles of guidance to draw distinctions in more difficult cases. These principles include the following:

1. *General Legal Authority.* Public health authorities may conduct activities pursuant to general legal authorization, which may justify classifying an activity as public health practice subject to additional analysis.
2. *Specific Intent.* The intent of human subjects research is to test a hypothesis and generalize findings or acquired knowledge beyond the activity's participants. Conversely, the intent underlying public health practice is to assure the conditions in which people can be healthy through public health efforts that are primarily aimed at preventing known or suspected injuries and diseases or promoting the health of a particular community.
3. *Responsibility.* Responsibility for the health, safety, and welfare of human participants in research falls upon a specific individual, typically the principal investigator. Public health practice, however, does not always vest responsibility for participants' welfare in individuals, but rather in government agencies or authorized partner entities.
4. *Participant Benefits.* Public health practice should contribute to improving the health of participants and populations. In contrast, research may, but does not necessarily, provide benefits to participants. Such is the nature of risk in research studies.
5. *Experimentation.* Research may involve introducing something nonstandard or experimental to human subjects or their identifiable health data. Public health practice is dominated by the use of standard, accepted, and proven interventions to address known or suspected public health problems.
6. *Participant Selection.* To reduce the possibility of bias in their studies, and to generalize their results, researchers may select humans for research at random. Participants in public health practice activities are self-selected persons with, or at risk of, an affected disease or condition who can benefit from the activity.

No set of principles will completely distinguish between human subjects research, public health practice, or other related activities. There will always be difficult examples of activities that do not fit neatly into either category. However, these principles may help resolve a majority of cases, provide consistency in decision making on a national basis, and help shape the level of confidentiality protections in research settings. It will remain important for public health authorities to follow ethical guidelines for data uses that do not fall within the Common Rule. The Centers for Disease Control and Prevention (CDC) is preparing additional ethical guidance for public health data uses outside of the research context.[41]

Conclusion

Health information privacy and confidentiality are vital to the legal and ethical performance of human subjects research. Research subjects expect that their identifiable health data will be kept confidential and that their use or disclosure will be limited to the purpose of the research. Theories of confidentiality and privacy are pervasive throughout the histories of medical ethics, human rights, and law. Modern conceptions of privacy support strong respect for the autonomy of individuals participating in research studies, offering significant protections for identifiable health data used in research studies and other settings. These protections, which continue to evolve, impact the design and performance of research studies by limiting some access to existing health databases, requiring specific written authorization (in many cases) of subjects to use their data for research purposes, and necessitating secure information practices to prevent breaches of confidentiality. Although modern protections clarify the privacy of research participants' data, additional challenges remain. Existing privacy laws do not protect research data uniformly. The focus of protections on individuals, but not the groups of which they are members, leads to infringements of group privacy. Conceptual difficulty in distinguishing research from public health activities creates significant potential for privacy violations. Addressing these and other challenges is essential to the performance of clinical research under ethical and legal norms that reflect responsible and dignified research data uses.

Acknowledgment

The authors thank Erin Fuse Brown, J.D., M.P.H., for her scholarly and research assistance on this chapter.

References

1. Beauchamp TL, Childress JF. *Principles of Biomedical Ethics*, 4th ed. New York, N.Y.: Oxford University Press; 1994.
2. Edelstein L. *The Hippocratic Oath: Text, Translation, and Interpretation.* Baltimore, Md.: Johns Hopkins Press; 1943.
3. Hodge JG, Gostin KG. Challenging themes in American health information privacy and the public's health: Historical and modern assessments. *Journal of Law, Medicine, and Ethics* 2005;32:670–9.
4. American Medical Association. *Code of Medical Ethics of the American Medical Association.* Chicago, Ill.: AMA Press; 1847. Chapter 1, Art. 1, § 2. [Online] Available: http://www.ama-assn.org/ama/upload/mm/369/1847code.pdf.
5. Faden RR, Beauchamp TL, with King NMP. *A History and Theory of Informed Consent.* New York, N.Y.: Oxford University Press; 1986.

6. Breckenridge AC. The right to privacy. In: Warren SD, Brandeis LD, eds. *The Right to Privacy.* Lincoln, Neb.: University of Nebraska Press; 1970.

7. The Nuremberg Code. In: *Trials of War Criminals Before the Nuremberg Military Tribunals Under Control Council Law No. 10. Volume 2.* Washington, D.C.: U.S. Government Printing Office; 1949: 181–2. [Online]. Available: http://www.hhs.gov/ohrp/references/nurcode.htm.

8. The National Commission for the Protection of Human Subjects of Biomedical and Behavioral Research. *The Belmont Report: Ethical Principles and Guidelines for the Protection of Human Subjects of Research.* Washington, D.C.: Department of Health, Education and Welfare; 1979. [Online] April 18, 1979. Available: http://www.hhs.gov/ohrp/humansubjects/guidance/belmont.htm.

9. National Social Welfare Assembly, Committee on Confidentiality. *Confidentiality in Social Services to Individuals: An Examination of Basic Concepts and Everyday Practices, With Suggestions for Overcoming Current Problems.* New York, N.Y.: National Social Welfare Assembly; 1958.

10. World Medical Association. *Declaration of Helsinki: Ethical Principles for Medical Research Involving Human Subjects.* Tokyo, Japan: WMA; October 2004. [Online] 2004. Available: http://www.wma.net/e/policy/b3.htm.

11. Council for International Organizations of Medical Sciences, in collaboration with the World Health Organization. *International Ethical Guidelines for Biomedical Research Involving Human Subjects.* Geneva, Switzerland: CIOMS and WHO; 2002. [Online] November 2002. Available: http://www.cioms.ch/frame_guidelines_nov_2002.htm.

12. Department of Health and Human Services, Office for Civil Rights. Standards for Privacy of Individually Identifiable Health Information, Title 45 (Public Welfare), Code of Federal Regulations, Part 160 (General Administrative Requirements). [Online] October 1, 2002. Available: http://www.access.gpo.gov/nara/cfr/waisidx_02/45cfr160_02.html.

13. Department of Health and Human Services, Office for Civil Rights. Standards for Privacy of Individually Identifiable Health Information, Title 45 (Public Welfare), Code of Federal Regulations, Part 164 (Security and Privacy). [Online] October 1, 2003. Available: http://www.access.gpo.gov/nara/cfr/waisidx_03/45cfr164_03.html.

14. Ware W. Lessons for the future: Dimensions of medical record keeping. In: Task Force on Privacy, Department of Health and Human Services. Health Records: Social Needs and Personal Privacy. Conference Proceedings, Washington, D.C.; February 11–12, 1993. [Online] Available: http://aspe.hhs.gov/pic/reports/ahrq/4441.pdf.

15. Department of Health and Human Services, National Institutes of Health, and Office for Human Research Protections. The Common Rule, Title 45 (Public Welfare), Code of Federal Regulations, Part 46 (Protection of Human Subjects). [Online] June 23, 2005. Available: http://www.hhs.gov/ohrp/humansubjects/guidance/45cfr46.htm.

16. General Accounting Office. *Medical Records Privacy: Access Needed for Health Research, but Oversight of Privacy Protections Is Limited.* Report to Congressional Requesters. GAO/HEHS-99-55. Washington, D.C.: GAO; 1999. [Online] February, 1999. Available: http://www.gao.gov/archive/1999/he99055.pdf.

17. Gostin L. Health information privacy. *Cornell Law Review* 1995;80;451–528.

18. Public Health Service Act. Title 42, United States Code, Chapter 6a—Public Health Service. [Online] January 5, 1999. Available: http://www.fda.gov/opacom/laws/phsvcact/phsvcact.htm.

19. Office for Human Research Protections, Department of Health and Human Services. *Guidance on Certificates of Confidentiality.* Washington, D.C.: DHHS; 2003. [Online] February 25, 2003. Available: www.hhs.gov/ohrp/humansubjects/guidance/certconf.htm.

20. Department of Health and Human Services, Office for Civil Rights. HIPAA Privacy Guidelines Guidance re: Research. [Online] April 3, 2003. Available: http://www.hhs.gov/ocr/hipaa/guidelines/research.rtf.

21. Rivara FP. Research and human subjects. *Archives of Pediatric and Adolescent Medicine* 2002;156:641–2.

22. Government Accountability Office. *Health Information Privacy: First-Year Experiences Under the Federal Privacy Rule.* Report to the Chairman, Committee on Health, Education, Labor, and Pensions U.S. Senate. GAO-04–965. Washington, D.C.: GAO; 2004. [Online] September 2004. Available: http://www.gao.gov/new.items/d04965.pdf.

23. Hodge JG, Gostin LO, with the Council of State and Territorial Epidemiologists Advisory Committee. *Public Health Practice vs. Research: A Report for Public Health Practitioners Including Cases and Guidance for Making Distinctions.* [Online] May 24, 2004. Available: http://www.cste.org/pdffiles/newpdffiles/cstephresrpthodgefinal.5.24.04.pdf.

24. Roper WL, et al. Effectiveness in health care: An initiative to evaluate and improve medical practice. *New England Journal of Medicine* 1988;318:1197–202.

25. Committee on Regional Health Data Networks, Institute of Medicine. *Health Data in the Information Age: Use, Disclosure, and Privacy.* Washington, D.C.: National Academy Press; 1994.

26. Sharrott D. Provider-specific quality-of-care data: A proposal for limited mandatory disclosure. *Brooklyn Law Review* 1992;58:85–150.

27. Gostin LO, Hodge JG, Calvo CM. *Genetics Law and Policy: A Report for Policymakers.* Denver, Colo.: National Conference of State Legislatures; 2001.

28. Annas GJ. Medical privacy and medical research—Judging the new federal regulations. *New England Journal of Medicine* 2002;346:216–20.

29. Melton LJ, III. The threat to medical-records research. *New England Journal of Medicine* 1997;337:1466–70.

30. Gostin LO, Hodge JG. Personal privacy and common goods: A framework for balancing under the national health information privacy rule. *Minnesota Law Review* 2002;6:1439–80.

31. Gwinn M, Khoury MJ. Research priorities for public health sciences in the post-genomic era. *Genetics in Medicine* 2002;4:410–1.

32. Nysteun A, et al. A cerebellar ataxia locus identified by DNA pooling to search for linkage disequilibrium in an isolated population from the Cayman Islands. *Human Molecular Genetics* 1996;5:525–31.

33. Escamillam M, et al. Use of linkage disequilibrium approaches to map genes for bipolar disorder in the Costa Rican population. *American Journal of Medical Genetics* 1996;67:244–53.

34. Macaulay AC, et al. Participatory research with native community of Kahnawake creates innovative code of research ethics. *Canadian Journal of Public Health* 1998;89:105–8.

35. Jonatansson H. Iceland's health sector database: A significant head start in the search for the biological grail or an irreversible error? *American Journal of Law and Medicine* 2000;26:31–67.

36. Streuwing JP, et al. The carrier frequency of the BRCA1 185 delAG mutation is approximately 1 percent in Ashkenazi Jewish individuals. *Nature Genetics* 1995;11:198–200.

37. Powers M. Justice and genetics: Privacy protection and the moral basis of public policy. In: Rothstein MA, ed. *Genetic Secrets.* New Haven, Conn.: Yale University Press; 1997.

38. Juengst ET. Groups as gatekeepers to genomic research: Conceptually confusing, morally hazardous, and practically useless. *Kennedy Institute of Ethics Journal* 1998;8:183–200.

39. Hodge JG, Harris ME. International genetics research and issues of group privacy. *Journal of Biolaw and Business* 2001;4(Annual Suppl.):15–21.

40. New York Public Health Law, Article 24-A, Protection of Human Subjects, §2441(2), Definitions (McKinney 2002). [Online] Available: http://public.leginfo.state.ny.us/menuf.cgi.

41. Fairchild A, et al. Public health data uses project: Ethical guidelines. Unpublished manuscript.

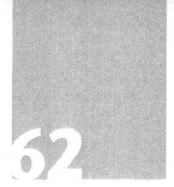

Wendy K. Mariner

Liability and Compensation for Injury of Research Subjects

Most clinical research with human subjects takes place out of public view without complaint or controversy. Yet the legal history of biomedical research highlights the occasional shocking catastrophe.[1,2] Scandals in particular periodically rouse public outrage, recommendations for law reform, and lawsuits, which refine the legal principles governing research. More than 30 years ago, revelations of the Tuskegee Syphilis study led to the adoption of federal regulations to protect research subjects in federally funded research.[3] More recently, the deaths of research subjects at renowned academic research institutions,[4,5] most famously that of 18-year-old Jesse Gelsinger at the University of Pennsylvania in 1999,[6] revived calls for reform.[7-11] So far, neither the legislation nor regulations governing research with human subjects has changed significantly, perhaps because public attention was diverted in the aftermath of September 11, 2001. However, lawsuits against researchers may have gained more visibility, both applying and refining fundamental legal principles.[12]

This chapter describes the major laws that define researchers' liability for harm to research subjects. Section 1 offers a thumbnail description of the sources of law governing clinical research. Sections 2 and 3 summarize the most important rights of research subjects and duties of investigators and the types of cases that have been adjudicated, noting areas of uncertainty that may encourage future legal claims and possible evolution in the law. Section 2 focuses on the subject's consent to participate in research and research with individuals who cannot or do not consent. Section 3 examines issues in the conduct of clinical trials. Section 4 notes the difficulty of determining the number and proportion of injuries experienced by research subjects, practical obstacles and defenses

to legal claims, and alternative ways to redress harm and compensate injured research subjects.

1. The Development and Sources of Law

All researchers are legally responsible to those enrolled in their clinical trials, just as physicians have been legally responsible to patients under their care for centuries.[13] Physicians have a duty to provide their patients with reasonable care in almost every type of legal system.[14] The Code of Hammurabi imposed penalties on physicians who failed to cure their patients 4,000 years ago, with the penalty increasing with the patient's status.[15] The American colonies brought English common law from England,[16] where court decisions finding that a physician could be liable for negligent harm to a patient were reported as early as 1374.[17] Historically, physicians who used experimental procedures were subject to malpractice liability for failing to employ accepted medical therapy.[18] Researchers have somewhat different duties than physicians, because research is not considered part of patient care, and researchers expose humans to investigational therapies and interventions that have not yet proved to be effective.

In the United States, the legal principles governing the rights of research subjects and the duties of physicians and researchers to research subjects are grounded primarily in the common law, or case law—the statements of rights and duties expressed in judicial opinions deciding specific lawsuits.[13] Legislation and regulations rarely addressed research until after World War II, when pharmacology and clinical trial methods began their modern development, and even then did not grant remedies to subjects.

The Nuremberg Code, which set forth 10 principles for research with humans, was the first international declaration of research ethics.[19] It qualifies as precedent under international common law, because it was part of the 1947 judgment issued by American judges in the tribunal established by the United States Military Government for Germany after World War II.[20] The Nazi physicians were convicted of crimes against humanity, including murder and torture, accomplished in the guise of medical experiments.[21-22] In the 1987 U.S. Supreme Court decision in *Stanley* v. *United States,* Justices William J. Brennan Jr. and Sandra Day O'Connor argued in dissenting opinions that subjecting people to experimentation without their knowledge or consent may violate a constitutional right to human dignity like that expressed in the Nuremberg Code.[23] Courts in the United States have not yet recognized such a specific constitutional right to human dignity and only recently have any courts applied the Nuremberg Code as precedent in American law.[24-26] The substance of the Code's principles, however, have been incorporated into statutes, regulations, and common law.[27] More recently, plaintiffs have used the Code's principles to support their claims, and some courts, even when declining to use the Code as precedent, have acknowledged its influence in what may be a harbinger of future application.[28-35]

The Declaration of Helsinki prescribes more detailed ethical standards for clinical research, and specifies in Article 5 that "[i]n medical research on human subjects, considerations related to the well-being of the human subject should take precedence over the interests of science and society."[36] Article 15 states, "The responsibility for the human subject must always rest with a medically qualified person and never rest on the subject of the research, even though the subject has given consent." The Declaration does not impose legal obligations, because it was adopted not by a legislature or court of law but by a private association of physicians as a statement of professional ethics.[37] Still, it may serve as evidence of minimum professional standards in legal determinations of the applicable standard of care. The same is true of the International Ethical Guidelines for Biomedical Research Involving Human Subjects, issued by the Council for International Organizations of Medical Sciences (CIOMS) in collaboration with the World Health Organization (WHO).[38] Despite physicians' widespread acceptance of both documents as more modern statements of research ethics, they are likely to remain a floor, not a ceiling, for legal duties, because courts are free to find that a professional standard is too low. Judge Learned Hand gave the classic statement of that principle in 1932, saying that

> in most cases reasonable prudence is in fact common prudence; but strictly it is never its measure; a whole calling may have unduly lagged in the adoption of new and available devices. It may never set its own tests, however persuasive be its usages. Courts must in the end say what is required; there are precautions so imperative that even their universal disregard will not excuse their omission.[39]

The Universal Declaration of Human Rights, adopted by the General Assembly of the United Nations in 1948, contains very general principles prohibiting "torture and cruel, inhuman or degrading treatment or punishment."[40] The International Covenant on Civil and Political Rights, adopted in 1966, contains a similar prohibition in Article 7, which also adds, "In particular, no one shall be subjected without his free consent to medical or scientific experimentation."[41] The United States is a signatory to both documents. U.S. companies sponsoring pharmaceutical research with humans may need to comply with international and regional conventions and guidelines on clinical research to obtain licensure of their products in signatory countries. For example, the Note for Guidelines on Good Clinical Practice (ICH/GCP Guidelines), issued following the International Conference on Harmonisation of Technical Requirements for the Registration of Pharmaceuticals for Human Use (ICH), requires that research sponsors provide insurance or indemnify investigators against claims arising from clinical trials.[42]

In the United States, formal regulations to supplement the common law were not adopted until the late 1970s after revelations of research with humans without their consent,[43] specifically the Tuskegee Syphilis Study,[3,44] which first prompted the study of ethical conduct of research by the National Commission for the Protection of Human Subjects of Biomedical and Behavioral Research.45[45] The National Commission's 1978 *Belmont Report* and recommendations[46] led to the promulgation of federal regulations, currently harmonized in the Common Rule, which apply to research with humans funded by or submitted to more than 20 federal departments and agencies, including, most recently the Department of Homeland Security.[47] Additional regulations followed from the work of the President's Commission for the Study of Ethical Problems in Medicine and Biomedical and Behavioral Research.[48]

The Common Rule requires an institution conducting research with humans to enter into an assurance agreement with the federal agency that it will comply with the regulations, including maintaining an institutional review board (IRB) to review and approve its research.[49] Although the Common Rule incorporates some basic common law requirements, such as informed consent to research, it does not preempt state, federal, or constitutional law.[50] Moreover, it does not grant individuals a personal remedy, such as compensation for injury, against researchers who violate the regulations.[51-52] Instead, the Office for Human Research Protections (OHRP) in the Department of Health and Human Services enforces compliance by suspending or terminating federal funding for an institution that fails to comply with the regulations. Courts have rejected a claim by research subjects that they were third party beneficiaries of an institution's general assurance and found that the regulations do not specifically authorize research subjects to enforce the contract.[53-54] Research subjects who seek a personal remedy must qualify under an independent common law or statutory rule. Some states have legislation regulating specific types of research, such as laws limiting research with fetuses, stem cells, or hazardous materials.[55-56] Such laws typically vest enforcement with a state agency and rarely grant a private right of action. In some cases, however, one who is injured may use the statute as evidence of the standard of care that an investigator should have followed.[57]

Despite periodic calls for reform, the law governing research with humans has changed little since the Common Rule regulations were first adopted almost 30 years ago. In contrast, the common law continues to evolve in response to new cases. Like state statutes, the Common Rule can be used as evidence of the standard of care accepted by investigators, but it does not exhaust the duties of researchers nor define the rights of research subjects themselves. Indeed, the Common Rule applies to institutions, not individual researchers, and does not apply to all research. Thus, the common law remains the primary source of rights and remedies for individuals who are injured while participating in research.[13]

2. Rights and Remedies for Research Subjects in the United States: Voluntary and Informed Consent

Unlike the Common Rule, which was adopted specifically to regulate certain research with humans, liability for injury is governed by generally applicable legal principles that apply to all individuals and organizations. The common law of torts is the primary source of researcher's duties, although the common law of contracts may apply in rare circumstances, and constitutional law may protect important liberty rights of research subjects.

Researchers who conduct clinical trials have three general types of duties to subjects: the duty to ensure that the trial itself is justified; the duty to ensure that the person participates voluntarily; and the duty to carry out the trial with reasonable care.[13] More specifically, under common law, researchers have the following duties:

- Determine that the research question to be answered is sufficiently important to justify the use of humans as research subjects.
- Properly design the clinical trial to ensure that it does not pose unnecessary, avoidable, or unreasonable risks to subjects.
- Ensure that the individuals invited to enroll as subjects are appropriate.
- Ensure that all subjects who enroll voluntarily agree to participate with full knowledge of the trial procedures and potential risks of participation.
- Ensure that all investigators are qualified to carry out their study functions.
- Conduct the trial with reasonable care so as to maximize the safety and welfare of subjects and minimize risks, including removing individuals from the trial or halting the trial when it endangers subjects.
- Provide appropriate information to subjects after the trial if necessary to protect their safety, health, or welfare.

Investigators are subject to liability to subjects who are injured as a result of their violation of any of these duties. Table 62.1 lists the possible legal claims (causes of action) for research subjects. In practice, lawsuits claiming research injuries typically assert all causes of action that fit the factual circumstances in order to avoid missing any potentially valid legal claim against a responsible party. A typical lawsuit today might include one or more claims of fraud, misrepresentation, negligence, assault, battery, intentional or negligent infliction of emotional distress, and possibly products liability, breach of contract, or violation of constitutional rights.[58] Each cause of action has somewhat different standards and possible remedies. A plaintiff may not recover more than the total amount of damages incurred for the same injury, regardless of the number of successful claims.

Historically, the majority of litigated cases arose from using people in research without their knowledge or consent.[13] Notorious examples of such research in the United States include the U.S. Public Health Service's Tuskegee Study of syphilis in poor, African American men,[44] the Willowbrook study of hepatitis B in mentally disabled children,[1] and the injection of cancer cells in patients at the Jewish Chronic Disease Hospital in 1963.[59-60] Yet none of those cases resulted in litigation. During the Cold War, the federal government exposed military personnel and civilians to radiation exposure without their knowledge,[26,61-64] and the Central Intelligence Agency gave LSD to unsuspecting personnel to study its effects.[23,65-66] Few of the Cold War experiments resulted in successful lawsuits, often because servicemen were precluded from suing the federal government.[67]

Battery

Using people in research without their consent violates fundamental principles of autonomy and self-determination, grounded in ancient English common law.[68-69] In 1891, the U.S. Supreme Court said that "no right is held more sacred, or is more carefully guarded, by the common law, than the right of every individual to the possession and control of his own person, free from all restraint or interference of others, unless by clear and unquestionable authority of law."[70] (More recently, the Supreme Court has suggested that this right is also part of individual liberty protected by the U.S. Constitution.[71-73]) Anyone who touches or causes an offensive or harmful contact with another person without the latter's consent commits a battery at common law, regardless of whether any injury results.[74,75] Individuals are entitled to recover at least nominal damages in battery—for the dignitary harm of invading the person's bodily integrity or inviolability of the person.[76] Substantial damages may be warranted when physical injury results.

Battery includes giving investigational drugs and devices to patients without disclosing the investigational nature of the intervention, as was the case with pregnant women who were given diethylstilbestrol (DES) to see whether it prevented miscarriage without telling them it was not part of the regular prenatal care they sought.[77] The use of an investigational drug or medical device without telling the patient that it was experimental continues to give rise to lawsuits.[78-84] For example, about 400 mostly indigent women with high-risk pregnancies at Tampa General Hospital were enrolled in a clinical trial beginning in 1986 to compare drug regimens for fetal respiratory distress syndrome.[31] Most signed consent forms while in pain or medicated with morphine because they were told the medicine was needed to save the baby's life. A class action on behalf of the women was settled in 2000 for $3.8 million.[85] In all these cases, the central violation was that people were involuntarily subjected to research.

Fraud and Misrepresentation

When an experiment is concealed entirely from those who are used as subjects, researchers can be liable for fraudulent concealment.[86-88] Several university studies of the effects of radiation exposure in the 1940s and 1950s hid the experiment from the subjects. For example, 829 pregnant women were given the radioactive isotope Iron 59 but told it was a vitamin or "sweet."[89] Their class action was settled in 1998 for $10.3 million.[90] Developmentally disabled children institutionalized at the Fernald School were fed Quaker Oats cereal with radioactive isotopes in the 1950s. A class action on behalf of the children was partially settled for $1.85 million in 1999.[91] The Human Radiation Experiments with cancer patients in the 1960s resulted in a class action settlement of $5.4 million in 1999.[26,92]

Research misrepresented as standard medical care may be actionable as fraud or misrepresentation, depending upon the investigator's intent. Negligent misrepresentation can occur when

Table 62.1
Federal and State Laws

Type	Causes of Action	Defenses
Federal	§1983 (violation of constitutional or federal rights) Federal Tort Claims Act Conspiracy RICO (Racketeer Influenced and Corrupt Organizations Act)	• Statute of limitations • Waiver, release • Sovereign immunity • Qualified immunity under §1983 • Government contractor immunity • Federal military action
State statutes	Tort claims against the state Wrongful death Statutes limiting research with the following: • Fetuses • Embryos • Institutionalized persons • Prisoners • Children Limitations on authority to consent to research	• Statute of limitations • Waiver, release • Sovereign immunity • Government contractor immunity • Charitable immunity • Federal preemption of state law • Contributory negligence • Comparative negligence
State common law	Tort law Intentional torts • Battery and assault • Fraudulent concealment • Fraudulent misrepresentation • Invasion of privacy • Breach of confidentiality • Conversion Unintentional torts • Negligence • Lack of informed consent • Negligent misrepresentation • Negligent research design • Negligent product design • Negligent conduct of research • Failure to notify of later-discovered risks/harms • Invasion of privacy • Breach of confidentiality Products liability • Design defect • Manufacturing error • Failure to warn of risks Contracts • Breach of contract • Breach of warranty • Third party beneficiary • Unjust enrichment	• Statute of limitations • Waiver, release • Consent, assumption of risk • Sovereign immunity • Government contractor immunity • Charitable immunity • Contributory negligence • Comparative negligence

*Note: Defenses are listed as an undifferentiated group and may apply to more than one cause of action.

an investigator fails to exercise reasonable care in communicating information or in ascertaining the accuracy of the information.[93] It is specifically applicable to professionals, like physicians and investigators, who have a duty to furnish information to patients and research subjects respectively. Fraud is more difficult to prove, because it requires evidence of false statements (written or oral) intended to induce a person to take action (or refrain from taking action), and proof that the plaintiff justifiably relied on such falsehoods and suffered injury as a result of such reliance.[94–95] The defendant must know or believe that his representation is false or at least that he does not have sufficient knowledge to make the representation.[95–96] Fraud may include the omission of information that one has a duty to disclose.[96] Researchers have a duty to

disclose any material information that might affect a person's decision about whether to enroll in a study.

Patients receiving medical care who are asked to participate in research may be especially susceptible to the therapeutic misconception—mistaking the research intervention for accepted medical therapy.[97–98] Both patients and researchers may hope that something "new" or "cutting edge" will turn out to help the patients. Physician-investigators are subject to an inherent conflict of interest between their patients' welfare and the trial protocol, and may experience psychological resistance to the idea that no benefit to the individual can be expected.[97] The opportunities for conflating research with therapy are growing with the number of clinical trials that enroll patients with medical conditions that have not responded satisfactorily to standard therapies, such as trials of devices like an artificial heart, gene transfer research, or cancer chemotherapy.[99,100] At least one study found that consent forms for Phase I cancer chemotherapy trials did not make clear that the trials were not designed for patient therapy.[101] Foremost among the problems that led the study coordinator for the University of Oklahoma's melanoma vaccine trials to seek assistance from the OHRP was her concern "that it had been coercive to promise subjects that the melanoma vaccine offered hope of a cure."[102] Those enrolled in that vaccine trial brought a lawsuit claiming that the investigational vaccine was misrepresented as a cure for cancer.[25] The university reached a settlement with some of the subjects in 2002.[103]

Those who believe they were misled may be more inclined to seek legal redress than those with a more informed and dispassionate view of research. Of course, disappointment, by itself, does not give rise to a cause of action for misrepresentation. However, investigators who mislead subjects, or encourage subjects to believe that an investigational intervention is standard therapy, or fail to correct a mistaken statement may be liable for misrepresentation.

Informed Consent

Today, clinical trials rarely hide their experimental purpose or proceed without seeking consent from subjects. The real question is whether the consent was informed, that is, meaningful enough to be valid and enforceable at law. The doctrine of informed consent, also required for medical treatment, requires investigators to provide prospective subjects with sufficient information about the proposed research to permit a knowledgeable decision about participation.[104–106] This includes the following:

- The fact that the person is being asked to participate in a research study, not medical treatment
- The purpose of the study, what will happen, and why
- What the subject will be asked to do and not do, where, and when
- The nature and potential risks of any investigational intervention, drug, or device
- The potential risks to the person of participation in the study
- The fact that participation is voluntary and that the person is free to withdraw from the study at any time
- What standard therapy exists for those who need therapy and choose not to participate

Beyond the minimum legal requirements, ethical guidelines and the Common Rule require telling prospective subjects about whether and what kind of compensation is available in case of injury.[36,38,107] In addition, the National Bioethics Advisory Commission and others recommend telling subjects whether they will have access to successful therapies after the trial.[108,109]

Detailed information about clinical trials became necessary when the risks of an intervention were no longer self-evident to the average person.[110] A person's consent to participate in research is meaningless, and of no legal effect, if that person does not understand what he or she is getting into. Thus, the law requires the party most knowledgeable about the trial—the researcher—to provide information that a person having only general knowledge would not ordinarily know. An investigator who fails to tell a prospective subject about facets of the trial that are material to that

person's decision breaches the duty of disclosure. This includes the foreseeable risks of harm, as well as the uncertainties inherent in the research, but does not include particular risks that are not foreseeable.[111] The breach is typically actionable as negligence—a failure to exercise reasonable care.

A cause of action in negligence requires the plaintiff to prove the following: the researcher had a duty (to disclose material information); the researcher breached the duty (by failing to disclose that information); the person was injured; and the breach of duty proximately caused that harm.[95,112] Proximate causation ordinarily requires proof that a reasonable person would not have enrolled (or continued) in the trial if the information had been disclosed. If the information is withheld in order to induce the person to enroll in the trial, it may be actionable as misrepresentation or even fraudulent concealment. Unlike battery, a negligence cause of action is not available unless the person has suffered cognizable physical injury.

The doctrine of informed consent allows written consent forms to be used as evidence of what subjects were told and what they agreed to, but consent documents are not conclusive.[113] Although federal regulations and some state statues require consent to be documented in writing, common law principles are directed at the content of oral communications.[114]

Several recent cases have claimed that researchers failed to obtain the subjects' informed consent.[31,115,116] For example, subjects in the University of Oklahoma melanoma vaccine trial claimed that no one was told that the investigational vaccine posed a risk of infection because it had not been manufactured in a sterile environment or tested for safety in animals.[25] The U.S. General Accounting Office (GAO, now the Government Accountability Office) found many instances of failure to obtain informed consent, as well as other problems, in the Department of Veterans Affairs (VA) research centers around the country, although few resulted in lawsuits.[117,118] Although individual investigators have the common law duty to obtain informed consent, a few courts have found that hospitals also assumed this duty by agreeing to comply with regulations governing research promulgated by the Food and Drug Administration (FDA) or the DHHS.[119–120]

The doctrine of informed consent was developed for individuals who are legally competent to make decisions; that is, free from coercion and capable of understanding and evaluating relevant information and making a voluntary decision.[114] All adults are presumed to be competent unless a court adjudicates them incompetent, either permanently (because of developmental disability, for example) or temporarily (as from medication, pain, or unconsciousness). Informed consent, then, requires the voluntary, informed and understanding decision of a competent adult.

Exceptions to the general rule have been made in practice. For example, the Common Rule permits an IRB to approve a study without all elements of informed consent (or waiving consent) when the "research could not practicably be carried out without the waiver or alteration" as long as the subjects will be informed after the study.[121] This waiver or alteration has been used in deception studies in psychology and behavioral research, when knowledge of the study's purpose or procedures would bias the responses and produce invalid results. Some deception studies can be controversial, but they rarely pose a risk of physical injury.[122–123] In addition, after the Gulf War, FDA regulations were amended to permit the president to authorize the use of investigational drugs and vaccines in armed forces personnel without consent for certain military operations.[124–125] Federal regulations have also adopted exceptions to the requirement for informed consent to permit research in life-threatening emergencies. However, the regulations do not trump state statutory or common law requiring informed consent. Clinical trials that study interventions intended to help people other than competent adults often raise questions about how to reconcile the need for scientific evidence with basic legal principles governing participation in research. These issues are discussed in the following section.

Research With Legally Incompetent Subjects

Clinical trials and other research studies sometimes use people who are not legally competent to consent to participate in research.[1,61,68,126] The law has not entirely confronted practice on this point. Questions about whether incompetent persons lawfully can be used in research, and, if so, in what circumstances, whether any form of surrogate authorization is necessary or sufficient to permit it, and the weight, if any, to be accorded federal regulations permitting such research, remain unsettled. Ethical principles may justify the use of incompetent persons in research when the goal of research is to discover the etiology or find a therapy for a disease or condition that affects only people who are not competent.[127–128] The need for research to help these groups, however, conflicts with the general principle prohibiting the use of individuals in research without their voluntary, competent, and informed consent.[129]

The doctrine of informed consent has been consistently applied to preserve the right of incompetent adults to refuse medical treatment.[71–72,130] Based on this reasoning, legal scholars and courts generally agree that incompetent adults also have the legal right to refuse to participate in research, and that their guardians can refuse on their behalf if that is what they would want or if the research would not be in their best interests.[131]

It is less clear whether the reverse is true. Few courts have considered whether a legal representative has the lawful authority to enroll an incompetent adult or child in a clinical trial. Several early reported decisions permitted an experimental procedure as part of treatment for a patient when no standard therapy was available, but did not address participation in a clinical trial.[13] The FDA adopted a similar exception by regulation allowing the immediate use of an investigational drug or device on a case-by-case basis in a life-threatening situation without the person's consent if that person cannot communicate or is otherwise not legally competent.[132] This exception allows the use of an investigational product not approved by the FDA for medical treatment, which otherwise would be prohibited by the Food, Drug and Cosmetic Act. The exception is not intended to set general standards for clinical trials. It applies only when the investigational product is immediately required to save the person's life, no alternative approved or generally recognized therapy offers an equal or better chance of saving the person's life, and there is no time to seek surrogate consent from the person's legal representative.

Federal Common Rule regulations governing research with mentally disabled adults have never been adopted.[126,129] Some states have statutes or regulations that prohibit research with residents of mental health institutions. Others permit research with incompetent adults in specific circumstances, including clinical trials.[133] In 1996, in response to concerns that therapies to save the lives of people in a life-threatening medical emergency could not be systematically evaluated because the patients' medical condition precluded them from giving consent to enroll in a clinical trial, the FDA adopted a rule authorizing certain types of emergency medical research without the consent of subjects.[134] This rule allows clinical trials of investigational emergency life-saving measures when "subjects are in a life-threatening situation, available treatments are unproven or unsatisfactory, and the collection of valid scientific evidence [including randomized placebo-controlled trials], is necessary to determine the safety and effectiveness of particular interventions;" and the intervention must be administered before any legal representative can make a decision.[134] Individual consent is not required for those who are unable "to give their informed consent as a result of their medical condition."[134] Those who are in a condition to make their own decision may not be enrolled without their informed consent. The rule itself does not expressly address whether individuals who lack competence when not in a medical emergency can be included in research.[135] In practice, it is unlikely that investigators in an emergency department will know who is or is not otherwise unable to consent solely because of their current medical emergency condition.

The emergency research rule contains additional conditions, including IRB review and approval and a somewhat ambiguous requirement for "consultation" with "representatives of the communities in which the clinical investigation will conducted and from which the subjects will drawn."[134] Public education about research has value in its own right. Community consultation, however, should not be confused with legal authorization of the research itself. A draft Guidance by the FDA confirms that the exception does not permit enrolling people without consent if state law precludes such research without consent.[136] Courts have never considered the decision to participate in research as belonging to anyone except the individual. In the absence of any court decision on the merits of the rule, it remains uncertain whether it would be upheld as a reasonable means of identifying effective emergency procedures or struck down as a violation of individual autonomy.

Two recent court decisions suggest that research with incompetent individuals may not be permitted unless it poses no more than minimal risk. A New York court struck down the state Office of Mental Health's regulations permitting research with mental health patients who were incapable of giving informed consent, because the regulations were not approved by the Commissioner of Health.[137] In part of its opinion that was considered advisory, because it was not necessary to decide the case, the court also noted, "It may well be that for some categories of greater than minimal risk nontherapeutic experiments, devised to achieve a future benefit, there is at present no constitutionally acceptable protocol for obtaining the participation of incapable individuals who have not, when previously competent, either given specific consent or designated a suitable surrogate from whom such consent may be obtained. The alternative of allowing such experiments to continue, without proper consent and in violation of the rights of the incapable individuals who participate, is clearly unacceptable."[137]

Although federal regulations and some state laws permit the use of children under certain conditions,[138–139] common law decisions concerning research with children have not yet reached consensus about whether parents or guardians have the legal authority to allow their children to participate in research.[139] Parents have a legal duty to safeguard their children and provide them with life-saving or essential medical care.[140–141] Parents have been permitted to consent to an individual experimental procedure when it offered a substantial probability of success and posed only minimal risks to the child.[139] Clinical trials may not be deemed to be in the best interest of the child, however, unless perhaps there is no standard medical therapy available for a life-threatening or very serious condition and the trial poses relatively minor risks. In 2001, Maryland's highest court found that parents and surrogate decision makers "cannot consent to the participation of a child or other person under legal disability in nontherapeutic research or studies in which there is any risk of injury or damage to the health of the subject."[32] Although the decision disconcerted some, it is a reminder that even practices that are presumed legitimate by many investigators and IRBs may not be found lawful when tested in court.[142] In a 2004 speech, Judge Dale R. Cathell, who issued the Maryland decision, warned investigators against assuming that the beneficial goals of research or compliance with federal regulations would protect them from liability for breaches of other legal duties: "In the tort litigation context, good intentions do not, even in the smallest degree, normally define duty and the breach of duty."[143]

Future studies of new ways to treat people in life-threatening circumstances could be challenged in litigation to resolve the question whether or when individuals can be used in research without their consent. Competent adults who have specific opinions about whether they wish to participate in research are free to execute powers of attorney authorizing a surrogate decision maker to consent or refuse on their behalf when they are not able to make their own decisions. Such documents may be analogous to health care proxies, but their legal validity has not yet been tested. One could reasonably argue that legal representatives and researchers who comply with a "research proxy's" instructions protect the person's rights by carrying out the person's wishes. It is possible, however, that such research proxies could be found to have no binding effect or perhaps not to apply with respect to research that poses significant risk.[144] Moreover, they would not resolve questions about children or adults who have never been competent.

The state has the power (*parens patriae*) to protect the safety and welfare of children and incompetent adults and could challenge their participation in research if parents or legal representatives fail to act in the best interests of their wards. Despite the need for clinical trials to evaluate interventions unique to children and incompetent adults, as well as federal regulations allowing such research in certain circumstances, the law governing their participation in research remains patchy and unsettled.

3. Rights and Remedies for Research Subjects in the United States: The Conduct of Research

Beyond ensuring that subjects are properly enrolled in a trial, investigators must carry out the research study in accordance with the protocol agreed to by the subjects. As with almost any endeavor, investigators have common law duties to prevent unlawful injury to subjects and to keep any promises made to subjects. The most relevant are summarized in this section.

Tort Claims

Although competent subjects who agree to participate in a clinical trial may assume the inherent risk of unexpected injury from an investigational intervention like a drug, they do not assume the risk of the researcher's own negligence or other wrongdoing in conducting the study. Here again, the general principles of law that require everyone to act with reasonable care to avoid foreseeable injury to others also apply to researchers. Investigators who violate their duties to design and carry out research properly and to protect subjects against foreseeable harms can be liable for injuries they cause.[13,145] Moreover, investigators, especially physician-investigators, are held to the standard of an expert in the field and must exercise the same degree of knowledge and skill that a similarly situated, qualified professional would exercise.

Examples of problems in carrying out clinical trials that have been cited in lawsuits include failing to seek IRB approval,[102] letting IRB approval lapse,[146] negligently or fraudulently enrolling ineligible persons in a trial,[25,102,117–118,147–149] using unapproved consent forms,[25,102,119] administering an incorrect dosage of an investigational drug contrary to the trial protocol,[150] performing other research interventions improperly or contrary to the trial protocol,[54,102,146] failing to stop a trial intervention that harms a subject,[145] failing to provide appropriate medical care to a person having an adverse reaction to a trial intervention,[97,120,145,150–152] and failing to tell subjects about risks discovered during or after the trial.[32,77,120,153–154] It should be noted that the federal regulations forbid researchers from requiring subjects to waive any of their legal rights or to release any responsible party from liability for negligence.[155]

Tort law holds employers vicariously liable (under the doctrine of *respondeat superior*) for the negligence of their employees in order to encourage employers to ensure that their employees act with reasonable care in performing their jobs.[156] Thus, universities, hospitals, and other organizations that carry out research may be vicariously liable for the unlawful acts and omissions of their employees and agents, regardless of the employer's own conduct.[25–26,32,77,157] Plaintiffs sometimes elect to sue the university or hospital if the individual researcher does not have sufficient assets to compensate the harm. This requires the plaintiff to prove not only that the individual researcher breached a duty of care to the research subject that was the proximate cause of injury, but also that the researcher was the employee or (actual or ostensible) agent of the organization.

Research organizations themselves may also act unlawfully and become liable for their own corporate (or direct) breaches of duty.[156] Organizations have a duty to use reasonable care in hiring, supervising, and terminating their research staff, just as hospitals have a duty to use care in granting and renewing physician privileges.[158] For example, an Illinois appellate court held that when the University of Chicago and Eli Lilly & Company learned that the children of women who were given DES had an increased risk of cancer, the corporation could be liable for failing to notify the former research subjects that they had been part of a DES experiment.[77]

Until recently, lawsuits have rarely targeted an IRB, even when subjects suspected that an IRB wrongfully approved a study, because most IRBs are an organizational component of a university or medical center, which would be the responsible legal entity. Members of IRBs have been named as defendants in a few cases in recent years, but no reported decision has even considered the possibility of IRB or IRB member liability, and there is no evidence that IRBs or IRB members have paid any damages to a plaintiff. In theory, perhaps, independently incorporated review organizations might be liable for their own unlawful actions.[149] However, it is doubtful that they would have any responsibility for injuries because IRBs do not control the conduct of research.

The Stratton Veterans Affairs Medical Center in Albany, N.Y., was recently accused of violating multiple duties to research subjects, including fraud, patient abuse, and carelessness, for a decade.[159] One researcher, Paul Kornak, pleaded guilty to criminal charges of making false statements, mail fraud, and criminally negligent homicide and was sentenced to 71 months in prison and payment of almost $640,000 in restitution to the VA and the drug companies.[160] Mr. Kornak reportedly changed medical records to enroll ineligible veterans in a clinical trial of cancer drugs, misrepresented himself as a physician, and continued to administer to subjects drugs with adverse reactions including premature death. Families of veterans also commenced a class action against the Department of Veterans Affairs and the individual researchers.[159]

Major research universities and medical centers have experienced similar problems of more or less severity, including the deaths of subjects in clinical trials. In 2003, a Detroit Veterans Affairs center administered a fatal overdose of drugs to a research subject.[159] In 1999, the Office for Protections from Research Risks (OPRR, now OHRP) suspended research at the West Los Angeles Veterans Affairs medical center for its history of failing to obtain informed consent and its careless conduct of research. The GAO found "a disturbing pattern of noncompliance" with regulations for the protection of human research subjects in eight Veterans Affairs centers.[161] A second GAO report several years later found little change.[118] OPRR found sufficient deficiencies in subject protection procedures to suspend federal funding at several medical centers, including Johns Hopkins University, Duke University, the University of Illinois at Chicago, Virginia Commonwealth University, and the University of Oklahoma.[162] In a few cases, the subjects' families commenced lawsuits against the institutions on multiple causes of action, ranging from negligence to intentional infliction of emotional distress and fraud.

Publicity about research scandals may increase public awareness of the risks and uncertainties inherent in research. It may also encourage injured research subjects and their families to bring claims for redress against researchers and their institutions. Jesse Gelsinger's father expressed surprise and anger at learning that James Wilson, who enrolled Jesse Gelsinger in a study, had founded a company to sell the rights to the vector for gene delivery that was tested in Jesse Gelsinger.[163] His lawsuit against the University of Pennsylvania and the investigators was settled within a month.[164] The fact that several recent lawsuits have targeted researchers who failed to disclose their financial connection with the studies they conducted suggests that research subjects are paying closer attention to researchers' financial ties. One study found that a majority of people surveyed believed that investigators and hospitals conduct clinical trials to make money and don't tell subjects all the risks involved.[165]

Some conflicts of interest may be inherent in research, but financial conflicts raise particular concerns.[166–170] Conflicts of interest may lead investigators to enroll ineligible subjects, resist finding that a trial intervention has harmed a subject, or to interpret, or even manipulate, data to support desired outcomes.[171,172] As universities rely on research funding for a growing proportion of their revenues, financial conflicts of interest can spread throughout the institution.[173] The DHHS issued new (interim) regulations on Feb. 3, 2005, to prevent possible conflicts of interest among research scientists at the National Institutes of Health (NIH).[174]

The final regulations apply only to senior employees and prohibit ownership of more than $15,000 of stock in any pharmaceutical, biotechnology, or medical device company (or $50,000 in the aggregate).[175] Senior NIH researchers also may not be employed by or receive compensation from such companies or health-care providers or insurers without prior NIH approval. Public opposition to such payments suggests that research conducted with conflicts of interest is peculiarly vulnerable to legal challenge.[176–178] Conflicts of interest may trigger legal claims against investigators and research institutions by injured research subjects or their representatives that might not otherwise have been brought. Financial conflicts of interest also may provide evidence for some claims if they influenced investigators to acts in ways that injure a subject. If the research is viewed as a business operation, wrongdoing might even be analogized to business fraud, when punitive damages might be allowed.[179]

Lawsuits sometimes function as the last resort for those who fail to achieve reform via the legislative or regulatory process. Thus, if research subjects or the general public believe that federal agencies, universities, or hospitals are not adequately investigating or penalizing research violations, those institutions may become the target of personal injury or even whistle-blower lawsuits.[180–181]

Studies using individually identifiable information qualify as research with humans, and investigators who collect such information have a duty to keep the information confidential and use it only as authorized by the subject.[114] Obtaining such private information without consent would ordinarily qualify as an invasion of privacy.[95,182] Misuse of confidential information in research is rare, and lawsuits based on such tort claims are virtually unheard of. The major risks to subjects from an invasion of privacy or breach of confidentiality are damage to reputation and economic costs, such as loss of insurance, employment, or housing, which are often too speculative to warrant legal action.[183] Research subjects concerned about privacy may seek new ways to control access to their information, such as contractually limiting information disclosure or even asserting a property interest in their information. Information technology has made it possible to link and manipulate large data sets, increasing both the value of information and the risk of unauthorized access.[184] The DHHS Privacy Rule, commonly known as the HIPAA (Health Insurance Portability and Accountability Act) Privacy Rule, has focused renewed attention on how medical information is used and disclosed.[185] Yet the Privacy Rule does not apply to researchers unless they are also considered to be a covered entity such as a physician or hospital employee who maintains regular records of medical care, and it does not preempt state privacy laws. A rash of reports about the loss of financial records may encourage public debate about medical as well as financial information, such as what types of studies count as research with humans and whether information collected for one purpose, such as cancer registries or public health surveillance, can be disclosed to others for research purposes without the individual's consent.[186]

Contract and Property Claims

Although most lawsuits claiming research harm have been based in tort law, the law of contract, property, or even intellectual property may be applied to certain research relationships in the future. The Maryland Court of Appeals has suggested that the consent form may be considered a contract between investigator and subject, which would permit a subject to recover damages for breach of contract in the event that an investigator failed to adhere to the terms of the agreement.[32]

Contract principles appear to be better suited to research with tissue samples, DNA, and other genetic material and information. Courts have generally accepted the presumption, which is consistent with general practice in the research community, that "donors" of such material relinquish any property interest in tissue (and related information) collected for a research study and that the material becomes the property of the investigator.[187] The only state supreme court decision on the issue of ownership dealt with a physician-patient relationship, not a research relationship. The Supreme Court of California found only that a physician had a duty to inform his patient, Moore, that he intended to develop and patent a cell line from Moore's tissue—Moore's spleen was removed as standard therapy for hairy cell leukemia.[188] Moore sued for conversion, arguing that the physician took (converted) his property (the spleen) without his knowledge or consent for the physician's own profitable use. The court denied Moore a share of the cell-line profits, finding that Moore had not expected to retain ownership of his spleen after its removal.

Although courts have not yet held that subjects have a property interest in tissue or DNA donated in research, there may be pressure to do so as genetic and genomic research increases and, with it, the promise of beneficial and commercially profitable results.[189–190] Two recent cases offer possible glimpses of the future. In the first, a group of parents of children with Canavan disease organized a foundation, recruited an investigator, and provided the tissue samples and genetic and pedigree information that made it possible to identify the gene and develop a test to detect it. When the discovery was patented and the foundation was asked to pay royalties for using the test, they sued the investigator and university for unjust enrichment, conversion, lack of informed consent, fraudulent concealment, breach of fiduciary duty, and misappropriation of trade secrets for failing to make the genetic test widely available, inexpensively or free.[191] A Florida court followed the reasoning in Moore, rejecting all but the unjust enrichment claim and found that the foundation and the research subjects did not retain any property interest in their tissue samples or genetic information. Before the last claim went to trial, the university holding the patent reached a settlement with the plaintiffs that allows certain research institutes and laboratories to use the test without a licensing fee.[192]

Parents of children with PXE (pseudoxanthoma elasticum) took a different approach to ensure their control over a genetic test for the disease. They, too, organized a foundation to collect tissue samples and genetic information. In addition, the foundation's founder participated directly in the research itself and was named as a coinventor on a successful patent application.[193] This approach allows the research subjects a measure of ongoing control over the use of the test.

The lesson of these cases may be that in the future, as a condition of participating in a study, subjects may insist on retaining ownership of any tissue or information used for commercial purposes or receiving a share of any profits from the research. Few subjects would qualify as an inventor for purposes of a patent application, but they may use contracts to require researchers to assign some or all resulting patent rights to them or to a representative organization. A contractual approach might also

be applied in the future to enable subjects to control the use of personally identifiable genetic or medical information, with or without related tissue samples.

Research subjects recently attempted to use contract principles to assert entitlement to products tested in clinical trials. Subjects in clinical trials of glial-derived neurotrophic factor (GDNF) for Parkinson's disease brought a lawsuit against the trial sponsor, Amgen Inc., seeking to compel Amgen to provide them with GDNF because they believed that it had helped them.[194] Amgen terminated the trials before their scheduled completion after finding cerebellar toxicity among primates and neutralizing antibodies in humans. The trial court found that the plaintiffs were not entitled to a preliminary injunction granting them access to GDNF because they had virtually no likelihood of succeeding on their claims: Their participation in the clinical trial did not create any contractual obligation on the sponsor's part to continue the trial or to provide GDNF, the sponsor had no fiduciary duty to the subjects, and the investigator had no authority to require the sponsor to provide GDNF. The court's legal analysis is consistent with current law. Investigators and sponsors of research generally retain the prerogative to terminate a study and to decline to distribute any investigational product. The case is notable because it demonstrates an attempt (albeit unsuccessful) to use litigation to obtain access to investigational products and perhaps a misunderstanding of clinical trials. Research is not a substitute for medical care, and researchers should not be put in the position of trying to compensate for the unavailability of health care elsewhere.

A related problem arises when people enroll in a clinical trial in order to obtain basic medical care that they cannot otherwise afford or which is not otherwise available.[195] AIDS research was pushed forward by advocates arguing that, in the absence of any proven therapy, clinical trials were the only treatment available to people with HIV infection.[196–198] However, if not carefully informed of the nature of the research, individuals under such pressures may enroll in inappropriate studies and experience harmful consequences. Many people enrolled in schizophrenia studies at more than a dozen medical schools in the 1980s and 1990s as a means to get basic health care.[97,199] Some became ill after being taken off their medication and brought legal claims against the investigators for failing to monitor their condition. These issues arise with particular sensitivity in clinical trials conducted by U.S. researchers in foreign countries, where an increasing proportion of clinical trials are conducted.[200–202] Those from other countries who believe that they have suffered harm while participating in research may be able to sue investigators in U.S. courts.[35,203] Although there is no legal obligation to provide the successful results of clinical trials to the study population or others, ethical principles increasingly recognize the need to do so.[36,199]

4. Estimating Research Injuries and Obtaining Redress

Millions of individuals are believed to have participated in clinical trials, but there is little comprehensive data on either the number of people or the number of injuries in research.[204,205] A 1996 U.S. GAO report found that the DHHS, which includes the NIH, spent about $5 billion to fund 16,000 studies involving humans each year.[206] OHRP data indicates that about 70 million people participated in research between 1990 and 2000, whereas institutions reported 8 deaths and fewer than 400 adverse events, suggesting to some that reporting may not be a reliable indicator of research injuries.[207] The increased number of trials and, presumably, research subjects may expand opportunities for error and injury, but the absence of empirical data makes estimating actual injuries speculative.

Despite the large number of clinical trials involving humans and the wide range of general laws that might apply to clinical trials, there have been few reported lawsuits on behalf of injured subjects.[13] It is often difficult to distinguish harms caused by the research from complications of illness or risks accepted as part of the study. Few attorneys are willing to take on personal injury cases that are difficult to prove or would recover damages less than the cost of litigation. In recent years, lawsuits may have become more visible because they can involve more parties on both sides. If there is a common problem in a large clinical trial, such as a systematic failure to advise subjects of risks or to perform research tasks properly, class action suits on behalf of all those harmed in the trial may be the most efficient form of lawsuit. By bringing together many people with a similar experience, class actions make litigation possible for individuals who could not otherwise afford it. They also put significant pressure on defendants to settle claims. Recent federal legislation places new restrictions on federal class actions, but state class actions remain possible.[208]

Alternative Remedies

Some commentators hope that litigation will improve the way research is conducted, as well as increase accountability on the part of investigators.[209] Although some lawsuits and publicity about claims, whether litigated to conclusion or not, have prompted institutions to improve their protections of research subjects, the common law has had less influence on the conduct of research than the Common Rule so far. Yet litigation may offer leverage for changing behavior in the future. Jesse Gelsinger's father, Paul, planned to use the settlement funds from the University of Pennsylvania to improve protections for research subjects.[164] Other litigants have used settlement agreements to forge new policies at research institutions. After the quiet settlement of a lawsuit by the family of Betsy Lehman, the *Boston Globe* reporter who died from an overdose of chemotherapy in a breast cancer trial at Dana-Farber Cancer Institute in Boston, the hospital created a new patient safety program to prevent medication and other errors, and the state created a broader program in her name.[210] In 2002, the University of South Florida Health Sciences Center and Tampa General Hospital agreed to new practices and procedures for research, including developing readable consent forms and training researchers in designing readable documents and tracking study subjects, as part of its settlement of a class action on behalf of indigent pregnant women who claimed they were enrolled in a clinical trial to compare drug regimens for fetal respiratory distress syndrome without their informed consent.[85]

If research subjects are unable to obtain equitable redress through litigation, their advocates may press for more stringent legislative penalties for researchers who violate the law. Paul Gelsinger was reportedly very disappointed in the Justice Department's settlement with the researchers, because it only forbade Wilson from leading research with humans until 2010, and fined

the University of Pennsylvania $517,496 and Children's National Medical Center $514,622.[211]

Defenses

Plaintiffs who have legitimate complaints may be precluded from bringing a lawsuit for several reasons. Statutes of limitations or repose limit the time in which a lawsuit may be commenced to several years after the injury occurred or should have been discovered. Time limits for negligence claims are typically three years, whereas fraud claims usually must be brought within six years. The vagaries of litigation are illustrated by *Heinrich* v. *Sweet*.[212] In 1997, the families of research subjects sued the Massachusetts Institute of Technology, the Massachusetts General Hospital, a New York association of universities, and the federal government, as well as the individual investigators, for conspiracy to conduct a boron neutron capture therapy experiment without their consent in the 1950s and 1960s. The study was to determine whether a boron compound injected into an artery would collect in a brain tumor and selectively attract radiation to eliminate the tumor without injuring other brain tissue. The subjects were patients with brain cancer. But the compound allegedly caused severe illness and premature death in many. The claims based on New York law were dismissed because they were brought after statutes of limitations had expired. The fraud claim under Massachusetts law was allowed to proceed, and the plaintiffs were awarded $13 million dollars, including $5 million in punitive damages, in 1999.[213] On appeal by defendants, however, the appeals court found that the doctrine of informed consent was not sufficiently established before 1970 to permit the plaintiff's claims, and vacated the judgment in 2002.[214] There is some irony in the ruling, because Massachusetts has had a law requiring consent to medical care since 1649.[215]

Sovereign immunity—based on the ancient notion that the king can do no wrong—can be a defense to tort claims brought against officials, employees, and agents of state and federal governmental institutions, such as state universities and city hospitals. Governments cannot be sued unless they waive sovereign immunity. The Federal Tort Claims Act waives federal sovereign immunity and permits tort suits against federal government agencies, like the NIH, in some circumstances.[216,217] Federal officials are also protected by qualified immunity from suit if they perform discretionary functions in their official capacity, unless they violate established constitutional rights.[218] States typically have similar statutes that waive sovereign immunity and permit tort claims against state entities, although the law often limits the dollar amount of liability to a maximum ($100,000 in Massachusetts).[219] Research subjects who are injured by government entities cannot sue the state unless their injuries fit the narrow causes of actions covered by a tort claims statute. Moreover, the U.S. Supreme Court has interpreted the 11th Amendment to forbid suits based on federal law to be brought in federal court against state government entities.[220–222] For nongovernment entities, some states continue to grant charitable immunity to nonprofit hospitals and educational institutions, limiting their tort liability for personal injury to a dollar amount ($20,000 in Massachusetts), although most states have abandoned such protection.

Products liability, a set of common law principles derived from both tort and contract law, is normally applicable to commercially marketed products, not investigational products still in clinical trials.[223] However, approved products being studied in postmarket trials may be subject to product liability claims based on a product defect. Some states grant manufacturers immunity from liability for personal injury caused by defective drugs if the FDA has approved the product at issue and the manufacturer has complied with FDA standards, unless it has withheld information from the FDA or acted fraudulently.

Compensation for Research Injuries

Compensation for research injuries is not systematically available in the United States outside the litigation system. Several national commissions and panels have given favorable consideration to or recommended compensating subjects for research injuries, but no formal, national mechanism has yet been adopted.[44,46,61,209,224–225] So far, compensation for injury remains voluntary, and institutions that provide it often limit it to providing remedial medical care.[203] Some hospitals and research institutes purchase liability insurance (products liability and clinical trials liability) to cover their payments to research subjects. However, these policies are typically limited to the cost of medical care and do not cover lost income or pain and suffering.[226]

International guidelines stop short of requiring compensation. The Council of Europe's Convention for the Protection of Human Rights and Dignity of the Human Being with regard to the application of Biology and Medicine has a chapter of general principles for the protection of subjects in scientific research.[227] Article 24 requires that "fair compensation" be provided to any subject who has suffered undue damage, by act or omission, but leaves the procedures and amounts to national law. The Council of Europe's recent additions to this Convention are virtually identical on the issue of fair compensation for research injuries (Article 31).[228]

Conclusion

The fundamental legal principles governing research with humans have changed little in the past half century. Although the Common Rule sets institutional standards for a substantial proportion of clinical trials, the common law remains the source of redress for injuries to subjects in research. Augmented by a growing body of statutory and constitutional jurisprudence, these general common law principles offer a comprehensive, but still evolving, description of the rights of research subjects and the obligations of investigators. As clinical trials increase in number and complexity, these principles will be applied and adapted to answer new research questions. Some causes of action little used in the past may become more prominent, such as dignitary harms inferred from constitutional provisions and international covenants. Lack of informed consent, the most prevalent complaint in published decisions, may center on the failure to disclose conflicts of interest or a research component of heath care. Litigation is sometimes used to obtain or encourage changes that neither private industry nor the legislature has yet adopted, as was the case with the tobacco litigation. If litigation fails to resolve disputes, people may be discouraged from participating in research unless they are made financial partners. If those enrolled in research are to be true *research participants*—the terminology that patient advocates now prefer—they may demand participation in the financial rewards as well as

the risks of research, as in the PXE case. Finally, it should be noted that criminal prosecution remains available for conduct that rises to the level of a criminal offense. Although criminal punishment does not compensate those who are injured, it often has a broader effect on national standards of conduct than civil law cases.

The relatively small number of published court decisions involving injuries to research subjects may be viewed either as reassuring evidence that research poses little serious risk to subjects or as a lack of adequate legal redress for hidden harms. More public attention to both the importance and uncertainties of research may encourage better protection against injuries and more public support for research.

References

1. Goldby S. Experiments at the Willowbrook State School. In: Katz J, with Capron AM, Glass ES, eds. *Experimentation With Human Beings.* New York, N.Y.: Russell Sage Foundation; 1972:1007–10.
2. Rothman DJ. *Strangers at the Bedside.* New York, N.Y.: Basic Books; 1991.
3. Jones J. *Bad Blood: The Tuskegee Syphilis Experiment,* new and expanded ed. New York, N.Y.: Free Press; 1993 [1981].
4. Weiss R. Boy's cancer prompts FDA to halt gene therapy experiments. *Washington Post* March 4, 2005:A2.
5. Levine S, Weiss R. Hopkins told to halt trials funded by U.S.; Death of Medical Volunteer prompted federal directive. *Washington Post* July 20, 2001:A1.
6. Fox JL. Gene-therapy death prompts broad civil lawsuit. *Nature Biotechnology* 2000;18:1136.
7. The Research Revitalization Act, S. 3060, 107th Congress, 2nd Session, 2002.
8. Shalala D. Protecting research subjects: What must be done? *New England Journal of Medicine* 2000;343:808–10.
9. Annas GJ. Why we need a national human experimentation agency. *Accountability in Research* 1999;7:293–302.
10. Office of Inspector General, Department of Health and Human Services. *Institutional Review Boards: A Time for Reform.* OEI-01-97-00193. Washington, D.C.: DHHS; 1998. [Online] June 1998. Available: http://oig.hhs.gov/oei/reports/oei-01-97-00193.pdf.
11. Office of Inspector General, Department of Health and Human Services. *Protecting Human Research Subject—Status of Recommendations.* OEI-01-97-00197. Washington, D.C.: DHHS; 2000. [Online] April 2000. Available: http://oig.hhs.gov/oei/reports/oei-01-97-00197.pdf.
12. Milford M. Lawsuits attack medical trials. *National Law Journal* August 27, 2001:A1.
13. Mariner WK. Human subjects research law, common law of human experimentation. In: Murray TJ, Mehlman MJ, eds. *Encyclopedia of Ethical, Legal and Policy Issues in Biotechnology.* New York, N.Y.: John Wiley & Sons, Inc.; 2000:654–75.
14. Dute J, Faure MG, Koziol H, eds. *Liability for and Insurability of Biomedical Research With Human Subjects in a Comparative Perspective.* New York, N.Y.: Springer-Verlag; 2004.
15. The Code of Hammurabi. [Online] Available: http://www.lawresearchservices.com/admin/CodeHam.htm.
16. Hughes G. Common law systems. In: Morrison AB, ed. *Fundamentals of American Law.* New York, N.Y.: Oxford University Press; 1996: 9–33.
17. *Stratton v. Swanlond,* Y.B. 48 Edw. III, fo. 6, pl. 11 (K.B.1374). In: Baker J, Milsom S, eds. *Sources of English Legal History: Private Law to 1750.* Stoneham, Mass.: Butterworth Legal Publishers; 1986: 360–2.

18. Burns CJ. Malpractice suits in American medicine before the Civil War. In: Burns CR, ed. *Legacies in Law and Medicine*. New York, N.Y.: Neale Watson Academic Publications, Inc.; 1977:107–22.

19. The Nuremberg Code. In: *Trials of War Criminals Before the Nuremberg Military Tribunals Under Control Council Law No. 10. Volume 2*. Washington, D.C.: U.S. Government Printing Office; 1949:181–2. [Online]. Available: http://www.hhs.gov/ohrp/references/nurcode.htm.

20. Drinan RF. The Nuremberg Principles in international law. In: Annas GJ, Grodin MA, eds. *The Nazi Doctors and the Nuremberg Code*. New York, N.Y.: Oxford University Press; 1992:174–82.

21. Lifton RJ. *The Nazi Doctors*. New York, N.Y.: Basic Books; 1986.

22. Proctor RN. *Racial Hygiene: Medicine Under the Nazis*. Cambridge, Mass.: Harvard University Press; 1988.

23. *Stanley v. United States*, 483 U.S. 669 (1987).

24. Annas GJ. The Nuremberg Code in U.S. courts: Ethics versus expediency. In: Annas GJ, Grodin MA, eds. *The Nazi Doctors and the Nuremberg Code*. New York, N.Y.: Oxford University Press; 1992: 201–22.

25. *Robertson v. McGee*, 2002 U.S. Dist. LEXIS 4072 (N.D. Okla. 2002).

26. In re *Cincinnati Radiation Litigation*, 874 F. Supp. 796, 820 (S.D. Ohio 1995).

27. Glantz LH. The influence of the Nuremberg Code on U.S. statutes and regulations. In: Annas GJ, Grodin MA, eds. *The Nazi Doctors and the Nuremberg Code*. New York, N.Y.: Oxford University Press; 1992:183–200.

28. *Hoover v. West Virginia Department of Health and Human Services*, 984 F. Supp. 978 (S.D. W.Va. 1997), aff'd 129 F.3d 1259 (11th Cir. 1997).

29. *White v. Paulsen*, 997 F. Supp. 1380 (E.D. Wash. 1998).

30. *Heinrich v. Sweet*, 62 F. Supp. 2d 282 (D. Mass. 1999).

31. *Diaz v. Hillsborough County Hospital Authority*, 2000 U.S. Dist. LEXIS 14061 (M.D. Fla. 2000).

32. *Grimes v. Kennedy Krieger Institute*, 366 Md. 29, 782 A.2d 807 (Md. 2001).

33. *Abdullah v. Pfizer, Inc.*, 2002 WL 31082956 (S.D.N.Y. September 17, 2002); 77 Fed. Appx. 48 (2003), on remand, 2005 U.S. Dist. LEXIS 16126 (2005).

34. *Ammend v. Bioport, Inc.*, 322 F. Supp. 2d 848 (W.D. Mich. 2004).

35. Annas GJ. Unspeakably cruel—Torture, medical ethics, and the law. *New England Journal of Medicine* 2005;352:2127–32.

36. World Medical Association. *Declaration of Helsinki: Ethical Principles for Medical Research Involving Human Subjects*. Tokyo, Japan: WMA; October 2004. [Online] 2004. Available: http://www.wma.net/e/policy/b3.htm.

37. *Hoover v. West Virginia Department of Health and Human Services*, 984 F. Supp. 978 (S.D. W.Va. 1997), aff'd 129 F.3d 1259 (11th Cir. 1997).

38. Council for International Organizations of Medical Sciences, in collaboration with the World Health Organization. *International Ethical Guidelines for Biomedical Research Involving Human Subjects*. Geneva, Switzerland: CIOMS and WHO; 2002. [Online] November 2002. Available: http://www.cioms.ch/frame_guidelines_nov_2002.htm.

39. The T.J. Hooper, 60 F.2d 737 (2d Cir. 1932).

40. United Nations. *Universal Declaration of Human Rights* (adopted by General Assembly resolution 217 A (III) of 10 December 1948). [Online] Available: http://www.un.org/Overview/rights.html.

41. United Nations. *International Covenant on Civil and Political Rights* (adopted by General Assembly Resolution 2200 A (XXI) of 19 December 1966). [Online] Available: http://www.unhchr.ch/html/menu3/b/a_ccpr.html.

42. Dute J, Nys H. International aspects of liability for and insurability of biomedical research involving human subjects. In: Dute J, Faure MG, Koziol H, eds. *Liability for and Insurability of Biomedical Research With Human Subjects in a Comparative Perspective*. New York, N.Y.: Springer-Verlag; 2004:351–8.

43. Beecher HK. Ethics in clinical research. *New England Journal of Medicine* 1966;74:1354–60.

44. Tuskegee Syphilis Study Ad Hoc Advisory Panel. *Final Report of the Tuskegee Syphilis Study Ad Hoc Advisory Panel*. Washington, D.C.: Department of Health, Education and Welfare; 1973. [Online] Available: http://biotech.law.lsu.edu/cphl/history/reports/tuskegee/tuskegee.htm.

45. National Research Act of 1974, 88 Stat. 342, codified, as amended, at 42 U.S.C. §§201–300aaa-13.

46. The National Commission for the Protection of Human Subjects of Biomedical and Behavioral Research. *The Belmont Report: Ethical Principles and Guidelines for the Protection of Human Subjects of Research*. Washington, D.C.: Department of Health, Education and Welfare; DHEW Publication OS 78-0012 1978. [Online] April 18, 1979. Available: http://www.hhs.gov/ohrp/humansubjects/guid-/guidance/belmont.htm.

47. Office of Science and Technology Policy. Federal Policy for the Protection of Human Subjects. *Federal Register* 1991;56(117): 28002–32.

48. President's Commission for the Study of Ethical Problems in Medicine and Biomedical and Behavioral Research. *Implementing Human Research Regulations: The Adequacy and Uniformity of Federal Rules and of their Implementation*. Washington, D.C.: U.S. Government Printing Office; 1983.

49. Department of Health and Human Services, National Institutes of Health, and Office for Human Research Protections. The Common Rule, Title 45 (Public Welfare), Code of Federal Regulations, Part 46 (Protection of Human Subjects). [Online] June 23, 2005. Available: http://www.hhs.gov/ohrp/humansubjects/guidance/45cfr46.htm.

50. 45 CFR §46.101(f); 45 CFR §46.116(e); 21 CFR §50.25.

51. 21 USC §337(a).

52. *Merrell Dow Pharmaceuticals, Inc. v. Thompson*, 478 U.S. 804 (1986).

53. *Klamath Water Users Protective Ass'n v. Patterson*, 204 F.3d 1206 (9th Cir.), cert. denied, 531 U.S. 812 (2000).

54. *Wright v. The Fred Hutchinson Cancer Research Center*, 269 F. Supp. 2d 1286 (W.D. Wash. 2002).

55. Committee on Guidelines for Human Embryonic Stem Cell Research, National Research Council. *Guidelines for Human Embryonic Stem Cell Research*. Washington, D.C.: National Academies Press; 2005.

56. *Dubont v. Cornell University*, 2002 Cal. App. Unpub. LEXIS 2187 (Ct. App. Cal., 4th Dist. 2002); unpublished opinion.

57. *Femrite v. Abbott Northwestern Hospital*, 568 N.W.2d 535 (Minn. App. 1997).

58. In *Robertson v. McGee*, 2002 U.S. Dist. LEXIS 4072 (N.D. Okla. 2002), plaintiffs alleged 122 counts against 21 defendants.

59. Fletcher JC. The evolution of the ethics of informed consent. In: Berg K, Tranoy KE, eds. *Research Ethics*. New York, N.Y.: Liss; 1983:187–228.

60. *Hyman v. Jewish Chronic Disease Hospital*, 15 N.Y.2d 317 (1965), rev'd 21 A.D. 2d 495 (2d Dept. 1964).

61. Advisory Committee on Human Radiation Experiments. *Final Report of the Advisory Committee on Human Radiation Experiments*. New York, N.Y.: Oxford University Press; 1996.

62. General Accounting Office. *Human Experimentation: An Overview of Cold War Era Programs* (Statement of Frank C. Conahan; Assistant Comptroller General; National Security and International Affairs Division). GAO/T-NSIAD-94–266. Washington, D.C.: U.S. Government Printing Office; 1994. [Online] September 28, 1994. Available: http://archive.gao.gov/t2pbat2/152601.pdf.

63. U.S. Congress, House of Representatives, Committee on Energy and Commerce, Subcommittee on Energy Conservation and Power. *American Nuclear Guinea Pigs: Three Decades of Radiation Experiments*

on U.S. Citizens, Report. Washington, D.C.: U.S. Government Printing Office; 1986.

64. Stephens M. *The Treatment: The Story of Those Who Died in the Cincinnati Radiation Tests.* Durham, N.C.: Duke University Press; 2002.

65. *Glickman v. United States,* 626 F. Supp. 171 (S.D.N.Y. 1985).

66. *Orlikow v. United States,* 682 F. Supp. 77 (D. D.C. 1988).

67. *Feres v. United States,* 340 U.S. 135 (1950).

68. Annas GJ, Glantz LJ, Katz BF. *Informed Consent to Human Experimentation: The Subject's Dilemma.* Cambridge, Mass.: Ballinger; 1977.

69. Capron AM. Informed consent in catastrophic disease research and treatment. *University of Pennsylvania Law Review* 1974;123:341–438.

70. *Union Pacific Railroad Co. v. Botsford,* 141 U.S. 250 (1891).

71. *Cruzan v. Director, Missouri Department of Health,* 497 U.S. 261 (1990).

72. *Vacco v. Quill,* 521 U.S. 793 (1997).

73. *Washington v. Harper,* 494 U.S. 210 (1990).

74. Faden RR, Beauchamp TL, with King NMP. *A History and Theory of Informed Consent.* New York, N.Y.: Oxford University Press; 1986.

75. American Law Institute. *Restatement (Second) of Torts.* Philadelphia, Penn.: American Law Institute; 1965, §13.

76. American Law Institute. *Restatement (Second) of Torts.* Philadelphia, Penn.: American Law Institute; 1965, §18.

77. *Mink v. University of Chicago,* 460 F. Supp. 713 (N. Dist. Ill. 1978).

78. *Ancheff v. Hartford Hospital,* 260 Conn. 785, 799 A.2d 1067 (Conn. 2002).

79. *Proctor v. Davis,* 291 Ill. App. 3d 265, 682 N.E. 2d 1203 (1997).

80. *Estrada v. Jaques,* 70 N.C. App. 627, 321 S.E. 2d 240 (N.C. App. 1984).

81. *Ahern v. Veterans Administration,* 537 F.2d 10989 (10th Cir. 1978).

82. *Monroe v. Harper,* 164 Mont. 23, 518 P.2d 788 (1974).

83. *Clemens v. Regents of the University of California,* 87 Cal. Rptr. 108 (Cal. Ct. App. 1970).

84. *Wilson v. Scott,* 412 S.W. 2d 299 (Tex. 1967).

85. Hanlon SF, Shapiro RS. Ethical issues in biomedical research: *Diaz v. Hillsborough County Hospital Authority. Human Rights* 2003;30:16–8. [Online] Available: http://www.abanet.org/irr/hr/spring03/biomedicalresearch.html.

86. *Stadt v. University of Rochester,* 921 F. Supp. 1023 (W.D.N.Y. 1996).

87. Dyer J. University issues apology for 1939 experiment that induced orphans to stutter. *San Jose Mercury News* June 14, 2001.

88. American Law Institute. *Restatement (Second) of Torts.* Philadelphia, Penn.: American Law Institute; 1977:§550.

89. *Craft v. Vanderbilt University,* 18 F.Supp. 2d 786 (M.D. Tenn. 1998).

90. $10.3 Million Settlement in Radiation Case. *Boston Globe* July 28, 1998:A5.

91. Verdicts and Settlements—Radioactive Isotope Experiments—Facility for Mentally Retarded Individuals, *Beaulieu v. Belmont. Massachusetts Lawyers Weekly* May 3, 1999:B6.

92. Judge approves $5 million settlement in radiation case. *Associated Press* May 5, 1999.

93. American Law Institute. *Restatement (Second) of Torts.* Philadelphia, Penn.: American Law Institute; 1977:§311.

94. Gregor R, et al. *American Jurisprudence,* 2nd ed. St. Paul, Minn.: Thomson-West; 2004:§23.

95. Keeton WP, Dobbs DB, Keeton RE, Owen DG. *Prosser and Keeton on the Law of Torts,* 5th ed. St. Paul, Minn.: West Publishing Co.; 1984:§105.

96. American Law Institute. *Restatement (Second) of Torts.* Philadelphia, Penn.: American Law Institute; 1977:§§526–551.

97. Katz J. Human experimentation and human rights. *St. Louis University Law Journal* 1993;38:7–54.

98. Appelbaum PS, et al. False hopes and best data: Consent to research and the therapeutic misconception. *Hastings Center Report* 1987;17(2):20–4.

99. *Karp v. Cooley,* 349 F. Supp. 827 (S.D. Tex. 1972).

100. Churchill LR, et al. Genetic research as therapy: Implications of "gene therapy" for informed consent. *Journal of Law Medicine and Ethics* 1998;26:38–47.

101. Horng S, et al. Descriptions of benefits and risks in consent forms for phase 1 oncology trials. *New England Journal of Medicine* 2002;347:2134–40.

102. Statement of Cherlynn Mathias, Hearing before the Subcommittee on Public Health, Committee on Health, Education, Labor, and Pensions, U.S. Senate, 107th Cong., 2d Sess. *Protecting Human Subjects in Research: Are Current Safeguards Adequate?,* S. Hrg. 107–424. Washington, D.C.: U.S. Government Printing Office; April 23, 2002:7–10.

103. Brown C. University of Oklahoma settles state lawsuit over melanoma study, other claims proceed. *BNA Health Law Reporter* 2002;11:1269–70.

104. *Canterbury v. Spence,* 464 F.2d 772 (D.C. Cir. 1972), cert. denied, 409 U.S. 1064 (1972).

105. *Cobbs v. Grant,* 8 Cal. 3d 229, 502 P.2d 1, 104 Cal. Rptr. 505 (1972).

106. President's Commission for the Study of Ethical Problems in Medicine and Biomedical and Behavioral Research. *Making Health Care Decisions.* Washington, D.C.: U.S. Government Printing Office; 1982.

107. Basic HHS Policy for Protection of Human Research Subjects, 45 CFR §46.116.

108. National Bioethics Advisory Commission. *Ethical and Policy Issues in Research Involving Human Participants.* Bethesda, Md.: NBAC; 2001. [Online] August, 2001. Available: http://www.georgetown.edu/research/nrcbl/nbac/human/overv011.pdf.

109. Glantz LH, Annas GJ, Grodin MA, Mariner WK. Research in developing countries: Taking "benefit" seriously. *Hastings Center Report* 1998;28(6):38–42.

110. Mariner WK. Informed consent in the post-modern era. *Law and Social Inquiry* 1988:385–406.

111. *Whitlock v. Duke University,* 637 F.Supp. 1463, 1471 (M.D. N.C. 1986), aff'd, 829 F.2d 1340 (4th Cir. 1987).

112. American Law Institute. *Restatement of the Law Third, Torts: Liability for Physical Harm.* Proposed Final Draft No. 1. Philadelphia, Penn.: American Law Institute; May 2005.

113. *Karp v. Cooley,* 493 F.2d 408 (5th Cir. 1974).

114. Annas GJ. *The Rights of Patients,* 3rd ed. Carbondale, Ill.: Southern Illinois University Press; 2004:124–6.

115. Wilson D, Heath D. Uninformed consent: What patients at the "Hutch" weren't told about the experiments in which they died. *Seattle Times* March 11, 2001:A1.

116. Reinert S. Doctor added to family's lawsuit; nurse died after lupus experiment. *The Patriot Ledger* (Quincy, Mass.) Nov. 7, 2002:12.

117. General Accounting Office. *VA Research: Protections for Human Subjects Need to Be Strengthened.* GAO/HEHS-00–155. Washington, D.C.: GAO; 2000. [Online] September 28, 2000. Available: http://www.gao.gov/new.items/he00155.pdf.

118. General Accounting Office. *VA Research: Actions Insufficient to Further Strengthen Human Protections* (Statement of Cynthia A. Bascetta; Director, Health Care—Veterans' Health and Benefits Issues). GAO-03–917T. Washington, D.C.: GAO; 2003. [Online] June 18, 2003. Available: http://www.gao.gov/new.items/d03917t.pdf.

119. *Kus v. Sherman Hospital,* 268 Ill. App. 3d 771 (1995).

120. *Lenahan v. University of Chicago,* 2004 WL 635570 (1st Dist. Ill. App. Ct. 2004).

121. 45 C.F.R. §46.116(c),(d).

122. Milgram S. *Obedience to Authority: An Experimental View.* New York, N.Y.: Harper & Row; 1974:193–202.

123. Humphreys L. *Tearoom Trade: Impersonal Sex in Public Places* (enlarged ed. with a retrospect on ethical issues). New York, N.Y.: Aldine de Gruyter; 1975:167–232.

124. 21 C.F.R. 50.23(d).

125. Annas GJ. Changing the consent rules for Desert Storm. *New England Journal of Medicine* 1992;326:770–3.

126. National Commission for the Protection of Human Subjects of Biomedical and Behavioral Research. *Research Involving Those Institutionalized as Mentally Infirm.* Washington, D.C.: Department of Health, Education and Welfare; 1978.

127. Moreno JD. Regulation of research on the decisionally impaired: History and gaps in the current regulatory system. *Journal of Health Care Law and Policy* 1998;1:1–21.

128. Field MJ, Berman RE, eds. *The Ethical Conduct of Research Involving Children.* Washington, D.C.: National Academies Press; 2004.

129. National Bioethics Advisory Commission. *Research Involving Persons with Mental Disorders That May Affect Decisionmaking Capacity, Volume I.* Rockville, Md.: NBAC; 1998. [Online] December 1998. Available: http://www.georgetown.edu/research/nrcbl/nbac/capacity/TOC.htm.

130. *Matter of Quinlan,* 70 N.J. 10, cert denied, 429 U.S. 922 (1976).

131. Capron AM. Ethical and human rights issues in research on mental disorders that may affect decision-making capacity. *New England Journal of Medicine* 1999;340:1430–4.

132. 21 C.F.R. §50.23(a)–(c).

133. *Trantafello v. Medical Center of Tarzana,* 227 Cal Rptr. 84 (Cal. Ct. App. 1976).

134. 21 C.F.R. §50.24.

135. Food and Drug Administration. Guidance for Institutional Review Boards and Clinical Investigators, 1998 Update. *Exception from Informed Consent for Studies Conducted in Emergency Settings: Regulatory Language and Excerpts from Preamble.* [Online] September 1998. Available: http://www.fda.gov/oc/ohrt/irbs/except.html.

136. Food and Drug Administration. *Draft Guidance for Institutional Review Boards, Clinical Investigators, and Sponsors: Exception from Informed Consent Requirements for Emergency Research.* [Online] March 30, 2000. Available: http://www.fda.gov/ora/compliance_ref/bimo/emrfinal.pdf.

137. *T.D. v. New York State Office of Mental Health,* 228 A.D.2d 95, 650 N.Y.S.2d 173 (1st Dept 1996), app. dism'd mem. opinion, 89 N.Y.2d 1029 (1997).

138. 45 C.F.R. §§46.404-.408; 21 C.F.R. §§50.51–50.54.

139. Grodin MA, Glantz LH, eds. *Children as Research Subjects.* New York, N.Y.: Oxford University Press; 1994.

140. Ross LF. *Children, Families, and Health Care Decision Making.* New York, N.Y.: Oxford University Press; 1998.

141. Mariner WK. Health care law. In: *Medical and Health Annual 1992.* Chicago, Ill.: Encyclopaedia Brittanica; 1991:312–6.

142. Hoffman DE, Rothenberg KR. Whose duty is it anyway?: The Kennedy Krieger opinion and its implications for public health research. *Journal of Health Care Law and Policy* 2002;6:109–47.

143. Cathell DR. Preserving research integrity: A researcher's legal duty to study participants. Speech presented at conference entitled "Research Integrity and Financial Conflicts of Interest in Clinical Research: Legal Issues and Regulatory Requirements," University of Virginia School of Medicine, October 15, 2004.

144. Karlawish JHT, Sachs GA. Research on the cognitively impaired: Lessons and warnings from the emergency research debate. *Journal of the American Geriatrics Society* 1997;45:474–81.

145. *Vodapest v. MacGregor,* 128 Wash. 2d 840, 913 P.2d 779 (1996).

146. *Sargon Enterprises, Inc. v. University of Southern California,* 2005 WL 435413 (2005); not officially published.

147. *Gelsinger v. University of Pennsylvania* (Pa. C. No. 001885), filed Sept. 18, 2000.

148. Fox JL. Gene-therapy death prompts broad civil lawsuit. *Nature Biology* 2000;18:1136.

149. Avery S. Psoriasis patient sues over drug trial. *News and Observer* (Raleigh, N.C.) July 11, 2003:B3.

150. Romano R. Fatal error becomes catalyst for reform. *Boston Globe* March 15, 1999:A11.

151. Willwerth J. Tinkering with madness. *Time Magazine* August 30, 1993.

152. Kong D. Study harmed mentally ill, agency reports. *Boston Globe* February 9, 1999:A8.

153. Insight Team of the Sunday Times of London. *Suffer the Children: The Story of Thalidomide.* New York, N.Y.: Viking Press; 1979:109.

154. Weiss R, Nelson D. Methods faulted in fatal gene therapy. *Washington Post* December 8, 1999:A1.

155. 45 C.F.R. §46.116.

156. Wing KR. Malpractice: Liability for negligence in the delivery and financing of health care. In: Wing KR. *The Law and the Public's Health,* 6th ed. Chicago, Ill.: Health Administration Press; 2003:294–302.

157. *Schwartz v. Boston Hospital for Women,* 422 F. Supp. 53 (S.D.N.Y. 1976).

158. *Darling v. Charlestown Memorial Hospital,* 33 Ill. 2d 326, 211 N.E.2d 253 (1965), cert. denied, 383 U.S. 946 (1966).

159. Sontag D. In harm's way—Abuses endangered veterans in cancer experiment. *New York Times* February 6, 2005:A1.

160. Virtanen M. Former VA researcher sentenced in drug trial scandal. Newsday.com November 21, 2005. [Online] Available (with subscription): http://www.newsday.com.

161. General Accounting Office. *VA Research: System for Protecting Human Subjects Needs Improvements* (Statement of Victor S. Rezendes; Assistant Comptroller General; Health, Education, and Human Services Division). GAO/HEHS-00-203. Washington, D.C.: GAO; 2000. [Online] September 28, 2000. Available: http://www.gao.gov/archive/2000/he00203t.pdf.

162. Steinbrook R. Protecting research subjects—The crisis at Johns Hopkins. *New England Journal of Medicine* 2002;346:716–20.

163. Stolberg SG. The biotech death of Jesse Gelsinger. *New York Times Magazine* November 28, 1999:137–151. [Online] Available: http://nytimes.com/library/magazine/home/19991128mag-stolberg.html.

164. Weiss R, Nelson D. Penn settles gene therapy suit. *Washington Post* November 4, 2000:A4.

165. Corbie-Smith G, et al. Distrust, race and research. *Archives of Internal Medicine* 2002;162:2458–63.

166. Lo B, Wolf LE, Berkeley A. Conflict-of-interest policies for investigators in clinical trials. *New England Journal of Medicine* 2000;343:1616–20.

167. Martin JL, Kasper DL. In whose best interest? Breaching the academic-industrial wall. *New England Journal of Medicine* 2000;343:1646–9.

168. McCrary SV, Anderson CB, Jakovljevic J, et al. A national survey of policies on disclosure of conflicts of interest in biomedical research. *New England Journal of Medicine* 2000;343:1621–6.

169. Ferris LE, Naylor CD. Physician remuneration in industry-sponsored clinical trials: The case for standardized clinical trial budgets. *Canadian Medical Association Journal* 2004;171:883–6.

170. Bodenheimer T. Uneasy alliance—Clinical investigators and the pharmaceutical industry. *New England Journal of Medicine* 2000;342:1539–44.

171. Montori VM, Jawschke R, Schünemann HJ, et al. User's guide to detecting misleading claims in clinical research reports. *British Medical Journal* 2004;329:1093–6.

172. Procyshyn RM, Chau A, Fortin P, Jenkins W. Prevalence and outcomes of pharmaceutical industry-sponsored clinical trials involving clozapine, risperidone, or olanzapine. *Canadian Journal of Psychiatry* 2004;49:601–6.

173. Barnes M, Florencio PS. Financial conflicts of interest in human subjects research: The problem of institutional conflicts. *Journal of Law Medicine and Ethics* 2002;30:390–402.

174. Department of Health and Human Services. Supplemental Standards of Ethical Conduct and Financial Disclosure Requirements for

Employees of the Department of Health and Human Services. *Federal Register* 2005;70(22):5543–65, codified at 5 CFR Parts 5501 and 5502.

175. 5 CFR §§5501.109–5501.110.

176. Steinbrook R. Standards of ethics at the National Institutes of Health. *New England Journal of Medicine* 2005;352:1290–2.

177. Willman D. Stealth merger: Drug companies and government medical research; some of the National Institutes of Health's top scientists are also collecting paychecks and stock options from biomedical firms. Increasingly, such details are kept secret. *Los Angeles Times* December 7, 2003:1.

178. Lenzer J. FDA to review "missing" drug company documents. *British Medical Journal* 2005;330:7.

179. Eisenberg T, LaFountain N, Ostrom B, Rottman D, Wells MT. Juries, judges, and punitive damages: An empirical study. *Cornell Law Review* 2002;87:743–80.

180. President's Commission for the Study of Ethical Problems in Medicine and Biomedical and Behavioral Research. *Whistleblowing in Biomedical Research: Policies and Procedures for Responding to Reports of Misconduct.* Washington, D.C.: U.S. Government Printing Office; 1982.

181. UAB pays feds $3.39M to settle whistleblower suits. *Birmingham Business Journal* April 14, 2005.

182. American Law Institute. *Restatement (Second) of Torts.* Philadelphia, Penn.: American Law Institute; 1965.

183. Rothstein MA, ed. *Genetic Secrets: Protecting Privacy and Confidentiality in the Genetic Era.* New Haven, Conn.: Yale University Press; 1999.

184. General Accounting Office. *Record Linkage and Privacy: Issues in Creating New Federal Research and Statistical Information.* GAO-01–126SP. Washington, D.C.: GAO; 2001. [Online] April 2001. Available: http://www.gao.gov/new.items/d01126sp.pdf.

185. Department of Health and Human Services. Standards for privacy of individually identifiable information. 45 CFR §§160, 164.

186. Mariner WK. Law and public health: Beyond emergency preparedness. *Journal of Health Law* 2005;38:247–85.

187. Marchant GE. Property rights and benefit-sharing for DNA donors? *Jurimetrics* 2005;45:153–78.

188. *Moore v. Regents of the University of California,* 51 Cal. 3d 120, 793 P.2d 479, 271 Cal. Rptr. 146 (1990), cert. denied, 499 U.S. 936 (1991).

189. Weir RF, Olick RS. *The Stored Tissue Issue: Biomedical Research, Ethics and Law in the Era of Genomic Medicine.* New York, N.Y.: Oxford University Press; 2004.

190. Mehlman MJ. *Wondergenes: Genetic Enhancement and the Future of Society.* Bloomington, Ind.: Indiana University Press; 2003.

191. *Greenberg v. Miami Children's Hospital, Inc.,* 264 F. Supp. 2d 1064 (S.D. Fla. 2003).

192. Canavan Foundation and Miami Children's Hospital Joint Press Release, September 29, 2003. [Online] Available: http://www .canavanfoundation.org/news2/09–03_miami.php.

193. Marshall E. Patient advocate named co-inventor on patent for PXE disease gene. *Science* 2004;305:5688.

194. *Suthers v. Amgen Inc.,* 05 Civ. 4158 (PKC), S.D.N.Y. June 6, 2005); slip opinion.

195. Kolata G, Eichenwald K. For the uninsured, drug trials are health care. *New York Times* June 22, 1999:1.

196. Delaney M. The case for patient access to experimental therapy. *Journal of Infectious Diseases* 1989;159:416–9.

197. Mariner WK. AIDS research and the Nuremberg Code. In: Annas GJ, Grodin MA, eds. *The Nazi Doctors and the Nuremberg Code.* New York, N.Y.: Oxford University Press; 1992:286–303.

198. Arno PS, Feiden KL. *Against the Odds: The Story of AIDS Drug Development.* New York, N.Y.: Harper Collins Publishers; 1992.

199. Whitaker R, Kong D. Doing harm: Research on the mentally ill. *Boston Globe* November 15–18, 1998.

200. National Bioethics Advisory Commission. *Ethical and Policy Issues in International Research: Clinical Trials in Developing Countries.* Bethesda, Md.: NBAC; 2001. [Online] April 30, 2001. Available: http://www.bioethics.gov/reports/past_commissions/nbac_international.pdf.

201. Annas, GJ. The right to health and the Nevirapine case in South Africa. *New England Journal of Medicine* 2003;348:750–4.

202. Washington Post Staff Writers. The body hunters (6-part series). *Washington Post* December 17–22, 2000.

203. 28 USC §1350.

204. Department of Health, Education and Welfare, Secretary's Task Force on the Compensation of Injured Research Subjects. *Report of the Task Force.* OS-77–003. Washington, D.C.: DHEW; 1977.

205. Institute of Medicine. *Responsible Research: A Systems Approach to Protecting Research Subjects.* Washington, D.C.: National Academies Press; 2002.

206. General Accounting Office. *Scientific Research: Continued Vigilance Critical to Protecting Human Research Subjects.* GAO/HEHS-96–72. Washington, D.C.: GAO; 1996. [Online] March 12, 1996. Available: http://www.gao.gov/archive/1996/he96072.pdf.

207. Shamoo AE. Adverse event reporting—The tip of an iceberg. *Accountability in Research* 2001;8:197–218.

208. Class Action Fairness Act. P.L. 109–2, 109th Cong., 1st Sess. February 18, 2005.

209. DeVille K. The role of litigation in human research accountability. *Accountability in Research* 2002;9:17–43.

210. Betsy Lehman Center for Patient Safety and Medical Error Reduction. [Online] Available: http://www.mass.gov/dph/betsylehman/.

211. Weiss R. U.S., researchers reach deal in '99 gene therapy case. *Washington Post* February 10, 2005:A03.

212. *Heinrich v. Sweet,* 62 F. Supp. 2d 282 (D. Mass. 1999).

213. *Heinrich v. Sweet,* No. 97–12134-WGY (D. Mass. October 15, 1999).

214. *Heinrich v. Sweet,* 308 F.3d 48 (1st Cir. 2002).

215. Colonial Laws of Massachusetts, Edition of 1660:17–18.

216. Federal Tort Claims Act, 28 USC §1346.

217. *Goodman v. United States,* 298 F.3d 1048 (9th Cir. 2002).

218. *Harlow v. Fitzgerald,* 457 U.S. 800 (1982).

219. Massachusetts General Laws, c. 258, §2.

220. U.S. Constitution, amend. XI.

221. *Hans v. Louisiana,* 134 U.S. 1 (1890).

222. *Seminole Tribe of Florida v. Florida,* 517 U.S. 44 (1996).

223. American Law Institute. *Draft Restatement of Torts, Third:* Products Liability §§1–3. Philadelphia, Penn.: American Law Institute; 2003.

224. President's Commission for the Study of Ethical Problems in Medicine and Biomedical and Behavioral Research. *Compensating for Research Injuries.* Washington, D.C.: U.S. Government Printing Office; 1982.

225. Kolberg R. RAC asks, who should pay for research injuries. *Journal of NIH Research* 1993;5:37–8.

226. *Federal Insurance Company v. Curon Medical, Inc.,* 2004 U.S. Dist. LEXIS 22365 (N.D. Cal. 2004).

227. Council of Europe, Directorate of Legal Affairs. *Convention for the Protection of Human Rights and Dignity of the Human Being With Regard to the Application of Biology and Medicine: Convention on Human Rights and Biomedicine.* Strasbourg, France; 1997. [Online] April 4, 1997. Available: http://conventions.coe.int/treaty/en/treaties/html/164.htm.

228. Council of Europe, Directorate of Legal Affairs. *Additional Protocol to the Convention on Human Rights and Biomedicine, Concerning Biomedical Research.* Strasbourg, France; 2005. [Online] January 25, 2005. Available: http://conventions.coe.int/treaty/en/treaties/html/195 .htm.

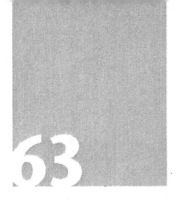

James V. Lavery

The Obligation to Ensure Access to Beneficial Treatments for Research Participants at the Conclusion of Clinical Trials

The conclusion of a clinical trial triggers a new set of ethical obligations to research participants. The way these obligations are conceptualized and fulfilled, particularly in clinical drug and device trials, can have a profound influence on the way research participants benefit from their participation in clinical research. In particular, the central question in many clinical trials is whether, at the conclusion of the trial, individual research participants should continue to be provided with drugs and devices that have benefited them during the trial. Although a solid consensus about this and related posttrial obligations has not yet emerged in the literature, several key ideas have been prominent and are beginning to influence research ethics guidelines and the practices of researchers and sponsors. Posttrial obligations can arise in any clinical research setting, but the ethical issues they raise have been particularly salient in research conducted in low- and middle-income countries by researchers and sponsors from high-income countries. As a result, analysis of international collaborative research has contributed a great deal to current thinking about these questions.

Posttrial obligations to research participants can be described under three broad headings: first, the obligation to avoid the exploitation of research participants by ensuring that they receive a fair distribution of research benefits along with the sponsors and investigators; second, the obligation to recognize the contribution of research participants, and third, the obligation to minimize the likelihood of feelings of loss or abandonment on the part of research participants whose continued access to a beneficial intervention might require special provisions beyond the planned clinical trial. Each of these obligations reflects a different ethical rationale, and these are discussed in greater detail below. Other

more controversial proposals have been made about posttrial obligations. For example, some commentators have argued that investigators also have an obligation to serve as advocates for therapies growing out of their research findings, particularly in some low- and middle-income countries in which bureaucrats and politicians may lack the knowledge and/or political will to utilize research findings in ways that may improve the health of their citizens.[1] Some of the implications of this type of expansion of the customary roles and responsibilities of investigators have also been explored.[2]

In this chapter, I describe the current thinking about obligations to research participants at the conclusion of a clinical trial, focusing on the three main obligations described above and emphasizing the issue of continued provision of beneficial drugs and devices. The chapter begins with a brief review of the current guidelines on posttrial obligations and then describes some of the current thinking about the ethical rationale and appropriate scope of posttrial obligations. It then explains what I call the "mechanics" of posttrial obligations, including specific mechanisms by which the obligations may be met. The chapter ends with three brief case examples of posttrial obligations in international research, the first of a successful funding partnership to ensure continued access to antiretroviral drugs for participants in HIV clinical trials in Thailand, the second of intermittent presumptive treatment (IPT) for malaria in a trial of infants in Kamasi, Ghana, and the third of a public-private partnership to develop a new antimalarial drug between the Medicines for Malaria Venture (MMV) and Bayer, which includes a comprehensive agreement about posttrial obligations for research.

Current Guidelines on Posttrial Obligations

A great deal of the recent debate about international research ethics has focused on how ethical obligations about highly complex matters should be articulated in international codes and guidelines. As with many other issues, the available guidance with respect to posttrial obligations is both limited and varied in ways that impede consensus, rather than promote it.

Declaration of Helsinki

One of the most controversial guidance statements related to posttrial obligations has been Paragraph 30 of the 2000 version of the World Medical Association's Declaration of Helsinki, which reads, "At the conclusion of the study, every patient entered into the study should be assured of access to the best proven prophylactic, diagnostic and therapeutic methods identified by the study."[3] Paragraph 30 has given rise to enormous controversy, although it has also played a formative role in laying out the contentious parameters of the posttrial obligations debate.

The first point is that posttrial obligations kick in "at the conclusion of the study." This seemingly simple observation has itself provoked considerable discussion. At issue is how to determine, for the purposes of posttrial obligations, when a trial has actually concluded. Historically, a great deal of international research—particularly drug trials—limited the amount of time spent in the host country. Once data collection has ended and appropriate procedures have been put in place for necessary follow-up, the investigators often return to their home countries, ending the effective presence of the trial in the host country. From the perspective of the host communities, then, this point might reasonably be thought to mark the conclusion of the trial. In fact, it is precisely this type of rapid departure that has fuelled sentiments of abandonment, which I discuss in greater detail below. But because Paragraph 30 goes on to emphasize interventions that have been "identified by the study" as satisfying (or not) the "best proven" criterion, the departure of the research team cannot serve as a reliable measure of a trial's conclusion.

A more promising, but still controversial, account of a study's conclusion is when the data analyses necessary to answer the primary research question(s) have been completed. But other problems quickly become apparent. How long does it take to prepare and analyze study data? What are the necessary analyses? Who should determine these? Taking this point even further, it can be argued that the conclusion of a trial follows the successful publication of the trial results, in other words, the point at which the trial has met the scientific requirement of peer review and the fair conclusions have been clarified and agreed upon by the study's investigators. But even this seemingly "hard" endpoint is now well known to be subject to gaming and manipulation by research sponsors and investigators. Depending on the favorability of the findings for their personal or corporate ends, sponsors and investigators may delay, or avoid completely, the responsibility of publishing their results, or may publish findings selectively.[4,5] In international collaborative studies, host country governments may also be reluctant to declare a specific trial (or necessary program of research) finished if the findings might suggest costly changes, such as the wholesale revision of a national malaria treatment and prevention program.[6] And yet, without a reliable marker of the conclusion of a trial, the remaining requirements of Paragraph 30 lack coherence.

Although the World Medical Association has long resisted calls for clarification of the intended meaning of the "best proven" requirement,[7] it remains a highly controversial standard in its own right.[8] All the more controversial, then, is Paragraph 30's implication that an individual study can provide definitive clarification of the status of the interventions it aims to compare. A cynical reading of this requirement is that it is simply impossible for an individual trial to clarify whether any given intervention is the "best proven," whatever the precise definition of that standard. A more forgiving reading would limit the scope of the claim to the results of the trial itself. If drug B proved to be better than drug A in a comparative trial, then it might be considered the "best proven" in the trial. If the trial met the ethical requirement of clinical equipoise, itself a highly controversial notion in the context of international research,[9] this would provide some indication that some judgment had been made about the adequacy of the care provided to participants in the trial. Although it may not clarify whether the selected standard of care is truly the *best proven* for the population and context of the trial,[10] it would at least offer some assurance that the appropriateness of the interventions being compared in the trial for the study population had been considered.

Paragraph 30 explicitly limits the applicability of posttrial obligations to "patients entered into the study." Although this approach is consistent with some of the justifications of posttrial obligations that I describe in more detail below, it also differs from other guidelines, such as those of the Council of International Organizations of Medical Sciences (CIOMS), which extend the obligation to communities and populations.

One of the most important of Paragraph 30's clauses is that patients should be "assured of access" to the best proven intervention. This requirement has also given rise to a great deal of debate and disagreement. Briefly, the debate relates primarily to the scope of the posttrial obligations, in other words, whether investigators and sponsors are required to assume the full responsibility for all aspects of the financing, procurement, approval, delivery, and oversight of the relevant interventions, or whether it is sufficient that they arrive at an appropriate agreement with other parties, including host country governments, about how these will be handled. These issues are also explored in greater detail below.

CIOMS

The other main driver for the debate about posttrial obligations has been the well-known "reasonable availability" clause of the 2002 version of the CIOMS International Ethical Guidelines for Biomedical Research Involving Human Subjects.[11] CIOMS Guideline 10 (Research in populations and communities with limited resources) states that "before undertaking research in a population or community with limited resources, the sponsor and the investigator must make every effort to ensure that the research is responsive to the health needs and the priorities of the population or community in which it is to be carried out, and any intervention or product developed, or knowledge generated, will be made reasonably available for the benefit of that population or community."[11]

As with the Declaration of Helsinki, the controversy surrounding the CIOMS guideline turns on several key points. First, the guideline makes explicit that plans to ensure the successful execution of posttrial obligations must be in place before researchers undertake the research, including means of ensuring that the research is responsive to the health needs and priorities of the population or community. In effect, this requires investigators, and other interested parties, to engage in planning and relationship-building activities that they might have little familiarity with, training for, or dedicated funding to support.[2] Second, the guideline implicates sponsors as well as researchers. Third, the guideline focuses on "ensuring" benefits, raising the same set of concerns as the "assured access" requirement of the Declaration of Helsinki.

The main thrust of the CIOMS guideline, however, is the "reasonable availability" requirement, which is meant to ensure that research avoids the exploitation of participants and communities by providing a mechanism for transferring benefits—when they are demonstrated in a clinical trial—to participants and populations. Because the reasonable availability requirement has played such a central role in the debate about exploitation in research,[12] I deal with it separately, and in more detail, below.

The 2002 revision of the CIOMS guidelines also includes an explicit statement about the ethical obligation of external sponsors to provide health-care services. Guideline 21 states that external sponsors should ensure the availability of "healthcare services that are essential to the safe conduct of the research . . . treatment for subjects who suffer injury as a consequence of research interventions . . . and healthcare services that are a necessary part of the commitment of a sponsor to make a beneficial intervention or product developed as a result of the research reasonably available to the population or community concerned."[11] This final requirement, though consistent with the intent of Guideline 10, reaches far beyond the idea of reasonable availability of products and/or knowledge. Like the "assured of access" statement in Paragraph 30 of the Declaration of Helsinki, Guideline 21 explicitly tags sponsors with the responsibility for ensuring that the entire health care infrastructure necessary to deliver a given intervention effectively, and safely, is put in place, along with the intervention itself.

There are two main complaints about this provision. First, Guideline 21 explicitly states that the products, knowledge, and necessary infrastructure must be provided "to the population or community concerned,"[11] as opposed to "every patient entered into the study," as specified in Paragraph 30 of the Declaration of Helsinki. The implications are obvious. First, there is the thorny problem of determining who the "population or community concerned" is in any given study.[13] An expansive interpretation of "population" or "community" could impose an enormous financial burden on research sponsors (public as well as private) that could have serious implications for their willingness and ability to fund international research. Although this might serve one interest of limiting "parachute" research by high-income country research sponsors that has limited value to low- and middle-income countries hosting the research, it might equally limit the feasibility, or desirability among sponsors, of funding and conducting research that is "responsive to the health needs and priorities of the population or community in which it is to be carried out," as required by Guideline 10.[11] Perhaps more to the point, it is not clear how such a standing obligation on the part of investigators and sponsors to ensure access to health care—even in a limited form—to all members of a community or population could be justified.

UNAIDS

One of the most challenging contexts for posttrial obligations has been preventive vaccine research, and the main focus of this type of research in recent years has been on the development of an effective vaccine for HIV/AIDS.[14] The UNAIDS Ethical Considerations in HIV Preventive Vaccine Research is similar in structure to the reasonable availability approach of the CIOMS guidelines.[15] UNAIDS Guidance Point 2 (Vaccine availability) states that "(a)ny HIV preventive vaccine demonstrated to be safe and effective, as well as other knowledge and benefits resulting from the HIV vaccine research, should be made available as soon as possible to all participants in the trials in which it was tested, as well as to other populations at high risk of HIV infection."[15]

The clause raises the now familiar litany of problems. What is a safe and effective vaccine? Is a 25% to 30% efficacy sufficient to trigger this obligation? What about a vaccine for rotavirus that causes a small number of serious side effects in children in the United States, but which is otherwise highly effective and could save millions of lives in low- and middle-income countries? Should it be considered safe?[16] Is the standard "as soon as possible" meant to take into account the real-world challenges of securing financing and political will for the administration of a vaccine to the target population? And how should "populations at high risk of HIV infection" be understood in vaccine trials in countries with huge populations, such as India and China?

Nuffield Council on Bioethics

The United Kingdom's Nuffield Council on Bioethics has issued two influential reports related to the ethics of research in developing countries: The first provided a rich overview of key issues,[1] and the second provided a report of a follow-up conference at which the initial report, and subsequent developments in the field, were considered.[17] Both reports addressed the issue of posttrial obligations to ensure continued provision of beneficial treatments to research participants at the conclusion of a clinical trial. The Council's recommendations direct researchers, sponsors, national health-care authorities, international agencies, and research ethics committees, prior to the initiation of a trial, to "clearly consider" provisions for monitoring possible long-term deleterious outcomes for an agreed period of time beyond the completion of the research. In addition, the Nuffield Council calls on these authorities to consider "the possibility of providing participants with the intervention shown to be best (if they are still able to benefit from it), for an agreed period of time."[1] The Council also endorses the position of the U.S. National Bioethics Advisory Commission[18] that proposals submitted for research ethics review should include an explanation of how proven interventions will be made available to research participants and an explicit justification if this is not seen to be feasible or relevant.

Wellcome Trust Position Statement

In light of sustained controversy in international research ethics, the Wellcome Trust issued a position statement and guidance notes for applicants to its research funding schemes for research involving people living in low- and middle-income countries.[19] Although it does not constitute a formal requirement for the receipt of funding from the Trust, the statement provides guidance to prospective investigators, including setting out "roles and responsibilities of the various parties involved." The Wellcome Trust position statement (Section 7) divides the issue of posttrial obligations into two separate categories, one for individual research participants and the other for the host country, region, and locality.[19] The statement makes clear that the Trust "may consider it an ethical requirement to guarantee post-research access to treatments to participants involved in research investigating chronic or progressive conditions."[19] It also cautions prospective applicants that the way in which they propose to handle these issues may affect the funding decision. Importantly, Section 11, on roles and responsibility, identifies both the investigator and her/his employing institution as sharing the responsibility for "engaging, where appropriate, in processes with relevant stakeholders (for example government ministries or pharmaceutical companies) to try and ensure post-research access to interventions demonstrated to be effective to host communities or populations."[19] Presumably, these obligations would apply as well to ongoing access for individual participants.

European Group on Ethics in Science and New Technologies

The European Group on Ethics in Science and New Technologies, an advisory body to the European Commission, issued an opinion on posttrial obligations in 2003: Opinion No. 17. Ethical Aspects of Clinical Research in Developing Countries.[20] Under Section 2.3 (Inequality), the opinion recognizes that scientific research alone cannot solve global inequalities, but it goes on to say that "[t]he public or private investigators who do their research in low- and middle-income countries have a moral duty to make a concrete contribution to overcome inequalities."[20] In this respect, the European Group directive is the most forceful of all the relevant guidance documents in stating the moral character of posttrial obligations.

Section 2.13 of the document begins with an important reference to practices in industrialized countries, in which the "free supply of a proven beneficial new drug to all participants of a trial after the trial is ended is the rule as long as it is not yet available through the normal health care system."[20] Section 2.13 continues, "In developing countries, the same rule must be applicable even if this implies supplying the drug for a lifetime if necessary. Moreover, there should be an obligation that the clinical trial benefits the community that contributed to the development of the drug. This can be e.g. to guarantee a supply of the drug at an affordable price for the community or under the form of capacity building."[20] The European Group guidelines avoid the CIOMS strategy of ambiguous language ("reasonable availability"), which was intended to facilitate deliberation and judgment in research ethics review rather than to prescribe a rigid position.

The European Group also directly challenges patent restrictions on publicly funded research. Its opinion states, "In order to avoid limitations due to patent rights when the research is carried out mainly with public funding, the results produced should be regarded as falling within the public domain, or else a system of compulsory licences for applications in developing countries should be considered."[20] This goes further than the other guidelines to throw down the gauntlet for research sponsors, which may

diminish their appetite for funding research in some circumstances that might ultimately have been of value to low- and middle-income countries. Whereas the Declaration of Helsinki, CIOMS, and UNAIDS guidelines are essentially voluntary standards,[21] the European Group directive could have a more direct influence because it may prove to be influential in terms of shaping the requirements for European Union funding schemes, including the EU transnational science and technology "Framework" funding initiatives.

Other Guidelines

Other influential guidelines, such as the World Health Organization (WHO) Good Clinical Practice Guidelines,[22] are widely used in clinical research, particularly by scientists in low- and middle-income countries, and address obligations to ensure continued provision of beneficial drugs at the conclusion of clinical trials. In 2005, UNESCO produced a Universal Declaration on Bioethics and Human Rights[23] that supports the basic moral thrust of posttrial obligations, namely that science and technology should improve the access of the world's poor "to quality health care and essential medicines, to adequate nutrition and water, improvements of living conditions and environment."[24] However, this effort has encountered severe criticism,[25] and it remains to be seen whether the UNESCO Declaration can exert any real influence on governments—particularly in low- and middle-income countries—to enhance their interest and participation in science funding, policy development, and health systems improvement. Increased attention to these issues in the laws and guidelines emanating from other countries, such as Brazil[26] and Uganda,[27] have helped to keep the issue high on the global health research policy agenda.

The Ethical Rationale for Posttrial Obligations

What is the ethical justification for obligations to provide medical care to research participants at the conclusion of a clinical trial? What principles provide the basis for policy and action on these issues? As noted above, the three broad ethical rationales for posttrial obligations are (1) avoiding exploitation in research, (2) recognizing the contribution of research participants, and (3) minimizing feelings of loss or abandonment on the part of research participants. Although avoiding exploitation and minimizing feelings of loss and abandonment can also be applied at the level of communities, in the sections below I will briefly outline the ethical rationale for these obligations for individual research participants, and the implications for research practice and policy.

The Obligation to Avoid Exploitation in Research

Posttrial obligations to ensure continued access to beneficial treatments for participants in clinical trials are now widely viewed as mechanisms for averting the exploitation of research participants. However, what constitutes exploitation in international research has proved to be surprisingly difficult to pin down. As a result, the topic has been the subject of sustained debate. Although most of the controversy has focused on what standard of care should be employed in clinical trials in resource-poor settings,[10] a recent account of exploitation in research has been targeted directly at deficiencies in the "reasonable availability" standard of the CIOMS guidelines.[28] Guidelines 10 and 21 of the 2002 CIOMS Guidelines lay out a framework for ensuring that the products and knowledge generated from the research become available for the benefit of participants and host country communities. But it has been argued recently that it is not the assurance of access to these *specific* benefits, so much as a fair distribution of the wider range of relevant benefits from research, including those that accrue to the investigators, that is the appropriate way to avoid exploitation in research. Several specific concerns with the CIOMS reasonable availability requirement have been noted in this regard.[12] Perhaps the most important of these is that limiting the eligible benefits to those specified in the reasonable availability clause can be viewed as inappropriately paternalistic, in that it privileges the views of the experts who drafted the CIOMS guidelines over the views of the host country participants as to what constitutes an appropriate benefit to warrant their participation in research.[12]

One rebuttal to this criticism of the reasonable availability approach is that it makes the determination of appropriate benefits a matter of negotiation. The worry is that existing differentials in power, influence, and resources between host country communities and organizations and the foreign researchers and sponsors might confer an unfair bargaining advantage to the foreign investigators, and that this might be manipulated to include inappropriate enticements to participate in research, rather than more meaningful contributions to the health of research participants.[10] The fair benefits model assumes that exploitation results from unfair distribution of benefits within particular agreements. Critics of the model dispute the claim that the terms of these agreements can be considered independent of the background economic conditions in the low- and middle-income countries hosting the research, which are widely perceived to be unjust.[29]

But given the poor record to date of transferring research-related benefits to communities in low- and middle-income countries, just how compelling these objections are, or how influential they should be in the posttrial obligations debate, is not clear. It is clear, however, that the skills and experience required to negotiate fair benefits effectively are not part of the typical training program for health researchers,[2] nor have these negotiations been deemed worthy of dedicated funding from research sponsors.

The Obligation to Recognize the Contribution of Research Subjects

Clinical trials, and the resulting gains for all interested parties, would simply not be possible without the willing participation of human subjects. Yet the formal recognition of the importance of their contribution is among the most poorly developed aspects of research and research ethics. The decision to participate in research, and to assume the associated risks, inconvenience, and inherent uncertainties, requires a commitment of trust on the part of research subjects. This feature of the relationship among the research subject, investigators, and research staff entails its own unique set of responsibilities, including the requisite trustworthiness of the investigators. What happens to research subjects once the trial is over can affect this relationship of trust between individual participants and investigators, and by extension, the overall level of trust in the research enterprise. There is a growing

recognition of the importance of respecting and protecting this public trust in the research enterprise.[30]

In light of these concerns the U.S. National Bioethics Advisory Commission (NBAC) in 2001 proposed an ethical justification for posttrial obligations in clinical research that it called "justice as reciprocity."[18] According to this model, justice or fairness requires some formal recognition of the essential contribution of research subjects to the research enterprise. In particular, some meaningful reciprocity is required of investigators and sponsors in return for research subjects' investment of time and energy, assuming personal risk—when it exists—in research, and in recognition of the fact that research subjects have ongoing interests in the findings, procedures, and impact of the research after their direct participation has ended.[18]

Justice as reciprocity goes beyond the basic ethical requirement that there be a favorable balance between the risks and potential benefits for research participants in a given trial—which some view as a sufficient guarantee of benefit. It involves a more holistic recognition that research participants represent a sine qua non of clinical research, and that the essential nature of their contribution warrants some special gratitude or recognition, over and above the potential benefits inherent in a given research design.

The Obligation to Minimize Feelings of Loss or Abandonment

Another contribution to thinking about posttrial obligations emanating from NBAC was the idea that the failure to recognize and implement posttrial obligations to research participants could result in a harmful loss for them.[18] For example, a research participant in a clinical drug trial is randomized to receive the experimental intervention, which turns out to have a beneficial clinical effect. If, at the conclusion of the trial, the sponsors and investigators were under no obligation to continue to provide this research participant with the experimental drug, or to take appropriate steps to ensure ongoing access to it—and if no other provisions for access have been made, such as approval and adoption within the public health system—then it is clear that the research participants would experience a significant loss and possibly a setback in health status. The psychology of this loss is also important ethically. When a research participant's involvement in a study ends abruptly, without any plan for continued communication or provision of information, and usually without any explicit show of gratitude, a range of dignitary harms become likely, including grief, frustration, and disappointment. As well, the experience could shake the participant's confidence in a fundamental aspect of personal security, in other words, the ability to count on the willing assistance of others in time of need. The obligation to avoid feelings of loss or abandonment among research participants might be thought of as a specific formulation of the principle of respect for persons in research. But given the background concerns about unfair distribution of the benefits of research, there is a strong rationale for treating this obligation as a special instance of this principle, deserving independent articulation.

In clinical research, a sense of loss is likely to be enhanced or exaggerated for research participants who mistakenly believe that a central aim of research is to serve their personal therapeutic goals, as opposed to the broader societal goal of knowledge-generation to improve treatment modalities. If, for whatever reason, research participants are operating on the assumption that their participation in a given research trial will result in improvements in their personal health—the "therapeutic misconception"[31]—without a deeper appreciation of the less predictable course of research, then the failure to provide mechanisms for some reasonable form of ongoing access to care at the conclusion of the trial is all the more likely to result in feelings of loss for these research participants, perhaps especially for those in low- and middle-income countries who may be less familiar with the aims and conventions of research.

Without fair and accurate accounts of what research participants should expect at the conclusion of a clinical trial, there are likely to be few justifications for the withdrawal of beneficial care by investigators or sponsors, especially when there are no other means to access the care. A more difficult question is whether disclosing to prospective participants that they can expect continued access to a beneficial therapy only for a specified period, or in a limited form, at the end of the trial is sufficient justification for discontinuing care after the trial. This question introduces the challenge of delineating the scope of posttrial obligations.

The Scope of Posttrial Obligations

Richard Ashcroft has outlined three possible positions on the scope of posttrial obligations: the *minimal* obligation position, the *maximal* obligation position, and a *more nuanced* approach.[32]

The Minimal Obligation Position

The minimal obligation position does not, under normal circumstances, require investigators to ensure research participants continued access to treatments from which they have benefited during the course of the clinical trial. This applies when the investigators have satisfied the usual requirements of ethical research,[33] including an honest account of what prospective participants can expect to happen to them during and after the trial and a favorable balance between risks and potential benefits. In this sense, the minimal obligation position might be viewed simply as a rejection of any posttrial obligations. It holds that as long as investigators and sponsors don't "withhold any normally available effective treatment,"[32] their actions can be considered fair, even in the absence of specific posttrial commitments. Ashcroft also emphasizes an economic reality to research funding and posttrial responsibilities that figures prominently in the minimal obligation position. In essence, research sponsors have a specific mandate that does not include paying for people's medical care outside the context of a specific trial. If funding agencies had limitless wealth, then clinical obligations to people who have previously participated in a clinical trial could be absorbed with no negative impact on the research mission. However, quite aside from the amount of available resources, many research funders, such as the U.S. National Institutes of Health, are prohibited by statute, or similar authority, from purchasing health-care services outside the normal confines of a clinical trial. The minimalist position, in essence, is a defense of the status quo and its clear demarcations between research and clinical care.

The Maximal Obligation Position

Economics figures prominently in the maximal obligation position as well. In this case, Ashcroft emphasizes the fact that research sponsors often derive enormous economic benefit from research, because the results of clinical trials can serve as the basis for regulatory approval of new drugs and devices that can then be sold within lucrative markets for enormous profits. This is an issue almost exclusively for private, for-profit, research sponsors, but because private sector research funding is now estimated at $30 billion a year globally (approximately 40% of global research funding),[34] and the profitability of the research-based pharmaceutical industry is well known,[35] it effectively applies to about half of the health research being conducted annually around the world.

The maximal position reflects key aspects of the "justice as reciprocity" rationale, described above. It is rooted in the simple observation that, although there could be no profits for new drugs without the voluntary participation of human subjects in research, these participants seldom even receive sufficient gratitude for their contributions, let alone a fair share of the gains. As well, research participants often assume some personal risks while making their contribution to research and this, too, deserves some appropriate recognition. Finally, in contrast to the minimal obligation position, which emphasizes clear boundaries between research and clinical care, the maximal obligation position recognizes that investigators do assume a duty of care for participants in a trial,[32,36] and that such a duty cannot simply be set aside because the data collection phase of a clinical trial has come to an end. Although it does not follow automatically from the maximal obligation position that research sponsors must provide treatment to participants following a clinical trial for the rest of their lives, it does not permit this conclusion to be dismissed out of hand.

A More Nuanced Approach

In recognition of the complex issues occupying the space between the minimal and maximal obligation positions, Ashcroft has proposed what he calls a "more nuanced position."[32] This approach incorporates features of the minimal and maximal positions with three main constraints: rationality, limited responsibility, and nonexploitation. These constraints dictate that posttrial obligations must not be arbitrary, but instead must take into account the prevailing circumstances in the countries and communities in which the trials take place, such as access to care and the research opportunity costs associated with various funding strategies for ongoing clinical care. As well, the more nuanced position recognizes that individual actors in these complex scenarios—sponsors and investigators—are limited in their ability to address these complex challenges, and it encourages an increased reliance on effective institutions and democratic process to achieve viable and ethically praiseworthy solutions. Finally, the more nuanced position requires that all of these other considerations must be met without falling back into the patterns of exploitation of communities in research that gave rise to these debates in the first place.[32]

Obligations to Research Participants in the Control Group of a Clinical Trial

The Nuffield Council report discusses some of the challenges related to ensuring ongoing access to beneficial treatments to members of the control group in a clinical trial, who might have received another, inferior, treatment or a placebo during the trial, depending on the study design.[1] Although there is little disagreement in principle that control group members should be provided with treatments demonstrated during the trial to be effective—in other words, either more effective than the treatment received by the control group or placebo, depending on the design of the trial—the Council's report highlights several circumstances that might justify exceptions. First, there may be circumstances, particularly in trials of longer duration, such as vaccine trials, in which some or all of the control group members are no longer at an age, or stage in disease progression, to benefit from the effective therapy. This situation may arise, for example, in vaccine trials involving children.

A critical issue in vaccine research is the duration and strength of protection from vaccination. The intensity of the immune response to the target disease pathogens often declines over time following vaccination, and generating a clear understanding of this attenuation requires a stable control group. Because the bulk of the attenuation occurs after the conclusion of a trial, a potential conflict arises between the obligation to provide effective treatments to the control group at the conclusion of the trial, and the obligation to maximize the scientific value of the trial by generating clear answers to questions such as the effective duration of the vaccine, which may be critical to the overall assessment of the vaccine's efficacy.[1] The Nuffield Council recommends that members of the control group should receive the vaccine at the conclusion of the trial, if it is deemed to be effective and if the group is still at risk of the disease against which the vaccine is targeted, but the Council recognizes that different conclusions may also be warranted, depending on the specific circumstances of the trial.[1] Another approach to this problem has been to provide the control group with an unrelated, though relevant, vaccine to ensure a benefit for the control group without undermining the overall integrity of the trial—for example, giving the control group in a malaria prevention trial a rabies vaccine instead of the experimental malaria vaccine.[37]

A closely related issue, which applies equally to members of the control group and the intervention group, is the responsibility to ensure that there is sufficient posttrial surveillance to detect treatment-related harms that might arise in the posttrial period, even if short-term testing suggests the treatment is safe. The Nuffield Council report describes the case of a high-titer measles vaccine trial in Guinea-Bissau and Senegal, in which children were provided high-titer vaccine at a younger age than the conventional measles vaccine. The children receiving the vaccine produced higher level of antibodies against measles than children receiving conventional measles vaccine, but long-term surveillance detected an increase in mortality among girls in the trial compared to girls receiving the conventional measles vaccine, several years after the end of the trial.[1] These examples help to illustrate the importance of long-term surveillance following clinical trials and the related challenge of ensuring fair provision of effective treatment for all trial participants.

Circumstances in Which Provision of Effective Treatment May Not Be Obligatory

The presumption underlying the obligation to ensure ongoing provision of treatment at the conclusion of a clinical trial is that the effective treatment will be beneficial to the research participants. Although this is a reasonable presumption, there are some cir-

cumstances in which this might not be the case. The clearest examples arise in clinical trials of chronic diseases, and malaria provides an excellent illustration of the problem in clinical trials in malaria-endemic countries. Acute, severe malaria kills more than 1 million children in low- and middle-income countries every year and now accounts for more than 10% of all childhood deaths in these countries.[38] Despite the high death rates from malaria, multiple infections with malaria parasites in childhood are also well known to confer protective immunity into adulthood. As a result, providing prophylaxis or treatments that might disrupt children's normal acquisition of immunity to malaria parasites beyond the conclusion of a clinical trial could have a detrimental effect on their later immunity and may increase their risk of illness or death in later life. This issue is discussed in more detail below.

The Mechanics of Posttrial Obligations

Mechanisms

To date, the principal mechanism for addressing posttrial obligations has been to capture the relevant interests and commitments of the various parties (e.g., sponsors, investigators, communities, governments) in a formal agreement that is finalized before the research is initiated. These *prior agreements,* as they have come to be known, reflect the constraints of Ashcroft's more nuanced position in that they treat the interests at stake as negotiable, which recognizes that the responsibilities of sponsors and investigators are limited, rather than absolute, and rational deliberations are required to achieve successful outcomes. Prior agreements also provide an avenue for the inclusion of other interests and responsibilities, such as the responsibilities of host country governments, which are often neglected in discussions of research ethics.

Alice Page has reviewed the use of prior agreements and has advocated their use in international research as a means of ensuring that benefits accrue to host country participants in research.[39] Page tackles six main criticisms that have been leveled against the use of prior agreements, ultimately concluding that none of these criticisms is sufficiently strong to warrant the abandonment of prior agreements. These criticisms reflect many of the same concerns that occupy the space between Ashcroft's minimal and maximal positions.

The first criticism is that prior agreements delay or prevent research. Page concedes that, even though this might be true in some circumstances, it is equally true that the benefits to host countries from their participation in international collaborative health research have been modest, making it difficult to gauge what is lost if research is delayed or prevented. Prior agreements, according to Page, open up space for innovative discussion about financing, underwriting, and delivering care posttrial, some of which has already given rise to benefits for host countries.[39]

The second criticism is that there are significant financial, logistical, and other practical obstacles to prior agreements. Again, Page argues that successful solutions and workable strategies will not be discovered without attempting some of these negotiations in practice, and she reemphasizes that these are surely worthy efforts if the central aim of prior agreements is sound.

The third criticism against requiring prior agreements is that it is not the prevailing international standard. As I have done, above,

Page reviews some of the ways that current international guidance documents deal with posttrial obligations and finds not only a general consistency with the main ethical thrust of prior agreements, but in some cases, such as in the UNAIDS guidance document and CIOMS Guideline 10, recognition of affirmative obligations. Similar affirmations of such obligations are present in the Human Genome Organization's Ethics Committee Statement on Benefit Sharing,[40] the WHO Operational Guidelines for Committees that Review the Ethics of Biomedical Research,[41] and numerous national guidelines issued by low- and middle-income countries.[26,27,42]

The fourth criticism is that researchers cannot realistically influence health policy. This criticism spans two related issues. The first, outlined briefly above, is that individual studies seldom provide clear direction for widespread policy adoption. The path is usually circuitous and prolonged. Although this may be a good reason to clarify the scope of obligations in international guidelines, it seems insufficient on its own to undermine the entire justification for posttrial obligations or the more specific emphasis on prior agreements.

The fifth criticism is that prior agreements would create a double standard with regard to clinical research conducted in the United States and other industrialized countries. This criticism seems flawed for two main reasons. First, prior agreements are already used to extend access to unapproved drugs and devices for research participants at the conclusion of clinical trials in high-income countries. These agreements are generally made among the regulatory authority, the drug or device manufacturer, and the trial sponsor(s), and provide limited access under clearly specified terms. These agreements may also extend to people who have not been participants in clinical trials, usually on compassionate grounds.[43,44] Second, rather than giving low- and middle income countries an unfair advantage, posttrial obligations and prior agreements actually aim to level the playing field by filling gaps in access to medical care that are, for the most part, better handled in high income countries.

The sixth, and final, criticism of prior agreements is that they can always be breached. This line of reasoning pays insufficient attention to the value of prior agreements as a way of structuring a negotiation about a complex set of interests, which might also serve as an important process for establishing the understanding and commitments that might make compliance with the terms of the prior agreements more likely than they would have been under a more informal agreement.

Sponsor Policies and Practices

The emphasis on posttrial obligations tends to obscure some important practical constraints on research sponsors. For example, the U.S. National Institutes of Health (NIH), the world's largest public funder of biomedical research, has a specific mission: to encourage and support research.[45] This mandate does not include the authority to purchase drugs or devices as health-care services, even as a continuation of the treatment tested in a clinical trial. In response to increasing pressure to ensure the continued provision of antiretroviral drugs at the conclusion of HIV/AIDS clinical trials, the NIH issued a guidance statement that clarified its mission and which recommended that "NIH-funded investigators work with host countries' authorities and other stakeholders to identify sources available, if any, in the country for the provision of antiretroviral treatment to antiretroviral treatment trial participants following their completion of the trial."[46] The NIH policy serves as an excellent illustration of how the policies and practices adopted by research sponsors—particularly the large, influential ones—can have a profound effect on the status of posttrial obligations.

A similar example comes from the United Kingdom's Wellcome Trust, another influential funder of global health research. Its position statement for research applicants establishes several important limits with respect to posttrial obligations. For example, Section 7 (Post-research access to interventions demonstrated to be effective), makes clear that "[t]he Wellcome Trust does not fund healthcare per se and considers the financial responsibility of providing successful interventions after research is over to fall outside its remit. It does, however, encourage grant applicants to consider how post-research access could be ensured."[19] Later in the same section, three main reasons are offered for these limits on the Trust's obligations for funding posttrial access: (1) that it "does not fall within the Wellcome Trust's remit and area of expertise," (2) that it "could divert funds away from supporting valuable research," and (3) that it "could render research prohibitively expensive for the Wellcome Trust."[19]

It is important to emphasize that these statements from health research funders do not indicate a lack of support for the notion of ensuring posttrial access to beneficial interventions. Instead, they illustrate the complexity and potential hazards associated with seemingly simple statements about the moral obligations of research sponsors in international guidelines. Posttrial obligations may serve as a useful illustration of the hazards of an overreliance on aspirational statements in international guidelines, which, although they may serve the intended purpose of establishing international expectations of ethical conduct, also may inadvertently impose complex requirements without offering further guidance about how these requirements might be applied. Although the stakes may be high for the research sponsors, investigators, and research participants alike, it is clear that we need more examples of workable posttrial agreements, and more innovation, in order to gain more confidence that declarations of posttrial obligations will produce the desired ethical results.

Public-Private Partnerships

The Nuffield Council on Bioethics recognized public-private partnerships (PPP) as an innovative and potentially powerful mechanism for addressing posttrial obligations in clinical research. PPPs are collaborative arrangements between public agencies and private entities to tackle problems related to global health. There is enormous diversity in the goals of PPPs, including distributing donated or subsidized products to control a specific disease, strengthening health services, educating the public, improving product quality or regulation, and new product development.[47,48] PPPs have been growing in importance in global health, including in the field of drugs and health products development. Although they are not mechanisms for posttrial obligations, per se, PPPs have several features that make them ideal contexts for exploring and implementing posttrial obligations. First, they allow public agencies to overcome constraints and limitations on their roles, authority, and resources. Second, they broaden the available sets of skills and experience that can be brought to bear on a problem, for example, by providing managers, administrators, and lawyers with extensive negotiating experience to assist investigators who may be inexperienced in these matters. And third, they can drastically expand the available pool of resources, or mechanisms for underwriting or financing complex initiatives, which can result in opportunities that would otherwise not be available to parties pursuing effective mechanisms for satisfying posttrial obligations. To date, most of the experiences with prior agreements and mechanisms for posttrial obligations have come from PPPs, and some of these are discussed in greater detail below.

Examples and Lessons

A great many factors influence the existence, nature, and success of posttrial obligations in research, beyond the nature of the research itself and the potential benefits to research participants. Not least among these factors are the prevailing economic and political forces globally, and their specific effects on research in low- and middle-income countries.[49] A recent example involved the antiretroviral drug Nevirapine, which is used to prevent mother-to-child transmission of HIV-1 and was tested in clinical trials on South African women, but whose distribution was severely limited by the South African government. A ruling by the South African Constitutional Court was required to establish that the restrictions constituted a barrier to the exercise of the right to health by South African women.[50] This ruling also removed a critical restriction that complicated posttrial agreements involving Nevirapine research in that country.

Support for posttrial obligations is not universal, as Ashcroft's minimal obligation position illustrates. Although most would agree that research is necessary to generate knowledge to address health problems in low- and middle-income countries, it is unrealistic and inappropriate for research to be viewed as a corrective for the widespread social injustice that characterizes most of the low- and middle-income world. Posttrial obligations arise at the murky interface between research and humanitarian assistance, a position that is best occupied with some trepidation. For example, Article 1.14 of the Canadian Tri-Council Policy Statement, the main national research ethics guidelines in Canada, states explicitly about research conducted outside Canada that "since researchers are not aid agencies, REBs [research ethics boards] should not try to force them to undertake aid work."[51] Similarly, the conscious negotiation for, and distribution of, benefits to research participants in clinical research that is required by posttrial agreements also holds enormous potential to create tension and unrest within communities.

Despite these challenges, posttrial obligations have been implemented successfully, and examples and lessons are beginning to emerge. In her review of prior agreements, Page describes several examples of how posttrial obligations have been approached in practice. These include prior agreements employed by the WHO with its industrial partners for new product development, by the International AIDS Vaccine Initiative (IAVI) with industry partners for vaccine development and with organizations such as the World Bank and low- and middle-income country governments to establish purchasing funds for vaccines, and in agreements negotiated around the first VaxGen Phase III HIV

vaccine efficacy trial in Thailand.[39] Here I will focus on three additional examples: first, the HIV Netherlands Australia Thailand Research Collaboration (HIV-NAT); second, a trial of intermittent presumptive treatment of infants for malaria in Kamasi, Ghana; and third, an industry partnership with a nongovernment organization (NGO) for the development of a new antimalarial drug.

The HIV Netherlands Australia Thailand Research Collaboration (HIV-NAT)

HIV-NAT was formed in 1996 as a partnership among the Thai Red Cross AIDS Research Centre, the Australian National Centre in HIV Epidemiology and Clinical Research, and the International Antiviral Therapy Evaluation Centre in Amsterdam. Its mandate was to undertake clinical trials of antiretroviral drugs and to ensure that participants in these trials continued to have access to the medications following the conclusion of the trials.[52] Initially, HIV-NAT negotiated access to antiretroviral drugs with drug companies in the context of "rollover protocols," in other words, studies that permit research participants to move directly from one study into an extension trial, either for different clinical trial phases or different outcome measures. But this practice became unsustainable as the population of trial participants in Thailand gained more and more experience with various antiretroviral drugs in clinical trials, which made it difficult to meet inclusion and exclusion criteria for the subsequent trials. Another HIV-NAT approach has been to negotiate with pharmaceutical companies that sponsor clinical trials either fixed-fund contributions to pay for, or commitments to provide, antiretroviral drugs for research participants.

Despite these mechanisms, in 2001 HIV-NAT anticipated a shortfall in antiretroviral drug supply for research participants completing clinical trials, and launched the HIV-NAT drug fund. About 85% of this fund is covered by overhead costs from running clinical trials, and about 15% from other revenues such as symposia and training programs. Since 2001, approximately 20% of research participants who have been unable to pay for their antiretroviral drugs, or who have been ineligible for other government-funded antiretroviral programs, have received support from the drug fund. The fund requires a monthly copayment from research participants, the amount of which is determined by a means test on admission to the fund. The fund has provided an important bridging mechanism during a period when the Thai government has been expanding its antiretroviral access program.[52]

Trials of Intermittent Presumptive Treatment of Malaria in Infancy

Intermittent presumptive treatment (IPT) of malaria involves the provision of an antimalarial drug or drugs during peak periods of vulnerability to infection in an effort to reduce morbidity and mortality from severe acute malaria. Because infants between 6 and 23 months of age represent a major component of the disease burden from malaria, IPT has been targeted primarily at pregnant women and infants.[53] For IPT of infants, the goal is to provide effective control of parasitemia and clinical episodes of malaria in children who are already infected, during the period when passive immunity acquired from the mother has declined, but before the immune advantages of acquired immunity to malaria parasites has had sufficient time to develop.[54] The rapid emergence of resistance to drugs used for IPT and the enormous scale of the disease burden from malaria globally have made the testing of different drugs and strategies for IPT a priority in malaria treatment, in both pregnant women and infants.

In several early clinical trials, IPT demonstrated improvements in morbidity and mortality in infants in the first year of life.[54] However, rapidly acquired resistance to preferred drugs for IPT, such as sulphadoxine-pyrimethamine (S-P), as demonstrated in a recent trial from Kamasi, Ghana,[55] has increased the urgency for further clinical trials to ensure that appropriate timing and duration of effective drug combinations are used in IPT to maximize its clinical benefits in both high- and low-transmission areas.[54]

Although IPT has been endorsed by WHO as part of the available arsenal of clinical tools to combat malaria,[56] recent findings about the rapid acquisition of S-P-resistant parasites, even after single dose administration of S-P, raised concerns about the long-term viability of S-P-based IPT programs. Yet the only way to determine effective solutions to these problems is through continued clinical testing of alternative IPT strategies.

In the Kamasi trial involving SP-resistance after a single dose administration of S-P, the placebo control group had fewer infections, fewer cases of parasitemia, and fewer cases of mild malaria than the S-P group.[55] The children enrolled in the trial had a mean age of 9 months at the beginning of the trial. Previous evidence had suggested that a course of S-P treatments at 2, 3, and 9 months, and amodiaquine treatments at 3, 5, and 7 months, reduce the incidence of malaria episodes and anemia.[57,58] Furthermore, there is concern that any additional treatment of asymptomatic children will lead to further selection of drug-resistant parasites that can result in increased morbidity and mortality by decreasing acquired immunity (the rebound effect).[53]

These IPT in infancy trials raise significant challenges for posttrial obligations to research participants. As described above, based on existing data, it may be that the children in both the placebo and control groups in the Kamasi trial have passed the critical window of opportunity for any further benefit from drug administration following the completion of the 26-week trial period. This might make continued provision of treatment of the infants at the conclusion of the trial impossible, or clinically inadvisable, given the serious nature of the associated risks. Similarly, given the rapid development of drug resistance to the frontline therapies used in IPT, fulfilling the obligation to ensure access to beneficial treatment for the infants in the Kamasi, and similar, trials also conflicts with the obligation not to contribute to increased drug-resistant strains of malaria parasites, which represent an enormous global health threat. In these circumstances, it is reasonable to conclude that the investigators still have an obligation to the infants in the trial, but that the obligation may best be met by careful clinical monitoring, as opposed to the administration of any specific treatment.

Bayer–Medicines for Malaria Venture Artemisone Deal

In their review of public-private partnerships for health, Kettler and White describe several case studies, including an agreement between Bayer Pharmaceuticals and the Medicines for Malaria Venture (MMV), for the development of a new malaria drug using Artemisone, a substance for which Bayer holds the patent.[48] This case serves as a useful example of how posttrial obligations can be addressed in the context of PPPs, an increasingly common approach to drug development, and therefore also an important context in which to consider posttrial obligations.[59] It also highlights efforts by MMV, a WHO initiative funded largely by the World Bank and private foundations, primarily the Bill and Melinda Gates Foundation, and a recognized global leader in PPP-driven drug discovery and development.[60]

There are four main players with recognized responsibilities in the Bayer–MMV deal, Bayer, MMV, WHO, and the host country health systems and patient groups. Under the terms of the agreement, Bayer has agreed to manufacture the Artemisone product for clinical trials and to fund the remaining preclinical and clinical studies. Later stage clinical development will receive guidance from WHO country teams and local health systems and patient groups. This is also the stage at which the details of ongoing access to Artemisone will be determined, if it proves to be beneficial for participants in current clinical trials. Bayer has agreed to make any beneficial product available at an "affordable price" to the partners of this agreement, to ensure ongoing access for all who need it.[48]

Summary

Posttrial obligations to research participants are intended to avoid the exploitation of research participants, to recognize the value of their contribution to the research enterprise, and to minimize the likelihood of feelings of loss or abandonment among research participants whose continued access to a beneficial intervention might require special provisions beyond the planned clinical trial. Major international research ethics guidelines, including the World Medical Association's Declaration of Helsinki and the Council of International Organizations of Medical Sciences guidelines, have offered controversial guidance on posttrial obligations, but the ensuing debate has been extremely influential in the development of current thinking about posttrial obligations.

Several positions have been proposed on the appropriate scope of posttrial obligations of researchers and sponsors, ranging from rejection of any specific posttrial obligations, beyond the usual demands of ethical research, to full responsibility to ensure access to needed interventions and even advocacy on behalf of research participants and their communities, especially in low- and middle-income countries.

Some special considerations are required in terms of ensuring access to effective treatment for members of the control group in clinical trials. There also are instances, such as some trials involving malaria and other chronic diseases, in which it may be impossible, or clinically inappropriate, to provide continued treatment, due to interference with the acquisition of natural immunity or contribution to the development of drug-resistant disease. These issues are illustrated by the Kamasi trial of intermittent presumptive treatment of malaria in infants.

The principal mechanism for addressing posttrial obligations to date has been *prior agreements* that reflect the key negotiated interests of sponsors, researchers, and research participants for a given clinical trial. Despite some important criticism, prior agreements remain the most common approach to ensuring that posttrial obligations are satisfied in practice.

Research sponsors have also been instrumental in the development of approaches to posttrial obligations. Private sponsors of research, including pharmaceutical companies and private foundations, are free to purchase and provide beneficial interventions to research participants at the conclusion of clinical trials, if the economic and humanitarian incentives are appropriate, but public research funding agencies are usually constrained from doing so by their mandates. Many sponsors, including the U.S. NIH and the U.K. Wellcome Trust, have established clear policies to reflect these constraints and have encouraged investigators to pursue posttrial obligations in their individual research activities. These policies do not indicate a lack of support for the notion of ensuring posttrial access to beneficial interventions. Instead, they illustrate the hazards and logistical challenges that posttrial obligations represent for research funders.

One innovative and powerful mechanism for addressing posttrial obligations is the public-private partnership, a collaborative arrangement between public agencies and private entities. Public-private partnerships allow public agencies to overcome constraints and limitations on their roles, authority, and resources; they broaden the available sets of skills and experience that can be brought to bear on a problem; and they can drastically expand the available pool of resources or mechanisms of underwriting or financing complex initiatives, which can result in opportunities that would otherwise not be available to parties pursuing effective mechanisms for satisfying posttrial obligations. The HIV Netherlands Australia Thailand Research Collaboration (HIV-NAT) and the Bayer–MMV deal to develop Artemisone are examples of how creative partnerships can ensure that posttrial obligations are satisfied in clinical trials.

References

1. Nuffield Council on Bioethics. *The Ethics of Research Related to Healthcare in Developing Countries.* London, England: Nuffield Council on Bioethics; 2002:122. [Online] Available: http://nuffieldbioethics.org/fileLibrary/pdf/errhdc_fullreport001.pdf.

2. Lavery JV. Putting international research ethics guidelines to work for the benefit of developing countries. *Yale Journal of Health Policy, Law, and Ethics* 2004;4:319–36.

3. World Medical Association. *Declaration of Helsinki: Ethical Principles for Medical Research Involving Human Subjects.* Tokyo, Japan: WMA; October 2004. [Online] 2004. Available: http://www.wma.net/e/policy/b3.htm.

4. Gotzsche PC, Hrobjartsson A, Johansen HK, et al. Constraints on publication rights in industry-initiated clinical trials. *JAMA* 2006; 295:1645–6.

5. Chan AW, Altman DG. Identifying outcome reporting bias in randomised trials on PubMed: Review of publications and survey of authors. *British Medical Journal* 2005;330:753–8.

6. Lang T, Hughes D, Kanyok T, et al. Beyond registration—Measuring the public-health potential of new treatments for malaria in Africa. *Lancet Infectious Diseases* 2006;6:46–52.

7. Frankish H. WMA postpones decision to amend Declaration of Helsinki. *Lancet* 2003;362:963.

8. Editorial. One standard, not two. *Lancet* 2003;362:1005.

9. London AJ. Equipoise and international human-subjects research. *Bioethics* 2001;15:312–32.

10. London AJ. The ambiguity and the exigency: Clarifying 'standard of care' arguments in international research. *Journal of Medicine and Philosophy* 2000;25:379–97.

11. Council for International Organizations of Medical Sciences, in collaboration with the World Health Organization. *International Ethical Guidelines for Biomedical Research Involving Human Subjects.* Geneva, Switzerland: CIOMS and WHO; 2002. [Online] November 2002. Available: http://www.cioms.ch/frame_guidelines_nov_2002.htm.

12. Participants in the 2001 Conference on Ethical Aspects of Research in Developing Countries. Moral standards for research in developing countries: From "reasonable availability" to "fair benefits." *Hastings Center Report* 2004;34(3):17–27.

13. Weijer C, Emanuel EJ. Protecting communities in biomedical research. *Science* 2000;289:1142–4.

14. Berkley S. Thorny issues in the ethics of AIDS vaccine trials. *Lancet* 2003;362:992.

15. Joint United Nations Programme on AIDS and World Health Organization. *UNAIDS Guidance Document: Ethical Considerations in HIV Preventive Vaccine Research.* Geneva, Switzerland: UNAIDS and WHO; 2000.

16. Weijer C. The future of research into rotavirus vaccine. *British Medical Journal* 2000;321:525–6.

17. Nuffield Council on Bioethics. *The Ethics of Research Related to Healthcare in Developing Countries: A Follow-Up Discussion Paper.* London, England: Nuffield Council on Bioethics; 2005. [Online] March 17, 2005. Available: http://www.nuffieldbioethics.org/fileLibrary/pdf/HRRDC_Follow-up_Discussion_Paper001.pdf.

18. National Bioethics Advisory Commission. *Ethical and Policy Issues in International Research, Vol. I.* Bethesda, Md.: NBAC; 2001. [Online] April 2001. Available: http://www.bioethics.gov/reports/past_commissions/nbac_international.pdf.

19. The Wellcome Trust. *Research Involving People Living in Developing Countries: Position Statement and Guidance Notes for Applicants.* London, England: The Wellcome Trust. [Online] Available: http://www.well-www.wellcome.ac.uk/doc_wtd015295.html.

20. European Group on Ethics in Science and New Technologies. *Opinion No. 17 to the European Commission: Ethical Aspects of Clinical Research in Developing Countries.* Brussels, Belgium: EGE; 2003. [Online] February 4, 2003. Available: http://ec.europa.eu/european_group_ethics/docs/avis17_en.pdf.

21. Lavery JV. The challenge of regulating international research with human subjects. SciDev.Net. [Online] June 10, 2004. Available: http://www.scidev.net/dossiers/index.cfm?fuseaction=policybrief&dossier=5&policy=52.

22. Idänpään-Heikkilä JE. WHO guidelines for good clinical practice (GCP) for trials on pharmaceutical products: Responsibilities of the investigator. *Annals of Medicine* 1994;26:89–94.

23. United Nations Educational, Scientific and Cultural Organization. Universal Declaration on Bioethics and Human Rights. Paris, France: UNESCO; 2005. [Online] Available: http://portal.unesco.org/shs/en/file_download.php/46133e1f4691e4c6e57566763d474a4dBioethicsDeclaration_EN.pdf.

24. Serra MC. UNESCO has given bioethics a human face. SciDev.Net. [Online] Dec. 1, 2005. Available: http://www.scidev.net/dossiers/index.cfm?fuseaction=dossierreaditem&dossier=5&type=3&itemid=453&language=1.

25. Faunce TA. Will international human rights subsume medical ethics? Intersections in the UNESCO Universal Bioethics Declaration. *Journal of Medical Ethics* 2005;31:173–8.

26. National Health Council. *Resolution No. 196/96 on Research Involving Human Subjects.* Brasilia, Brazil: NHC, 1996; Addition: Resolution No. 251, 1997; Addition: Resolution No. 292, 1999.

27. Uganda National Council of Science and Technology (UNCST). *Guidelines for the Conduct of Health Research Involving Human Subjects in Uganda.* Kampala, Uganda: UNCST; 1998:32.

28. Participants in the 2001 Conference on Ethical Aspects of Research in Developing Countries. Fair benefits for research in developing countries. *Science* 2002;298:2133–4.

29. Arras JD. Fair benefits in international medical research. *Hastings Center Report* 2004;34(3):3.

30. DeAngelis CD. Conflict of interest and the public trust. *JAMA* 2000;284:2237–8.

31. Appelbaum PS, Lidz CW, Grisso T. Therapeutic misconception in clinical research: Frequency and risk factors. *IRB: Ethics and Human Research* 2004;26(2):1–8.

32. Ashcroft R. After the trial is over: What are the sponsor's obligations? SciDev.Net. [Online] May, 2005. Available: http://www.scidev.net/dossiers/index.cfm?fuseaction=policybrief&dossier=5&policy=63.

33. Emanuel EJ, Wendler D, Grady C. What makes clinical research ethical? *JAMA* 2000;283:2701–11.

34. Global Forum for Health Research. *Monitoring Financial Flows for Health Research 2001.* Geneva, Switzerland: Global Forum for Health Research; 2001.

35. Angell M. Excess in the pharmaceutical industry. *Canadian Medical Association Journal* 2004;171:1451–3.

36. Zimmerman SV. Translating ethics into law: Duties of care in health research involving humans. *Health Law Review* 2005;13(2&3):13–8.

37. Bojang KA, Milligan PJ, Pinder M, et al., and the RTS, S Malaria Vaccine Trial Team. Efficacy of RTS, S/AS02 malaria vaccine against *Plasmodium falciparum* infection in semi-immune adult men in The Gambia: A randomised trial. *Lancet* 2001;358:1927–34.

38. Lopez AD, Begg S, Bos E. Demographic and epidemiological characteristics of major regions, 1990–2001. In: Lopez AD, Mathers CD, Ezzati M, Jamison DT, Murray CJL, eds. *Global Burden of Disease and Risk Factors.* New York, N.Y.: Oxford University Press; 2006:17–44.

39. Page AK. Prior agreements in international clinical trials: Ensuring the benefits of research to developing countries. *Yale Journal of Health Policy, Law, and Ethics* 2002;3:35–66.

40. Human Genome Organisation Ethics Committee. Statement on Benefit Sharing. London, England: HUGO; 2000. [Online] April 9, 2000. Available: http://www.hugo-international.org/Statement_on_Benefit_Sharing.htm.

41. World Health Organization. *Operational Guidelines for Ethics Committees That Review Biomedical Research.* Document TDR/PRD/ETHICS/2000.1. Geneva, Switzerland: WHO; 2000. [Online] Available: http://www.who.int/tdr/publications/publications/pdf/ethics.pdf.

42. Indian Council of Medical Research. *Ethical Guidelines for Biomedical Research on Human Subjects.* New Delhi, India: ICMR; 2000. [Online] Available: http://www.icmr.nic.in/ethical.pdf.

43. Center for Drug Evaluation and Research, Food and Drug Administration. Access to Unapproved Drugs. [Online] Available: www.fda.gov/cder/cancer/access.htm.

44. Health Canada. Special Access Programme—Drugs. [Online] Available: http://www.hc-sc.gc.ca/dhp-mps/alt_formats/hpfb-dgpsa/pdf/acces/sapfs_pasfd_2002_e.pdf.

45. U.S. Congress. Public Health Service Act. Title 42 (Public Health and Welfare), United States Code, Chapter 6A (Public Health Service). [Online] January 5, 1999. Available: http://www.fda.gov/opacom/laws/phsvcact/phsvcact.htm.

46. National Institutes of Health. Guidance for addressing the provision of antiretroviral treatment for trial participants following their completion of NIH-funded HIV antiretroviral treatment trials in developing countries. Bethesda, Md.: National Institutes of Health; March 18, 2005. [Online] Available: http://grants.nih.gov/grants/policy/antiretroviral/guidance.doc.

47. Widdus R. Public-private partnerships for health: Their main targets, their diversity, and their future directions. *Bulletin of the World Health Organization* 2001;79:713–20.

48. Kettler H, White K. Valuing industry contributions to public-private partnerships for health product development. In: Davey S, ed. *Initiative on Public-Private Partnerships for Health, Global Forum for Health Research.* Geneva, Switzerland: The Initiative on Public-Private Partnerships for Health; 2003.

49. Flory JH, Kitcher P. Global health and the scientific research agenda. *Philosophy and Public Affairs* 2004;32:36–65.

50. Annas GJ. The right to health and the Nevirapine case in South Africa. *New England Journal of Medicine* 2003;348:750–4.

51. Canadian Institutes of Health Research, the Natural Sciences and Engineering Research Council of Canada, and the Social Sciences and Humanities Research Council of Canada. *Tri-Council Policy Statement: Ethical Conduct for Research Involving Humans,* Article 1.14. [Online] 1998 (with 2000, 2002, and 2005 amendments). Available: http://www.pre.ethics.gc.ca/english/policystatement/policystatement.cfm.

52. Ananworanich J, Cheunyam T, Teeratakulpisarn S, et al. Creation of a drug fund for post-clinical trial access to anti-retrovirals. *Lancet* 2004;364:101–2.

53. Breman JG, O'Meara WP. Intermittent preventive treatment for malaria in infants: Moving forward cautiously. *Journal of Infectious Diseases* 2005;192:1869–71.

54. White NJ. Intermittent preventive treatment for malaria: A better understanding of the pharmacodynamics will guide more rational policy making. *PLoS Medicine* 2005;2(1):e3.

55. Marks F, von Kalckreuth V, Kobbe R, et al. Parasitological rebound effect and emergence of pyrimethamine resistance in *Plasmodium falciparum* after single-dose sulfadoxine-pyrimethamine. *Journal of Infectious Diseases* 2005;192:1962–5.

56. World Health Organization. World Malaria Report 2005. Geneva, Switzerland: WHO; 2005. [Online] Available: http://www.rbm.who.int/wmr2005/.

57. Schellenberg D, Menendez C, Kahigwa E, et al. Intermittent treatment for malaria and anaemia control at time of routine vaccinations in Tanzanian infants: A randomised, placebo-controlled trial. *Lancet* 2001;357:1471–7.

58. Massaga JJ, Kitua AY, Lemnge MM, et al. Effect of intermittent treatment with amodiaquine on anaemia and malarial fevers in infants in Tanzania: A randomized placebo-controlled trial. *Lancet* 2003;361:1853–60.

59. Sharp D. Not-for-profit drugs—No longer an oxymoron? *Lancet* 2004;346:1472–4.

60. Nwaka S, Ridley RG. Virtual drug discovery and development for neglected diseases through public-private partnerships. *Nature Reviews: Drug Discovery* 2003;2:919–28.

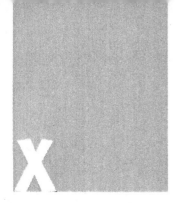

Multinational Research

Ruth Macklin

Appropriate Ethical Standards

Wherever research involving human beings may be conducted, it must adhere to appropriate ethical standards. Yet despite universal agreement on this fundamental requirement, interpreting and applying the concept of ethical standards has produced a surprising amount of vagueness, ambiguity, and even disagreement. Even more vexing is the need to determine the appropriate ethical standards for multinational research.

A thorough analysis of this topic requires examination of conceptual as well as ethical issues. At least the following questions must be addressed: Are all ethical aspects of research with human subjects properly considered *standards*? Should standards be universally applicable or are variations permissible according to economic, political, or cultural differences among nations? When different ethical standards are potentially applicable, to which ones should researchers adhere? How should disagreements about ethical standards in research be adjudicated or resolved?

In multinational research, these questions have given rise to debates over so-called double standards. Are double standards acceptable in multinational research, or should researchers adhere to a single ethical standard, regardless of differences among nations or cultural groups? It is impossible to assess opposing positions in this debate without clarifying just what counts as an ethical standard, and what are the criteria for determining when standards are appropriate.

History and Current Guidelines

The first known regulations governing research involving human beings were promulgated in 1900 in Prussia, addressed to the directors of clinics, polyclinics, and similar establishments. A somewhat later code in Germany was the Circular of February 28, 1931, of the Reich Minister of the Interior, about two years before the start of the Nazi era.[1] Under a more informal policy of disclosure to the subjects and their consent to participate, the U.S. Army carried out experiments on healthy subjects for decades, beginning with Walter Reed's yellow fever experiments in the early 1900s.

However, scholars have concluded that the 1947 Nuremberg Code is almost certainly the first *international* code.[2] Therefore, the history of ethical standards for research in the international context can be said to begin with the Nuremberg Code and to proceed through the Declaration of Helsinki in 1964, revisions in the Helsinki Declaration from 1975 to 2000, and International Ethical Guidelines issued by the Council for International Organizations of Medical Sciences (CIOMS), culminating in the 2002 revision. (See Part 2 of this volume for discussion of these and other codes, declarations, and guidelines.)

However, the term *standards* appears only in rare instances in these documents, and when it does appear, there is no explanation of precisely what the term means. The 1964 Declaration of Helsinki said, "It must be stressed that the standards as drafted are only a guide to physicians all over the world. Doctors are not relieved from criminal, civil, and ethical responsibilities under the laws of their own countries."[3] These same sentences appear, with no other explicit references to ethical standards, in amended versions of the Declaration in 1975, 1983, 1989, and 1996. The substantially revised version of the Declaration in 2000 includes the following sentence: "Medical research is subject to ethical standards that promote respect for all human beings and protect their health and rights."[4] These brief mentions of standards in the Declaration of Helsinki could refer to some or all of the provisions in the document.

The CIOMS International Ethical Guidelines make explicit reference to standards in both the 1993 version and the 2002 revision. Guideline 15 of the 1993 version is entitled "Externally Sponsored Research" and includes the following provision: "An external sponsoring agency should submit the research protocol to ethical and scientific review according to the standards of the country of the sponsoring agency, and the ethical standards applied should be no less exacting than they would be in the case of research carried out in that country."[5]

Guideline 3 of the 2002 version has only a slight change in wording and includes an additional requirement, but the reference to standards is the same: "An external sponsoring organization and individual investigators should submit the research protocol for ethical and scientific review in the country of the sponsoring organization, and the ethical standards applied should be no less stringent than they would be for research carried out in that country. The health authorities of the host country, as well as a national or local ethical review committee, should ensure that the proposed research is responsive to the health needs and priorities of the host country and meets the requisite ethical standards."[6]

The concept of ethical standards remains unanalyzed. This vagueness in the concept gives rise to two problems. The first is failure to distinguish between principled ethical standards, on the one hand, and ethically necessary procedural mechanisms, which are sometimes referred to as standards, on the other. The second problem is uncertainty whether ethical standards for research should be universally applicable or whether they may be relative to cultural norms and other differences among countries. The answer to both questions depends on what counts as an *ethical standard*. Does the level of treatment provided to research participants who acquire a disease in the course of a trial constitute an ethical standard? Does the clinical treatment provided to a control group in randomized, controlled trials—often referred to as *standard of care*—count as a standard? (See Chapter 66.) Are the requirements for the manner in which informed consent is obtained and documented ethical standards? Or are they procedures, to be properly distinguished from standards?

Ethical Standards: Universal or Relative?

It is difficult to find a clear statement of a universal standard for research ethics. One candidate might be the following: *If it is unethical to carry out a particular research project in a developed country, it is unethical to do that same research in a developing country.* However, this formulation is flawed because it fails to recognize that particular circumstances can be so different that some research that could not be conducted in a developed country could still be ethically acceptable in a developing country.

Another flawed statement of a universal view, which its authors call the "Uniform Care Requirement," states that all participants in research "should receive the level of care they would receive in a developed country."[7] Adherence to this requirement would make it impossible to do research designed to develop treatments for tropical diseases in remote, rural areas of developing countries, which lack the facilities of tertiary care hospitals in industrialized countries. However, most proponents of a universal standard would not claim that such research is ethically unacceptable.

The Uniform Care Requirement seeks to protect vulnerable populations from exploitation, implying that decision makers in those countries might agree to research that would be rejected in industrialized countries because of high risk to participants or other ethical concerns. An expression of this position is an opinion issued by the European Group on Ethics in Science and New Technologies (EGE) in 2003. The opinion, entitled "Ethical Aspects of Clinical Research in Developing Countries," states the following:

> [R]esearch activities involving human subjects cannot exclusively be assimilated to an economic activity subject to market rules. On the contrary, in the context of solidarity, regarding health as a public good, rather than a commodity, it needs to be regulated according to fundamental principles. The general approach chosen within this Opinion is that fundamental ethical rules applied to clinical trials in industrialized countries are to be applicable everywhere. Even if some difficulties may arise in their implementation, a weakening of the standards would be in contradiction to the fundamental principles of human rights and dignity and their universal guarantee and protection.[8]

A different view—in effect, a form of ethical relativism—holds that rules governing research practices may vary according to the cultural norms accepted in the country in which the research is carried out. Respect for diversity underlies this form of ethical relativism, which rejects the notion that a single set of ethical standards for research should prevail in our culturally diverse world. Still another consideration, different from cultural variation, is the economic disparity between industrialized countries and resource-poor countries. This disparity has been used to justify some research in developing countries that could not be conducted in industrialized countries, based not on cultural factors but rather on different needs in resource-poor and wealthier countries.

One proposed analysis intends to show the possibility of accepting universal ethical standards for research while permitting differences in what is provided to research subjects in developed and developing countries.[9] The key to this analysis lies in distinguishing the ethical *principles* that apply to particular research endeavors from other aspects, such as the research design. The relevant ethical principles embody the well-known and widely accepted requirements of informed consent, reasonable risks in light of potential benefits and minimization of risk. As long as these universal ethical principles are fulfilled, according to this argument, the research can be judged ethically acceptable. What permits a research design to be different in an industrialized country and a resource-poor country is the difference in local circumstances—in particular, in economic resources. According to Orentlicher, "It does not follow that, if a research study is unethical in the United States, it is also unethical in Kenya." Under this approach, the determination of whether a double standard exists depends on whether research in different countries adheres to the same ethical principles, not whether a particular study could be conducted in one country but not in another.

This analysis has a certain appeal. The key to accepting it, however, lies in whether the economic circumstances of industrialized and resource-poor countries should count as a morally relevant factor in assessing the ethics of a particular research design. If a study is designed and conducted by Kenyan researchers, funded only by Kenyan resources, with no collaboration or sponsorship by the pharmaceutical industry or an industrialized country, then a good case can be made for accepting the moral relevance of the local economic circumstances. If the Kenyan researchers *cannot* provide expensive drugs or laboratory equipment to carry out a particular study design, then it makes no sense to say they *ought* to do so. However, in the type of research most commonly carried out in developing countries, there is an external sponsor or an industrialized country collaborator. These external sponsors or collaborators could afford to supply the same costly drugs that they would provide for participants if similar research were conducted in the industrialized country.

Some people reject the idea that different economic conditions in rich and poor countries can justify conducting research in the poor country that could not be ethically conducted in the rich country. Greco contends that "It is clear that the pressures to lower the ethical standards set by the DoH [Declaration of Helsinki] are primarily economic—it costs less to run a trial where you do not have to provide for medical care. . . . So let us push to keep the highest ethical standards applied everywhere."[10]

Other commentators maintain that economic factors do constitute a relevant difference between industrialized and resource-poor countries, and that this difference can justify the use of different standards. For example, Resnik contends:

We . . . should not expect a single standard of research to govern all study designs. There are a variety of ethical principles that apply to research on human subjects, and they sometimes conflict. . . . In order to achieve an optimal balance of these different ethical standards, we need to take into account various social, cultural economic, political, as well as scientific factors. . . . One might even argue that it is unjust, unfair, and insensitive to demand that the exact same standards of research that govern study designs in developed nations should also be implemented in developing countries.[11]

Countries in Europe and North America have for many years had detailed laws and regulations governing research involving human subjects. More recently, developing countries such as Brazil, South Africa, and India have introduced laws or policies with requirements that are equally stringent. However, many countries still have the only barest minimum of such controls or none at all. Conflicts are bound to arise when a country in which research is being carried out lacks norms or mechanisms that have become accepted standards in the sponsoring country or agency. If researchers in developing countries must adhere to regulations promulgated by industrial countries, this is sometimes characterized as ethical imperialism. But if researchers in some countries can ignore ethical standards widely accepted elsewhere, the door would be open to a regime of ethical relativism allowing virtually any standard a country desired. The key to resolving this apparent dilemma lies in distinguishing between ethical principles and procedural mechanisms.

Distinguishing Ethical Standards From Procedures

The 2000 report of the U.S. National Bioethics Advisory Commission (NBAC) on international research makes a useful dis-

tinction between substantive and procedural ethical requirements.[12] Substantive ethical requirements, the NBAC says, are those embodied in the fundamental principles of bioethics stated in the *Belmont Report*: respect for persons, beneficence, and justice[13] (see Chapter 14). These substantive principles constitute ethical *standards,* and should be applied universally. They give rise to such requirements as obtaining informed consent individually from each adult participant, disclosing adequate information about the research maneuvers to be performed, and fully informing participants of the risks and anticipated benefits of those interventions. Procedural requirements, on the other hand, may vary according to cultural and other differences in multinational research. For example, the requirement that informed consent documents be signed can hardly be applied in a country with low literacy rates, and the composition of ethical review committees in urbanized communities may not be appropriate in a heavily rural society. Distinguishing between substantive and procedural ethical requirements can make it possible to apply the same ethical standards across national borders, while permitting differences in specific procedures to respect cultural variations. On the other hand, failure to distinguish between substantive standards and procedures may give rise to a perception of ethical conflicts when none really exist.

In order to determine whose ethical standards should be adopted when there is an appearance of conflict, it is necessary to agree on what constitutes ethical *standards.* For example, the 1993 CIOMS Guidelines included a provision intended to prevent exploitation of host countries in externally sponsored research. This guideline required scientific and ethical review of proposed research to be carried out "according to the standards of the country of the sponsoring agency, and the ethical standards applied should be no less exacting than they would be in the case of research carried out in that country." This provision prompted the criticism by Christakis and Levine that the guidelines reflected a "Western bias" because of "the assumption that the circumstances . . . in the developed world are the norm. Thus, the developed world is envisioned as more advanced, not only technologically but also morally."[14]

This criticism is not shared by any of the developing countries that by 2005 had enacted laws or adopted ethical guidelines governing research. Most provisions in these regulations and guidelines replicate the CIOMS guidelines and the Declaration of Helsinki. In particular, all adhere to the ethical *standard* that informed consent be obtained from each individual research participant, yet they permit certain *procedures* in obtaining consent to diverge from the U.S. requirement for written, signed, informed consent forms.

Informed Consent: Standards Versus Procedures

Confusion between ethical standards and procedures has even given rise to debates over the necessity of obtaining individual informed consent from research participants. Differences among cultures—especially with regard to the primacy of the individual—have prompted some to argue that the concept of informed consent is understandable and applicable in the West but is irrelevant to social and cultural norms in Africa and Asia. For example, when the CIOMS first presented its Proposed International Ethical Guidelines for Human Experimentation at a conference sponsored by the World Health Organization in December 1980, Emily Miller, a U.S. participant, described the guidelines as "essentially based on American standards of ethical review as well as on the international codes"—the Nuremberg Code and the Declaration of Helsinki.[15] This concern was also voiced by some participants from developing countries, who objected to elements of the proposed guidelines on grounds of ethical imperialism. As Miller reported, "How far, they wondered, can Western countries impose a certain concept of human rights? In countries where the common law heritage of individuality, freedom of choice, and human rights do not exist, the . . . guidelines may seem entirely inappropriate."[15]

The idea that respect for human rights applies only to Western countries is surely peculiar, in light of the numerous United Nations treaties and covenants ratified by almost all countries, including those in Africa, Asia, and the Middle East. However, the only direct reference to human rights in the context of research is Article 7 of the International Covenant on Civil and Political Rights: "No one shall be subjected to torture or to cruel, inhuman or degrading treatment or punishment. In particular, no one shall be subjected without his free consent to medical or scientific experimentation." Although this passage may at first appear to equate research involving human beings with "inhuman or degrading treatment," it is not medical or scientific experimentation itself but rather the absence of voluntary, informed consent that constitutes inhuman or degrading treatment.

The requirement for individual, informed consent is by now enshrined in laws and guidelines of many non-Western countries. The South African guidelines state two rules regarding informed consent: "i. research subjects should know that they are taking part in research; ii. research involving subjects should only be carried out with their consent." Yet these guidelines also say, "It can be proper for research involving less than minimal risk and which is easily comprehended to proceed on the basis of oral consent given after an oral description of what is involved."[16] Similarly, the guidelines issued by the Indian Council of Medical Research require that informed consent be obtained from each individual subject. But the guidelines also say that the nature and form of the consent may depend on a number of different factors.[17]

In some developing countries, a substantial proportion of the population is illiterate or semiliterate. Requiring written, signed consent documents when the research participants are illiterate is clearly inappropriate. For semiliterate participants, a written consent document may be appropriate, especially because family members whom the participant may wish to involve in the consent process may be literate.

It is important to distinguish between the requirement that a written document be provided to a prospective participant and the requirement that the participant sign the document. In some countries, the meaning of signing a document is quite different from what it is in North America or Western Europe. Even when the need for individual, informed consent is fully acceptable, it would be ethically appropriate to waive the requirement of a signature on a consent document if the country has a history of oppressive regimes or if people are fearful, based on their experience, that a signed document might be used against them in some manner. This can pose a problem for multinational research involving drugs for which approval will be sought from the U.S. Food and Drug Administration (FDA). FDA regulations require written, signed informed consent documents in research that in-

volves more than minimal risk. All clinical trials testing investigational new drugs are likely to be categorized as involving more than minimal risk.

In addition, researchers who conduct clinical trials in developing countries often confront practices that depart from the requirements of informed consent in the United States and other industrialized countries. For example, in many developing countries, physicians routinely withhold information from patients with certain diseases. Even if this custom might be defended in ordinary medical practice, it poses a severe challenge to the disclosure required for research involving human participants. Adherence to local practices could require withholding diagnoses from patients who become research participants and concealing key elements of the research design, such as the use of placebo controls, the process of randomizing subjects into different groups in a clinical trial and the expected efficacy (or lack of efficacy) of a method being tested.[18,19] Withholding information also might promote the mistaken assumption—known as the therapeutic misconception—that the purpose of research is to benefit participants by providing them with a known, effective treatment for their medical condition (see Chapter 58).

Potential participants cannot make an informed decision without knowing that they may not receive a proven treatment that will benefit them. To enroll individuals who are not provided with such key items of information would deviate from the substantive ethical standard of disclosure required for adequate informed consent.

In a randomized clinical trial of adjuvant treatment for breast cancer conducted in Vietnam, the principal investigator, Richard R. Love, "found himself uncertain about the application of American standards of informed consent in the Vietnamese setting," according to an article he coauthored in the *Journal of Investigative Medicine*.[20] After consultation with Vietnamese immigrants in the United States (including physicians, a sociologist, and several women), Love concluded that "American standards would not be acceptable to Vietnamese physicians, political leaders in Vietnam, or the vast majority of Vietnamese patients."[20]

The researcher told the institutional review board (IRB) at his U.S. medical school that in Vietnam, patients do not participate in medical decision making, but look to their physicians to tell them the appropriate treatment. As a result, he contended that he needed to withhold any elements of the consent process that would suggest uncertainty on the part of the treating doctor. Specifically, he wanted to avoid discussion of alternative therapies, and he did not want to reveal that the proposed treatment had been determined by randomization. After many months of deliberation and considerable negotiation, the IRB approved a consent form that did include the key elements of informed consent, "though with somewhat less detail than is typical in a U.S. consent form," Love and his coauthor reported. Love and Fost stated that it is unclear whether the women in the study understood that their treatment was determined by randomization. However, a small survey of the participants in the study suggested that the women actually did understand randomization to a degree comparable with studies in industrialized countries.

Multinational research requires adherence to internationally accepted standards, one of which is disclosure to research participants—even if similar disclosure to patients is not the norm in a host country's practice of medicine. Reluctance to disclose a physician's uncertainty about the best treatment rests on customary medical practice in such countries. The authors of the article describing the breast cancer study in Vietnam argued that "trying to force [the U.S. mode of] consent on the physicians [in Vietnam] risked losing their cooperation with the project because of the tone of cultural imperialism that it would convey."

During its study of international research, the NBAC heard evidence confirming that in many cultures, a diagnosis of cancer is made not to the patient but instead to the patient's family. The question is whether practices common in the clinical setting should be acceptable in the research setting, especially when local or national cultural practices depart significantly from international standards of informed consent in research.

The NBAC report contains two recommendations that address this issue:

Recommendation 3.1: Research should not deviate from the substantive ethical standard of voluntary informed consent. Researchers should not propose, sponsors should not support, and ethics review committees should not approve research that deviates from this substantive ethical standard.[12]

Recommendation 3.2: Researchers should develop culturally appropriate ways to disclose information that is necessary for adherence to the substantive ethical standard of informed consent, with particular attention to disclosures relating to diagnosis and risk, research design, and possible post-trial benefits.[12]

A report by the United Kingdom's Nuffield Council on Bioethics essentially agrees with the NBAC recommendations, affirming that "obtaining genuine consent to research from participants is vital in ensuring that respect for persons is promoted."[21]

A different problem arises when research participants are unacquainted with the concepts and methods of modern science or biomedical research. In this situation, the NBAC urges researchers to seek creative ways of presenting information, such as by analogies readily understood by the local population. It is not sufficient simply to present the information. An important component of the process is determining whether the prospective subjects adequately understand what they have been told. To this end, the NBAC recommends the following:

Recommendation 3.4: Researchers should develop procedures to ensure that potential participants do, in fact, understand the information provided in the consent process and should describe those procedures in their research protocols.[12]

Recommendation 3.5: Researchers should consult with community representatives to develop innovative and effective means to communicate all necessary information in a manner that is understandable to potential participants. When community representatives will not be involved, the protocol presented to the ethics review committee should justify why such involvement is not possible or relevant.[12]

In cross-cultural contexts, some commentators consider it problematic to require that informed consent be obtained from each individual recruited as a research participant. Christakis and Levine claim that to do so is "philosophically and practically difficult."[14] Some Asian and African cultures lack the individualistic concept of a person to which the Western world adheres, so how to apply the principle of respect for the person becomes problematic.

Some ethicists hold that researchers should adhere to local customs and traditions, and that insisting on Western requirements for individual informed consent in other cultures is ethical imperialism.[22] Others maintain that individual informed consent should not be eliminated or altered. "We see no convincing arguments for a general policy of dispensing with, or substantially modifying, the researcher's obligation to obtain first-person consent in biomedical research conducted in Africa," said IJsselmuiden and Faden.[23]

The 2002 Nuffield Council report calls for requiring informed consent:

[W]e cannot avoid the responsibility of taking a view when the two aspects of respect—respect for culture and respect for persons—come into conflict with one another. We are of the view that the fundamental principle of respect for persons requires that participants who have the capacity to consent to research should never be subjected to research without such consent.[21]

Those who would subordinate the principle of respect for persons to other considerations have not identified a competing ethical principle that deserves a higher ranking. The unstated assumption that culture outranks respect for persons places respect for cultural tradition on a par with the three most widely acknowledged principles of ethical research: respect for persons, beneficence, and justice. No one argues against the ethical requirement that researchers should be culturally sensitive. But a limit is reached when a cultural practice violates an internationally accepted principle of research ethics.

A different sort of problem arises when it is necessary to obtain permission from a community leader or tribal chief in order to enter the community to embark on research. That requirement has to be respected, but it is no different in principle from the need in Western culture to obtain permission to enter the premises from the head of a workplace or a school principal. Permission from a tribal chief or village leader may be required, but should not serve as a substitute for individual informed consent obtained from each potential participant. The NBAC report contains the following recommendation:

Recommendation 3.6: Where culture or custom requires that permission of a community representative be granted before researchers may approach potential research participants, researchers should be sensitive to such local requirements. However, in no case may permission from a community representative or council replace the requirement of a competent individual's voluntary informed consent.[12]

Considerably more problematic is the need to obtain individual informed consent from women in cultures in which the husband or father of an adult woman normally grants permission for her participation in activities outside the home. The NBAC's recommendation on this point calls for a presumption that men and women should be treated equally in the informed consent process, but it would give men the power to say "No" in cultures in which that seems necessary.

Recommendation 3.9: Researchers should use the same procedures in the informed consent process for women and men. However, ethics review committees may accept a consent process in which a woman's individual consent to participate in research is supplemented by permission from a man if all of the following conditions are met:

a. it would be impossible to conduct the research without obtaining such supplemental permission; and
b. failure to conduct this research could deny its potential benefits to women in the host country; and
c. measures to respect the woman's autonomy to consent to research are undertaken to the greatest extent possible.

In no case may a competent adult woman be enrolled in research solely upon the consent of another person; her individual consent is always required.[12]

Here, as in other recommendations, the NBAC leaves the ultimate decision on controversial matters to the discretion of an ethics review committee.

Unlike the NBAC recommendation, the CIOMS 2002 Guidelines do not permit a departure from the need to obtain individual informed consent only from the woman. The commentary under CIOMS' Guideline 16 states the following:

> [Only] the informed consent of the woman herself is required for her participation. In no case should the permission of a spouse or partner replace the requirement of individual informed consent. If women wish to consult with their husbands or partners or seek voluntarily to obtain their permission before deciding to enroll in research, that is not only ethically permissible but in some contexts highly desirable. A strict requirement of authorization of spouse or partner, however, violates the substantive principle of respect for persons.[6]

In this, as in other areas of multinational research, what some people take to be ethical imperialism, others consider proper adherence to universally applicable ethical standards.

Adherence to U.S. Rules: Appropriate Standards or Ethical Imperialism

U.S. federal regulations require that research using federal funds conducted outside the United States must be reviewed by an IRB that has been approved by the U.S. Office for Human Research Protections (OHRP). The CIOMS International Ethical Guidelines require scientific and ethical review in both the sponsoring and the host country. Some commentators contend that this is precisely the right mechanism for adequate protection of human participants. Others argue that approval of proposed research by a U.S. IRB should be sufficient, and still others argue that a research ethics committee in the developing country should suffice. Between these positions are a variety of views about how flexible a sponsoring country's regulations should be when research is conducted elsewhere, and whether requiring strict adherence to the sponsoring country's rules is another instance of ethical imperialism or "colonialism" in the conduct of research. In a study commissioned by the NBAC, 77 percent of U.S. and 85 percent of developing country researchers surveyed recommended the use of international guidelines instead of U.S. regulations to cover joint projects.[12]

In 2002, OHRP issued new rules for non-U.S. institutions seeking authorization as sites for research by U.S. investigators or others using U.S. funds. The technical name for this authorization is Federalwide Assurance for International (non-U.S.) Institutions. The foreign institution must indicate on the application whether the Declaration of Helsinki or some other statement of ethical principles governs it in protecting the rights and welfare of human participants in research. If the box marked "Other" is checked and other principles are named, a copy of those principles must be submitted with the application.

Adherence to a statement of ethical principles is not sufficient, however. The institution applying for this authorization also must comply with U.S. regulations or with alternative regulatory standards that are considered to be generally consistent with the U.S. Common Rule—the U.S. policy for the protection of human subjects in federally sponsored research (see Chapter 15). In addition, the international institution must obey any additional regulations that may be imposed by a federal agency involved in or funding the research. OHRP listed the following as acceptable international regulations:

a. The U.S. Federal Policy for the Protection of Human Subjects, known as the Common Rule (e.g., Subpart A) or the U.S. Department of Health and Human Services (DHHS) regulations at 45 CFR 46 and its Subparts A, B, C, and D;
b. The May 1, 1996, International Conference on Harmonization E-6 Guidelines for Good Clinical Practice (ICH-GCP-E6), Sections 1 through 4;
c. The 1993 Council for International Organizations of Medical Sciences (CIOMS) International Ethical Guidelines for Biomedical Research Involving Human Subjects;
d. The 1998 Medical Research Council of Canada Tri-Council Policy Statement on Ethical Conduct for Research Involving Humans;
e. The 2000 Indian Council of Medical Research Ethical Guidelines for Biomedical Research on Human Subjects; or
f. Other standard(s) for the protection of human subjects recognized by U.S. Federal Departments and Agencies which have adopted the U.S. Federal Policy for the Protection of Human Subjects.[24]

It is much easier to agree to comply with ethical principles than to succeed in conforming to detailed regulations governing research. Ethical principles are stated in general terms and often require interpretation for each situation to which they are applied; regulations are normally quite specific and cover a wealth of topics in minute detail.

There is, however, a gray area in which procedures become so important that they shade into ethical principles. An example is the requirement for due process in legal or ethical proceedings, in which the rights of accused individuals are protected by procedural safeguards. If the procedural mechanisms for protecting the rights and welfare of human subjects of research in developing countries are equivalent to the protections in place in the United States and other industrialized countries, then it would surely be paternalistic to insist on ethical review of proposed research by a committee sitting in the United States. Nevertheless, it may be difficult to ascertain that procedural mechanisms are equivalent simply by examining rules of procedure, such as the rules governing an IRB in a developing country. If the members of the IRB are inexperienced, if they have not been educated in research ethics, or if members have serious conflicts of interest, these shortcomings will not be reflected in the committee's procedural rules.

Additional questions surround the mechanism of committee review, including at least the following: Must ethics committees in developing countries have the same composition and rules of procedure as U.S. IRBs? When research proposals are reviewed by an IRB in both countries, how should any disagreements between the two committees be resolved?

Available evidence suggests that, at least in the United States, IRBs rarely if ever try to communicate with host country ethics review committees. United States IRBs do not seek pertinent information from the developing country committee, nor even ascertain whether a qualified committee exists. In a 2003 review of international clinical research, Fitzgerald, Wasunna, and Pape proposed the following:

> IRBs from a wealthy sponsor country should ensure that a viable local ethics committee in the proposed host country will review the protocol. . . . A viable local IRB should be viewed as a critical resource for IRBs in sponsor countries. . . . Better communication between the sponsor country IRB and the local IRB could help resolve [any] disagreements. . . . Further, the sponsor country IRB and the local IRB may possess complementary expertise and may be able to carry out a better review working together than either could working alone.[25]

If U.S. IRBs were to adopt this novel recommendation, they would raise the review of multinational research to a new level, improving both the quality of the review process and the protection of the rights and welfare of research participants in developing countries.

The Debate Over Double Standards

Some commentators have maintained that identical standards should be employed the world over, whereas others contend that different standards are required because different circumstances obtain. But does *different* necessarily mean *lower*?

Rothman argues that "there are strong practical as well as principled reasons for Americans to follow American ethical standards when they do research abroad.[26] He contends that U.S. IRBs have "too little familiarity with developing countries to set different standards." Angell agrees that ethical standards should not depend on where the research is performed. "The nature of investigators' responsibility for the welfare of their subjects should not be influenced by the political and economic conditions of the region" she writes. ". . . [A]ny other position could lead to the exploitation of people in developing countries, in order to conduct research that could not be performed in the sponsoring countries."[27]

Resnik, however, contends that we "should not expect a single standard of research to govern all study designs. There are a variety of ethical principles that apply to research on human subjects, and they sometimes conflict."[11] And Mbidde, a Uganda Cancer Institute researcher, strongly defends research in his country that could not have been conducted in the United States or Western Europe:

> Ugandan studies are responsive to the health needs and the priorities of the nation. . . . [T]he appropriate authorities, including the national ethics review committee, have satisfied

themselves that the research meets their own ethical requirements. With these requirements met, if Ugandans cannot carry out research on their people for the good of their nation, applying ethical standards in their local circumstances, then who will?[28]

This consideration puts a different twist on the matter. In the absence of research conducted in developing countries, the inhabitants are denied the potential benefits that may result. In many such countries, a majority lacks access to treatments available in industrialized countries or, for that matter, any treatment at all. If research is not conducted in developing countries, the public health benefits that could result may never be available to the population. Still, the Ugandan researcher's comments hark back to the concern about the quality of protection of research participants in developing countries. Are the procedural mechanisms for protecting the rights and welfare of human subjects adequate in those countries?

If there is something inherently unjust about allowing a double standard of ethics in research—one for industrialized countries, another for resource-poor countries—what are the options for arriving at a single standard, applicable wherever human beings are enrolled as research participants? Some commentators justify a double standard because of the undeniable differences in wealth and other resources that exist in the world. Those who hold this view point to the vast array of activities, outside the sphere of human subject research, in which inequalities exist. Further, they contend, rectifying inequalities among nations, or even among subpopulations within nations, will not be accomplished by imposing obligations on the sponsors of biomedical research.

This argument rests on the view that different economic conditions can justify different standards for providing care and treatment to research participants. The argument begins with the premise (1) that the world is filled with inequalities in resources, which is true; adds a second premise, also true (2) that striving for a single standard in research will do nothing to rectify the larger number of existing inequalities; inserts an implicit premise (3) that research involving human subjects should be treated no differently from other international endeavors; and concludes (4) that double standards in research are ethically acceptable.

The validity of this argument turns on premise (3), which is not a factual statement but an *ought* statement. To accept it is to consider biomedical research and health care as just another commodity in a market-driven world. However, if one views health care, medical benefits, and the research that yields these services as a special sort of social good, it is possible to reject the idea that research involving human subjects should be treated no differently from other activities driven by market forces.[8]

Opponents of the single-standard position might argue that they start from a quite different set of premises. They contend that insisting on one standard in research will not reduce inequalities among rich and poor nations, but that adjusting ethical standards to reflect differing real-world conditions will, in fact, reduce these inequalities. They conclude, therefore, that there is an obligation to insist on different standards of research. The plausibility of this argument depends on empirical facts and circumstances in specific cases. There is probably no way to adjudicate the general arguments in defense of single or double standards without the factual details necessary for reaching sound conclusions.

International ethical codes and guidelines will not resolve all questions or conflicts that may arise in the design and conduct of multinational research. Any differences in judgments made by two or more committees that review a research protocol will have to be negotiated. On some points, codes and guidelines may be insufficiently specific. On other issues, provisions in codes or guidelines that address the same point may vary in minor or even major respects. For example, existing guidelines differ over the use of placebo controls and the level of care and treatment to be provided to research subjects during and after a clinical trial (see Chapters 25, 65, and 66). As long as unresolved differences remain among parties committed to conducting research according to the highest ethical standards, it is open to question whether ethical codes or guidelines should attempt to settle the conflict by imposing an unequivocal rule.

References

1. Annas GJ, Grodin MA, eds. *The Nazi Doctors and the Nuremberg Code: Human Rights in Human Experimentation.* New York, N.Y.: Oxford University Press; 1992.

2. Perley S, Fluss SS, Bankowski Z, Simon F. The Nuremberg Code: An international overview. In: Annas GJ, Grodin MA, eds. *The Nazi Doctors and the Nuremberg Code: Human Rights in Human Experimentation.* New York, N.Y.: Oxford University Press; 1992:149–73.

3. World Medical Association. *Code of Ethics of the World Medical Association: Declaration of Helsinki.* Helsinki, Finland: WMA; June 1964. *British Medical Journal* 1964;2:177.

4. World Medical Association. *Declaration of Helsinki: Ethical Principles for Medical Research Involving Human Subjects.* Tokyo, Japan: WMA; October 2004. [Online] 2004. Available: http://www.wma.net/e/policy/b3.htm.

5. Council for International Organizations of Medical Sciences, in collaboration with the World Health Organization. *International Ethical Guidelines for Biomedical Research Involving Human Subjects.* Geneva, Switzerland: CIOMS and WHO; 1993.

6. Council for International Organizations of Medical Sciences, in collaboration with the World Health Organization. *International Ethical Guidelines for Biomedical Research Involving Human Subjects.* Geneva, Switzerland: CIOMS and WHO; 2002. [Online] November 2002. Available: http://www.cioms.ch/frame_guidelines_nov_2002.htm.

7. Killen J, Grady C, Folkers GK, Fauci AS. Ethics of clinical research in the developing world. *Nature Reviews/Immunology* 2002;2:210–5.

8. European Group on Ethics in Science and New Technologies. *Opinion No. 17 to the European Commission: Ethical Aspects of Clinical Research in Developing Countries.* Brussels, Belgium: EGE; 2003. [Online] February 4, 2003. Available: http://ec.europa.eu/european_group_ethics/docs/avis17_en.pdf.

9. Orentlicher D. Universality and its limits: When research ethics can reflect local circumstances. *Journal of Law, Medicine, and Ethics* 2002;30:403–10.

10. Greco DB. Revising the Declaration of Helsinki: Ethics vs. economics or the fallacy of urgency. *Canadian HIV/AIDS Policy and Law Review* 2000;5(4):94–7.

11. Resnik DB. The ethics of HIV research in developing nations. *Bioethics* 1998;12:286–306.

12. National Bioethics Advisory Commission. *Ethical and Policy Issues in International Research.* Washington, D.C.: NBAC; 2001. [Online] April 30, 2001. Available: http://www.georgetown.edu/research/nrcbl/nbac/clinical/V011.pdf.

13. The National Commission for the Protection of Human Subjects of Biomedical and Behavioral Research. *The Belmont Report: Ethical Principles and Guidelines for the Protection of Human Subjects of Research.* Washington, D.C.: Department of Health, Education and Welfare; DHEW Publication OS 78-0012 1978. [Online] April 18, 1979. Available: http://www.hhs.gov/ohrp/humansubjects/guidance/belmont.htm.

14. Christakis NA, Levine RJ. Multinational research. In: Reich WT, ed. *Encyclopedia of Bioethics,* 2nd ed. New York, N.Y.: Simon & Schuster Macmillan; 1995.

15. Miller E. International trends in ethical review of medical research. *IRB: A Review of Human Subjects Research* 1981;3(8):9–10.

16. South Africa Medical Research Council. *Guidelines on Ethics in Medical Research.* Tygerberg, South Africa: South Africa Medical Research Council; 1993. [Online] Available: http://www.mrc.ac.za/ethics/consent.htm.

17. Indian Council of Medical Research. *Ethical Guidelines for Biomedical Research on Human Subjects.* New Delhi, India: Indian Council of Medical Research; 2000. [Online] Available: http://icmr.nic.in/ethical.pdf.

18. Kass N, Hyder AA. Attitudes and experiences of U.S. and developing country investigators regarding U.S. human subjects regulations. In: National Bioethics Advisory Commission. *Ethical and Policy Issues in International Research: Clinical Trials in Developing Countries, Vol. II.* Bethesda, Md.: NBAC; 2001:B-1–B-220. [Online] Available: http://www.georgetown.edu/research/nrcbl/nbac/clinical/V012.pdf.

19. Sugarman J, Popkin B, Fortney J, Rivera R. International perspectives on protecting human research subjects. In: National Bioethics Advisory Commission. *Ethical and Policy Issues in International Research: Clinical Trials in Developing Countries, Vol. II.* Bethesda, Md.: NBAC; 2001:E-1–E-30. [Online] Available: http://www.georgetown.edu/research/nrcbl/nbac/clinical/V012.pdf.

20. Love RR, Fost NC. Ethical and regulatory challenges in a randomized control trial of adjuvant treatment for breast cancer in Vietnam. *Journal of Investigative Medicine* 1997;45:423–31.

21. Nuffield Council on Bioethics. *The Ethics of Research Related to Healthcare in Developing Countries.* London, England: Nuffield Council on Bioethics; 2002. [Online] April 2002. Available: http://www.nuffieldbioethics.org/fileLibrary/pdf/errhdc_fullreport001.pdf.

22. Newton L. Ethical imperialism and informed consent. *IRB: A Review of Human Subjects Research* 1990;12(3):10–1.

23. IJsselmuiden CB, Faden RR. Research and informed consent in Africa—Another look. *New England Journal of Medicine* 1992;326:830–3.

24. Department of Health and Human Services, National Institutes of Health, and Office for Human Research Protections. The Common Rule, Title 45 (Public Welfare), Code of Federal Regulations, Part 46 (Protection of Human Subjects). [Online] June 23, 2005. Available: http://www.hhs.gov/ohrp/humansubjects/guidance/45cfr46.htm.

25. Fitzgerald DW, Wasunna A, Pape JW. Ten questions for institutional review boards when reviewing international clinical research protocols. *IRB: Ethics and Human Research* 2003;25(2):14–8.

26. Rothman DJ. The shame of medical research. *New York Review of Books* Nov. 30, 2000;47(19):60–64.

27. Angell M. Investigators' responsibilities for human subjects in developing countries. *New England Journal of Medicine* 2000;342:967–9.

28. Mbidde EK. Letter to the editor. *New England Journal of Medicine* 1997;338:836.

Ezekiel J. Emanuel

Benefits to Host Countries

One of the major ethical issues in biomedical research relates to access to drugs and other interventions after a trial has been completed. If the ultimate purpose of research studies is to improve health, then somehow ensuring access to interventions proven safe and effective would seem to be a necessary step. Yet, as is well documented, adoption of any new intervention or technology is haphazard at best.[1] In part this is because after research studies, the drugs or devices might not be submitted for regulatory approval or, if submitted, might not be approved. In addition, health-care providers might not implement the interventions because of inertia or lack of training. And, in both developing and developed countries, the high cost of the interventions might preclude access to these interventions. Historically, a commonly identified problem—which may or may not have been common— has been so-called helicopter or "briefcase" research. The researchers, concerned about the data and publication, came, conducted their study, obtained the relevant data, and left the research area, unconcerned about what subsequently transpired for the research participants and their community.

Beginning in the early 1990s, concern about such helicopter research led to the articulation of a new ethical principle to ensure that the community in which the research was conducted benefited from the research. This became known as the *reasonable availability* requirement. It is important to understand the fundamental purpose of this requirement, the nature of the requirement, criticisms of the requirement, and three different alternatives.

Benefits of Biomedical Research

Although biomedical research may have intrinsic merit in expanding understanding of human biological systems, it is fundamentally a practice with instrumental value. The ultimate aim of biomedical research is not just to increase knowledge but to improve human health and well-being.[2–4] The fundamental ethical challenge is that the people and communities that participate in research are assuming risks and burdens, whereas the benefits of the knowledge gained from research can extend to many other people who have not assumed any risks or burdens. That some might benefit because others are exposed to risks raises the specter of exploitation[5] (see Chapter 20).

This risk of exploitation is inherent in all biomedical research that might benefit people beyond those actually enrolled in the research study.[6,7] It is particularly worrisome in situations in which those who participate as subjects in the research are less likely to actually benefit from the research itself or the results of the research. They might not benefit because they are poor and cannot afford the intervention, because they live in communities that lack the infrastructure or health-care personnel to deliver the intervention, or because their community is poor and the companies marketing the intervention might not deem it financially worthwhile to have the intervention licensed and distributed there. These are conditions that are more frequent in developing countries.[8] Consequently, the concern about ensuring that participants and communities benefit from research has arisen most forcefully and consistently in relationship to research conducted in developing countries.[9]

In order to avoid or minimize the possibility of exploitation, those who assume the risks and burdens of research should be assured of receiving fair benefits from the research.[5,7] This notion is embedded in the ethical requirement that biomedical research has social value. The challenge is how to fulfill this requirement of ensuring that the research participants and community who bear the burdens and risks actually benefit. In what follows, I will present and critically assess the reasonable availability requirement and three alternate accounts.

Reasonable Availability

The most influential attempt at ensuring that participants and communities, especially those in developing countries, benefit from participating in biomedical research has been the reasonable availability requirement.[10] The Council for International Organizations of Medical Sciences (CIOMS) proposed this requirement in its 1993 *International Ethical Guidelines for Biomedical Research Involving Human Subjects*. In the commentary to Guideline 8, "Research involving subjects in underdeveloped communities," CIOMS argued the following:

> As a general rule, the sponsoring agency should ensure that, at the completion of successful testing, any product developed will be made reasonably available to inhabitants of the underdeveloped community in which the research was carried out; exceptions to this general requirement should be justified, and agreed to by all concerned parties before the research is begun.[10]

This requirement was reemphasized in the commentary to Guideline 15, "Obligations of sponsoring and host countries," which stated,

> As a general rule, the sponsoring agency should agree in advance of the research that any product developed through such research will be made reasonably available to the inhabitants of the host community or country at the completion of successful testing.[10]

Furthermore, the 2002 revision of the CIOMS Guidelines reemphasized this requirement. Reasonable availability was not just included in a commentary but made part of Guideline 10 which requires that

> [b]efore undertaking research in a population or community with limited resources, the sponsor and the investigator must make every effort to ensure that . . . any intervention or product developed, or knowledge generated, will be made reasonably available for the benefit of that population or community.[11]

In the commentary on this Guideline, CIOMS justified this requirement by stating that it was necessary to avoid exploitation:

> If the knowledge gained from the research in such a country is used primarily for the benefit of populations that can afford the tested product, the research may rightly be characterized as *exploitative* and, therefore, unethical. . . . In general, if

there is good reason to believe that a product developed or knowledge generated by research is unlikely to be reasonably available to, or applied to the benefit of, the population of a proposed host country or community after the conclusion of the research, it is unethical to conduct the research in that country or community [emphasis added].[11]

In the years since its original formulation, many individuals and groups have supported the reasonable availability requirement as necessary for ethical research in developing countries. For instance, Crouch and Arras:

> agree with the Council for International Organizations of Medical Sciences (CIOMS) guidelines and with many observers that in order to be judged ethical and non-exploitative in the final analysis, such research must not only address local problems, but the results must also be made reasonably available to local populations.[12]

The chair and executive director of the National Bioethics Advisory Commission (NBAC) in the United States argued that

> [i]f the intervention being tested is not likely to be affordable in the host country or if the health care infrastructure cannot support its proper distribution and use, it is unethical to ask persons in that country to participate in research, since they will not enjoy any of its potential benefits.[13]

And NBAC argued in its report on the topic, *Ethical and Policy Issues in International Research: Clinical Trials in Developing Countries,*

> NBAC concludes that at the end of a clinical trial that results in an effective intervention, research participants should be provided with this intervention. In addition, NBAC concludes that before initiation of a research project, researchers or sponsors should consider how they might make benefits, if any, available to others in the host country with the understanding that appropriate host country decisionmakers must be meaningful and essential participants in making such arrangements.[14]

The second point in the UNAIDS guidance document entitled *Ethical Considerations in HIV Preventive Vaccine Research* states,

> Any HIV preventive vaccine demonstrated to be safe and effective, as well as other knowledge and benefits resulting from HIV vaccine research, should be made available as soon as possible to all participants in the trials in which it was tested, as well as to other populations at high risk of HIV infection. Plans should be developed at the initial stages of HIV vaccine development to ensure such availability.[15]

The guidance document's elaboration of this point states that "making a safe and effective vaccine reasonably available to the population where it was tested is a basic ethical requirement."[15] Thus, the authors of the UNAIDS document make clear that they think reasonable availability is a fundamental ethical requirement beyond debate.

Similarly, the health law and bioethics group at Boston University has strongly advocated reasonable availability:

> In order for research to be ethically conducted [in a developing country] it must offer the potential of actual benefit to

the inhabitants of that developing country. . . . [F]or under-developed communities to derive potential benefit from re-search, they must have access to the fruits of such research.[16]

And the Boston University bioethicists argue that without rea-sonable availability, the participants and community will be exploited:

> Unless the interventions being tested will actually be made available to the impoverished populations that are being used as research subjects, developed countries are simply *exploiting* them in order to quickly use the knowledge gained from the clinical trials for the developed countries' own benefit [em-phasis added].[17]

Although avoiding the phrase *reasonable availability,* even the 2000 revision of the Declaration of Helsinki seems to endorse something like the requirement in paragraph 19:

> Medical research is only justified if there is a reasonable likelihood that the populations in which the research is car-ried out stand to benefit from the results of the research.[18]

Specification of the Reasonable Availability Requirement

Although widely supported, the reasonable availability require-ment is vague. CIOMS acknowledges in its 2002 guidelines that "the issue of reasonable availability is complex and will need to be determined on a case-by-case basis" and then lists myriad "rele-vant considerations."[11] Four main issues require specification: (1) the nature of the commitment; (2) who is responsible for ful-filling the requirement; (3) what constitutes making something reasonably available; and (4) who must have access (see Table 65.1). On each of these issues there has been a very wide range of answers. Thus, despite agreement on the very general reasonable availability requirement, there is substantial disagreement on how it should be specified and actually put into practice.[19]

First, how strong or explicit should the commitment to pro-vide the drug or vaccine be at the initiation of the research trial? CIOMS seems to require an explicit, almost contract-like mecha-nism, agreed to before the trial. CIOMS's guidelines state that this commitment should be "[a]greed to by all concerned parties be-fore the research is begun" and that the "[s]ponsoring agency should agree in advance of the research."[11] The 2000 revision of the Declaration of Helsinki endorses a much less explicit and stringent guarantee; it does not require availability to be ensured in advance.[18] Conversely, NBAC goes further than CIOMS, not only requiring "agreements" but also requiring that mechanisms to ensure affordability and infrastructure to "support [the new in-tervention's] proper distribution and use" are in place.[14] Some commentators go further still, arguing that reasonable availability means more than "the mere assertion that the interventions will be feasible for use in the developing countries." Rather, prior to be-ginning a study there needs to be "a real plan as to how the in-tervention will actually be delivered," and this includes "identified funding" for upgrades to health-care infrastructure and roads if necessary.[16,17]

Second, the original 1993 CIOMS requirement placed re-sponsibility for ensuring reasonable availability on the sponsoring agency: "As a general rule, the sponsoring agency should en-sure. . . ."[10] The 2002 version expands this responsibility to in-clude "the sponsor and investigator."[11] NBAC suggests that the responsibility for the plan be on "researchers or sponsors," al-though it is unclear who has responsibility for the actual provi-sion.[14] Conversely, the Declaration of Helsinki fails to specify who is responsible for guaranteeing reasonable availability.[18] Im-portantly, the UNAIDS document suggests that the responsibility for fulfilling this requirement is broad-based, encompassing not just "health and research communities" but also "representatives from the executive branch, health ministry, local health authori-ties, and relevant scientific and ethical groups" in the host coun-try.[15] And still others seem to lay responsibility on "developed countries" without specifying any particular actors. Interestingly, although both CIOMS and NBAC suggest that host country de-cision makers be participants in negotiations about providing the

Table 65.1
Issues Involved in the Reasonable Availability Requirement

Source	How Strong and Explicit a Commitment?	Who Is Responsible?	When Is Access Reasonably Available?	Who Should Be Guaranteed Reasonable Availability?
CIOMS[11]	"Agree in advance of the research"	Sponsors and investigators	Unspecified	"Inhabitants of underdeveloped community in which the research was carried out" "Host community and country"
NBAC[14]	"Negotiations and agreements" preceding the start of research, which include provisions for enhancing infrastructure	"Researchers or sponsors"	Unspecified	"Host country"
Helsinki[18]	Does not require specific prior agreement	Unspecified	Unspecified	"Population in which the research is conducted"
Annas, Grodin, et al.[16,17]	Requires definitive commitments, including "funding identified"	Developed world	"Proper distribution and use"	"Host country"

interventions, almost none of the guidelines or commentators place *responsibility* for making drugs and other interventions available on the governments of developing countries.

Third, when is access reasonably available? Does going through the host country's regulatory process and licensing a new drug or technology qualify as making it reasonably available? Can the drug or intervention be priced at a market price, or does it have to be free to be reasonably available? What if it is provided at a subsidized price but is not free? If a new drug is provided at a subsidized price but many people still cannot afford it, is it reasonably available? None of the guidelines or commentators seems to accept licensing with the price set at a market rate as sufficient to satisfy "reasonable availability." However, neither do any of the guidelines or commentators specify how this issue should be resolved or offer a rationale for resolving it.

Fourth, to whom should the drug or other intervention be made reasonably available? The range of possibilities extends from the research participants, their local community, the region of the country from which they come, the entire country in which the research was conducted, the geographic region of the continent where the research was conducted, finally to every person who needs the intervention in the world. The choice obviously has substantial financial and logistical implications. Indeed, it may also influence the selection of research sites. If the sponsor or researchers have responsibility for providing the intervention to the host country, then there will be bias against conducting research projects in populous countries such as India or Indonesia, in favor of less populous countries such as The Gambia. CIOMS clearly suggests that the requirement extends beyond the research participants to the "host community or country."[11] But CIOMS does not specify what the parameters of the "host community" are, whether they are limited to villages, neighborhoods of cities, entire cities, or provinces. The Declaration of Helsinki also seems to suggest that the requirement extends beyond the research participants but uses the ambiguous phrase, the "population in which the research is carried out."[18] NBAC seems to endorse the "host country."[14] Annas and Grodin also contend that the entire "host country" must have the drug or intervention reasonably available.[17] However, these guidelines and commentators do not offer a principled justification why they select the group they do.

Criticisms of the Reasonable Availability Requirement

Although ambiguity of the reasonable availability requirement is a problem, there have been other challenges. Nine distinct criticisms have been articulated challenging the very notion that reasonable availability is an ethical requirement for research in developing countries[20] (see Table 65.2).

First, and most important, critics argue that the reasonable availability requirement mistakes how to properly address exploitation.[20] Reasonable availability focuses on guaranteeing a *particular type* of benefit, but the fundamental requirement for addressing exploitation is to ensure a *fair level* of benefits, given the burdens and risks someone assumes as a research participant and the benefits others obtain.[5] The key to exploitation is not *what* item people get, but *how much* they get.[21] Another way to put this is that reasonable availability is like requiring that the baker gets access to bread rather than ensuring the baker is paid a fair amount of money.

Critics claim that CIOMS and others fail to understand the nature of exploitation and therefore miss the appropriate solution. Guaranteeing that a drug or other intervention is made available to the local community may correspond to the fair level of benefits sometimes, by chance, but at other times it may not correspond to the fair level of benefits.[20] For instance, for a very risky study, reasonable availability may not be fair because it is too little. Conversely, for a very safe trial, such as a vaccine trial, the reasonable availability requirement may necessitate providing too much benefit. A better approach is to calibrate the benefits to the burdens, rather than to guarantee a particular type of benefit.

Second, critics argue that the reasonable availability requirement seems to embody a very narrow notion of benefits. Everyone agrees that to avoid exploitation, participants and the community bearing the burden must receive a fair level of benefits.[5,20,21] However, critics argue that the reasonable availability requirement seems to count only availability of the drug or intervention as a benefit. There are many benefits from the both the conduct and results of research beyond availability of the drug or other intervention: training of health-care personnel, construction of health-care facilities or other physical infrastructure, provision of health-care services beyond those required in the research study, and even declines in disease prevalence, such as drops in HIV, from educating the population about health care. These, too, must be considered in the evaluation of whether the research benefits the participants and larger community. Yet these are completely ignored by the reasonable availability requirement.[20,21]

Third, the various conceptions of the reasonable availability requirement provide no justification for who should receive the benefits. The requirement is meant to minimize the chance of exploitation. Therefore, the requirement should be directed at those who are at risk of exploitation. This is not likely to be the entire host community and certainly should not include the whole country in which the research is being conducted.[20,21] Critics argue that those who would require the entire country to receive reasonable availability to the drug in order to avoid exploitation, such as the Boston University group,[16,17] have a mistaken notion of exploitation.

In the context of research, exploitation occurs when those who bear the risks and burdens of research are not provided sufficient benefits.[5,20] Ethics requires ensuring that the research participants who clearly bear burdens receive benefits. The local community should benefit, to the extent it bears any burdens of the research. This suggests that the benefits should focus on the research participants and the host community to the degree that they bear risks and benefits. Because the entire country is unlikely to bear risks, it is not ethically entitled to benefits in order to avoid exploitation.

Fourth, the Nuffield Council on Bioethics argues that the reasonable availability requirement fails to acknowledge the actual process of translating research results into practice.[22] Few drugs, vaccines, or other interventions are introduced into use based on the results of a single trial. As the Council notes,

A fundamental problem that must be acknowledged is that current guidance fails to reflect the reality that only rarely does a single research study lead to the discovery of a new intervention that can be introduced promptly into routine care. For example, before mefloquine was registered as an antimalarial medicine, the [World Health Organization] WHO

Table 65.2

Nine Criticisms of Reasonable Availability

Criticism	Explanation
Mistaken conception of exploitation	Reasonable availability focuses on a type of benefit but exploitation focuses on a fair level of benefits. It is not what people get but how much they get.
Narrow conception of benefits	Reasonable availability counts only access to a drug, vaccine, or intervention as a benefit, and ignores other benefits, such as training, infrastructure, or health services.
Excessively wide group of beneficiaries	Reasonable availability requires access for host community or country. But addressing exploitation requires benefits only for those bearing risks or burdens of research, with no justification for conferring benefits on a whole country that does not bear a burden of research.
No single trial is definitive	Reasonable availability requires access to a drug, vaccine, or intervention after a single trial. But often it takes multiple confirmatory trials to prove the safety and effectiveness of an intervention.
Reasonable availability of knowledge undermines benefit	2002 CIOMS revision suggests obligation can be met by reasonable availability of "knowledge generated." This dilutes importance of requirement.
Uncertainty of benefit	Reasonable availability requires benefit after successful testing. But in Phase III trials, equipoise holds that only half of new interventions are successful. Thus, new drug will be made available only in half of trials.
Misplaces responsibility for implementation	Reasonable availability places responsibility for providing drug onto sponsors and researchers who are not responsible for drug or vaccine regulatory approval and lack authority to provide development aid for provision of drugs or vaccines.
Unrealistic timeline for implementation	Reasonable availability requires rapid implementation. But even if not immediately implemented, some interventions can be implemented over time as prices fall and data on utility accumulates.
Providing one drug may be "golden handcuff"	Reasonable availability secures a particular drug, vaccine or other intervention. But if research proves another intervention is better, the community may be guaranteed the old drug not the newer, more effective one.

Special Programme for Research and Training in Tropical Diseases (TDR) conducted 18 studies on three continents.[22]

Such a situation seems to be occurring regarding circumcision for prevention of HIV.[23] Despite one "successful" trial showing the efficacy of circumcision, many people are awaiting data from several confirmatory trials before evaluating whether this intervention should be recommended.[24] This is the natural process of evaluating health-care interventions. It means that it may be impossible from scientific and health policy standpoints to actually approve a medication after one or even a few "successful" trials. Data from other confirmatory trials might be necessary before an intervention can and should be made available.

Fifth, CIOMS changed the reasonable availability requirement in a way that undercut its impact. Between 1993 and 2002, CIOMS altered its requirement from reasonable availability of drugs and interventions to "ensuring that any intervention or product developed, *or knowledge generated*, will be made reasonably available for the benefit of the population or community [emphasis added]"[10,11] Questions have been raised about whether adding this knowledge clause actually undermines the requirement.

Initially, the requirement seemed to be written with the idea that every research trial would result in a successful new drug or intervention that could then be distributed to the community. But it seemed to ignore or overlook early Phase I research that does not prove the effectiveness of a drug or other intervention but may only assess safety. In the 1993 requirement, CIOMS prohibited Phase I and II trials from being conducted in the developing countries to ensure that research did produce proven interventions that could be made reasonably available: "Phase I drug studies and Phase I and II vaccine studies should be conducted only in developed communities of the country of the sponsor."[10] How-

ever, this limitation was attacked by representatives of developing countries who objected to the restriction and demanded that Phase I and II studies be conducted in their countries. But Phase I and many Phase II research trials do not generate proven drugs or interventions that can be made reasonably available.

To address this problem, the 2002 CIOMS guideline included reasonable availability of the knowledge generated from the study.[11] Critics claim that CIOMS's phrasing is problematic. It is not clear what making knowledge *reasonably available* means. Does this mean publishing it? Translating the data in the local language? More importantly, if interpreted as actually written, with the crucial word "or,"—that is, requiring that "any intervention or product developed, *or* knowledge generated, will be made reasonably available [emphasis added]"—then a sponsor could choose to provide *either* the product *or* the knowledge. Obviously providing the knowledge—the study data—is relatively easy and cheap and would obviate the need to provide the actual intervention. This phrasing seems to dilute the importance of the reasonable availability requirement.

Sixth, it has been argued that even in Phase III studies, the reasonable availability requirement provides an uncertain benefit to the community because it makes benefits dependent on whether the trial is a "successful testing" of a new product. If there is true clinical equipoise prior to the initiation of a Phase III trial conducted in a developing country, then the new intervention should be proven more effective in only about half of the trials.[25] Consequently, reliance on the reasonable availability requirement to provide benefits implies that the host community will receive sufficient benefits from only half or so of all Phase III studies. This is a very limited benefit.

Seventh, some critics argue that CIOMS is wrong in placing the responsibility for reasonable availability on researchers and sponsors. They are researchers, not health policy makers or de-velopment funders. As the Nuffield Council argued,

> [T]here is general agreement that researchers have some re-sponsibilities regarding the provision of an effective inter-vention after a trial has ended, but disagreement about how far that responsibility extends. Certainly, the main function of the researchers is to undertake research. They cannot be ex-pected to adopt a leading role in making effective interven-tions available.[22]

Others have concurred, noting that it is often beyond the legal authority of researchers and some sponsors to guarantee reasonable availability. For instance, the National Institutes of Health (NIH) in the United States and the Medical Research Council (MRC) in Britain do not control drug approval processes in their own coun-tries, much less in developing countries.[20] Further, the NIH and the MRC are legally limited to funding research and prohibited from funding development or health-care provision. Budgets for development and health-care services are usually in different gov-ernment agencies, such as the U.S. Agency for International De-velopment, and different departments, such as the Department of State, and are subject to different requirements than are medical research grants. Researchers and even sponsors usually have lim-ited influence over the priorities of those agencies. The reasonable availability requirement, critics argue, is naïve and unrealistic about the actual workings of governments and foreign aid.

Eighth, critics have argued that the reasonable availability requirement implies too short a time horizon for implementation of interventions. The requirement fails to acknowledge that an intervention may be costly just after completion of the research, but that costs may drop—often substantially—over time, thereby expanding opportunities to implement the intervention and im-prove health. The Nuffield Council mentions the Hepatitis B vaccine and an integrated package of interventions to improve child mortality that had high initial costs.[22] But over time the costs fell substantially, and host governments became more willing to allocate resources to the interventions. The Council warns that by implying that the intervention must be made available within a short time, the requirement might forestall its subsequent adoption:

> [T]he costs of some interventions shown to be successful may not decline significantly until some time after the conclusion of the research. To describe all such research as therefore unethical may lead to the loss of [subsequent] opportunities to improve health care.[22]

Finally, there is a worry that in the dynamic world of bio-medical research, a pledge of reasonable availability of a single drug or intervention might become a "golden handcuff."[20] Agreement to receive a specific drug, vaccine, or other interven-tion proven in the trial, rather than cash or some other transferable benefit, commits the population to using the specific intervention tested in the trial. But what happens if another drug, vaccine, or other intervention is proven more effective but in a different com-munity? Pharmaceutical companies might be willing to provide their own drug directly, but would be unwilling to provide the product of a competitor. So the original community becomes tied to an outmoded intervention. This scenario is not so implausible. Such quick changes have occurred in the best drugs for prevention of maternal-fetal HIV transmission.

Some argue that an agreement guaranteeing reasonable avail-ability could have an escape clause, requiring that if a more ef-fective intervention is developed, the sponsor would provide money to the host community so that it could purchase the new, more effective intervention. It seems highly unlikely that any sponsor would consent to such an arrangement. Moreover, this response seems to recognize that the real benefit is not reasonable availability to the specific proven intervention but resources—the money—to purchase a set of benefits that the community deems valuable, which itself may evolve. Indeed, the idea that the com-munity could have a clause requiring the sponsor to pay instead of making the drug, vaccine, or other intervention available under-mines the ethical justification of the reasonable availability re-quirement itself. Once a specific proven drug is not deemed an indispensable benefit, the rationale for the reasonable availability requirement is negated.

Nuffield Council on Bioethics

One alternate account of providing benefits to host countries is that of the Nuffield Council. The Council does not endorse the reason-able availability requirement, but unfortunately has not offered an integrated alternative requirement. The Council seems to suggest that six actions are ethically necessary.[22] First, participants in the trial should be monitored for possible long-term deleterious out-comes of the research beyond the completion of the trial. Second, members of both the control group and the intervention group should be provided "the intervention shown to be best (if they are still able to benefit from it) for an agreed period of time." Third, the availability or unavailability of treatment beyond the end of the trial should be clearly explained to prospective participants during the consent process. Fourth, explorations should be made whether the treatment shown to be better can be introduced in a sustainable manner to the whole community or the country where the research was conducted. Fifth, the Nuffield Council endorses the NBAC's recommendation that proposals submitted to institutional review boards (IRBs) or other research ethics committees (RECs) should include provisions for making new proven interventions available to some or all of the host country population, or should explain why the research should be done even if this is impossible.[22] Finally, the Council requires that all research strengthen the capacity of devel-oping countries to conduct health research: "Genuine partnerships should be promoted in order to strengthen expertise in research and institutional development and to maximize opportunities for the transfer of skills and knowledge."[22]

Fair Benefits Framework

Probably the most developed and detailed alternative to the rea-sonable availability requirement is the fair benefits framework.[20,21] This view was elaborated by a widely representative group of re-searchers, IRB members, bioethicists, and others from the United States, Europe, and eight African countries at a conference in Malawi in 2001.

The fair benefits framework makes two fundamental as-sumptions. First, the key to avoiding exploitation is ensuring that the people who bear the risks and burdens of research receive fair benefits through the conduct and/or results of research. Second, all types of benefits that might flow from research, not just access to a tested drug, must be considered in determining the fair benefits. The population at risk for exploitation is the relevant group to receive benefits; this includes the participants in the research study as well as any members of the community who might also bear burdens and risks for carrying out the research.

The fair benefits framework supplements the usual conditions for the ethical conduct of research. In this sense, it applies in addition to ensuring that the research has social value, that participants are selected fairly, that the research study has been subject to independent review by an IRB or REC, and that individual participants provide informed consent.[6,7] Most importantly, the fair benefits framework is in addition to the risk-benefit evaluation of the particular study. The risk-benefit ratio of the study must be favorable; the benefits to individual prospective participants must outweigh the risks, or the net risks must be acceptably low.

To these widely accepted principles for evaluating the ethics of individual research studies, the fair benefits framework adds three additional principles for ensuring that study participants and others who bear burdens of the research get a fair share of the benefits of the research (see Table 65.3).

Principle 1: Fair Benefits. There should be a comprehensive delineation of tangible benefits to the research participants and the population from both the conduct and the results of research. These benefits can be of three types: (1) benefits to research participants during the research, (2) benefits to the population during the research, and (3) benefits to the participants and/or the population after completion of the research. It is not necessary to provide each of these types of benefits. The ethical imperative is for a fair level of benefits. As the burdens on the participants and the community increase, so the benefits must increase. Similarly, as the benefits to the sponsors, researchers, and others outside the population increase, the benefits to the host population should also increase.

Principle 2: Collaborative Partnership. The population being asked to enroll determines whether a particular array of benefits is sufficient and fair. Just as there is no agreement on what constitutes a fair wage, there is no shared international standard of fairness in terms of benefits from a study; reasonable people disagree.[26] More importantly, only the host population can determine the value of the benefits for itself. Outsiders are likely to be poorly informed about the health, social, and economic context in which the research is being conducted, and they are unlikely to fully appreciate the importance of the proposed benefits to the population.

The population's choice to participate in the research must be free and uncoerced; refusing to participate in the research study must be a realistic option. Although there can be controversy about who speaks for the population being asked to enroll, this is a problem that is not unique to the fair benefits framework. Even—or especially—in democratic processes, unanimity of decisions cannot be the standard; disagreement is inherent in democracy. But how consensus is determined in the absence of an electoral process is a complex question in democratic theory beyond this framework to resolve.

Principle 3: Transparency. Because equity is determined by comparisons with similar interactions, fairness is relative. Therefore,

Table 65.3
Principles and Benchmarks of the Fair Benefits Framework

Principles	Benchmarks for Determining Whether the Principle Is Honored

Fair benefits	• Benefits to participants during the research
	   1. *Health improvement*: Health services that are essential to the conduct of the research that improve the health of the participants
	   2. *Ancillary health services*: Health services beyond those essential to the conduct of the research that are provided to the participants
	• Benefits to participants and population during the research
	   1. *Ancillary health services*: Health services provided to the population
	   2. *Public health measures*: Additional public health measures provided to the population
	   3. *Employment and economic activity*: The provision of jobs for the local population that stimulate local economic activity
	• Benefits to population after the research
	   1. *Availability of the intervention*: Provision of the intervention if it is proved safe and effective
	   2. *Capacity development*: Improvements in the health-care infrastructure, training of health-care and research personnel, and training of research personnel in research ethics
	   3. *Public health measures*: Additional public health measures provided to the population
	   4. *Long-term collaboration*: Development of additional research projects with the population
	   5. *Financial rewards*: Sharing of the financial rewards or intellectual property rights related to the intervention being evaluated

Collaborative partnership	• *Free, uncoerced decision making*: The population is capable of making a free and uncoerced decision; it can refuse participation in the research. • *Population support*: When it has understood the nature of the research trial, the risks and benefit to individual participants, and the benefits to the population, the population decides that it wants the research to proceed.
Transparency	• *Central repository of benefits agreements*: An independent body creates a publicly accessible repository of all formal and informal benefits agreements. • *Community consultation*: Forums with populations may be invited to participate in research, informing them about previous benefits agreements.

transparency—like the full information requirements for ideal market transactions—is necessary to allow comparisons with similar transactions. A population in a developing country is likely to be at a distinct disadvantage, relative to a sponsor from a developed country, in determining whether a proposed level of benefits is fair. To address these concerns, a publicly accessible repository of all benefits agreements should be established and operated by an independent body, such as the World Health Organization (WHO). Such a repository would permit independent assessments of the fairness of various benefits agreements by populations, researchers, governments, and others, such as nongovernmental organizations. Such a repository would facilitate the development of a *case law* set of standards of fairness that can evolve out of a number of agreements.

Along with the usual eight requirements for ethical research,[6,7] the principles of the fair benefits framework ensure that (1) the population has been selected for a good scientific reason; (2) the research poses few net risks to the research participants; (3) there are sufficient benefits to the research participants and population; (4) the population is not coerced into participation; (5) the population freely decides whether to participate and whether the level of benefits is fair given the risks and burdens to the population of the research; and (6) there is an opportunity for comparative assessment of the fairness of the benefits agreements.

Criticism of Fair Benefits Framework

There has been limited criticism of the fair benefits framework, possibly because only a relatively short amount of time has elapsed since its delineation. Three main criticisms have been leveled.

First, the fair benefits framework accepts "the status quo in the host community as normative baseline for assessing research."[27] This creates unequal bargaining, with the researchers from developed countries having more power to wait or go to alternative research venues. Thus researchers impose their agenda on developing countries. Second, using the status quo as the baseline means it is possible that "each party [can secure] a net benefit [and yet] the distribution of those benefits is hugely disproportionate."[27] Finally, the fair benefits framework fails to delve into "root causes" of ill health but concentrates on the "symptomatic manifestations of deeper problems." In this regard, it leads to a "piecemeal and ad hoc approach to the needs of those in the developing world."[27] It focuses on health but does not explore other social structures that might improve health, such as the power distribution in a community, education of women, and so forth. Despite permitting benefits in many different sectors, from economic improvements to education, the fair benefits framework does not offer an integrated, unified approach to solving the problems of developing countries.

Importantly, these criticisms seem to apply not just to the fair benefits framework but also to the reasonable availability requirement. After all, the reasonable availability requirement accepts the status quo as the baseline for determining that availability to a new drug should be required. Moreover, its focus is decidedly piecemeal and partial. It considers benefits only in one sector—availability of drugs, vaccines, or other health-related interventions. By contrast, the fair benefits framework requires that in determining fair benefits, all sectors be assessed—ranging from economic conditions to education to public health measures.

The criticisms seem to miss the fact that the fairness of agreements is not determined just by bargaining. The purpose of the transparency principle is to provide an external check that independently assesses the fairness of agreements.

Human Development Approach

Yet another procedure for achieving fairness for research participants is known as the human development approach, proposed by Alex London.[27] It has only been outlined in the most general of ways. Importantly, it does not attempt to address just the problem of exploitation by researchers from developed countries conducting research in developing countries. Rather, it seeks to address global injustice. Further, the particular conception of justice involved is one that calls on people in developed countries—including researchers—to establish and foster "basic social structures that guarantee to community members [in developing countries] the fair value of their most basic human capacities."[27]

This is a very abstract claim. Its elucidation seems to imply two specific obligations. First, researchers must target "rudimentary health problems that can impede the ability of community members to function . . . [including] literacy and education . . . providing basic nutrition and rudimentary health care."[27]

Second, researchers must "expand the capacity of the basic social structures of that community to better serve the fundamental interests of that community's members." Furthermore, collaborative research initiatives "must directly and indirectly expand the capacity of the host community's basic social structures either to meet the distinctive health priorities of that community's members or to meet their basic health needs under distinctive social or environmental circumstances."[27]

It is a bit unclear what this means in a practical sense, but it does suggest that the emphasis must be on capacity development in the broadest sense. Indeed, the only specific suggestion to researchers from the human development approach is the following:

> The imperative to try to make the results of successful research available within the host community increases in inverse proportion to the capacity of that community's basic social structures to translate those results into sustainable benefits for community members. To the extent that the host community cannot translate the results into sustainable benefits for its population on its own, an imperative exists either to build partnerships with groups that would be willing to augment the community's capacity to do so, or *to locate the research within a community with similar health priorities and a more appropriate health infrastructure*. Similarly, the imperative to provide an array of ancillary benefits to community members increases in inverse proportion to the community's capacity to treat or ameliorate the ancillary health problems that researchers are likely to encounter [emphasis added].[27]

Criticism of the Human Development Approach

The abstract nature and vagueness of the human development approach makes it difficult to be certain what it requires. But five preliminary criticisms seem plausible.

First, it mistakes the problem that ensuring benefits to host countries is meant to address. Most people accept that global injustice and exploitation are major ethical problems in the world. However, the purpose of specifying the extent of the obligation to provide benefits to developing countries that participate in biomedical research projects is to minimize the possibility of exploitation by developed country researchers and sponsors. Such benefits are not meant to address underlying background global injustice. The human development approach is thus speaking to a different issue from that being addressed by the reasonable availability requirement or fair benefits framework. There is a disconnect between the ethical challenges posed by conducting research trials in developing countries and the issues the human development approach takes itself to be addressing.

Second, the human development approach seems most relevant in helping to specify what research questions are being pursued in developing countries, rather than the benefits that flow from specific research protocols. That researchers should target "rudimentary health problems" that impede function seems to define the research agenda. It is not helpful in specifying what and how much benefits—in health, economic conditions, capacity development, and so forth—researchers or sponsors owe to the host community based on the specific projects to be initiated.

Third, depending on interpretation, the human development approach is too demanding, too undemanding, or too abstract and vague to be action-guiding. On one interpretation, the requirement to "expand the capacity of the host community community's basic social structure to better serve the fundamental interests of that community's members" is too expansive. This requirement seems to entail changing the entire fabric of a developing country's society. Such an imperative is way beyond the legitimate requirements than can be asked of researchers or sponsors who are trying to conduct trials of prospective malaria or HIV vaccines. Conversely, if the requirement is simply to increase, by any amount, the capacity of a community's health-care system, then this seems even more minimalist than the reasonable availability requirement or the fair benefits framework. Almost anything a developed country research team might do—train some local people to help with the project, build a clinic, provide economic stimulus—would count as expanding the capacity of the social structures. That such contradictory interpretations seem possible suggests that this requirement is too amorphous to specify for a researcher, or a sponsor, or an IRB what exactly must be done to fulfill the requirement.

Fourth, the *inverse proportion* standard seems unjustified. The human development approach seems to require researchers to provide ancillary benefits not based on what the researcher does, but based on the community's preexisting needs. This raises many problems. Practically, this would create a huge disincentive to conduct research in very poor settings, because the obligations on researchers would be greater. Ethically, obligations typically depend on what one party owes, which is independent of the needs of the party to whom the obligation is owed. But under the human development approach, the extent of the obligation seems independent of the kind or magnitude of the researchers' study. The same obligation seems to exist whether the researcher is conducting a small Phase I study or a massive Phase III vaccine trial. In addition, this approach seems to increase researchers' obligations if others shirk their duty. If the obligations of researchers depend upon the extent of poverty or the inadequacy of community social

structures, the researchers' obligations seem to depend upon whether others are fulfilling their duties.[28] A community could have terrible poverty or poor community social structure because its rulers are terribly corrupt. Why should a researcher's obligations to provide benefits then increase? Obligations to help the poor of the world should not increase because their poverty is made worse by the shirking of obligations by others or by corruption or by problems of the community's own making.[28]

Finally, there is a deep contradiction in the human development approach's recommendations. The only specific requirement from the human development approach seems to be that researchers ensure that the community where a trial is conducted can "translate those [research] results into sustainable benefits for community members." This seems to mean that researchers must augment the community's capacities to help its population. But if the community lacks the capacity to "translate those results," then the researchers have no obligation with respect to it. According to the human development approach, the researchers should go somewhere else; they should conduct their research in a community "with similar health priorities [as the researcher] and a more appropriate health infrastructure." This seems to suggest that researchers do not have obligations to help poorer communities but can pick and choose the community they conduct their research in. They can minimize their obligations by going to better off communities that already have the appropriate infrastructure. Thus, the specific guidance from the human development approach directly contradicts its ethical foundation, namely that "claims of justice cannot be limited to the boundaries of the contemporary nation-state" and that obligations go to enhancing the "most basic human capacities," not just those of people in countries that have appropriate infrastructure. Indeed, the specific practical recommendation of the human development approach seems to mesh with one interpretation of the reasonable availability requirement, namely, that research is ethical only if there is already sufficient infrastructure to make the proven drug, vaccine, or other intervention available.

Conclusion

There is widespread agreement that to avoid exploitation, researchers must ensure that the participants and host community in which the research is conducted benefit from the research. The people and the host community could benefit from the conduct of the research and/or its results. Disagreement focuses on how they should benefit. Four different approaches have been offered. The reasonable availability requirement claims they must benefit by being given the drug or other intervention proven effective in the trial; that is the only ethically appropriate way for them to benefit. The Nuffield Council seems to think that providing the actual participants the intervention and providing capacity development to the larger community is sufficient. The fair benefits framework requires the participants and host community receive a fair level of benefits chosen from a collection of ten potential types of benefits. Finally, the human development approach requires enhancement of basic human capacities of host communities, with the level of enhancement determined by the level of deprivation of the community. Over time, the implications of these various approaches will be evaluated with appropriate refinements made.

Disclaimer

The views expressed are those of the author alone and do not represent any position or policy of the U.S. National Institutes of Health, the Public Health Service, or the Department of Health and Human Services.

References

1. Black N. Evidence based policy: Proceed with care. *British Medical Journal* 2001;323:275–8.
2. Levine RJ. *Ethics and Regulation of Clinical Research,* 2nd ed. New Haven, Conn.: Yale University Press; 1988: chapter 1.
3. Freedman B. Scientific value and validity as ethical requirements for research. *IRB: A Review of Human Subjects Research* 1987;9(6):7–10.
4. Vanderpool HY, ed. *The Ethics of Research Involving Human Subjects.* Frederick, Md.: University Publishing Group; 1996.
5. Wertheimer A. *Exploitation.* Princeton, N.J.: Princeton University Press; 1996.
6. Emanuel EJ, Wendler D, Grady C. What makes clinical research ethical? *JAMA* 2000;283:2701–11.
7. Emanuel EJ, Wendler D, Killen J, Grady C. What makes clinical research in developing countries ethical? The benchmarks of ethical research. *Journal of Infectious Diseases* 2004;189:930–7.
8. Benatar SR. Avoiding exploitation in clinical research. *Cambridge Quarterly of Healthcare Ethics* 2000;9:562–5.
9. Wilmshurst P. Scientific imperialism: If they won't benefit from the findings, poor people in the developing world shouldn't be used in research. *British Medical Journal* 1997;314:840–1.
10. Council for International Organizations of Medical Sciences, in collaboration with the World Health Organization. *International Ethical Guidelines for Biomedical Research Involving Human Subjects* Geneva, Switzerland: CIOMS and WHO; 1993.
11. Council for International Organizations of Medical Sciences, in collaboration with the World Health Organization. *International Ethical Guidelines for Biomedical Research Involving Human Subjects.* Geneva, Switzerland: CIOMS and WHO; 2002. [Online] November 2002. Available: http://www.cioms.ch/frame_guidelines_nov_2002.htm.
12. Crouch RA, Arras JD. AZT trials and tribulations. *Hastings Center Report* 1998;28(6):26–34.
13. Shapiro HT, Meslin EM. Ethical issues in the design and conduct of clinical trials in developing countries. *New England Journal of Medicine* 2001;345:139–42.
14. National Bioethics Advisory Commission. *Ethical and Policy Issues in International Research: Clinical Trials in Developing Countries.* Bethesda, Md.: NBAC; 2001. [Online] April 2001. Available: http://www.bioethics.gov/reports/past_commissions/nbac_international.pdf.
15. Joint United Nations Programme on HIV/AIDS (UNAIDS). *Ethical Considerations in HIV Preventive Vaccine Research.* Geneva, Switzerland: UNAIDS; 2000. [Online] May 2000. Available: http://data.unaids.org/Publications/IRC-pub01/JC072-EthicalCons_en.pdf.
16. Glantz LH, Annas GJ, Grodin MA, Mariner WK. Research in developing countries: Taking "benefit" seriously. *Hastings Center Report* 1998;28(6):38–42.
17. Annas GJ, Grodin MA. Human rights and maternal-fetal HIV transmission prevention trials in Africa. *American Journal of Public Health* 1998;88:560–3.
18. World Medical Association. *Declaration of Helsinki: Ethical Principles for Medical Research Involving Human Subjects.* Tokyo, Japan: WMA; October 2004. [Online] 2004. Available: http://www.wma.net/e/policy/b3.htm.
19. Macklin R. After Helsinki: Unresolved issues in international research. *Kennedy Institute of Ethics Journal* 2001;11:17–36.
20. Participants in the 2001 Conference on Ethical Aspects of Research in Developing Countries. Moral standards for research in developing countries: From "reasonable availability" to "fair benefits." *Hastings Center Report* 2004;34(3):17–27.
21. Participants in the 2001 Conference on Ethical Aspects of Research in Developing Countries. Fair benefits for research in developing countries. *Science* 2002;298:2133–4.
22. Nuffield Council on Bioethics. *The Ethics of Research Related to Healthcare in Developing Countries.* London, U.K.: Nuffield Council on Bioethics; 2002. [Online] Available: http://nuffieldbioethics.org/fileLibrary/pdf/errhdc_fullreport001.pdf.
23. Beukes L. Caution on circumcision cuts South Africa's AIDS researchers. *Nature Medicine* 2005;11:1261.
24. Auvert B, Taljaard D, Lagarde E, et al. Randomized, controlled intervention trial of male circumcision for reduction of HIV infection risk: The ANRS 1265 trial. *PLoS Medicine* 2006;2(11):e298.
25. Chalmers I. What is the prior probability of a proposed new treatment being superior to established treatments? *British Medical Journal* 1997;314:74–5.
26. Pogge T. *World Poverty and Human Rights.* Cambridge, U.K.: Polity Press; 2002: chapters 1, 4.
27. London AJ. Justice and the human development approach to international research. *Hastings Center Report* 2005;35(1):24–37.
28. Murphy LB. *Moral Demands in Nonideal Theory.* New York, N.Y.: Oxford University Press; 2000: chapter 5.

Søren Holm   John Harris

66

The Standard of Care in Multinational Research

Introduction and History

Although the issue concerning *standard of care* has become prominent in the controversy concerning HIV/AIDS research in developing countries, it is not a new problem, nor is it a problem that only occurs in relation to multinational research.

Any biomedical research project in which the research protocol envisages that a group of, or all of, the research participants will receive a level of treatment that is less than the ordinary standard of care raises the issue of whether this is ethically justified. It is thus an issue that occurs in all randomized trials with a placebo group, if there is a known effective treatment.

The nature of the standard of care discussion has been influenced by the debate over the perinatal HIV transmission studies in the late 1990s and the historical development and the specific wording of the World Medical Association's (WMA's) Declaration of Helsinki[1] and the Guidelines of the Council of International Organizations of Medical Sciences (CIOMS)[2] (see Chapters 13 and 16). We will therefore initially present a short outline of the case that opened the standard of care debate and of the development of the regulatory instruments, in particular the Declaration of Helsinki. (Various national regulations also cover this issue, but we have decided not to include them in this analysis because of their great variability and limited relevance outside of their national context.)

In 1994, the AIDS Clinical Trial Group 076 study established that treating HIV-infected mothers with AZT during the last trimester of pregnancy, intravenously during delivery, and treating the newborn child for six weeks after birth dramatically reduced perinatal HIV transmission, but at a cost of about US $800 per pregnancy.[3] This made the 076 regimen unaffordable in all of sub-Saharan Africa, in countries with the highest number of perinatal transmissions. The regimen was also logistically difficult to implement as part of routine prenatal care in other high prevalence countries. There was therefore an urgent need to develop affordable and feasible alternatives for these countries, and a number of trials with shorter versions of the regimen were initiated. All of these, except one trial in Thailand, used placebo in the control group. These studies led to a fierce debate about whether it is ever justified to use a lesser standard of care for the control group, in this case placebo, rather than the state of the art intervention, in this case the 076 regimen.

Although there was some criticism of the placebo studies in the literature from 1995,[4] not much happened until the Public Citizen Health Research Group criticized the trials in a congressional hearing on bioethics in May of 1997.[5] There were a number of news reports of these hearings, but they went largely unnoticed by the general media until Marcia Angell criticized the trials in a 1997 editorial in the *New England Journal of Medicine*.[6] The editorial was accompanied by a Sounding Board article by Peter Lurie and Sidney Wolfe of the Public Citizen Health Research Group.[7] They argued that the placebo-controlled trials were unethical because the control group was denied a proven beneficial treatment. According to section II.3 of the 1996 and then current version of the Declaration of Helsinki, all the participants "should be assured of the best proven diagnostic and therapeutic method."[8] Lurie and Wolfe also claimed that a placebo trial might not require fewer subjects nor would it take longer to get the necessary results. They rejected the argument that because the standard of care in developing countries was no treatment at all, research subjects in the placebo group would not be denied the treatment available *in that country*. They pointed out that the reason for this standard of care is economic, rather than medical. However, it would not be difficult for economic reasons to provide the participants in the study with AZT in the required amount: this would not add much to the cost of the study. Lurie and Wolfe recognized that it may not be justifiable to provide more expensive forms of care, such as treatment in coronary care units.

The respective directors of the U.S. National Institutes of Health (NIH) and the Centers for Disease Control and Prevention (CDC), Harold Varmus and David Satcher, defended the trials by arguing that placebo control was essential to the purpose of the trials:

> The most compelling reason to use a placebo-controlled study is that it provides definite answers to questions about safety and value of an intervention in the setting in which the study is performed, and these answers are the point of research. . . . Comparing an intervention of unknown benefit—especially one that is affordable in a developing country—with the only intervention with a known benefit (the 076 regimen) may provide information that is not useful to patients. If the affordable intervention is less effective than the 076 regimen—not an unlikely outcome—this information will be of little use in a country where the more effective regimen is unavailable. Equally important, it will still be unclear whether the affordable intervention is better than nothing and worth the investment of scarce resources.[9]

The Declaration of Helsinki and the Standard of Care Debate

The Declaration of Helsinki was first promulgated by the WMA in 1964, but it was only with the 1975 revision, often referred to as Helsinki II, that it achieved the status of an internationally recognized basic document in research ethics. The 1964 version contained no paragraph relating directly to the standard of care, although one might interpret paragraph II.2 to contain the germ of a standard of care idea: "The doctor can combine clinical research with professional care, the objective being the acquisition of new medical knowledge, only to the extent that clinical research is justified by its therapeutic value for the patient."[10] In the 1975 revision, paragraph II.3 reads, "In any medical study, every patient—including those of a control group, if any—should be assured of the best proven diagnostic and therapeutic method."[11] And this was amended in 1996 to read, "In any medical study, every patient—including those of a control group, if any—should be assured of the best proven diagnostic and therapeutic method. This does not exclude the use of inert placebo in studies in which no proven diagnostic or therapeutic method exists."[8]

The final official steps in the development of the standard of care doctrine were in the last major revision of the Declaration, adopted by the WMA's 52nd General Assembly in Edinburgh, Scotland, in October 2000, along with a Note of Clarification of paragraph 29 added by the WMA General Assembly in Washington, D.C., in 2002.[1] The work on this revision was started in 1997 when the American Medical Association proposed a significantly altered version of the Declaration of Helsinki. During the very long revision process that followed, the standard of care issue was one of the most discussed.[12] A proposed revision that was put forward in 1999, but rejected, contained this paragraph 18:

> In any biomedical research protocol every patient-subject, including those of a control group, if any, should be assured that he or she will not be denied access to the best proven diagnostic, prophylactic or therapeutic methods *that would otherwise be available to him or her*. This principle does not exclude the use of placebo or no-treatment control groups if such are justified by a scientifically and ethically sound research protocol [emphasis added].[13]

This would have significantly weakened the standard of care rule.

In the text of this revision as finally approved, the term "best proven diagnostic and therapeutic method" from the 1975 revision was superseded by "best current prophylactic, diagnostic, and therapeutic methods." This terminology may imply a slightly stricter standard, but the text (now paragraph 29 of the 2000 version) is otherwise very similar to the 1996 revision:

> The benefits, risks, burdens and effectiveness of a new method should be tested against those of the best current prophylactic, diagnostic, and therapeutic methods. This does not exclude the use of placebo, or no treatment, in studies where no proven prophylactic, diagnostic or therapeutic method exists.[1]

After the publication of the 2000 revision, this paragraph provoked substantial criticism and controversy. In 2002, the meeting of the WMA General Assembly in Washington, D.C., issued the Note of Clarification reaffirming the strict interpretation of paragraph 29:

> The WMA hereby reaffirms its position that extreme care must be taken in making use of a placebo-controlled trial and that in general this methodology should only be used in the absence of existing proven therapy. However, a placebo-controlled trial may be ethically acceptable, even if proven therapy is available, under the following circumstances:
>
> - Where for compelling and scientifically sound methodological reasons its use is necessary to determine the efficacy or safety of a prophylactic, diagnostic or therapeutic method; or
> - Where a prophylactic, diagnostic or therapeutic method is being investigated for a minor condition and the patients who receive placebo will not be subject to any additional risk of serious or irreversible harm.
>
> All other provisions of the Declaration of Helsinki must be adhered to, especially the need for appropriate ethical and scientific review.[1]

The corresponding section in the CIOMS Guidelines reads:

> Guideline 11: Choice of control in clinical trials
>
> As a general rule, research subjects in the control group of a trial of a diagnostic, therapeutic, or preventive intervention should receive an established effective intervention. In some circumstances it may be ethically acceptable to use an alternative comparator, such as placebo or "no treatment."

Placebo may be used:

- when there is no established effective intervention;
- when withholding an established effective intervention would expose subjects to, at most, temporary discomfort or delay in relief of symptoms;
- when use of an established effective intervention as comparator would not yield scientifically reliable results and use of placebo would not add any risk of serious or irreversible harm to the subjects.[2]

The use of "established effective intervention" makes the CIOMS Guidelines slightly less stringent than the Declaration of Helsinki, but not much. (The 1993 version of the CIOMS Guidelines had no specific guideline concerning this issue, but part of the commentary on Guideline 14 read, "If there is already an approved and accepted drug for the condition that a candidate drug is designed to treat, placebo for controls usually cannot be justified."[14]) CIOMS added five pages of commentary to Guideline 11 showing an awareness of the complications involved in specifying exactly when the three exceptions in the guideline apply. The commentary touches on many of the issues discussed below, but wavers between an analysis on the level of research participants and an analysis on the level of states or societies.[15]

It has recently been argued by Reidar Lie and colleagues that the Declaration of Helsinki is in conflict with the international consensus on the standard of care issue, but this is disputed.[16]

Core Conception of "Standard of Care"

The core of the concept of "standard of care" is that there is, for each particular medical condition, a set of recognized treatments and care interventions that constitute the present "standard of care" for that condition. For different conditions this may range from no treatment at all, because there is no effective treatment or because no treatment is needed, to highly complex and expensive treatment regimens. The standard of care is the baseline against which other treatment regimens can be compared. Over time the standard of care for a given condition will often change as new research-based therapies supersede older and now obsolete treatments.

This core conception of standard of care is, however, not unproblematic on epistemological and normative grounds.[17,18] There may be disagreement in the scientific community concerning which of two or more treatment modalities is the best (or most appropriate), and therefore there may be more than one particular treatment that has the status of the standard of care. This disagreement may occur within one country and one medical community, but it may also occur between countries.

There also may be disagreement concerning the criteria for identifying the standard of care. Is it (1) the best available treatment? (2) the most commonly used treatment? (3) the treatment that is promoted by the relevant authorities? (4) the treatment advocated by the common textbooks? (5) a treatment that is "good enough," and so forth? For each of the options, there are further questions about the exact meaning of the criterion, for example, what do best and available mean in "best available treatment"?

The borders may be fuzzy and ill defined, and there may be large gray areas, but this does not preclude our distinguishing between clear cases. (The problem in identifying the "standard of care" is in many ways analogous to the problem in identifying whether or not there has been negligence in malpractice suits.) In many instances we can identify whether a particular treatment falls within or outside the standard of care. If in a study of a new treatment for duodenal ulcer, a physician plans to give his or her control group placebo instead of proton pump inhibitors and antibiotics, the control group will be given something that is less than the current standard of care.

The ability to determine whether a particular proposed treatment falls below the standard of care critically depends on the identification of the relevant treatment universe. The standard of care for duodenal ulcer described above is valid in the United Kingdom or the United States, but it may not be valid in the rural areas of the most economically deprived countries in Africa.

One major determinant of the level of treatment offered as standard in a given health care system is the economic resources available to the health-care system. The standard of care issue is often most urgent in research being carried out in a health-care system with fewer resources than the health care system from which the researchers originate or in which the results are to be used. These resource differences can be very large, but it is important to note that disparities occur not only between countries but also within countries when there is tiered provision of health care.

To What Does Acceptance of the Standard of Care Commit Us?

The core ethical rationales for maintaining a standard of care restriction in the planning or assessment of research projects falls into three not mutually exclusive categories. The first possible rationale is the idea that people should be predictably (ex ante) worse off by participating in a biomedical research project than they would have been if they had not participated. The second is the idea that research participation should not cause predictable harm by deprivation of known effective treatment. The third is that it would be against the researchers' professional obligations as medical doctors (or other health-care professionals) to treat any of their patients in a way that is not in the patients' best interests.

Society permits people to participate in research that involves some level of risk, pain, and inconvenience for no therapeutic benefit. Consistency suggests society should allow similar negative effects caused by deviations from the standard of care. Therefore, the real standard of care issue is not whether any deviations from the standard of care can be justified, but whether and under what conditions large deviations from the standard of care can be justified.[19–21]

An important question in this regard is: What is or is not in someone's interests?[19,22] What is or is not in a particular individual's interests is an objective matter, despite the fact that the person's subjective preferences codetermine these interests. Although the choice of the preferences is subjective, once they are chosen their fulfillment can be objectively assessed. Although research participants have a special role to play in determining this, we also know that human beings frequently act against their own interests. Indeed the idea of respect for persons, which underpins these guidelines, has two clear and sometimes incompatible elements, namely, concern for welfare and respect for autonomy. Because people often have self-harming preferences, well illustrated by smoking, drug abuse, overeating, or selfless altruism, they are sometimes bad judges of their own interests.

Individuals benefit from—or have a chance of living in—a society and, indeed, in a world in which medical research is carried out and that uses the benefits of past research. Medical research is of benefit both to patients and to research participants; it is in their interests to be in a society that pursues and actively accepts the benefits of research and in which research and its fruits are given a high priority. All individuals also benefit from the knowledge that research into diseases or conditions from which they do not currently suffer but to which they might succumb is ongoing. It enhances security and gives people hope for the future, for themselves and their descendants, and others for whom they care.

If this is correct, then each individual should have a strong general interest that there be research, and that there be well-founded research—not excluding but not exclusively on their condition or on conditions that are likely to affect them. All such research is also of clear benefit to everyone in the society. (This argument relies on the implicit premise that there is some realistic chance that some of the benefits of medical research have flowed or will flow to each person or persons that they care for.) A narrow interpretation of the requirement that research be of benefit to the subject of the research is therefore perverse.[23]

The interest of the participant *cannot* be the only consideration, nor can it automatically take precedence over other interests of comparable moral significance. Claims that the patient's interest must always take precedence involve a straightforward mistake: Being or becoming a research participant is not the sort of act that could conceivably, in itself, augment either someone's moral claims or their rights. Any principle of equality would emphasize that *all* people are morally important and, with respect to one another, each has a claim to equal consideration. No one has a claim to overriding consideration. To say that the interests of the participant must take precedence over the interests of others must be understood either as a way of reasserting that a researcher's narrowly conceived professional interests must not have primacy over the human rights of research participants. It might emphasize some specific contractual duties. Or it might recognize that some, but importantly only some, research participants will attract merit by voluntarily shouldering significant burdens. However, as a general remark about the obligations of the research community, the health-care system, society, or indeed of world community, it is not sustainable.

Obligations of Researchers to Participants in Trials

What should be the obligations of researchers to their subjects? The strongest obligations to research participants are derived from a more general obligation to refrain from harming others. This is a specific instance of the obligation of nonmaleficence, which is the obverse of the obligation of beneficence.[24,25] Such obligations are no more stringent to research participants than they are to anyone in similar need. That said, it will look like special pleading to reject the requirements of the Declaration of Helsinki.

Barry Bloom has produced a *reductio ad absurdum* of the standard of care we are discussing. He points out,

> Few, if any, clinical trials in developing countries have evaluated whether simple, inexpensive interventions, such as aspirin and beta-blockers, will reduce mortality from heart attacks and strokes, as they do in the industrialized world. . . . Were the standard of "best proven therapeutic method" to be literally invoked in such a trial, many study subjects suffering heart attacks would have to be provided with either angioplasty or coronary artery bypass surgery, which are hardly "reasonably available" in countries where per capita expenditures for health are $10 per year or less.[26]

Bloom is here using the wording of an earlier version of the Declaration of Helsinki, but the idea is for all practical purposes the same. Although Bloom's reminder is important, it cannot follow that because researchers cannot do everything that they are then permitted to do nothing. The question must be, what standard of care is appropriate given all the circumstances of the study, including all the costs involved? The impossibility of providing everything that might be interpreted as "best current prophylactic, diagnostic and therapeutic methods" does not lead to the conclusion that the only alternative is "local standards of care." However, Bloom's *reductio* argument does at least show that the provisions of the Declaration of Helsinki cannot, as written, be universally applied.

Other things being equal, it is not justifiable to let people suffer when physician-researchers could protect them, nor is it normally ethical to leave people with poorer standards of care than could reasonably be provided for them.[27,28] However, it is necessary to look more closely at the equality of other factors and at how to determine "what could reasonably be provided."

The moral obligation that researchers try to ensure that others are not made unduly worse off applies to *all* others, not simply to the subjects of any trial. Therefore, when researchers are considering the others whom they must try not to make unduly worse off, they must also include those who may benefit from the results of the trial. Thus the argument that supports the best standard of care for those in the trial also supports the best standard of care for those who would benefit from the trial. No one would be made worse off by such a policy, and some will be made better off.

It merits insistence that leaving people no worse off than they would have been had no trial taken place is a minimum standard of care. The relevant question is not, will the participants be no worse off than they would have been? Rather it is, what obligations do researchers have toward people to protect them from avoidable harm?

What are the obligations of investigators to those who enter a drug or vaccine trial? The investigators' obligations are of course in part determined by what protections participants are judged to be entitled to. These obligations may also involve our conception of the professional obligations of medical practitioners or other investigators, which derive from their special role or responsibilities. More basically this question raises fundamental issues about the justifications for a particular research project and indeed the research enterprise more generally.

There is a difference between deciding what research is acceptable and should be done in the abstract—at the planning stage, when all people involved are unknown—and acting according to researchers' professional obligations when confronted with the individual research participant. It is generally assumed that health professionals in particular have specific and overriding obligations to those they deal with in their professional capacity. This is clearly a rule that works well in many situations. However, it is not an absolute rule. There are many circumstances in which it is routinely broken—for instance, in balancing the home life of health professionals against their obligations to patients. Such balancing is also necessary in clinical research, as is the realization that the researcher is actually fulfilling two roles at the same time: in a health professional-patient relationship, and also in a researcher-voluntary research participant relationship.

When a person benefits from research but refuses to participate in it, that person clearly is acting unfairly. He or she is free-riding on the back of the contribution of others. When people volunteer to participate in research, they are doing what any reasonable, decent person should be willing to do if he or she wishes and expects to receive the benefits of research—at least when the risks and dangers to research participants are minimal or low. The level of protection required to render the risks of participation minimal is a question of fact, or at least of judgment, in each case.

Moreover, it is widely recognized that there is sometimes an obligation to make sacrifices for the community, or that sometimes the community is entitled to deny autonomy and even violate bodily integrity in the public interest. This obligation is recognized and accepted in a number of areas, including the following: control of dangerous drugs, control of road traffic, compulsory vaccination and screening tests, quarantine for communicable disease, compulsory military service, detention under mental health acts, and compulsory attendance for jury service at criminal trials.[29] Most of these involve some denial of autonomy and some imposition of public standards. However, these are clearly exceptional cases in which overriding moral considerations take precedence over individual autonomy.

If medical research is a public good shared by large numbers of people, then a number of conclusions may be said to follow:

- It should not simply be assumed that people would not wish to act in the public interest, at least when the costs and risks involved are minimal. In the absence of specific evidence to the contrary, if any assumptions are made, they should be that people are public-spirited and would wish to participate.
- It may be reasonable to presume that people would not consent to do things contrary to their own and to the public interest unless misinformed or coerced. The reverse is true when—as in vaccine trials—participation is in both personal and the public interest.
- If it is right to claim that there is a general obligation to act in the public interest, then there is less reason to challenge consent and little reason to regard participation as actually or potentially exploitative. We do not usually say, "Are you quite sure you want to?" when people fulfill their moral and civic obligations. We do not usually insist on informed consent in such cases. We are usually content that they merely consent or simply acquiesce.

Reexamining the Declaration of Helsinki's Requirements

The two requirements of the 2000 Declaration of Helsinki related to standard of care are "A.5: In medical research on human subjects, considerations related to the well-being of the human subject should take precedence over the interests of science and society" and "C.29: The benefits, risks, burdens and effectiveness of a new method should be tested against those of the best current prophylactic, diagnostic, and therapeutic methods."[1] A narrow interpretation of the first requirement is unwarranted. In the case of research, a clear distinction cannot be sustained between the interests of the participants and the interests of other people who are equally entitled to concern, respect, and protection. The same arguments and the same ethical principles that require researchers to assure the best proven therapies to those in a study also require that those therapies be assured to *all who stand in need of them*.

What then would be a reasonable and ethical balance between these interests? Researchers must weigh carefully and compassionately what is reasonable to ask of potential participants in a trial for their free and unfettered consideration. However, provided potential research participants are given full information, and are free to participate or not as they choose, then the only remaining question is whether it is reasonable to permit people to choose to participate, given the risks and the sorts of gains and benefits that are likely. Is it reasonable to ask people to run whatever degree of risk is involved, to put up with the inconvenience and intrusion of the study in all the circumstances of the case? These circumstances will include both the benefits to them personally of participating in the study and the social value that will flow from the study to other persons, persons who are of course equally entitled to our concern, respect, and protection. Putting the question in this way makes it clear that the standards of care and levels of protection to be accorded to research participants who have full information must be, to a certain extent, study-relative.

The powerful moral reasons for conducting vaccine and drug trials are not drowned by the powerful reasons we have for protecting research participants. There is a balance to be struck here, but it is not a balance that must always and inevitably be loaded in favor of the protection of research participants. Research participants are entitled to the concern, respect, and protection of researchers, to be sure, but they are no more entitled to it than are the people who are threatened or are dying from HIV/AIDS or other major diseases.

It seems unethical to stand by and watch around 3 million people die each year of AIDS alone[30] and to avoid taking steps to prevent such loss—steps that will not put lives at risk and that are taken only with the fully informed consent of those who participate. Fully informed consent, although not foolproof, is the best guarantor of the interests of research participants. Residual dangers—for example, difficulties of constructing suitable consent protocols and supervising their administration in rural and isolated communities in populations that may have low levels of formal education—must be balanced against the dangers of not conducting the trial, which include the massive loss of life that diseases cause.

Researchers' Obligations of Beneficence and Justice

Nonmaleficence is not all of morality. We also have obligations of beneficence toward each other and obligations to act justly. We therefore have to consider the implications of the researcher's obligation of beneficence toward the potential and actual research participants. If the researcher is a health-care professional, his or her professional obligations may also come into play.

Many of the instances in which the standard of care issue becomes most acute involve resource-rich researchers and resource-poor participants. It is at least arguable that if persons deliberately place themselves in a situation in which they will be in contact with needy people, they also place themselves in a situation in which they will have to take their obligation of beneficence seriously. The standard argument that obligation of beneficence can and should not be discharged impartially—it is claimed to be impossible to benefit everyone—does not "protect" researchers who bring themselves in contact with a limited number of needy people whom they could benefit, it they chose to do so. The defense that "It is not my responsibility to help these people" is of questionable validity even when applied to the average citizen in a rich Western country.

The researchers could try to claim that their role as researchers limits their obligation of beneficence, but this is unconvincing. If a research participant collapses on the floor, there is clearly a duty to help him or her; and if the researcher discovers a serious but easily treatable condition unrelated to the research, there would be a moral duty to treat this condition, even if the participant could not pay.

However, this argument based on beneficence is quite general. It does not show that the researchers' positive obligations should be discharged only within the research project, or only toward the research participants. Although we can therefore conclude that researchers cannot insulate themselves from obligations of beneficence, this has no direct bearing on the standard of care issue. The obligations can be discharged in many ways other than through changing the standard of care.

Effective Research Oversight

At this point it is important to enter a few caveats. First, not all research projects have a realistic chance of generating important new knowledge. Some ask uninteresting or trivial questions, and some are so badly designed that they cannot generate valid knowledge. The prospective research participant may not be in a position to discover this, and there is a need for prior research oversight to ensure that no one is asked to participate in research that is not likely to generate collective benefit.

Second, whereas it is true that we all have a personal interest in the progress of medical research—in order not to be a free rider, and to further my own interests and those of people I care about—it is not necessarily true that we all have the same kind of interest. In each specific research project, the benefits may simply be too remote from us. Therefore, the conclusion that a researcher has a right to ask for consent does not entail the further conclusion that any particular research participant has an obligation to give consent. For instance, the potential research participant may already have "done his bit for society" by contributing to other important social activities.

Third, a research oversight system for the real world has to take into account that researchers may have strong self-interested reasons for promoting certain research projects and that the rules that are formalized (for instance, concerning standard of care) have to strike the right balance between rigidity and flexibility. If the rules are too rigid, valuable research will be hindered; if they are too flexible, unscrupulous researchers will exploit them.

Is There a Larger Issue of Exploitation?

Until now, we have mainly focused on the question of whether research participants are exploited, but is there an issue of systemic exploitation? Two dimensions of this question need to be considered: (1) Are high-income countries exploiting low-income countries by performing research that follows the priorities or serves the interests of those societies or their people? (2) Is some of this research being conducted in a way that would not be allowed within the borders of the researchers' own countries?

To take the first question first—whether low-income countries are exploited by research that does not serve their own interests—is not settled by that fact alone. As we have seen when considering the obligations of individual research participants, in societies there may be a duty on all of us to participate in research, primarily or even exclusively for the benefit of others. A claim of exploitation would have to rely on showing unfairness or some other asymmetrical wrongdoing in the overall "exchange" involved in the research.

The second question is more difficult. Here we can attempt only gestures toward a satisfactory answer. There are many reasons for which societies set limits for research that may be undertaken within their borders. And even if certain research is considered morally wrong in one country, it does not follow that it is unethical to carry out such research in other countries. It might, however, become wrongful if the other countries allow the research not because they have carefully considered the situation and decided to allow it, but instead because they are unable or unwilling to enforce suitable research ethics regulation.

A related issue is whether research sponsored by high-income countries and firms in those countries distorts the priorities of the health-care systems of low-income countries by focusing on "the wrong issues." This is an important consideration, but it is not directly related to the standard of care. Research according to high-income priorities may respect standard of care restrictions, however specified, and research according to low-income priorities may breach them.

Study Design Implications

If we accepted the idea that true, uncoerced, informed consent is a sufficient condition for recruiting a person into a research project, the standard of care issue would disappear because it could be argued that the person in question had accepted a particular standard of care.

It is, however, the case that all national and international research ethics regulations of which we are aware conceptualize informed consent as a necessary but not sufficient condition. It is therefore necessary to include considerations of standard of care in the planning and design of biomedical research projects.

What are the implications of standard of care considerations for study design? The wording of the most important international documents is, unfortunately, ambiguous, and it is therefore not possible to derive precise design guidelines directly from these documents. Let us, nevertheless, analyze the relevant sections in the most recent Declaration of Helsinki and CIOMS Guidelines (the relevant sections have been reproduced above).

A few conclusions can be drawn with near certainty:

1. If an effective treatment for the condition in question is generally available in the locality in which the research takes place, this treatment or a treatment of similar effectiveness has to be offered to all research participants, if the condition in question is more than minor.

2. In research taking place in a locality with a different local standard of care than the standard of care in the locality of the researcher or research sponsor, the use of the lower standard of care will require justification either in terms of the research question to be answered or because of strong methodological necessity.

Rather more tentatively, it can be suggested that negative deviations from the local standard of care may be easier to justify when the local standard of care is high. The Note of Clarification to paragraph 29 of the Declaration of Helsinki is centrally concerned with the need to allow placebo-controlled trials for regulatory or pharmaceutical industry-related purposes. Because the regulatory demands are primarily imposed by regulatory agencies in affluent countries, consistency would require them to allow this kind of relaxation of the standard of care in their own jurisdictions.[15]

Furthermore, the design question is complicated by the fact that the standard of care issue is often intertwined with other issues in the ethical evaluation of a research project. A larger deviation from the standard of care may be justifiable if the project is aimed at solving an important research question, or a deviation may be more problematic if consent procedures are questionable.

A New Principle of Research Ethics

It is always encouraging to be able to end on a positive note. We therefore propose the following addition to the Declaration of Helsinki:

> Biomedical research involving human subjects cannot legitimately be neglected, and is therefore permissible, when the importance of the objective is great and the risks to and the possibility of exploitation of fully informed and consenting subjects is small.[19]

The recognition that the obligation to do justice applies not only to research subjects but also to those who will benefit from the research must constitute an advance in thinking about international standards of research ethics.

How would our conclusions apply to specific questions that often arise in the context of research? Let's see:

> 1. Does one have an obligation to provide the best current treatment to participants in a trial, when one could easily do so in the context of the trial and the results of the trial will benefit not the host country but the sponsoring country?

Here the answer is clear and simple. When the best current treatment could be offered easily in the context of the trial, obviously it should be offered, and the question of where eventual benefits will be felt is irrelevant.

> 2. Does one have an obligation to provide the best current treatment to participants in a trial when the best current

treatment is a life-saving intervention not available to the participants outside the research context, and when withholding that treatment is necessary for methodological reasons in order to identify improved interventions for patients in the host country?

To this, the answer is equally clear but more complicated. This question asks whether research participants may agree to enter a trial that can take place only if they are not given the best current treatment—a life-prolonging therapy not otherwise available to them, and one that would, if given, render the trial pointless. Here it seems to us that so long as the trial participants are clear and wish to go ahead on this basis, knowing that the benefits to themselves of entering the trial will be small but knowing also that they are helping in the development of a treatment that may help them or their compatriots later, they should be free to choose whether or not they wish to participate. Because by hypothesis they would not receive the life-prolonging therapy outside the context of the trial, and it could not be provided within that context because the trial could not then take place, they are not worse off than they would otherwise be, and they have a chance (albeit a small one) of being personally better off later, and a larger chance of contributing to the development of a therapy that will benefit others including those in their own country. Would our feelings about the ethics of their decision be altered if they knew that the primary beneficiaries would be foreigners rather than compatriots? We hope no one would be so mean-spirited as to think so.

Finally,

> 3. Are there limits to the obligation to run risks or forgo benefits for the sake of research, if the only beneficiaries are people in rich countries, and those who forgo the benefits are the poor?

The business about rich and poor countries can in a sense be seen as an irrelevance. It might, for instance, be only the poor in the rich countries that benefit. The fundamental question is more general: Can some people validly consent to enter trials from which they themselves will derive little or no benefit, primarily for the sake of others? Remember, the obligation we are talking of must be fully voluntary; there is no question of compulsion or coercion. In such a case, there seems no reason why people should not choose to benefit others even if those others are strangers, foreigners, or whatever. And the fact that the people who are most likely to benefit are strangers seems not to be made much worse by the fact that they are likely also to be foreigners.

Maybe what is hiding underneath the question above is not a question about the location of beneficiaries, but about regulatory hypocrisy. If a country will not allow a certain kind of research to take place within its jurisdiction because such research is seen to be morally problematic—for example, if it would not allow its own poor and untreated to participate in the research—but still wants to conduct the research elsewhere and reap its benefits, then the country is prima facie inconsistent and hypocritical. There is clearly a link between the wealth of a country and its ability to develop and enforce research ethics regulations, and if rich countries exploit weak regulatory systems in poor countries that may be a problem, but it is not primarily a problem about standard of care.

References

1. World Medical Association. *Declaration of Helsinki: Ethical Principles for Medical Research Involving Human Subjects.* Tokyo, Japan: WMA; October 2004. [Online] 2004. Available: http://www.wma.net/e/policy/b3.htm.

2. Council for International Organizations of Medical Sciences, in collaboration with the World Health Organization. *International Ethical Guidelines for Biomedical Research Involving Human Subjects.* Geneva, Switzerland: CIOMS and WHO; 2002. [Online] November 2002. Available: http://www.cioms.ch/frame_guidelines_nov_2002.htm.

3. Conner EM, Sperling RJ, Gelber R, et al. Reduction of maternal-infant transmission of human immunodeficiency virus type 1 with zidovudine treatment. *New England Journal of Medicine* 1994;331:1173–80.

4. Cohen J. Bringing AZT to poor countries. *Science* 1995;269:624–6.

5. Cohen J. Ethics of AZT studies in poorer countries attacked. *Science* 1997;276:1022.

6. Angell M. The ethics of clinical research in the third world. *New England Journal of Medicine* 1997;337:847–9.

7. Lurie P, Wolfe SM. Unethical trials of interventions to reduce perinatal transmission of the human immunodeficiency virus in developing countries. *New England Journal of Medicine* 1997;337:853–6.

8. World Medical Association. *Declaration of Helsinki: Recommendations Guiding Physicians in Biomedical Research Involving Human Subjects.* Somerset West, Republic of South Africa: WMA; October 1996. *JAMA* 1997;277:925–6.

9. Varmus H, Satcher D. Ethical complexities of conducting research in developing countries. *New England Journal of Medicine* 1997;337:1003–5.

10. World Medical Association. *Code of Ethics of the World Medical Association: Declaration of Helsinki.* Helsinki, Finland: WMA; June 1964. *British Medical Journal* 1964;2:177.

11. World Medical Association. Declaration of Helsinki: *Recommendations Guiding Medical Doctors in Biomedical Research Involving Human Subjects.* Tokyo, Japan: WMA; October 1975. *Medical Journal of Australia* 1976;1:206–7.

12. Theme issue: Revising the Declaration of Helsinki: A fresh start. *Bulletin of Medical Ethics* 1999;150.

13. World Medical Association. Proposed revision of the Declaration of Helsinki: WMA document 17.C/Rev1/99. *Bulletin of Medical Ethics* 1999;150:18–22.

14. Council for International Organizations of Medical Sciences, in collaboration with the World Health Organization. *International Ethical Guidelines for Biomedical Research Involving Human Subjects.* Geneva, Switzerland: CIOMS and WHO; 1993.

15. Macklin R. *Double Standards in Medical Research in Developing Countries.* New York, N.Y.: Cambridge University Press; 2004.

16. Lie RK, et al. The standard of care debate: The Declaration of Helsinki versus the international consensus opinion. *Journal of Medical Ethics* 2004;30:190–3.

17. Hyder AA, Dawson L. Defining standard of care in the developing world: The intersection of international research ethics and health systems analysis. *Developing World Bioethics* 2005;5:142–52.

18. London AJ. The ambiguity and the exigency: Clarifying 'standard of care' arguments in international research. *Journal of Medicine and Philosophy* 2000;25:379–97.

19. Harris J. Ethical genetic research on human subjects. *Jurimetrics* 1999;40:77–92.

20. Harris J. Research on human subjects, exploitation and global principles of ethics. In: Lewis ADE, Freeman M, eds. *Law and Medicine: Current Legal Issues, Vol. 3.* New York, N.Y.: Oxford University Press; 2000:379–99.

21. Harris J, Holm S. Why should doctors take risks? Professional responsibility and the assumption of risk. *Journal of the Royal Society of Medicine* 1997;90:625–9.

22. Harris J. Scientific research is a moral duty. *Journal of Medical Ethics* 2005;31:242–8.

23. Harris J. The ethics of clinical research with cognitively impaired subjects. *Italian Journal of Neurological Sciences* 1997;18:9–15.

24. Harris J. *Violence and Responsibility.* London, England: Routledge and Kegan Paul; 1980.

25. Beauchamp TL, Childress JF. *Principles of Biomedical Ethics,* 4th ed. New York, N.Y.: Oxford University Press; 1994.

26. Bloom BR. The highest attainable standard: Ethical issues in AIDS vaccines. *Science* 1998;279:186–8.

27. Harris J. The Marxist conception of violence. *Philosophy and Public Affairs* 1974;3:192–221.

28. Harris J. *The Value of Life.* London, England: Routledge and Kegan Paul; 1985.

29. Harris J. Ethical issues in geriatric medicine. In: Tallis RC, Fillit HM, eds. *Brocklehurst's Textbook of Geriatric Medicine and Gerontology,* 6th ed. London, England: Churchill Livingstone; 2003.

30. UNAIDS. Q&A I: Facts about the AIDS epidemic and its impact. [Online] Available: http://data.unaids.org/pub/GlobalReport/2006/20060530-Q-A_PartI_en.pdf.

Alex John London

Responsiveness to Host Community Health Needs

There is near universal agreement within the scientific and ethics communities that a necessary condition for the moral permissibility of cross-national, collaborative research is that it be responsive to the health needs of the host community. It has proven difficult, however, to leverage or capitalize on this consensus in order to resolve lingering disputes about the ethics of international medical research. This is largely because different sides in these debates have sometimes provided different interpretations of what this requirement amounts to in actual practice.

The goal of the discussion that follows is to clarify the nature of this important moral requirement. The first section explains the requirement for responsiveness to host community health needs in the context of international medical research. The second section examines various formulations of this requirement as they are enunciated in some of the core consensus documents in research ethics. The third section then defends a particular interpretation of this requirement, and the final sections examine more liberal alternatives with the aim of highlighting points of agreement and assessing the significance of areas of disagreement.

Responding to the Developing World's Health Needs

The health inequalities that currently divide the developed from the developing world are not morally neutral. As the Ad Hoc Committee on Health Research Relating to Future Health Interventions of the World Health Organization (WHO) has noted, "The health of the world's peoples has improved more in the past four generations than in the whole of their history." [1] However, the size

and extent of these gains have differed radically between populations of economically developed countries and impoverished nations of the developing world. In 1990, for example, more than a third of the global disease burden could be attributed to a handful of conditions that are virtually unknown in affluent nations of the developed world. These conditions include communicable childhood diseases such as pneumonia, diarrheal diseases, malaria, and various vaccine-preventable infections, as well as malnutrition and high rates of maternal and infant mortality arising from poor reproductive health. [1] Not only are these conditions more likely to occur in circumstances of social and economic deprivation, they are also more difficult to treat under such circumstances; and the devastating toll that they take on the populations in which they are endemic only reinforces the very conditions of deprivation in which such health problems flourish. As a result, the staggering health problems that plague many communities of the developing world play a major role in perpetuating a cycle of impoverishment, premature mortality, and underdevelopment.

The distinctive health problems of the developing world are inextricably bound up with poverty and other forms of social and political deprivation. Recently, however, the attention of scientists, ethicists, and policy makers has focused on what is increasingly viewed as a form of deprivation that occurs in the context of medical research. What is sometimes called the *10/90 disequilibrium* or the *10/90 gap* refers to the statistic that roughly 90% of the global burden of premature mortality can be attributed to diseases that primarily affect populations of the developing world, but only 10% of the annual global research budget of $50 billion to $60 billion is targeted at those diseases. Instead, 90% of the money spent each year on medical research across the globe focuses on the health needs of populations in the developed world, which account for only 10% of the global burden of premature mortality.[1-3] To some degree, therefore, wealthy populations of the developed world have been able to use the fruits of scientific inquiry to safeguard and to secure their health needs so effectively because their needs have been the direct focus of the overwhelming majority of scientific inquiry.

Recognizing the morally problematic nature of the 10/90 gap has generated support for increasing collaborative research activities in the developing world. At the same time, however, such support is tempered by the awareness that too often in the past, when communities in the developing world have participated in research activities, they have not benefited from the fruits of those efforts. Instead, these benefits have been enjoyed primarily by more affluent populations of the developed world.[4] Such practices are now widely regarded as exploitative and, therefore, unethical. As a result, efforts to increase the involvement of the developing world in medical research have had to grapple with the difficult issue of how to achieve this goal while preventing the exploitation of those populations in the process.

One requirement that is intended to facilitate both of these goals is that cross-national collaborative research must be conducted in such a manner as to leave the host community better off than it was, or at least not worse off. This requirement supports another, namely, that international medical research must be responsive to the health needs and priorities of the host community. Together, these conditions constitute important moral constraints on permissible research, as well as substantive moral ideals toward which research should strive. Nevertheless, different interpretations of key concepts in these requirements have at times produced conflicting views about what these requirements amount to in actual practice.

Different Expressions of the Requirement

Perhaps the clearest statement of the requirement that collaborative international research be responsive to the health needs of the host community is presented by the Council for International Organizations of Medical Sciences (CIOMS), in collaboration with the WHO, in its International Ethical Guidelines for Biomedical Research Involving Human Subjects[5] (see Chapter 16). Guideline 3 of the 2002 text governs "ethical review of externally sponsored research" and states in part, "The health authorities of the host country, as well as a national or local ethical review committee, should ensure that the proposed research is responsive to the health needs and priorities of the host country and meets the requisite ethical standards." The phrase *health needs and priorities* introduces two key concepts and raises the question of their relationship. In order to understand what this guideline requires, it is necessary to clarify (a) what constitute the *health needs and priorities* of the host community and (b) what is required to show that a research initiative is sufficiently "responsive" to the host community's health needs and priorities, so understood.

To begin with, *health needs* are concerns that are particularly important or urgent because of their close relationship to the ability of persons to be free from medical conditions that shorten their lives or prevent them from functioning in ways that are basic or fundamental to their pursuit of a reasonable life plan.[6] In this respect, health needs stand in contrast to health-related wants or

desires, when these terms refer to things that may help to improve the functionality of persons but which lack this urgency.

Among the various health needs that exist within a community, some may be viewed as more urgent or important than others. For instance, prostate cancer and breast cancer may be health needs that are *represented* in a resource-poor community in the sense that a significant cohort of people may suffer from these conditions. Nevertheless, finding new means of treating these afflictions may not be a health priority of such a community if significantly larger numbers of people suffer and die much earlier in life from conditions such as malaria, tuberculosis, or HIV. When this is the case, the latter conditions might constitute health needs that are also health priorities of such communities. In other communities, however, finding new means of treating prostate or breast cancer may constitute important health priorities. Communities can differ, therefore, in their health priorities even when significant members of their populations have common health needs.

Every community is constrained to use its finite social, economic, and human resources to meet a wide range of basic needs of community members. As a result, communities may differ in their social priorities, giving greater or lesser priority to different needs, depending on their broader social circumstances. For example, fostering economic development through job growth may be a top priority in a community with high rates of unemployment and low per capita income levels. So might be expanding the country's infrastructure or improving national security. Different communities may therefore view health-related issues, such as preventing the spread of HIV and providing a wide range of childhood vaccinations, as more or less of a priority than other social or economic concerns.

These rudimentary distinctions raise an important question about the requirement for responsiveness to host community health needs: Should the requirement be understood in a fairly restrictive way, according to which collaborative research initiatives should be required to focus on health needs that are also health priorities of the host community? Or should it be understood in a more liberal way, according to which it is sufficient for research to focus on a health need that is represented in the host community, even if it is not necessarily a health priority, so long as the research is adequately responsive to other priorities of the host community?

Perhaps the most natural reading of CIOMS Guideline 3 is that it requires research to be responsive to those health needs *that are also health priorities* of the host community. In this view, it is not sufficient to establish that the health need in question is merely represented in the host community. Rather, the health need in question must be sufficiently urgent or important that finding the means of addressing it represents a judicious use of the community's scarce social resources.

On the other hand, a literal reading of Guideline 10 of the 2002 text appears to be consistent with the more liberal or permissive interpretation of this requirement. This guideline governs "research in populations and communities with limited resources," and holds the following:

> Before undertaking research in a population or community with limited resources, the sponsor and the investigator must make every effort to ensure that:
>
> • the research is responsive to *the health needs and the priorities* of the population or community in which it is to be carried out [emphasis added]; and

- any intervention or product developed, or knowledge generated, will be made reasonably available for the benefit of that population or community.

Because "the health needs" of the host community do not necessarily fall under the scope of "the priorities" of that community in this statement, a literal reading of this guideline is consistent with the more liberal view.

To illustrate the importance of the difference between these two positions, consider the double-blind, randomized, placebo-controlled trial proposed in 2001 by the pharmaceutical company Discovery Laboratories. This trial would have compared the company's new surfactant agent, Surfaxin, against a placebo in impoverished communities of Latin America. Surfactants are substances that are essential to the ability of the lungs to absorb oxygen, and roughly half a dozen surfactant agents are commonly used to save the lives of premature infants in countries of the developed world. In return for hosting this study, Discovery Labs offered to upgrade and modernize the intensive care units in which the study would take place, increasing the ability of host communities to provide neonatal care to premature infants. This study, however, provoked an outcry over its use of a placebo control, which critics charged violated the current standard of care for treating premature infants. But this study also raises a more profound question that must be addressed prior to concerns about standards of care. Namely, was this proposed project sufficiently responsive to the health needs of host community members?

The most natural reading of CIOMS Guideline 3 supports the verdict that this research was not morally permissible because it did not target a health need that was also a health priority of the host community. Several effective surfactant agents are already widely used in developed counties, but these agents are not available in the impoverished communities that would host this trial. Moreover, Surfaxin was not specifically designed for use in the developing world. It therefore did not have properties that would make it more likely to be deployed in the developing world or more likely to be effective in that context than existing surfactants.

According to the weaker requirement that is at least consistent with a literal reading of Guideline 10, however, this research could be seen as permissible. It targeted a health need that was represented in the host community, and supporters argued that it was responsive to other priorities of the host community—such as strengthening the health-care infrastructure, training and educating medical personnel, and perhaps also fostering economic activity that would result from hosting the research.

Each of these views represents a different way of trying to satisfy the requirement in CIOMS that "the research project should leave low-resource countries or communities better off than previously or, at least, no worse off." In fact, the requirement for responsiveness to host community health needs can itself be viewed as emanating from the imperative in CIOMS that host countries should be left "at least, no worse off." As a result, the core consensus documents in research ethics have been more concerned with the relationship between access to benefits and the *responsiveness* clause in this requirement than with clarifying the relationship between the health needs and the priorities of the host community.

Similar tensions exist within the responsiveness clause of this requirement, however. In the CIOMS guidelines, under the section, "General Ethical Principles," for example, we are told that research in low-resource countries or communities, "should be responsive to their health needs and priorities *in that* any product developed is made reasonably available to them, and as far as possible [should] leave the population in a better position to obtain effective health care and protect its own health [emphasis added]". Here, responsiveness is equated with ensuring that the fruits of any successful research initiatives are made reasonably available in the host community. This statement also emphasizes the important role that medical research can play in helping communities safeguard their own health by discovering new diagnostic or therapeutic modalities. As I argue below, the requirement to ensure reasonable availability seems most appropriate when combined with the requirement that such research actually focus on health needs that are also health priorities of that community.

On the other hand, not all medical research is designed to vindicate a new diagnostic or treatment modality. Similarly, not all research that has this end succeeds in achieving its goal. However, research initiatives can be designed in such a way as to ensure that they provide host communities with indirect or ancillary benefits of various kinds.[7,8,3] For instance, researchers can provide vaccinations or rudimentary medical care to community members. They can train and educate local medical personnel and thereby contribute to enriching local research capacity. In this regard, the commentary on Guideline 10 again appears to be consistent with a more liberal view. There we are told, "It is not sufficient simply to determine that a disease is prevalent in the population and that new or further research is needed: the ethical requirement of 'responsiveness' can be fulfilled only if successful interventions *or other kinds of health benefit* are made available to the population [emphasis added]". Here it appears that the requirement of responsiveness can be met by providing other kinds of health benefits to the host community. As I argue below, this view seems most reasonable when conjoined to the somewhat weaker requirement that research need only focus on health needs that are represented in the host community as long as that enterprise is responsive to other priorities of that community. I will return to this point in the following section.

In some of the core consensus documents in research ethics the reasonable availability requirement eclipses entirely the debate over what is required in order to be adequately responsive to the health needs of the host population. The Declaration of Helsinki, for example, does not explicitly state that medical research must be responsive to the health needs of the host population (see Chapter 13). Paragraph 19, however, does state, "Medical research is only justified if there is a reasonable likelihood that the populations in which the research is carried out stand to benefit from the results of the research."[9] This paragraph, however, is often cited by commentators as an instance of the requirement that research be responsive to the health needs of the host community.[4,10]

In its report, *Ethical and Policy Issues in International Research: Clinical Trials in Developing Countries*, the National Bioethics Advisory Commission (NBAC) affirmed that "Clinical trials conducted in developing countries should be limited to those studies that are responsive to the health needs of the community."[11] The NBAC derives the requirement of responsiveness to host population health needs from the values of beneficence and justice. Following the Belmont Report[12] and the U.S. Department of Health and Human Services' Common Rule, the NBAC holds that the requirement of beneficence is satisfied when the risks to research participants are reasonable in light of the prospect that the research initiative will generate either of two possible benefits: tangible benefits to trial participants or increases in the "fund of human knowledge" (see Chapters 14 and 15). The NBAC then views the value of justice as requiring that "some of the benefits must accrue to the group from which the research participants are selected."[11]

According to the NBAC's justification of the requirement for responsiveness to host community health needs, some members of the host community must benefit either from the increases in the fund of human knowledge generated by the research or from tangible benefits that come from research participation. Both interpretations of the responsiveness requirement outlined above, however, can be viewed as interpretations of the argument that the NBAC offers. Nevertheless, the NBAC finds that researchers and their sponsors have an obligation to take steps prior to initiating a research initiative to ensure that the fruits of any successful research will be made reasonably available to the host population. As I argue below, however, this requirement seems most reasonable when combined with an interpretation of responsiveness to host community health needs that requires research to focus on health priorities of the host community.

The Nuffield Council on Bioethics displays the clearest grasp of the existence of, and conflict between, the two views outlined above concerning the requirement for responsiveness to host community health needs. In paragraph 2.24 of its 2002 report, *The Ethics of Research Related to Healthcare in Developing Countries,* the Council notes that "in countries where nearly all research related to healthcare is externally funded, the priorities for research have been largely set by the external sponsors." [3] It also notes the existence of the 10/90 disequilibrium, or 10/90 gap, mentioned earlier. This leads the Nuffield Council to affirm, in paragraph 4.8, that there is a general moral duty to alleviate suffering; and this moral duty creates a more specific moral obligation to conduct research that deals with the health problems in developing countries. However, the Council stops short of requiring all externally funded research to target health needs that fall within the nationally defined health priorities of the host community. Its reason for this, articulated in paragraph 2.31, is that even research that does not target a local health priority can "offer considerable indirect benefits to host countries in the developing world because of the potential for strengthening the national capacity in research, in the form of improved infrastructure and training." At paragraph 2.32, the Council therefore emphasizes that although it is important to encourage research that does advance local health priorities, this is not a necessary requirement because "all research contributes to the development of local skills and expertise in research, quite apart from the inherent value in diversity of research."[3]

The Nuffield Council, therefore, explicitly recognizes the moral permissibility of externally sponsored, international research that does not focus on a health priority of the host community. Presumably, such research is morally permissible only to the extent that it targets a health need that is represented in the host community and conveys sufficient indirect benefit to the host community that it can be seen as advancing other priorities of that community, such as strengthening the local research capacity.

Focus on Health Needs That Are Health Priorities

The survey of core consensus documents presented in the previous section reveals two salient dimensions along which alternative positions concerning the responsiveness to host community health needs requirement can be distinguished. For our present purposes, the most important distinction concerns whether international research initiatives are required to target health needs that that are also health priorities of the host community or whether it is sufficient to target health needs that are simply represented in the host community, as long as the research is sufficiently responsive to other priorities of the host community. This distinction is represented by the rows in the matrix in Table 67.1. I have labeled the top row *Restrictive* and the bottom row *Permissive* to indicate that not only do views that fall into the lower row permit all research that would be permitted by views in the top row, they permit a wider range of research as well. Within each row, views may then be distinguished as more or less restrictive depending on whether they also endorse the reasonable availability requirement.

Because it is sometimes difficult to tell exactly which combinations of these views are being advocated in some consensus documents, it is worth briefly exploring the merits of these positions in their own right. The top row of the matrix in Table 67.1 represents a variety of views that have been defended by numerous commentators.[13–17] Although these positions differ in significant ways, they share several basic tenets.

One shared tenet of views that occupy this row in the matrix is that an adequate understanding of a community's health needs must consider the important connections that exist between the health status of people and the operation of a variety of basic social structures. One social structure that is particularly salient in this regard is a community's local health-care system. As Jha and colleagues have emphasized, strengthening the *close-to-client* health system in developing countries would significantly increase the ability of local populations to access the effective medical interventions that already exist for some 90 percent of the avoidable mortality in low- and middle-income countries.[18]

The health status of individuals is also deeply affected by the way in which other basic social structures in their community allocate fundamental rights, such as who has access to literacy and education, including access to information about individual and public health; who has access to the means of productive employment; whose freedom of speech and association is protected; and whose sovereignty over their own person is respected. Whether or not the fundamental institutions of a community are directed at providing these social determinants of health can have a tremendous impact on the nature and extent of the health problems that members of that community face—as well as on the opportunities that are available to individuals to deal effectively

Table 67.1

Matrix of Models of Responsiveness to Health Needs

	Reasonable Availability Is Required	Reasonable Availability Is Not Required
Must target health needs that are also health priorities	Most restrictive	Less restrictive
May target health needs that are not health priorities	Less permissive	Most permissive

with those conditions that do arise. Communities that use their scarce social resources to invest in the basic capacities of community members have significantly greater success in staving off famine and epidemic disease. Those that do not direct community resources to these ends often create conditions in which starvation and disease flourish, sometimes on a massive scale.[19,20]

At the same time, sickness and disease themselves threaten important interests of individuals and communities alike. On the one hand, they impede the ability of individuals to function on an equal standing with others by restricting the full range of social opportunities that are available to them and often shortening their lives. In turn, the inability of individuals to take effective advantage of the full range of the social and economic opportunities available to them can significantly impact the ability of communities to advance important social and political goals such fostering education and economic growth.[21]

In light of these interrelationships, one of the views that occupies the top row of the matrix, the human development model, holds that various parties from developed countries, including government officials and the citizens they represent, have a duty to aid those in the developing world. It also holds that the duty to aid should be understood as a duty to assist those populations in developing and maintaining fair and equitable social structures that serve to safeguard and to advance the basic interests of community members.[17] What is required in order to discharge this general duty will differ for various stakeholders depending on their ability to influence different aspects of the social structures in developing countries. For example, the citizens of developed countries have a duty to support efforts to make better use of existing knowledge, resources, and interventions that could make a significant impact on the lives of those in the developing world. However, this view recognizes that even when a greater share of existing resources are directed toward advancing this goal, scientific research still has an important role to play in this process.

When this general duty to aid is applied to researchers and to research sponsors, therefore, the human development model translates the duty into an obligation to ensure that scientific research is responsive to host community health needs in a particular way. The model assumes that research can function as a powerful engine for creating the understanding and the interventions that are necessary to bridge gaps between the basic interests of community members and the ability of that community's basic social structures to safeguard and advance those interests. In order to bridge such gaps, clinical research must focus on health problems of developing-world communities that cannot be met more effectively or efficiently through the application of existing resources. Such health needs may be novel in the sense that there are no known means of treating or ameliorating them, or they may be health needs that have to be met under novel circumstances. That is, effective interventions may exist, but it may not be possible to deploy them within the host community on a sustainable basis. As a result, inquiry may be necessary in order to ascertain how to best to meet those needs under conditions that are attainable and sustainable within the host community. By focusing on health needs that cannot be met more effectively or efficiently through the application of existing knowledge or resources, and by doing so in a way that seeks to bridge the gaps between important health needs of community members and the ability of basic social structures in that community to meet those needs, collaborative

research represents an important avenue through which the more general duty to aid may be discharged.

This view of the duty to aid, and the role of scientific research in advancing its goals, provides important guidance for selecting the criteria for determining which of a community's health needs should be given priority for research purposes. In particular, such criteria should be responsive to (a) the significance of the impact of a health need on the ability of individuals to access the full range of social opportunities that would otherwise be open to them, including their ability to cooperate in advancing important social goals, (b) the impact of these needs on equity and social justice in the host community, (c) the prevalence of these needs in the host population, and (d) whether they can be more effectively or efficiently met through the application of existing knowledge and resources. Some important steps have recently been taken in this regard by a variety of communities that have sought to define their national health priorities so that research can focus on what has been termed *essential national health research,* or ENHR.[1-3] ENHR refers to a strategy of systematic priority setting within which research questions can be identified and prioritized according to factors such as economic impact, cost effectiveness, effects on equity, social justice, and their contribution to strengthening research capacity in the host community.

Medical research that focuses on such health priorities has several important moral properties. Such research can make a strong prima facie claim to represent a just use of the host community's scarce social, economic, and human resources and to having significant social value because (a) these resources are being used to generate the knowledge, methods, and interventions necessary to expand the capacity of important social structures in the host community—such as the close-to-client health system—to address significant health needs of that community's members and (b) these needs could not be met more effectively or efficiently through the application of existing knowledge or resources.[17] As a result, such criteria represent a valuable means of identifying research questions that are essentially directed at closing the so-called 10/90 gap.

Although these criteria provide general constraints on what can count as a health priority in the research context, the actual health priorities of a community must be identified through the collaborative efforts of a number of parties. It is essential, therefore, that the process of identifying these priorities be transparent and open to public scrutiny. Similarly, it is essential that this process involve the participation of community representatives from local as well as national levels, including representatives of relevant minority groups. In this way, research can be responsive to on-the-ground factors that influence the prevalence of the condition in question, as well as factors that influence the ability to effectively treat those who are afflicted with it. The goal of these requirements is to ensure accountability and legitimacy as well as scientific and social responsibility.

The importance of ensuring such a transparent and legitimate process of democratic consultation has recently been emphasized by what is known as the fair benefits approach to international research.[7,8] This approach has also been a leading critical force in challenging the requirement of reasonable availability. Exploring the details of this approach and some of its possible variants will provide a clear context within which to evaluate positions that might fall into the cells in the Table 67.1 that are labeled "less restrictive," "less permissive," and "more permissive."

Less Restrictive Criteria for Permissible Research

The fair benefits approach has been critical of positions that require pretrial assurances of reasonable availability on the grounds that such requirements are overly restrictive and may actually work against the interests of developing world populations. This critical view of the reasonable availability requirement grows out of several concerns.

First, the fair benefits approach emphasizes that the reasonable availability requirement is relevant only to Phase III research. However, communities in the developing world might want to host Phase I or Phase II studies, or epidemiological studies, which are not designed to vindicate novel therapeutic or diagnostic modalities. Like the Nuffield Council, this approach also recognizes that there are numerous direct and indirect ways in which hosting a research initiative can benefit host communities. Such benefits might include the training of medical personnel, creating economic opportunities for employment, providing medical care, enhancing the local infrastructure, or enacting public health measures such as providing clean water. In fact, this approach holds that it might be possible for host communities to derive indirect benefits from hosting a research initiative that are more directly responsive to the larger priorities of that community than is the prospect of receiving access to the particular intervention being evaluated within that study. If this is the case, then requiring researchers and their sponsors to ensure reasonable availability puts an arbitrary roadblock in the way of research that might provide real benefits to developing world communities. It also paternalistically restricts the ability of host communities to bargain for the kind and amount of benefits that they desire most from a research initiative.

In its basic structure, therefore, the fair benefits approach represents an explicit defense of the more liberal version of the requirement for responsiveness to host community health needs identified in our survey of core consensus documents. Like those documents, this approach permits only medical research that is consistent with the values of beneficence and nonmaleficence. Research is permissible, therefore, only if there is a reasonable likelihood that it will leave the host community better off than it was, or at least not worse off. However, because the fair benefits approach views the reasonable availability requirement as overly restrictive, it adopts instead a mechanism of open deliberation and bargaining to achieve an exchange of benefits that is sufficient to leave the host community better off. Research initiatives must address "a health problem of the developing country population," and they must ensure that host communities receive a fair share of the benefits that are generated from research participation. Of course, decisions about how much of which kinds of benefits make hosting research worthwhile depend crucially on the priorities of the host community. So such questions are left for members of the host community to decide. These decisions would be subject to public debate, and a record of previous agreements would be used as a benchmark for fairness. Using this deliberative process to identify which kinds of benefit constitute a "fair" share in light of the host community's needs and priorities is meant to respect the autonomy of host community members and to ensure that the research has social value.

Because this approach requires that host community members receive a fair share of benefit from research that addresses "a health problem of the developing country population" without clarifying whether the problem must be a health priority of the host community, several different versions of this position can be constructed. If "a health problem of the developing country population" is understood as referring to a health priority of the host community—which would place it in the top row of the matrix in Table 67.1—then it can provide a rationale for what I have labeled a "less restrictive" approach to international research. It is less restrictive in the following sense: In addition to permitting all of the research that is permitted by positions in the "more restrictive" cell, it also permits research that targets a health priority of the host community without requiring pretrial assurances that any fruits of that study—if there are any—will be made reasonably available to members of the host community. Such projects are morally permissible, however, only as long as they do provide members of the host community with a fair package of ancillary benefits.

This version of the fair benefits approach overlaps to a considerable degree with the human development approach. Both require research to focus on a health priority of the host community but this version of the fair benefits approach rightly emphasizes the importance of ensuring that the indirect benefits that can attend research participation are coordinated so as to be responsive to priorities of the host community. This is especially important in cases in which the research is not designed to vindicate a new diagnostic or therapeutic modality. After all, Phase III research must often build on prior epidemiological research and on Phase I and Phase II studies. When it is appropriate to carry out such studies in the developing world, the research should be justified according to the requirements of this version of the fair benefits approach. Here, too, the criteria outlined above for prioritizing a community's health needs might also be used within the context of democratic consultation with host community members to determine which of the indirect benefits of research would best advance the community's larger social priorities.

Tensions arise between this version of the fair benefits approach and other views that occupy the most restrictive cell in the matrix in the context of Phase III research. Proponents of the fair benefits approach worry that research sponsors and other funding agencies will be unwilling to commit themselves to funding interventions whose therapeutic or diagnostic properties have not been clearly established. They therefore worry that such reticence may hinder the conduct of valuable research.

In contrast, proponents of the reasonable availability requirement worry that without prior commitments, the knowledge that is gained from collaborative research will not have a material impact on the health needs of host community members. For instance, many commentators who were critical of the short-course AZT trials in the developing world were explicitly rejecting a view that would fall into the "less restrictive" area of the matrix in Table 67.1. In particular, they argued that it is not sufficient for research to target a health priority of the host community if members of that community never benefit from the application of the knowledge generated by such trials. After all, effective interventions exist for many of the most pressing health problems in the developing world, and many of these interventions were vindicated by research that was carried out in such populations. Nevertheless, many of these interventions have not made a significant impact on disease burdens in these communities because they are largely unavailable there. As a result, critics hold that the position labeled "less restrictive" does not go far enough toward advancing the health interests of developing world populations.[4]

To a large degree, such tensions reflect the difference between pragmatic and aspirational approaches to international research. The pragmatic approach gives priority to generating knowledge that can be used to advance the health needs of developing world populations, leaving the problem of how to make these advances materially available to be dealt with later. The more aspirational approach emphasizes that host community members will benefit from medical research only to the extent that the fruits of that enterprise are used to expand the capacity of local social structures to meet the needs of the community. From this standpoint, one component of the requirement for responsiveness to host community health needs includes having reasonable assurance that the research enterprise is part of a social division of labor in which the knowledge that it generates will actually be applied to advance the interests of host community members.

Careful consideration of the criteria for responsiveness that were articulated in the previous section can mitigate the tensions that exist between these views. In particular, within the human development model, a fundamental part of identifying research initiatives that are capable of closing gaps between the basic health needs of a community's members and the capacity of basic social structures in that community to meet those needs is identifying target interventions that can be effectively deployed under conditions that are attainable and sustainable in the host community.[22] An important aspect of advance research planning, therefore, should be matching communities with research initiatives with the goal of ensuring that (a) the research target represents a health priority of the host community, (b) when research is designed to vindicate a therapeutic or diagnostic modality, there is a strong likelihood that any fruits of the research could be integrated into the basic social structures of the host community, and (c) the research initiative can provide an anchor for indirect benefits that are responsive to the broader priorities of the host community.

In all cases, research protocols should be accompanied by an assessment of the likelihood that the study intervention could be implemented in the host community, including an assessment of conditions that would need to be in place in order to increase this likelihood. Evaluations of whether pretrial assurance of reasonable availability is necessary should involve an explicit assessment of the likelihood that any knowledge generated could be used to expand the capacity of social structures in the host community to meet the basic health needs of community members—including an assessment of the extent to which the support of governmental, nongovernmental, or private entities is necessary to attain and sustain the conditions required for this goal.

Weakening the Criteria for Permissible Research

Significantly more liberal approaches to international research can be generated if the requirement in the fair benefits approach that research address "a health problem of the developing country population" is interpreted as permitting research that focuses on a health need that is merely *represented* in the host population. In such a view, as long as the ancillary or indirect benefits associated with the research are viewed as a fair return by members of the host community, then this position views positions that occupy the top row of the matrix as overly restrictive of important medical research and as paternalistically limiting the ability of developing world populations to advance their various interests and priorities.

Of the two cells in the permissive row, the less permissive view is conceptually unstable and perhaps incoherent. From the standpoint of the human development approach, it represents an inefficient way of advancing the fundamental interests of host community members, because it requires local governments and other funding agencies to spend scarce resources on interventions that do not necessarily address priority health problems of the host communities. From the standpoint of the "most permissive" view, the requirement of ensuring reasonable availability would only serve to prevent some research from taking place that would have otherwise offered benefits to host community members that they would have been willing to accept.

Although it seems clearly problematic in the abstract, this ad hoc approach is what appears to result from simply imposing the requirement of reasonable availability on all international research. As the Nuffield Council points out, most externally sponsored research in the developing world is driven by the priorities of the sponsoring entities. To the extent that the consensus documents canvassed earlier endorse the requirement of reasonable availability without clearly requiring research to focus on a health priority in the host community, these documents leave themselves open to withering criticisms from both more permissive and more restrictive perspectives.

The "most permissive" interpretation of the fair benefits approach is internally coherent and rationally compelling. It permits all the research that is permitted by views that occupy other cells in the matrix, while also permitting any research initiative that addresses a health need that is represented in the host community—so long as the host population receives what it views as a fair package of benefits in return. From this standpoint, hosting clinical research that generates significant indirect benefits for the host community, but which targets a disease problem that is not a priority in the host community might be seen as analogous to hosting a commercial plant that produces products that are enjoyed primarily by members of another community but which provides significant indirect benefits to the host community.

This view, however, raises a number of troubling concerns. To begin with, it is so liberal that it permits the continued use of developing world populations to answer questions that primarily address the health goals and priorities of the developed world. In this respect, it threatens to perpetuate or even to exacerbate the 10/90 gap. Second, the ancillary or indirect benefits that can be generated from research are unlikely to address root causes of disease in the developing world in a sustainable way. In particular, the disparities in bargaining power between research sponsors and host communities, combined with constant pressures to limit the costs associated with individual research projects, make it likely that there will remain a fairly low ceiling on the kind and extent of indirect benefits that host communities can access through the bargaining process.

Third, although it is true that medical research should be carried out so as to produce important indirect benefits, its most significant value lies in its ability to discover information necessary to improve the capacity of important social structures to minister to the health needs of community members. One of the critical reasons for the sharp gains in longevity and quality of life in the developed world over the past four generations has been the success of these nations in understanding health problems from a scientific standpoint and integrating that understanding not just into their respective health-care systems, but into the education and lives of community members more generally.[1] In light of the profoundly urgent and pervasive health needs of the developing world, combined with the disparities in research representation represented by the 10/90 gap, strong reasons support changing funding priorities and creating incentives for governmental, nongovernmental, and private entities to focus more directly on priority health problems of developing world populations.[13–17] This process can be guided, at various stages, by understanding the requirement for responsiveness to host community health needs as holding that clinical research (a) must take health needs that constitute health priorities of the host community as the occasion for inquiry, and (b) must function as part of a social division of labor in which the fruits of such increased understanding have a high likelihood of being used to expand the capacity of that community's health-related social structures to meet the most pressing needs of community members.

Conclusion

When properly planned, scientific research can be a conduit for myriad direct and indirect benefits to host community members. The true social value of scientific research, however, emanates from its capacity to generate the knowledge, methods, and interventions necessary to enhance the ability of important social structures in the host community to address the most significant health needs of that community's members. Collaborative research initiatives should therefore be required to justify their responsiveness to host community health needs in these terms.

Acknowledgment

This chapter was written with the generous support of a New Directions Fellowship from the Andrew W. Mellon Foundation.

References

1. World Health Organization. *Investing in Health Research and Development: Report of the Ad Hoc Committee on Health Research Relating to Future Intervention Options.* Geneva, Switzerland: WHO; 1996. [Online] Available: http://www.who.int/tdr/publications/publications/investing_report.htm.
2. Commission on Health Research for Development. *Health Research: Essential Link to Equity in Development.* New York, N.Y.: Oxford University Press; 1990.
3. Nuffield Council on Bioethics. *The Ethics of Research Related to Healthcare in Developing Countries.* London, England: Nuffield Council on Bioethics; 2002. [Online] Available: http://nuffieldbioethics.org/fileLibrary/pdf/errhdc_fullreport001.pdf.
4. Annas GJ, Grodin MA. Human rights and maternal-fetal HIV transmission prevention trials in Africa. *American Journal of Public Health* 1998;88:560–3.
5. Council for International Organizations of Medical Sciences, in collaboration with the World Health Organization. *International Ethical Guidelines for Biomedical Research Involving Human Subjects.* Geneva, Switzerland: CIOMS and WHO; 2002. [Online] November 2002. Available: http://www.cioms.ch/frame_guidelines_nov_2002.htm.
6. Daniels N. *Just Health Care.* New York, N.Y.: Cambridge University Press; 1985.
7. The Participants in the 2001 Conference on Ethical Aspects of Research in Developing Countries. Moral standards for research in developing countries: From "reasonable availability" to "fair benefits." *Hastings Center Report* 2004;34(3):17–27.
8. Participants in the 2001 Conference on Ethical Aspects of Research in Developing Countries. Fair benefits for research in developing countries. *Science* 2002;298:2133–4.
9. World Medical Association. *Declaration of Helsinki: Ethical Principles for Medical Research Involving Human Subjects.* Tokyo, Japan: WMA; October 2004. [Online] 2004. Available: http://www.wma.net/e/policy/b3.htm.
10. Macklin R. After Helsinki: Unresolved issues in international research. *Kennedy Institute of Ethics Journal* 2001;11:17–36.
11. National Bioethics Advisory Commission. *Ethical and Policy Issues in International Research: Clinical Trials in Developing Countries.* Bethesda, Md.: NBAC; 2001:iii,7–8. [Online] Available: http://www.bioethics.gov/reports/past_commissions/nbac_international.pdf.
12. The National Commission for the Protection of Human Subjects of Biomedical and Behavioral Research. *The Belmont Report: Ethical Principles and Guidelines for the Protection of Human Subjects of Research.* Washington, D.C.: Department of Health, Education and Welfare; DHEW Publication OS 78-0012 1978. [Online] April 18, 1979. Available: http://www.hhs.gov/ohrp/humansubjects/guidance/belmont.htm.
13. Benatar SR. Global disparities in health and human rights: A critical commentary. *American Journal of Public Health* 1998;88:295–300.
14. Attaran A. Human rights and biomedical research funding for the developing world: Discovering state obligations under the right to health. *Health and Human Rights* 1999;4:27–58.
15. Benatar SR, Daar AS, Singer PA. Global health ethics: The rationale. *International Affairs* 2003;79:107–38.
16. Flory JH, Kitcher P. Global health and the scientific research agenda. *Philosophy and Public Affairs* 2004;32:36–65.
17. London AJ. Justice and the human development approach to international research. *Hastings Center Report* 2005;35(1):24–37.
18. Jha P, et al. Improving the health of the global poor. *Science* 2002;295:2036–9.
19. Sen A. *Poverty and Famines.* Oxford, England: Clarendon Press; 1981.
20. Sen A. *Development as Freedom.* New York, N.Y.: Anchor Books; 1999.
21. Bloom D, Canning D. The health and wealth of nations. *Science* 2000;87:1207–9.
22. London AJ. Equipoise and international human-subjects research. *Bioethics* 2001;15:312–32.

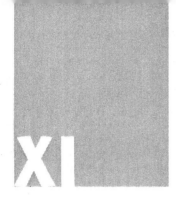

XI

Clinical Investigator Behavior

Trudo Lemmens

Conflict of Interest in Medical Research

Historical Developments

The topic of conflict of interest in medical research has become one of the standard issues in any textbook on research ethics and, particularly in the past decade, has also become a core component of the medical and bioethics literature. More than half of the articles on this subject published in the medical literature since 1966 were published since 1999. The significant increase in the number of such publications is undoubtedly related to the growing role of financial interests in the biomedical research enterprise. Particularly, since the 1980s, following the passage of the Bayh-Dole Act in the United States, which explicitly allowed the commercialization of federally funded research and promoted the patenting of biomedical inventions,[1] the pharmaceutical and biotechnology industries have taken on a more important role in biomedical research. Their influence has expanded through increased industry sponsorship of academic research and as a result of the growth in industry-organized research. The increase in the volume of conflict of interest commentaries, analyses, and policies is the most striking development, but there has also been noticeable shift in focus. Although the conflict of interest debate has historically focused on the conflicts faced by individual investigators, increasing attention is being paid to larger institutional and professional pressures that result from the commercialization of research and of academia. But the issue of conflict of interest is not new and is not exclusively associated with the context of commercialized research.

The Physician-Researcher and Conflict of Interest

Many of the historical examples of research controversies described earlier in this textbook can be seen as illustrations of a fundamental tension that exists between researchers' commitment to scientific inquiry and their obligations, as health-care professionals, to promote the health and well-being of their patients. Significantly, most of the troublesome historical scandals took place in the context of governmentally sponsored research in which financial interests played little or no role. One only has to recall, for example, how researchers involved in the infamous Tuskegee syphilis study were so committed to gathering information on the physical progression of the disease in African American patients that they continued to observe the patients' decline until 1972, 29 years after effective medication for treating the condition became available[2,3] (see Chapter 8). The physicians involved did not seem to appreciate how they were violating their primary obligation to their patients, an obligation imposed on them as members of the medical profession. Nor did they seem to recognize in the context of their study a moral duty to prevent harm. Their interest in research affected their professional judgment as clinicians and their commitment to their primary obligation to care for the sick.

Tuskegee and other research controversies illustrate well what conflict of interest is about. Few will suggest that the researchers involved in these studies consciously and purposely harmed their research subjects. Yet their clinical judgment and moral sensitivity were clouded by a blind focus on obtaining research results. In fact, in the context of conflict of interest, we often can see only in retrospect that people were likely blinded by a particular focus. We cannot enter the minds of people to determine their real motivation, but we deduce from what happened that their judgment was skewed by a focus on secondary interests.

The legacy of these historical controversies underlies the strong emphasis on the primary obligation to protect patients in various guidelines and regulations dealing with conflicts of interest. They highlight, in a very blunt way, how devastating the consequences of an overzealous focus of medical researchers on obtaining research results can be.

The more subtle debate around the notion of clinical equipoise can also be seen as recognition of the crucial tension between the differing duties of researchers and clinicians (see Chapter 24). Indeed, the concept of clinical equipoise aims at sketching the conditions under which clinicians can ethically justify proposing participation in a clinical trial to their patient. The quandary that Charles Fried[4] and later commentators such as Benjamin Freedman[5] tried to solve is precisely the potential clash between the primary obligation of physicians to provide the best available individualized care and the primary obligation of researchers to conduct a medically important study—a study that involves research procedures that differ from individualized patient care. The limits placed on clinical research by clinical equipoise—for example, in its imposition of strict limits on placebo-controlled trials, or in its imposition of stopping rules—reflect an understanding that the obligations of clinicians can clash with the obligations of researchers; and that when this happens, there is a clear hierarchy between the interests of clinicians and the interests of researchers: the former trump the latter.

The U.S. National Commission for the Protection of Human Subjects of Biomedical and Behavioral Research, which was established in the wake of significant post–World War II research calamities, recognized in its 1978 report that researchers "are always in a position of potential conflict by virtue of their concern with the pursuit of knowledge as well as the welfare of the human subjects of their research."[6] This fundamental conflict of individual investigators is the primary reason why agencies such as the National Commission recommended an independent review of research protocols by research ethics committees (RECs) or institutional review boards (IRBs). (I will use the term REC, which is the term used in the Guidelines of the International Conference on Harmonization of Good Clinical Practice. The term IRB is confusing when used in the context of private review boards.)

Financial Conflicts of Interest

The recent literature on conflicts of interest focuses nevertheless very much on the impact of financial conflicts. There is a reason why it is appropriate to focus on financial conflicts of interest and to regulate these conflicts in more detail. Financial interests are objective, fungible, and quantifiable; they can easily be measured.[7] Moreover, they can be dealt with more easily than many other types of influence that are inherent to any human endeavor. Evidence supports the claim that financial interests have an impact on the behavior of many physicians and researchers, as they do on many other people, and that such interests ought to be regulated more efficiently. Finally, the commercial boom in medical research also creates specific pressures that raise ethical and regulatory issues. Although IRB review of research protocols seemed in the 1970s an appropriate remedy for dealing with the fundamental conflict that exists in clinical research, it may no longer be sufficient to deal with different challenges to research raised in the modern research context.

The growing financial interests in drug development have led to a boom in the conduct of clinical trials.[8,9] With more drugs in the pipeline, and commercial pressure to get new medicines quickly onto the market, competition among pharmaceutical companies to find researchers and patients to participate in research has significantly increased over the past two decades. In 1998, 30,000 more physicians were involved in clinical trials in the United States than in 1988, an increase of 600%.[10] Over the same period, there was a 60% increase in the number of community-based clinical trials.[11] Community-based physicians, most often remunerated through monetary incentives, are increasingly competing with researchers based in academic institutions for access to research participants.[8] The conduct of clinical trials is shifting from the teaching hospitals of academic institutions to the offices of private physicians and contract research organizations.[9] Whereas in 1994, 63% of clinical trials were taking place in academia, in 2004 that percentage had shrunk to 26%.[12]

As a result of the boom in research activities, more participants are also involved in medical research, increasing pressures on recruitment. There are no systematic national or international data on the total number of people who participate in research, but the available information suggests that that number is large. A 2005 investigative report published in *Bloomberg Markets* states that in the United States, industry annually spends $14 billion to test experimental substances on humans and that "3.7 million people have been human guinea pigs," but this report does not contain more details as to the period covered.[13] In Canada, the Health Products and Food Branch reviewed more than 800 applications for clinical drug trials in 1998 and predicted an average 20% annual increase in clinical trials conducted in the country, which also suggests that the number of research subjects keeps climbing.[14]

Although there is no official information on how many people participate in clinical trials, the high number of drugs under development suggests that research participants are in high demand and that such research increasingly takes place in a highly competitive environment. In this environment, research participants have become a scarce and valuable commodity.[15] One industry expert stated that recruitment of participants is the industry's number one challenge in clinical research.[16]

Pressure to recruit participants exists not only because of the increase in the number of clinical trials being undertaken but also because of the competitive market environment, in which the speed of trials has significant financial implications. When an experimental drug or device has considerable medical and market potential, corporate sponsors of research and researchers themselves are under enormous pressure to ensure that the research is undertaken as efficiently and as quickly as possible. This explains why the use of financial recruitment incentives has become so important. Financial recruitment incentives are used both to stimulate patient recruitment among physicians and to entice patients or healthy research subjects to enroll in clinical trials.

At the same time, industry also is increasingly sponsoring academic research and creating closer ties to the academic research community. Corporate contributions to academic research are steadily increasing, particularly in many reputable institutions.[17] Academic research institutions are increasingly part of the competitive research environment and are thus confronted with similar issues. The growing conflicts of interest in academia raise an additional concern—the potential disappearance of a truly independent and critical academic sector that could provide a counterbalance to commercially motivated research.[18]

Various Forms of Financial Conflicts of Interest

There are various ways in which researchers can have financial interests in research. Companies and contract research organizations often pay researchers incentives to recruit patients or to recruit them more quickly. Researchers may receive significant amounts of money in the context of research. As a result, some clinicians may be tempted to engage in clinical research because of the financial rewards offered. In the year 2000, the Office of Inspector General of the U.S. Department of Health and Human Services (DHHS) issued a report documenting various recruitment activities and confirming a growing interest in the lucrative aspects of conducting clinical trials. The report illustrates, for example, how a private family practice markets potential access to its patients for Phase I to Phase IV trials to sponsors of clinical trials.[19]

Financial conflicts can also be created by industry sponsorship of research projects and research centers. Institutional conflicts of interest created by large corporate donations can affect the attitude of individual researchers within the institution.[20] Research positions often depend on ongoing industry funding. In many academic institutions, clinical researchers have to find their own source of funding for at least part of their salaries. Industry funding is often easier to obtain than funding through granting agencies. Endowed chairs, even if they are established without any conditions attached, may create an expectation that the chair and/or junior faculty positions associated with the donation of the chair will be loyal to the donor.[21]

Researchers sometimes receive research-related rewards, for example in the form of expensive research equipment, books, or payment for participation at conferences. Some become members of speaker bureaus of pharmaceutical sponsors and receive payments for lecturing, or they are indirectly rewarded by receiving nominations to paid positions on corporate and expert advisory boards.

Financial interests also are increasingly created through the provision of investments and stock. Researchers may obtain stock or other direct financial interests in a company or in a product that is developed as a result of their research. For example, researchers and institutions involved in the Canadian Stem Cell Network can receive stock in the company that has been set up to commercialize research conducted by members of the network. Researchers or their family members may also independently buy equity in the producers of pharmaceutical products that can be affected by their research.

The growing commercial interests in research are perhaps best demonstrated by an apparent increase in insider trading in the context of research. A recent study by Overgaard and colleagues seems to confirm earlier anecdotal reports that insider trading is indeed occurring in medical research.[22] The study suggests that some people with inside knowledge about ongoing research projects are treating these projects as opportunities for financial gain. Interestingly, two recent publications raise the specter of insider trading by volunteer research participants, who may obtain valuable information about the likely success of a new compound because of their involvement in the research.[23]

Concerns

Concerns about the impact of financial interests in research can be divided in two broad categories, and each of these categories can be associated with specific types of controversies. First, some controversies have highlighted how financial interests may affect the safety and well-being of human subjects by influencing the way researchers recruit subjects and how they treat subjects in the course of a clinical trial. Commercialization also may threaten the integrity of the research process, the production of data, and the publication and sharing of results. When commercial interests threaten to influence behavior in a way that affects the safety and well-being of human research subjects, the nature of the conflict is clear. It is a conflict between a secondary financial interest and the primary obligation of physician-researchers to protect the well-being of research subjects.

The impact of commercial interests on the integrity of research reveals a potential conflict between the primary duty of investigators to obtain scientifically valid results and the secondary interest of financial gain. This primary duty to conduct valid research is connected to the idea that there is, indeed, a higher calling to

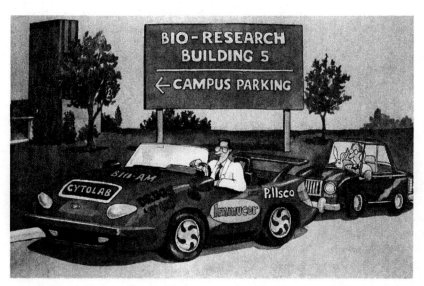

Figure 68.1. Financial Conflict of Interest (Artist's Impression). Source: Andy Myer (artist) and Bruce Agnew. Reproduced with permission.

scientific inquiry than simply providing a set of positive results. Medical research aims at contributing to scientific progress and ultimately at promoting the health and well-being of patients and of the public at large. Even within an entirely commercial research setting, it is important to recognize that there is a public purpose to the research endeavor, that of providing a safe and effective product to the public; and a public interest in making sure that financial interests do not cloud the judgment of those who have a commercial interest in the outcome of the research. When research subjects are involved, the ethical obligation of respect for persons entails an obligation to conduct research that is valid and has value.[24] Antal E. Solyom invokes statements of the American Medical Association (AMA) about the important role of physicians to ameliorate suffering and promote well-being and argues that they imply that "clinical research is a *social good.*"[25]

Financial Conflicts of Interest and the Well-Being and Safety of Research Subjects

Increased competition for access to research subjects has led to recruitment practices that can create significant conflicts of interests for researchers. Many more physicians outside academic research centers now participate in medical research—often not because of their interest in the study nor because of the intrinsic value of the study, but because of the financial rewards for recruiting patients and for participating in the research.

The fact that physicians are paid to provide service is hardly a new issue. Physicians in clinical practice are paid by patients, health insurers, or the public health-care system, generally on a fee-per-service basis. Although arguments have been made that this may create a conflict of interest, it is a fundamental aspect of clinical practice and not unique to the research setting, even if it does create problems of potential overuse. However, remuneration in the context of research takes forms different from remuneration in the clinical context. Some forms of remuneration resemble the fee-per-service model that physicians normally use in their clinical practice. Researchers are often paid the same amount as they would have earned for spending the same time with a patient or for performing the same clinical tasks, such as drawing blood, conducting specific diagnostic tests, or filling out forms. In those circumstances, the conflict of interest, although it clearly can create problems, is no different than those faced by clinicians who are paid for practicing medicine.[26] In fact, the AMA, in a general opinion on conflicts of interest, indicates that researchers' remuneration by sponsors that is "commensurate with the efforts of the researcher on behalf of the company" is acceptable.[27] The Canadian Medical Association, in a policy on interactions with the pharmaceutical industry, states that physicians ought to accept remuneration for participation in research "only if such activity exceeds their normal practice patterns," and it suggests that remuneration can replace lost income.[28]

Despite the existence of these guidelines, more significant financial incentives are frequently offered to physicians in the context of clinical research. As the DHHS Office of Inspector General reported in 2000, research sponsors are increasingly encouraging health-care professionals to recruit subjects by offering recruitment incentives—often paying for the mere fact of referring a patient to a clinical trial, usually referred to as finder's fees.[18] Finder's fees ranging between $2,000 and $5,000 per patient have

been reported in industry-sponsored research.[29] Other incentives include an extra payment for each 20 patients recruited; or, during the recruitment process, sponsors may offer bonuses when recruitment is not going fast enough, to induce competition among participating researchers. Payments may also be offered to reward researchers for managing to keep their patients enrolled in a clinical trial until the end of the trial. If part of a physician's remuneration is dependent on keeping research subjects in a trial, decisions to remove participants who are not doing well from the study can be negatively affected.

Recruitment incentives may not always be clearly identifiable. They may sometimes be hidden in general payments to physician-researchers. For that reason, it may be difficult for IRBs to evaluate whether the money offered to researchers for participating in research is reasonable in relation to what they are expected to do. Access to the research project's budget and a good understanding of its provisions are required to fully appreciate whether payments are of the nature of recruitment incentives, or constitute appropriate compensation.

When researchers have significant financial interests, there are concerns that their decisions may be influenced in a way that affects the safety and well-being of their research subjects, as well as the public at large. Delays in conducting the research can affect the profit margins of both the sponsor and the researchers, since they delay commercialization of the product. Researchers may perceive risks in the research to be less significant and may be inclined to move more quickly in trying a new compound on human subjects.

The 1999 Jesse Gelsinger case is often considered a paradigm case that highlights how significant financial interests of investigators and institutions in companies that are funding the research may be perceived as undermining the protection of the safety and well-being of human subjects in research[30,31] (see Chapter 10). In that case, the lead investigator's interests in the company involved were as high as $13.5 million, an amount that he allegedly received for his 30 % share when the company was sold a couple of years after Gelsinger's death.[31] Various other investigators, institutional officials, and the University of Pennsylvania itself also had significant financial interests. A Food and Drug Administration (FDA) letter following Gelsinger's death cited various problems with the gene transfer trial and violations of the FDA regulations.[32] The FDA alleged that inclusion criteria were disrespected, that side effects had been underreported and that the regulatory authorities and the IRB had not been adequately informed of various important events and changes to the protocol. A picture emerges of investigators who may have been all too eager to push the trial along, notwithstanding indications of significant risks, and without appropriate consent.[29] Scientific zeal or the desire for public recognition and/or academic fame for curing a disease through gene therapy may have been a contributing factor.

In fact, there is no direct and unequivocal evidence in the Gelsinger case that investigators were driven by financial interests. We cannot enter the minds of those who have such interests and therefore cannot know for sure why researchers acted the way they did. In addition, researchers may often be unconsciously influenced by the lure of monetary benefits. It is therefore impossible to establish clear empirical evidence of a *causal* relation between financial interests and the behavior of researchers or the outcome of the study.

But the extent of the financial interests in the Gelsinger case and the nature of the misconduct together clearly created a perception that the financial interests may have played a role. Not surprisingly, the death of Jesse Gelsinger fueled development of further conflict of interest policies by various regulatory agencies and professional organizations.[30] In 2000, for example, the American Society of Gene Therapy adopted a policy prohibiting researchers who are involved in obtaining informed consent, selecting participants, or clinical management of a trial from having any equity, stock options, or comparable financial arrangements with the trial sponsors.[33]

Neither the lead investigator, James Wilson, nor any of the other investigators involved was ever formally convicted for the alleged fraud and other violations. In February 2005, the FDA announced that it had reached a civil settlement with the institutions involved and with Wilson. Under the agreement, the University of Pennsylvania and the Children's National Medical Center agreed to pay a total of over $1 million. In addition, Wilson and two other investigators accepted restrictions on their research activities, including a five-year prohibition for Wilson to function as a sponsor of an FDA-regulated clinical trial.[34]

Conflicts of Interest and Research Integrity

Threats to the validity of medical research are the second major concern associated with conflicts of interest. Since 2000, various agencies and official organizations, including the DHHS, the Association of American Medical Colleges (AAMC), and the Institute of Medicine (IOM) have explicitly cited the threat created by financial interests as a reason to consider major reforms into how research is organized and reviewed.[30,35–37]

If the scientific validity of a study on which clinical practice will be based is flawed, consumers and patients can be harmed. In addition, public trust in medical research can be affected if it becomes apparent that conflicts of interest have undermined the reliability of data.

The integrity concerns can be divided into two broad categories. First, financial interests may have a subtle impact on the design of the study, the conduct of the study itself, and the interpretation of research data. Second, reports of various recent controversies reveal cases of outright manipulation and increasing control by industry over research questions and over dissemination of results through selective publication of data and ghostwriting. A detailed discussion of all of these aspects related to commercialized research exceeds the context of conflict of interest. Nonetheless, the nature of these controversies must be mentioned, to the extent that they show how some researchers have been influenced either because they have financial interests in the research or because commercial sponsors, by manipulating researchers' secondary interests, tempt them to act inappropriately.

There is a statistically significant association between source of funding for medical research and research outcome: Industry-funded studies are more likely to reach industry-friendly conclusions than studies that are not funded by industry (see Chapter 71). In addition, medical journals have a publication bias: Positive studies are more likely to be published than negative studies. This is not necessarily associated with financial conflicts of interest. Reports have shown an overall tendency of overrepresentation of positive studies in the medical literature. One recent study highlights the bias toward publication of positive results in clinical trials funded by the Canadian Institutes of Health Research.[38]

Although this reflects a general problem associated with scientific publications, industry interests may add to the problem.

The studies on the relation between funding source and outcome raise at least a perception that financial interests can affect the conduct and interpretation of research. Other secondary interests beyond financial ones come into play, such as the interest academic researchers have in reporting to their academic superiors that they obtained significant research funding, and the interest in authoring publications. Indeed, researchers may be reluctant to protest against decisions of research sponsors not to publish studies, or to present only a selected set of research results, out of a concern to keep good relations with the sponsor for the purpose of future funding.[21] They may also act on the basis of their own personal interest in obtaining easy publications and in enhancing their academic record.

The issue of authorship brings us to another phenomenon associated with the increased commercialization of medical research. Sponsors may hire medical service agencies to analyze and write up the final research results, and often offer the nearly finished manuscript as an easy publication to established academics in the field.[9] The sponsor's motive is that academic authorship gives credibility to the research and helps to get the studies published in the most respected medical journals. Academic researchers may be happy that they can add a prestigious publication to their curriculum vitae. A 1998 article in the *Journal of the American Medical Association* reported that up to 11% of articles published in six leading academic journals used ghost authors.[39] A 2003 article in the *British Journal of Psychiatry* discusses in detail the publication strategy by a medical service agency, including the use of ghost authors, for the promotion of the drug sertraline.[40]

Concerns about ghost writing and lack of access to the results of a study are at the core of another controversy surrounding selective serotonin reuptake inhibitors (SSRIs), which culminated in a lawsuit by New York State's attorney general against GlaxoSmithKline.[41,42] The company was accused of "persistent and repeated fraud" related to its alleged encouragement to sales agents to misrepresent crucial safety and efficacy information in their dealings with physicians. The lawsuit charged that in 1990, a research unit of GlaxoSmithKline had conducted several studies focusing on the safety and efficacy of its blockbuster drug Paxil for the treatment of depression in children and adolescents. While the studies revealed an increased risk of suicidality, suicidal ideation, and agitation, and did not indicate significant efficacy, the company coordinated the publication of only a selection of positive results of one of the three studies in the *Journal of Child and Adolescent Psychiatry*.[43] Authors of the article included several prominent academic researchers. The lawsuit was settled out of court after the company agreed to pay a fine and publicize research results on a publicly accessible web site.

These controversies are connected to academia and involve academic researchers. Robert Steinbrook mentions that gag clauses remain common in clinical trial agreements signed by academic investigators.[12] Under such agreements, investigators cannot analyze the data without agreement from the sponsor and cannot publish any results without obtaining the consent of the sponsor. There is no uniformity in the approach taken by various U.S.-based academic centers with respect to contractual publication agreements.[44] Many academic institutions still allow provisions that give sponsors the right to interfere in one way or another in the publication of the research results, for example, by giving them the right to draft the manuscript, control access to the data, or insert their own statistical analysis.

The phenomena of ghost authorship and publication restrictions have their place in a discussion of conflict of interest in medical research. The use of ghost authors is a clear violation of authorship guidelines of the International Committee of Medical Journal Editors[45] and of established research standards. When researchers submit themselves to publication restrictions they undermine their primary commitment to research integrity, which is among the core professional obligations of researchers. They make their primary obligation as researchers subordinate to the interests of the company that sponsors the research and to their secondary interest to add another publication to their CV.

Those who agree to become authors of a publication without any real involvement violate their primary obligation as researchers. Researchers who participate in the formulation of scientific arguments for publication normally require access to the full data and personal involvement in the analysis. If not, they can be considered to violate their primary obligation to have a full understanding of research results before participating in publication of the results. They also violate their primary obligation as researchers when they sign confidentiality agreements that put them in a position whereby they may not be allowed to publicize research results that were obtained in a trial.

Researchers fulfill other crucial functions in the research enterprise. Many are members of influential expert committees that provide advice to drug regulatory agencies or that develop clinical practice guidelines. They also often function as peer reviewers for scientific journals and write review articles describing the state of science in their area of specialization. Financial interests in companies whose profitability can be affected by their expert or review work may interfere with researchers' primary obligations in these positions. Many researchers realize this, although they may have a tendency to think that financial interests are more of a problem for other researchers than for themselves. A study on conflicts of interest among authors of clinical practice guidelines reveals that 89% of the authors of such guidelines had some form of financial relationship with companies whose interests might be affected by their recommendations.[46] When asked whether financial interests had affected the recommendations made in these guidelines, 19% of the respondents thought that financial interests had influenced their coauthors, but only 7% acknowledged that they themselves could be influenced.

One can argue also that researchers who participate in practices that undermine the integrity of medical research violate a primary commitment to society. Being able to conduct research, particularly when it involves human subjects, ought to be seen as a privilege that comes with societal obligations. Researchers have a professional commitment to conduct research with integrity and with a commitment to search for truth.

Historical Development of Remedies

Conflicts of interest can be dealt with through various means: disclosure, declaration to a hierarchical authority, regulatory review, increased monitoring, reorganization of the research setting, and outright prohibition. Disclosure is the most basic and historically most invoked mechanism to deal with conflicts of interest. The idea behind disclosure is that when people divulge the

interest they have, others can take this into consideration when judging the value of the research being conducted, the arguments put forth by researchers, or the potential impact that the interest may have on the researchers' actions.

Disclosure is used as a remedial tool at various levels. In clinical care, disclosure is seen as an important part of the fiduciary obligations of physicians. Trust is a crucial element of a fiduciary relationship, and those who are acting as fiduciaries must divulge any possible personal interest that could impact on their ability to act for the benefit of the other party.

In the context of research, there is disagreement as to whether researchers are in a fiduciary relationship with their research subjects. Support for a strict disclosure requirement based on the fiduciary relation between a physician-researcher and a patient can be found in the famous 1990 California Supreme Court case of *Moore* v. *Regents of the University of California*.[47] More recently, a U.S. district court in Florida found that a researcher who collected tissue samples to study Canavan disease did not have a fiduciary obligation toward donors and refused to recognize that researchers had an obligation to disclose their financial interests when collecting the samples; however, the court did leave open the possibility that research subjects could invoke unjust enrichment to challenge the financial gain made by researchers or sponsors based on the contribution of research subjects.[48]

But even without a clear fiduciary relationship, it seems reasonable to argue that research subjects should be informed of any significant financial interests that researchers may have.[10] The basis for this duty can be found in the ethical requirements of respect for persons, autonomy, and in beneficence.[49]

Official reports and guidance documents do not always speak in one voice. The Council on Ethical and Judicial Affairs of the AMA emphasizes that any potential commercial applications of research involving human tissue must be disclosed to subjects and that human tissue should not be used for commercial purposes without the informed consent of the donor.[50] Conversely, recent conflict of interest guidance documents issued by the DHHS and by the AAMC do not endorse a strict disclosure obligation to participants. They give institutional authorities or IRBs and RECs leeway in determining when and to what extent financial interests ought to be disclosed.[35,37] It is interesting to note that a 2004 study suggests that research subjects want to be informed of financial conflicts of interest.[51]

Disclosure is also a standard remedy to promote the integrity of the research process itself. Most established medical journals now require that authors of manuscripts submit a form in which they declare any potential conflicts of interest. The "uniform requirements" of the International Committee of Medical Journal Editors (ICMJE), an influential group consisting of the editors of the major medical journals, requires that authors disclose "all financial and personal relationships that might bias their work."[45] The Committee does not explicitly require that all conflicts also be printed, but it suggests that "[i]f doubt exists, it is best to err on the side of publication."[45] Although the most influential medical journals have taken the approach that conflicts of interest have to be explicitly declared in publications, many major science journals continue to hold that disclosure to readers is not necessary. A 2001 analysis of science and medical journals revealed that only about 13% of these journals had conflict of interest policies.[52]

Several leading medical journals have followed a more stringent conflict of interest approach for review articles and editorials, specifying that authors of such articles should have no financial ties to the producers of products or therapies that are discussed in the article, nor to their competitors. However, it tells us something about the commercialization of medical research that in 2002, the *New England Journal of Medicine* felt the need to soften its very strict "no-financial-interest" policy toward editorialists and review authors because the editors could no longer find sufficient authors without such interests, particularly in the context of clinical drug trials.[53] According to its new policy, only significant financial interests are prohibited, and less significant financial interests are evaluated on a case-by-case basis.

Disclosure is also the basis of other regulatory review mechanisms. As early as 1995, two U.S. agencies involved in medical research funding, the Public Health Service[54] and the National Science Foundation,[55] introduced regulations requiring disclosure of financial conflicts of interest in grant applications if researchers have an interest of more than $10,000 or more than 5% ownership in a commercial entity.[30] In 1998, the FDA also adopted financial conflict of interest regulations that require disclosure of equity interests of more than $50,000, and disclosure of payments to investigators unrelated to the costs of research if they amount to more than $25,000.[56]

Most academic institutions require researchers to disclose internally on an annual basis any external sources of income. While the purpose of these reporting obligations is often to verify whether employees are accepting external work that could interfere with their internal professional obligations, in the context of medical research they also aim at detecting conflicts of interest that could affect researchers' ability to be independent in their research. Several institutions have set up specialized conflict of interest committees to scrutinize whether financial interests are of such nature that they may inappropriately impact research activities. In recent reports and guidance documents, the DHHS and the AAMC endorse the establishment of such specialized committees.[35,37] In addition to emphasizing the need for IRBs or RECs to determine whether researchers with a conflict of interest should be allowed to conduct research involving human subjects, the AAMC recommends that conflict of interest committees collaborate with the IRBs or RECs and communicate information about any financial interests of researchers who submit protocols for review. The AAMC also recommends in both of its reports that conflicts of interest be subsequently disclosed by the IRB or REC to the research subjects.[36,37]

It indeed seems important that IRBs or RECs are informed of financial interests that could inappropriately affect how researchers deal with research subjects, or how they conduct the research and analyze the results, so that research subjects can be informed of these interests. In institutions where no conflict of interest committees exist, IRBs or RECs should take the initiative to collect all relevant information about conflicts of interest. Many research ethics guidelines, such as the Canadian Tri-Council Policy Statement on Ethical Conduct for Research Involving Humans, explicitly mandate the REC to evaluate conflicts of interest.[57] Inasmuch as there is sufficient evidence to support the claim that financial interests often negatively affect research, it seems appropriate to treat them as a risk factor to be taken into consideration when evaluating a protocol. After the REC has weighed each conflict of interest and has determined that it does not disqualify the researchers from conducting the research, it is also appropriate that financial interests be divulged to research subjects.[58]

Although RECs and institutional conflict of interest committees are playing an increasingly important role, there still is reason to be concerned about their ability to deal appropriately with conflicts of interest. First of all, RECs are already overburdened and understaffed. Second, in institutions without conflict of interest committees, RECs may not have members with the appropriate expertise to fully understand and appreciate the financial intricacies of research contracts and sponsorship agreements. Third, commentators have pointed out that RECs in academic centers are located within the institution in which research takes place and are staffed with people who often have close relationships with those submitting protocols for review.[30] REC members may have their own conflicts of interest, for example, when reviewing research projects submitted by their departmental superiors. In addition, their institution's growing financial interest in research may contribute to potential institutional pressure on RECs.

As pointed out earlier, the majority of clinical trials are now undertaken outside of academic institutions. These clinical trials are reviewed by private RECs. Some of these private RECs are proprietary, in other words, set up by a company to review its own research, whereas the majority are separate, for-profit ventures, set up to review research protocols in exchange for payment of a review fee. These private commercial RECs face even more substantial conflicts of interest.[59] First, they are part of the commercialized clinical trials scene and owe their very existence to a lucrative research business. They are clearly more closely connected to industry interests than are academic RECs. REC members know that the context in which they operate is a for-profit one. Members of proprietary RECs are aware that their rejection of a protocol directly affects the profit margin of the company that determines their employment. A private REC's decision to reject a protocol can have repercussions for future contracts because their revenue is based on clients' willingness to use their services. Nothing in the regulatory structure in the United States or Canada prohibits clients from going to another private REC, even with the same protocol, although drug regulatory agencies now request that they be informed of any REC review and rejection by other RECs.

Notwithstanding the fundamental conflict of interest faced by for-profit RECs, particularly in a system that does not prohibit forum shopping, drug regulatory agencies rely very much on private RECs for the review of clinical trials. Some of them have become key players in the industry. According to a *Bloomberg Markets* report, the most successful U.S. private IRB, Western IRB, reviews more than half of the new drug submissions to the FDA.[13] In light of IRBs' significant public role, the lack of tight regulation is surprising and seems inappropriate.

New Developments: Toward More Stringent and Structural Conflict of Interest Policies

More stringent as well as more structural approaches to remedying conflicts of interest have gained much support in the last decade. A common thread in many of these recommendations is a move away from reliance on case-by-case measures that focus on the integrity of individual researchers and toward more regulatory and structural interventions. This seems directly related to the realization that individual investigators' conflicts of interest have increased, and that growing commercial pressures on the research sector as a whole need to be addressed. It no longer seems reasonable to argue that conflict of interest issues can be sufficiently addressed by focusing on individual researchers in isolation and by relying on mere disclosure procedures. Various controversies in the context of drug development have highlighted the growing power of the industry to influence the conduct and outcome of research and to control the flow of information resulting from clinical research. Legislative initiatives such as the Bayh-Dole Act, as well as funding initiatives encouraging commercialization of academic research, have made it harder for individual academic researchers to avoid conflict of interest situations.[60] Remedies that focus on individual behavior do not address the underlying causes of the demise of scientific integrity and the commercial pressure on researchers and institutions.[20]

Since 2000, the need to deal with conflicts of interest more widely has been recognized explicitly by various organizations and committees. The National Bioethics Advisory Commission emphasized in its 2001 report, *Ethical and Policy Issues in Research Involving Human Participants,* that institutions ought to develop appropriate policies on financial conflicts of interests and that reliance on IRB review is insufficient.[61] The IOM in 2003 produced similar recommendations about the need for a systematic and specialized review of both individual and institutional conflicts of interest. Interestingly, the IOM report also specifically recommended that institutions develop policies to assess the conflicts of interest of IRB members.[30] The AAMC issued a report on individual conflicts of interest in 2001, followed the next year by a report on institutional conflicts of interest. In 2003, the DHHS launched a consultation process to develop new guidelines on financial relationships in research,[62] which resulted in a 2004 Guidance Document for IRBs, investigators, and institutions.[35] The Guidance Document emphasizes, as does the 2002 AAMC report, that financial conflicts of interest can create institutional pressures that have to be addressed at an institutional level.

Both the AAMC report and the DDHS Guidance Document suggest that individual or institutional financial interests in research may sometimes be so significant that the research should not take place in that institution. They further point out that institutional responsibilities for research activities should be separated from the management of the financial interests of the institution. The AAMC also clearly relinquishes disclosure as the primary mechanism to deal with conflicts of interest. The Association introduces a stringent—albeit rebuttable—presumption in the context of individual conflicts of interest that those with a financial interest in research should not participate in that research, unless the REC determines that there are special reasons why the researcher should be allowed to be involved.[36] Special reasons would include the special expertise of the researcher or specific institutional technology or knowledge that is not readily available elsewhere. Other recommended options include the establishment of special monitoring programs for both the informed consent procedures and for the conduct of research itself.

Other prominent organizations also are exploring ways to strengthen conflict of interest policies. After media reports revealed that several influential researchers at the U.S. National Institutes of Health (NIH) had significant financial interests in companies that could benefit from research undertaken by the NIH, and that systematic exceptions had been permitted to the existing conflict of interest rules,[63,64] NIH Director Elias Zerhouni proposed stringent conflict of interest regulations in February 2005, which would have significantly restricted outside activities of NIH officials with "entities substantially affected by NIH programs, policies, or operations."[65] Under the proposed regulations, NIH researchers and their immediate family members were, for example, not allowed to have any financial interests in companies whose activities could benefit from their NIH-related activities. The proposed regulations were the subject of intense debate and were criticized, particularly from within the organization, as being too stringent.[66] New standards were subsequently published in August 2005 to accommodate the expressed concerns.[67] The new standards permit certain outside activities that seemed to be prohibited under the initial proposal, such as class lectures, serving on data and safety monitoring boards, and participating in grant and peer review committees. The new standards also limit the restriction on holding financial interests in substantially affected organizations to senior NIH employees and their immediate families and allow these people to have investments in such companies that do not exceed $15,000.

Professional organizations, academia, journal editors, and health policy analysts have argued strongly for other, more systemic measures to combat some of the phenomena discussed earlier. Many of their recommendations in that context do not directly target individual conflicts of interest but rather aim to alter underlying structures and conditions under which researchers may be enticed by financial rewards or hindered by financial interests of sponsors.

Journal editors, for example, have taken several steps in an attempt to restore the credibility of scientific publications. In the past decade, most journals have introduced more detailed authorship forms, in which they explicitly ask authors to confirm that, in line with the criteria introduced by the by the ICMJE, they (1) have made substantial contributions to the conception and design, or acquisition of data, or analysis and interpretation of data, (2) have drafted the article or revised it critically for important intellectual content, and (3) have approved the final version.[45] Although this measure relies very much on the honesty of the submitting authors, it constitutes a confirmation of the importance of access to data and of genuine authorship. It forces researchers to take personal responsibility for their actions. Journals are also considering strengthening the requirements of disclosing conflicts of interest. One journal announced in 2005, for example, that authors who do not disclose conflicts of interest when submitting an article will be banned from submitting other articles in the future.

In addition to taking measures to disclose some authors' financial interests and promote genuine authorship, the ICMJE has recently endorsed a new policy requiring registration of clinical trials before the start of the trial, as a precondition for the subsequent publication of trial results in their journals.[45,68] The idea behind this requirement is that when trials are registered, it becomes harder to hide results that do not provide interesting or positive results for sponsors. The registration of clinical trials promotes openness and makes it more likely that results will be scrutinized and challenged. Transparency of the research process promotes accountability and can also put pressure on researchers to be more critical when being invited to join a research project that is coordinated or even controlled by sponsors. In addition, it may give academic authors who have participated in commercially funded research a stronger argument when they insist that the results of the study should be published.

Even before the ICMJE introduced this system as a precondition for submission, registration of clinical trials had been promoted in the United States, for example through the NIH's establishment in 2000 of a clinical trials databank: ClinicalTrials.gov.[69] In 2002, the FDA issued a guidance document imposing an obligation for all clinical trials involving serious and life-threatening diseases to be registered with this databank. This requirement notwithstanding, a recent study indicated that of 127 cancer protocols sponsored by industry that met the inclusion criteria, only 47% were in fact submitted to ClinicalTrials.gov for registration.[70,71]

Public registration of clinical trials has been recommended by various other organizations and groups. In 2005, a group of 9 research organizations and 131 international researchers signed the Ottawa Statement, which called for the introduction of a stringent, mandatory, and universal registration requirement for clinical research.[72,73]

This idea of setting up a worldwide mandatory registration system for clinical trials has been formally endorsed by the World Health Organization (WHO), following recommendations made by the International Clinical Trials Registry Platform (ICTRP), a WHO working group that consulted extensively with various stakeholders.[74] Although the research community and industry[75] agreed on the importance of introducing some form of registration, there had been significant disagreement about how much detail should be provided in this public registry and about the timing of the release of specific information about the trials, such as scientific title, primary and secondary outcomes, and sample size.[76] The ICTRP concluded that detailed registration is essential and provided an extensive list of required registration entries. Registration of clinical trials is clearly seen as a first step. A new working group is now evaluating the need to develop a registry of research results.[77]

Other commentators have called for more drastic measures to curb the potential negative impact of industry's control over medical research. Marcia Angell and Sheldon Krimsky both argue in recent books that it is crucial to separate those conducting medical research and those who have a financial interest in the outcome of the research.[17,78] They both recommend that a new drug testing agency be established that would control the development and conduct of clinical trials. The agency would determine, in dialogue with the company that submits a request, the appropriate design of a clinical trial aimed at testing efficacy and safety of a new compound. An independent accredited drug testing center would then conduct the trial and analyze the results. Although Angell and Krimsky do not elaborate on this further, it is appropriate to think about how academic research units could be involved in such a newly designed clinical trials process coordinated through a government drug testing agency. Instead of negotiating directly with industry, and thereby facilitating the use of financial incentives that can create significant conflicts of interest, academic researchers would be involved in clinical trials through an intermediate governmental structure. Various conflict of interest issues discussed above, for example those related to the use of recruitment incentives and to the phenomenon of ghost authorship, would be more tightly controlled and could likely be avoided.

Wayne A. Ray and C. Michael Stein have come up with a more detailed proposal for regulatory reform of the drug regulatory system that addresses several of the problems discussed earlier.[79] They recommend the establishment of three new independent centers: a center for new drug approval, a center for postmarketing studies, and a center for drug information. The center for new drug approval would be more independent from industry funding and would be better informed of all ongoing clinical trials. The center for postmarketing studies would fund independent studies to evaluate the long-term efficacy and safety of drugs that are introduced on the market. The center for drug information would more tightly control how research results and data are presented to the public.

Conclusion

The establishment of one or more new independent clinical trials agencies is among the most drastic measures that have been proposed to curb the impact of conflicts of interest. The proposal fits within an overall trend over the past two decades toward a more systemic approach to conflicts of interest. A new clinical trials agency would obviously not solve all of medicine's conflict of interest woes. Indeed, conflicts of interest can also exist when researchers work for government agencies. In addition, clinician-researchers have to reconcile inherent conflicting interests within clinical research. And even if an independent agency is established, industry interests in other areas of medical research will likely remain. Increased vigilance, informed by continuing empirical evaluation of the potential impact of structural relations between sponsors and medical researchers, is crucial in the context of the growing commercialization of medical research. Promotion of integrity through educational initiatives, disclosure of conflicts of interest, changes to academic evaluation criteria, and administrative review of conflicts of interest within various institutional settings remain valuable tools to improve research integrity. But the proposal for a more fundamental separation between those who conduct research and those who have an interest in its outcome reflects an understanding that the growing commercial interest in research cannot be addressed by reliance on traditional disclosure policies, review by research ethics boards, or the very divergent reporting obligations organized within academic institutions. More structural changes are needed to restore the public trust in medical research. Better regulatory control over conflicts of interest would constitute recognition of the fact that medical research is a vital activity of crucial public importance and that protecting the integrity of medical research is crucial to protect trust in medicine itself.

References

1. Eisenberg R. Patents, product exclusivity, and information dissemination: How law directs biopharmaceutical research and development. *Fordham Law Review* 2003;72:477–91.

2. Goliszek A. *In the Name of Science: A History of Secret Programs, Medical Research, and Human Experimentation.* New York, N.Y.: St. Martin's Press; 2003:79–84.

3. Jones JH. *Bad Blood: The Tuskegee Syphilis Experiment,* new and expanded ed. New York, N.Y.: Free Press; 1993 [1981].

4. Fried C. *Medical Experimentation: Personal Integrity and Social Policy.* Amsterdam, The Netherlands: North-Holland Publishing; 1974.

5. Freedman B. Equipoise and the ethics of clinical research. *New England Journal of Medicine* 1987;317:141–5.

6. National Commission for the Protection of Human Subjects of Biomedical and Behavioral Research. *Institutional Review Boards: Report and Recommendations.* Washington, D.C.: U.S. Government Printing Office; 1978.

7. Thompson DF. Understanding financial conflicts of interest. *New England Journal of Medicine* 1993;329:573–6.

8. Larkin M. Clinical trials: What price progress? *Lancet* 1999;354:1534.

9. Bodenheimer T. Uneasy alliance—Clinician investigators and the pharmaceutical industry. *New England Journal of Medicine* 2000;342:1539–44.

10. Morin K, et al. Managing conflicts of interest in the conduct of clinical trials. *JAMA* 2002;287:78–84.

11. Rettig RA. The industrialization of clinical research. *Health Affairs* 2000;19(2):129–46.

12. Steinbrook R. Gag clauses in clinical-trial agreements. *New England Journal of Medicine* 2005;352:2160–2.

13. Evans D, Smith M, Willen L. Special report: Big Pharma's shameful secret. *Bloomberg Markets* December 2005. [Online] Available: http://www.bloomberg.com/specialreport/bigpharma.html.

14. Regulations Amending the Food and Drug Regulations (1024—Clinical Trials), P.C. 2001–1042, *Canada Gazette* 2001.II.1116.

15. Lemmens T, Miller PB. The human subjects trade: Ethical and legal issues surrounding recruitment incentives. *Journal of Law, Medicine, and Ethics* 2003;31:398–418.

16. Lemmens T, Miller PB. Regulating the market in human research participants. *PLoS Medicine* 2006;3(8):e330.

17. Krimsky S. *Science in the Private Interest: Has the Lure of Profits Corrupted Biomedical Research?* Lanham, Md.: Rowman & Littlefield; 2003.

18. Brown JR. Self-Censorship. In: Lemmens T, Waring DR, eds. *Law and Ethics in Biomedical Research: Regulation, Conflict of Interest, and Liability.* Toronto: University of Toronto Press; 2000: 82–94.

19. Office of Inspector General, Department of Health and Human Services. *Recruiting Human Subjects: Pressures in Industry-Sponsored Clinical Research.* OEI-01-97–00195. Washington, D.C.: DHHS; 2000. [Online] June 2000. Available: http://oig.hhs.gov/oei/reports/oei-01-97–00195.pdf.

20. Emanuel EJ, Steiner D. Institutional conflict of interest. *New England Journal of Medicine* 1995;332:262–7.

21. Tereskerz PM. Research accountability and financial conflicts of interest in industry-sponsored clinical research: A review. *Accountability in Research* 2003;10:137–58.

22. Overgaard CB, et al. Biotechnology stock prices before public announcements: Evidence of insider trading? *Journal of Investigative Medicine* 2000;48:118–24.

23. Helft PR, Ratain MJ, Epstein RA, Siegler M. Inside information: Financial conflicts of interest for research subjects in early phase clinical trials. *Journal of the National Cancer Institute* 2004;96:656–61.

24. The National Commission for the Protection of Human Subjects of Biomedical and Behavioral Research. *The Belmont Report: Ethical Principles and Guidelines for the Protection of Human Subjects of Research.* Washington, D.C.: Department of Health, Education and Welfare; DHEW Publication OS 78-0012 1978. [Online] April 18, 1979. Available: http://www.hhs.gov/ohrp/humansubjects/guidance/belmont.htm.

25. Solyom AE. Ethical challenges to the integrity of physicians: Financial conflicts of interest in clinical research. *Accountability in Research* 2004;11:119–39.

26. Choudhry S, Choudhry NK, Brown AD. Unregulated private markets for health care in Canada? Rules of professional misconduct, physician kickbacks and physician self-referral. *Canadian Medical Association Journal* 2004;170:1115–8.

27. American Medical Association, Council on Ethical and Judicial Affairs. Conflicts of interest: Biomedical research. Opinion E-8.031. Chicago, Ill.: AMA; 1998. [Online] Available: http://www.ama-assn.org/ama/pub/category/3840.html.

28. Canadian Medical Association. CMA Policy: Physicians and the Pharmaceutical Industry (Update 2001). Ottawa, Canada: CMA; 2001. [Online] Available: www.caro-acro.ca/caro/new/caro/press/physicians_industry.pdf.

29. Goldner JA. Dealing with conflicts of interest in biomedical research: IRB oversight as the next best solution to the abolitionist approach. *Journal of Law, Medicine, and Ethics* 2000;28:379–404.

30. Committee on Assessing the System for Protecting Human Research Participants, (Federman DD, Hanna KE, Rodriguez LL, eds.). *Responsible Research: A Systems Approach to Protecting Research Participants.* Washington, D.C.: National Academies Press; 2003.

31. Gelsinger PL. Uninformed Consent: The Case of Jesse Gelsinger. In Lemmens T, Waring DF, eds. *Law and Ethics in Biomedical Research: Regulation, Conflict of Interest, and Liability.* Toronto: University of Toronto Press; 2006: 12–32.

32. Letter from Dennis E. Baker, Associate Commissioner for Regulatory Affairs, Center for Biologics Evaluation and Research, Food and Drug Administration to James Wilson, Institute for Human Gene Therapy, University of Pennsylvania. [Online] Available: http://www.fda.gov/foi/nooh/Wilson.htm.

33. American Society of Gene Therapy. Policy of the American Society of Gene Therapy: Financial Conflicts of Interest in Clinical Research. [Online] April 5, 2000. Available: http://www.asgt.org/position_statements/conflict_of_interest.html.

34. United States Attorney's Office, Eastern District of Pennsylvania. United States Attorney's Office News Release: U.S. settles case of gene therapy study that ended with teen's death. [Online] February 9, 2005. Available: http://www.usdoj.gov/usao/pae/News/Pr/2005/feb/UofPSettlement%20release.html.

35. Department of Health and Human Services. Final Guidance Document: Financial Relationships and Interests in Research Involving Human Subjects: Guidance for Human Subject Protection. [Online] May 5, 2004. Available: http://www.hhs.gov/ohrp/humansubjects/finreltn/fguid.pdf.

36. Association of American Medical Colleges, Task Force on Financial Conflicts of Interest in Clinical Research. *Protecting Subjects, Preserving Trust, Promoting Progress: Policy and Guidelines for the Oversight of Individual Financial Conflict of Interest in Human Subjects Research.* Washington, D.C.: AAMC; 2001. [Online] December 2001. Available: http://www.aamc.org/research/coi/firstreport.pdf.

37. Association of American Medical Colleges, Task Force on Financial Conflicts of Interest in Clinical Research. *Protecting Subjects, Preserving Trust, Promoting Progress II: Principles and Recommendations for Oversight of an Institution's Financial Interests in Human Subjects Research.* Washington, D.C.: AAMC; 2002. [Online] Available: http://www.aamc.org/research/coi/2002coireport.pdf.

38. Chan AW, et al. Outcome reporting bias in randomized trials funded by the Canadian Institutes of Health Research. *Canadian Medical Association Journal* 2004;171:735–40.

39. Flanagin A, et al. Prevalence of articles with honorary authors and ghost authors in peer-reviewed medical journals. *JAMA* 1998;280:222–4.

40. Healy D, Cattell D. Interface between authorship, industry and science in the domain of therapeutics. *British Journal of Psychiatry* 2003;183:22–7.

41. *Eliot Spitzer, Attorney General of the State of New York v. Glaxo SmithKline.* [Online] February 13, 2003. Available: http://www4.dr-rath-foundation.org/pdf-files/nyglax021303cmp.pdf.

42. Marshall E. Antidepressants and children: Buried data can be hazardous to a company's health. *Science* 2004;304:1576–7.

43. Keller M, et al. Paroxetine in major depression [letter]. *Journal of the American Academy of Child and Adolescent Psychiatry* 2003;42:514–5.

44. Mello MM, Clarridge BR, Studdert DD. Academic medical centers' standards for clinical-trial agreements with industry. *New England Journal of Medicine* 2005;352:2202–10.

45. International Committee of Medical Journal Editors. *Uniform Requirements for Manuscripts Submitted to Biomedical Journals: Writing and Editing for Biomedical Publication.* [Online] February 2006. Available: http://www.icmje.org/.

46. Choudhry NK, Stelfox HT, Detsky AS. Relationships between authors of clinical practice guidelines and the pharmaceutical industry. *JAMA* 2002;287:612–7.

47. *Moore v. Regents of the University of California.* 793 P.2d 479 (Cal. 1990).

48. *Greenberg v. Miami Children's Hospital.* 264 F. Supp. 2d 1064 (S.D. Fla. 2003).

49. Resnik D. Disclosing conflicts of interest to research subjects: An ethical and legal analysis. *Accountability in Research* 2004;11:141–59.

50. American Medical Association, Council on Ethical and Judicial Affairs. Commercial Use of Human Tissue, Opinion 2.08. In: AMA. *Code of Medical Ethics: Current Opinions.* Chicago, Ill.: AMA; 1998:21.

51. Kim S, et al. Potential research participants' views regarding researcher and institutional financial conflict of interest. *Journal of Medical Ethics* 2004;30:73–9.

52. Krimsky S, Rothenberg LS. Conflict of interest policies in science and medical journals: Editorial practices and author disclosures. *Science and Engineering Ethics* 2001;7:205–18.

53. Drazen JM, Curfman GD. Financial associations of authors. *New England Journal of Medicine* 2002;346:1901–2.

54. Public Health Service, Department of Health and Human Services. Title 42 (Public Health), Code of Federal Regulations, Part 50 (Policies of General applicability), Subpart F: Responsibility of Applicants for Promoting Objectivity in Research for Which PHS Funding Is Sought. [Online] October 1, 2000. Available: http://grants.nih.gov/grants/compliance/42_CFR_50_Subpart_F.htm.

55. National Science Foundation. Investigator Financial Disclosure Policy. *Federal Register* 1995;60(132):35820–3.

56. Food and Drug Administration, Department of Health and Human Services. Title 21 (Food and Drugs), Code of Federal Regulations, Part 54 (Financial Disclosure by Clinical Investigators). [Online] April 1, 2006. Available: http://www.access.gpo.gov/nara/cfr/waisidx_06/21cfr54_06.html.

57. Canadian Institutes of Health Research, Natural Sciences and Engineering Research Council of Canada, Social Sciences and Humanities Research Council of Canada. *Tri-Council Policy Statement: Ethical Conduct for Research Involving Humans,* section 4.1. [Online] 1998 (with 2000, 2002 and 2005 amendments). Available: http://www.pre.ethics.gc.ca/english/policystatement/policystatement.cfm.

58. Waring DR, Lemmens T. Integrating values in risk analysis of biomedical research: The case for regulatory and law reform. *University of Toronto Law Journal* 2004;54:249–90.

59. Lemmens T, Freedman B. Ethics review for sale? Conflict of interest and commercial research ethics review boards. *Milbank Quarterly* 2000;78:547–84.

60. Lemmens T. Leopards in the temple: Restoring integrity to the commercialized research scene. *Journal of Law, Medicine, and Ethics* 2005;32:641–57.

61. National Bioethics Advisory Commission. *Ethical and Policy Issues in Research Involving Human Participants.* Bethesda, Md.: NBAC; 2001:59. [Online] August 2001. Available: http://www.georgetown.edu/research/nrcbl/nbac/human/overv011.pdf.

62. Department of Health and Human Services. Draft: Financial Relationships and Interests in Research involving Human Subjects: Guidance for Human Subject Protection. *Federal Register* 2003;68(61):15456.

63. Willman D. Stealth merger: Drug companies and governmental medical research. *Los Angeles Times* December 7, 2003.

64. Willman D. Curbs on outside deals at NIH urged. *Los Angeles Times* August 9, 2004.

65. Department of Health and Human Services. 5 CFR 5501 and 5502: Supplemental Standards of Ethical Conduct and Financial Disclosure Requirements for Employees of the Department of Health and Human Services. *Federal Register* 2005;70(22):5543–65.

66. Resnik DB. Conflicts of interest at the NIH: No easy solution. *Hastings Center Report* 2005;35(1):18–20.

67. National Institutes of Health. Conflict of Interest Information and Resources. [Online] Available: http://www.nih.gov/about/ethics_COI.htm.

68. DeAngelis CD, et al. Clinical trials registrations: A statement from the International Committee of Medical Journal Editors. *JAMA* 2004;292:1363–4.

69. National Institutes of Health. ClinicalTrials.gov. [Online] Available: http://www.clinicaltrials.gov/.

70. Derbis J, Toigo T, Woods J, Evelyn B, Banks D. FDAMA section 113: Information program on clinical trials for serious and life-threatening diseases [poster]. Ninth Annual FDA Science Forum, Washington, D.C., April 24, 2003.

71. Turner EH. A taxpayer-funded clinical trials registry and results database: It already exists within the U.S. Food and Drug Administration. *PLoS Medicine* 2004;1(3):e60.

72. Krleža-Jerić K, et al. Principles for international registration of protocol information and results from human trials of health related interventions: Ottawa Statement (part 1). *British Medical Journal* 2005;330:956–8.

73. Ottawa Group. Ottawa Statement on Trial Registration. [Online] Available: http://ottawagroup.ohri.ca/.

74. World Health Organization. International Clinical Trials Registry Platform. [Online] Available: http://www.who.int/ictrp/en/.

75. International Alliance of Pharmaceutical Associations. Joint position on the disclosure of clinical trial information via clinical trial registries and databases. [Online] 2005. Available: http://www.ifpma.org/Documents/NR2205/joint%20position_clinical%20trials.PDF.

76. Krleža-Jerić K. Clinical trial registration: The differing views of industry, the WHO, and the Ottawa Group. *PLoS Medicine* 2005;2(11):e378.

77. Lemmens T, Bouchard R. Mandatory clinical trial registration: Rebuilding trust in medical research. In: Global Forum for Health Research, *Global Forum Update on Research for Health, Vol. 4. Equitable Access: Research Challenges for Health in Developing Countries.* London, UK: Pro-Book Publishing; 2007:40–46.

78. Angell M. *The Truth About the Drug Companies: How They Deceive Us and What to Do About It.* New York, N.Y.: Random House; 2004.

79. Ray WA, Stein CM. Reform of drug regulation—Beyond an independent drug-safety board. *New England Journal of Medicine* 2006;354:194–201.

Ezekiel J. Emanuel   Dennis F. Thompson

The Concept of Conflicts of Interest

As the practice of medicine and the conduct of biomedical research have become increasingly commercialized, the risk that financial or other similar interests could improperly influence the conduct of physicians, researchers, and other professionals has correspondingly risen.[1] This risk is at the root of the problem of conflict of interest that now confronts all professionals who seek to pursue the venerable goals of their profession while responding to the new and appealing demands of the marketplace. Prominent among the professionals who must deal with these potential conflicts are clinical researchers. Especially since passage of the Bayh-Dole Act in 1980, industry has become increasingly involved in clinical research. Commercial considerations are playing a greater role in decisions about research, even in academic and other not-for-profit institutions. In response to this growing influence of commercial interests, there has been a corresponding increase in the number and scope of regulations designed to control conflicts between these interests and the core goals of research. Despite the greater attention that conflicts of interest are now receiving, uncertainty persists about what constitutes a conflict of interest, why such conflicts should be regulated, and what standards should guide their regulation.

Brief History

In the 1970s the ability to use recombinant technologies to splice DNA and create microorganisms that produced proteins spawned the biotechnology industry. Although this development did not create the problem of conflicts of interest in biomedical research, it dramatically changed its emphasis and scope.[2] New biotechnology companies, such as Genentech and Biogen, were founded by academics to commercialize their scientific innovations. The new enterprises created more intimate links between industry and academia than had existed before. At the same time, traditional pharmaceutical companies began investing in biomedical research centers, donating large sums to academic institutions in exchange for the right to turn the discoveries into profitable applications. In 1974, Harvard Medical School signed a $23 million, 12-year agreement with Monsanto, which supported laboratory research into antiangiogenesis factors.[3] Monsanto received the rights to an exclusive worldwide license for all inventions created as part of the research it supported. Soon thereafter Harvard signed an agreement with DuPont for $5 million to support a new genetics department at the medical school. In 1980, Hoechst AG donated tens of millions of dollars over 10 years to fund a Department of Molecular Genetics at the Massachusetts General Hospital in exchange for receiving exclusive licenses for all commercially exploitable discoveries.[4]

The Bayh-Dole Act in 1980 significantly accelerated the trend toward closer links between industry and academia. The Act permitted universities and other research institutions to hold and license patents on discoveries funded with federal grants. The law stimulated large and steady increases in industry-academic collaborations . The number of patents granted to universities increased. The sources of funding for biomedical research shifted. Although earlier more than half came from the federal government, now nearly 60% comes from private industry[5] (see Figure 69.1).

There were early attempts to control the conflicts of interest to which these collaborations gave rise. After the creation of biotechnology companies closely linked with university research

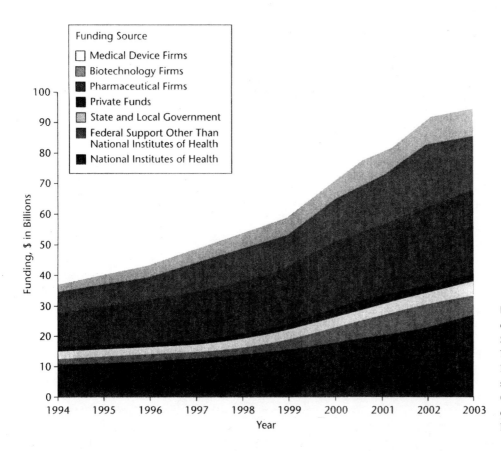

laboratories in the early 1980s, California required professors in its state colleges and universities to disclose any financial interests they had in such companies.

A major scandal at the Harvard-affiliated Massachusetts Eye and Ear Infirmary (MEEI) in 1988 gave greater prominence to the problem and stimulated further reform. An ophthalmology fellow there, Scheffer C.G. Tseng, developed a vitamin A-based ointment for dry eye syndrome, a painful condition in which the eye cannot maintain a tear film.[6,7] After preliminary positive findings, Tseng sold the rights for the treatment to Spectra Pharmaceutical Services for $310,000. At the time Tseng also owned 530,000 shares in the company, which, as an article in *Nature* noted, "hoped to market the very same vitamin A-enriched jelly that Tseng was smearing onto the eyeballs of his patients."[7] One senior physician at the MEEI who was Tseng's adviser also owned shares in Spectra and had contributed to early research on the treatment.

In a clinical trial of Tseng's treatment, the protocol was changed numerous times in ways that seemed to be dictated more by commercial than by scientific interests. For instance, the protocol had originally called for 50 patients, but 250 patients ended up being treated. After Spectra received orphan-drug status for the vitamin A treatment, it sold stock to the public, and Tseng sold some shares at a substantial profit. However, the research was beginning show that the jelly was no more effective than a placebo. Because of concerns about the changes in protocol and conflict of interest, the study was stopped and subjected to external investigation by Harvard and MEEI. Although the investigation found that no scientific misconduct had occurred and no patients had been harmed, the possibility of more serious abuse in the future had become clear. Harvard Medical School appointed a committee

to examine the risks and to propose new conflict of interest rules.[8,9]

In the mid-1980s, the leading general medical journals began requiring authors to disclose financial conflicts of interest. In 1984, the *New England Journal of Medicine* started to include notes indicating funding sources for the studies it published, as well as "direct business associations by a corporation that has financial interest in the work being reported."[10,11] The *Journal* asked authors to voluntarily submit a statement of financial interests to the editors, who would then determine whether to include the information along with the article. In 1985, *JAMA* adopted a similar policy, which was recently revised.[12] In 1988, the International Committee of Medical Journal Editors adopted a policy that requested that authors voluntarily disclose financial interests related to the article.[13]

Beginning in the mid-1990s, concerns about financial conflicts of interest among academic researchers led to the creation of new rules and the strengthening of existing rules in the biomedical research community. Some professional societies began requiring their own officers and authors who submitted abstracts to their annual meetings or articles to their journals to disclose any conflicts of interest.

Another impetus to the regulation of conflicts in clinical research came from publicity following the death of Jesse Gelsinger in September 1999 (see Chapter 10). The 18-year-old Gelsinger had taken part in an experimental gene transfer study at the University of Pennsylvania. Shortly after one of the treatments, he died. His death—the first reported death ever directly attributable to a gene transfer experiment—triggered an avalanche of revelations. There were questions about the quality of informed consent at the university. There were charges that the university had failed to promptly report both animal data showing toxicities and toxic side effects with previous patients that could have suspended, if not closed, the study.

In response to a query from the National Institutes of Health (NIH), gene transfer researchers all over the country revealed more than 650 dangerous adverse reactions they had also previously kept secret, including several deaths. In addition to these problems, the case highlighted the dangers of conflicts of interest. James M. Wilson, one of the lead investigators, had founded Genovo, Inc., a biotechnology company focused on gene transfer technologies. He and his family held 30 percent of the company's stock while Genovo supported his gene transfer research with millions of dollars a year. The university itself held 3.2 percent of the company's stock. Although the causal relationship between Wilson's and the university's financial interests and the research violations that ultimately lead to Gelsinger's death is controversial, this case prompted calls for stricter conflict of interest rules not only at the university but at other research institutions.

Soon thereafter, in a decision closely watched in medical schools throughout the country, the Harvard Medical School faculty rejected a proposal, which had been supported by some of its own prominent faculty and researchers in other schools, that would have liberalized its conflict of interest policies.[14] In October 2002, after two years of study, the Association of American Medical Colleges issued a comprehensive analysis of conflict of interest and proposed recommendations for stricter rules.[15] Other professional societies also further strengthened their conflict of interest rules.[16]

But by 2004, some observers began to worry that pressure for stronger conflict of interest rules had led to overreactions in some institutions.[17] They feared that charges of conflict of interest were being made irresponsibly, and that rules were being expanded indiscriminately. Press and congressional revelations about relationships between NIH researchers and biomedical companies led the new NIH director to propose new and tougher rules.[18] But many scientists both within and outside of the NIH criticized these rules as overbroad and draconian.[19] They cited the proposed rule that prohibited secretaries and food handlers from holding stock worth more than $15,000 as an inappropriate expansion of the idea of conflict of interest, and argued that these extreme measures would discredit the legitimate applications of the idea. They also criticized charges of conflict of interest for researchers who provided investment advice as mistaken.[20] As a consequence of these criticisms, the regulations were modified in 2005.[21]

Fundamental Elements

A conflict of interest is a set of circumstances or conditions in which professional judgment of a primary interest, such as the integrity and quality of research, tends to be unduly influenced by a secondary interest, such as personal financial gain.[22,23] Three elements of this definition require further explanation: the two kinds of interest and the nature of the conflict.

The Primary Interest

All professionals have a primary interest, which creates obligations defined by the goals of their profession. For teachers, it is to educate their students; for judges, it is to render justice; for physicians, it is to promote the health of their individual patients. The primary interest of biomedical researchers is to conduct and disseminate research that generates knowledge that can—directly or through additional research—lead to understanding of biological systems and improvements in human health.

Exactly identifying the primary interest may sometimes be controversial, but there is usually agreement that, whatever it is, it should have decisive weight in the professional decisions an individual or institution makes. An individual researcher should be primarily interested in the integrity of the research, not income or reputation, and not even the welfare of potential patients who may be affected by the research. A medical or research institution should be primarily interested in maintaining the quality of the research, not in maximizing its endowment or burnishing its reputation.

The Secondary Interest

Beyond their primary interest in the integrity of research, researchers have secondary interests, which are both professional and personal. The other professional interests include receiving recognition for their scientific contributions, obtaining grant support, mentoring research fellows, and doing their part as citizens of their research institutions.[24] In addition to their role as biomedical researchers, they may have other professional responsibilities as clinical physicians, department chairs, interviewers for medical school or residency admissions, and leaders of professional societies. Like other professionals, researchers also have personal responsibilities in such roles as parents, family breadwinners, community leaders, and political activists. From the perspective of the professional role as a researcher, all of these activities create secondary interests. None is usually illegitimate in itself, and some are even a necessary and desirable part of the professional practice of researchers. After all, research requires financial support, and profitable research can save lives. The secondary interests are objectionable only under circumstances in which they tend to have greater weight than the primary interest.

Conflict of interest rules typically focus on financial gain, not because it is more potent or corrupting than the other interests but because it is relatively more objective, fungible, and quantifiable.[22] Money can be measured, and it can be traded for other goods. In addition, monetary conflicts may be easier for people to understand and thus are more likely to undermine public trust in the research enterprise.[25] Furthermore, there is usually little controversy over whether financial interests should be secondary, and thus should not influence the integrity of a professional's judgment, whereas some other interests, such as professional reputation, might be regarded as a competing primary interest. It is therefore a mistake to object to the regulation of financial conflicts by pointing to the many other kinds of potential conflicts. Because it is not feasible to regulate most of these other interests, it is all the more important to control financial conflicts.

Financial interests come in many different forms. Financial interests that benefit the researchers personally include stock holdings and options, consulting fees, honoraria for speaking, payments for serving as an expert witness, and licensing fees if distributed to the individual researcher. The financial interests of the researcher's spouse and dependent children must also be considered. The financial rewards of a spouse who might consult for a drug company could influence the researcher's judgment.

The most common and difficult interests to regulate are not directly personal in these ways. Direct financial support for a research protocol or program and in-kind gifts, such as specialized reagents or equipment, may be useful or even necessary for the research, but if they come from sources with a strong interest in the outcome of the research, they may still be suspect. If such support constitutes only a fraction of the total funding for a research project or program, it is less problematic.

The Conflict

It is important to understand that a conflict of interest refers to a *tendency*, not an occurrence. Experience, common sense, and some psychology research data demonstrate that in certain circumstances some individuals and institutions may let secondary interests have excessive weight in their professional decisions and thereby distort their professional judgment. Rules that control this tendency, even if the threat is actualized in relatively few cases, are intended to protect against this risk. Therefore, a conflict exists whether or not a particular individual or institution is actually unduly influenced by the secondary interest. It exists if the individual or institution is making decisions under circumstances that, based on past experience, tend to lead to distortions in judgment. When a researcher owns substantial shares of stock in the company that is the sole funder of the research on a new drug, there is reason to believe that the conclusions are more likely to favor the drug, or more likely to remain unpublished. Preventing dissemination of research results can be an even more dangerous form of distortion than publication of false results, which can potentially be checked by peer review.

When there is no chance that individuals can affect a primary interest—that is, when they do not have decision-making authority regarding a primary interest—then they cannot have a conflict of interest. For example, in biomedical research, if staff members do not have authority or power to determine how a study will be designed, conducted, interpreted, or disseminated, then they do not have a conflict of interest with respect to that study.

In determining whether a conflict exists, why not consider particular decisions or cases instead of general tendencies or circumstances? First, it is usually impracticable to conduct the kind of investigation that would be necessary to determine what actually motivates professional decisions in individual cases. Second, it would often be impossible to do so. Usually there are multiple considerations that could affect judgment. For researchers, relevant considerations that influence their judgment often include the absolute and relative importance of a scientific question compared with competing projects, the speed with which the research can be accomplished, the availability and commitment of potential collaborators, and the cost of the research in terms of time and money. It is often difficult if not impossible for the decision makers themselves to determine how much various considerations affected their judgment.

Third and most importantly, citizens who are affected by the research and others to whom the researchers are ultimately accountable are often not in a position to assess the motives of researchers in individual cases. It is neither possible nor desirable that the process of research should be regularly open to the kind of invasive investigation that would be necessary to determine individual motives. We therefore need general rules to govern conflicts, even if they are overly broad and prohibit some conduct that, if it could be fully investigated, would be perfectly legitimate.

These considerations also show that the common distinctions between *potential* or *perceived* conflicts and *actual* conflicts of interest are not helpful. All conflicts of interest are potential because they refer to tendencies. And all conflicts involve perceptions or appearances because they are specified from the perspective of people who do not have sufficient information to assess the actual motivations of a decision maker and the effects of these motives on his or her judgment.

Contrasting an actual conflict with a perceived conflict leads to two opposite but equally unhelpful conclusions. First, it encourages the mistaken idea that, though perhaps one should try to avoid even the appearance of a conflict, the appearance is not as bad as the actual conflict; it is, after all, a "mere" appearance. This neglects the fact that the prohibited conflict is in fact already an appearance, a perception in the sense described above, and therefore cannot be a lesser offense simply because it is an appearance. The effect of insisting on the distinction is to undermine the basic rationale for prohibiting any conflict of interest; it makes a conflict seem not so serious unless we can point to evidence that a person was actually motivated to favor secondary over primary interests. When a researcher's judgment is *actually* distorted by acceptance of a gift or the prospect of royalties, the violation is no longer simply a conflict of interest but rather is the victory of the wrong interest. It becomes another, different kind of offense, one that may involve negligence, abuse of power, or even dishonesty and bribery.

The second unhelpful conclusion goes in the opposite direction. It encourages overly broad and excessively subjective rules, which can be used to raise questions about conduct or agreements that are perfectly proper. With a loose notion of perception or appearance, circumstances that cause anyone to be suspicious—even uninformed citizens or muckraking reporters—come to count as conflicts of interest. It is therefore important to limit conflicts to circumstances specified by rules grounded in past experience and interpreted by reasonable persons on the basis of relevant and publicly available facts. Those facts include such considerations as whether the person with the alleged conflict has decision-making authority, and the extent to which the secondary interest is related to the primary interest.[26]

Finally, conflicts should not be taken to include all the conflicting interests that researchers may confront in practice. There is a tendency to treat conflicts of interest as just another kind of choice between competing values, such as the familiar dilemmas that arise from the use of patients in research. However, in these clinical trial dilemmas, both of the conflicting interests (for example, the safety of the subjects and the integrity of the research) might be considered primary. Both have a presumptive claim to priority, and the problem is to decide which to choose. Accordingly, these are often called conflicts of commitments as distinct from conflicts of interest. In conflict of interest cases, one or both of the primary interests are assumed to have priority, and the problem is to ensure that the secondary interest—such as financial return—does not dominate. This asymmetry between the interests is a distinctive characteristic of conflict of interest problems.

Paradigmatic Examples

The classic case of a conflict of interest involves a researcher who owns stock in or consults for a pharmaceutical company, and who also serves as the principal investigator in a clinical trial evaluating whether a drug manufactured by that company is safe and effective. In such a case, the researcher's primary interest should be in designing a rigorous and valid trial, conducting the trial responsibly, collecting data thoroughly and accurately, interpreting the data objectively, and disseminating the data widely. The researcher's financial interest might distort judgments at any one or all of these stages of the process. The researcher might design a trial comparing the pharmaceutical company's drug to a competitor's drug used at a less than effective dose or designate an outcome measure that is of marginal clinical relevance; the researcher might overlook relevant outcomes or stop data collection prematurely; the researcher might overinterpret the results; and, if the study's findings are adverse, the researcher might not publish them or, if they are favorable to the company's drug, might publish them multiple times in different formats.

The case becomes somewhat more complex if the researcher does not hold stock in the company whose drug is being evaluated in the trial, but holds stock in or consults for a pharmaceutical company that produces a rival drug. Even if the trial is not a direct comparison with this competitor's drug, the researcher may still have a conflict of interest because he or she has a financial interest in having the research trial fail.

Similarly, members of institutional review boards (IRBs) or research ethics committees (RECs) can have financial conflicts of interest if they hold stock in, consult for, or receive honoraria to speak for a pharmaceutical or device manufacturer, and the IRB or REC reviews a protocol that is evaluating a drug or device made by the manufacturer. In this case, the member's primary obligation is to rigorously evaluate the ethics of the research protocol. The member's personal financial interest in the company could lead to overestimating the social value of the research, inadequately assessing the scientific validity of the design, or underestimating the risks while overstating the benefits of the research.

Conversely, individuals may have financial interests, such as owning stock in a pharmaceutical company or receiving honoraria for speaking engagements, that do not constitute conflicts of interest. If a principal investigator who conducts clinical research on vaccines owns stock in a pharmaceutical company that manufacturers no vaccines and conducts no research on vaccines, there is no conflict of interest. Without a financial interest related to vaccines, the researcher's judgment regarding the design, conduct, interpretation, and dissemination of clinical trials of vaccines cannot be distorted by any interest arising from owning the stock. The value of the pharmaceutical company's stock will not be affected by the results of the vaccine research.

Similarly, a researcher conducting a clinical trial on a drug may, without creating a conflict of interest, accept an honorarium from potential investors who wish to learn about the trial.[27] Because the honorarium is not contingent on the choice of a particular trial design or result, it is unlikely to influence judgments regarding the conduct, interpretation, or dissemination of the results. There are serious ethical and legal concerns when clinical researchers offer paid advice to investors.[28] However, these involve the risks of insider trading, breaches of confidentiality, and the exploitation of special medical knowledge for the exclusive benefit of people who are willing or able to pay. These risks are distinct from those produced by conflict of interest, though they may be equally or more harmful.

Accepting honoraria from investors should be distinguished from cases in which the researcher is paid to speak about the trial by the pharmaceutical company whose drug is being evaluated. This is obviously improper if data are presented in a biased way. But it is a conflict of interest even if the data are presented objectively, because of the circumstances.

People involved in a research trial may have financial interests that do not constitute conflicts of interest. For instance, the secretary for the principal investigator might hold stock in the pharmaceutical company whose drug is being studied by the investigator. This does not constitute a conflict of interest because the secretary has no decision-making authority over the design, conduct, interpretation, or dissemination of the research related to the drug. The secretary cannot decide what outcomes to assess, whether the results indicate the drug is clinically beneficial, or whether and where to publish a paper about the trial results. A harder case is the research fellow who has no authority but might have some power to affect the results by changing how the data are collected or analyzed.

Conflicts of interest arise not only for individual researchers but also for research institutions, including universities and affiliated hospitals. These institutions have primary responsibilities for overseeing the research conducted by their faculty Research institutions might license patents, collect milestone and royalty payments, hold stock or options in pharmaceutical, biotechnology, device, or other biomedical companies, and might receive donations or other payments from companies whose products are the subject of research at the institution. Such financial interests could induce university officials to be less aggressive in in monitoring the research conducted at their institutions.

A former university president, Derek Bok, has observed, "Universities do not come to the task [of controlling conflict of interest in research] with entirely clean hands, for they, too, may have financial interests that could conceivably bias the results."[29] He noted that the principal purpose of the consortia that some universities, such as Columbia and Duke, have formed to bid for contracts from pharmaceutical firms to test new drugs is not to support cutting-edge research, but rather to earn money. Schools that benefit from these consortia have a large stake in preserving the relationships with the companies whose products they test. "To that extent, they have an incentive to avoid results that will disappoint their corporate sponsors."[29] That they put their financial gains to other good uses does not eliminate the conflict. It may make the conflict more insidious. Furthermore, such financial interests may affect IRB or REC review, making these panels reluctant to judge industry-sponsored studies as lacking in value or having biased designs.

Purposes of Safeguards

A common criticism of conflict of interest rules is that they unfairly punish ethical researchers for the misdeeds of the few unethical ones. Rules regulating conflicts in research are a "serious insult to the integrity of scientists" who have any financial connection with industry, a prominent critic writes.[30] "To ascribe a conflict of interest automatically in such situations amounts to an assumption that the sponsor's interests have influenced the investigator . . . and that the research findings are different from what they would otherwise have been."[30] Criticisms of this kind reflect a widely held view of conflict of interest rules, but the view derives from a mistaken understanding of the purposes of the rules.

The first purpose of the rules is to maintain the integrity of professional judgment. The rules seek to minimize the influence of secondary interests, such as personal financial gain, that are irrelevant to the merits of decisions about the conduct of research. The rules do not assume that any researcher will necessarily let financial gain influence his or her judgment. They assume only that there is uncertainty about motives—that it is often difficult if not impossible to know with the required degree of confidence what has influenced decisions. Given the general difficulty of discovering the real motives on which people in complex situations act, it is safer to decide in advance to remove, as far as possible, factors that could distract anyone from concentrating on the primary goals of research.

Judging the results of decisions is not an adequate substitute for guarding against improper motives, as some commentators seem to assume. Peer review admittedly offers some protection against mistaken or fraudulent results presented for publication. But the integrity of a particular piece of published research is not the only concern. The possibility that the results of a particular research project might turn out differently because it is funded by an interested party is only one danger against which conflict of interest rules are directed. The decision not to disseminate negative results is usually not reviewed by anyone other than the researcher and the sponsor. More generally, we should also be concerned about influences on the direction of the research and the choice of topics—for example, the tendency of industry-sponsored researchers at academic institutions to put more emphasis on commercially useful research than on basic research.[31]

The second purpose of conflict of interest rules depends even less on the assumption that a researcher will produce biased results because of a conflict of interest. That purpose is to maintain confidence in professional judgment. Here the point is to minimize conditions that would cause reasonable persons to suspect that professional judgment has been improperly influenced, whether or not it has. Maintaining confidence in professional judgment is partly a matter of prudence. To the extent that the public and public officials distrust the profession, they are likely to demand greater external regulation of research, and are likely to supply fewer resources for its support. Because of these possible effects, the purpose is also distinctly ethical. Since the actions of individual researchers can affect public confidence in the whole profession, individuals have an obligation to other people—specifically, a duty to make sure that their own conduct does not impair their colleagues' capacity to conduct research.[32]

The purposes of conflict of interest rules should not be diluted by stretching the rules beyond their appropriate limits. They are not intended to capture the whole range of improper conduct in which researchers may engage. The rules do not seek to prevent other kinds of unethical conduct, such as fraud or deception, or unprofessional conduct, such as incompetence or negligence.

Standards

Standards for assessing conflicts of interest identify factors that make conflicts of interest more or less severe. The severity of a conflict depends on (1) the *likelihood* that professional judgment in the relevant circumstances will tend to be unduly influenced by a secondary interest, and (2) the *seriousness* of the harm or wrong that is likely to result from such influence (see Table 69.1).

In assessing the likelihood, we may reasonably assume that within a certain range, the greater the value of the secondary interest—the larger the financial gain—the more likely its influence on researchers' judgments. Below a certain value, the gain is likely to have no effect on judgments. This is why, for example, *de minimis* standards are appropriate for gifts. The value should also generally be measured relative to typical income for the relevant class of researchers, and relative to the scale of the research project. For instance, $10,000 in value is likely to have more effect on a research fellow with a lower income than on a senior principal investigator with a substantially larger income.

The scope of the conflict refers to the duration and depth of the relationship of the researcher and the commercial entity. Longer and closer associations increase the scope. A continuing relationship as a member of the board or chief scientific officer of a company, for example, creates a more serious problem than the acceptance of a one-time grant or gift. Consulting agreements that extend for years or honoraria that cover years of speaking are more problematic than one-time arrangements. Likewise, serving on a company's scientific advisory board, which intimately ties the researcher to the fate of the company, is more likely to affect the researcher's judgment than occasionally speaking for the company.

The extent of discretion—how much latitude a researcher enjoys in the exercise of professional judgment—partly determines the likelihood that a financial interest will influence the research. The more closely the research methods follow conventional practice, the less room there is for judgment, and hence for improper influence. Similarly, the less independent authority the professional has in a particular case, the less latitude there is for improper influence. A conflict involving a lab technician, for example, is generally less severe than one involving a principal investigator. A researcher also may enjoy less independent authority if he or she is part of a large team overseeing a research trial and is subject to oversight by a data safety and monitoring board (DSMB), rather than being responsible only for external auditing of the data collection. In assessing the extent of the researcher's discretion, however, it is important to consider the independence of other members of the executive committee, DSMB, and other oversight bodies. If some of the other individuals also have relevant financial interests, then independence of judgment might well be compromised.

In assessing the seriousness of a conflict, we should consider first the value of the primary interest: the integrity of research. The potential effects of a conflict include not only the possibility of direct harm to the research project, but also the indirect harm that results from a loss of confidence in the judgment of the individual researcher and the integrity of future research.

The greater the scope of consequences, the more serious is the conflict. Beyond its impact on the research of a particular individual, a conflict may have effects on the research of colleagues. Questions such as these should be considered: Will the fact that this drug company is sponsoring this research project tend to undermine confidence in the results of the work of other researchers in the institution? Will it undermine their ability to raise funds from other sources? Claims of academic freedom should not be allowed to obscure the fact that the actions of any

Table 69.1
Likelihood and Seriousness in Evaluating Conflicts of Interest

Standard	Considerations	Examples
Likelihood	Value of the secondary interest	• The size of the investment relative to the overall income of a researcher or an institution
		• The structure of the incentives
		• The importance to the research
	Scope of conflict	• Is the arrangement a one-time interaction or a continuing relationship? A single payment for research support is not as risky as an ongoing investment in the company.
	Extent of discretion	• How much room there is for influence of secondary factors? The greater the number and importance of researchers' judgments the higher the likelihood of conflict.
Seriousness	Value of the primary interest	• The more central the research, the more risk if there is a conflict.
		• To what degree does a conflict affect the trust in other researchers?
	Scope of consequences	• What types of harms might result for research participants, the integrity of the study, or approval of a product?
		• What are the effects on the profession as a whole, or on research funding in general?
		• Will an institution's arrangements encourage others to do the same and further erode professional standards?
	Extent of accountability	• Are the potentially harmful outcomes discoverable by others and reversible?
		• Is there review by independent researchers or an outside body?

particular researcher may substantially affect the independence or freedom of colleagues.

Institutional Safeguards

Disclosure

The most common safeguard against conflicts of interest is disclosure. Disclosure operates by giving people who may be affected by the results of the research, or who may otherwise need to assess the risks of distorted judgment, the information they need to make a decision about the integrity of the research. By knowing about the financial interest, the readers of an article or the reviewers of a research protocol can make their own decisions about the likelihood and seriousness of a distorted judgment in the conduct of the research.

The disclosure may be made to any of a variety of groups: (1) conflict of interest committees established by institutions to oversee faculty conflicts, (2) IRBs reviewing particular research protocols, (3) journal editors, (4) readers of research abstracts and journal articles and audience members at oral presentations, and (5) participants in research trials. There is wide agreement about the appropriateness of disclosure to groups 1 through 4. But even

here, there is reason to question whether the disclosures that are typically given to these groups are as accurate and complete as they should be. Some researchers evidently do not even understand the requirements for disclosure imposed by journals or even their own institutions.[33] Some institutions have established training programs to try to remedy this problem. Some journals no longer simply ask researchers whether they have conflicts of interest but prompt them to specify their financial interests in detail.

What should be disclosed? The *de minimis* level of financial interest, below which there is no need for disclosure, varies considerably. Many organizations and research institutions have adopted the levels advocated by the Association of American Medical Colleges suggesting that below $10,000 in value, disclosure is not required.[15] The U.S. Food and Drug Administration (FDA) has an even higher *de minimis* threshold for clinical researchers. Conversely, other organizations, such as the American Society of Clinical Oncology (ASCO), argue there should be no *de minimis* threshold. ASCO maintains that all financial interests, no matter their current value, should be disclosed to journal editors, readers of the society's journal and abstract book, and audience members at its meetings.[16]

As for research participants, the fifth group listed above, the requirements of disclosure are more controversial. Many people believe that research participants are entitled to information about the researcher's conflicts because they are bearing the risks of the interventions. To withhold the information is at best to treat them paternalistically and at worst to exploit them without their consent. Others argue that disclosure serves more to protect the researcher from criticism than the research participants from risks. It is merely a way of evading responsibility—shifting the burden of making the decision to the participants, who are usually not well-placed to assess the significance of any conflicts. Unlike fellow physicians and researchers reading a journal article, most participants do not have sufficient background to make independent evaluation of the disclosure. If the participants must for medical reasons participate in the research study—or if it is strongly in their interest, given their disease and other options—then the information about financial interests is not especially helpful. The disclosure may increase the anxiety of these participants and decrease the trust of the public in the research enterprise.

There are other problems with disclosure. It leaves the financial interest intact, giving the impression that the researchers are ethically approved and do not have to be further concerned about their entanglements with industry. Importantly, if disclosure to research participants is not standard, then other methods of protecting against conflict of interest become even more necessary. More generally, when disclosure only reveals a problem, without providing any guidance or means for resolving it, we should seek other ways—either as a substitute or a supplement—to deal with the conflict of interest.

In the case of institutional conflicts of interest, it is difficult to see how disclosure alone could be an effective remedy. Individual researchers are typically expected to disclose their conflicts to the institution itself through its conflict of interest or ethics committee or IRB. To whom should the institution disclose? An external body could be authorized to oversee the actions of the institution regarding any research in which it has a financial interest. But whether such a body can be truly independent and effective is questionable if, as is usually the case, the institution creates and sustains the body. Nevertheless, if the conflict of interest cannot be eliminated, and the institution's expertise is essential for the research, then the establishment of such an external body may be the best remedy, provided its members are substantially independent.

Management

A second safeguard would create procedures for managing the conflict of interest. Potential mechanisms include assigning a colleague without a conflict to obtain the informed consent from research participants, establishing an independent external audit of the data, and instituting a separate DSMB to evaluate the study's data. Why try to manage rather than prohibit conflicts? Management techniques are necessary when other safeguards, such as divestiture or blind trusts, are unavailable. Such techniques might also be preferable when the participation of the conflicted researcher is necessary for the project. For example, the inventor of a new technology, who holds a patent on it and has founded or served as a scientific adviser to a company that licensed it, may have irreplaceable skills needed in the early phase of the clinical research. Management rather than prohibition might also be appropriate when the research involves a rare disease, and the particular researcher may be in a unique position to conduct the actual research because of expertise, access to appropriate patients, or a specialized referral network.

Prohibition

Finally, prohibition may be necessary to guard against some types of conflicts. In all the types of prohibition, a researcher with a financial interest related to the research is either prevented from engaging in the research itself or required to forgo all financial gains related to the research. Prohibition must usually operate in conjunction with disclosure. We do not know what to prohibit until the financial interests are revealed at least to an ethics committee, IRB, or some other authority in a position to issue the prohibition. Unlike either disclosure or management, prohibition ensures that a financial interest cannot create a conflict of interest.

Prohibition has been used in major clinical trials. An instructive example is the post-CABG (post-coronary artery bypass graft surgery) clinical trial, a multicenter randomized, double-blind study to determine whether lowering cholesterol and antithrombotic treatments lowers the subsequent development of blockage of the venous grafts to heart arteries. The investigators and members of their immediate families in this study were not permitted to

buy, sell, or hold stock or stock options in any of the companies providing or distributing medication under study for the following periods: from the time the recruitment of patients for the trial begins until funding for the study in the investigator's unit ends and the results are made public; or from the time the recruitment of patients for the trial begins until the investigator's active and personal involvement in the study or the involvement of the institution conducting the study (or both) ends.[34]

Further, the investigators were prohibited from serving as paid consultants to the companies during the same period.

The rules also applied to "all key investigators, not just the principal investigator."[34] They provided that "people who provide primarily technical support or who are purely advisory—with no direct access to the trial participants or data—[are] not be subject to these policies unless they are in a position to influence the study's results or have privileged information on the outcome."[34] Thus the policy applied to physicians who merely enrolled patients but did not influence the design, interpretation, or dissemination of the study findings.

Other organizations that have prohibited researchers from having financial interests in their research have drawn the circle to whom the prohibitions apply more narrowly. For instance, ASCO's rules prohibit principal investigators from having any personal financial interest, such as consulting fees or honoraria or equity, in the research in which they are participating.

According to this policy, physicians who merely enroll patients in a study are not prohibited from having financial interests in the study because they do not control the design, overall conduct, interpretation, or dissemination of the research.

Conclusion

The problem of conflict of interest in clinical research has become more challenging as the conduct of the research has become more dependent on commercial support and the products of research have become more profitable for commercial enterprise. The need for a better understanding of the nature of conflicts of interest and a clearer formulation of rules to govern those conflicts are therefore even more necessary than in the past. A firmly grounded policy for regulating conflicts can support greater confidence in the profession of research and the results it produces. It can enable researchers and research institutions better to pursue their main mission It can help them to concentrate more resolutely on their primary interest in conducting research that respects the highest standards of scientific integrity as they produce knowledge for the benefit of society.

References

1. Rodwin M. *Medicine, Money and Morals.* New York, N.Y.: Oxford University Press; 1993.
2. Kenney M. *Biotechnology: The University-Industrial Complex.* New Haven, Conn.: Yale University Press; 1986.
3. Culliton BJ. Harvard and Monsanto: The $23 million alliance. *Science* 1977;195:759–63.
4. Culliton BJ. The Hoechst department at Mass General. *Science* 1982; 216:1200–3.
5. Moses H III, Dorsey ER, Matheson DHM, Thier SO. Financial anatomy of biomedical research. *JAMA* 2005;294:1333–42.
6. Booth W. Conflict of interest eyed at Harvard. *Science* 1988;242: 1497–9.
7. Shulman S. Conflict of interest over Harvard drug. *Nature* 1988;335: 754.
8. Faculty of Medicine, Harvard University. *Faculty Policies on Integrity in Science* January 2, 1992.
9. Faculty of Medicine, Harvard University. *Faculty Policies on Integrity in Science* February 1996.
10. Relman AS. Dealing with conflicts of interest. *New England Journal of Medicine* 1984;310:182–3.
11. Flanagin A. Conflict of interest. In: Jones AH, McLellan F, eds. *Ethical Issues in Biomedical Publication.* Baltimore, MD: Johns Hopkins University Press; 2000:137–65.
12. Knoll E, Lundberg GD. New instructions for *JAMA* authors. *JAMA* 1985;254:97–8.
13. International Committee of Medical Journal Editors. Uniform requirements for manuscripts submitted to biomedical journals. *Annals of Internal Medicine* 1988;108:258–65. [Online] February 2006. Available: http://www.icmje.org/.
14. Martin JB, Kasper DL. In whose best interest? Breaching the academic-industrial wall. *New England Journal of Medicine* 2000;343: 1646–9.
15. Association of American Medical Colleges, Task Force on Financial Conflicts of Interest in Clinical Research. *Protecting Subjects, Preserving Trust, Promoting Progress: Policy and Guidelines for the Oversight of Individual Financial Interests in Human Subjects Research.* Washington, D.C.: AAMC; 2001. [Online] December 2001. Available: http://www.aamc.org/research/coi/firstreport.pdf.
16. American Society of Clinical Oncology. Revised conflict of interest policy. *Journal of Clinical Oncology* 2003;21:2394–6.
17. Stossel TP. Regulating academic-industrial research relationships—Solving problems or stifling progress? *New England Journal of Medicine* 2005;353:1060–5.
18. Department of Health and Human Services. Supplemental standards of ethical conduct and financial disclosure requirements for employees of the department of health and human services. Interim final rule with request for comments. *Federal Register* 2005;70(22): 5543–65.
19. The Executive Committee of the NIH Assembly of Scientists. Prohibiting conflicts of interest at the NIH. *The Scientist* 2005;19(10):10.
20. Hampson L, Emanuel EJ. Physicians advising investment firms [letter]. *JAMA* 2005;294:1897.
21. Department of Health and Human Services. Supplemental standards of ethical conduct and financial disclosure requirements for employees of the Department of Health and Human Services. *Federal Register* 2005;70(168):51559–74.
22. Thompson DF. Understanding financial conflicts of interest. *New England Journal of Medicine* 1993;329:573–6.
23. Emanuel EJ, Steiner D. Institutional conflicts of interest. *New England Journal of Medicine* 1995;332:262–8.
24. Levinsky NG. Nonfinancial conflicts of interest in research. *New England Journal of Medicine* 2002;347:759–61.
25. Davidoff F, et al. Sponsorship, authorship, and accountability. *Lancet* 2001;358:854–6.
26. American College of Physicians. Physicians and the pharmaceutical industry. *Annals of Internal Medicine* 1990;112:624–6.
27. Topol EJ, Blumenthal D. Physicians and the investment industry. *JAMA* 2005;293:2654–7.
28. Editors. Insider trading versus medical professionalism. *Lancet* 2005;366:781.
29. Bok D. *Universities in the Marketplace: The Commercialization of Higher Education.* Princeton, N.J.: Princeton University Press; 2003.
30. Rothman K. The ethics of research sponsorship. *Journal of Clinical Epidemiology* 1991;44:S25–S28.
31. Blumenthal D, Gluck M, Louis KS, Stoto MA, Wise D. University-industry research relationships in biotechnology: Implications for the university. *Science* 1986;232:1361–6.
32. Kassirer JP. Medicine at center stage. *New England Journal of Medicine* 1993;328:1268–9.
33. Boyd EA, Cho MK, Bero LA. Financial conflict-of-interest policies in clinical research: Issues for clinical investigators. *Academic Medicine* 2003;78:769–74.
34. Healy B, Campeau L, Gray R, et al. Conflict-of-interest guidelines for a multicenter clinical trial of treatment after coronary-artery bypass graft surgery. *New England Journal of Medicine* 1989;320:949–51.

Lindsay A. Hampson   Justin E. Bekelman   Cary P. Gross

70

Empirical Data on Conflicts of Interest

The clinical research landscape changed dramatically during the final two decades of the twentieth century. Unprecedented investment in both basic and clinical research led to a six-fold increase in biomedical research expenditures. In 2001, industry funded 60% of biomedical research expenditures, compared to 32% in 1980, with industry providing a majority of funding by the mid-1990s[1,2] (see Figure 70.1). This shift in funding sources was fueled in large part by the passage of the Bayh-Dole Act in 1980.[3] The act encouraged universities and medical schools to commercialize research conducted with government funds by providing them the exclusive patent rights.[3] The potential revenues from these arrangements, combined with decreasing clinical revenues, resulted in a substantive growth partnership between academic medical centers and industry.[4]

However, the evolution in the scope and nature of clinical research has not been without controversy.[4,5] Recent media attention has increased public awareness about conflicts of interest in research.[6,7] Initial events involved individual researchers reporting difficulties with disseminating the results of their industry-sponsored research.[8,9] The deaths of several participants in research led by investigators with apparent financial conflicts of interest also raised media attention.[7,10,11] More recently, widely used drugs such as cerivastatin and rofecoxib were removed from the market because of safety concerns amid worries about whether clinical trial data were suppressed by industry sponsors.[12-16] Public trust in research has therefore waned, as prospective trial participants and clinicians have become concerned about the financial conflicts of interest inherent in industry-sponsored research.[17,18]

Industry sponsorship has been an engine of innovation; however, it has also been associated with both real and perceived ethical lapses in the conduct of research. In this chapter, we describe financial conflicts of interest (COIs), provide data demonstrating how financial COIs can promote bias, and present details about approaches for managing COIs.

Types and Prevalence of Conflicts of Interest

Three types of financial conflicts of interest can affect clinical research: project-specific, researcher-specific, and institutional.

Project-Specific Conflicts

Project-specific COIs refer to industry funding that supports the design and conduct of an individual study. The majority of clinical research conducted in the United States now involves this type of conflict, because industry sponsorship of clinical research is more than double government spending. In 2002, companies that were members of the Pharmaceutical Research and Manufacturers of America (PhRMA), the industry's trade association, spent $18 billion on Phase I, II, and III clinical trials, whereas the National Institutes of Health (NIH) spent only $8 billion (see Figure 70.1).[19,20]

The prevalence of project-specific financial conflicts also becomes apparent in reviews of published manuscripts. Recent analyses of disclosed conflicts of interest in randomized controlled trials published in leading medical journals found that approximately

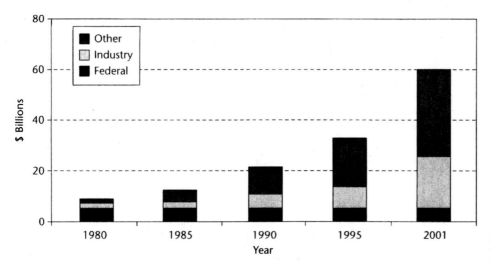

Figure 70.1. National Biomedical Research Expenditures

two-thirds of Phase III trials were sponsored either completely or partially by industry.[21-23]

Researcher-Specific Conflicts

In addition to industry support of a specific study, investigators may have personal interests in either the study sponsor or the agent being investigated. The data show that these relationships are relatively common; it is estimated that one-third of investigators at academic institutions have some type of personal financial relationship with industry sponsors[24-27] (see Table 70.1). Krimsky et al. cross-referenced a database of 789 published manuscripts with authors' affiliations and patent applications and found that 34% of manuscripts had at least one author with a financial interest.[26] Among authors of randomized controlled trials published in high-impact general medical journals, the most common types of financial disclosures appear to be employment (30%), consultancies and honoraria (22%), and grants (18%).[28] Less common types of financial ties include serving on an educational or speaker's bureau (7%) and serving on an advisory board. Notably, the financial ties that receive the most attention, namely royalties from patents (1% of conflicts) and stock ownership (7%), are actually among the least common types of ties.

Institutional Conflicts

Institutional conflicts of interest arise when institutions or institutional decision makers have financial interests that might influence or appear to influence the conduct or oversight of research involving human subjects.[29,30] The institution as a corporation may have financial interests in the form of royalty or equity interests in companies that sponsor research or whose value could be affected by ongoing research in institutional departments. Institutional decision makers, such as trustees or board members, senior officers of the institution, or members of institutional bodies responsible for research oversight—that is, institutional review boards (IRBs) or conflict of interest committees—may also have a variety of research-related financial interests, including consulting fees, speaking honoraria, corporate board membership, or equity holdings. A 2005 survey of 893 IRB members at academic insti-

tutions found that 36% reported having at least one industry relation in the past year.

The prevalence of institutional conflicts of interest has not been assessed in a systematic manner.[25,31] Only one study investigated the prevalence of equity ownership among both non-medical and medical academic institutions. The Association of University Technology Managers found in 2003 that 61% of U.S. member institutions reported forming at least one start-up company, receiving equity in 67% of start-up companies formed.[32] The prevalence of other types of institutional financial interests or personal financial ties held by institutional decision makers has not been examined.

Conflicts of Interest and Their Influence on Research

Concern about conflicts of interest in research is centered mostly (though not exclusively) on worries that such financial ties might compromise or have a negative influence on research and the way it is conducted. In this section, we will present data about the effect of financial interests on various parts of the research process: (1) research topic choice, (2) study design, (3) study conduct, (4) data interpretation, (5) data reporting and dissemination, (6) study outcome, and (7) research participant safety (see Table 70.2).

Research Topic Choice

Even before a research study is designed or conducted, critics warn that researchers could already be influenced by financial ties.[27,33,34] One study found that researchers with commercial support were significantly more likely than those without such support to report taking for-profit considerations into account when choosing a research topic (35% vs. 14%, $p < 0.001$), reporting that their choice of topic was affected "somewhat or greatly by the likelihood that the results would have a commercial application."[27] Another study, which surveyed investigators conducting research studies on antianginal therapies, found that although most researchers conducted their clinical trials because of interest in the topic, 45% of the researchers reported that they

Table 70.1

Prevalence of Conflicts of Interest

Study	Study Sample	Financial Interaction	Results
University Scientists			
Blumenthal (1996),[27] Campbell (1998)[135]	Faculty members in the life sciences at the 50 U.S. universities receiving the most funding from the NIH	Industry sponsorship of research	28% of faculty received industry research funds. 43% of faculty received research-related gifts (equipment, biomaterials, discretionary funds).
Boyd (2000)[76]	Positive disclosure forms submitted from 1980 to 1999 by faculty at the University of California, San Francisco	Consultantship, gifts, personal funds, equity interest	7.6% of faculty investigators reported financial ties with sponsors, including speaking fees (34%), consulting (33%), advisory board positions (32%), or equity (14%).
Published Manuscripts			
Krimsky (1998)[24]	Published manuscripts	Technology transfer, new venture formation	34% of articles had at least one author with a personal financial interest in the results.
Gross (2003)[28]	Published randomized controlled trials	Study funding source	37% of RCTs published in leading medical journals were industry-sponsored.
Buchkowsky (2004)[150]	Published clinical ttrials	Study funding source, author affiliation with study sponsor	Among 100 trials published in 1997–2000: 62% had sole or partial industry funding, and 66% of industry-sponsored studies had at least one author with industry affiliation.
Perlis (2005)[151]	Published clinical trials (psychiatry)	Study funding source, author conflicts	60% of 397 studies published in leading psychiatric journals in 2001–2003 received industry funding. 47% included at least one author with a financial conflict.
Ridker (2006)[152]	Published superiority trials in cardiovascular medicine	Study funding source	66% of 303 studies that were published in leading medical journals in 2000–2005 and disclosed funding source were sponsored by industry.
Institutions			
Stevens (2004)[32]	Members of the Association of University Technology Managers	Technology transfer, new venture formation	61% of institutions had formed at least one start-up company. 67% of institutions had received equity in start-up companies formed. 94% (30 of 32) of responding U.S. hospitals had formed start-up companies.
Other			
Ashar (2004)[136]	Practicing internists	Involvement in industry-sponsored trials	22% of surveyed internists in Maryland reported that they engage in industry-sponsored clinical trials.
Choudhry (2002)[137]	Professional society guideline authorship committee members		87% of guideline authors had industry relations. 58% reported industry research support. 38% served as consultants/employees.
Campbell (2006)[153]	Institutional Review Board (IRB) members at academic institutions	Financial relation with industry in the prior year	22.6% received research funding from industry. 14.5% served as a paid industry consultant. 36.2% reported ANY financial relation.

Table 70.2

The Effects of Financial Conflicts of Interest on Research

Research Process	References	Issues
Choice of topic	Massie (1984)[33]	Almost half of researchers report that they would not have conducted their clinical trials without industry funding.
	Blumenthal (1986),[34] Blumenthal (1996)[140]	Researchers with commercial support are more likely to report taking for-profit considerations into account when choosing a research topic.
Study design	Anderson (1991),[42] Cho (1996),[43] Djulbegovic (2000),[44] Kjaergard (1999),[45] Liebeskind (1999)[46]	Industry-sponsored research is of higher quality compared to nonindustry sponsored research.
	Clifford (2002),[36] Davidson (1986),[37] Djulbegovic (1999),[38] Jadad (1996),[39] Neumann (2000),[41] Knox (2000)[142]	Industry-sponsored research is equivalent in methodologic quality to nonindustry sponsored research.
	Bero (1992),[47] Rochon (1994)[48]	RCTs published in industry-sponsored supplements were generally of lower quality than those published in the parent journals.
Study conduct	CONVINCE trial (2003)[138] Apotex's deferiprone trial (1996)[8]	Case examples of trials that were stopped early for "commercial reasons."
Data interpretation	Stelfox (1998)[143]	Researchers are more likely to recommend the use of a drug if they have financial ties to industry.
	Barnes (1998)[52]	Researchers are less likely to talk about the negative effects of smoking if they have an affiliation with tobacco companies.
Data reporting and dissemination	Melander (2003),[57] Whittington (2004)[62]	Industry favorable results are more likely to be published than results not favorable to industry.
	CLASS (2000),[61] Friedberg (1999)[144]	An example of biased reporting: the CLASS study published results of only 6 months of a yearlong study in which clinical implications of the results were different.
	Chan (2004)[70]	Biased reporting is not associated with industry funding.
	Rochon (1994)[146]	Biased reporting is associated with industry funding.
	Olivieri-Apotex case (1998/99)[8] Dong-Boots case (1997)[9,66] Spitzer-GSK case (2004)[67] Bayer case (1999)[16]	Cases of industry withholding data.
	ICMJE (2004)[68]	Publication bias at peer-reviewed journals can select against publication of negative clinical trial results.
	Blumenthal (1997)[147]	Researcher publication delay associated with industry relationships and engagement in commercial activity.
Study outcome	Various[25,37,43,44,48,52,53,55,76,77,81,143,144,148,149]	Industry-funded clinical research leads to pro-industry results more frequently than nonindustry funded research.
Participant safety	Jesse Gelsinger case at University of Pennsylvania[10,11]	Case of research participant being enrolled in a study in which researchers had significant financial interests. Participant was not eligible and researchers had not notified the FDA of severe side effects experienced by prior subjects or four animals that had died after undergoing similar treatment.
	Fred Hutchinson Cancer Research Center bone marrow transplant protocol[7]	Researchers with significant financial interests enrolled participants in a study in which 80/82 participants died of various causes while participating in the study. No evidence implicating COI in patient safety.

would not have conducted their trials had they not had funding from the pharmaceutical industry.[33] Results such as these indicate that industry relationships may influence researchers in their choice of research topic.[27] However, little else is known about the influence that financial considerations or commercial viability have on researchers' choices of research topic, and there are many motives and factors that make this determination.

Study Design

To measure the methodological rigor of published trials, researchers utilize quality assessment grading systems that have evolved over nearly 45 years.[35] These comprise selected methodologic criteria addressing key components of quality, such as randomization, blinding, and predetermination of sample size.

Several studies demonstrate that industry-sponsored research appears to be of similar methodologic quality to nonindustry-sponsored research. Using various quality assessment tools, 11 studies have reported that industry-sponsored research is either of equivalent[36–41] or better[42–46] methodologic quality than nonindustry-sponsored studies. However, two studies found that randomized clinical trials (RCTs) published in industry-sponsored supplements were generally of lower quality compared with RCTs published in parent journals.[47,48]

Although methodologic grading is an important component of quality assessment, it falls short of determining a study's overall quality.[35] Evaluation of study design (that is, the relevance of the question asked or the use of appropriate control therapies) is absent from these grading systems and may contribute to bias in important but subtle ways.

Several studies have investigated the relation between sponsorship and the choice of comparison agents. Two studies found that industry-sponsored studies were significantly more likely to use inactive controls (i.e., placebo or no-therapy controls) than were nonindustry-sponsored studies.[44,45] Another study found that industry-sponsored RCTs of oral fluconazole for systemic fungal infections tended to use poorly absorbed oral drugs as comparison agents, thus favoring the success of fluconazole.[49] Finally, two reviews of clinical trials suggested that the dose of the industry-associated drug tended to be higher than that of the comparison agent in industry-sponsored studies.[50]

Data Analysis and Interpretation

Once data from clinical trials have been collected, researchers must interpret and synthesize the data. There has been some concern that researchers' conflicts of interest could bias this process within individual studies, as well as when authors collect and summarize the body of evidence in a given field. The VIGOR study of the anti-inflammatory pain medication rofecoxib (Vioxx) raised such concerns; critics have suggested that the cardiovascular risks associated with Vioxx were obscured. The analysis of cardiovascular events reportedly employed a different termination date than was used for the cardiovascular outcome, effectively removing three myocardial infarctions from the Vioxx group. Further, trial data suggesting that Vioxx was associated with important adverse events such as arterial thrombosis were not included in the study manuscript.

One study demonstrated that authors' financial ties could be associated with their interpretation of a body of evidence surrounding a specific clinical question. Stelfox et al. reviewed all studies published in 1995 and 1996 on the debated topic of the safety of calcium channel blockers to treat hypertension and ischemic heart disease and classified conclusions as supportive, neutral, or critical.[51] They found that 96% of the supportive authors had financial relationships with manufacturers of calcium-channel antagonists, as compared with 60% of the neutral authors and 37% of the critical authors ($p < 0.001$). Perhaps even more surprising, this trend held true for those researchers who had a financial interest in any manufacturer. When the results were stratified by type of financial tie, the same trend was observed for researchers receiving honoraria, support for educational programs, and research funding, but did not hold true for those researchers who served as consultants or were employed by manufacturers.[51]

Another area of research where apparent bias in data synthesis can be observed is in articles discussing the health effects related to tobacco. In one study of 106 review articles on the health effects of passive smoking, 37% of the reviews concluded that passive smoking is not harmful to health. The authors found that 94% of reviews conducted by tobaccoindustry–affiliated authors reported that passive smoking was not harmful, while only 18% of reviews conducted by non-affiliated authors reached that conclusion.[52] After controlling for article quality, the only factor that predicted a review's conclusion was whether or not the author had received funding from or participated in activities sponsored by a tobacco company (odds ratio, 88.4; 95% CI, 16.4–476.5; $p < 0.001$). Examples such as these caution that one should be concerned not only about the financial ties of researchers involved in the trials themselves, but also about the financial interests of authors who synthesize or integrate existing data to make clinically relevant recommendations.

Data Reporting and Dissemination

It has been suggested that conflicts of interest could also bias the manner in which the data are presented and reported.[52–57] Clinical research that produces results favorable to the drug or device being studied is more likely to be published than clinical research that produces results that are not favorable.[57,58] As a result, the published body of evidence available to clinicians, or to authors of clinical guidelines, would favor the industry's therapeutic agent. This problem can be further exacerbated by duplicate publications of studies demonstrating favorable outcome.[59] Conversely, adverse events associated with the experimental agent may be minimized or underreported.[60,61]

There are several recent examples of this bias, most notably in the use of selective serotonin reuptake inhibitors (SSRIs) to treat depression in children. One study conducted an analysis of 42 placebo-controlled trials of SSRI drugs submitted to Swedish drug regulators.[57] Of the 21 studies in which the experimental drug was found to be more effective than placebo, the results of 19 (90.5%) were published, whereas of the 21 studies in which the experimental drug was not more effective than placebo, only 6 (28.6%) were published. Furthermore, the data from three of the studies with industry-favorable results were published multiple times, resulting in duplicate publications; none of the studies with nonindustry-favorable results gave rise to duplicate publication.

In a second example, researchers from the United Kingdom conducted a meta-analysis of data from randomized trials that evaluated five different SSRIs against placebo.[62] The authors reviewed articles that were either published in peer-reviewed journals or unpublished and reviewed by the U.K. Committee on the Safety of Medicines. When published data alone were considered, it appeared that there was a positive risk-benefit ratio for all five of the drugs studied. However, when unpublished data were also considered, the data indicated that the risks outweighed the benefits for four out of the five drugs studied. This discrepancy raises concern, because the results of studies such as these are likely to affect the prescribing habits of doctors.[63]

However, it is unknown what caused the failure to publish results. This publication bias could be due to (1) industry withholding trial data, (2) the bias against publishing negative studies at peer-reviewed journals, or (3) researchers delaying or withholding data, whether because of a lack of interest in publishing negative results or due to the influence of industry ties.[8,9,37,58,63–65]

Industry Data Withholding

There have been several high-profile attempts by industry to prevent publication of negative data.[8,9] One such case involved Betty Dong, a researcher at the University of California at San Francisco (UCSF) who was conducting a study sponsored by Boots Pharmaceuticals to compare Boots' brand name version of levothyroxine with three competing products.[9] Dong found that the four preparations were bioequivalent; Boots blocked publication of her results, claiming that the study was flawed. A UCSF independent investigation found that the study had been conducted according to rigorous scientific and ethical standards. When Dong submitted her results for publication in 1994, Boots forced her to withdraw the study, citing a confidentiality clause in her contract. Under pressure from the Food and Drug Administration (FDA), the results were finally published in 1997.[66]

In another example, a study that surveyed leading life science companies, 56% of company representatives reported that the research conducted in universities is "often or sometimes kept confidential beyond the time required to file a patent."[27]

In 2004, New York Attorney General Eliot Spitzer sued GlaxoSmithKline (GSK), charging that the company violated New York State law by withholding negative data about one of its drugs, Paxil, used to treat depression in children.[67] Spitzer charged that GSK had conducted at least five studies on the use of Paxil in treating depression in children, yet the results of only one of those studies were published. In the studies that were not published, the results failed to demonstrate efficacy of the drug and, further, demonstrated a possible increased risk of suicidal intention. Spitzer's complaint cited a 1998 internal GSK memo, which states that the company must "manage the dissemination of these data in order to minimi[z]e any potential negative commercial impact."[67] The lawsuit was settled when GSK agreed to establish a public database including summaries of all GSK-sponsored studies involving a GSK drug.

Journal Publication Bias

In a recent statement, the International Committee of Medical Journal Editors (ICMJE) acknowledged that medical journal bias is a problem.[68] "Unfortunately, selective reporting of trials does occur, and it distorts the body of evidence available for clinical decision making," the ICMJE said.[68] It noted that at least some selection bias occurs because journal editors are "generally more enthusiastic" about publishing trials with positive results and "typically are less excited" about publishing those with negative results.[68]

Researcher Publication Delay or Data Withholding

Publication of results—including positive results—can be delayed by other factors as well. One study that surveyed over 2,000 life sciences faculty members found that one-fifth of respondents had delayed publication for more than six months during the past three years to allow for patent application/negotiation, to resolve intellectual property rights disputes, to protect their scientific lead over competitors, or to slow the distribution of undesired results.[64]

Delays in publication were associated with participation in a research relationship with industry (OR 1.34; 1.07–1.59) and engagement in commercial activities (OR 3.15; 2.88–3.41).[64] Results such as these suggest that financial relationships could lead to researchers delaying the dissemination of their research results. It must be noted that these data were collected from life science researchers and not researchers conducting clinical research.

There have, however, been examples of this reporting bias seen in the dissemination of clinical research data. One example of this is seen in the published article in *JAMA* of the Celecoxib Long-term Arthritis Safety Study (CLASS). In the published trial, which compared the use of celecoxib with traditional nonsteroidal antiinflammatory drugs (NSAIDs) in the treatment of osteoarthritis and rheumatoid arthritis, the investigators concluded that celecoxib "was associated with a lower incidence of symptomatic ulcers and ulcer combinations combined" than traditional NSAIDs.[69]

However, this conclusion was reached from an analysis that took into account only the first 6 months of data from a study that was designed for a 12-month endpoint. The complete 12-month study data—which were not published but were available to the FDA—showed no proven safety advantage for celecoxib over NSAIDs in reducing ulcer complications, a direct contradiction of the published 6-month results.[14,15] The editors of *JAMA* were not told of the complete study data at the time the article was published.[12,13] In addition, an author of an accompanying favorable editorial published with the CLASS study had not been provided with the full 12-month study data either. "I am furious. . . . I wrote the editorial. I looked like a fool. But . . . all I had available to me was the [6-month] data presented in the article," the author, M. Michael Wolfe, was quoted as saying in the *Washington Post*.[12]

Data regarding the association between differential reporting and industry sponsorship, however, show a mixed picture. In one cohort study including 99 clinical trials (half of which were industry-funded), Chan et al. looked for unreported and incompletely reported trial outcomes in these trials, comparing published trial results with study protocols and protocol amendments.[70] Although both unreporting and incomplete reporting of efficacy outcomes (71% and 92% prevalence, respectively) and harm/safety outcomes (60% and 81% prevalence, respectively) were found, there was no significant statistical association between this reporting differential and the presence of industry funding. Many studies suggest that occurrences of differential reporting are probably due to selective reporting of trial data, often due to outcomes not being statistically significant.[65,71–75]

However, other studies and case examples have found that industry sponsorship was associated with reduced reporting of unfavorable results.[12–15,56] One study, which reviewed original research articles on cost or cost-effectiveness analyses of six oncology drugs, found that studies sponsored by the investigational drugs' manufacturers were less likely than nonprofit-sponsored studies to report qualitative conclusions that were unfavorable to the drug being studied (5% vs. 38%, $p = .04$), whereas overstatements of quantitative results were not significantly different (30% vs. 13%, $p = .26$).

Regardless of why, it is apparent that differential reporting and dissemination *does* occur, and this phenomenon could explain—at least in part—the preponderance of pro-industry results among published industry-sponsored studies.[53,55]

Study Outcome

Data suggest that industry-funded clinical research leads to pro-industry results more frequently than does nonindustry-funded research.[25,37,43,44,51–53,55,56,76–81] This could be a result of several factors that have already been raised: problems related to data dissemination, study designs that favor pro-industry results, issues related to study conduct, or biased reporting of trial results.

To attempt to quantify the impact of financial conflicts of interests on biomedical research, a meta-analysis of eight articles, which together evaluated 1,140 original studies, assessed the relation between industry sponsorship and outcome in original research. Aggregating the results of these articles showed a statistically significant association between industry sponsorship and pro-industry conclusions, in that the odds of a positive study outcome were about 3.6 times higher for industry-sponsored than for nonindustry-sponsored studies (OR 3.60; 95% confidence interval, 2.63–4.91).[25] Subsequent analyses have demonstrated consistent findings among different samples of trials and after adjusting for study quality and sample size.[23,77]

However, studies such as these do not necessarily demonstrate biased or compromised studies; these data could be explained by an industry "pipeline" issue. That is, industry is likely to commit resources only to clinical research that is likely to yield positive results.[25,37,79] In addition, industry could preferentially support trial designs that favor positive results.[44]

Participant Safety

Although safety is probably the most important aspect of research, there are no data about whether financial interests compromise the safety and well-being of trial participants. This gap is mostly a result of the lack of data on the overall safety of clinical research in general. However, there have been multiple cases in which critics charge that conflicts of interest threatened the safety of research participants.

One such example is the Jesse Gelsinger case. Gelsinger, an 18-year-old research participant, died in a gene transfer study at the University of Pennsylvania in 1999. After Gelsinger's death, the FDA concluded that he had been placed on the protocol and given an infusion of genetic material despite the fact that his liver was not functioning at the minimum level required by study criteria. Additionally, the researchers had not notified the FDA of severe side effects experienced by prior subjects, nor of four monkeys that had died after undergoing similar treatment, information that the FDA claimed would have resulted in halting the study. The researchers conducting the study had significant financial ties to the company sponsoring the study. After investigations by the FDA and an outside panel appointed by the University of Pennsylvania, three of the researchers were sanctioned and two institutions were fined[10,11] (see Chapter 10).

In a second case, 83 out of 85 research subjects who were enrolled in a 12-year bone marrow transplant protocol at Fred Hutchinson Cancer Research Center in Seattle died of various causes while participating in the study; an independent investigation found that researchers and the institution had almost $300 million worth of holdings in a company sponsoring part of the study.[7,82] Although this information provoked a lawsuit charging that conflicts of interest compromised participant safety, one must be careful not to draw unsubstantiated conclusions. The individuals enrolled in this study had terminal cancers and the study was conducted over 12 years, thus it is difficult to use survival as a meaningful outcome for this type of study. In fact, the researchers were cleared of conflict of interest allegations in the lawsuit that was brought against them by some participants' families.[83,84] Thus although there have been cases in which the safety of clinical research appears to have been compromised, it is difficult to draw any concrete conclusions about whether these errors were caused by the influence of financial ties on researcher judgment, especially due to the lack of data about the safety of clinical research in general.

Protections Against Conflict of Interest

Having examined the influences that financial conflicts of interest can have on research, it is necessary to understand what sort of protections are in place. There are three main types of protection: disclosure, management, and prohibitions.

Disclosure

Disclosure of researchers' financial ties to industry is the most widely used protection. Researchers are required to disclose their financial ties to a variety of audiences, including COI and other institutional committees, journal publications, and research participants. The rationale for disclosure as a mechanism for mitigating the potential adverse effects of conflicts of interest is that end-users of the scientific data should be informed about the nature and scope of the conflicts involved with a particular study and its investigators, so that they can weigh this information when they assess the validity of the research.

Disclosure in Journals

With the rise of controversy over conflicts of interest in research, medical journals have increasingly adopted disclosure policies.[24,85] In the 1980s, some journals began implementing voluntary conflict of interest disclosure policies that encouraged researchers to disclose financial relationships and research funding; but studies published in the mid-1990s found that only about one in four journals had adopted such policies.[24,86] Although ICMJE guidelines state that the source of study support and the role of industry sponsors must be disclosed by authors, a 2003 study of 268 articles found that adherence to these guidelines was variable; overall, 89% of articles disclosed the source of study support but only 8% of industry-sponsored studies disclosed the role of the study sponsor.[28]

One study published in 1995 found that 26% of editors who participated in a survey required authors to disclose funding sources,[87] and another study found that as of 1997, only 15.8% of 1,396 scientific and biomedical journals had an explicit conflict of interest policy in place.[86]

Disclosure to Research Participants

The idea of requiring disclosure of individual and institutional COIs to research participants has attracted increasing attention.[88–90] Some bioethicists and researchers assert that such disclosures would help participants make informed decisions when considering participation in a research study and would maintain public trust and transparency in the research enterprise.[88,89,91–93] In addition, disclosure of conflicts to participants could potentially limit the extent to which researchers and institutions engage in financial relationships with industry.[89]

The 2000 revision of the Declaration of Helsinki mandates that "in any research on human beings, each potential subject must be adequately informed of . . . the sources of funding, any possible conflicts of interest, [and the] institutional affiliations of the researcher."[94] Other groups, including the American Medical Association, have also recommended disclosure to research participants.[95–98]

Although disclosure of COIs to participants may have a face validity, the strategy has been criticized as well. Some critics have expressed concern that participants may not be in the best position to interpret the disclosed information or recognize their options (other than not participating in the research study).[88,89,92] Others have suggested that disclosure to participants places responsibility on them, rather than on researchers and institutions, thereby putting the onus on the least powerful group.[89,99] Furthermore, one author has asserted that disclosure of relatively inconsequential conflicts of interest may disrupt the relationship between the physician and the patient (or the researcher and the participant).[89] However, a 2005 survey of 253 cancer trial participants found that over 90% expressed little or no worry about financial ties that researchers might have with pharmaceutical companies.[154] Additionally, the majority of respondents indicated that they would still have enrolled in the trial even if their researcher owned stock (76%) or could potentially receive royalty payments (70%).

Management

COI management strategies can be conceived of as a continuum that encompasses all strategies for reducing the impact of COI beyond disclosure and short of outright prohibition. Management of COIs can be conceptualized as an attempt to ensure the safety and autonomy of potential participants, the objectivity of science, and the transparency of the entire scientific process. There are several distinct approaches to management, including clinical trial registration, data safety and monitoring boards, independent consent monitors, and mechanisms to ensure investigator independence.

Clinical Trial Registration

There have been recent calls to implement a clinical trials registry in response to concerns about selective reporting of clinical trials. One approach to ensure access to trial data has involved reframing the concept of nondisclosure from a scientific and ethical issue into a legal one: A case filed by then New York State Attorney General Elliot Spitzer charged GlaxoSmithKline (GSK) with fraud for not disclosing all clinical trial results concerning the safety of depression medications in children. As part of the subsequent settlement, GSK developed a publicly accessible clinical trials registry containing the results of all GSK-sponsored studies.[67,100] Fewer than than three years later, the newly available GSK clinical trial registry was used as a key data source in a high-profile meta-analysis questioning the safety of the diabetes medication rosiglitazone. The validity of this analysis was questioned, in part

because it was based on the only type of data available to the authors—pooled data, rather than patient-level data that would allow for more robust statistical analysis. Large clinical trials are still underway, and the final word on rosiglitazone's safety is still to be determined. Yet this incident reinforces both the potential advantages of transparency—allowing independent assessment of drug safety—and the the disadvantages of only partial transparency. The lack of access to primary data led to decreased methodologic rigor.

The ICMJE confronted this issue in 2004, stating that "honest reporting begins with revealing the existence of all clinical studies, even those that reflect unfavorably on a research sponsor's product."[68] As such, ICMJE members agreed to adopt a clinical trials registration policy, requiring investigators to register their trials in a free public registry as a condition for consideration for publication. All clinical trials, defined by the ICMJE as "any research project that prospectively assigns human subjects to intervention or comparison groups to study the cause-and-effect relationship between a medical intervention and a health outcome," must be registered as or before participants are enrolled; this definition explicitly excludes Phase I trials that assess toxicity and pharmacokinetics.[68] The registry must include—at a minimum—the 20 criteria specified by the World Health Organization.[68] Notably, the ICMJE clinical trial registry does not require that results be included in the registry.

Institutional Conflict of Interest Policies

An important difference exists between oversight of investigator and oversight of institutional conflicts of interest. In the former case, an institutional committee oversees investigators, whereas in the latter case the institution is overseeing itself.[30] The execution of such self-regulation and oversight is challenging. Although several models have been proposed for both internal and external oversight of institutional conflicts of interest, little is known about which methods are used in practice.[2,30,101–103]

Regulatory agencies and professional societies have issued guidance documents on the management of institutional conflicts of interest.[96,104–107] Suggested strategies focus largely on ensuring a "firewall" between institutional officials who oversee research efforts and those responsible for technology transfer and investment decisions. Additionally, institutional decision makers who hold personal financial interests in matters that come under their oversight are expected to recuse themselves or divest their holdings. IRB members, who are charged by the university with overseeing research, are specifically required by DHHS (45 CFR 46.107(e))[108] and FDA (21 CFR 56.107(e))[109] regulations to recuse themselves from participating in any deliberations concerning protocols in which they have conflicting interests. However, adherence to these policies was called into question by a recent national survey of IRB members. Of the IRB members who reported having financial conflicts pertaining to a protocol that had come before their IRB, about one third indicated that they rarely or never disclosed the relationship to an IRB official.

Authorship and Accountability Requirements

In response to concerns about the integrity of publications resulting from industry-sponsored clinical research, the ICMJE in 2001 established criteria for authorship and accountability in publications reporting on clinical trials.[110] These standards require authors to reveal the sponsor's role in the study, and some journals have implemented a requirement for the responsible author to sign a statement stating that "he or she accepts full responsibility for the conduct of the trial, had access to the data, and controlled the decision to publish."[110] To ensure investigator independence, ICMJE standards also state that articles in which the sponsor had sole control over the trial data or decision to publish trial results will not be published.

Some journals have implemented more stringent requirements in order to ensure independence in data interpretation. In 2005, JAMA issued a new conflict of interest policy requiring industry-sponsored studies to give the raw study data to an independent statistician for a second, independent statistical analysis in order to be considered for publication.[63] This statistician must be given the raw study data, "along with the study protocol and the pre-specified plan for data analysis" and must "verify the appropriateness of the analytic plan and conduct an independent analysis of the raw data."[63] JAMA's policy also requires industry-sponsored studies to have at least one investigator with full access to study data who is not employed by any commercial funding source.[63]

Prohibition

Finally, the strictest protection for conflicts of interest is prohibition. Prohibitions can be against types of conflicts of interest (e.g., industry consultation is not allowed), or amounts of financial interests (e.g., cannot have financial ties that total over $10,000 per year), or can require researcher divestiture to be a part of a study or removal of a researcher from a study. For example, the NIH has implemented new policies regarding the conflicts of interest of its employees. As a result of allegations that NIH researchers allowed consulting fees to influence research decisions involving the companies' products, the Department of Health and Human Services and the Office of Government Ethics issued new conflict of interest regulations. The new policy, which stands in contrast to past policies in which ties with industry were widely accepted, includes prohibition of employment, consulting, and speaking for a *substantially affected organization* (SAO)—although exceptions can be allowed—as well as prohibitions against senior employees and their dependents owning more than $15,000 worth of stock in an SAO.[111,112]

Challenges to Implementing Effective Safeguards

Implementing policies that are effective in regulating conflicts of interest is a challenging process for both government and private institutions. The challenges include promoting consistency of conflict of interest policies and maintaining awareness and adherence to these policies.

First, although disclosure is considered the most widely used protection, there are no consistent standards for disclosure, and thus requirements vary widely between institutions and journals and often lack specificity.[25,87,125–128] One study, conducted in 2001 by the U.S. General Accounting Office (now the Government Accountability Office, GAO), examined the disclosure policies of five major research institutions and found that their rules regarding disclosure and prohibitions of financial interests differed considerably.[129] The study found that the five universities had different threshold amounts for disclosure, different disclosure

timelines, and different processes for managing disclosed conflicts of interest. Another study that examined the 100 institutions receiving the most NIH funding in 1998 found that 55% of policies required all faculty members to disclose, whereas 45% required only the principal investigator or those conducting the research to disclose.[128] This study also found that only 19% of the policies specified limits on the extent of researchers' financial ties and only 12% specified limits on the acceptable amount of delay in publication of research results.[128] The authors of this study caution that variability in conflict of interest policies could cause "unnecessary confusion among industrial partners or competition among universities for corporate sponsorship" and could ultimately weaken public confidence in university research.[128]

Second, even if institutions do have conflict of interest policies, researchers are not necessarily aware of or well informed about these policies.[128,130] For example, a survey of UCSF and Stanford researchers found that 58% were not able to accurately describe the conflict of interest policy at their institution.[130] Also, even if conflict of interest information is disclosed, the disclosed information may not necessarily be well recorded or readily available to those who need it, such as IRBs. Problems such as these indicate that research institutions need not only to implement coherent conflict of interest policies, but also to educate faculty members in order to make these policies useful.

Furthermore, data suggest that even if conflict of interest policies are in place, adherence to these policies may be deficient. One study examined adherence to the ICMJE's 1997 uniform requirements for manuscripts submitted to biomedical journals.[28,131] Only 69% of articles reporting on an industry-sponsored trial disclosed the nature of the relationship between the authors and the study sponsor, and only 8% reported the role of the study sponsor in the methods section.[28] Furthermore, only 89% of studies disclosed the source of study support as required by the uniform requirements.

Even with heightened awareness of the need for disclosure, authors may still fail to disclose to the extent required by journals. When several authors failed to disclose to JAMA in 2006 *any* potential conflicts of interest (beyond conflicts related to the study under review), the journal published letters of apology from the authors to readers and wrote an editorial response to emphasize the seriousness of this omission.[23,132]

Finally, variations in the contractual provisions within clinical trial agreements may allow industry sponsors to exert influence over industry-funded research despite the best intentioned conflict of interest policies. Clinical trial agreements are one of the legal tools by which relationships between institutions and industry are regulated. However, clinical trial agreements infrequently delineate protective provisions, such as requirements that results be published, and frequently allow for restrictive provisions, such as prohibitions against allowing researchers to share information with third parties after trial completion.[133,134] Given the heterogeneity in clinical trial agreements among academic medical centers, there is also concern that companies could "shop for" the most permissive settings in which to sponsor research.[134]

Conclusion

With the increased involvement of the pharmaceutical industry in the clinical research enterprise, financial conflicts of interest in clinical research have presented a fundamental challenge to ensuring objectivity and independence in research conduct. Financial conflicts of interest appear to be common, whether in the form of industry sponsorship of clinical research studies or through personal financial ties between researchers and pharmaceutical companies.

It is important to note that conflict of interest is not synonymous with bias. The vast majority of researchers and institutions carry on credible and ethical research regardless of whether a conflict of interest is present. However, data strongly suggest that financial conflicts can threaten the integrity of the research process through several mechanisms, such as influencing the choice of research topic, selection of control agents, research conduct, and outcome, as well as the interpretation, reporting, and dissemination of clinical research data.

In order to protect against the negative consequences of any conflicts of interest, there are three main types of protections in place: disclosure, management, and prohibitions. Recently, medical journals have been at the forefront of instituting disclosure and management policies, requiring the creation and use of publicly accessible clinical trial databases, and ensuring objectivity by the use of independent statisticians to review industry-sponsored trial data. In addition, the federal government and many professional organizations have imposed stricter regulations on the involvement and financial ties that researchers, such as those at the National Institutes of Health, can have with industry organizations.

There still remain several barriers to ensuring the independence and objectivity of clinical researchers in the face of conflicts of interest. Nationally, conflict of interest policies vary widely, and data regarding the awareness of and adherence to such policies remain less than ideal. Furthermore, contracts between clinical researchers and industry sponsors are presenting even greater challenges.

In order to avoid biased judgment of researchers and institutional decision makers, conflict of interest policies need to be augmented and made more uniform, and institutions must make sure that safeguards for preventing the negative influences of conflicts of interest are in place. The involvement of industry in the clinical research enterprise is important, but precautions must be taken to ensure that clinical research continues to be conducted in an objective and ethical manner.

References

1. National Institutes of Health. *National Institutes of Health Extramural Data and Trends.* Bethesda, Md.: NIH; 2000.
2. Moses L. Measuring effects without randomized trials? Options, problems, challenges. *Medical Care* 1995;33:AS8–AS14.
3. U.S. Congress. Patent and Trademark Law Amendments Act of 1980 (Bayh-Dole Act). Pub. L. 96–517, 96th Congress, 2nd Session, Title 35 (Patents), United States Code, Chapter 30.
4. Angell M. Is academic medicine for sale? *New England Journal of Medicine* 2000;342:1516–8.
5. Kassirer JP. *On The Take: How Medicine's Complicity With Big Business Can Endanger Your Health.* New York, N.Y.: Oxford University Press; 2004.
6. Goldner JA. Dealing with conflicts of interest in biomedical research: IRB oversight as the next best solution to the abolitionist approach. *Journal of Law, Medicine, and Ethics* 2000;28:379–404.
7. Wilson D, Heath D. Uninformed consent: What patients at the "Hutch" weren't told about the experiments in which they died. *Seattle Times* March 11, 2001:A1.
8. Nathan DG, Weatherall DJ. Academic freedom in clinical research. *New England Journal of Medicine* 2002;347:1368–71.
9. Rennie D. Thyroid storm. *JAMA* 1997;277:1238–43.
10. Check E. Sanctions agreed over teenager's gene-therapy death. *Nature* 2005;433:674.
11. Couzin J, Kaiser J. Gene therapy: As Gelsinger case ends, gene therapy suffers another blow. *Science* 2005;307:1028.
12. Okie S. Missing data on Celebrex; Full study altered picture of drug. *Washington Post* August 5, 2001:A11.
13. Egger M, et al. Value of flow diagrams in reports of randomized controlled trials. *JAMA* 2001;285:1996–9.
14. Hrachovec JB, Mora M. Reporting of 6-month vs. 12-month data in a clinical trial of celecoxib [letter]. *JAMA* 2001;286: 2398.
15. Wright JM, et al. Reporting of 6-month vs. 12-month data in a clinical trial of celecoxib [letter]. *JAMA* 2001;286:2398–400.
16. Psaty BM, et al. Potential for conflict of interest in the evaluation of suspected adverse drug reactions: Use of cerivastatin and risk of rhabdomyolysis. *JAMA* 2004;292:2622–31.
17. Kim SY, et al. Potential research participants' views regarding researcher and institutional financial conflicts of interest. *Journal of Medical Ethics* 2004;30:73–9.
18. Chaudhry S, et al. Does declaration of competing interests affect readers' perceptions? A randomised trial. *British Medical Journal* 2002;325:1391–2.
19. Pharmaceutical Research and Manufacturers of America (PhRMA). Pharmaceutical Industry Profile 2004. Washington, D.C.: PhRMA; 2004.
20. Turman R. NIH spending on clinical research; 2004.
21. Brody BA, Anderson C, McCrary SV, et al. Expanding disclosure of conflicts of interest: The views of stakeholders. *IRB: Ethics and Human Research* 2003;25(1):1–8.
22. Perlis RH, et al. Industry sponsorship and financial conflict of interest in the reporting of clinical trials in psychiatry. *American Journal of Psychiatry* 2005;162:1957–60.
23. Ridker PM, Torres J. Reported outcomes in major cardiovascular clinical trials funded by for-profit and not-for-profit organizations: 2000–2005. *JAMA* 2006;295:2270–4.
24. Krimsky S, Rothenberg L. Financial interest and its disclosure in scientific publications. *JAMA* 1998;280:225–6.
25. Bekelman JE, Li Y, Gross CP. Scope and impact of financial conflicts of interest in biomedical research: A systematic review. *JAMA* 2003;289:454–65.
26. Krimsky S, et al. Financial interests of authors in scientific journals: A pilot study of 14 publications. *Science and Engineering Ethics* 1996;2:395–410.
27. Blumenthal D. Ethics issues in academic-industry relationships in the life sciences: The continuing debate. *Academic Medicine* 1996;71:1291–6.
28. Gross CP, Gupta AR, Krumholz HM. Disclosure of financial competing interests in randomised controlled trials: Cross sectional review. *British Medical Journal* 2003;326:526–7.
29. Emanuel EJ, Steiner D. Institutional conflict of interest. *New England Journal of Medicine* 1995;332:262–7.
30. Johns MM, Barnes M, Florencio PS. Restoring balance to industry-academia relationships in an era of institutional financial conflicts of interest: Promoting research while maintaining trust. *JAMA* 2003;289:741–6.
31. Barnes M, Florencio PS. Financial conflicts of interest in human subjects research: The problem of institutional conflicts. *Journal of Law, Medicine, and Ethics* 2002;30:390–402.

32. Stevens A, Toneguzo F. Survey Summary of Technology Licensing (and Related) Performance and U.S. and Canadian Academic and Nonprofit Institutions, and Technology Investment Firms. Northbrook, Ill.: Association of University Technology Managers; 2004.

33. Massie BM, Rothenberg D. Impact of pharmaceutical industry funding of clinical research: Results of a survey of antianginal trials [abstract]. *Circulation* 1984;70(Supp1.2):390S.

34. Blumenthal D, Gluck M, Louis KS, et al. University-industry research relationships in biotechnology: Implications for the university. *Science* 1986;232:1361–6.

35. Berk PD, Sacks HS. Assessing the quality of randomized controlled trials: Quality of design is not the only relevant variable. *Hepatology* 1999;30:1332–4.

36. Clifford TJ, Barrowman NJ, Moher D. Funding source, trial outcome and reporting quality: Are they related? Results of a pilot study. *BMC Health Services Research* 2002;2:18.

37. Davidson RA. Source of funding and outcome of clinical trials. *Journal of General Internal Medicine* 1986;1:155–8.

38. Djulbegovic B, et al. The quality of medical evidence in hematology-oncology. *American Journal of Medicine* 1999;106:198–205.

39. Jadad AR, et al. Assessing the quality of reports of randomized clinical trials: Is blinding necessary? *Controlled Clinical Trials* 1996;17:1–12.

40. Bennett C, et al. Clinical trials: Are they a good buy? *Journal of Clinical Oncology* 2001;19:4330–9.

41. Neumann P, et al. Are pharmaceuticals cost-effective? A review of the evidence. *Health Affairs* 2000;19:92–109.

42. Anderson JJ, Felson DT, Meenan RF. Secular changes in published clinical trials of second-line agents in rheumatoid arthritis. *Arthritis and Rheumatism* 1991;34:1304–9.

43. Cho MK, Bero LA. The quality of drug studies published in symposium proceedings. *Annals of Internal Medicine* 1996;124:485–9.

44. Djulbegovic B, et al. The uncertainty principle and industry-sponsored research. *Lancet* 2000;356:635–8.

45. Kjaergard LL, Nikolova D, Gluud C. Randomized clinical trials in Hepatology: Predictors of quality. *Hepatology* 1999;30:1134–8.

46. Liebeskind DS, Kidwell CS, Saver JL. Empiric evidence of publication bias affecting acute stroke clinical trials. *Stroke* 1999;30:268.

47. Bero LA, Galbraith A, Rennie D. The publication of sponsored symposiums in medical journals. *New England Journal of Medicine* 1992;327:1135–40.

48. Rochon PA, et al. Evaluating the quality of articles published in journal supplements compared with the quality of those published in the parent journal. *JAMA* 1994;272:108–13.

49. Johansen HK, Gotzsche PC. Problems in the design and reporting of trials of antifungal agents encountered during meta-analysis. *JAMA* 1999;282:1752–9.

50. Heres S, et al. Why olanzapine beats risperidone, risperidone beats quetiapine, and quetiapine beats olanzapine: An exploratory analysis of head-to-head comparison studies of second-generation antipsychotics. *American Journal Psychiatry* 2006;163:185–94.

51. Stelfox H, et al. Conflict of interest in the debate over calcium channel antagonists. *New England Journal of Medicine* 1998;338:101–5.

52. Barnes DE, Bero LA. Why review articles on the health effects of passive smoking reach different conclusions. *JAMA* 1998;279:1566–70.

53. Als-Nielsen B, et al. Association of funding and conclusions in randomized drug trials: A reflection of treatment effect or adverse events? *JAMA* 2003;290:921–8.

54. Davey Smith G, Egger M. Meta-analysis: Unresolved issues and future developments. *British Medical Journal* 1998;316:221–5.

55. Kjaergard LL, Als-Nielsen B. Association between competing interests and authors' conclusions: Epidemiological study of randomised clinical trials published in the BMJ. *British Medical Journal* 2002;325:249.

56. Monette J, et al. Physician attitudes concerning warfarin for stroke prevention in atrial fibrillation: Results of a survey of long-term care practitioners. *Journal of the American Geriatrics Society* 1997;45:1060–5.

57. Melander H, et al. Evidence b(i)ased medicine—Selective reporting from studies sponsored by pharmaceutical industry: Review of studies in new drug applications. *British Medical Journal* 2003;326:1171–3.

58. Dickersin K, et al. Publication bias and clinical trials. *Controlled Clinical Trials* 1987;8:343–53.

59. Tramèr MR, et al. Impact of covert duplicate publication on meta-analysis: A case study. *British Medical Journal* 1997; 315:635–40.

60. Curfman GD, Morrissey S, Drazen JM. Expression of concern: Bombardier et al., Comparison of upper gastrointestinal toxicity of rofecoxib and naproxen in patients with rheumatoid arthritis. *N Engl J Med* 2000;343:1520–8. *New England Journal of Medicine* 2005;353:2813–4.

61. Silverstein FE, et al. Gastrointestinal toxicity with celecoxib vs. nonsteroidal anti-inflammatory drugs for osteoarthritis and rheumatoid arthritis: The CLASS study: A randomized controlled trial. Celecoxib Long-Term Arthritis Safety Study. *JAMA* 2000; 284:1247–55.

62. Whittington CJ, et al. Selective serotonin reuptake inhibitors in childhood depression: Systematic review of published versus unpublished data. *Lancet* 2004;363:1341–5.

63. Fontanarosa PB, Flanagin A, DeAngelis CD. Reporting conflicts of interest, financial aspects of research, and role of sponsors in funded studies. *JAMA* 2005;294:110–1.

64. Campbell E, Weissman J, Blumenthal D. Relationship between market competition and activities and attitudes of medical school faculty. *JAMA* 1997;278:222–6.

65. Krzyzanowska MK, Pintilie M, Tannock IF. Factors associated with failure to publish large randomized trials presented at an oncology meeting. *JAMA* 2003;290:495–501.

66. Dong BJ, et al. Bioequivalence of generic and brand-name levothyroxine products in the treatment of hypothyroidism. *JAMA* 1997;277:1205–13.

67. Office of New York State Attorney General Eliot Spitzer. Settlement sets new standard for release of drug information. Albany, N.Y.: Department of Law, New York State Capitol; 2004. [Online] August 24, 2004. Available: http://www.oag.state.ny.us/press/2004/aug/aug26a_04.html.

68. DeAngelis CD, et al. Clinical trial registration: A statement from the International Committee of Medical Journal Editors. *JAMA* 2004;292:1363–4.

69. Silverstein FE, Faich G, Goldstein JL, et al. Gastrointestinal toxicity with celecoxib vs. nonsteroidal anti-inflammatory drugs for osteoarthritis and rheumatoid arthritis. The CLASS study: A Randomized Controlled Trial. *JAMA* 2000;284:1247–55.

70. Chan AW, et al. Empirical evidence for selective reporting of outcomes in randomized trials: Comparison of protocols to published articles. *JAMA* 2004;291:2457–65.

71. Hahn S, Williamson PR, Hutton JL. Investigation of within-study selective reporting in clinical research: Follow-up of applications submitted to a local research ethics committee. *Journal of Evaluation in Clinical Practice* 2002;8:353–9.

72. Hahn S, et al. Assessing the potential for bias in meta-analysis due to selective reporting of subgroup analyses within studies. *Statistics in Medicine* 2000;19:3325–36.

73. Williamson PR, et al. Individual patient data meta-analysis of randomized anti-epileptic drug monotherapy trials. *Journal of Evaluation in Clinical Practice* 2000;6:205–14.

74. Mills JL. Data torturing. *New England Journal of Medicine* 1993; 329:1196–9.

75. Pocock SJ, Hughes MD, Lee RJ. Statistical problems in the reporting of clinical trials: A survey of three medical journals. *New England Journal of Medicine* 1987;317:426–32.

76. Boyd EA, Bero LA. Assessing faculty financial relationships with industry: A case study. *JAMA* 2000;284:2209–14.

77. Bhandari M, et al. Association between industry funding and statistically significant pro-industry findings in medical and surgical randomized trials. *Canadian Medical Association Journal* 2004; 170:477–80.

78. Yaphe J, et al. The association between funding by commercial interests and study outcome in randomized controlled trials. *Family Practice* 2001;18:565–8.

79. Friedberg M, et al. Evaluation of conflict of interest in economic analyses of new drugs used in oncology. *JAMA* 1999;282: 1453–7.

80. Turner N, et al. Cancer in old age—Is it inadequately investigated and treated? *British Medical Journal* 1999;319:309–12.

81. Swaen GM, Meijers JM. Influence of design characteristics on the outcome of retrospective cohort studies. *British Journal of Industrial Medicine* 1988;45:624–9.

82. Marshall E. Clinical research; Fred Hutchinson Center under fire. *Science* 2001;292:25.

83. Stromberg I. Clinical trials beat the rap. *Wall Street Journal* Apr. 12, 2004:A18.

84. Marshall E. Hutchinson's Mixed Win. *Science* 2004;304:371.

85. van Kolfschooten F. Conflicts of interest: Can you believe what you read? *Nature* 2002;416:360–3.

86. Krimsky S, Rothenberg L. Conflict of interest policies in science and medical journals: Editorial practices and author disclosures. *Science and Engineering Ethics* 2001;7:205–18.

87. Wilkes MS, Kravitz RL. Policies, practices, and attitudes of North American medical journal editors. *Journal of General Internal Medicine* 1995;10:443–50.

88. Lawton MP, Brody EM. Assessment of older people: Self-maintaining and instrumental activities of daily living. *Gerontologist* 1969;9: 179–86.

89. Foster RS. Conflicts of interest: Recognition, disclosure, and management. *Journal of the American College of Surgeons* 2003;196: 505–17.

90. Finkel MJ. Should informed consent include information on how research is funded? *IRB: A Review of Human Subjects Research* 1991;13(5):1–3.

91. de Lissovoy G, et al. Cost for inpatient care of venous thrombosis: A trial of enoxaparin vs. standard heparin. *Archives of Internal Medicine* 2000;160:3160–5.

92. Jellinek MS, Levine RJ. IRBs and pharmaceutical company funding of research. *IRB: A Review of Human Subjects Research* 1982;4(8): 9–10.

93. Roizen R. Why I oppose drug company payment of physician/ investigators on a per patient/subject basis. *IRB: A Review of Human Subjects Research* 1988;10(1):9–10.

94. World Medical Association. *Declaration of Helsinki: Ethical Principles for Medical Research Involving Human Subjects.* Tokyo, Japan: WMA; October 2004. [Online] 2004. Available: http://www.wma.net/e/ policy/b3.htm.

95. Association of American Medical Colleges, Task Force on Financial Conflicts of Interest in Clinical Research. *Protecting Subjects, Preserving Trust, Promoting Progress: Policy and Guidelines for the Oversight of Individual Financial Interests in Human Subjects Research.* Washington, D.C.: AAMC; 2001. [Online] December 2001. Available: http://www.aamc.org/research/coi/firstreport.pdf.

96. Task Force on Research Accountability, Association of American Universities. *Report on Individual and Institutional Financial Conflict of Interest.* Washington, D.C.: AAU; 2001. [Online] Available: http:// www.aau.edu/research/COI.01.pdf.

97. Council on Ethical and Judicial Affairs, American Medical Association. Managing conflicts of interest in the conduct of clinical trials. Chicago, Ill.: American Medical Association; 2000.

98. Department of Health and Human Services. Financial Relationships and Interests in Research Involving Human Subjects: Guidance for Human Subject Protection. *Federal Register* 2003;68(61): 15456–60.

99. Angell M. Remarks of Marcia Angell, M.D., in HHS Conference on Financial Conflicts of Interest, 2000. Bethesda, Md., August 26.

100. Gibson L. GlaxoSmithKline to publish clinical trials after US lawsuit. *British Medical Journal* 2004;328:1513.

101. Martin JB, Kasper DL. In whose best interest? Breaching the academic-industrial wall. *New England Journal of Medicine* 2000;343:1646–9.

102. Gelijns AC, Thier SO. Medical innovation and institutional interdependence: Rethinking university-industry connections. *JAMA* 2002;287:72–7.

103. Duval G. Institutional conflicts of interest: Protecting human subjects, scientific integrity, and institutional accountability. *Journal of Law, Medicine, and Ethics* 2004;32:613–25.

104. Association of American Medical Colleges, Task Force on Financial Conflicts of Interest in Clinical Research. *Protecting Subjects, Preserving Trust, Promoting Progress II: Principles and Recommendations for Oversight of an Institution's Financial Interests in Human Subjects Research.* Washington, D.C.: AAMC; 2002. [Online] Available: http://www.aamc.org/research/coi/2002coireport.pdf.

105. Pharmaceutical Research and Manufacturers of America (PhRMA). PhRMA Principles on Conduct of Clinical Trials and Communication of Clinical Trial Results. [Online] 2002 (revised June 2004). Available: http://www.phrma.org/files/Clinical%20Trials.pdf.

106. Office of Human Research Protections, Department of Health and Human Services. Draft Interim Guidance: Financial Relationships in Clinical Research: Issues for Institutions, Clinical Investigators, and IRBs to Consider When Dealing With Issues of Financial Interests and Human Subjects Protection. Bethesda, Md.: OHRP; 2001.

107. National Human Research Protections Advisory Committee, Letter to the Honorable Tommy G. Thompson, Secretary of Health and Human Services, Re: HHS Draft Interim Guidance: Financial Relationships in Clinical Research: Issues for Institutions, Clinical Investigators and IRBs to Consider When Dealing With Issues of Financial Interests and Human Subject Protection, 2001.

108. Department of Health and Human Services, National Institutes of Health, and Office for Human Research Protections. The Common Rule, Title 45 (Public Welfare), Code of Federal Regulations, Part 46 (Protection of Human Subjects). [Online] June 23, 2005. Available: http://www.hhs.gov/ohrp/humansubjects/guidance/45cfr46.htm.

109. Food and Drug Administration, Department of Health and Human Services. Title 21 (Food and Drugs), Code of Federal Regulations, Part 56 (Institutional Review Boards). [Online] April 1, 2006. Available: http://www.gpo.gov/nara/cfr/waisidx_06/21cfr56_06 .html.

110. Davidoff F, et al. Sponsorship, authorship, and accountability. *Lancet* 2001;358:854–6.

111. Steinbrook R. Protecting research subjects—The crisis at Johns Hopkins. *New England Journal of Medicine* 2002;346:716–20.

112. Department of Health and Human Services. 5 CFR Parts 5501 and 5502. Supplemental Standards of Ethical Conduct and Financial Disclosure Requirements for Employees of the Department of Health and Human Services; Interim final rule with request for comments. *Federal Register* 2005;70(22):5543–65.

113. Leith CP, et al. Acute myeloid leukemia in the elderly: Assessment of multidrug resistance (MDR1) and cytogenetics distinguishes

biologic subgroups with remarkably distinct responses to standard chemotherapy. A Southwest Oncology Group study. *Blood* 1997; 89:3323–9.

114. Weiss R. NIH will restrict outside income. *Washington Post*, February 2, 2005;A1.

115. Knight J. Accusations of bias prompt NIH review of ethical guidelines. *Nature* 2003;426:741.

116. Check E. NIH urged to rewrite rules on consultancies. *Nature* 2004;429:119.

117. Ein D. NIH at the brink; America's research excellence at stake. *Washington Times* June 2, 2004.

118. Editorial. Double dipping at NIH. *Washington Post* July 5, 2004:A16.

119. Kaiser J. Biomedical research: Feeling the heat, NIH tightens conflict-of-interest rules. *Science* 2004;305:25–6.

120. Agres T. NIH sees fight on ethics rules. *The Scientist* February 25, 2005;6.

121. Kaiser J. NIH intramural scientists unite. *ScienceNOW* November 15, 2004.

122. Wadman M. NIH workers see red over revised rules for conflicts of interest. *Nature* 2005;434:3–4.

123. Editorial. Unhealthy ethics. *Washington Post* April 6, 2005:A18.

124. Heil E. Senators say NIH ethics policies are now too stringent. *Congress Daily* Apr. 6, 2005:5–6.

125. Bero LA. Disclosure policies for gifts from industry to academic faculty. *JAMA* 1998;279:1031–2.

126. Lo B, Wolf LE, Berkeley A. Conflict-of-interest policies for investigators in clinical trials. *New England Journal of Medicine* 2000; 343:1616–20.

127. McCrary SV, et al. A national survey of policies on disclosure of conflicts of interest in biomedical research. *New England Journal of Medicine* 2000;343:1621–6.

128. Cho MK, et al. Policies on faculty conflicts of interest at US universities. *JAMA* 2000;284:2203–8.

129. General Accounting Office. *Biomedical Research: HHS Direction Needed to Address Financial Conflicts of Interest*. GAO-02–89. Washington, D.C.: GAO; 2001. [Online] November 2001. Available: http://www.aau.edu/research/gao.pdf.

130. Boyd EA, Cho MK, Bero LA. Financial conflict-of-interest policies in clinical research: Issues for clinical investigators. *Academic Medicine* 2003;78:769–74.

131. International Committee of Medical Journal Editors. Uniform requirements for manuscripts submitted to biomedical journals. *JAMA* 1997;277:927–34.

132. Kurth T, et al. Unreported financial disclosures in a study of migraine and cardiovascular disease. *JAMA* 2006;296:653–4.

133. Mello MM, Clarridge BR, Studdert DM. Academic medical centers' standards for clinical-trial agreements with industry. *New England Journal of Medicine* 2005;352:2202–10.

134. Schulman KA, et al. A national survey of provisions in clinical-trial agreements between medical schools and industry sponsors. *New England Journal of Medicine* 2002;347:1335–41.

135. Campbell EG, Louis KS, Blumenthal D. Looking a gift horse in the mouth: Corporate gifts supporting life sciences research. *JAMA* 1998;279:995–9.

136. Ashar BH, et al. Prevalence and determinants of physician participation in conducting pharmaceutical-sponsored clinical trials and lectures. *Journal of General Internal Medicine* 2004;19:1140–5.

137. Choudhry NK, Stelfox HT, Detsky AS. Relationships between authors of clinical practice guidelines and the pharmaceutical industry. *JAMA* 2002;287:612–7.

138. Black HR, et al. Principal results of the Controlled Onset Verapamil Investigation of Cardiovascular End Points (CONVINCE) trial. *JAMA* 2003;289:2073–82.

139. Psaty BM, Rennie D. Stopping medical research to save money: A broken pact with researchers and patients. *JAMA* 2003; 289:2128–31.

140. Blumenthal D, et al. Participation of life-science faculty in research relationships with industry. *New England Journal of Medicine* 1996;335:1734–9.

141. Djulbegovic B, Bennet CL, Lyman GH. Violation of the uncertainty principle in conduct of randomized controlled trials (RCTs) of erythropoietin (EPO). *Blood* 1999;94(Suppl.1):399A.

142. Knox KS, et al. Reporting and dissemination of industry versus nonprofit sponsored economic analyses of six novel drugs used in oncology. *Annals of Oncology* 2000;11:1591–5.

143. Stelfox HT, et al. Conflict of interest in the debate over calcium-channel antagonists. *New England Journal of Medicine* 1998;338: 101–6.

144. Friedberg M, et al. Evaluation of conflict of interest in economic analyses of new drugs used in oncology. *JAMA* 1999;282: 1453–7.

145. Juni P, Rutjes AW, Dieppe PA. Are selective COX 2 inhibitors superior to traditional non steroidal anti-inflammatory drugs? *British Medical Journal* 2002;324:1287–8.

146. Rochon PA, et al. A study of manufacturer-supported trials of non-steroidal anti-inflammatory drugs in the treatment of arthritis. *Archives of Internal Medicine* 1994;154:157–63.

147. Blumenthal D, et al. Withholding research results in academic life science: Evidence from a national survey of faculty. *JAMA* 1997;277:1224–8.

148. Turner C, Spilich GJ. Research into smoking or nicotine and human cognitive performance: Does the source of funding make a difference? *Addiction* 1997;92:1423–6.

149. Yaphe J, et al. The association between funding by commercial interests and study outcome in randomized controlled drug trials. *Family Practice* 2001;18:565–8.

150. Buchkowsky SS, Jewesson PJ. Industry sponsorship and authorship of clinical trials over 20 years. *Annals of Pharmacotherapy* 2004;38: 579–85

151. Perlis RH, Perlis CS, Wu Y, Hwang C, Joseph M, Nierenberg AA. Industry sponsorship and financial conflict of interest in the reporting of clinical trials in psychiatry. *American Journal of Psychiatry* 2005;162(10):1957–60.

152. Ridker PM, Torres J. Reported outcomes in major cardiovascular clinical trials funded by for-profit and not-for-profit organizations: 2000–2005. *JAMA* 2006;295(19):2128–31.

153. Campbell EG, Weissman JS, Vogeli C, et al. Financial relationships between institutional review board members and industry. *New England Journal of Medicine* 2006;355:2321–9.

154. Hampson LA, Agrawal M, Joffe S, Gross CP, Verter J, Emanuel EJ. Patients' views on financial conflicts of interest in cancer research trials. *New England Journal of Medicine* 2006;355(22):2330–7.

Eric G. Campbell   David Blumenthal

Industrialization of Academic Science and Threats to Scientific Integrity

Historical Perspective

Relationships between academia and industry have existed since the early 1900s, when more than half of all trustees of U.S. universities were from the industrial sector.[1] However, academic-industry relationships (AIRs) and commercialization began in earnest when chemical and pharmaceutical companies began to undertake research and sought university help in solving scientific problems. Commercialization of research got another boost as universities established independent organizations to commercialize the results of faculty research. The earliest of these was the Research Corporation, which was formed in 1912 to manage pollution technology developed at the University of California.[1] A similar technology transfer organization was created in 1925 when the University of Wisconsin formed the Wisconsin Alumni Research Foundation (WARF) to commercialize a patent on the technology for irradiating dairy products to instill vitamin D in them—a process that virtually eliminated rickets as a childhood disease.[2] The purpose of organizations like WARF and the Research Corporation was to keep commercial activities "at arm's length" out of fear that they would compromise the integrity of the academic research enterprise. Despite the fact that these firms conferred great benefit on the public, their creation met with considerable angst within the halls of the academy.

In the late 1970s and 1980s, events in the fields of science, law, and public policy converged to fuel an upsurge in the commercialization of academic research in the life sciences.[3] This revolution began in the then nascent field of biotechnology and resulted from the 30-year investment by the federal government in science following the Second World War. Perhaps the most important scientific breakthrough was the discovery and subsequent commercialization of recombinant DNA technologies by Stanley Cohen and Herbert Boyer in the early 1970s, along with parallel breakthroughs in monoclonal antibody technologies, fermentation technologies, genetic sequencing, and genetic synthesis.[4] These discoveries emerging from the field of biology would soon overtake the field of chemistry as the source of new drugs—a concept that pharmaceutical companies clearly recognized and that motivated them to establish relationships with academic based researchers and organizations to take advantage of the biological revolution occurring in academia.

The biotechnology revolution occurred alongside a series of public policy developments that facilitated AIRs. As a result of economic concerns driven by rising oil prices and stagnant corporate productivity, elected officials began to explore policy changes that would stimulate the U.S. economy. Policy makers saw academia as a rich, untapped source of new technologies that could jump start the sagging corporate sector and ultimately the economy as a whole. One problem identified by officials was the lack of motivation on the part of academic scientists and their institutions to aggressively exploit the commercial potential of their research—much of which was funded by the federal government through the National Institutes of Health (NIH), the National Science Foundation (NSF), and the Department of Defense. A watershed event in this regard was the 1980 passage of the Bayh-Dole Act, which allowed universities and individual researchers to claim ownership of the intellectual property resulting from federally funded research, which then could be licensed to companies.[5] In essence, Bayh-Dole stoked the fires of academic commercialization by creating a new and potentially large stream of revenues flowing to academia from the commercial sector.

A third development, this time in patent law, added additional fuel to the fires of academic commercialization. As a result of the U.S. Supreme Court's 1980 ruling in the *Diamond v. Chakrabarty* case, it became possible to patent new life forms resulting from biological manipulation.[6] Many of the most promising technologies for drug development were emerging from the creation of novel cells and the substances these cells produced, but companies needed a way to protect the commercial value of these discoveries. The *Chakrabarty* decision provided such protection and ultimately reassured universities and industry that commercial ventures based on biotechnology could be economically viable.

As a result of these tri-part changes in science, policy, and law, a number of large, high-profile relationships between academic institutions and industry developed. One of the highest profile relationships was a 1980 agreement between the Massachusetts General Hospital (MGH) and a German chemical and drug company, Hoechst AG. Hoechst funded not only research at the MGH, but also the creation of a new Department of Molecular Genetics and the construction of a research building.[7] Other relationships were established between Harvard Medical School and the DuPont Co, Washington University at St. Louis and Monsanto, Yale University and Bristol Meyers, and the University of California at Berkeley and Novartis, among others. At the same time, new start-up companies founded by university faculty and located proximal to major universities emerged in Massachusetts and California, including Amgen, Novartis, Genentech, and Chiron. Overall, from 1980 to 1990 it was estimated that university faculty participated in the founding of 500 life science companies in the United States.[7] Further, in 2001 the journal *Nature* reported that one-third of all the biotechnology companies in the world had been founded by faculty members at the University of California.[8]

The 1980s and 1990s witnessed a virtual gold rush of activity among academics, universities, and industry via the patent system, a surge dominated by the life sciences (see Figure 71.1). In the 1970s, patent awards to academic institutions were in the range of 250 to 350 per year. In 1980, awards totaled 390, whereas in 2000, they reached 3,087, a nearly eight-fold increase in just 20

years.[9] Almost one-half of those patents were in the life sciences, up from 15% in 1980.

Over the decade of the 1990s, university technology transfer activities increased at a tremendous rate. For example, the number of professional staff devoted to university research commercialization activities increased more than three-fold from approximately 438 full-time employees to more than 1,300 full-time employees.[9]

At the turn of the 21st century, the commercial activities of academic faculty and institutions again gained national prominence. Numerous studies detailing the nature, extent, and consequences of academic-industry relationships,[11–14] including case studies of alleged conflicts of interest in clinical research,[1] drew critical press attention.

At the urging of the newly created Office for Human Research Protections and the Secretary of Health and Human Services, the federal government aggressively promoted the need for government to assist universities in the identification and management of relationships with industry through a draft interim guidance.[15] The goal of the guidance was to help university administrators with academic-industry relationships without imposing any specific prohibitions. Organizations representing medical schools and universities pressed the federal government to hold off making the guidance final, asking for an opportunity to create their own task forces to make recommendations.

Core Conception

AIRs are defined as arrangements in which academic scientists carry out research or provide intellectual property in return for financial compensation in the form of cash, equities, and other considerations. Table 71.1 provides a conceptualization of the various types of AIRs.

Ethical Issues

The academic life science research enterprise in the United States rests on at least four, and perhaps more, fundamental assumptions

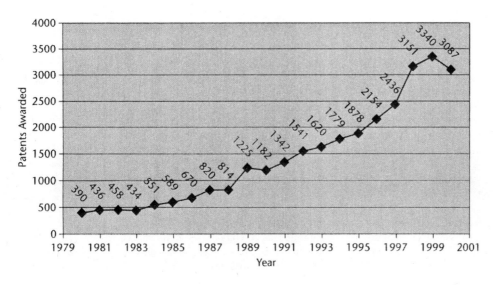

Figure 71.1. Trends in University Patents (1979–2001).[10] (Data from U.S. Patent and Trademark Office.)

Table 71.1

Conceptualization of AIRs

Type of Relationship	Definition	Comments
Research	Industry support of a scientist's university-based research, usually in the form of a grant or a contract.[12]	Institutions benefit financially because research grants support salaries and facilities that otherwise would have to be supported by the institution, fund raising, or other grants.
Consulting	Provision of advice, service, or information by an academic faculty member to commercial organizations.[16]	Individual scientists can retain funds from these activities over and above their institutional salaries. Institutions can benefit financially in cases in which faculty could use these funds to support professional activities that otherwise would be charged to the institution.
Licensing	Granting industry the rights to commercialize university-owned technologies.	These relationships are often negotiated and managed by an office of technology transfer located within the universities, medical schools, and independent hospitals, and research facilities.[17] In most universities, faculty share some of the financial benefits of licensing relationships with their institutions.
Equity	Participation by academic scientists in the founding and/or ownership of new companies commercializing university-based research, especially in biotechnology.	Often new companies, which are cash-poor, provide equity or options to purchase equity as compensation for relationships such as the consulting and licensing relationships described above.[18] This equity may be held by individual scientists as well as academic institutions.
Training	Companies provide support for graduate students or postdoctoral fellows, or contract with academic institutions to provide various educational experiences (such as seminars or fellowships) to industrial employees.[11]	Institutions benefit because these relationships defray the costs of graduate training. For example, in 2005 the Massachusetts General Hospital accepted $6.5 million from industry to dramatically expand its graduate medical education programs including live lectures in 24 cities, teleconferences, and webcasts.[19]
Gifts	The transfer of scientific or nonscientific resources, independent of an institutionally negotiated research grant or contract, between industry and academic scientists.[20]	Examples of gifts include equipment, biomaterials, discretionary funding, support for travel to professional meetings, and entertainment-related items such as tickets to sporting events, cultural events and dinners.

regarding what is considered to be appropriate and/or inappropriate conduct in science. The first assumption is based on the ideal of truth in the pursuit, generation, transmission, and application of knowledge.[21] That is, science should above all be completely free from any form of dishonesty, bias, or distortion. Many worry that relationships between academics and industry could motivate scientists to report findings that are not true, ignore other results, or mislead people while giving talks at professional meetings.

A second fundamental assumption is that scientific information, data, and materials should be shared in the scientific community. Robert Merton, a leading sociologist of science, described this assumption as "communism" in which the results of science are owned by the community and the individual scientist's rights are limited to the honor and fame that may come from a discovery.[22] Open sharing of scientific results is believed to contribute to the most efficient advance of science by preventing scientists from wasting effort and other scarce resources in repeating past work, and by enabling them to build on colleagues' success. Sharing also creates a sense of shared purpose among scientists. However, although developments in public policy, law, and science have brought about increased relationships with industry, these changes may also have increased the amount of secrecy in science primarily associated with protecting intellectual property rights through the patent system.

The third fundamental assumption is related to the safety of those who serve as research participants. Investigators are required to ensure that the risks to participants in human research are minimized. Many fear that relationships with industry may encourage investigators to inappropriately enroll patients in trials, which might increase the chances that research participants suffer negative health outcomes, despite the fact that there are no data beyond anecdote and speculation to support this concern.[23]

The fourth assumption is self-regulation. The primary responsibility to ensure that members of the scientific community honor the assumptions of the ethical contract described above rests with the scientific community itself and the organizations that comprise it: universities, professional associations, and nonprofit institutes.[24,25] Of course, numerous governmental encouragements and restrictions have been enacted to supplement the scientific community's own efforts—such as institutional review boards and NIH conflict of interest rules. But the scientific community assumes and jealously protects an inherent professional right and responsibility to regulate itself. The assumption of self-regulation related to relationships with industry is reflected in a complex web of university- and hospital-based institutional reporting systems, conflict of interest committees, and other mechanisms in the scientific infrastructure that are designed to disclose and manage relationships with industry. This self-regulation is designed to ensure that universities have the flexibility to adapt to their unique situations related to relationships between industry and their faculty.

Empirical Data

The most recent nationally representative data regarding the prevalence and magnitude of AIRs in the life sciences stem from surveys of industry representatives and life science faculty conducted in the mid-1990s.[11,12] In 1994, senior level executives at life science companies in the United States were surveyed. Based on industry reports, it was estimated that 88% of companies employed academic faculty members as consultants. A survey of basic scientists at the 50 most research-intensive U.S. universities found that 60% of respondents had consulted in the three preceding years (35.2% with a privately held company and 24.5% for a public company).[11]

More than half of surveyed companies supported university-based research either through research grants or contracts. Among faculty members, 28% of respondents reported receiving research support for their university-based research from industrial sources. The prevalence of support was greater for researchers in clinical departments (36%) than for those in nonclinical departments (21%). Characteristics of industry funding in the life sciences suggested that grants tended, on average, to be small in size and short in duration. Industry respondents indicated that 71% of company-supported projects in 1994–1995 were funded at less than $100,000 a year. Only 6% of responding firms provided annual funding of $500,000 or more. For 84% of the firms that had relationships with academia, the typical relationship lasted two years or less.[11] Industrial support also constituted a relatively small proportion of the total research funding to universities in the mid-1990s, about 12% of the total.

Another commonly reported form of industrial support of academic scientists is through research gifts.[20] Among life science faculty in the 50 most research-intensive universities, almost half (43%) received research gifts, independent of a grant or a contract from industry, in the three years preceding the study. The most widely reported gifts received from industry were biomaterials (24%), discretionary funds (15%), research equipment (11%), trips to professional meetings (11%), and support for students (9%). Of those receiving a gift, 66% reported the gifts were important to their research.

There are limited national data on the frequency of equity or licensing relationships among faculty. In 1992 Krimsky and colleagues found that as many as 34% of lead authors of articles published in 14 major biological and medical journals had a financial interest in a company with activities related to their published research. Krimsky also found that 15% of lead authors from Massachusetts institutions had personal financial interests in a company supporting their research.[26] A study of disclosures at a single research institution, the University of California at San Francisco, found that 7.6% of clinical principal investigators had some form of personal financial ties to industry.[14] A third of these reported temporary speaking engagements for companies, a third involved the investigator holding a paid position on a scientific advisory board or board of directors, and 14% related to the ownership of equity in a firm.[14]

Relationships Between AIRs and Bias of Reporting

In recent years, a significant body of research and commentary has suggested that relationships between academic scientists and industry have an impact on the content of scientific reports emerging from industry-supported research.[8,25,27–29] The most comprehensive study to date is an analysis of 23 studies of the impact of academic-industry relationships on the outcomes of

science that was published in 2003. This analysis found "a statistically significant relationship between industry sponsorship and pro-industry conclusions."[30] In other words, industry-funded studies are significantly more likely to yield results that favor industrial sponsors than would be expected by chance alone. Examples of scientific areas in which industry-funded studies reached pro-industry conclusions included randomized clinical trials in multiple myeloma, economic analyses of oncology drugs, studies of nicotine and cognitive performance, nonsteroidal anti-inflammatory drugs, and calcium channel blockers.

That is not to say that all industry-funded studies are intentionally biased. It may be that industry selectively funds research that is most likely to yield favorable conclusions, or that industry-funded studies address different questions than nonindustry-funded studies. Others have suggested that there are a number of reasons why some pharmaceutical funded studies are more likely to yield pro-industry results. These reasons include the following:

1. Selecting a comparison drug that is known to be inferior to the sponsor's drug
2. Selecting an inappropriate dose of the comparison drug
3. Using multiple endpoints for the study and selecting the endpoint that presents the sponsor's drug in the best light for publication
4. Doing multicenter trials and selecting results for publication from centers that are most favorable
5. Selectively presenting results from subgroup analyses[31]

At the time of this writing, no study had been published exploring researchers' beliefs and experiences regarding these phenomena.

Relationships Between AIRs and Data Withholding/Secrecy

A significant body of empirical evidence dating from the mid-1990s demonstrates that relationships with industry are associated with secrecy in science. A 1996 survey of life science faculty in the 50 most research-intensive U.S. institutions found that 14.5% of those with funding from industry reported engaging in trade secrecy compared with 4.7% of those without funding from industry.[12] In addition, a 2002 study found that those with research funding from industry were significantly more likely to delay publication of their research results by more than six months to allow for the commercialization of their research.[32]

Relationships Between AIRs and Protection of Human Research Participants

There are no systematic data regarding the impact of AIRs on the protection of human research participants. However, industry relationships have been associated with concerns about the treatment of human research participants. Perhaps the best known case involved the death of a 19-year-old, Jesse Gelsinger, in a gene transfer study at the University of Pennsylvania in 1999[1] (see Chapter 10). A subsequent investigation of the case found that James Wilson, one of the principal investigators and the director of the University's Institute for Human Gene Therapy, which conducted the study, held patents on various aspects of the study's procedures. In addition, Wilson and the University of Pennsylvania held stock in a company that stood to benefit if the study was successful. Despite Gelsinger's death, the company was eventually sold, and Wilson's and the University of Pennsylvania's equity stakes were valued at $13.5 and $1.4 million, respectively.[1]

Concern has also arisen about IRB members' relationships with industry. Because IRBs are charged to protect human subjects in clinical research studies, the behavior of its members is crucial to the safety of research at their institution. A recent survey of faculty members serving on IRBs found that consulting relationships with industry are common, with about half (47%) of all faculty IRB members having served as a consultant to industry in the previous three years.[33] It is possible that relationships with companies could impact members' IRB-related activities and attitudes, and such ties clearly raise issues related to conflicts of interest.

Concern regarding conflicts of interest and IRBs erupted in 1999 at Duke University when at least 2,000 studies involving human research participants were suspended after the federal government determined that Duke did not adequately protect patients involved in such studies.[34] Among the 20 deficiencies cited by the Office for Protection from Research Risks—predecessor of the Office for Human Research Protections—was the suggestion that conflicts of interest on the part of senior-level administrators at Duke had compromised the ability of Duke's IRBs to make independent and unbiased decisions regarding research protocols. Although this is far from conclusive, the inspector general of the Department of Health and Human Services concluded, "There has been no progress in insulating IRBs from conflicts that can compromise their mission in protecting human subjects."[35]

University Disclosure and Management

For the most part, the primary responsibility for the disclosure and management of relationships with industry has been vested in the university and faculty, as a form of professional self-regulation. Because there is wide variation in universities in terms of their size, research intensity, history, culture, and ownership status (public/private), it is not surprising that there is wide variation in university policies and procedures related to the reporting, oversight, and management of relationships with industry. A content analysis of the conflict of interest policies at the 100 universities that received the most funding from the NIH in 1998 found that disclosure policies varied widely across institutions. For example, 55% of the policies required disclosures from all faculty members, whereas 45% required only faculty who were principal investigators to disclose. Also, less than 20% of institutional policies specified limits on faculty financial relationships with industry, and 12% provided specific limits on the amount of time publication may be delayed.[13] However, the fact that universities have policies and practices about the disclosure and management of relationships does not mean these policies are enforced or that they are effective in preventing misconduct. For example, a survey of the conflict of interest policies at U.S. institutions receiving more than $5 million in funding from the NIH or the NSF found that the management of conflicts and penalties for nondisclosure were almost universally discretionary.[36]

Policy Implications

The data presented above have numerous policy implications for academia and industry. First, policy attention is needed to address inconsistencies in the disclosure of industry relationships. Full disclosure constitutes a minimally acceptable response to the demonstrated risks posed by industry relationships. As a result, a minimum set of uniform disclosure policies and practices related to industry relationships should be adopted by all universities, associated teaching hospitals, and academic clinical facilities. These policies and procedures should be developed by an independent organization with significant input from the academic community, such as the National Academy of Sciences.

Currently, there is wide variation regarding which individuals are required to disclose their relationships with industry. Because evidence clearly indicates that AIRs exist related to the education, research, and patient care missions of universities, it is necessary that all individuals holding faculty appointments and all academic administrators at the level of department chair and above (even if they do not hold faculty appointments) should disclose their own and their immediate family members' relationships with industry on an annual basis.

However, reliance on disclosure alone in addressing the risks associated with AIRs is inadequate for a number of reasons.[29,37] First, although disclosure is intended to bolster public confidence in the integrity of the research enterprise, it may have the opposite effect of raising widespread concern and promoting calls for reform. Second, disclosure is perceived as accusatory and carries negative connotations—particularly in academic settings that tend to have more participatory governance structures. Third, in many cases, individuals and institutions to which disclosures are made may not have the skills or authority to use the information to manage conflicts of interest. Further, universities have no mechanism to verify the accuracy of faculty disclosures and thus could easily be deceived by inaccurate or incomplete disclosures. According to one commentator, "The net effect of all of these reservations is that open disclosure is of extremely limited value."[29] Disclosure may be necessary; universities and government cannot manage relationships they don't know about. But it is not sufficient.

Beyond disclosure, it is essential to maintain the autonomy of individual institutions regarding the review and management of relationships with industry once they are disclosed along important dimensions such as research intensity, public/private status, and institutional size. For example, we believe it should be left to the institution to decide which relationships are acceptable and which are not, which relationships require additional monitoring by the institution and which do not, and the form such monitoring or oversight should take (such as oversight by a single individual or a committee). Although the federal government may be able to provide guidance on such issues, we believe it is imprudent at this time to vest the absolute authority regarding these issues in any single institution or organization. Additional recommendations regarding the management of relationships with industry can be found in our published work and will not be repeated here.[38]

Implications for Study Design

In designing studies funded or influenced by industry, scientists should keep the risks associated with these relationships in mind. Regarding the risk of industry bias, studies should be designed and executed to test hypotheses that are carefully selected to avoid favoring one outcome or another. The responsibility for ensuring the integrity of the scientific enterprise rests solely with the investigative team and is embodied in the choice of appropriate study endpoints, comparison drugs, dosing levels, data analyses, and reporting procedures.

Regarding secrecy, academic researchers should not accept any contractual provisions or make any noncontractual agreements that delay publication of results beyond the time needed to file a patent application. Nor should they accept contract provisions that prohibit the sharing of information, data, and materials with other scientists who wish to replicate published work. Further, all publications describing the results of scientific experiments should include sufficient detail about the way an experiment was done to allow for replication of the published research.

Regarding the protection of human research participants, IRBs or other similar institutional bodies or groups can assist in protecting human participants related to the risks of relationships with industry discussed above. In all proposals sent to the IRB, scientists should disclose whether they or one of their family members have any relationship with the study sponsor(s). When relationships exist, the complete details of the relationships should be fully disclosed to the IRB. Once the study is in progress, scientists should notify the IRB if a relationship changes or if a new industry relationship is formed that is related to the study.

Unresolved Issues and Data Requirements

Numerous aspects of academic-industry relationships could benefit from the collection of additional empirical data. There are no current, comprehensive, publicly available data on faculty members' or government scientists' relationships with industry or commercial activities. At the institutional level, there are no comprehensive data on the nature, extent, and consequences of universities,' medical schools,' and hospitals' relationships with industry and commercial activities. Even when data on commercialization and industry relationships are collected by individual institutions, the data rarely delve deeply into details of the relationships and are rarely shared with individuals outside of the institution, especially private institutions.

In addition to a much more extensive data collection effort, we believe it is necessary that the debate about AIRs and commercialization be balanced and fair. Though we have focused in this chapter on the problems associated with AIRs, we acknowledge that these relationships also have benefits that are important to preserve and promote.[38] For example, relationships with industry provide scientists with resources to conduct research, write papers, attend conferences, support students, and develop new products and services that likely would not be supported from nonindustrial sources. There can be little doubt that these activities result in scientific advance and innovation in health care. The critical challenge is to find a way to manage the risks of AIRs while preserving their many benefits.

Disclaimer

The views expressed are those of the authors alone and do not necessarily represent the views of Harvard Medical School, Partners HealthCare, the Massachusetts General Hospital, or the Institute for Health Policy.

References

1. Washburn J. *University Incorporated: The Corruption of Higher Education*. New York, N.Y.: Basic Books, 2005.
2. Blumenthal D, Epstein S, Maxwell J. Commercializing university research: Lessons of the WARF experience. *New England Journal of Medicine* 1986;314:1621–6.
3. Blumenthal D, Campbell EG. Academic-industry relationships in biotechnology: Overview. In: Mehlman MJ, Murray TH, eds. *Encyclopedia of Ethical, Legal and Policy Issues in Biotechnology*. New York, N.Y.: John Wiley & Sons, Inc.; 2000:1–9.
4. Cohen SN, et al. Process for producing biologically functional molecular chimeras. U.S. Patent #4,237,224, December 2, 1980. [Online] Available: http://www.uspto.gov/patft/index.html.
5. *Diamond v. Chakrabarty,* 477 U.S. 303 (1980).
6. Bayh-Dole Act, Pub. L. 96–517, 1980.
7. M. Kenney. *Biotechnology: The University-Industry Complex*. New Haven, Conn.: Yale University Press; 1988.
8. Krimsky S. *Science in the Private Interest: Has the Lure of Profits Corrupted Biomedical Research?* Lanham, Md.: Rowman and Littlefield; 2003.
9. Powers J, Campbell EG. The commodification of academic science: Ethical implications and policy concerns. Unpublished manuscript, 2005.
10. U.S. Patent and Trademark Office, Office of Electronic Information Products, Patent Technology Monitoring Division. U.S. Colleges and Universities—Utility Patent Grants, Calendar Years 1969–2000. [Online] Available: http://www.uspto.gov/web/offices/ac/ido/oeip/taf/univ/cls_gr/all_univ_clg.htm.
11. Blumenthal D, Causino N, Campbell EG, Louis KS. Relationships between academic institutions and industry in the life sciences—An industry survey. *New England Journal of Medicine* 1996;334:368–73.
12. Blumenthal D, Campbell EG, Causino N, Louis KS. Participation of life-science faculty in research relationships with industry. *New England Journal of Medicine* 1996;335:1734–9.
13. Cho MK, Shohara R, Schissel A, Rennie D. Policies on faculty conflicts of interest at U.S. universities. *JAMA* 2000;284:2203–8.
14. Boyd E, Bero L. Assessing faculty financial relationships with industry: A case study. *JAMA* 2000;284:2209–14.
15. National Human Research Protections Advisory Committee, Department of Health and Human Services. Draft Interim Guidance: Financial Relationships in Clinical Research: Issues for Institutions, Clinical Investigators, and IRBs to Consider When Dealing With Issues of Financial Interests and Human Subject Protection. [Online] January 10, 2001. Available: http://www.hhs.gov/ohrp/nhrpac/mtg12–00/finguid.htm.
16. Jones LM. *The Commercialization of Academic Science: Conflict of Interest for the Faculty Consultant*. Doctoral Dissertation, University of Minnesota, 2000.
17. Panel of Advisors on the Life Sciences, Ewing Marion Kauffman Foundation. *Accelerating Technology Transfer and Commercialization in the Life and Health Sciences*. Kansas City, Mo.: Ewing Marion Kauffman Foundation; 2003. [Online] August 2003. Available: http://www.kauffman.org/pdf/TechTranPanel_Report.pdf.
18. Bowie N. *University-Business Partnerships: An Assessment*. Lanham, Md.: Rowman & Littlefield; 1994.
19. Kowalczyk L. Psychiatry funding questioned; drug firms aid Mass. General. *Boston Globe* May 14, 2005:A1.
20. Campbell EG, Blumenthal D, Louis KS. Looking a gift horse in the mouth: Corporate gifts that support life sciences research. *JAMA* 1998;279:995–9.
21. Bulger RE, Heitman E, Reiser SJ, eds. *The Ethical Dimensions of the Biological and Health Sciences*, 2nd ed. New York, N.Y.: Cambridge University Press; 2002.
22. Merton RF. *Social Theory and Social Structure*. New York, N.Y.: The Free Press; 1968.

23. Bodenheimer T. Uneasy alliance: Clinical investigators and the pharmaceutical industry. *New England Journal of Medicine* 2000;342:1539–44.

24. Blumenthal D. Doctors in a wired world: Can professionalism survive connectivity? *Milbank Quarterly* 2002;80:525–46.

25. The Medical Professionalism Project. Medical professionalism in the new millennium: A physicians' charter. *Lancet* 2002;359:520–2.

26. Krimsky S, Rothenberg LS. Conflict of interest policies in science and medical journals: Editorial practices and author disclosures. *Science and Engineering Ethics* 2001;7:205–18.

27. Bok D. *Universities in the Marketplace: The Commercialization of Higher Education*. Princeton, N.J.: Princeton University Press; 2003.

28. Angell M. *The Truth About Drug Companies: How They Deceive Us and What to Do About It*. New York, N.Y.: Random House; 2004.

29. Kassirer JS. *On the Take: How Medicine's Complicity With Big Business Can Endanger Your Health*. New York, N.Y.: Oxford University Press; 2005.

30. Bekelman JE, Li Y, Gross CP. Scope and impact of financial conflicts of interest in biomedical research: A systematic review. *JAMA* 2003; 289:454–65.

31. Smith R. Medical journals and pharmaceutical companies: Uneasy bedfellows. *British Medical Journal* 2003;326;1202–5.

32. Campbell EG, Clarridge BR, Gokhale M, et al. Data withholding in academic genetics: Evidence from a national survey. *JAMA* 2002; 287:473–81.

33. Campbell EG, Weissman JS, Clarridge B, et al. Characteristics of faculty serving on IRBs: Results of a national survey of medical school faculty. *Academic Medicine* 2003;78:831–7.

34. Kaplan S, Brownlee S. Duke's hazards: Did medical experiments put patients needlessly at risk? *U.S. News and World Report* 1999; 126(20):66–8,70.

35. Office of Inspector General, Department of Health and Human Services. *Protecting Human Research Subject—Status of Recommendations*. OEI-01–97–00197. Washington, D.C.: DHHS; 2000. [Online] April 2000. Available: http://oig.hhs.gov/oei/reports/oei-01–97–00197.pdf.

36. McCrary SV, et al. A national survey of policies on disclosure of conflicts of interest in biomedical research. *New England Journal of Medicine* 2000;343:1621–6.

37. Thompson DF. Understanding financial conflicts of interest. *New England Journal of Medicine* 1993;329:573–6.

38. Campbell EG, Powers JB, Blumenthal D, Biles B. Inside the triple helix: Government, university and industry technology transfer and commercialization in the life sciences. *Health Affairs* 2004;23: 64–77.

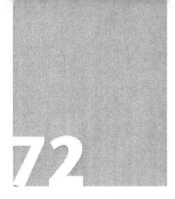

David B. Resnik

Fraud, Fabrication, and Falsification

Honesty is one of the core values of science, but for many years there have been concerns about dishonesty and deception in research. In 1830, the mathematician and inventor Charles Babbage (1791–1871) wrote about unethical practices that he had observed in British science. He discussed examples of hoaxing, forging, trimming, and cooking data. Hoaxing and forging occur when one makes up data; trimming occurs when one clips off pieces of data that do not agree with one's hypothesis; and cooking occurs when one manipulates data in order to make them appear to be more accurate than they really are.[1] In 1847, the American Medical Association (AMA) was formed to promote professionalism in medical practice and research. In 1849, the AMA formed a board to analyze quack remedies and debunk fraudulent claims made by snake oil salesmen.[2]

Dishonest practices in research have been described as "fraud" or "research misconduct." There are two different senses of fraud: the ordinary meaning of the word and a precise, legal meaning. Fraud, in the ordinary sense of the word, connotes dishonesty, deception, trickery, forgery, and related concepts. The *American Heritage Dictionary* defines fraud as "[a] deception deliberately practiced in order to secure unfair or unlawful gain."[3] Although data alteration would seem to fit this definition, the ordinary meaning of the word *fraud* lacks the precision that is needed for a clear discussion of data alteration in science. Dishonest activities in science may involve complex manipulations of data that can be difficult to distinguish from honest activities.

The legal meaning of fraud also does not adequately describe some of the dishonesty that one finds in science. *Black's Law Dictionary* defines fraud as "a knowing or reckless misrepresen-

tation of a material fact that induces a person to act to his or her detriment."[4] A researcher who misrepresents the truth or conceals a material fact in an official communication with the U.S. government, such as a grant application or progress report to a granting agency, could face legal liability for fraud under contract law, tort law, or the False Claims Act (FCA). If the government wins an FCA lawsuit, the defendant must repay the money he has fraudulently obtained and pay treble damages. Under the *qui tam* provisions of the FCA, individuals may bring lawsuits on behalf of the government and win up to 30% of the award if the lawsuit is successful. A half dozen misconduct cases have resulted in lawsuits against research institutions under the FCA.[5]

Although this legal definition of fraud is useful in understanding dishonest activities in science that are also illegal, it is not very helpful in understanding data fabrication or falsification. First, many actions that do not fit the legal definition of fraud would still be considered highly unethical in research. For example, fabrication or falsification of an immaterial (or irrelevant) fact in a scientific paper would be considered misconduct in science, even though it would not fit the legal definition of fraud. Second, some actions that fit the legal definition of fraud might not be considered to be research misconduct. For example, a person who makes a reckless misrepresentation that induces others to act their detriment would commit fraud, but this action might be considered an honest error in science. Misconduct involves intentional deception.[6] Errors, even reckless ones, are unintentional. An error in research may constitute negligence—even gross negligence—but not misconduct.

To avoid confusions that may occur by using the term fraud to describe dishonest actions in science, this chapter will focus on research misconduct instead of research fraud.

What Is Research Misconduct?

Since the 1980s, different governments and funding agencies have used different definitions of research misconduct. The U.S. government used several different definitions of research misconduct during that time.[7] After several years of debate, in 2000 the White House Office of Science and Technology Policy (OSTP) developed a federal definition of misconduct that has been adopted by all federal agencies that support intramural or extramural research, including the National Institutes of Health (NIH) and National Science Foundation (NSF). The policy was implemented in 2005. According to the OSTP definition,

> [r]esearch misconduct is defined as fabrication, falsification, or plagiarism in proposing, performing, or reviewing research, or in reporting research results. Fabrication is making up data or results and recording or reporting them. Falsification is manipulating research materials, equipment, or processes, or changing or omitting data or results such that the research is not accurately represented in the research record. . . . Plagiarism is the appropriation of another person's ideas, processes, results, or words without giving appropriate credit. Research misconduct does not include honest error or differences of opinion.[8]

There are several important points to consider about this definition. The definition limits research misconduct to three types of misdeeds: fabrication, falsification, and plagiarism—known unofficially by the acronym FFP. Other definitions of misconduct, such as those used by other governments or some earlier federal definitions, are broader than the categories of fabrication, falsification, and plagiarism. In 1989, the Public Health Service (PHS), which oversees the NIH, used a definition of research misconduct that included FFP as well as "other practices that seriously deviate from those that are accepted in the scientific community."[9] The Wellcome Trust, the largest biomedical research charity in the United Kingdom, has developed a definition of misconduct that is broader that the OSTP definition. Under the Wellcome Trust definition, misconduct includes "deliberate, dangerous, or negligent deviations from accepted practices in carrying out research" and "failure to follow established protocols if this failure results in unreasonable risk or harm to humans, other invertebrates, or the environment."[10] The OSTP chose a narrower definition of misconduct for several reasons: (1) Most researchers regard fabrication, falsification, and plagiarism as serious offenses because they all involve dishonesty in science; (2) it is more difficult to define and adjudicate ethical problems, such as "serious deviations from accepted practices in carrying out research"; and (3) research institutions complained that a broader definition was unnecessary and unmanageable.[7] Most research institutions have policies and procedures that address other types of unethical or illegal conduct not covered by the OSTP definition, such as harassment, violations of human or animal research regulations, theft, mismanagement of funds, and so forth (see Tables 72.1 and 72.2).

It is important to note that the OSTP definition of misconduct encompasses many research activities beyond publication, such as

Table 72.1

Definition of Research Misconduct

- *Research misconduct*: Fabrication, falsification, or plagiarism in research. Honest errors and disagreements are not research misconduct.
- *Fabrication*: Making up data or results and recording or reporting the fabricated material.
- *Falsification*: Manipulating research materials, equipment, or processes, or changing or omitting data or results such that the research is not accurately represented in the research record.
- *Plagiarism*: The appropriation of another person's ideas, processes, results, or words without giving appropriate credit.

proposing, performing, or reviewing research. For example, misconduct includes fabrication or falsification of data on an application for a federal grant; it also includes plagiarism of ideas from a grant application.

Honest errors or differences of opinion are not classified as misconduct. This limitation is important, because error and disagreement are common in scientific research. Indeed, one might argue that scientific progress cannot occur without them.[6]

Conflicts of interest also are not classified as misconduct. Although conflicts of interest can undermine the integrity and trustworthiness of research, they are not ethically or legally equivalent to fabrication, falsification, or plagiarism. Scientists with a conflict of interest can still conduct good research, provided that they do not allow their financial or personal interests to bias their scientific judgment. Moreover, conflict of interest is covered by other federal rules aimed at eliminating or managing conflicts (see Chapters 68–71).

Even though the definition of research misconduct is fairly straightforward, it may be difficult to apply in some borderline cases involving manipulation of data or images. Most researchers exclude erroneous or anomalous data points, such as statistical outliers, from their analysis of the data. Indeed, it is seldom the case that researchers report the results of every single experiment related to a particular project. However, although some trimming and editing of data is common in scientific research, deceptive trimming—especially trimming that affects the overall results of research—can be considered falsification of data.[6] Problems can also arise in the manipulation of digital images of biological structures, which play an important role in many different fields including cytology, genetics, genomics, pathology, anatomy, and virology. Researchers can use software such as Photoshop to cut, paste, amplify, reverse, soften, blur, brighten, or darken various features of digital images. Some alteration of digital images is acceptable in research, provided that it is used to help the audience better understand data and it is not used to mislead. But image manipulation that affects the interpretation of data may constitute data fabrication or falsification.[11]

The OSTP definition of misconduct now applies to all biomedical research funded by the U.S. government. Research institutions that receive federal contracts or grants are responsible for the initial investigation and adjudication of allegations of scientific misconduct. Most research institutions have developed their own policies that define research misconduct and procedures for investigating and adjudicating misconduct allegations. These procedures should conform to requirements recommended by the OSTP, such as fairness, confidentiality, protection of whistle blowers, and due process. Before institutions conduct formal

Table 72.2
Research Misconduct and Serious Deviations From Accepted Research Practices

	Unethical	Illegal*
Research Misconduct		
Fabrication (making up data)	Yes	Yes
Falsification (changing data)	Yes	Yes
Plagiarism	Yes	Yes
Serious Deviations From Accepted Research Practices		
Inadequate record keeping	Yes	No
Refusing reasonable requests to share data, materials, or methods	Maybe**	Maybe**
Gross negligence in research	Yes	No
Destruction or theft of property	Yes	Yes
Using statistical techniques to misrepresent data	Yes	No
Interfering with a misconduct inquiry or investigation	Yes	Yes
Making a false accusation of misconduct	Yes	No
Exploitation or poor supervision of students or subordinates	Yes	No
Undeserved or inappropriate authorship	Yes	No
Duplicate publication	Maybe**	No
Breaching confidentiality in peer review	Yes	No
Violations of laboratory safety rules	Maybe**	Yes
Violations of rules for the protection of human subjects	Maybe**	Yes
Violations of rules for research on laboratory animals	Maybe**	Maybe**
Failure to disclose conflicts of interest	Maybe**	Maybe**
Misuse of funds	Yes	Yes
Financial fraud	Yes	Yes
Sexual or other harassment	Yes	Yes

* *Illegal* means "violation of United States government statutes or regulations."
** *Maybe* means "depends on the situation/circumstances."

investigations into misconduct allegations, they conduct inquiries to determine whether the allegations are frivolous or lack merit. Institutional sanctions for misconduct range from censure, reduction in privileges or salary, to loss of employment. Institutions are also responsible for reporting misconduct investigations and findings to sponsoring agencies, which have the option of conducting their own investigations and implementing their own sanctions. Federal sanctions for research misconduct range from supervision in the future use of federal funds in research to debarment from eligibility to receive federal funds for research. From 1994 to 2003, the PHS took 133 administrative actions against researchers who were found to have committed misconduct.[12]

Notable Cases of Misconduct or Alleged Misconduct in Biomedical Research

Throughout history, biomedical researchers have had a reputation for honesty and integrity. However, there are some notable episodes in which even the most prominent researchers have committed, or appeared to have committed, data falsification or fabrication, plagiarism, and other misdeeds (see Table 72.3). The

founder of the modern theory of heredity, Austrian monk and botanist Gregor Mendel (1822–1884), has been accused of research misconduct. In 1936, statistician R. Fisher published a paper analyzing the data that Mendel reported in his paper on the genetics of plant hybrids. Fisher found that the data Mendel reported agreed more closely with his hypotheses than would be expected if the data had been generated from natural experiments, which would have some random fluctuations. Fisher concluded that "the data of most, if not all, of the experiments have been falsified so as to agree closely with Mendel's expectations."[13] According to some estimates, Mendel's data were so close to the values predicted by his hypotheses that the odds were 33,000 to 1 against his actually having obtained the data from his observations.[14]

Even though the evidence appears to support the view that Mendel was either exceedingly lucky or falsified some of his data to conform to his expectations, this conclusion is not consistent with his character. Mendel was a very careful scientist with a reputation for thoroughness and integrity.[14] His scientific peers did not recognize his work, but he was convinced of its importance. One would not expect someone like him to alter data to fit his theories. However, in his will, Mendel made the unusual request that his laboratory notebooks be destroyed after his death. One could speculate that he made the request in order to secure

Table 72.3
Well-Known Cases of Alleged Misconduct in Biomedical Research

Case, Date(s)	Issues	Outcome
Gregor Mendel, 1865	Data falsification	No resolution
Piltdown Man, 1908–1953	Fabrication	Fabrication found
Cyril Burt, 1970s	Fabrication, falsification, plagiarism	No resolution
William Summerlin, 1973	Fabrication	Admission of guilt
John Darsee, 1981	Fabrication	Fabrication found
E.A.K. Alsabati, 1980s	Plagiarism	No admission of guilt
Thereza Imanishi-Kari, 1986	Fabrication, falsification	Exonerated
Stephen Breuning, 1983–1988	Fabrication, falsification	Fabrication, falsification found
Roger Poisson, 1993	Falsification	Falsification found
Bernard Fisher, 1994	Falsification	Exonerated
Eric Poehlman, 1995–2005	Falsification	Admission of guilt
Woo Suk Hwang, 2005	Fabrication	Fabrication found

his reputation after death, but the scientific community will probably never know for certain why he made this request or whether he falsified data.[13]

One of the most infamous episodes of data fabrication in the history of biology occurred in the beginning of the 20th century. After Charles Darwin (1809–1882) published his *On the Origin of Species* in 1859, scientists who accepted his theory of natural selection were interested in finding evidence in the fossil record linking humans and apes. In 1908, an amateur geologist and a prominent British paleontologist claimed to have found the skull of a "missing link" between man and apes in a gravel bed at Piltdown, England. For many years, researchers accepted the skull as authentic, because it was consistent with their anthropological and archeological theories. By the 1930s, doubts about the authenticity of the skull began to arise when it was found to be inconsistent with other hominid fossils. In 1953, physical and chemical tests proved that the skull was a fake: the upper part of the skull was a fossil that had been artificially aged to appear older than it was, and the lower jaw was not even a fossil.[15]

In the 1970s, the famous psychologist Cyril Burt (1883–1971) was accused of fabricating and falsifying data in his studies of identical twins, fabricating data on declining levels of intelligence in the United Kingdom, falsely claiming relationships with collaborators, and falsely claiming to be the originator of factor analysis in psychology.[15] Burt, who held the chair of psychology at University College London for 20 years and was the official psychologist of the London City Council, argued that intelligence was strongly genetically determined. Burt's defenders claimed that he did not falsify or fabricate data, and that the problems with his data were due poor record keeping or errors. Because these allegations were made after he was dead, only Burt's defenders responded to these charges.

Another famous fabrication incident took place in 1974 at the prestigious Sloan-Kettering Institute in New York. In 1973, William Summerlin joined Robert Goode's transplantation immunology laboratory at Sloan-Kettering. Summerlin, who was a well-known immunologist, had been studying organ transplantation. Summerlin believed that organ rejection could be prevented by culturing organs in a tissue culture for days or weeks before

transplantation. Other scientists were having difficulty replicating Summerlin's work. To prove his hypothesis, Summerlin conducted some experiments that he claimed involved the transplantation of tissue between genetically unrelated strains of mice. In the experiments, Summerlin cultured and then "transplanted" patches of skin from black-haired mice onto white-haired mice. He hoped to prove that his hypothesis was correct by showing that the white-haired mice would not reject the patch of skin with black hair.

A laboratory assistant who was in charge of taking care of the mice noticed that alcohol could wash away the black color on the white mice. The assistant reported this finding to Goode, who suspended Summerlin from his work so that a committee could investigate the incident. Summerlin soon confessed to using a black felt tip pen to produce patches of black hair on the white mice. The committee examined Summerlin's other experiments and determined that Summerlin and several collaborators had fabricated data relating to the "transplantation" of corneas in rabbits. The committee also found that Summerlin was probably suffering from an emotional illness. The committee recommended that Summerlin be granted a medical leave of absence, correct the irregularities in his work, and publish retractions. Summerlin claimed that he fabricated data because he was under a great deal of personal and professional stress. The scandal ruined the career of Goode, who was one of the top immunologists in the country at the time.[16]

In 1981, John Darsee, a highly productive postdoctoral fellow at Harvard Medical School, was accused of fabricating and falsifying data in a dozen papers and abstracts. Darsee's supervisor was cardiologist Eugene Braunwald, who was chair of medicine at Brigham and Women's Hospital and Harvard Medical School. A committee investigating the incident found that Darsee committed misconduct in five of the papers that he published with faculty at Harvard, including Braunwald, and eight papers that he published with faculty at Emory Medical School, where he was a doctoral student. The committee also found that Darsee had fabricated data in two undergraduate papers that he published while at Notre Dame. Although the committee did not find that the coauthors had committed misconduct, it raised serious questions about their responsibilities as coauthors, because many of the fabrications in

Darsee's published papers would be obvious to an expert in his field upon a careful reading of those papers. Eventually, 17 papers and 53 abstracts coauthored by Darsee were retracted. Even though this episode ended Darsee's career as a biomedical scientist, he went on to pursue a career in clinical medicine.[17]

Infamous cases of plagiarism also occurred in the 1980s. In one case, E.A.K. Alsabati, a Jordanian biologist, republished in his own name articles by others that had previously appeared in obscure, small-circulation journals. In some cases, he simply retyped the articles and submitted them for publication. Although Alsabati never admitted any wrongdoing, several scientific journals, including *Nature* and the *British Medical Journal,* published excerpts from the original articles right next to Alsabati's articles.[15]

In 1983, two science journalists, William Broad and Nicholas Wade, published *Betrayers of Truth: Fraud and Deceit in the Halls of Science.*[18] The book raised the public's and media's awareness of unethical conduct in science. Broad and Wade also accused Isaac Newton, Robert Millikan, and Gregor Mendel of manipulating data to produce sought-after results.

The Baltimore Affair

From 1986 to 1996, a scandal took place that had a major impact on science policy in the United States. The scandal, which became known as the Baltimore affair, centered on a paper published in the journal *Cell* in 1986. The paper had six coauthors, including the Nobel laureate David Baltimore.[19] The paper reported that inserting a single antibody gene from another strain of mice can induce a mouse's own antibodies to change their molecular structure, suggesting a new mechanism of immunity. The experiments, which were funded by the NIH, were conducted at the Whitehead Institute, a research center associated with the Massachusetts Institute of Technology (MIT) and Tufts University. Margot O'Toole, who was a postdoctoral fellow working under the supervision of Assistant Professor Thereza Imanishi-Kari, one of the paper's authors, became suspicious when she found 17 pages from Imanishi-Kari's lab notebooks that she believed contradicted the results reported in the paper. After failing in her attempt to reproduce these results, O'Toole informed review boards at Tufts and MIT about her suspicions of possible fabrication or falsification.[20]

Internal investigations by committees at Tufts and MIT found some errors in the research but no evidence of misconduct. The NIH's Office of Scientific Integrity (OSI) reviewed these findings and launched its own investigation. In April 1988, Representative John Dingell (D-Mich.), chairman of the House Commerce Committee's Oversight and Investigations Subcommittee, held several hearings on fraud in science, including the Baltimore case. The Secret Service assisted in the investigation by seizing and analyzing Imanishi-Kari's notebooks. Baltimore testified before the House subcommittee and defended the research. He described the investigations conducted by the NIH and Congress as a "witch hunt."[20]

The scandal continued to generate headlines during the early 1990s. Baltimore resigned from his position as president of Rockefeller University in 1992 due to his involvement in the scandal. In 1994, the Office of Research Integrity (ORI), formerly the OSI, concluded that Imanishi-Kari had fabricated and falsified data. Tufts asked Imanishi-Kari to take a leave of absence after the

ORI issued its findings. However, an appeals panel at the Department of Health and Human Services (DHHS) exonerated Imanishi-Kari in 1996. The panel concluded that the evidence against her was unreliable or uncorroborated. To this day, Imanishi-Kari maintains her innocence in the affair. She admits to poor record keeping but she denies that she ever falsified or fabricated data. Most researchers with knowledge of the case believe that Imanishi-Kari was not guilty of fabrication or falsification and that Baltimore was unfairly tainted by the scandal that now bears his name. Many researchers were also concerned that some members of Congress may have used the case for political gain.[20]

In the 1980s and 1990s there were several other high-profile misconduct scandals in the biomedical sciences. The House subcommittee that reviewed the Baltimore case also impugned Stephen Breuning, a psychologist who had been accused of misconduct in 1983, on charges of falsifying reports to the National Institute of Mental Health (NIMH). In 1987, the NIMH found that Breuning reported nonexistent patients, fabricated data, and falsified data on grant applications. In 1988, Breuning was convicted of criminal fraud and sentenced 60 days of imprisonment and five years' probation. He also had to pay $11,352 in restitution to the University of Pittsburgh.[6]

In 1993, the ORI concluded that Roger Poisson, a Canadian surgeon conducting research as part of the National Surgical Adjuvant Breast and Bowel Project (NSABP), had falsified data on 117 patients from 1977 to 1990. In one instance, Poisson falsified an informed consent document. Poisson admitted that he subscribed to a loose interpretation of the NSABP's inclusion and exclusion criteria for the study and said that he tried to admit as many patients as possible to the study so that they would have a chance of qualifying for advanced treatment methods.[21] The House subcommittee also held hearings on the case and learned that Bernard Fisher, chairman of the NSABP and a University of Pittsburgh cancer researcher, who discovered the misconduct, had published several papers containing the falsified data.[22] The ORI ordered Fisher to reanalyze the data. The results of the reanalysis showed that the falsified data had no effect on the research results. The reanalysis, which was published in the *New England Journal of Medicine,* showed that lumpectomies are effective at treating breast cancer tumors less than 4 cm in diameter.[23] Fisher claimed that he was forced to resign his position at the University of Pittsburgh to appease Congress and the National Cancer Institute, which sponsored the NSABP. Even though the ORI found that Fisher did not commit misconduct, he sued the government for damaging his reputation. The NIH had labeled 93 of Fisher's papers with the warning "scientific misconduct—data to be reanalyzed" on its computerized databases.[21]

In 1996, a reviewer for the journal *Oncogene* challenged a paper submitted by a graduate student working in the lab of Francis Collins, the director of the National Human Genome Research Institute and head of the Human Genome Project. The reviewer questioned the data in the paper and accused the student of misconduct. Collins examined the student's research records and determined that the student had committed misconduct. The student confessed, and Collins retracted five papers the student had published with coauthors and wrote a letter to more than 100 scientists advising them of problems with the papers. Although Collins handled this episode well, he was concerned that neither he nor his senior scientists had detected problems with these papers before they were submitted for publication. He described the entire ordeal as the most devastating experience of his life.[17]

Two Stunning Cases in 2005

One of the most expensive cases of research misconduct occurred in 2005, when Eric Poehlman, a well-known expert on menopause, aging, and metabolism, admitted to falsifying data on 15 federal grant applications and 17 publications. The NIH and the Department of Agriculture had awarded Poehlman $2.9 million worth of grants based on falsified data. Poehlman, who had held an academic appointment at the University of Vermont College of Medicine, was barred for life from receiving any federal research funding and retracted 10 papers. Poehlman also agreed to pay the federal government $180,000 to settle a civil lawsuit; he could have received a $250,000 fine and up to five years' imprisonment. Poehlman's scam began to unravel in 2000, when research assistant Walter DeNino discovered inconsistencies in a longitudinal study of aging. According to DeNino, Poehlman switched some data points to make it appear that some of his subjects were becoming sicker over time. DeNino filed a complaint against Poehlman, and an investigative committee at the University of Vermont found that Poehlman had falsified data in several papers. In one of those papers, a highly cited study on menopause published in the *Annals of Internal Medicine* in 1995, most of the experimental subjects did not exist. In 2001, before the investigation ended, Poehlman left the University of Vermont and took a position at the University of Montreal. He left the University of Montreal in January 2005.[24]

Another high-profile case occurred in 2005, when South Korean scientist Woo Suk Hwang admitted to fabricating data used to support a groundbreaking article published in *Science* in February 2005, which purported to demonstrate the derivation of 11 embryonic stem cell lines using nuclear transfer techniques (i.e., therapeutic cloning). A panel at Seoul National University, where Hwang conducted the research, found that none of the DNA in the 11 cell lines reported in the article matched the DNA in the cell lines of the human subjects used in the experiment. The panel also determined that Hwang faked data in a paper he published in 2004 on therapeutic cloning, and that coauthorship on the 2005 paper had been awarded for merely procuring eggs. The panel did not challenge Hwang's claim to have produced the world's first cloned dog, Snuppy.[25] Hwang, who had become a national hero, resigned from his position and faced up to 10 years in prison if convicted of fraud. In another ethical twist, the world also learned that two of the egg donors for the 2005 article, junior researchers working in Hwang's laboratory, may have been coerced.[25] Had Hwang's work been valid, it would have indicated that one of the main goals of stem cell research, therapeutic cloning, is achievable. Researchers have sought to develop therapeutic cloning because the stem cells produced by this process would be genetically identical to those of the patient, because they contain the patient's own DNA. Organs and other tissue grown from these stem cells would be less likely to be rejected by the patient's immune system than tissue produced by other techniques. The South Korean scandal dealt a severe blow to embryonic stem cell research, and gave ammunition to critics of therapeutic cloning.[26]

Regulatory Responses to Research Misconduct

The misconduct scandals in federally funded biomedical research in the 1980s had a major impact on U.S. government policies. In 1989, the PHS formed two agencies, OSI and the Office of Scientific Integrity Review (OSIR), to review misconduct allegations against PHS-funded researchers and provide information and support for research institutions. In 1992, the PHS replaced these two agencies with the ORI, which is located with the DHHS. The ORI oversees all research integrity activities for the PHS, which oversees NIH research. The ORI investigates allegations of research misconduct and sponsors educational and research activities;[27] it has sponsored conferences on research integrity and has funded grants to conduct research on research integrity. Other federal agencies have their own structures for dealing with research ethics issues. For example, the National Science Foundation's (NSF's) Office of Inspector General (OIG) oversees research integrity activities for that agency. The Food and Drug Administration's (FDA) Office of Regulatory Affairs deals with research integrity problems related to privately funded research submitted to the FDA. The ORI has the authority to investigate allegations involving FDA research if the research is partly supported by the PHS.[28]

In 1989, the NIH began requiring institutions that receive training grants to meet training requirements for education in responsible conduct of research (RCR) for graduate students funded by NIH grants. Universities have taken a variety of approaches to fulfilling this NIH requirement, ranging from formal courses in RCR, to RCR seminars or workshops, to RCR training incorporated into existing courses in research methods. In 2000, the NIH began requiring its intramural researchers to receive education in RCR. The NIH now requires intramural researchers to take an online, introductory course in RCR as well as to receive annual updates. In the fall of 2000, the ORI mandated that all personnel receiving PHS grants also receive instruction in nine core topics in RCR, which included data management, authorship and publication, peer review, mentoring, collaboration, research misconduct, conflict of interest, research animals, and research with humans. When the George W. Bush administration came to power in 2001, the PHS suspended the mandate on the grounds that the ORI had not followed proper procedures for issuing formal administrative rules. As of 2007, the policy was in limbo.[6]

The National Academy of Sciences (NAS) has issued two major reports related to research ethics. The first report, published in 1992, examined misconduct in science.[29] It developed a definition of scientific misconduct, attempted to estimate the incidence of misconduct, and examined some of the causes of misconduct. The second report, published in 2002, focused on promoting integrity in scientific research. The report stressed the importance of education in research ethics, mentoring and leadership, and institutional self-assessment.[30] In 1989, the NAS also published *On Being a Scientist,* a useful handbook on research ethics. The handbook, which was revised in 1995, is available on the web.[31]

Empirical Data on Research Misconduct

Estimates of the incidence of misconduct in research vary greatly.[32] In one of the most reliable surveys, 6%–9% of students and faculty reported direct knowledge of fabrication, falsification, or plagiarism.[33] However, estimates based on 200 confirmed misconduct cases reported to ORI over a 20-year period yield a rate of one misconduct episode per 100,000 researchers per year.[32] One of the difficulties with estimates based on this sort of analysis is that misconduct is probably underreported. The ORI is interested in gathering more evidence about the incidence of misconduct and has sponsored research to try to address this issue.

Even if one supposes that the misconduct rate is quite low, this does not mean that misconduct is not a serious problem for researchers. Fabrication, falsification, plagiarism, and other highly unethical research activities can negatively affect the integrity and reliability of the published research record, destroy cooperation and trust among researchers, and undermine public support for science. Additionally, fabrication or falsification in clinical research can cause harm to human research participants or the public health.[21] For example, if clinical researchers falsify data concerning adverse events in human studies, then agencies that oversee research, such as the FDA and institutional review boards, may lack the information they need to protect other research subjects from harm. If clinical researchers fabricate or falsify data pertaining to the safety or a new drug, and the FDA approves the drug on the basis of erroneous data, then the drug could severely harm or kill people. However, it is worth noting that most of the well-known cases of misconduct in biomedicine have involved basic research, not clinical research. In the NASBP case, Poisson's misconduct did not have an impact on the overall results of clinical recommendations.

Since the 1980s, there have been two prevailing explanations for research misconduct.[6] Some scientists and researchers claim that misconduct is committed by individuals who are morally corrupt, mentally unstable, or under great financial or emotional pressure. If they are right, misconduct is a rare event that results from a few bad apples. However, most organizations and scholars who have studied that problem argue that misconduct is due to the institutional, social, and economic factors in the research environment, such as financial and proprietary interests in research, problems with the supervision of subordinates, the mentoring relationship, tenure and promotion policies, the pressure to publish, careerism, the need to recruit patients for clinical trials, and publication practices. Although money does not automatically corrupt researchers, there is a growing concern about the influence of financial interests in science.[34] One commentator has described conflicts of interests as risk factors for misconduct.[35] It is worth noting, however, that most of the well-known misconduct cases have occurred in publicly funded research instead of privately funded research, which would suggest that factors other than money, such as ambition or arrogance, play a greater role in causing misconduct. However, the fact that most of the well-known cases of misconduct have occurred in government-funded research does not prove that private research is more ethical than public research. One very simple explanation for the fact that the private sector has fewer misconduct cases is that we generally know more about publicly funded research than we know about privately funded research. In public research, government agencies publish their findings of misconduct. In private research, misconduct can occur beneath the cloak of trade secrecy. Obviously, these issues merit further study.

Conclusion: Education and Oversight

A commitment to honesty lies at heart of the research enterprise. Honesty plays an important role in every step in the process of research, from designing the experiment, to recording data, to analyzing and interpreting data. Although honesty seems like a fairly straightforward issue in scientific research, this is far from the case. Scientists often must make complex judgments and decisions concerning the conduct of research that have an important effect on the objectivity, reliability, and integrity of their data and results. To promote honesty in science and prevent research misconduct, researchers and institutions should take the following steps:

- Senior researchers (or mentors) should help junior researchers (or students) learn how to strive for honesty and integrity in science. They should teach junior researchers how to design experiments, collect and record data, and analyze and interpret data. They should teach their students about the importance of honesty in all aspects of scientific communication, including not only research but also grant writing, peer review, publication, and expert testimony. This education can take place in research methods courses, research ethics courses, or during informal discussions in a laboratory or office.
- In addition to educating junior researchers, senior researchers should properly supervise junior researchers. They should establish protocols and standard operating procedures to provide guidance for junior researchers. They should also communicate directly with junior researchers on a regular basis about their research obligations and responsibilities.
- Universities and research organizations should support efforts to educate junior researchers about the ethical conduct of research. They should provide money and staff for courses, workshops, seminars, lectures, or other activities designed to enhance the research ethics curriculum.
- Universities and research organizations should also develop policies and procedures related to honesty in science, which should address research misconduct, fabrication, falsification, plagiarism, supervision of subordinates, and data management.
- Universities and research organizations should establish clear and fair procedures for investigating and adjudicating allegations of misconduct, including protection for whistle blowers, protection of the rights of the accused, and confidentiality.

Acknowledgment

This article was supported by intramural program of the National Institute of Environmental Health Sciences, National Institutes of Health. It does not represent the views of the National Institute of Environmental Health Sciences or the National Institutes of Health.

References

1. Babbage C. *Reflections on the Decline of Science in England.* New York, N.Y.: Augustus Kelley; 1970 [1830].

2. American Medical Association. AMA History. [Online] Available: http://www.ama-assn.org/ama/pub/category/1923.html.

3. *The American Heritage Dictionary of the English Language,* 4th ed. New York, N.Y.: Houghton Mifflin; 2000.

4. *Black's Law Dictionary,* 7th ed. St. Paul, Minn.: West Publishing; 1999.

5. Kalb P, Koehler K. Legal issues in scientific research. *JAMA* 2002;287:85–91.

6. Shamoo A, Resnik D. *Responsible Conduct of Research.* New York, N.Y.: Oxford University Press; 2003.

7. Resnik D. From Baltimore to Bell Labs: Reflections on two decades of debate about scientific misconduct. *Accountability in Research* 2003;10:123–35.

8. Office of Science and Technology Policy, Executive Office of the President. Federal Policy on Research Misconduct; Preamble for Research Misconduct Policy; Notification of Final Policy. *Federal Register* 2000;65(235):76260–4. [Online] Available: http://www.ori.dhhs .gov/policies/fed_research_misconduct.shtml.

9. Public Health Service, Department of Health and Human Services. 42 CFR Part 50: Responsibilities of Awardee and Applicant Institutions for Dealing With and Reporting Possible Misconduct in Science; Final Rule. *Federal Register* 1989;54(151):32446–51.

10. Koenig B. Scientific misconduct: Wellcome rules widen the net. *Science* 2001;293:1411–2.

11. Rossner M, Yamada K. What's in a picture? The temptation of image manipulation. *Journal of Cell Biology* 2004;166:11–5.

12. Medical schools conflict of interest policies improve; Additional improvements suggested. *Office of Research Integrity Newsletter* 2004; 13(1):4. [Online] Available: http://www.ori.dhhs.gov/documents/ newsletters/v0113_n01.pdf.

13. Fisher R. Has Mendel's work been rediscovered? In: Stern C, Sherwood E, eds. *The Origin of Genetics.* San Francisco, Calif.: W. H. Freeman; 1990:164.

14. Nissani M. Psychological, historical, and ethical reflections on the Mendelian paradox. *Perspectives in Biology and Medicine* 1994;37: 182–96.

15. LaFollette M. *Stealing Into Print: Fraud, Plagiarism and Misconduct in Scientific Publishing.* Berkeley, Calif.: University of California Press; 1992.

16. Hixson J. *The Patchwork Mouse.* Garden City, N.J.: Doubleday; 1976.

17. Ryan K. Research misconduct in clinical research. *Acta Ontologica* 1999;38:93–7.

18. Broad W, Wade N. *Betrayers of the Truth: Fraud and Deceit in the Halls of Science.* New York, N.Y.: Simon and Schuster; 1982.

19. Weaver D, Reis M, Albanese C, Costantini F, Baltimore D, Imanishi-Kari T. Altered repertoire of endogenous immunoglobulin gene expression in transgenic mice containing a rearranged MY heavy chain gene. *Cell* 1986;45:247–59.

20. Kevles D. *The Baltimore Case: A Trial of Science, Politics, and Character.* New York, N.Y.: Norton; 1998.

21. Buyse M, Evans S. Fraud in clinical trials. In: Colton T, Redmond CK, eds. *Biostatistics in Clinical Trials.* New York, N.Y.: John Wiley & Sons; 2001:432–69.

22. Resnik D. Data falsification in clinical trials. *Science Communication* 1996;18(1):49–58.

23. Fisher B, Anderson S, Redmond C, et al. Reanalysis and results after 12 years of follow-up in a randomized clinical trial comparing total mastectomy with lumpectomy with or without irradiation in the treatment of breast cancer. *New England Journal of Medicine* 1995; 333:1456–61.

24. Kinitisch E. Researcher faces prison for fraud in NIH grant applications and papers. *Science* 2005;307:1851.

25. Cyranoski D. Verdict: Hwang's human stem cells were all fakes. *Nature* 2006;439:122–3.

26. Normile D, Vogel G. Korean university will investigate cloning paper. *Science* 2005;310:1749–50.

27. Pascal C. The history and future of the office of research integrity: Scientific misconduct and beyond. *Science and Engineering Ethics* 1999;5:183–98.

28. Office of Research Integrity. Handling Misconduct. [Online] Available: http://ori.dhhs.gov/misconduct/PHS_offices.shtml.

29. Panel on Scientific Responsibility and the Conduct of Research, Committee on Science, Engineering, and Public Policy, National Academy of Sciences. *Responsible Science, Vol. 1. Ensuring the Integrity of the Research Process.* Washington, D.C.: National Academy Press; 1992.

30. Committee on Assessing Integrity in Research Environments, Board on Health Sciences Policy and Division of Earth and Life Studies, Institute of Medicine. *Integrity in Scientific Research: Creating an Environment That Promotes Responsible Conduct.* Washington, D.C.: National Academies Press; 2002.

31. Committee on Science, Engineering, and Public Policy, National Academy of Sciences. *On Being a Scientist: Responsible Conduct in Research,* 2nd ed. Washington, D.C.: National Academy Press; 1995. [Online] Available: http://www.nap.edu/readingroom/ books/obas/.

32. Steneck N. Assessing the integrity of publicly funded research. Proceedings from the Office of Research Integrity Conference on Research on Research Integrity. Washington, D.C.: ORI; 2000:1–16.

33. Swazey J, Anderson M, Louis K. Ethical problems in academic research. *American Scientist* 1993;81:542–3.

34. Krimsky S. *Science in the Private Interest.* Lanham, Md.: Rowman and Littlefield; 2003.

35. Bodenheimer T. Conflicts of interest in clinical drug trials: A risk factor for scientific misconduct. Office of Human Research Protections, Conference on Conflicts of Interest in Research, August 15, 2000, Washington, D.C. [Online] Available: http://www.hsph .harvard.edu/bioethics/uae/BodenheimerCOI.html.

Drummond Rennie

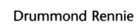

The Obligation to Publish and Disseminate Results

For better or for worse, publication is the medium by which the scholar's work is distributed and judged. Thus much of a scholar's reputation depends upon what, where, and how much he or she publishes, and on how that work is received publicly by others.[1]
—Donald Kennedy

The Ethical Basis for Scientific Publication

The job of a scientist was summarized by Benjamin Franklin (1706–1790) as "[t]o study, to finish, to publish." Michael Faraday later wrote much the same thing.[2] Both recognized that scientific work cannot exist until it is published. Only then can fellow scientists have the full details in order to judge the worth of the science and attempt replication or refutation. To quote the National Academy of Sciences' report *Responsible Science,* "Science is a cumulative activity in which each scientist builds on the work of others. Publication of results is an integral and essential component of research because it enables others to gain access to each scientist's contribution."[3] Research institutions that receive public money, including almost all major universities, receive public esteem, support, and tax advantages because it is generally acknowledged that they exist for the public good. If research is locked up within the institutions, the health of the public cannot be served. It is for this reason that university regulations include the unfettered right to publish.[4] It is for this reason that clinical scientists, whether they work in academe or in commercial

organizations, have the obligation to publish. To be a researcher implies being an author, and to be an author implies publication, and so dissemination.

The individual who agrees to participate in research as a subject in a clinical trial takes on the hardships and risks for the benefit of mankind, and the pact between participant and researcher implies that the results will be broadly known. Few would undertake this altruistic task if they thought that their results would remain hidden or be held as trade secrets. Clinical scientists, therefore, have a particular obligation to publish, governed by the Declaration of Helsinki (see Chapter 13). Article 11 states, "Medical research involving human subjects must conform to generally accepted scientific principles, be based on a thorough knowledge of the scientific literature, other relevant sources of information, and on adequate laboratory and, where appropriate, animal experimentation."[5] If results are not published, the scientific literature will be deficient, and it will be impossible to meet the standard of Article 19: "Medical research is only justified if there is a reasonable likelihood that the populations in which the research is carried out stand to benefit from the results of the research." Finally, Article 27 states in part, "Both authors and publishers have ethical obligations. In publication of the results of research, the investigators are obliged to preserve the accuracy of the results. Negative as well as positive results should be published or otherwise publicly available. . . . Reports of experimentation not in accordance with the principles laid down in this Declaration should not be accepted for publication."[5]

What Constitutes Work Deserving of Publication?

Investigators alone have to judge when a piece of their study is mature enough for publication. In the field of clinical trials, they must guard against premature publication of reports that can directly affect the treatment of patients. Though there are no rigid rules, the aim of publication must be to convey the most useful information in the most efficient form, and each publication should be a substantive contribution. Investigators lose the respect of their colleagues if they are perceived as merely advancing their own self-interest by slicing their work into numerous fragments ("salami publication" of "least publishable units") to maximize the number of their publications.[6–8] This tactic greatly decreases the value of the combined publications to the reader, who must search multiple sources, each inevitably containing much repetitious material. A similar inappropriate practice, called the "meat extender" tactic, is to keep publishing the same study with the addition of small amounts of data in each article.[9] Each paper should contain sufficient information for the reader to assess its validity and replicate the results.

What Constitutes Publication and Dissemination?

Publication of a clinical study is the action of making it publicly known. Strictly speaking, this would include sticking a manuscript on a bulletin board; but because that would so limit the spread of the information compared with printing it in a journal, publication is not considered to have occurred unless the information has also been disseminated ("spread abroad, diffused") to more than a few colleagues or, say, outside a sponsoring company. Roughly half of conference abstracts result in later published articles. Lectures, conference abstracts and posters are all forms of dissemination. By and large, journals approve of such presentations as working papers, even if they are in print before conferences, and do not disqualify the later, fully refined manuscripts on the basis of duplication. Until the last decade, publication and dissemination have almost invariably denoted appearance in print. The majority of journals now appear in both print and electronic versions, whereas some are entirely electronic. The general standards for publication and dissemination in either medium are the same.

Additional Databases or Trial Banks

Print journals are expensive to produce and wasteful of natural resources, so they usually have strict limits on the space available for articles. This forces the authors to select what data to present, and these data must be sufficient to buttress all the authors' conclusions. There may be large amounts of background information that readers might request, and which the editors assume as a condition of acceptance that the authors will provide. Electronic publication expands the ability of the authors and the journals to provide databanks of information, for example *trial banks* of data on clinical trials they publish. Such systems are still being developed and assessed.

Redundant (Duplicate) Publication and Prior Publication

Medical journals strongly discourage duplicate submission to different journals for publication lest two journals "unknowingly and unnecessarily undertake the work of peer review and editing of the same manuscript, and publish (the) same article," both claiming the right to publish and to own the copyright.[8] The guidelines of the International Committee of Medical Journal Editors (ICMJE) define *redundant* or *duplicate* publication as "publication of a paper that overlaps substantially with one already published in print or electronic media." The guidelines go on to state, "The bases of this position are international copyright laws, ethical conduct, and cost-effective use of resources. Duplicate publication of original research is particularly problematic, since it can result in inadvertent double counting or inappropriate weighting of the results of a single study, which distorts the available evidence."[8]

If repetition of previously published data is necessary, as von Elm et al. write, "authors must acknowledge the main article overtly by using a cross-reference."[10] Moreover, these authors caution, "Covert duplicate publication has been widely disapproved. This practice is wasteful of the time and resources of editors, peer reviewers, and readers, and it is misleading because undue weight is given to observations that are being reported repeatedly. When duplicates are inadvertently included in a systematic review, the conclusion of that systematic review may change."[10,11] Finally, covert duplicate publication is dishonest and undermines the integrity of science.[10,12,13]

Journal editors frequently have to make judgments about the extent of overlap between two or more of the authors' manuscripts or their published work. Prior publication may be judged to have occurred if substantially the same article has appeared in conference proceedings that were circulated, on paper or electronically, to more than a very few people, and authors are advised to check the policies of the journal to which they propose to submit their work. Editors are helped when prospective authors enclose copies of related, possibly overlapping manuscripts either to be submitted elsewhere or in press. Because the discovery of deception results in publication of a notice, or even a retraction, there are reasons beyond correct scientific behavior for authors to be open about parallel manuscripts. The standards for acceptable secondary publication are listed by the ICMJE.[8]

The Author's Obligation to the Reader: To Maintain Trust

As readers, we must be skeptical, but we must start with the assumption that, though the authors might be mistaken, their report is a fair representation of what they observed. We are forced to accord them trust because we cannot be in their institutions, checking their work. This implies that, as Lederberg has said, "Above all, the act of publication is an inscription under oath, a testimony."[14] Authors make an unseen pact with their readers which require authors to be accountable. Authors have the duty to respond openly and promptly when questions are raised that challenge their findings. This may, for example, involve the provision of unpublished data, whether or not this is required as a condition of their funding.[3] Without this acceptance of accountability, authorship is meaningless, and the trust that binds authors and readers is broken. It is for this reason that the idea of anonymous science, popular 300 years ago, was abandoned: Trust could not be expected or granted. Authorship may bring credit; it invariably carries responsibility. This, rather than glory or priority, is what gives authorship both meaning and importance.

The Social Role of Authorship

Published articles are not merely the means whereby new work is communicated between scientists. They also serve a crucial social role in establishing priority, reputation, and standing. Publications are necessary for the correct attribution of credit for scientific discovery, and they constitute the coins by which academics proceed along the toll road of promotion.[15] The number and worth of publications, and the prestige of the journals in which they have appeared, may constitute the most important factors in assessments for academic tenure and promotion.

History and Definition of Authorship

The present discussion is limited to modern clinical research. The standards for authorship in, for example, particle physics, in which scores or hundreds of coauthors are common, or for philosophy, in which the single-authored paper still persists, may differ markedly from those governing authorship of clinical studies and trials. The standards for other professions may vary even more widely. For example, in the legal profession, an opinion written by law clerks, when published, carries the name of the judge alone;[16] movie screen writers operate under still another system.[17]

The term *author* derives, like the word *augment,* from the Indo-European base *aug-* (to multiply) and the Latin *augere* (to increase, to originate or grow). The word has been used in England since the 14th century as denoting "[o]ne who sets forth written statements; the composer or writer of a treatise or book."[18] As Vickers points out, "The author emerged as a professional writer in the sixth century B.C., and many of the attributes we associate with authorship—a sense of individual identity, in style, attitude, literary structure; a hatred of plagiarism; a respected role in society—were already found in abundance in Greco-Roman antiquity."[19] In literature, we may argue whether there was a real person called Homer, or whether his works were the product of an oral tradition carried on by many tellers of tales. Or we can dispute whether John Fletcher wrote more than half of the *Henry VIII* that we usually attribute to Shakespeare.[19] But it is our expectation that in fiction, now as in the past, there is usually only one author. That author is expected to take responsibility if, for example, plagiarism or libel are alleged.

Scientific Authorship

Terms change. As science grew and branched into a separate series of disciplines, it was proposed in the 1830s at the British Association for the Advancement of Science, whose members seemed uncomfortable being called *savants* or *philosophes,* that those who practiced science, by analogy with artists, be called *scientists.*[18] The

members adopted the word at the suggestion of their cofounder, William Whewell, who in 1833 had invented the word at the request of the poet Coleridge.[20] In the century or so that it took for this word to take hold, it continued to be assumed that investigator-scientists, when they wrote up their observations, were to be called *authors,* so no new term evolved simultaneously. The concept of an author developed when cooperative work was rare and the author of a scientific article, like that of a novel, was almost invariably one person. In science, it was not until around 1955 that the average number of authors per scientific article rose above two, and this has occurred in numerous clinical disciplines.[21–24]

Since then, the total number of scientists has multiplied, as has their total number of publications[25] and the number of authors per publication.[26] The cause was the increasing need for specialists to invite scientists in other disciplines to collaborate with them. As the proportion of one- and two-author publications fell, the proportion with three, four, or more authors rose.[21] One scientist, Yury Struchkov, published one article every 3.9 days for 10 years, whereas 20 researchers worldwide published at least once every 11.3 days throughout the decade of the 1980s.[27] More than half of these researchers were biomedical investigators who ran medium-to-large laboratories.[27] Over the last half of the 20th century, the average number of authors per published article has grown exponentially.[26,28]

One factor remained constant, however: It was usually impossible to link the job title of the coauthor to the job he or she had actually done in the research. Team research, introduced to manage the increasing complexity of research, had brought with it problems in assigning both credit and responsibility. A notable example of team research is the clinical trial, and the number of clinical trial reports with more than 100 authors began to climb, also exponentially, after 1990.[29]

The Obligations of Coauthors to Each Other

When they submit manuscripts, scientific authors have obligations to their patients, institutions, journals, and readers. Some of these are symbolized in the forms and checklists that journals require them to sign. But coauthors are also accountable to each other. The severe consequences on the lives and careers of the innocent coauthors of a fraudulent researcher serve as reminders that each individual on the byline has to take responsibility for something more than his or her own narrow contribution, and that each has the duty to help assure the integrity of the whole article. Each author must be willing to support the general conclusions of a study, and assist in answering questions after publication[7] (see Boxes 73.1–73.3).

Why Is Credit for Authorship So Key?

At the deepest level, the author wants to be heard and acknowledged. "Most books are not valuable 'properties'; they're voices, laying perpetual claim to their authors' existence," wrote the poet Thomas Mallon, whose book *Stolen Words* tells the story of how a serial plagiarist robbed him of his work and took over his life.[30] This has been so from the earliest times, and there are many accounts of the anger authors have expressed when their work was plagiarized.[19] In science, there are other factors that make authorship credit so coveted. A place on the byline is properly earned by the contribution of the author to the research, and the community, broadly speaking, recognizes that. Indeed, given the fact that publications are the product of working researchers, the place publications have in our system of rewards, and the ease with which an investigator's publications may be counted, it is no surprise to find how strenuously scientists fight for that place.

Authorship Disputes

It is because credit for authorship has taken on such an important social and professional role that scientists view authorship with so much anxiety and passion, and it is for these reasons that disputes about authorship are so frequent, so wasteful of time, and so badly resolved. Though scientists as diverse as Newton and Freud have expressed concerns about correct attribution of credit, their issues were largely with researchers who were not their collaborators. But an inevitable consequence of increasing the number of coauthors is that it becomes harder to form the one-to-one relationships necessary to secure trust among the authors,[31] and it should be no surprise that disputes between authors are increasing exponentially.[32] Vagueness as to roles and responsibilities among coauthors has resulted in a failure to examine and disclose uncollegial or even fraudulent behavior. Though scores of articles have been written on the problem and many solutions advanced, such disputes still arise frequently and until recently, we were little further in achieving consensus on how to resolve them. Indeed, at present the Department of Health and Human Services' Office of Research Integrity does not even consider authorship disputes, leaving these cases for their institutions to tackle.[33]

The Two-Sided Coin of Authorship

The coin of academic advancement is authorship.[15] That coin has two sides, credit and accountability. When there is one author, there is rarely any problem with assigning responsibility. But the expansion in numbers of authors per paper to an average of about six has led to a tendency to dilute responsibility while seeming not to diminish credit. To medical editors, one of the consequences of coauthorship seems to be the excessive credit that may be assumed by each of the coauthors. Whether that is true or not, responsibility certainly becomes diluted, and a consequence of coauthorship seems to be that the greater the number of coauthors, the less responsibility any will take for the whole. The result is that coauthors of fraudulent scientists have insistently denied knowing anything about the fabrications or, indeed, almost anything about the offending papers.[34–38] When questions have arisen about the integrity of published papers, too often the wretched editor has been told in effect that the paper was an orphan. Yet if coauthors cannot assure quality and detect problems, the reader is entitled to ask, Who can?[34]

Misuse of the Current System of Credit

From the mid-1970s on, coincident with the growth of multiple authorship, there has been a steady accumulation of problems due to practices destructive of the trust between authors and their readers. Coauthors showed themselves unwilling or unable to assure themselves of the integrity of their colleagues' work. In several cases, prominent journals published entirely fabricated data concerning imaginary series of patients, yet the coauthors had never bothered to satisfy themselves as to the existence of patients or data.[15,34,36,38–40] Other authors have failed to disclose highly relevant data bearing directly on the efficacy and harms of drugs.[41–46] In several instances, the sponsors of studies that produced unfavorable results have taken the data, analyzed them in misleading ways, and published the slanted analyses in order to preempt the investigators.[4,47,48] In order to increase apparent support for new therapies, the same results in the same trials have been reported numerous times in different journals under different authors' names.[13,49]

Two widespread and pernicious practices further distance those who reap the credit from appearing on the byline from accountability for their articles: in the first case by having spurious authors on the byline, and in the second by omitting those who wrote the article from the byline. The first is *honorary* or *guest* authorship, usually bestowed on senior colleagues who did nothing to justify authorship, in order to gratify them and to lend the articles an aura of authority.[15,50] There have been numerous instances in which the coauthors of fabricating authors have had to suffer public humiliation, so being invited in as a guest author has its dangers.[34,36,38, 51] The second unethical practice is *ghost* authorship.[52,53] Hiding the names and affiliations of the real authors is a deception practiced on the reader, often in order to achieve greater sales. Whole companies make their living by ghostwriting articles,[54] and in the case of research reviews, in which bias in selection is easily introduced, the academics who are paid to have their names as the sole authors may have been asked to give only the most cursory glance at the contents.[55] Their willing participation in such a practice is unethical.

Disagreement About Who Is Responsible for the Content of an Article

Cases of gross scientific misconduct have revealed disagreement in the scientific community about who is responsible for each part of an article when there are several authors, each brought in because they have different areas of expertise. It is fairly simple when, as has happened, the authors turn out to have been so ignorant of their own publication that they did not have the expertise to realize their published figure was factitious.[56] However, three prominent cases have caused controversy. In the first (Box 73.1), when a researcher at the University of California, San Diego (UCSD) was found to have fabricated and falsified research, his university conducted a close examination of all his 137 publications and declared 60 of them to be fraudulent or questionable. The university found many of the coauthors guilty of a culpable degree of carelessness, while recognizing that it might be unfair to hold all coauthors responsible for all parts of an article.[36]

In the second (Box 73.2), a National Institutes of Health (NIH) inquiry found two researchers at Stanford University guilty of scientific misconduct in relation to several multiauthored articles.[39,40] Stanford held that all the coauthors shared responsibility for the whole of each of their articles, whereas the NIH panel decided that this was too high a standard and "not feasible in

Box 73.1
The Slutsky Case

Robert Slutsky, a cardiologist at the University of California, San Diego (UCSD), resigned in 1985 when a member of a promotion committee noticed apparent duplications of results in 2 of his published articles.[36,102] Slutsky's lawyer asked that 15 of his articles, published in 8 journals, be retracted. However, over 7 years Slutsky had published 137 articles (one every 13 working days), which left a cloud over a large amount of published work. UCSD took this extremely seriously. Over a year, 10 faculty members investigated Slutsky's 137 articles, and finally declared that 77 were valid, 48 "questionable," and 12 "fraudulent." In November 1987, the UCSD committee investigating the affair published its full results in the *New England Journal of Medicine.*[36]

The investigating committee also examined the role of the co-authors. The members asked, "In multi-authored papers, can one expect, for example, the statistician to know personally how the data were collected?" The committee concluded,

> An unrealistic standard cannot be applied in judging the culpability of coauthors. But the standards should be higher than that of many of Slutsky's coauthors . . . many have been careless about verifying the accuracy of publications that carry their names. We believe this to be a culpable degree of carelessness. Acceptance of gift authorship (in which no scientific contribution was made) is also a culpable act of deliberate misrepresentation.

Unhappily, this remarkably determined effort to hold coauthors responsible and to clean up the literature is not the norm.

Box 73.2
The Stanford Case

In 1987, Philip Berger, director of the Stanford University Mental Health Clinical Research Center, resigned after an audit of research funds turned up problems with the research itself.[103] The university investigative panel found that in studies of neurotransmitters, cerebrospinal fluid from senile patients had been included among the "normal" controls; that 10 published articles contained analyses based on these controls; and that in 3, exclusion of these control values invalidated the conclusions of the articles.[103] At Stanford's request, all the authors wrote letters of correction or retraction to the journals. The university report held all the coauthors to be responsible, though the university provost, noting that at that time there were no generally accepted standards for the amount of responsibility to be borne by each co-investigator, asked the university faculty to formulate such guidelines.[103]

The National Institute of Mental Health (NIMH), which had been prodding Stanford into a deeper investigation, decided to review the case and held its own inquiry.[39] NIMH's report was issued in June 1989—before the creation of the NIH Office of Scientific Integrity and, later, the Public Health Service Office of Research Integrity, to oversee such investigations.

The NIMH report concluded that the members of its panel "did not believe that all the coauthors share responsibility for a paper. However, the panel believed that the responsibility is necessarily and properly focused on each coauthor's area of expertise." The panel concluded that "the burden of responsibility lies with the senior clinical coauthors Drs. Berger and Stahl." The report further noted,

> The panel believed it was doubtful that inspections by the coauthors would have revealed the errors in the data base. To have identified these errors, the coauthors would have had to be made aware of the circumstances of recruitment for all the normal control subjects and would have had to have access to each patient's medical records. The panel believed that this detailed and in-depth level of knowledge by all collaborators is not feasible in contemporary multidisciplinary research.[39]

Unlike Stanford, the NIMH panel vindicated all but the two senior authors.[104]

---

contemporary multidisciplinary research."[39] Correspondence in *Science* revealed the depth of disagreement after another case of misconduct, ranging from the view that all authors must share credit and blame equally, to the counter view that such a requirement would raise the risks of collaboration to suicidal levels and was unrealistic.[57–63]

More recently, in the Schön case (Box 73.3), in which nearly two dozen articles had to be retracted, a committee of inquiry created by Schön's employer found his collaborators guiltless and unaccountable, despite the fact that they had received widespread public acclaim at the time the work had been published.[37,64]

The lesson taught by numerous cases of fraudulent, frivolous, confused, and deceptive authorship is that authors have often concentrated solely on the credit that accrues to them, and that action must be taken by researchers, institutions, and journals to make accountability an equally essential component of authorship.

Initiatives to Promote Good Publishing Practices

The answer to the frivolous way in which some scientists have regarded their trusted position as authors is to link credit closely to accountability. Perhaps sensing the need for accountability as coauthors have increasingly crowded onto bylines over the years, authors have assumed that they were conveying information about who was responsible for the article by the way collaborators' names were ordered on the byline. Scientists have been dogmatic in giving their views about what each position in the sequence of authors

should mean to the reader—but these views are inconsistent. They range from the contention that the first author is always the junior fellow, the last the most senior individual, and the second the senior statistician or the physician who entered most patients, to the view that all positions are equal and names should be arranged alphabetically—a practice that some journals adopted until they found themselves avoided by authors late in the alphabet.[65–67] Surveys, however, have shown that although everyone is sure what the order means, everyone else, even in the same subspecialty, has a different reading.[68] The information, then, is broadcast in an idiosyncratic code, and the reader is never allowed into the secret, which is why Davies et al. found great variability in ways of assessing authorship, say, for promotion.[69] Davis and Gregerman proposed that allocation of credit could be indicated by assigning each author a numerical fraction corresponding to the work done.[70] The names were to be ordered according to this fraction. Perhaps because this seriously meant article was written in a humorous way, no one took them up on the idea.

Box 73.3
The Schön Case

Jan Hendrik Schön, a highly productive solid-state physicist working at Bell Laboratories, published over 90 articles in four years, most listing him as first author. In 2001, he published 1 paper every 8 days, most of them describing important advances in a number of fields. His sensational results attracted close scrutiny, and when several researchers noted republication and manipulation of his figures, an inquiry was held in 2002.[105] A panel of independent experts assembled by Bell Laboratories examined allegations concerning 25 separate articles in which Schön had had a total of 20 coauthors.[37,105] The panel noted that "if valid, the work he and his coauthors report would represent a remarkable number of major breakthroughs in condensed-matter and sold-state physics."

The investigating panel (the Beasley Committee) found Schön guilty of scientific misconduct and he was fired by Bell Laboratories. At the same time, the panel members noted that "all device fabrication, physical measurement, and data processing . . . were carried out (with minor exceptions) by Hendrik Schön alone, with no participation by any coauthor or other colleague. None of the most significant physical results was witnessed by any coauthor or other colleague."[37] Finding "no evidence that the laboratory practices of any coauthor of Hendrik Schön . . . are outside the accepted practices of their fields," the committee "completely cleared" the coauthors of scientific misconduct. However, it devoted a section of its report to the coauthors' professional responsibility. "By virtue of their coauthorship," it noted, "they implicitly endorse the validity of the work."[37]

"The Committee found this to be an extremely difficult issue, which the scientific community has not considered carefully," the report said. "Therefore, no clear, widely accepted standards of behavior exist." Central to collaborative research, the committee said, lay

> the question of professional responsibility [that] involves the balance between the trust necessary in any collaborative research and the responsibility all researchers bear for the veracity of results with which they are associated. The Committee does not endorse the view that each coauthor is responsible for the entirety of a collaborative endeavor: the relative responsibility of researchers with very different expertise, seniority and levels of participation must be considered.

The Committee concluded that the coauthors had "in the main, met their responsibilities."

Following the report, the American Physical Society revised its ethical guidelines. No longer were all coauthors to be held to a standard of equal responsibility. The new guidelines stated that all authors shared some degree of responsibility for the whole, but only some have responsibility for the entire paper.[106] In a correspondence following the Schön decision, I pointed out that to find all the coauthors guiltless of misconduct and of failure to meet their professional responsibilities effectively meant that they can have contributed nothing that merited authorship to the research.[64]

The International Committee of Medical Journal Editors Statements

Over the years, the International Committee of Medical Journal Editors (a.k.a., the Vancouver Group) has developed the following criteria:

> Authorship credit should be based on (1) substantial contributions to conception and design, or acquisition of data, or

analysis and interpretation of data; (2) drafting the article or revising it critically for important intellectual content; and (3) final approval of the version to be published. Authors should meet conditions 1, 2, and 3.

- Acquisition of funding, collection of data, or general supervision of the research group, alone, does not justify authorship.
- All persons designated as authors should qualify for authorship, and all those who qualify should be listed.
- Each author should have participated sufficiently in the work to take public responsibility for appropriate portions of the content.[8]

These criteria have been widely adopted in biomedicine. In addition, journals have become much more helpful in publishing their criteria and what they expected of authors. Unfortunately, abuses continue, and several studies have shown widespread ignorance of these criteria by authors, or when they did know, extensive flouting of the rules.[71,72]

Efforts to Limit the Number of Authors

Arguing that in any group, only a few can truly carry out all the functions that would qualify them as authors,[28] editors have tried to limit the number on the byline. These efforts have been doomed partly because they were arbitrary, partly because there are good scientific reasons for groups to form for a common purpose, and partly because the editors kept having to make exceptions to their own rules. The ICJME decreed initially that no more than three authors should be listed, but increased this to six in 1994. Molecular biologists have persuaded the National Library of Medicine to list 25, and we can expect these numbers to increase.

The Concept of Contributorship

Things began to change with the realization that abuses of authorship were at the root of many of the problems medical editors encountered, and the editors held a conference on authorship in Nottingham, England, in 1996. A proposal by myself and my colleagues was debated and largely approved, and was published the next year.[40] The essence of the proposal was as follows: Instead of concentrating on credit, everyone should focus on strengthening the trust necessary for the author-reader relationship. Authors (who should satisfy the ICMJE criteria) should, before sending in their manuscripts to journals, decide who had contributed what—the job each researcher had actually done, rather than the official position each occupied. They should then list the contributions of each author, in rough order of perceived importance of contribution, and editors should publish this information for the readers. Each part of the work would be attributed to one or more of the author/contributors on the byline. Further, one or more of the authors would take formal responsibility for the integrity of the whole, acting as *guarantor*. If questions later arose, it would be easy to tell who was responsible for answering them.

It was noted at the time that the system was descriptively precise, and, being transparent, in the best traditions of science. It is fair, and discourages ghost and guest authorship. It might even discourage fraud by making lying harder.[73] It also removed a curious anomaly. The custom had long been that those who contributed least, namely those acknowledged for their help, had their contributions specified for the reader, whereas the contributions of the individuals on the byline remained vague. The new system would still acknowledge individuals, but now authors would also reveal their contributions. An important benefit might prove to be to improve the system of academic promotions and appointments, because panels would be able to rely on the explicit statements of candidates at the time the articles were published, instead of their later recollections. The original proposal suggested that for scientific articles, the term *author* be dropped completely in favor of *contributor*, in order to make the point. This proved too radical for the community to swallow.

The system was adopted rapidly by a number of journals, led by *The Lancet*[74] and *BMJ* (formerly the *British Medical Journal*). It was shown to be simple to manage and to take up little page space.[75] It was subsequently debated at three retreats held by the Council of Science Editors, and endorsed by them and by the World Association of Medical Editors. In 2003, the two largest general scientific journals, *Nature* and *Science,* adopted the policy,[76] as did the NIH.[77] The ICMJE statement now reads, "Some journals now request and publish information about the contributions of each person named as having participated in a submitted study, at least for original research. Editors are strongly encouraged to develop and implement a contributorship policy, as well as a policy on identifying who is responsible for the integrity of the work as a whole."[8]

As the statement rightly points out, "While contributorship and guarantorship policies obviously remove much of the ambiguity surrounding contributions, it [sic] leaves unresolved the question of the quantity and quality of contribution that qualify for authorship."[8] This is why the ICMJE criteria for authorship remain important.

As more journals adopt the system of disclosing contributions, as transparency and clarity are achieved, and as attention is focused on guaranteeing the integrity of the whole, the controversies over who is responsible for what part of the research when allegations of misconduct arise following publication should die down.

Naturally, it has taken a long time for this innovation to diffuse to the thousands of biomedical journals. However, now that the disclosure of contributions of authors has become the standard, it is interesting to note that in 1941, the inventors of penicillin fully disclosed their individual contributions to this seminal study in a footnote to their article in *The Lancet.*[78]

The Problem of Large Trials

Large, multicenter trials have been the first to face up to the issue of indicating which of the investigators did what. A good example is given by the report of the fourth ISIS trial, published in 1995. This listed 2,000 "members," conveniently divided into committees for writing, data monitoring, and so on, and with a detailed description of the tasks of the unit overseeing the research.[79] However, the 1993 Ig Nobel prize was accepted by the *New England Journal of Medicine* on behalf of the 972 GUSTO investigators listed as coauthors for one article, at two words per author.[80,81] Clearly, not everyone satisfied the conditions necessary

to claim authorship. Some editors tried to decree limits, and clinical researchers naturally objected, arguing that if we are not to penalize those who take the trouble to conduct large, multicenter trials, while rewarding those who publish small, uncontrolled trials, such editorial limits on the number of authors were self-defeating.[15,82] It is becoming accepted that the core group who design and direct the study, analyze the data, and write the article should be named on the byline as authors, writing for the others who are bundled together in the study's name thus: "for the XYZ Investigators." Their names are then listed fully in the acknowledgments. Once again, it is important that all those who appear as named authors on the byline satisfy the ICMJE criteria and have their individual contributions listed for the reader. For a fuller treatment of the problems of indexing and citation when there is group authorship, and for discussion of the issue of authorship for research groups, see Flanagin et al., 2002.[83,84]

The ICMJE recommendations for authorship of trials are as follows:

> When a large, multi-center group has conducted the work, the group should identify the individuals who accept direct responsibility for the manuscript. These individuals should fully meet the criteria for authorship defined above and editors will ask these individuals to complete journal-specific author and conflict of interest disclosure forms. When submitting a group author manuscript, the corresponding author should clearly indicate the preferred citation and should clearly identify all individual authors as well as the group name. Journals will generally list other members of the group in the acknowledgements. The National Library of Medicine indexes the group name and the names of individuals the group has identified as being directly responsible for the manuscript.[8]

Investigation and Retraction

The obligations of the authors require that some of them take part in audit of their trials, to ensure the integrity of the data. The obligations authors undertake also require prompt investigation of allegations of fraudulent behavior. If a retraction is advised after a finding by a properly constituted investigative panel, it is the duty of all the coauthors to correct the literature with a retraction linked prominently to the original article.[8] There are excellent models provided for this by Weiss and his colleagues of the Cancer and Leukemia Group B[85] and by Hoeksema et al.[86] Such an audit system uncovered the fabrications of the South African researcher Werner Bezwoda,[87] and, in contrast to cases in which retraction has failed to occur,[36] has helped patients and their physicians.

Ethical Requirements of Authors and Journals Introduced by Commercial Sponsorship

Article 27 of the Declaration of Helsinki states in part, "Negative as well as positive results should be published or otherwise publicly available. Sources of funding, institutional affiliations and any possible conflicts of interest should be declared in the publication."[8] In the area of clinical trials, the obligation to publish, clearly laid out in the Declaration of Helsinki, may be at odds with the wishes of the commercial entities that have sponsored a study.

The sponsors may insist that they own the data, and may want to exercise full control over the clinical researchers, suppress unfavorable results, and proceed legally against researchers who try to publish.[4,47,48,88,89]

There are several ways in which a literature biased in favor of commercial products may occur. Prudent investment of resources will limit manufacturers to sponsor trials of products for which they have strong prior evidence that the result will be favorable for their product, and, for regulatory approval, sponsors will demand rigorous conduct of the trials. There is some evidence that sponsors will try to influence the analysis and reporting of those trials they allow to be published. For example, both the VIGOR and CLASS COX-2 inhibitor studies were incompletely reported, with the effect that in the former report, a toxic effect was concealed, and in the latter, the fact there was no advantage to the new drug was concealed.[90] Failure to report outcomes, and so bias trial reports, is common, and particularly in the reporting of harms, is associated with commercial funding.[91,92] There is overwhelming evidence that sponsors will try to control dissemination of results.

Clinical researchers, particularly when they work in universities, in which publication is not merely a privilege and a right but also a duty, face severe conflicts unless their contract with a sponsor ensures them an unfettered right to publish, full access to all the data, and control over the analyses. Because of recent scandals, there is a strong movement, based on scientific, ethical, and legal principles, to forbid restrictive contracts and allow full dissemination of trial results. For example, on December 10, 2004, the Association of American Medical Colleges issued a statement "strongly supporting the elimination of restrictive confidentiality clauses in clinical trial contracts between pharmaceutical companies and academic or physician researchers."[93]

So many episodes of deceptive behavior have occurred associated with the widespread takeover of clinical trials by industry, and the resulting secrecy and bias, that editors and reviewers no longer instinctively trust the authors to present a faithful account of the work.[49,94–97] The reputation of a journal, which is what attracts authors, is inevitably bound up with that of the authors and their articles. Medical editors are naturally solicitous of their journals' reputations, not least because circulation and income depend on those reputations. To this concern is added the wider consideration that it is the editor's duty to publish information valuable for the public's health, and there are numerous studies to show that financial ties bias reporting in ways that act to the detriment of optimal patient care.

As a direct consequence of very many scandals associated with commercial and financial influences on the behavior of researchers, and the extensive and well-documented bias in reporting,[99] journal editors have, over the past 25 years, introduced a wide range of assurances to be sought from authors to try to bolster the editors' faith in the integrity of the work. As a result, to fulfill the ethical and practical requirements of authorship in most large medical journals, authors must expect to attest to the editor, and disclose to the reader, several sorts of information. These will vary between journals, and potential authors should always check with the specific journal's instructions for authors.

In general, authors must disclose their affiliations and the names, research institutions, and sites of all members of the research group. They must provide information, to be published, on all possible relevant financial ties, and their funding and support. They must provide a statement about the role of the sponsor,

particularly an assurance that they, the authors, had complete freedom to publish and had control over, and access to, all the data. If there is any doubt about this and about their freedom to analyze the data (for example, if the statistical analysis was done by someone paid by the sponsors), the journal may demand independent statistical analysis and review of all the data as a condition of acceptance. Readers seeking an example of this should look at the disclosures in a report of a trial by Gallant et al., in which the contributions of the authors are also disclosed.[98]

Events in 2004 and 2005 associated with trials of COX-2 inhibitors and selective serotonin reuptake inhibitors have underscored the crucial clinical importance of publication of all trials and, equally essential, the registration of trials at inception.[83,94] This is an ethical duty that falls on the authors, and the editors of journals are now insisting that they will not publish trials unless the authors provide evidence that their trials have been registered, preferably at inception, with a large, easily accessible register.[94,99] The ICMJE published a statement on this in September 2004.[8]

Finally, in order to help to ensure the ethical conduct of research, each publication should note that the trial was approved by an institutional review board or other ethical committee and that informed consent was obtained from all participants. These items are often left out, especially when the article is a secondary publication from a trial whose main results have already been published.[100]

Policy Implications and Unresolved Ethical Issues and Requirements

The massive publicity during 2004 following the revelations of unpublished trials on antidepressants in children and COX-2 inhibitors in adults threw a spotlight on serious ethical deficiencies in the conduct of corporate sponsors of trials, who have dragged their feet for years on the issue of trial registration and publication. It also reflected badly on the many clinical researchers whom the manufacturers sponsored, and who had written the reports (or acquiesced in their suppression), many of whom had multiple financial ties.[46,94] The behavior of both groups was unethical, and the community of clinical researchers should note that this failure of investigators and their sponsors to take the responsibilities of authorship seriously was directly contrary to the words and intent of the Declaration of Helsinki. It took a lawsuit to move industry to reluctant acquiescence.[101] The subject also was being considered in the U.S. Congress, but the issue would go away if authors behaved ethically. In the meantime, it is urgent that researchers be reminded of the ethical responsibilities that author/investigators take on when they conduct and report trials.

References

1. Kennedy D. *Academic Duty*. Cambridge, Mass.: Harvard University Press; 1997:208.
2. Rennie D. Guarding the guardians: A conference on editorial peer review. *JAMA* 1986;256:2391–2.
3. Panel on Scientific Responsibility and the Conduct of Research; Committee on Science, Engineering, and Public Policy; National Academy of Sciences; National Academy of Engineering; and,

Institute of Medicine. *Responsible Science—Ensuring the Integrity of the Research Process, Vol. I.* Washington, D.C.: National Academy Press; 1992.

4. Rennie D. Thyroid storm. *JAMA* 1997;277:1238–43.

5. World Medical Association. *Declaration of Helsinki: Ethical Principles for Medical Research Involving Human Subjects.* Tokyo, Japan: WMAl October 2004. [Online] 2004. Available: http://www.wma.net/e/policy/b3.htm.

6. Broad WJ. The publishing game: Getting more for less. *Science* 1981;211:1137–9.

7. Scientific Directors, Intramural Research Programs, National Institutes of Health. *Guidelines for the Conduct of Research in the Intramural Research Programs at NIH,* 3rd ed. Bethesda, Md.: NIH; 1997. [Online] January 1997. Available: http://www.nih.gov/news/irnews/guidelines.htm.

8. International Committee of Medical Journal Editors. Uniform Requirements for Manuscripts Submitted to Biomedical Journals: Writing and Editing for Biomedical Publication. [Online] October 2005. Available: http://www.icmje.org/index.html#top.

9. Huth EJ. Irresponsible authorship and wasteful publication. *Annals of Internal Medicine* 1986;104:257–9.

10. von Elm E, Poglia G, Walder B, Tramèr MR. Different patterns of duplicate publication—An analysis of articles used in systematic reviews. *JAMA* 2004;291:974–80.

11. Anon. Definition of "sole contribution." *New England Journal of Medicine* 1969;281:676–7.

12. Tramèr MR, Reynolds DJM, Moore RA, McQuay HJ. Impact of covert duplicate publication on meta-analysis: A case study. *British Medical Journal* 1997;315:635–40.

13. Huston P, Moher D. Redundancy, disaggregation, and the integrity of medical research. *Lancet* 1996;347:1024–6.

14. Lederberg J. Communication as the root of scientific progress. *The Scientist* 1993;7(3):10–4.

15. Rennie D, Flanagin A. Authorship! Authorship! Guests, ghosts, grafters, and the two-sided coin. *JAMA* 1994;271:469–71.

16. Anon. U.S. Judge rejects claim of plagiarism. *New York Times* May 4, 1988:B4.

17. Friend T. Credit grab: How many writers does it take to make a movie? *New Yorker* October 20, 2003:160–9.

18. Weiner E, ed. *Oxford English Dictionary.* [CD-ROM]. 2nd ed. New York, N.Y.: Oxford University Press; 1992.

19. Vickers B. *Shakespeare, Co-Author: A Historical Study of Five Collaborative Plays.* Oxford, England: Oxford University Press; 2002: 527.

20. Snyder LJ. William Whewell. In: Zalta EN, ed. *The Stanford Encyclopedia of Philosophy* (Spring 2004 edition). [Online] Available: http://plato.stanford.edu/archives/spr2004/entries/whewell/.

21. The rise and rise of collaborative writing. *New Scientist* 1990;126–31.

22. Drenth JP. Multiple authorship: The contribution of senior authors. *JAMA* 1998;280:219–21.

23. Mussurakis S. Coauthorship trends in the leading radiological journals. *Acta Radiologica* 1993;34:316–20.

24. Sobal J, Ferentz KS. Abstract creep and author inflation. *New England Journal of Medicine* 1990;323:488–9.

25. Price de Solla DJ. *Little Science, Big Science.* New York, N.Y.: Columbia University Press; 1993.

26. Strub RL, Black FW. Multiple authorship. *Lancet* 1976;2:1090–1.

27. Anderson C. Writer's cramp. *Nature* 1992;355:101.

28. Huth EJ. Editors and the problems of authorship: Rulemakers or gatekeepers? In: Council of Biology Editors, Editorial Policy Committee. *Ethics and Policy in Scientific Publication.* Bethesda, Md.: Council of Biology Editors; 1990.

29. Regalado A. Multiauthor papers on the rise. *Science* 1995;268:25.

30. Mallon T. *Stolen Words: Forays Into the Origins and Ravages of Plagiarism.* New York, N.Y.: Penguin Books Ltd.; 1991.

31. Rennie D. Who did what? Authorship and contribution in 2001. *Muscle and Nerve* 2001;24:1274–7.

32. Wilcox LJ. Authorship: The coin of the realm, the source of complaints. *JAMA* 1998;280:216–7.

33. Commission on Research Integrity, Department of Health and Human Services. *Integrity and Misconduct in Research.* Washington, D.C.: DHHS; 1995. [Online] Available: http://ori.dhhs.gov/documents/report_commission.pdf.

34. Stewart WW, Feder N. The integrity of the scientific literature. *Nature* 1987;325:207–14.

35. Relman AS. Lessons from the Darsee affair. *New England Journal of Medicine* 1983;308:1415–7.

36. Engler RL, Covell JW, Friedman PJ, Kitcher PS, Peters RM. Misrepresentation and responsibility in medical research. *New England Journal of Medicine* 1987;317:1383–9.

37. Beasley MR, Datta S, Kogelnik H, Kroemer H, Monroe D. *Report of the Investigation Committee on the Possibility of Scientific Misconduct in the Work of Hendrik Schön and Coauthors.* Bell Labs, Lucent Technologies; 2002. [Online] September 2002. Available: http://www.lucent.com/news_events/pdf/researchreview.pdf.

38. Broad W, Wade N. *Betrayers of the Truth: Fraud and Deceit in the Halls of Science.* New York, N.Y.: Simon and Schuster; 1982.

39. Report of the Investigative Panel, National Institute of Mental Health for the Stanford University Mental Health Clinical Research Center. Panel to investigate possible misconduct in science under grant MH-30854 May 24, 1989. Washington, D.C.: DHHS; 1989.

40. Rennie D, Yank V, Emanuel L. When authorship fails: A proposal to make contributors accountable. *JAMA* 1997;278:579–85.

41. Rennie D. Editors and auditors. *JAMA* 1989;261:2543–5.

42. Potkin SG, Cannon HE, Murphy DL, Wyatt RJ. Monoamine oxidase in schizophrenia. *New England Journal of Medicine* 1978;298:1150–2.

43. Hrachovec JB, Mora M, Wright JM, Perry TL, Bassett KL, Chambers GK, Silverstein F, Simon L, Faich G. Reporting of 6-month vs. 12-month data in a clinical trial of celecoxib [Letters]. *JAMA* 2001;286:2398–2400.

44. Bombardier C, Laine L, Reicin A, et al., for the VIGOR Study Group. Comparison of upper gastrointestinal toxicity of rofecoxib and naproxen in patients with rheumatoid arthritis. *New England Journal of Medicine* 2000;343:1520–8.

45. Dieppe PA, Ebrahim S, Martin RM, Jüni P. Lessons from the withdrawal of rofecoxib. *British Medical Journal* 2004;329:867–8.

46. Topol EJ. Failing the public health—Rofecoxib, Merck, and the FDA. *New England Journal of Medicine* 2004;351:1707–9.

47. Kahn JO, Gherng DW, Mayer K, Murray H, Lagakos S, for the 806 Investigator Team. Evaluation of HIV-1 immunogen, an immunologic modifier, administered to patients infected with HIV having 300 to 549 x 106/L CD4 cell counts. *JAMA* 2000;284:2193–2202.

48. Thompson J, Baird P, Downie J. *The Olivieri Report.* Toronto, Canada: James Lorimer and Co. (Canadian Association of University Teachers series); 2001.

49. Rennie D. Fair conduct and fair reporting of clinical trials. *JAMA* 1999;282:1766–8.

50. President of Royal College resigns. *British Medical Journal* 1994;309:1530.

51. LaFollette MC. *Stealing Into Print: Fraud, Plagiarism, and Misconduct in Scientific Publishing.* Berkeley, Calif.: University of California Press; 1992.

52. Flanagin A, Carey LA, Fontanarosa PB, Phillips SG, Pace BP, Lundberg GD, Rennie D. Prevalence of articles with honorary authors and ghost authors in peer-reviewed medical journals. *JAMA* 1998; 280:222–4.

53. Flanagin A, Rennie D. Acknowledging ghosts. *JAMA* 1995;273:73.

54. Healy D, Cattell D. Interface between authorship, industry and science in the domain of therapeutics. *British Journal of Psychiatry* 2003;183:22–7.

55. Hornbein T, Bero L, Rennie D. The publication of commercially supported supplements statement. *Anesthesia and Analgesia* 1995;81:887–8.

56. Relman AS. Responsibilities of authorship: Where does the buck stop? *New England Journal of Medicine* 1984;310:1048–9.

57. Marshall E. Fraud strikes top genome lab. *Science* 1996;274:908–10.

58. Wooley CF. "Struck" by fraud. [Letter]. *Science* 1996;274:1593.

59. de Sa P, Sagar A. "Struck" by fraud. [Letter]. *Science* 1996;274:1593.

60. Gilson MK. Responsibility of coauthors. [Letter]. *Science* 1997; 275:14.

61. Baskin TI. Responsibility of coauthors. [Letter]. *Science* 1997;275:14.

62. Pasachoff JM. Responsibility of coauthors. [Letter]. *Science* 1997; 275:14.

63. Loehle C. Responsibility of coauthors [Letter]. *Science* 1997;275:14.

64. Rennie D. A proposal for transparency [Letter]. *Science* 2002; 298:1554.

65. Garfield E. *Essays of an Information Scientist.* Philadelphia, PA: ISI Press; 1983.

66. Burman KD. Hanging from the masthead: Reflections on authorship. *Annals of Internal Medicine* 1982;97:602–5.

67. Over R, Smallman S. Citation idiosyncrasies. *Nature* 1970;228:1357.

68. American Association for the Advancement of Science. Survey of journals conducted by the American Association for the Advancement of Science. Internal document. 1995.

69. Davies HD, Langley JM, Speert DP, for the Pediatric Investigators' Collaborative Network on Infections in Canada. Rating authors' contributions to collaborative research: The PICNIC survey of university departments of pediatrics. *Canadian Medical Association Journal* 1996;155:877–82.

70. Davis PJ, Gregerman RI. Parse analysis: A new method for the evaluation of investigators' bibliographies. *New England Journal of Medicine* 1969;281:989–90.

71. Drenth JP. Proliferation of authors on research reports in medicine. *Science and Engineering Ethics* 1996;2:469–80.

72. Squires BP. Authors: Who contributes what? *Canadian Medical Association Journal* 1996;155:897–8.

73. Benson K. Science and the single author: Historical reflections on the problem of authorship. *Cancer Bulletin* 1991;43:324–30.

74. Horton R. The signature of responsibility. *Lancet* 1997;350:5–6.

75. Yank V, Rennie D. Disclosure of researcher contributions: A study of original research articles in *The Lancet. Annals of Internal Medicine* 1999;130:661–70.

76. Kennedy D. Multiple authors, multiple problems. *Science* 2003; 301:733.

77. BECON 2003 Symposium Committee. *Catalyzing Team Science: Report From the 2003 BECON Symposium.* Bethesda, Md.: NIH; June 23–24, 2003. Available: www.becon1.nih.gov/symposia_2003/becon2003_symposium_final.pdf.

78. Abraham EP, Chain E, Fletcher CM, Gardner AD, Heatley NG, Jennings MA, Florey HW. Further observations on penicillin. *Lancet* 1941;2:177–188.

79. Fourth International Study of Infarct Survival Collaborative Group. ISIS-4: A randomised factorial trial assessing early oral captopril, oral mononitrate, and intravenous magnesium sulphate in 58,050 patients with suspected myocardial infarction. *Lancet* 1995;345:669–85.

80. Nadis S. Ig Nobel prizes reward fruits of unique labour. *Nature* 1993;365:599.

81. The GUSTO Investigators. An international randomized trial comparing four thrombolytic strategies for acute myocardial infarction. *New England Journal of Medicine* 1993;329:673–82.

82. Carbone PP. On authorship and acknowledgments. [Letter]. *New England Journal of Medicine* 1992;326:1084.

83. Dickersin K, Scherer R, Suci E, Gil-Montero M. Problems with indexing and citation of articles with group authorship. *JAMA* 2002;287:2772–4.

84. Flanagin A, Fontanarosa PB, DeAngelis CD. Authorship for research groups. *JAMA* 2002;288:3166–8.

85. Weiss RB, Vogelzang NJ, Peterson BA, Panasci LC, Carpenter JT, Gavigan M, Sartell K, Frei E 3rd, McIntyre OR. A successful system of scientific data audits for clinical trials. A report from the Cancer and Leukemia Group B. *JAMA* 1993;270:459–64.

86. Hoeksema HL, Troost J, Grobbee DE, Wiersinga WM, van Wijmen FCB, Klasen EC. Fraud in a pharmaceutical trial. *Lancet* 2000; 356:1773.

87. Weiss RB, Rifkin RM, Stewart FM, Theriault RL, Williams LA, Herman AA, Beveridge RA. High-dose chemotherapy for high-risk primary breast cancer: An on-site review of the Bezwoda study. *Lancet* 2000;355:999–1003.

88. Stryker J. Who owns the data? Conflicts in privately funded research. California Healthline. [Online] December 11, 2000. Available: http://www.californiahealthline.org/index.cfm?Action=dspItem&itemID=102361&ClassCD=CL126.

89. Trinkl A, O'Brien J. University of California, San Francisco responds to inaccurate claims by company. UCSF Press Release, November 1, 2000. [Online] Available: http:www.ucsf.edu/pressrel/2000/11/110101.html.

90. Fontanarosa PB, Rennie D, DeAngelis CD. Postmarketing surveillance—Lack of vigilance, lack of trust. *JAMA* 2004;292:2647–50.

91. Chan A-W, Hróbjartsson A, Haahr MT, Gøtzsche PC, Altman DG. Empirical evidence for selective reporting of outcomes in randomized trials. *JAMA* 2004;291:2457–65.

92. Chan A-W, Altman DG. Identifying outcome reporting bias in randomised trials on PubMed: Review of publications and survey of authors. *British Medical Journal* 2005;330:753–6.

93. Association of American Medical Colleges. AAMC endorses call for less restrictive research contracts. Press release, December 10, 2004. [Online] Available: http://www.aamc.org/newsroom/pressrel/2004/041210.htm.

94. Rennie D. Trial registration—A great idea switches from ignored to irresistible. *JAMA* 2004;292:1359–62.

95. Callahan D. *What Price Better Health?: Hazards of the Research Imperative.* Berkeley and Los Angeles, Calif.: University of California Press; 2003.

96. Kassirer JP. *On the Take: How Medicine's Complicity With Big Business Can Endanger Your Health.* New York, N.Y.: Oxford University Press; 2005.

97. Angell M. *Science on Trial.* New York, N.Y.: W.W. Norton & Company, Inc.; 1996.

98. Gallant JE, Staszewski S, Pozniak AL, et al. Efficacy and safety of tenofovir DF vs. stavudine in combination therapy in antiretroviral-naive patients: A 3-year randomized trial. *JAMA* 2004;292:191–201.

99. Dickersin K, Rennie D. Registering clinical trials. *JAMA* 2003; 290:516–23.

100. Yank V, Rennie D. Reporting of informed consent and ethics committee approval in clinical trials. *JAMA* 2002;287:2835–8.

101. The People of the State of New York, by Eliot Spitzer, Attorney General of the State of New York, against GlaxoSmithKline. In: Supreme Court of the State of New York County of New York; filed June 2, 2004; 2004.

102. Whitely WP, Rennie D, Hafner AW. The scientific community's response to evidence of fraudulent publication: The Robert Slutsky case. *JAMA* 1994;272:170–3.

103. Barinaga M. All collaborators held to be responsible for errors. *Nature* 1988;336:3.

104. Barinaga M. NIMH assigns blame for tainted studies. *Science* 1989;245:812.

105. Service RF. Bell Labs fires star physicist found guilty of forging data. *Science* 2002;298:30–1.

106. Brumfiel G. Physics guidelines drop equal-responsibility clause. *Nature* 2002;420:258.

Credits and Permissions

1. Bruce Agnew
   - Conflict of interest cartoon. Reproduced in Chapter 68 as Figure 68.1 with permission.

2. Tom L. Beauchamp
   - Photograph of members of the National Commission for the Protection of Human Subjects of Biomedical and Behavioral Research, 1977. Reproduced in Chapter 14 as Figure 14.1 with permission.

3. Linda Bryder
   - Figure 1. Standardized Death Rates from Tuberculosis (All Forms and Pulmonary) per 100,000 Population, England and Wales, and Scotland, 1850–1950. In: Linda Bryder, *Below the Magic Mountain,* New York, NY: Clarendon Press, 1988, p. 7. Reproduced in Chapter 4 as Figure 4.1 with permission.

4. Paul Gelsinger and Mickie Gelsinger
   - Photograph of Jesse Gelsinger, June 22, 1999. Reproduced in Chapter 10 as Figure 10.2 with permission.

5. Seiichi Morimura
   - Aerial photograph of Unit 731. Reproduced in Chapter 3 as Figure 3.1 with permission.

6. Guido Sauter
   - Photograph of tissue sample repository. Reproduced in Chapter 28 as Figure 28.1 with permission.

We thank and acknowledge the following copyright holders for permission to reproduce the following materials.

1. *The American Medical Association*
   - Figure 1. Funding for Biomedical Research by Source, 1994–2003, in: Moses H 3rd, Dorsey ER, Matheson DHM, Thier SO. Financial anatomy of biomedical research. *Journal of the American Medical Association* 2005;294:1333–42. Copyright © 2005, American Medical Association. All rights reserved. Reproduced in Chapter 69 as Figure 69.1 with permission.

2. *The American Philosophical Society*
   - Application form for membership in the Walter Reed Society, from the Thomas M. Rivers Papers, American Philosophical Society, Philadelphia, Penn. Reproduced in Chapter 1 as Figure 1.3 with permission.

3. *American Thoracic Society*
   - Figure 7, in: Feldman WH, Hinshaw HC, Mann FC. Streptomycin in experimental tuberculosis. *American Review of Tuberculosis* 1945;52:269–98. © American Thoracic Society. Reproduced in Chapter 4 as Figure 4.5 with permission.

4. *Cambridge University Press*
   - Emanuel EJ, Grady C. Four paradigms of clinical research and research oversight. *Cambridge Quarterly of Healthcare Ethics* 2007;16(1):82–96. Copyright © 2007

Cambridge University Press. Reproduced as Chapter 11 with permission.

5. *Chemical Engineering*
   - Photograph of final stage of deep fermentation of streptomycin. In: Porter RW. Streptomycin: Engineered into commercial production. *Chemical Engineering*, Vol. 53, No. 10, pp. 94–8 and 142–5 (1946). Reproduced in Chapter 4 as Figure 4.3 with permission.
   - Photograph of streptomycin distillation towers in Elkton, Va. In: Porter RW. Streptomycin: Engineered into commercial production. *Chemical Engineering*, Vol. 53, No. 10, pp. 94–8 and 142–5 (1946). Reproduced in Chapter 4 as Figure 4.4 with permission.
   - Schematic diagram of the streptomycin manufacturing process. In: Porter RW. Streptomycin: Engineered into commercial production. *Chemical Engineering*, Vol. 53, No. 10, pp. 94–8 and 142–5 (1946). Reproduced in Chapter 4 as Figure 4.7 with permission.

6. *Frederick L. Ehrman Medical Library Archives, New York University School of Medicine*
   - Photograph of Saul Krugman. Reproduced in Chapter 7 as Figure 7.1 with permission.

7. *Elsevier*
   - Part of Table I: CHARM mortality results at each interim analysis and at study closeout. In: Pocock S, Wang D, Wilhelmsen L. The data monitoring experience in the Candesartan in Heart Failure morbidity (CHARM) program. *American Heart Journal* 2005;149(5):939–43. Reproduced in Chapter 53 as Table 53.2, with permission from Elsevier.

8. *Eyedea Presse*
   - Photograph of a Nazi freezing experiment at Dachau, September, 1942. (A 1172/14–21.2223, neg. 00977). Reproduced in Chapter 2 as Figure 2.2 with permission.

9. *Juvenile Diabetes Research Foundation*
   - Photograph of Mary Tyler Moore testifying at a Senate hearing, 2003. Reproduced in Chapter 23 as Figure 23.2 with permission.

10. *Klinik für Psychiatrie und Psychotherapie, Akademisches Lehrkrankenhaus der Charité—Universitätsmedizin Berlin.*
    - Photograph of Nazi neuropathologist, Berthold Ostertag (1895–1975). Reproduced in Chapter 2 as Figure 2.1 with permission.

11. *Lance Armstrong Foundation*
    - Photograph of Lance Armstrong addressing an audience in front of the U.S. Capitol Building. Reproduced in Chapter 23 as Figure 23.1 with permission.

12. *March of Dimes*
    - Photograph of Jonas Salk inoculating his son, Jonathan, May 16, 1953. © March of Dimes Birth Defects Foundation. Reproduced in Chapter 5 as Figure 5.1 with permission.

- Basil O'Connor, A Message to Parents. Thomas Francis Papers, Manual of Suggested Procedures for the Conduct of the Vaccine Field Trial in 1954, Bentley Historical Library, University of Michigan. © March of Dimes Birth Defects Foundation. Reproduced in Chapter 5 as Figure 5.3 with permission.

13. *Oxford University Press*
    - Figure 1. Standardized Death Rates from Tuberculosis (All Forms and Pulmonary) per 100,000 Population, England and Wales, and Scotland, 1850–1950. In: Linda Bryder, *Below the Magic Mountain*, New York, N.Y.: Clarendon Press; 1988:7. Reproduced in Chapter 4 as Figure 4.1 with permission.

14. *Photo Researchers, Inc.*
    - Scanning electron micrograph (SEM) of Anopheles stephensi. Reproduced in Chapter 26 as Figure 26.1 with permission.
    - Scanning electron micrograph (SEM) of a human embryo at the 10-cell stage on the tip of a pin. Reproduced in Chapter 46 as Figure 46.1 with permission.

15. *Royal College of Physicians (London), Heritage Collections*
    - Photograph of Sir Geoffrey Marshall. In: *Munk's Roll*, Volume VII, p. LIII. Reproduced in Chapter 4 as Figure 4.6 with permission.

16. *Rutgers University Libraries, Special Collections and University Archives*
    - Photograph of Albert Schatz and Selman Waksman at Martin Hall, New Jersey College of Agriculture, circa 1944. Reproduced in Chapter 4 as Figure 4.2 with permission.

17. *Temple University, Urban Archives*
    - Photograph of Solomon McBride and prisoner/research subject in Holmesburg Prison, Philadelphia, Penn. Reproduced in Chapter 43 as Figure 43.1 with permission.

18. *United States Holocaust Memorial Museum*
    - Photograph of Nazi neuropathologist, Berthold Ostertag (1895–1975). Reproduced in Chapter 2 as Figure 2.1 with permission.
    - Photograph of Karl Brandt and his fellow defendants in the dock at the Nuremberg Doctors Trial. Reproduced in Chapter 12 as Figure 12.1 with permission.

19. *University of Virginia Library, Special Collections*
    - Illustrated depiction of Walter Reed's yellow fever experiment, from the Papers of Jefferson Randolph Kean, MSS 628, Special Collections, University of Virginia Library. Reproduced in Chapter 1 as Figure 1.1 with permission.

20. *Wiley-Liss, Inc.*
    - Figure 1, Overview of Family-Based Recruitment Methods, in: Beskow LM, et al. Ethical issues in identifying and recruiting participants for familial genetic

research. *American Journal of Medical Genetics* 2004;130A:424–31. © 2004 Wiley-Liss, Inc. Reproduced in Chapter 29 as Figure 29.2 with permission.

21. *Wyeth*
   • Dean Cornwell's *Conquerors of Yellow Fever,* 1939. Reproduced in Chapter 1 as Figure 1.2 with permission.

Other images that are in the public domain have been reproduced throughout the volume. Source information for these is indicated beneath each image.

Index

Figures and tables are indicated with *f* and *t*.